Y0-AAQ-900

NURSING DRUG REFERENCE:
A PRACTITIONER'S GUIDE

Editor

MARILYN W. EDMUNDS, M.S.
University of Maryland
Graduate School of Nursing
Department of Primary Care
Baltimore, Maryland

BRADY COMMUNICATIONS COMPANY, INC. ● BOWIE, MARYLAND 20715
A Prentice-Hall Publishing Company

Publishing Director: David Culverwell
Acquisitions Editor: Richard A. Weimer
Production Editor: Janis K. Oppelt
Art Director: Don Sellers, AMI
Assistant Art Director: Bernard Vervin
Manufacturing Director: John A. Komsa

Typesetter: Harper Graphics, Waldorf, Maryland
Printer: Fairfield Graphics, Fairfield, Pennsylvania
Typeface: Century Schoolbook (text); Antique Olive (display)

DISCLAIMER

Every effort has been made to check the accuracy of the contents of this book, with particular attention paid to dosage schedules. Because of the rapid advances in pharmacology, we also strongly urge practitioners to consult the latest drug product package inserts in order to obtain the most accurate and up-to-date information regarding drugs included here.

Nursing Drug Reference: A Practitioner's Guide

Library of Congress Cataloging in Publication Data
Main entry under title:

Nursing drug reference.

  Includes index.
   1. Drugs. 2. Pharmacology. 3. Nurse practitioners.
I. Edmunds, Marilyn W. [DNLM: 1. Drugs—Nursing texts.
2. Nurse practitioners—Nursing texts. QV 55 P895]
RM300.N88 1985   615'.1   83-21562

ISBN 0-89303-764-8

Prentice-Hall of Australia, Pty., Ltd., *Sydney*
Prentice-Hall Canada, Inc., Scarborough, *Ontario*
Prentice-Hall Hispanoamericana, S.A., *Mexico*
Prentice-Hall of India Private Limited, *New Delhi*
Prentice-Hall International, Inc., *London*
Prentice-Hall of Japan, Inc., *Tokyo*
Prentice-Hall of Southeast Asia Pte. Ltd., *Singapore*
Editora Prentice-Hall Do Brasil LTDA., *Rio de Janeiro*
Whitehall Books, Limited, Petone, *New Zealand*

Printed in the United States of America

85 86 87 88 89 90 91 92 93 94 95   1 2 3 4 5 6 7 8 9 10

CONTENTS

CONTRIBUTORS

Kathleen Awalt, R.N., M.S., P.N.P.-C., Instructor, University of Maryland School of Medicine, Baltimore, Maryland

Geraldine Polly Bednash, R.N., B.S.N., M.S.N., A.N.P.-C., Assistant Professor, George Mason University and Dewitt Army Hospital Family Practice Residency Program Consultant, Fairfax, Virginia.

Molly Craig Billingsley, R.N., Ed.D., A.N.P.-C., Associate Professor, George Mason University, Fairfax, Virginia. Formerly Senior Nurse Practitioner, The Teen Health Service, St. Johns Hospital, Lowell, Massachusetts.

Mary Ann Bolter, R.N., M.S., A.N.P.-C., Formerly Nurse Practitioner, Group Health Association, Bethesda, Maryland.

Carol P. Burke, R.N., M.S., A.N.P.-C., Nurse Practitioner, University of Maryland, Baltimore County Student Health Center, Baltimore, Maryland.

Marilyn Winterton Edmunds, R.N., M.S.N., A.N.P.-C., Assistant Professor, University of Maryland, Primary Care Department, Baltimore, Maryland.

Sheila T. Fitzgerald, R.N., M.S.N., A.N.P.-C., Doctoral Student, Occupational Health, The Johns Hopkins University, Baltimore, Maryland.

Marsha E. Goodwin, R.N., M.S.N., M.A., A.N.P.-C., Office of Geriatrics and Extended Care, Veterans Administration, Washington, D.C.

Doreen C. Harper, R.N., Ph.D., A.N.P.-C., Chairperson, R.N. Program, University of Maryland School of Nursing, Baltimore County Campus, Catonsville, Maryland.

Carole A. Hill, R.N., M.S., A.N.P.-C., Director of Nursing, Charlestown Community Inc., Catonsville, Maryland.

L. Colette Jones, R.N., Ph.D., A.N.P.-C., Associate Professor, University of Maryland School of Nursing, Primary Care Department, Baltimore, Maryland.

Irene McCrea, R.N., M.S., A.N.P.-C., Instructor, Howard Community College, Columbia, Maryland.

Candis Morrison, R.N., M.S., A.N.P.-C., Community College of Baltimore Health Service, and Private Practice, Baltimore, Maryland.

Patricia H. Newton, R.N., B.S., A.N.P.-C., Private Practice, Alexandria, Virginia.

Mary Fry Rapson, R.N., Ph.D., A.N.P.-C., Acting Associate Dean for Undergraduate Studies, University of Maryland School of Nursing, Baltimore, Maryland.

Linda Ross, R.N., M.A., P.N.P.-C., Instructor, Georgetown University Hospital, Dept. of Pediatrics, School of Medicine, Child Development Center, Washington, D.C.

Marna Justice Ross, R.N., M.S., A.N.P.-C., Formerly Nurse Practitioner, Planned Parenthood of Maryland, Baltimore, Maryland.

Joann Sabados-Carolina, R.N., M.S., A.N.P.-C., Nurse Practitioner, Community Health, Patient Care, West Orange, New Jersey.

Maren Stewart, R.N., M.S., A.N.P.-C., Community Health Nurse, Prince Georges County Health Department, Maryland.

Carol C. Sylvester, R.N., M.S., A.N.P.-C., Gerontologic Practitioner in Foster Care Program for the Frail Elderly, The Johns Hopkins Hospital, Baltimore, Maryland.

Carol Ann Vittek, R.N., M.S., A.N.P.-C., Nurse Practitioner, Adult Emergency Department, The Johns Hopkins Hospital, Baltimore, Maryland.

Barbara Sommer Wieferich, R.N., M.S., A.N.P.-C., formerly of Church Hospital, Baltimore, Maryland.

Carol Wilson, R.N., M.S.N., P.N.P.-C., Nurse Practitioner, Rosemont Community Doctors Center, Baltimore, Maryland.

Bonnie Keegan Winterton, R.N., A.N.P.-C., formerly of Brigham Young University Student Health Center, Provo, Utah.

FOREWORD

The nurse practitioner movement is now nearly two decades old. At its inception no, much thought was given to the necessity for a new level of knowledge of pharmacology for nurse practitioners. Early practitioner education programs were short. They tended to focus primarily on the diagnostic process with brief coverage of treatment using written protocols. The view of the nurse practitioner role was more circumscribed than it is now, and there seemed to be an assumption that nurse practitioners might somehow lean upon the scientific knowledge base of their physician colleagues.

However, as the nurse practitioner movement matures it seems obvious that one profession cannot lean upon the knowledge base of another. Our patients are safe only if we are competent, and our level of competence involves understanding not only what to do but also why we do it. This does not mean that nurse practitioners cannot ask for consultation or refer patients with complex problems to physicians and other health professionals, but it does mean that we need to treat ordinary illnesses in a safe fashion and to make intelligent referrals.

Thus, as the nurse practitioner role became more clearly defined, it has become apparent that a good basic knowledge of clinical pharmacology is needed and that understanding necessarily predicated on a suitable textbook. Traditional nursing texts tend to be limited to the information that is needed to safely administer and monitor drugs for adverse side effects. While this data is important, it is insufficient for making decisions about prescribing. Traditional medical texts tend to focus on pharmacokinetics, with less emphasis on the clinical application of knowledge. They also fail to emphasize patient teaching, which is such a central focus of the nurse practitioner role.

This text was designed to fill that gap between the medical and nursing texts. The plan for the work was formulated by Marilyn W. Edmunds, a nurse practitioner faculty member, and it was written by her in conjunction with 23 other contributing authors, all of whom are nurse practitioners. These clinicians understood the needs of this new field. The text they have produced furnishes the important scientific background about drugs that is needed for decision-making, yet retains the nursing concerns for patient teaching and comfort.

This work is particularly important in this era of controversy over prescription writing privileges. This function is handled in a variety of ways in state laws and regulations. Moreover, many states are contemplating changes in the law to give nurse practitioners and nurse midwives more responsibilities. Yet before they make these changes, legislators want to be assured that nurses are competent to prescribe. This is a time of testing of the nurse practitioner role and a high level of performance is called for. This book should help supply one of the tools upon which a strong clinical practice base may be built.

Bonnie Bullough, R.N., Ph.D., FAAN
Certified Pediatric Nurse Practitioner
and Family Nurse Practitioner
Dean, School of Nursing
State University of New York at Buffalo

PREFACE

With the expanding role of nurses has come commensurate expanding responsibility in regard to medications. While nurses have always had significant obligation in implementing physician medication orders, the character of the medication tasks nurses undertake has continued to evolve. With the advent of the nurse practitioner role, nurses have been gradually gaining legal authority to prescribe medications. Even in states in which practitioners do not prescribe medications, nurses have accepted more and more responsibility for the medication monitoring of clients with chronic disease. While the legal sanction for nurses varies from state to state in both its scope and degree of implementation, the challenges for nurses practicing in the expanded role to accurately assess client needs, match the best medication to the clinical problem, and monitor the therapeutic effects becomes more obvious.

The degree of freedom which nurses should have with regard to prescribing medications is not uniform, and the debate over this issue has been most intense from those groups interested in limiting this authority. The suggestion has been made that no new group of non-physician drug prescribers should be introduced into the health care system until they can carry out their responsibilities as well as or better than current drug prescribers. If one were to accept this criteria, it would be obvious that a variety of techniques should be adopted to help prescribers become as effective as possible in implementing their new task. One of the resources which has been developed to assist the new practitioners is this reference manual.

The skeleton of this book developed from the desire to find a pharmacology reference book which is congruent in philosophy with accepted nursing practice. Every component of the book has been influenced in development by the nursing process format and the pressures placed on clinical practice by expanded role performance of the nurse. What has emerged is a true nursing product.

This book was written primarily as a reference manual for the nurse practicing in an expanded role, regardless of title, and has an ambulatory, out-patient orientation. It is anticipated that nurse practitioners, nurse midwives, mental health therapists, and other staff clinicians will make up the bulk of the reading audience. However, because of the nursing process format, the book should appeal to the total spectrum of nursing clinicians from the advanced nursing student to the skilled practitioner. The nurse in occupational health settings, nursing homes, student health centers, Hospice care units, as well as more traditional sites may benefit from this information. Students in particular should be able to easily find and use the information presented. While the "nursing process", as such, is familiar to nurses, other non-nursing personnel may recognize within it the basic elements of the standard problem-solving approach. Thus, physician's assistants, psychiatric social workers, school health aides, psychologists, dieticians, etc. may also benefit from utilizing the information this book provides.

This manual has been written by experienced nursing clinicians who have blended together academic knowledge and practical experience needed to prescribe medication and/or monitor the therapeutic effects of common medications. They have synthesized the information which they as clinicians have found important in achieving meaningful results with clients taking these products. The success of their experience with patients has been substantial and their qualifications to speak with authority are high.

As an educator, I have experienced constant frustration in assembling all the information which nurse practitioners should know for safe drug prescribing. Most nurse practitioners rely heavily upon an assembly of medical, pharmacologic and nursing texts, sifting through several texts to find a group of coherent facts to guide clinical practice. The medical texts often brush over the parameters which should be assessed and monitored, while the pharmacologic texts get lost in the pharmacokinetics and biological interactions. The traditional nursing texts remain too general for the prescribing of specific medications. None seem to stress the patient teaching components which are so crucial to the nurse practitioner-patient relationship.

With the nurse's involvement in the prescribing of medications, nursing moves beyond the appropriateness of simple "nursing implications" sections found in traditional drug books to guide practice. The whole gamut of the prescribing process becomes enmeshed with the nursing process, where assessment, plan, implementation, and evaluation are fundamental to effective practice. Consequently, within the framework of this book, the nurse's responsibility in regard to medications is intertwined with the prescribing and monitoring process. In the first section of each drug monograph, nursing and medical information important in the assessment process, are outlined. This includes assessment of both the subjective and objective problems of the patient and a discussion of the action and usual indications for the drug. The purpose of this section, then, is to allow the nurse the opportunity to assess the match between patient complaints and actions of the medication.

The second phase of the nursing process, planning, includes specific contraindications, warnings, and precautions which the nurse must be aware of if this medication is to be utilized. This information should be examined in light of the specific clinical status of the individual client, and the medication plan should be thoroughly outlined.

In the third phase of the nursing process, implementation, cautions regarding drug interactions are included. General information about the dosage schedule and administration techniques is presented, and specific implementation considerations are outlined. Information which the patient needs to know about taking this medication is presented. This section is written in lay terminology and should be presented to the patient, in either written form (preferably) or through verbal teaching sessions. A large number of research studies have indicated that more than 50% of medications are taken in error by clients at home and that compliance can be increased and drug errors decreased through the use of written instructions. These facts make this section of patient teaching information especially important. Nurses have traditionally excelled in patient teaching and counseling, and this section was developed to serve as the core of teaching information which, when passed on to patients, should help in achieving better therapeutic responses.

The fourth component of the nursing process, evaluation, includes adverse reactions which might be prompted by the medication, signs and symptoms of overdosage, and specific parameters for the nurse to monitor while the patient is taking this drug. These include when the patient should be seen again, what laboratory work should be obtained, and changes in client status which would indicate either the appropriate therapeutic response or that the drug should be discontinued.

The medications which have been selected for inclusion in this manual are ones which will be of the widest use to the variety of clinicians it is to serve, although the focus on outpatient ambulatory medications does exclude some products. Attempts have been made to include both generic standards of therapy and new and promising medications just appearing on the market.

Many students and professional colleagues have generously provided helpful comments on and criticisms of sections of this book. The staff of Brady Communications Company were invaluable in their assistance during the preparation of this text. I would particularly like to thank my editors Laura Marcy, Dave Culverwell, and Richard Weimer, for their assistance. Production editors Karen Zack and Janis Oppelt have earned my greatest admiration and friendship for their conscientious attention to detail on this long and complex project. I value greatly the encouragement of Allan Rosenbaum Ph.D., Virginia Ruth D.P.H, Mary Rapson Ph.D., and Alyce Edmunds during the trying times of the editing process.

This book is dedicated with love to Omni and Carma Winterton, whose abundant faith and confidence made the whole thing possible, and to my husband, Cliff, and children Michael, Christopher, Clark, and Megan, who sacrificed much that this book might come to be.

HOW TO USE THIS BOOK

This book is divided into 10 major chapters reflecting major categories of drugs. Each section can be readily found by consulting the key to the chapters on the inside cover of the front or back of the book.

Each of the 10 major sections of this book contain drug monographs outlining important information about individual drugs or groups of related drugs. Each section begins with an outline which refers the reader directly to product information.

For example:

Amebicides (page 2)
Anthelmintics (page 8)
Antibiotics (page 23)
Antifungals (page 76)
Anti-infectives (Misc) (page 84)
Antimalarials (page 90)
Antitubercular Drugs (page 103)
Antiviral Drugs (page 133)
Sulfonamides (page 139)

Each drug monograph begins with an introductory explanation regarding drug action followed by four major sections of information, organized according to the "Nursing Process." These four sections, *Assessment, Plan, Implementation,* and *Evaluation,* contain standard drug information as well as information integrated throughout which the nurse needs to be aware of before prescribing this drug or assuming responsibility for monitoring the care of patients receiving this medication. Information of particular importance for the nurse to be aware of is printed in green.

When consulting the section on *Assessment,* the usual indications for use of the drug will be found, as well as subjective and objective complaints presented by patients who might be candidates for this medication. Wherever indicated, suggestions for patient assessment are included. This section is designed to allow the practitioner to assess the fit of the drug to the specific patient problem.

ASSESSMENT:

INDICATIONS: Used as the primary therapy for intestinal or extraintestinal amebiasis. Choice of drug depends upon the location of the infection. The most common extraintestinal infection is hepatic abscess. Due to the toxicity and complexity of extraintestinal infections it might be wise to consult the Parasitic Disease Division, Centers for Infectious Diseases, Centers for Disease Control, Atlanta, Georgia 30333 (telephone 404-329-3670) prior to treatment. While it is doubtful that nurse practitioners would prescribe some of these medications, they often assume responsibility for monitoring the progress of patients placed on this therapy.

Diiodohydroxyquin and metronidazole are also used in the treatment of *Trichomonas vaginalis* (see section on vaginal anti-infectives). Chloroquine phosphate, primarily an antimalarial agent, is also used for amebiasis and rheumatoid arthritis. (See antimalarial section.)

SUBJECTIVE: History of diarrhea, vomiting, weight loss. Also, history of travel to or living in areas with a low standard of hygiene.

OBJECTIVE: Presence of amebas or cysts in the stool.

The *Plan* section contains drug contraindications, warnings, and precautions as suggested by various drug manufacturers. The standard information in this portion of the monograph assists the practitioner in developing a medication plan for individual patients, particularly those patients who may be very young, the elderly, pregnant or breast-feeding women, or patients with particular organ dysfunction or impairment.

PLAN:

CONTRAINDICATIONS: There are five major drugs which are used as amebicides. The contraindications are somewhat different according to the drug chosen:

Chloroquine phosphate: Do not use if the patient has a history of visual or retinal changes, porphyria, or hypersensitivity to 4-aminoquinoline compounds.

Diiodohydroxyquin: Do not use if the patient has a history of hypersensitivity to 8-hydroxyquinoline compounds or iodine, hepatic or renal disease, optic neuropathy, or severe thyroid disorders.

WARNINGS: Due to the toxicity of these drugs, exercise care in determining the need for such treatment. Do not exceed recommended dosages. If subsequent treatments are needed, allow proper time interval prior to second treatment. Use metronidazole with discretion as it has been proven carcinogenic in mice.

PRECAUTIONS: Monitor for signs of toxicity. If severe symptoms appear that are not attributable to the disorder, discontinue the drug.

Patients receiving emetine HCl should live sedentary life styles during the time of treatment. This drug may cause ECG changes which persist for weeks after therapy is discontinued. The ECG changes are similar to those of myocardial infarction. Emetine may also decrease potassium levels.

The *Implementation* section contains valuable information obtained from recently reported studies and clinical experience which assists the practitioner in safe and accurate drug administration. The latest information on drug interactions, general administration, and dosage is provided. If the drug monograph contains information on only one individual drug, the specific product information and dosage schedules are included here.

IMPLEMENTATION:

DRUG INTERACTIONS: With the exception of metronidazole, there are no significant drug interactions. Combining metronidazole with alcohol can produce headache, flushing, cramps, nausea and vomiting. If combined with disulfiram, acute psychoses may result.

ADMINISTRATION AND DOSAGE SPECIFICS: The choice of the drug depends upon the location of the infection. Some of these drugs are specific for extraintestinal infections. Due to the toxicity of these drugs, the decision for treatment must be weighed carefully. When prescribing any of these drugs, use the smallest therapeutic dosage possible for the shortest duration of time. If the initial drug is ineffective and the alternative is more hazardous, a repeat treatment with the initial drug may be advisable. Table 1-1 shows a suggested protocol of treatment for amebiasis. (See individual product sections for dosage schedule.)

This section also contains considerations for implementing the therapeutic regimen as outlined for the practitioner in a step-by-step format. These items include relevant history to obtain from the patient, specific items to stress in patient teaching, other treatment modalities which might be considered, as well as reminders about key drug actions, adverse reactions, or drug storage and handling information.

IMPLEMENTATION CONSIDERATIONS:

—Obtain a complete health history including the presence of hypersensitivity to drugs, concurrent use of alcohol or disulfiram, underlying systemic renal, cardiac, thyroid or liver disease which may be a contraindication to use of these drugs, and possibility of pregnancy.

—Document the presence of amebae.

—Order baseline complete blood count, electrolytes, kidney and liver function tests, and ECG. Do audiometric and ophthalmologic examinations if specific drug for therapy could affect these systems.

What the patient needs to know when taking the preparation is also presented in this section. This information should always be shared with the patient when drug therapy with the particular product is begun. It is, therefore, written in second person and in a simpler language so that it can be duplicated directly and given to patients, or utilized by the nurse as the core of patient-teaching sessions.

WHAT THE PATIENT NEEDS TO KNOW:

—Take all medication as prescribed. Do not skip doses or double medication doses. Do not stop taking medication without being advised by health practitioner to do so.

—Taking this drug with or after meals will decrease the chances of stomach upset.

—Some patients experience side effects from this medication. Be certain to report any new or troublesome symptoms to your health care practitioner.

—The gastrointestinal system (mouth) is the point of entry for these infections. Usually infection results from fecal contamination of foods, or by hand-mouth contamination. Careful washing of food before eating, and washing of hands after going to the bathroom and before preparing food is important to avoid spreading infection.

—After drug therapy has been completed, it is essential that periodic stool examination be performed to look for reinfection or for people who may still have amebiasis but are not symptomatic.

The *Evaluation* section lists both alphabetically and by body systems major adverse reactions which have been reported by patients using these products. The most commonly reported reactions are printed in green in order to provide a proper perspective for practitioners when they view the list.

EVALUATION:

ADVERSE REACTIONS: Chloroquine Phosphate: *CNS:* convulsions, dizziness, fatigue, headache, irritability, neuromyopathy, nightmares, psychic stimulation. *Dermatologic:* pigmentary changes of skin and mucosa, pruritus.
EENT: ototoxicity, tinnitus, vertigo, visual disturbances. *Gastrointestinal:* abdominal cramps, anorexia, diarrhea, nausea, vomiting. *Hematopoietic:* agranulocytosis.

Diiodohydroxyquin: *CNS:* agitation, ataxia, headache, neurotoxicity, peripheral neuropathy, retrograde amnesia, vertigo. *Dermatologic:* discoloration of hair and nails, papular and pustular eruptions, pruritus, urticaria. *EENT:* loss of vision, optic atrophy, optic neuritis. *Gastrointestinal:* abdominal cramps, anal irritation and pruritus, anorexia, constipation, diarrhea, epigastric discomfort, gastritis, nausea, vomiting. *Hematopoietic:* agranulocytosis. *Other:* chills, fever, hair loss, thyroid enlargement.

Emetine HCl: *Cardiovascular:* cardiac dilatation, congestive failure, dyspnea, ECG abnormalities, gallop rhythm, hypotension, myocarditis, pericarditis, precordial pain. *CNS:* central or peripheral nerve function changes, dizziness, headache, mild sensory disturbances, neuromuscular symptoms. *Dermatologic:* urticarial, pur-

---

Information regarding signs, symptoms, and treatment of overdosage are also outlined. The final evaluation material focuses on particular parameters which the practitioner should monitor while the patient is taking the medication. Baseline data which should be obtained and laboratory data or clinical signs which should be monitored are identified. Information which guides the practitioner in determining whether the proper therapeutic response is being achieved, or whether therapy should be terminated, are included. Specific follow-up stuides which may be required and how often the patient should be seen are also presented when relevant.

OVERDOSAGE: Chloroquine toxicity might produce headache, drowsiness, visual disturbances, ototoxicity and cardiovascular collapse which could result in respiratory and cardiac arrest. Diiodohydroxyquin overdosage is usually due to the iodine in this drug. These symptoms include headache, fever, chills, rhinitis, sore throat, dermatitis and furunculosis. Optic neuritis and loss of vision could also develop. When emetine is the drug of treatment, toxicity to the cardiac muscle may be indicated by an increase in pulse and a decrease in blood pressure. Sudden cardiac failure could develop. Metronidazole can produce CNS toxicity, which may be heralded by confusion, irritability, paresthesia, ataxia or tremors. Paromomycin overdosage could result in ototoxicity, nephrotoxicity or malabsorption syndrome.

PARAMETERS TO MONITOR: Prior to initiating therapy, carefully screen patients by obtaining complete history and physical examination. Screen for visual, hearing, hematologic, cardiovascular, hepatic, kidney or thyroid disorders. Obtain baseline audiometry and ophthalmologic examinations, liver function tests, electrolytes, kidney function tests, complete blood count, blood pressure, pulse and weight. Observe for therapeutic and adverse effects. With emetine, ECG monitoring is also mandatory. All or some of these tests may be repeated during and following drug therapy, as indicated. After drug therapy, periodic stool examinations are necessary to ascertain that the disease has been eliminated. These examinations may be done on a monthly basis for up to a year after therapy.

When the general drug monograph describes a group of related drugs, specific product information is presented at the end of the monograph. Each generic drug is listed alphabetically, with specific product listings (including trade name, dosage forms and strengths) whether product is available over the counter, drug administration and specific dosage schedules. Considerations for the practitioner continue to be integrated throughout the specific product information content.

CHLOROQUINE PHOSPHATE

PRODUCTS (TRADE NAME):
Aralen Phosphate (Available in 25 mg tablets equivalent to 150 mg chloroquine base.) **Chloroquine Phosphate** (Available in 250 mg tablets, equivalent to 150 mg chloroquine base.)

DRUG SPECIFICS: Avoid use in patients with visual or retinal changes. Watch for ototoxicity. Obtain baseline audiometry tests. This is a drug used primarily in combination with other ambecides in treatment of hepatic abscess.

ADMINISTRATION AND DOSAGE SPECIFICS:
Hepatic Abscess:
Adults: Following treatment by emetine (1 mg/kg per day IM for up to 5 days), give 600 mg base (1 gm) daily for two days, then 300 mg base (500 mg) daily for 2-3 weeks. At the same time give diiodohydroxyquin 650 mg three times daily for 20 days.
Children: Following treatment by emetine (1 mg/kg IM per day in two doses for up to 5 days), give 10 mg base/kg per day (maximum 300 mg base daily) for 2-3 weeks. At the same time give diiodohydroxyquin 30-40 mg/kg daily in three doses for 20 days.

A complete index is included in the back of the book, with drugs listed by major category, generic and trade names.

A special appendix has been developed for assisting the student, the clinician, and new non-physician drug prescribers. Various tables which might assist in interpreting or writing prescriptions and calculating drug conversion dosages are included in this final section.

1

ANTI-INFECTIVES

AMEBICIDES

ACTION OF THE DRUG: The main action of an amebicide is the destruction of the invading ameba which may be located within the intestinal lumen or at an extraintestinal site. The exact mechanism of action is unknown.

ASSESSMENT:

INDICATIONS: Used as the primary therapy for intestinal or extraintestinal amebiasis. Choice of drug depends upon the location of the infection. The most common extraintestinal infection is hepatic abscess. Due to the toxicity and complexity of extraintestinal infections it might be wise to consult the Parasitic Disease Division, Centers for Infectious Diseases, Centers for Disease Control, Atlanta, Georgia 30333 (telephone 404-329-3670) prior to treatment. While it is doubtful that nurse practitioners would prescribe some of these medications, they often assume responsibility for monitoring the progress of patients placed on this therapy.

Diiodohydroxyquin and metronidazole are also used in the treatment of *Trichomonas vaginalis* (see section on vaginal anti-infectives). Chloroquine phosphate, primarily an antimalarial agent, is also used for amebiasis and rheumatoid arthritis. (See antimalarial section.)

SUBJECTIVE: History of diarrhea, vomiting, weight loss. Also, history of travel to or living in areas with a low standard of hygiene.

OBJECTIVE: Presence of amebas or cysts in the stool.

PLAN:

CONTRAINDICATIONS: There are five major drugs which are used as amebicides. The contraindications are somewhat different according to the drug chosen:

Chloroquine phosphate: Do not use if the patient has a history of visual or retinal changes, porphyria, or hypersensitivity to 4-aminoquinoline compounds.

Diiodohydroxyquin: Do not use if the patient has a history of hypersensitivity to 8-hydroxyquinoline compounds or iodine, hepatic or renal disease, optic neuropathy, or severe thyroid disorders.

Emetine Hydrochloride: Do not use for those patients that have been treated with this drug less than 6 weeks previously, elderly persons, children, or in the presence of cardiac or renal disorders or pregnancy.

Metronidazole: Do not give in the presence of hypersensitivity to the drug, history of retinal or visual changes, blood dyscrasias, CNS disorder, pregnancy or to nursing mothers. Do not give to patients who are unreliable in eliminating alcohol intake during therapy, or those currently taking disulfiram (Antabuse).

Paromomycin: Do not give in the presence of hypersensitivity, intestinal obstruction or impaired renal function.

WARNINGS: Due to the toxicity of these drugs, exercise care in determining the need for such treatment. Do not exceed recommended dosages. If subsequent treatments are needed, allow proper time interval prior to second treatment. Use metronidazole with discretion as it has been proven carcinogenic in mice.

PRECAUTIONS: Monitor for signs of toxicity. If severe symptoms appear that are not attributable to the disorder, discontinue the drug.

Patients receiving emetine HCl should live sedentary life styles during the time of treatment. This drug may cause ECG changes which persist for weeks after therapy is discontinued. The ECG changes are similar to those of myocardial infarction. Emetine may also decrease potassium levels.

IMPLEMENTATION:

DRUG INTERACTIONS: With the exception of metronidazole, there are no significant drug interactions. Combining metronidazole with alcohol can produce headache, flushing, cramps, nausea and vomiting. If combined with disulfiram, acute psychoses may result.

ADMINISTRATION AND DOSAGE SPECIFICS: The choice of the drug depends upon the location of the infection. Some of these drugs are specific for extraintestinal infections. Due to the toxicity of these drugs, the decision for treatment must be weighed carefully. When prescribing any of these drugs, use the smallest therapeutic dosage possible for the shortest duration of time. If the initial drug is ineffective and the alternative is more hazardous, a repeat treatment with the initial drug may be advisable. Table 1-1 shows a suggested protocol of treatment for amebiasis. (See individual product sections for dosage schedule.)

IMPLEMENTATION CONSIDERATIONS:

—Obtain a complete health history including the presence of hypersensitivity to drugs, concurrent use of alcohol or disulfiram, underlying systemic renal, cardiac, thyroid or liver disease which may be a contraindication to use of these drugs, and possibility of pregnancy.

—Document the presence of amebae.

—Order baseline complete blood count, electrolytes, kidney and liver function tests, and ECG. Do audiometric and ophthalmologic examinations if specific drug for therapy could affect these systems.

Table 1-1. DRUG PROTOCOL FOR TREATMENT OF AMEBIASIS

Site of Infections	*Choice of Drug*	*Alternate Drug*
Intestinal		
Asymptomatic	Diiodohydroxyquin	Paromomycin
Mild to moderate	Metronidazole and diiodohydroxyquin	Paromomycin
Severe	Metronidazole and diiodohydroxyquin	Emetine HCl and diiodohydroxyquin
Extraintestinal		
hepatic abscess	Metronidazole and diiodohydroxyquine	Emetine HCl followed by chloroquine phosphate and diiodohydroxyquin

—Diet should be high calorie, low residue during therapy. Increase intake of fluids. Monitor intake and output during therapy.

—Teach patient about the method of infection and review specific methods of personal hygiene to prevent reinfection and to reduce the risk of spreading infection to others.

—Good rapport with patient should promote compliance.

—It will be important to obtain follow-up stool specimens to document effective treatment.

WHAT THE PATIENT NEEDS TO KNOW:

—Take all medication as prescribed. Do not skip doses or double medication doses. Do not stop taking medication without being advised by health practitioner to do so.

—Taking this drug with or after meals will decrease the chances of stomach upset.

—Some patients experience side effects from this medication. Be certain to report any new or troublesome symptoms to your health care practitioner.

—The gastrointestinal system (mouth) is the point of entry for these infections. Usually infection results from fecal contamination of foods, or by hand-mouth contamination. Careful washing of food before eating, and washing of hands after going to the bathroom and before preparing food is important to avoid spreading infection.

—After drug therapy has been completed, it is essential that periodic stool examination be performed to look for reinfection or for people who may still have amebiasis but are not symptomatic.

EVALUATION:

ADVERSE REACTIONS: Chloroquine Phosphate: *CNS:* convulsions, dizziness, fatigue, headache, irritability, neuromyopathy, nightmares, psychic stimulation. *Dermatologic:* pigmentary changes of skin and mucosa, pruritus.

EENT: ototoxicity, tinnitus, vertigo, visual disturbances. *Gastrointestinal:* abdominal cramps, anorexia, diarrhea, nausea, vomiting. *Hematopoietic:* agranulocytosis.

Diiodohydroxyquin: *CNS:* agitation, ataxia, headache, neurotoxicity, peripheral neuropathy, retrograde amnesia, vertigo. *Dermatologic:* discoloration of hair and nails, papular and pustular eruptions, pruritus, urticaria. *EENT:* loss of vision, optic atrophy, optic neuritis. *Gastrointestinal:* abdominal cramps, anal irritation and pruritus, anorexia, constipation, diarrhea, epigastric discomfort, gastritis, nausea, vomiting. *Hematopoietic: agranulocytosis. Other:* chills, fever, hair loss, thyroid enlargement.

Emetine HCl: *Cardiovascular:* cardiac dilatation, congestive failure, dyspnea, ECG abnormalities, gallop rhythm, hypotension, myocarditis, pericarditis, precordial pain. *CNS:* central or peripheral nerve function changes, dizziness, headache, mild sensory disturbances, neuromuscular symptoms. *Dermatologic:* urticarial, purpuric lesions. *Gastrointestinal:* abdominal cramps, diarrhea, loss of taste, nausea, vomiting. *Local:* aching and muscle weakness at injection site, tenderness. *Metabolic:* decreased serum potassium levels. *Other:* edema.

Metronidazole: *Cardiovascular:* ECG changes (T wave flattening). *CNS:* ataxia, confusion, depression, fatigue, headache, incoordination, insomnia, irritability, neuromyopathy, paresthesias of extremities, sleepiness, vertigo. *Dermatologic:* flushing, pruritus. *EENT:* blurred vision, nasal congestion. *Gastrointestinal:* abdominal cramps, anorexia, constipation, diarrhea, nausea, proctitis, vomiting. *Genitourinary:* cystitis, decreased libido, dysuria, dyspareunia, incontinence, pelvic pressure, polyuria, pyuria. *Hematopoietic:* leukopenia, neutropenia. *Other:* fever, metallic taste, overgrowth of nonsusceptible organisms.

Paromomycin Sulfate: *CNS:* headache, vertigo. *Dermatologic:* pruritus, rash. *EENT:* Ototoxicity. *Gastrointestinal:* abdominal cramps, anal pruritus, anorexia, constipation, diarrhea, epigastric discomfort, malabsorption syndrome, nausea, steatorrhea, vomiting. *Genitourinary:* hematuria, nephrotoxicity. *Hematopoietic:* eosinophilia. *Other:* overgrowth of nonsusceptible organisms.

OVERDOSAGE: Chloroquine toxicity might produce headache, drowsiness, visual disturbances, ototoxicity and cardiovascular collapse which could result in respiratory and cardiac arrest. Diiodohydroxyquin overdosage is usually due to the iodine in this drug. These symptoms include headache, fever, chills, rhinitis, sore throat, dermatitis and furunculosis. Optic neuritis and loss of vision could also develop. When emetine is the drug of treatment, toxicity to the cardiac muscle may be indicated by an increase in pulse and a decrease in blood pressure. Sudden cardiac failure could develop. Metronidazole can produce CNS toxicity, which may be heralded by confusion, irritability, paresthesia, ataxia or tremors. Paromomycin overdosage could result in ototoxicity, nephrotoxicity or malabsorption syndrome.

PARAMETERS TO MONITOR: Prior to initiating therapy, carefully screen patients by obtaining complete history and physical examination. Screen for visual, hearing, hematologic, cardiovascular, hepatic, kidney or thyroid disorders. Obtain baseline audiometry and ophthalmologic examinations, liver function tests, electrolytes, kidney function tests, complete blood count, blood pressure, pulse and weight. Observe for therapeutic and adverse effects. With emetine, ECG monitoring is also mandatory. All or some of these tests may be repeated during and following drug therapy, as indicated. After drug therapy, periodic stool examinations are necessary to ascertain that the disease has been eliminated. These examinations may be done on a monthly basis for up to a year after therapy.

CHLOROQUINE PHOSPHATE

PRODUCTS (TRADE NAME):
Aralen Phosphate (Available in 25 mg tablets equivalent to 150 mg chloroquine base.) **Chloroquine Phosphate** (Available in 250 mg tablets, equivalent to 150 mg chloroquine base.)
DRUG SPECIFICS: Avoid use in patients with visual or retinal changes. Watch for ototoxicity. Obtain baseline audiometry tests. This is a drug used primarily in combination with other ambecides in treatment of hepatic abscess.

ADMINISTRATION AND DOSAGE SPECIFICS:

Hepatic Abscess:

Adults: Following treatment by emetine (1 mg/kg per day IM for up to 5 days), give 600 mg base (1 gm) daily for two days, then 300 mg base (500 mg) daily for 2-3 weeks. At the same time give diiodohydroxyquin 650 mg three times daily for 20 days.

Children: Following treatment by emetine (1 mg/kg IM per day in two doses for up to 5 days), give 10 mg base/kg per day (maximum 300 mg base daily) for 2-3 weeks. At the same time give diiodohydroxyquin 30-40 mg/kg daily in three doses for 20 days.

DIIODOHYDROXYQUIN OR IODOQUINOL

PRODUCTS (TRADE NAME):

Iodoquinol (Available in 650 mg tablets.) **Moebiquin** (Available in 650 mg tablets.) **Yodoxin** (Available in 210 mg tablets or 25 gm powder.)

DRUG SPECIFICS: Diiodohydroxyquin is the drug of choice in asymptomatic intestinal amebiasis. It is also used as adjunctive therapy with other amebecides. It is also effective in the treatment of trichomonas vaginalis infections.

ADMINISTRATION AND DOSAGE SPECIFICS:

Asymptomatic Intestinal Amebiasis:

Adults: 630 to 650 mg po three times daily for 20 days.

Children: 30-40 mg/kg/day po in 3 doses for 20 days.

Mild or moderate Intestinal Amebiasis:

Adults: In addition to metronidazole (750 mg three times daily for 5-10 days) give 630 to 650 mg po three times daily for 20 days.

Children: In addition to metronidazole (35-50 mg/kg/day in three doses for 10 days) give 30-40 mg/kg po per day in 3 doses for 20 days.

Severe Intestinal Amebiasis:

Adults: As an alternative to metronidazole and diiodohydroxyquin, may give emetine (1 mg/kg per day (maximum 60 mg daily) IM for up to 5 days) plus 630 to 650 mg diiodohydroxyquin po three times daily for 20 days.

Children: As an alternative to metronidazole and diiodohydroxyquin, may give emetine (1 mg/kg per day in 2 doses [maximum 60 mg day] IM for up to 5 days) plus 30-40 mg/kg/day diiodohydroxyquin po in 3 doses for 20 days.

Hepatic Abscess:

Adults: In addition to metronidazole (750 mg/three times daily for 5-10 days) give diiodohydroxyquin 630 to 650 mg three times daily for 20 days. May also give in combination with emetine (1 mg/kg per day [maximum 60 mg daily] IM for up to 5 days, followed by chloroquine phosphate (600 mg base [1 gm] daily for two days then 300 mg base [500 mg] daily for 2-3 weeks and at the same time give 630 to 650 mg diiodohydroxyquin three times daily for 20 days.

Children: In addition to metronidazole (35-50 mg/kg daily in three doses for 10 days) give 30-40 mg/kg diiodohydroxyquin per day in three doses for 20 days. May also give with emetine (1 mg/kg per day in two doses (maximum 60 mg daily) IM for up to 5 days), followed by chloroquine phosphate (10 mg base/kg per day (maximum 300 mg base daily) for 2-3 weeks and 30-40 mg/kg diiodohydroxyquin daily in three doses for 20 days.

EMETINE HCL

PRODUCTS (TRADE NAME):
  Emetine HCl (Available in 65 mg/ml for injection.)
DRUG SPECIFICS: This product is used as alternative drug therapy in severe intestinal or extraintestinal amebiasis therapy. Because of its effects on the heart, ECG monitoring is mandatory while patient is taking this product and patient should be as sedentary as possible during treatment period.
ADMINISTRATION AND DOSAGE SPECIFICS:
  Severe Intestinal Amebiasis:
  Adults: Give 1 mg/kg per day (maximum 60 mg daily) IM for up to 5 days. Also give 630 to 650 mg diiodohydroxyquin three times daily for 20 days.
  Children: Give 1 mg/kg per day in 2 doses (maximum 60 mg daily) IM for up to 5 days. At the same time give 30-40 mg/kg per day diiodohydroxyquin in 3 doses for 20 days.
  Hepatic Abscess:
  Adults: Give 1 mg/kg per day (maximum 60 mg daily) IM for up to 5 days. Follow with chloroquine phosphate (600 mg base [1 gm] daily for two days, then
    300 mg base [500 mg]) daily for 2-3 weeks) and 630 to 650 mg diiodohydroxyquin three times daily for 20 days.
  Children: Give 1 mg/kg per day in two doses (maximum 60 mg daily) IM for up to 5 days. Follow with chloroquine phosphate (10 mg base/kg/day [maximum 300 mg base daily] for 2-3 weeks) and 30-40 mg/kg diiodohydroxyquin daily in three doses for 20 days.

METRONIDAZOLE

PRODUCTS (TRADE NAME):
  Flagyl (Available in 250 and 500 mg tablets. **Metronidazole, Metryl, Protostat, Satric** (Available in 250 and 500 mg tablets.)
DRUG SPECIFICS:
  Drug of choice used in mild to severe intestinal amebiasis and in treatment of hepatic abscess. Patient should not take alcohol while on this medication or use with disulfiram. Because it has been found to be carcinogenic in rats, unnecessary use should be avoided.
ADMINISTRATION AND DOSAGE SPECIFICS:
  Mild, moderate and severe intestinal amebesiasis:

Adults: Give 750 mg three times daily for 5-10 days plus diiodohydroxyquin 630 to 650 mg three times daily for 20 days.

Children: Give 35-50 mg/kg per day in three doses for 10 days, plus diiodohydroxyquin 30-40 mg/kg per day in 3 doses for 20 days.

Hepatic Abscess:

Adults: 750 mg three times daily for 5-10 days, plus diiodohydroxyquin 630 to 650 mg three times daily for 20 days.

Children: 35-50 mg/kg daily in three doses for 10 days, plus 30-40 mg/kg diiodohydroxyquia per day in three doses for 20 days.

PAROMOMYCIN

PRODUCTS (TRADE NAME):

Humatin (Available in 250 mg capsules and 125 mg/5 ml syrup.)

DRUG SPECIFICS:

Used as alternative drug therapy for asymptomatic intestinal amebiasis and mild to moderate infections. May cause ototoxicity and baseline audiometry tests should be obtained. Give medication with meals.

ADMINISTRATION AND DOSAGE SPECIFICS:

Asymptomatic intestinal amebiasis:

Adults and children: As alternative to diiodohydroxyquin, give 25-30 mg/kg per day in three doses for 7 days.

Mild to Moderate Intestinal Amebiasis:

Adults and children: Give 25-30 mg/kg per day in 3 doses for 7 days.

Mary Ann Bolter

ANTHELMINTICS

DIETHYLCARBAMAZINE CITRATE

ACTION OF THE DRUG: The exact mechanism of action of diethylcarbamazine citrate as an anthelmintic is not known. It is theorized that it acts on microfilariae and sensitizes the parasite's cuticle to allow phagocytosis by the mixed macrophages of the host's reticuloendothelial system.

ASSESSMENT:

INDICATIONS: This drug is used mostly in tropical areas, or in patients who have been in areas where these filariae are endemic. The drug would be prescribed by a physician; however non-physicians may frequently have responsibility for monitoring the progress of a patient on this drug. It is used in the treatment of filariasis due to *Wuchereria bancrofti* (a nematode parasite found in tropical and subtropical countries, transmitted by Culex mosquitoes, mites or flies, and producing obstruction of the lymphatic ducts leading to elephantiasis), malayan filariasis, dipelalonemiasis or loiasis (an infection caused by a filarial worm dwelling in tumors in subcutaneous connective tissue and often affecting the eyes).

SUBJECTIVE-OBJECTIVE: The person may be asymptomatic or present with listlessness, fatigue, irritability, abdominal pain, diarrhea and weight loss. Persons may present with edema, especially of the lower extremities, and discharge from the eyes.

PLAN:

CONTRAINDICATIONS: Avoid giving this preparation to pregnant women because it may promote uterine contractions. Do not give if hypersensitivity to drug is present.

WARNINGS: Patients with recent history of malaria should be treated with an antimalarial agent before administration of this drug to help prevent a relapse.

PRECAUTIONS: Use with care in patients with hypertension, severe hepatic, renal or cardiac disease, or in patients with ocular onchocerciasis. It is not used in children under 1 year of age.

IMPLEMENTATION:

PRODUCTS (TRADE NAME):
Hetrazen (Available in 50 mg tablet.)

ADMINISTRATION AND DOSAGE SPECIFICS: Start this oral medication at lowest recommended dose and then gradually increase dosage as needed.

Wuchereriasis: 2.0 mg/kg tid after meals for 3-4 weeks.

Loiasis: 2.0 mg/kg after meals tid for 3-4 weeks.

Onchocerciasis: 2.0 mg/kg after meals tid for 3-4 weeks.

IMPLEMENTATION CONSIDERATIONS:

—Obtain a health history to determine presence of hypertension, severe hepatic, renal or cardiac disease, ocular onchocerciasis, malaria, or hypersensitivity to drug. Also determine possibility of pregnancy.

—Concomitant administration of antihistamines or corticosteroids may be necessary to reduce allergic effects, particularly in the treatment of ocular onchocerciasis.

—This preparation is often used in hospitalized patients so patient can be kept recumbent for 48 hours after treatment.

—Systemic corticosteroids should be given 7-10 days after treatment.

—Patients may develop allergic reactions to the dead microfilaria and may need symptomatic treatment.

—Keep tablets in a tightly closed container.

—Start patient with a low dosage and gradually increase it.

WHAT THE PATIENT NEEDS TO KNOW:
—It is important to take this medication as ordered.
—Take the medication after meals.
—Store tablets in a tightly closed container.
—Good personal hygiene is essential in preventing reinfection. Important

habits include properly washing and cooking food, washing hands after using toilet and before preparing food.

—Report any unusual or uncomfortable side effects from the drug to your health care provider.

EVALUATION:

ADVERSE REACTIONS: *CNS:* depression, dizziness, headache, weakness. *Gastrointestinal:* anorexia, nausea, vomiting. *Other:* arthralgia, lassitude, malaise, myalgia, skin rash. Allergic reactions may occur due to the dead microfilaria and may be expressed as fever, lymphadenitis, pruritus and pedal edema.

PARAMETERS TO MONITOR: Observe for compliance with therapy schedule, and suppression of the organism. Diagnosis should be made from a stool specimen. Follow-up stool specimens should be obtained after treatment. An ophthalmologic examination should be obtained if patient is being treated for ocular onchoceriasis.

Linda Ross

MEBENDAZOLE

ACTION OF THE DRUG: Mebendazole blocks the glucose uptake of helminths.

ASSESSMENT:

INDICATIONS: Mebendazole is used in single or mixed infections for the treatment of pinworm, roundworm, hookworm and whipworm.

SUBJECTIVE: The person may be asymptomatic or present with listlessness, fatigue, irritability, abdominal pain, diarrhea and weight loss. Persons with pinworms may complain of itching around the anus, especially at night, which causes painful scratching and restless sleep.

OBJECTIVE: Severe hookworm infestations may produce anemia and even retardation of growth and development. Diagnosis rests upon laboratory examinations of stools in which eggs, cysts or portions of the helminths are found. Applying scotch tape to the anal area of a child once he or she has gone to sleep may trap pinworms outside the body for confirmation of infection.

PLAN:

CONTRAINDICATIONS: Do not give in the presence of hypersensitivity to the drug, in children younger than 2 years and in pregnant women.

IMPLEMENTATION:

PRODUCTS (TRADE NAME):
Vermox (Available in 100 mg chewable tablet.)

ADMINISTRATION AND DOSAGE SPECIFICS: No special diets, fasting or purgation prior to administration is necessary. Medication is taken orally, by chewing, crushing, and/or mixing with food. Due to easy transmission of parasites, it is suggested that all immediate family members be treated.

Adults and children:

Pinworms: 100 mg po single dose.

Roundworms, hookworms, and whipworms: 100 mg po bid (morning and evening) for 3 days. Repeat treatment in 3-4 weeks if infestation not cleared.

IMPLEMENTATION CONSIDERATIONS:

—Obtain a complete health history to determine whether there is any hypersensitivity to the drug, or possibility of pregnancy.

—Learn the signs and symptoms of the various helminths infestations.

—Teach the patient hygienic techniques that will be needed by the patient and other family members in order to halt reinfestation.

—It is important to obtain a follow-up stool specimen after treatment is completed to document absence of helminths.

—Since pinworm infections are easily transferred from person to person all family members may have to be treated.

WHAT THE PATIENT NEEDS TO KNOW:

—It is important to take this medication as ordered. Therapy usually involves an initial treatment which should kill all worms, but in some cases a second course must be taken. It is important to report any symptoms which do not disappear after treatment.

—Worms which are passed in bowel movements are still alive and capable of infecting others. Care must be used to avoid transmission. During the next week you should:

a. Wash the toilet seat daily with soap and water.

b. Boil sheets and underwear twice with water and disinfectant.

c. Use special precautions in handling food or drink around others.

—Good personal hygiene is essential in preventing reinfection. Some worms are transmitted through improperly cooked meat or fish; through eating unwashed fruit or vegetables; or through fecal contamination of food or water. Children who go barefoot may become infected with hookworm from animal droppings. Proper preparation and cooking of food and washing of hands after using the toilet and before preparing food are important habits to develop.

—Worm infestations are easily transmitted and all family members may need to be tested for their presence.

—Some people experience diarrhea and abdominal discomfort associated with taking the medication.

EVALUATION:

ADVERSE REACTIONS: This drug is practically free of side effects. Transient diarrhea and abdominal pain may be produced by massive infestation and expulsion of the helminths rather than from the drug itself. Fever has been reported.

PARAMETERS TO MONITOR: Obtain a stool specimen to confirm diagnosis. Obtain a repeat stool specimen after therapy is concluded to document absence of worms.

Linda Ross

PIPERAZINE

ACTION OF THE DRUG: Piperazine paralyzes the muscles of parasites by blocking the effects of acetylcholine at the neuromuscular junction and the parasite is expelled by normal peristalsis.

ASSESSMENT:

INDICATIONS: This product is used in the treatment of roundworms and pinworms.

SUBJECTIVE: Patient may be asymptomatic or present with listlessness, fatigue, and irritability. Persons with pinworms may complain of itching around the anus especially at night, which causes painful scratching and restless sleep.

OBJECTIVE: Diagnosis rests upon laboratory examinations of stools in which eggs, cysts or portions of the helminth are found. Presence of pinworms is often documented by applying scotch tape to anus at night, since worms migrate outside the rectum through the relaxed anus to lay eggs.

PLAN:

CONTRAINDICATIONS: Do not give in the presence of hypersensitivity to the drug or its salts, renal or hepatic disease, severe malnutrition or anemia. Do not use in patients with convulsive disorders.

WARNINGS: This drug has potential neurotoxicity; therefore prolonged or repeated treatment in excess of the recommended dosage should be avoided, especially in children. Safety during pregnancy has not been established.

PRECAUTIONS: This drug may produce severe CNS, gastrointestinal or hypersensitivity reactions.

IMPLEMENTATION:

DRUG INTERACTIONS: Pyrantel pamoate and piperazine are antagonistic. Concurrent use with chlorpromazine may provoke convulsions. Piperazine can produce a false or decreased uric acid value, a clastogenic effect to the bone marrow and leukocytes, and EEG changes.

PRODUCTS (TRADE NAME):

Antepar (Available in 500 mg tablet and 500 mg/5 ml syrup.) **Piperazine** (Available in 500 mg/5 ml syrup, and 250 and 500 mg tablets.) **Vermizine** (Available in 500 mg/5 ml syrup.)

ADMINISTRATION AND DOSAGE SPECIFICS:
Roundworm (Ascariasis) Infections:
Adults: Single daily oral dose of 3.5 gms for 2 consecutive days.
Children: Single daily oral dose of 75 mg/kg; maximum daily dose 3.5 gm. Give for two consecutive days.

In severe infections treatment course may be initiated again after a one-week interval.
Pinworm (Enterobiasis) Infections:
Adults and children: Single daily oral dose of 65 mg/kg; maximum daily dose 2.5 gm. May be administered for 7 consecutive days.

IMPLEMENTATION CONSIDERATIONS:
—Obtain a complete health history to determine the presence of renal or hepatic disease, severe malnutrition or anemia, convulsive disorders, or hypersensitivities.

—Learn the signs and symptoms of roundworms and pinworms.

—Teach the patient hygienic techniques that will be needed by the patient and other family members in order to halt reinfestation.

—It is important to obtain a follow-up stool specimen after treatment is completed to document absence of helminths.

—Since pinworm infections are easily transferred from person to person all family members may have to be treated.

—No special preparation of the patient is needed prior to administering the drug.

—Development of neurologic complications provides a sufficient reason for abandoning this medication and using an alternative.

—Store syrup and tablets in tightly closed containers to avoid evaporation.

—Liquid preparations are more acceptable for children.

—Medication is usually administered in the morning before breakfast.

WHAT THE PATIENT NEEDS TO KNOW:
—It is important to take this medication as ordered. Therapy usually involves an initial dosage which should kill all worms, but in some cases a second course must be taken.

—Worms which are passed in bowel movements are still alive and capable of infecting others. Care must be used to avoid transmission. During the next week you should:

a. Wash the toilet seat daily with soap and water.

b. Boil sheets and underwear with water and disinfectant. Change sheets daily.

c. Use special precautions in handling food or drink around others.

d. Vacuum bedroom or use a wet mop on tile. Do not sweep.

e. Shower immediately upon rising in the morning, and put on clean underwear.

—Good personal hygiene is essential in preventing reinfection. Some worms are transmitted through improperly cooked meat or fish; through eating unwashed fruit or vegetables; or through fecal contamination of food or water.

Proper preparation and cooking of food, washing of hands after using toilet and before preparing food are important habits to develop.

—Worm infestations are easily transmitted and all family members may need to be tested for their presence.

—Alert your health provider if you develop any signs of headache, tremors, muscle weakness, blurred vision or an eye which deviates and does not align properly with the other eye.

—Keep this drug out of the reach of children and all others for whom it is not prescribed.

EVALUATION:

ADVERSE REACTIONS: *CNS:* large doses may cause blurred vision, incoordination, vertigo. *Dermatologic:* urticaria. *Gastrointestinal:* abdominal cramps, diarrhea, nausea, vomiting.

OVERDOSAGE: *Signs and symptoms:* Convulsions and respiratory depression.

PARAMETERS TO MONITOR: Monitor for therapeutic effect. Diagnosis is made with a stool specimen, and a repeat stool specimen should be examined after treatment is concluded. Re-treatment is indicated if infestation has not cleared up. Observe for side effects from the drug.

Linda Ross

PYRANTEL PAMOATE

ACTION OF THE DRUG: Pyrantel pamoate has a nerve blocking effect which results in spastic paralysis of parasites. This drug is also an inhibitor of cholinesterases. The paralyzed parasite is then expelled by normal peristalsis.

ASSESSMENT:

INDICATIONS: This drug is used in the treatment of roundworm, pinworm and hookworm infestations.

SUBJECTIVE: Person may be asymptomatic or present with listlessness, fatigue, irritability, abdominal pain, diarrhea and weight loss. Persons with pinworms may complain of itching around the anus, especially at night, which causes painful scratching and restless sleep.

OBJECTIVE: Hookworm infestation may produce anemia, and if severe enough it may produce retardation of growth and development. Diagnosis rests upon laboratory examination of stools in which eggs, cysts or portions of the helmintic are found. The presence of pinworms may be documented by applying scotch tape to anus at night as pinworms often migrate outside the relaxed anus to lay eggs.

PLAN:

CONTRAINDICATIONS: Do not use in presence of hypersensitivity to the drug or in pregnancy.

WARNINGS: Safety in children under two is not established.

PRECAUTIONS: Use with caution in patients with liver dysfunction, severe malnutrition or anemia.

IMPLEMENTATION:

DRUG INTERACTIONS: Pyrantel pamoate and piperazine are mutually antagonistic. This drug may produce elevated SGOT levels.

PRODUCTS (TRADE NAME):

Antiminth (Available in a 50 mg/ml oral suspension.)

ADMINISTRATION AND DOSAGE SPECIFICS: Medication can be administered as a single dose for treating roundworms and pinworms. For hookworms it requires longer therapy. No special fasting or diet is necessary before taking medication. Taking drug with fruit juice or milk may make it more palatable.

Roundworm and Pinworm Therapy:

Adults and children: Single dose of 11 mg/kg; maximum dose 1 gm. This dose should be repeated after 2 weeks for pinworms.

Hookworms: (This therapy is still investigational.)

Adults and children: 11 mg/kg for three consecutive days. Treatment should be repeated after 1 month if necessary.

IMPLEMENTATION CONSIDERATIONS:

—Obtain a complete health history to determine underlying medical problems, hypersensitivity, or possibility of pregnancy.

—Learn the signs and symptoms of the various helminth infestations.

—Teach the patient hygienic techniques that will be needed by the patient and other family members in order to halt reinfestation.

—It is important to obtain a follow-up stool specimen after the treatment is completed (4-6 weeks for roundworms; 2 weeks later for hookworms) to document absence of helminths.

—Since pinworm infections are easily transferred from person to person all family members may have to be treated.

—If treatment is for hookworms, patient may have an iron deficiency anemia and may require an iron supplement plus a diet rich in iron and vitamins.

WHAT THE PATIENT NEEDS TO KNOW:

—It is important to take this medication as ordered. Therapy usually involves an initial dosage which should kill all worms. In some cases a second course must be taken.

—Worms which are passed in bowel movements are still alive and capable of infecting others. Care must be used to avoid transmission. During the next week you should:

a. Wash the toilet seat daily with soap and water.

b. Boil sheets and underwear twice with water and disinfectant.

c. Use special precautions in handling food or drink around others.

—Good personal hygiene is essential in preventing reinfection. Some worms are transmitted through improperly cooked meat or fish; through eating unwashed fruit or vegetables; or through fecal contamination of food or water. Children who go barefoot may become infected with hookworms from animal droppings. Proper preparation and cooking of food and washing of hands after using toilet and before preparing food are important habits to develop.

—Worm infestations are easily transmitted, and all family members may need to be tested for their presence.

—Iron supplements and a diet rich in iron may be required if you are being treated for hookworm.

EVALUATION:

ADVERSE REACTIONS: *CNS:* dizziness, drowsiness, headache, and insomnia. *Gastrointestinal:* abdominal cramps, anorexia, diarrhea, nausea, tenesmus and vomiting. *Other:* skin rashes and weakness.

PARAMETERS TO MONITOR: Monitor for relief of symptoms and therapeutic effect. If being treated for hookworm, do baseline blood work to determine if therapy with iron is indicated. This should be repeated after treatment is finished. In all cases of worms, diagnosis is made with a stool specimen, and a repeat stool specimen should be examined after treatment is concluded. Re-treatment is indicated if infestation has not cleared up. Observe for side effects from drugs.

Linda Ross

PYRVINIUM PAMOATE

ACTION OF THE DRUG: Pyrvinium pamoate is a cyanine dye which inhibits oxygen intake in aerobic parasites and prevents the utilization of exogenous carbohydrates.

ASSESSMENT:

INDICATIONS: This drug is used primarily in pinworm infestations. It is also being used investigationally in the treatment of strongyloidiasis.

SUBJECTIVE: Patients may be asymptomatic or present with listlessness, fatigue, and irritability. Persons with pinworms may complain of itching around anus especially at night which causes painful scratching and restless sleep.

OBJECTIVE: Diagnosis rests upon laboratory examination of stools in which eggs or portions of the helminth are found. Pinworms may be documented by applying scotch tape to anus at night, since pinworms migrate outside the rectum through the relaxed anus to lay eggs.

PLAN:

CONTRAINDICATIONS: Do not use in patients with hypersensitivity to the drug, intestinal obstruction, inflammatory bowel diseases, renal or hepatic disease.

WARNINGS: Safe use during pregnancy and breast feeding has not been established. Children weighing less than 10 kg are also at greater risk. The patient needs to be warned that urine, stool and emesis will be red.

PRECAUTIONS: Gastrointestinal reactions are more likely to occur in older children and adults who have received large doses.

IMPLEMENTATION:

PRODUCTS (TRADE NAME):
Povan (Available in 10 mg/ml oral suspension and 50 mg film-coated tablet.)
ADMINISTRATION AND DOSAGE SPECIFICS:
Adults and children: 5 mg/kg as a single dose. Repeat in 2 or 3 weeks if necessary. 350 mg (7 tablets) is the maximum dose.
IMPLEMENTATION CONSIDERATIONS:
—Obtain a health history to determine whether there are any underlying medical problems, hypersensitivity or possibility of pregnancy that would pose a problem in taking this medication.
—Learn the signs and symptoms of pinworm infestation.
—Teach the patient hygienic techniques that will be needed by the patient and other family members in order to halt reinfestation.
—It is important to obtain a follow-up stool specimen after treatment is completed to document absence of helminths.
—Since pinworm infections are easily transferred from person to person all family members may have to be treated.
—Emesis occurs more frequently with suspension than with the tablets.
—Drug has staining properties; therefore warn patient to be careful not to spill it. Drinking through a straw may help prevent staining of teeth.

WHAT THE PATIENT NEEDS TO KNOW:
—It is important to take this medication as ordered. Therapy usually involves an initial dosage which should kill all worms, but in some cases a second course must be taken. It is important to report any symptoms which do not disappear after treatment.
—The medication is a red dye and therefore urine, stool, emesis and teeth will be stained from it.
—If taking the liquid product, use a straw which will decrease staining of the teeth. The staining effects are not permanent.
—Swallow tablets whole. Give with meals or milk to avoid stomach upset.
—Store medication in a tight container and protect it from light.
—Worms which are passed in bowel movements are still alive and capable of infecting others. Care must be used to avoid transmission. During the next week you should:

a. Wash the toilet seat daily with soap and water.

b. Boil sheets and underwear twice with water and disinfectant.

c. Use special precautions in handling food or drink around others.

—Good personal hygiene is essential in preventing reinfection. Some worms are transmitted through improperly cooked meat or fish; through eating unwashed fruit or vegetables; or through fecal contamination of food or water. Children who go barefoot may become infected with hookworms from animal droppings. Proper preparation and cooking of food, washing of hands after using toilet and before preparing food are important habits to develop.

—Worm infestations are easily transmitted and all family members may need to be tested for their presence.

—Avoid too much sun or use of a sun lamp when beginning treatment and for a few days after.

EVALUATION:

ADVERSE REACTIONS: *CNS:* dizziness. *Gastrointestinal:* abdominal cramps, diarrhea, nausea, and vomiting. *Other:* photosensitivity, skin rash.

PARAMETERS TO MONITOR Monitor for therapeutic effect. Diagnosis is made with a stool specimen and a repeat stool specimen should be examined after treatment is concluded. Re-treatment is indicated if infestation has not cleared up. Observe for side effects from drug.

Linda Ross

QUINACRINE HCL

ACTION OF THE DRUG: Quinacrine HCl is used in treatment of tapeworm infestations. It causes the scolex of the cestode to temporarily detach from the intestinal wall, thereby dislodging and expelling the intact worm.

ASSESSMENT:

INDICATIONS: This drug is used in the treatment of cestodiasis (tapeworm infestation); however, niclosamide and paromomycin have mainly replaced this drug. It is the drug of choice for giardiasis, a protozoa infestation.

SUBJECTIVE: Often there are no symptoms. In severe infestations tapeworms may produce diarrhea, abdominal cramps, flatulence, distention and nausea. In giardiasis, abdominal pain and a mucous diarrhea which produces weight loss are the predominant symptoms.

OBJECTIVE: Presence of tapeworm segments may be found in clothing or bedding. Abdominal tenderness and weight loss may be present.

Diagnosis rests upon laboratory examination of stools in which eggs, cysts or portions of the tapeworm are found.

PLAN:

CONTRAINDICATIONS: Do not give with hypersensitivity to the drug, in patients with G-6-PD deficiency, or in pregnant women.

WARNINGS: Quinacrine HCl may precipitate severe attacks of psoriasis. Porphyria may also be exacerbated.

PRECAUTIONS: Use with caution in adults over 60 years, or children younger than 1 year; in patients with severe renal or cardiac disease, or a history of psychosis and/or alcoholism.

IMPLEMENTATION:

DRUG INTERACTIONS: Quinacrine increases the toxicity of primaquine. It also inhibits aldehyde dehydrogenase, thus producing a disulfiram type of reaction. MAO inhibitors potentiate the adverse effects of the drug. Quinacrine inhibits the anticoagulant activity of heparin. Alkalinizing agents such as sodium bicarbonate tend to potentiate the drug and produce toxicity if given in large doses over a period of time. Quinacrine may also cause an apparent increase in urine and plasma cortisol, plasma 11-hydroxycorticosteroid levels.

PRODUCTS (TRADE NAME):
Atabrine HCl (Available in 100 mg tablets.)
ADMINISTRATION AND DOSAGE SPECIFICS:
Giardiasis: Take drug after meals with a full glass of water, tea or fruit juice.
Adults: 100 mg po three times daily for 5-7 days.
Children: 7 mg/kg po daily in three divided doses (maximum 300 mg/day) after meals for 5 days.

Cestodiasis: For the treatment of cestodes, the preparation of the patient includes eating a bland, low-residue or liquid diet one to two days before treatment. The patient should remain fasting after the evening meal. A saline or soap suds enema may or may not be given the evening before treatment. In the morning, omit breakfast and give the medication. The pulverized tablets may be administered with jam or honey to disguise the bitter taste. The medication may be taken orally or through a duodenal tube. After one to two hours give a saline cathartic to flush out the worm. If the worm is expelled, it will be stained yellow. If a duodenal tube is used, dissolve the total dose in 100 ml of warm water and give the total amount. Then flush the tube with additional water. Give the cathartic 30 minutes later and then remove the tube.

Adults and children 14 years or older: Give 4 doses of 200 mg, ten minutes apart, accompanied by 600 mg of sodium bicarbonate with each dose.

Children 11-14 years: Give a total of 600 m in 3-4 doses, ten minutes apart, with 300 mg sodium bicarbonate with each dose.

Children 5-10 years: Give a total of 400 mg. Saline cathartic is given 1-2 hours after treatment.

IMPLEMENTATION CONSIDERATIONS:
—Obtain a complete health history including presence of cardiac, renal disease or hypersensitivity to medication, concurrent use of primaquine or MAO inhibitors.

—Learn the signs and symptoms of the various helminth infestations.

—Teach the patient hygienic techniques that will be needed by the patient and other family members in order to halt reinfestation.

—Treatment may be repeated in 2 weeks if found to be ineffective.

—It is important to obtain a follow-up stool specimen after treatment is completed to document absence of helminths. If scolex is not found, stools should be examined periodically. They must be free of worm eggs or segments for three to six months to be certain of cure.

—Sodium bicarbonate may be given before the drug to help reduce nausea and vomiting.

—The drug imparts a reversible yellow color to skin and urine.

—Periodic complete ophthalmologic examinations will be necessary if the patient is receiving prolonged therapy.

WHAT THE PATIENT NEEDS TO KNOW:

—It is important to go through the preparation period and take the medication exactly as ordered. Therapy usually involves an initial dosage which should kill all worms, but in some cases a second course must be taken two weeks later.

—Worms are present in cysts passed in bowel movements and are capable of infecting others. Care must be used to avoid transmission. During the next two weeks you should:

a. Wash the toilet seat daily with soap and water.

b. Boil sheets and underwear twice with water and disinfectant

c. Use special precautions in handling food or drink around others.

—Good personal hygiene is essential in preventing reinfection. Some worms are transmitted through improperly cooked meat or fish or through fecal contamination of food or water. Proper preparation and cooking of food, washing of hands after using toilet and before preparing food are important habits to develop.

—Report any visual disturbances to your health care provider.

—This medication produces a temporary yellow color to skin and urine.

—A skin rash may occur while taking this drug.

—Nail pigmentation, along with blue and black skin, may also occur.

—Do not drink any alcoholic beverages while taking this medication or you will become very nauseated and vomit.

—Boil water or use iodine-treated water if source water is known to be contaminated.

—Keep this product out of the reach of children and all others for whom it is not prescribed. Improper dosage is dangerous.

EVALUATION:

ADVERSE REACTIONS: *CNS:* aggressive behavior, anxiety, CNS stimulation, convulsions, confusion, emotional change, euphoria, headache (usually associated with chronic administration), irritability, nervousness. *Gastrointestinal:* nausea, vomiting. *Hematopoietic:* blood dyscrasias, hepatitis. *Other:* contact dermatitis, corneal edema or deposits (reversible), exfoliative dermatitis, psychosis (transient), urticaria, yellowish discoloration of the skin.

OVERDOSAGE: *Signs and symptoms of acute toxicity:* Cardiovascular: cardiac arrhythmias, hypotension, shock. CNS: convulsions, insomnia, psychic stimulation, restlessness. GI: abdominal cramps, diarrhea, nausea, vomiting. Other: yellow skin pigmentation. *Treatment:* Symptomatic. Promote emesis or refer to physician for gastric lavage. Convulsions should be controlled. Tracheal intubation may be necessary to support respirations. To promote urinary excretion of drug, increase hydration and acidification of the urine by administration of ammonium chloride. Observe for at least 6 hours.

PARAMETERS TO MONITOR: Obtain baseline CBC and liver function studies. A baseline ophthalmologic examination may be indicated in patients with questionable eye history also. Obtain stool specimen for diagnosis, and repeat specimens at three and six months. Monitor for improvement of symptoms, appearance of side effects.

Linda Ross

THIABENDAZOLE

ACTION OF THE DRUG: The exact action of thiabendazole is not known, but it is thought to interfere with the metabolic pathways essential for a variety of helminths. Some sources suggest the enzyme fumarate reductase is inhibited.

ASSESSMENT:

INDICATIONS: This is the drug of choice for cutaneous larva migrans (creeping eruption), pinworms, roundworms, *Strongyloides* and mild cases of hookworm.

SUBJECTIVE: Person may be asymptomatic or present with listlessness, fatigue, irritability, abdominal pain, diarrhea and weight loss. Persons with pinworms may complain of itching around the anus, especially at night, which causes painful scratching and restless sleep. Tapeworms may produce diarrhea, abdominal cramps, flatulence, distention and nausea. Presence of tapeworm segments may be found in clothing or bedding.

OBJECTIVE: Larva migrans is a peculiar eruption occurring in a changing pattern on the skin, due to migration beneath its surface of a fly larva. Hookworm infection may produce anemia, retardation of growth and development.

Diagnosis rests upon laboratory examinations of stools in which eggs, cysts or portions of the helminth are found. Pinworms may also be documented by applying scotch tape to the anus at night, since pinworms frequently migrate outside the rectum through the relaxed anus to lay eggs.

PLAN:

CONTRAINDICATIONS: Do not give in the presence of hypersensitivity to the drug.

WARNINGS: Activities requiring mental alertness should be avoided. Safety for use in pregnancy and breast-feeding has not been established.

PRECAUTIONS: Use with care in patients with impaired liver or renal function and patients with severe malnutrition or anemia. Due to limited clinical experience with the drug in children who weigh less than 15 kg, the possible risk should be weighed against the benefits.

IMPLEMENTATION:

PRODUCTS (TRADE NAME):
Mintezol (Available in 500 mg/5 ml liquid suspension and in 500 mg chewable tablets.)

ADMINISTRATION AND DOSAGE SPECIFICS: Chew tablets well before swallowing. Take drug after meals.

Adults and children over 150 lb: 1.5 gm po.

Adults and children under 150 lb: 10 mg/lb po.

Pinworms (enterobiasis): Give two doses in one day; repeat regimen in 7 days.

Cutaneous larva migrans: Give two doses per day for 2 days. If active lesions are still present after completion of therapy, a second course should be administered.

Roundworms (ascariasis), Strongyloides and hookworms: Give 2 doses per day for 2 days.

IMPLEMENTATION CONSIDERATIONS:

—Obtain a health history to determine whether there are any underlying medical problems or hypersensitivities that contraindicate use of the medication.

—Learn the signs and symptoms of the various helminth infestations.

—Teach the patient hygienic techniques that will be needed by the patient and other family members in order to halt reinfestation.

—It is important to obtain a follow-up stool specimen after treatment is completed to document absence of helminths.

—Since pinworm infections are easily transferred from person to person all family members may have to be treated.

—If treatment is for hookworm, patient may have an iron deficiency anemia and therefore may need added iron supplement and a diet rich in iron and vitamins.

—In the treatment of cutaneous larva migrans, severe itching may take place and a concomitant administration of an anti-inflammatory agent may be necessary.

WHAT THE PATIENT NEEDS TO KNOW:

—It is important to take this medication as ordered. Therapy usually involves an initial dosage which should kill all worms, but in some cases a second course must be taken to ensure killing new worms that have just been hatched. It is important to report any symptoms which do not disappear after treatment.

—Tablets must be chewed thoroughly before swallowing, and taken after meals.

—Worms which are passed in bowel movements are still alive and capable of infecting others. Care must be used to avoid transmission. During the next week you should:

a. Wash the toilet seat daily with soap and water.
b. Boil sheets and underwear twice with water and disinfectant.
c. Use special precautions in handling food or drink around others.

—Good personal hygiene is essential in preventing reinfection. Some worms are transmitted through improperly cooked meat or fish; through eating unwashed fruit or vegetables, or through fecal contamination of food or water. Children who go barefoot may become infected with hookworm from animal droppings. Proper preparation and cooking of food, washing of hands after using toilet and before preparing food are important habits to develop.

—Worm infestations are easily transmitted and all family members may need to be tested for their presence.

—Medication may cause an asparagus-like odor of the urine. Skin may also have an unusual odor.

—This medication may cause drowsiness or dizziness; therefore use caution in driving or performing tasks requiring alertness.

EVALUATION:

ADVERSE REACTIONS: The incidence of side effects increases with increasing dosages and length of treatment. *CNS:* dizziness, drowsiness, headache. *Gastrointestinal:* anorexia, diarrhea, nausea, vomiting. *Other:* abnormal liver function, enuresis, hyperirritability, hypotension, jaundice, tinnitus, yellowish tinge to vision (these all occur only rarely).

PARAMETERS TO MONITOR: Monitor for extent of symptoms, and for therapeutic effect. If being treated for hookworm, do baseline blood work to determine if therapy with iron is indicated. This should be repeated after treatment is finished. In all cases of worms, diagnosis is made with a stool specimen, and a repeat stool specimen should be examined after treatment is concluded. Re-treatment is indicated if infestation has not cleared up. Observe for side effects from drugs.

Linda Ross

ANTIBIOTICS

AMINOGLYCOSIDES

ACTION OF THE DRUG: The main action of the aminoglycosides is the inhibition of ribosomal protein synthesis. Since they are poorly absorbed, the primary action is on gastrointestinal bacterial flora.

ASSESSMENT:

INDICATIONS: Drug choice is dependent on the identification of the infectious organism by appropriate cultures or smears, or based on the clinical picture. Aminoglycosides are broad-spectrum antibiotics effective in the treatment of gram negative infections. Non-physician health providers would only rarely prescribe these drugs, but may be responsible for monitoring the progress of patients on this type of medication.

SUBJECTIVE-OBJECTIVE: The patient in need of antibiotic therapy may present in any number of ways ranging from asymptomatic to severely ill. Keep in mind common infectious indicators such as fever, inflammation, erythema, edema or pain.

PLAN:

CONTRAINDICATIONS: Do not use in the presence of hypersensitivity to aminoglycosides or in patients with intestinal obstruction.

WARNINGS: Significant renal toxicity, which is usually reversible, has been reported with drug use. Risk of toxicity increases in patients with renal impairment. Use with discretion in the elderly. Significant auditory and vestibular ototoxicity may occur in patients on prolonged therapy or taking higher than recommended dosages. There is an increased risk in patients with pre-existing renal or auditory diseases. Concurrent use of anesthesia or muscle relaxants with aminoglycosides may result in neuromuscular blockade with resultant respiratory paralysis. Neuromuscular blockade may also occur in aminoglycoside treatment with myasthenia gravis. Discretion should be used during treatment in pregnant and nursing mothers since the drugs cross the placental barrier and are secreted in breast milk.

PRECAUTIONS: Cross allergenicity has been noted among the aminoglycosides. Aminoglycosides are excreted through the urinary system in high concentrations. An increased risk of toxicity exists in therapy of premature babies, infants and the elderly. Superinfection may occur with treatment.

IMPLEMENTATION:

DRUG INTERACTIONS: An increased risk of toxicity exists with concurrent use of ototoxic, neurotoxic, nephrotoxic or potent diuretic drugs (amikacin, cephaloridine, colistin, ethacrynic acid, furosemide, gentamicin, kanamycin, mannitol, meralluride sodium, neomycin, paromomycin, polymyxin B, sodium mercaptomerin, streptomycin, tobramycin, vancomycin or viomycin). Concurrent use of anesthesia or muscle relaxants with aminoglycosides may result in neuromuscular blockade with resultant respiratory paralysis. Dimenhydrinate may mask ototoxicity of the drug. Aminoglycosides may alter laboratory values in the following manner: increased CSF proteins, urinary glucose and protein, BUN, creatinine, bilirubin; a positive Coombs' test; decreased serum haptoglobin.

ADMINISTRATION AND DOSAGE: Aminoglycosides should be used with discretion because of toxic effects. Risk of toxicity is low in patients with normal renal function and if dosage is not exceeded. Patient must be well hydrated.

IMPLEMENTATION CONSIDERATIONS:
—Obtain a thorough health history: history of hypersensitivity to aminoglycosides, other medications which may interact with the drug, history of renal impairment, auditory impairment or myasthenia gravis, pregnancy or breast feeding.
—Inform anesthesiologist that the patient is on aminoglycosides.
—Discontinue drug if patient notes diminished hearing, tinnitus or if audiogram denotes perception loss.
—Due to drug toxicity, all patients must be under strict observation for toxicity or adverse reactions.
—Follow patients with serum drug levels.
—Keep patients well hydrated.

WHAT THE PATIENT NEEDS TO KNOW:
—Take the medication exactly as ordered. Do not stop taking medication once symptoms have disappeared. Do not save medication.
—Some patients experience side effects with this drug. Be certain to notify your health provider if any new or troublesome symptoms develop. Particularly watch for ringing in the ears (tinnitus), a feeling that the room is spinning, or a decrease in urine output.
—Bathe daily and brush teeth regularly. Watch for signs of infection in mouth, anal and vaginal areas.

EVALUATION:

ADVERSE REACTIONS: *CNS:* headache, dizziness, vertigo, numbness, tingling, ototoxicity, paresthesia, convulsions. *Gastrointestinal:* nausea, vomiting, anorexia, weight loss, stomatitis. *Hematopoietic:* altered reticulocyte count, leukopenia, thrombocytopenia, pancytopenia, anemia. *Hypersensitivity:* rash, purpura, pruritus, urticaria, anaphylaxis. *Other:* hepatomegaly, hepatic necrosis, myocarditis, pseudotumor cerebri, splenomegaly, hypotension, hypertension, arthralgia, nephrotoxicity, respiratory depression.
OVERDOSAGE: If toxicity or overdosage occurs, peritoneal dialysis or hemodialysis is indicated for removal of the toxin.
PARAMETERS TO MONITOR: Monitor for therapeutic effects. Obtain baseline audiogram, repeat audiogram during therapy. In renal impairment, renal studies should be obtained prior to initiation of therapy and repeated during therapy. Obtain serum drug levels for long-term therapy.

AMIKACIN SULFATE

PRODUCTS (TRADE NAME):
Amikin (Available as 100 mg/2ml, 500 mg/2 ml, 1 gm/4 ml for injection.)

DRUG SPECIFICS:

Parenteral medication effective in the treatment of the following susceptible organisms: *Enterobacter aerogenes, E. coli, Klebsiella, Acinetobacter, Proteus, Providencia, Pseudomonas, Serratia marcescens* and penicillinor methicillin-resistant staphylococci. May be used in the treatment of unidentified infections before results of sensitivity tests are known. Used in the treatment of neonatal sepsis. Do not mix with other drugs. Monitor renal function.

ADMINISTRATION AND DOSAGE SPECIFICS:

Adults and children: 7.5 mg/kg/day IM or IV infusion every 12 hours. Do not exceed 1.5 mg/day. Usual course is 7-10 days.

Neonates: 10 mg/kg loading dose followed by 7.5 mg/kg every 12 hours. IM or IV infusion for 7 to 10 days as needed.

GENTAMICIN SULFATE

PRODUCTS (TRADE NAME):

Apogen, Bristogen, Garamycin, Gentamicin Sulfate, U-Gencin (Available as 0.1% cream, 40 mg/ml and 60 mg/1.5 ml injection, 0.1% ointment, 3 mg/mg ophthalmic ointment, 3 mg/ml ophthalmic solution, 10 mg/ ml for pediatric injection.)

DRUG SPECIFICS:

Parenteral medication effective in the treatment of the following susceptible organisms: *Enterobacter aerogenes, E. coli, Klebsiella pneumoniae, Proteus, Pseudomonas aeruginosa, Salmonella, Serratia marcescens or Shigella.* May be used in combination with penicillin or cephalosporins in the treatment of unidentified infections before results of sensitivity tests are known. However, do not mix with carbenicillin. There is reported synergistic nephrotoxicity with concurrent use of amphotericin B or cephalothin.

ADMINISTRATION AND DOSAGE SPECIFICS:

Adults: 1 mg/kg every 8 hours. May use up to 5 mg/kg/day in 3-4 divided doses parenterally.

Children: 2-2.5 mg/kg every 8 hours.

Neonates over 1 week and infants: 2.5 mg/kg every 8 hours.

Premature and neonates: 2.5 mg/kg every 12 hours.

KANAMYCIN SULFATE

PRODUCTS (TRADE NAME):

Kantrex, Klebcil (Available as 500 mg capsules, 500 mg/2ml and 1 gm/3 ml injection, and 75 mg/2 ml pediatric injection.)

DRUG SPECIFICS:

All oral aminoglycosides exhibit poor systemic absorption. Effective in the suppression of bacterial flora in the gastrointestinal tract before surgery. (Use with mechanical cleansing and low residue diet.) Contraindicated in the presence of intestinal obstruction. Use with discretion in patients with ulcerative bowel lesions. Also effective in the treatment of hepatic coma by reducing the ammonia-forming bacteria in the gastrointestinal tract. (In hepatic coma, avoid concomitant diuretic use and dietary protein.)

ADMINISTRATION AND DOSAGE SPECIFICS:

Adults: 7.5 mg/kg every 12 hours IM or IV.

Children: 7.5 mg/kg every 12 hours IM or IV.

Suppression of intestinal bacteria: 1 gm po every hour for 4 hours, followed with 1 gm po every 6 hours for the next 36-72 hours.

Hepatic coma: 8-12 gm/day po in divided doses.

NEOMYCIN SULFATE

PRODUCTS (TRADE NAME):

Mycifradin Sulfate (Available in 500 mg tablet and 125 mg/5 ml oral solution.) **Neobiotic, Neomycin Sulfate** (Available as 500 mg tablets.)

DRUG SPECIFICS:

Effective in the treatment of enteropathogenic diarrhea due to *E. coli*. Also used as preoperative preparation for surgery. Do not continue treatment for longer than 10 days. Do not exceed 1 gm/day.

All oral aminoglycosides exhibit poor systemic absorption. Neomycin sulfate is effective in the suppression of bacterial flora in the gastrointestinal tract before surgery. It is contraindicated in the presence of intestinal obstruction. Use with caution in patients with ulcerative bowel lesions. It is also effective in the treatment of hepatic coma by reducing the ammonia-forming bacteria in the gastrointestinal tract. Effective in the treatment of diarrhea due to *E. coli*. Reported to inhibit the gastrointestinal absorption of digoxin, decreases the absorption of 5-fluorouracil (oral form), reduces the absorption of methotrexate (oral), decreases the absorption of penicillin V, and decreases the absorption of cyanocobalamin (vitamin B12).

ADMINISTRATION AND DOSAGE SPECIFICS:

Suppression of Intestinal Bacteria: 24 hours before surgery give 40 mg/lb/day po in 6 divided doses. Use with mechanical cleansing and low residue diet.

Hepatic Coma:

Adults: 4-12 gm/day po in divided doses.

Children: 50 to 100 mg/kg/day in divided doses.

Infectious Diarrhea:

Adults: 3 gm/day as needed.

Children: 50 mg/kg/day in divided doses for 2-3 days.

PAROMOMYCIN SULFATE

PRODUCTS (TRADE NAME):
  Humatin (Available as 250 mg capsules.)
DRUG SPECIFICS:
  All oral aminoglycosides exhibit poor systemic absorption. They are contrain-
dicated in the presence of intestinal obstruction. Use with discretion in patients
with ulcerative bowel lesions. Also effective in the treatment of hepatic coma by
reducing the ammonia-forming bacteria in the gastrointestinal tract.
ADMINISTRATION AND DOSAGE SPECIFICS:
  Intestinal Amebiasis: 25-35 mg/kg/day po in 3 divided doses for 5-10 days with
meals.
  Hepatic Coma: 4 gm/day po in divided doses for 5-6 days.

STREPTOMYCIN SULFATE

PRODUCTS (TRADE NAME):
  Streptomycin Sulfate (Available in 400 mg and 500 mg/ml injection.)
DRUG SPECIFICS:
  Available in parenteral form. Effective in the treatment of granuloma inguinale, tularemia, plague, enterococcal endocarditis (with penicillin), tuberculosis (with
anti-tuberculosis therapy), and bacterial endocarditis (with penicillin). Treatment
for the plague may produce a Herxheimer reaction. Although non-physicians would
only rarely prescribe this, they often have the responsibilty for monitoring the status
of a patient on this drug. Administer deep IM in large muscle mass.
ADMINISTRATION AND DOSAGE SPECIFICS:
  Alpha and nonhemolytic streptococcus endocarditis:
  Adults: 1st week: 1 gm parenterally twice a day with penicillin; 2nd week: 0.5
gm parenterally twice a day with penicillin.
  Enterococcal endocarditis:
  Adults: 1 gm parenterally twice a day for 2 weeks and 0.5 mg twice daily with
penicillin for 4 weeks.
  Plague:
  Adults: 2-4 gm/day in divided doses parenterally until the patient is afebrile.
  Tuberculosis:
  Adults: 1 gm/day parenterally with anti-tuberculosis therapy.
  Tularemia:
  Adults: 1-2 gm/day parenterally in divided doses for 7-10 days until the patient
is afebrile for 5-7 days.
  Children: 40 mg/kg/day parenterally in 2 divided doses.
  Premature and newborn: 20-30 mg/kg/day parenterally in 2 divided doses.

TOBRAMYCIN SULFATE

PRODUCTS (TRADE NAME):
Nebcin (Available as 40 mg/ml powder for injection, 10 mg/ml vials for pediatric injection and 40 mg/2 ml and 60 mg/1.5 ml and 80 mg/2 ml disposable syringes.)

DRUG SPECIFICS:
Effective in the treatment of infections due to the following susceptible organisms: *Citrobacter, E. coli, Klebsiella, Enterobacter, Serratia marcescens, Proteus, Providencia, Pseudomonas aeruginosa*. May be used in combination with penicillin or cephalosporin in the treatment of unidentified infections before results of sensitivity tests are known. Do not pre-mix with other drugs. Avoid serum concentrations greater than 12 mcg/ml.

ADMINISTRATION AND DOSAGE SPECIFICS:
Adults and children: 3 mg/kg/day IM every 8 hours for 7 to 10 days.

Neonates under 1 week: 4 mg/kg/day in 2 divided doses every 8 hours for 7 to 10 days.

Joann Sabados-Carolina

BACITRACIN

ACTION OF THE DRUG: Bacitracin in a bactericidal drug that inhibits muco-peptide cell wall synthesis.

ASSESSMENT:

INDICATIONS: Drug choice is dependent on the identification of the infectious organism by appropriate cultures or smears or based on the clinical picture. Due to the nephrotoxic effect of bacitracin, the drug should be restricted to use in severe illness. Non-physicians would rarely prescribe this drug but are often responsible for evaluating the status of the patient on this drug. Bacitracin is effective in the treatment of staphylococcal pneumonia or empyema in infants.

SUBJECTIVE-OBJECTIVE: The patient in need of antibiotic therapy may present in any number of ways, ranging from asymptomatic to severely ill. Keep in mind common infectious indicators such as fever, inflammation, erythema, edema or pain.

PLAN:

CONTRAINDICATIONS: Do not use in the presence of hypersensitivity to this drug.

WARNINGS: Renal failure due to tabular and glomerular necrosis has been reported. Do not exceed recommended dosage.

PRECAUTIONS: Superinfection may occur with treatment.

IMPLEMENTATION:

DRUG INTERACTIONS: Concurrent use of bacitracin with nephrotoxic drugs may produce an additive effect. Avoid concurrent use with colistimethate sodium, kanamycin, neomycin, polymyxin-B, streptomycin and viomycin. Avoid concurrent use with anesthetics, neuromuscular blocking agents or drugs with neuromuscular blocking activities since they may produce an additive effect.

PRODUCTS (TRADE NAME):
Bacitracin (Available in 10,000 units/vial and 50,000 units/vial for injection and as topical ointment.)

ADMINISTRATION AND DOSAGE:
Infants under 2.5 kg: 900 units/kg/day IM in two to three divided doses.
Patients over 2.5 kg: 1,000 units/kg/day IM in two to three divided doses.

IMPLEMENTATION CONSIDERATIONS:
—Obtain a complete health history: previous history of renal impairment, other medications that may produce drug interactions, hypersensitivity to bacitracin.
—Notify anesthesiologist that patient is taking this drug before surgery.
—The patient or guardian should be informed of the possible toxicity associated with drug usage, especially nephrotoxicity.
—Monitor intake and output.
—Watch for superinfections.

WHAT THE PATIENT NEEDS TO KNOW:
—Notify health care provider if decreased urinary output occurs.
—Medication should be given exactly as ordered.
—Any unusual symptoms should be reported promptly to health care provider.

EVALUATION:

ADVERSE REACTIONS: *Gastrointestinal:* nausea, vomiting. *Renal:* nephrotoxicity, increased serum drug levels without an increase in drug dosage. *Other:* pain, rash with intramuscular injection.

PARAMETERS TO MONITOR: Observe for therapeutic effect of drug. Obtain baseline renal studies and continue to monitor throughout therapy. Observe for signs of nephrotoxicity. Monitor intake and output.

Joann Sabados-Carolina

CEPHALOSPORINS

ACTION OF THE DRUG: A bacteriostatic and bactericidal preparation that is structurally and pharmacologically related to the penicillins. The main action is the inhibition of mucopeptide synthesis of the bacterial cell wall.

ASSESSMENT:

INDICATIONS: Drug choice is dependent on the identification of the infectious organism by appropriate cultures or smears, or based on the clinical picture. This category represents broad-spectrum drugs that may be used as an alternative therapy in susceptible organisms. These drugs should only be used when the benefits will outweigh the risks of therapy. Drugs may be classified as first, second, or third generation agents, differentiated primarily by their antibacterial spectrum. In general, second and third generation drugs are progressively more effective than first generation agents against a broad group of gram-negative organisms, while progressively less effective against gram-positive organisms. Third generation agents also show more efficacy against resistant organisms, have increased resistance to beta-lactamase inactivation, but with greater cost. Differences between drugs within categories is primarily pharmacokinetic. Effective in susceptible strains of *Escherichia coli, Clostridium, Neisseria gonorrhoeae* (when penicillin or tetracycline is not indicated), *Haemophilus influenzae, Klebsiella* (non-hospital acquired), *Proteus mirabilis* (non-hospital acquired), *Staphylococcus* (penicillin sensitive and penicillinase producing), group A beta-hemolytic streptococci, *Streptococcus pneumoniae* and *Treponema pallidum* (when a penicillin or tetracycline is not indicated) are effective in the prophylaxis of postoperative infection, treatment of intra-abdominal infections, bone or joint infection, or gonorrhea.

SUBJECTIVE-OBJECTIVE: The patient in need of antibiotic therapy may present in any number of ways, ranging from asymptomatic to severely ill. Keep in mind common infectious indicators such as fever, inflammation, erythema, edema or pain.

PLAN:

CONTRAINDICATIONS: Do not use in the presence of hypersensitivity to any cephalosporins.

WARNINGS: Partial cross-allergenicity may exist in patients hypersensitive to the penicillins. Use with extreme caution in patients reporting any previous allergy to penicillin. Nephrotoxicity has been reported and is greater in the elderly and in individuals with impaired renal function. Caution should be observed in pregnant and nursing mothers.

PRECAUTIONS: Treatment for group A beta-hemolytic streptococci should last for a minimum of 10 days. In the treatment of gonorrhea, the patient must be evaluated for syphilis, since the drug may mask signs and symptoms of syphilis. Before initiation of therapy for gonorrhea, suspicious lesions should be evaluated with a dark-field exam. Monthly serologic followups should continue for 3 months after therapy. Superinfection may occur with treatment.

IMPLEMENTATION:

DRUG INTERACTIONS: Bacteriostatic agents may antagonize the bactericidal action of the drug. Probenecid and sulfinpyrazone may inhibit renal tubular secretion. Avoid concurrent use of other nephrotoxic drugs such as amikacin, colistin, ethacrynic acid, furosemide, gentamicin, kanamycin, neomycin, polymixin B and tobramycin. Some Cephalosporins may enhance the activity of oral anticoagulants. Cephalosporins may cause the following alterations in laboratory tests: false positive for glucose in Benedict's and Fehling's solution or Clinitest tablets, false positive direct Coombs' test, true indirect and direct positive Coomb's test transient increase in SGPT, SGOT, BUN, creatinine or potassium.

ADMINISTRATION AND DOSAGE: Dosage is dependent on the severity of the illness and the specific product. See specific product information for further information. Complete listing of medications according to generation is found in Table 1-2 although many of the products which would be used for hospitalized patients are not discussed in this book.

IMPLEMENTATION CONSIDERATIONS:

—Obtain a thorough health history: prior hypersensitivity to this drug or to penicillin; history of renal impairment; other medications which may interact with medication.

—Close supervision of the elderly patient is necessary because of the natural decline in renal function.

—Use Clinistix or Tes-Tape to test urine if patient is diabetic.

TABLE 1-2, FIRST, SECOND, AND THIRD GENERATION CEPHALOSPORINS

First Generation Drugs	Cefadroxil
	Cefazolin
	Cephalexin
	Cephradine
	Cephapirin
	Cephalothin
Second Generation Drugs	Cefaclor
	Cefamandole
	Cefoxitan
	Cefuroxime
Third Generation Drugs	Cefotaxime
	Ceftizoxime
	Cefoperazone
	Moxalactam

—Watch for superinfections.
—Discuss with patient possible adverse effects.

WHAT THE PATIENT NEEDS TO KNOW:
—Medication should be taken exactly as ordered.
—Oral dosage is best taken on an empty stomach, one hour before or two hours after meals. Take with a full glass of water.
—Some patients experience side effects with this drug. Therefore, notify your health provider if you notice any new or uncomfortable symptoms.
—Allergic reactions, decreased urinary output, severe and prolonged diarrhea should be reported to health provider immediately.
—Bathe daily and brush teeth regularly. Observe for signs of infection in mouth, oral and anal areas.
—Use Clinistix or Tes-Tape if you are checking your urine for glucose.

EVALUATION:

ADVERSE REACTIONS: *CNS:* dizziness, headache, malaise, vertigo. *Gastrointestinal:* anorexia, abdominal pain, diarrhea, dyspepsia, glossitis, heartburn, nausea, tenesmus, vomiting. *Hematopoietic:* hemolytic anemia (rare), leukopenia, neutropenia, thrombocytopenia. *Hypersensitivity:* anaphylaxis, eosinophilia, fever, rash, urticaria. *Other:* dyspnea, dysuria, pain with IM administration, thrombophlebitis with IV therapy.

OVERDOSAGE: Abdominal cramps, diarrhea, nausea, vomiting may occur.

PARAMETERS TO MONITOR: Draw baseline hepatic and renal studies. Continue to monitor hepatic and renal function in the impaired and elderly. Develop a flowchart to help document therapeutic effect or adverse reactions. Closely observe for decreased urinary output, proteinuria, rising BUN, rising creatinine clearance, severe and persistent diarrhea, hypersensitivity or superinfection. Following IV administration, monitor for thrombophlebitis.

CEFACLOR

PRODUCTS (TRADE NAME):
Ceclor (Available in 250 and 500 mg capsules and 125 mg/5 ml and 250 mg/5 ml oral suspension.)

DRUG SPECIFICS:
Used in upper and lower respiratory tract infections, otitis media and, skin and urinary tract infections. Effective against *S. pneumoniae, H. influenzae and S. pyogenes, S. aureus, E. coli, P. mirabilis, Klebsiella* and coagulase-negative staphylococci.

ADMINISTRATION AND DOSAGE SPECIFICS:
Adults: 250 mg every 8 hours. Give 500 mg every 8 hours in severe infections or with resistant organisms. Do not exceed 4 gm/day.
Children: Give 20 mg/kg/day in divided doses every 8 hours. Dosage may be doubled in severe infections. Do not exceed 1 gm/day.

CEFADROXIL

PRODUCTS (TRADE NAME):
Duricef, Ultracef (Available as 500 and 1000 mg tablets or capsules; 125 mg/ 5 ml, 250 mg/5 ml and 500 mg/5 ml oral suspension).
DRUG SPECIFICS:
Current literature suggests there is questionable advantage to use of this drug because of risk of nephrotoxicity and expense. It is effective in the treatment of urinary tract infections caused by *E. coli, Klebsiella, Proteus mirabilis*. It is also used in the treatment of *staphylococcus* or *streptococcus* skin infections, or in group A beta-hemolytic streptococcal infections. Oral dosage is best administered on an empty stomach.
ADMINISTRATION AND DOSAGE SPECIFICS:
Adults: 1-2 gram po every day or 500 mg po twice a day.
Children: 30 mg/kg/day in divided doses every 12 hours.

CEPHALEXIN

PRODUCTS (TRADE NAME):
Keflex (Available as 250, 500 mg capsules, 1 gm tablets, and 125 mg/5 ml,250 mg/5 ml oral suspension and 100 mg/ml pediatric drops).
DRUG SPECIFICS:
Effective in the treatment of infections due to *E. coli*, (acute prostatitis), *Haemophilus influenzae, Klebsiella* (acute prostatitis), group A beta-hemolytic streptococci, *Streptococcus pneumoniae, Staphylococcus* (skin and soft tissue infection). Renal studies indicated with prolonged therapy. Shake oral suspension and pediatric drops well. Diarrhea is less common than with other cephalosporins.
ADMINISTRATION AND DOSAGE SPECIFICS:
Adults: 1-4 grams/daily po in divided doses every 4-6 hours.
Children: 25-100 mg/kg/day po in four divided doses.

CEPHAPIRIN SODIUM

PRODUCTS (TRADE NAME):
    Cefadyl (Available as 500 mg, 1 gm, or 2 gm/vial for injection, 1, 2, 4 gm piggyback vials).
DRUG SPECIFICS:
    Effective in the treatment of infections caused by *E. coli* (urinary tract infections), *Haemophilus influenzae, Klebsiella* (urinary tract infections), *Proteus mirabilis* (urinary tract infections), *Staphylococcus* (skin and soft tissue infections), alpha *Streptococcus viridans,* group A beta-hemolytic streptococci, *Streptococcus pneumoniae.* For IM administration, inject into large muscle mass. For IV administration, alternate veins to prevent thrombophlebitis.
ADMINISTRATION AND DOSAGE SPECIFICS:
    Adults: 500 mg-1 gm parenterally every 4-6 hours. Up to 12 gm/day may be necessary for severe infections.
    Children: 40-80 mg/kg/day parenterally in four divided doses; not recommended for infants under 3 months old.

CEPHRADINE

PRODUCTS (TRADE NAME):
    Anspor (Available as 250 and 500 mg capsules, and 125 and 250 mg oral suspension.) **Velosef** (Available as 250, 500 and 1000 mg capsules, or 250, 500 mg, 1 gm/vial for injection, 2 gm in 100 ml vial, 2 gm in 200 ml vial, and 4 gm in 100 ml vial; 125 mg/5 ml and 250 mg/5 ml oral suspension.)
DRUG SPECIFICS:
    Effective in the treatment of infections due to *E. coli,* (prostatitis, urinary tract infections), *Haemophilus influenzae, Klebsiella* (prostatitis, urinary tract infections), *Proteus mirabilis* (prostatitis, urinary tract infections), *Staphylococcus* (skin and soft tissue infection), group A beta-hemolytic streptococci, *Streptococcus pneumoniae.* Do not mix with lactated Ringer's solution or antibiotics. Shake oral suspension well before using.
ADMINISTRATION AND DOSAGE SPECIFICS:
    Adults: 250-500 mg po every 6 hours; 2-4 gram/day in four divided doses parenterally. Maximum dose 8 gram/day.
    Children: 25-50 mg/kg/day po in equally divided doses every 6-12 hours; 75-100 mg/kg/day in equally divided doses every 6-12 hours for otitis media caused by *Haemophilus influenzae.* Maximum dose 4 gram/day. Or 50-100 mg/kg/day parenterally in four divided doses. May use up to 300 mg/kg/day safely.
    In patients with impaired renal function, give an initial loading dose of 750 mg followed by:

Creatinine Clearance (ml/min)	Dose
over 20	500 mg every 6-12 hours
15-19	500 mg every 12-24 hours
10-14	500 mg every 24-40 hours
5-9	500 mg every 40-50 hours
under 5	500 mg every 50-70 hours

Joann Sabados-Carolina

CHLORAMPHENICOL

ACTION OF THE DRUG: The main action of the drug is to inhibit protein synthesis in susceptible microorganisms.

ASSESSMENT:

INDICATIONS: Drug choice is dependent on the identification of the infectious organism by appropriate cultures or smears, or based on the clinical picture. Although this is a broad-spectrum drug, it should only be used in situations where the benefits outweigh the potential risks. It is a drug that should not be prescribed by anyone other than a physician. However, nurse practitioners and other health providers may often monitor the progress of a patient receiving chloramphenicol. It is the drug of choice for *Salmonella typhi* (typhoid fever). It is useful in serious infections due to *Haemophilus influenzae* (ampicillin resistant), *Lymphogranuloma, Chlamydia psittaci, Rickettsia* and *Salmonella*. It is used for meningitis due to *Neisseria meningitidis* or in infections with *Streptococcus pneumoniae* in individuals allergic to penicillin.

SUBJECTIVE-OBJECTIVE: The patient in need of antibiotic therapy may present in any number of ways, ranging from asymptomatic to severely ill. Keep in mind common infectious indicators such as fever, inflammation, erythema, edema or pain.

PLAN:

CONTRAINDICATIONS: Do not use in the presence of hypersensitivity or toxicity to this drug. Not indicated in the treatment of an infection that will respond to a less toxic drug.

WARNINGS: Only to be used in serious infections where other drugs have failed. Patient is usually hospitalized, where adequate monitoring of status can take place. Severe blood dyscrasias (rare), including aplastic anemia, have been reported with short- and long-term therapy. Discretion should be used during treatment in pregnant and nursing mothers since the drug crosses the placental border and is secreted in breast milk. Use with caution in premature babies, neonates, and infants. Gray syndrome of the newborn has been reported with drug when excessive doses are given.

PRECAUTIONS: Severe and fatal blood dyscrasias have been reported occasionally after short-term and long-term therapy. Irreversible bone marrow depression has been reported after therapy. Dosage should be decreased in impaired hepatic or renal function. Superinfection may occur with treatment.

IMPLEMENTATION:

DRUG INTERACTIONS: May antagonize the bactericidal effects of the penicillins, cephalosporins, clindamycin, erythromycin and lincomycin. Concurrent use of bone marrow depressants should be avoided. May affect the metabolism of oral anticoagulants. In anemic patients, may decrease the effect of vitamin B_{12}, folic acid and iron preparations. May prolong the half-life of chlorpropamide, dicumarol, phenobarbital, phenytoin, sulfonylureas and tolbutamide. Diuretics may increase urinary excretion.

PRODUCTS (TRADE NAME):
Chloramphenicol, Chloromycetin, Amphicol, Mychel, Chloromycin Palmitate (Available as 250 and 500 mg capsules, 1% cream, 1% ophthalmic ointment, 5 mg/15 ml otic solution, and 150 mg/5 ml oral suspension.) **Chloramphenicol Sodium Succinate** (Available in 100 mg/ml powder for injection.)

ADMINISTRATION AND DOSAGE: Patient is often hospitalized to monitor toxicity of drug. Lower doses may be indicated in individuals with impaired hepatic or renal function. Use with caution in the elderly.

Shake oral preparation well before administration. Oral dosage should be administered on an empty stomach. Switch from IV to oral form as soon as possible.

Chloramphenicol sodium succinate is only effective if administered IV and not to exceed 100 mg/ml. Administer over 1-2 minute interval. Avoid repeated courses of therapy.

Adults: 50-100 mg/kg/day in four divided doses.
Children: 50 mg/kg/day in four divided doses.
Neonatal over 2 weeks: 50 mg/kg/day in four divided doses.
Neonatal under 2 weeks: 25 mg/kg/day in four divided doses.

IMPLEMENTATION CONSIDERATIONS:
—Obtain a thorough health history: prior history of renal or hepatic impairment, prior history of hypersensitivity or toxicity to the drug, medicines that may interact with chloramphenicol.

—Be alert to the possibility of bone marrow depression after therapy is completed. Watch for bruising, petechiae, sore throat or weakness.

—Check for superinfection in the oral, vaginal or rectal areas.

—Premature babies, newborns, and infants should be monitored closely for the possibility of Gray syndrome. Watch for abdominal distention, cyanosis, irregular respirations or vasomotor collapse.

WHAT THE PATIENT NEEDS TO KNOW:
—Medication should be taken exactly as prescribed.
—This medicine may interfere with urine testing for glucose if Clinitest is used.
—There are some serious side effects which may be associated with the use of this drug. Therefore it is important that any new symptoms or discomfort be brought to your health provider's attention promptly.
—Bathe daily, brush teeth regularly, and observe for signs of infection which may develop in mouth, anal or vaginal areas.

EVALUATION:

ADVERSE REACTIONS: *CNS:* mild depression, headache, mental confusion, optic neuritis, peripheral neuritis. *Gastrointestinal:* nausea, vomiting, diarrhea, stomatitis, black hairy tongue, enterocolitis. *Hematopoietic:* There are two types of bone marrow depression that may occur: (1) A reversible depression is characterized by a vacuolization of erythroid precursors and an increased cellularity of bone marrow. This is dose related and reversible with discontinued use. (2) An irreversible depression which is not dose related and may occur weeks to months after therapy. This may lead to a fatal aplastic anemia with a risk factor of 1:24,000 to 1:50,000. Other blood dyscrasias include agranulocytosis, leukopenia, neutropenia and thrombocytopenia. *Hypersensitivity:* fever, rash, urticaria, angioedema, anaphylaxis. *Other:* Gray syndrome of newborn. During therapy for typhoid fever, a Jarisch-Herxheimer reaction may occur.

OVERDOSAGE: Possible nausea, vomiting or diarrhea.

PARAMETERS TO MONITOR: Baseline blood work should be done prior to the initiation of therapy. This blood work should evaluate the function of the hematopoietic system, hepatic and renal function. Follow-up blood studies should be obtained every 2-3 days during therapy. Discontinue drug use if blood dyscrasias develop—anemia, leukopenia, pancytopenia, reticulocytopenia, thrombocytopenia. Careful monitoring of premature babies, newborns and neonates for Gray syndrome is necessary. Particularly monitor hepatic and renal function in those with impairment, and the elderly patient. Serum drug levels may be obtained in the elderly. Develop a flow chart to follow signs and symptoms of the infection, and to evaluate therapeutic effect of the drug. Also record signs of adverse reactions or superinfections.

Joann Sabados-Carolina

CLINDAMYCIN

ACTION OF THE DRUG: Clindamycin is a bacteriostatic drug that inhibits ribosomal protein synthesis.

ASSESSMENT:

INDICATIONS: Drug choice is dependent on the identification of the infectious organism by appropriate cultures or smears or based on the clinical picture. Clindamycin is only to be used in severe infections due to streptococci, pneumococci, staphylococci or anaerobic bacteria when penicillin or erythromycin is contraindicated. It is not indicated in the treatment of meningitis, since the drug does not adequately diffuse into cerebrospinal fluid.

SUBJECTIVE-OBJECTIVE: The patient in need of antibiotic therapy may present in any number of ways, ranging from asymptomatic to severely ill. Keep in mind common infectious indicators such as fever, inflammation, erythema, edema or pain.

PLAN:

CONTRAINDICATIONS: Do not use in the presence of hypersensitivity to clindamycin or lincomycin.

WARNINGS: Clindamycin has been reported to cause severe and fatal colitis characterized by abdominal cramps, diarrhea and rectal passage of blood and mucus. These symptoms may not appear until after treatment is completed. Discontinue drug if severe and persistent diarrhea occurs. If drug is not discontinued, follow-up with large bowel endoscopy is indicated. Discretion should be used during therapy in pregnancy and in nursing mothers since the drug crosses the placental barrier and is secreted in breast milk. Safety has not been established for newborn use. Severe anaphylactoid reactions have occurred.

PRECAUTIONS: Use with caution in patients with gastrointestinal disease, especially colitis, due to toxicity and in patients with a history of asthma, multiple allergies or tartrazine sensitivity. Diarrhea associated with drug usage is not tolerated well in patients over 60 years of age with severe illness. Discretion should be used in treatment of patients with renal disease. Superinfection may occur with treatment.

IMPLEMENTATION:

DRUG INTERACTIONS: Concurrent use may enhance the effects of neuromuscular blocking agents. Antidiarrheals with kaolin and pectin will decrease the oral absorption about 90%. Use of erythromycin or chloramphenicol may produce antagonistic effects with concurrent use of lincomycin. Antiperistaltic antidiarrheals have the ability to delay removal of the toxin from the colon, thus prolonging diarrhea. Clindamycin may alter laboratory tests in the following manner: increased serum levels of SGPT, SGOT, alkaline phosphatase and bilirubin; bromsulphalein retention; decreased platelet count.

PRODUCTS (TRADE NAME):
Cleocin HCl, Cleocin Pediatric, Cleocin Phosphate (Available in 75 mg and 150 mg capsules, 75 mg/5 ml granules for pediatric use, 300 mg/2 ml ampule and 600 mg/4 ml ampule for IM or IV injection.)

ADMINISTRATION AND DOSAGE: Give intramuscular medication deep in large muscle mass. Single intramuscular injections that total 600 mg or greater are not recommended. For intravenous therapy, do not administer as bolus. Intravenous clindamycin phosphate must be diluted before administration. For oral administration, take on empty stomach with a full glass of water.

Adults: 150-300 mg every 6 hours po, with more severe infections requiring 300-450 mg every 6 hours po; 600-1,200 mg/day parenterally in 2-4 divided doses, with more severe infections requiring 1,200-2,700 mg/day in 2-4 divided doses.

Children: 8-16 mg/kg/day po in 3-4 divided doses, with more severe infections requiring 16-20 mg/kg/day po in 3-4 divided doses; 15-25 mg/kg/day parenterally in 3-4 divided doses, with more severe infections requiring 25-40 mg/kg/day parenterally in 3-4 divided doses.

IMPLEMENTATION CONSIDERATIONS:
—Obtain a complete health history: history of hypersensitivity to clindamycin or lincomycin, history of gastrointestinal disorders (particularly colitis), history of renal impairment, history of asthma, multiple allergies or tartrazine sensitivity, other medications that may cause drug interactions, pregnancy or breast-feeding.
—Watch for superinfections in the oral or perineal area.
—Be aware that clindomycin therapy may alter values of some laboratory tests.

WHAT THE PATIENT NEEDS TO KNOW:
—Medication should be taken exactly as prescribed. Do not stop taking medication once symptoms disappear. Do not save medication.
—Medicine is best absorbed on a empty stomach, 1 hour before or 2 hours after meals, with a full glass of water.
—Some patients experience side effects when taking this drug. Therefore it is especially important to notify your health care provider if you have any new or troublesome symptoms.
—Bath daily and brush teeth regularly. Watch for infections in mouth, anal or vaginal areas.
—Notify health care provider if you have severe or persistent diarrhea, abdominal cramps or blood/mucus in stools.

EVALUATION:

ADVERSE REACTIONS: *Gastrointestinal:* abdominal pain, colitis, diarrhea, esophagitis, nausea, vomiting. *Hematopoietic:* agranulocytosis, eosinophilia, neutropenia (transient), thrombocytopenia. *Hypersensitivity:* anaphylaxis, maculopapular rash, erythema multiforme (rare), Stevens-Johnson syndrome (rare). *Other:* abnormal liver function studies, jaundice, polyarthritis (rare). *After intramuscular injection:* pain, induration, sterile abscess. *After intravenous administration:* thrombophlebitis.
OVERDOSAGE: Nausea, vomiting, diarrhea or abdominal cramps occur.
PARAMETERS TO MONITOR: Monitor therapeutic effect of drug. Observe for indications of colitis: severe diarrhea, abdominal cramps, bloody/mucoid stools. In severe and persistent diarrhea, monitor hydration status: intake, output, state of mucous membranes, weight, skin turgor. In extended therapy, monitor hepatic, renal and hematologic studies. In intravenous therapy watch for thrombophlebitis. Observe for adverse reactions and superinfection.

Joann Sabados-Carolina

COLISTIMETHATE SODIUM

ACTION OF THE DRUG: Colistimethate sodium is a bactericidal drug that alters the lipoprotein cell membrane.

ASSESSMENT:

INDICATIONS: Drug choice is dependent on the identification of the infectious organism by appropriate cultures or smears, or based on the clinical picture. Colistimethate sodium is effective in the treatment of the following susceptible organisms: *Enterobacter aerogenes, E. coli, Klebsiella pneumoniae, Pseudomonas aeruginosa.* Drug should be used with discretion because of possible toxicity.

SUBJECTIVE-OBJECTIVE: The patient in need of antibiotic therapy may present in any number of ways, ranging from severely ill to asymptomatic. Keep in mind common infectious indicators such as fever, inflammation, erythema, edema or pain.

PLAN:

CONTRAINDICATIONS: Hypersensitivity to colistimethate sodium.

WARNINGS: Transient neurologic disturbances have been reported. Discretion should be used during treatment in pregnancy and nursing mothers since the drug crosses the placental border and is secreted in breast milk.

PRECAUTIONS: Use with caution in patients with impaired renal function and in the elderly.

IMPLEMENTATION:

DRUG INTERACTIONS: Colistimethate sodium may enhance the activity of surgical neuromuscular blocking agents or antibiotics with neuromuscular blocking properties such as: decamethonium, gallamine triethiodide, kanamycin, neomycin, polymyxin B, streptomycin, succinylcholine or tubocurarine. Avoid concurrent use with other nephrotoxic drugs.

PRODUCTS (TRADE NAME):
Coly-Mycin M (Available as 150 mg/vial for injection).

ADMINISTRATION AND DOSAGE:
Adults and children: 2.5-5 mg/kg/day parenterally in 2-4 divided doses. Do not exceed 5 mg/kg/day in patients with normal renal function. Dosage must be altered in patients with impaired renal function.

IMPLEMENTATION CONSIDERATIONS:
—Obtain a thorough health history: renal impairment, hypersensitivity to colistimethate sodium, other medications which may cause drug interactions, pregnancy or breast feeding.

—Observe for decreased output, increased BUN, increased serum creatinine.

—Side effects are transient and disappear when drug is discontinued.

WHAT THE PATIENT NEEDS TO KNOW:
—Medication should be taken exactly as prescribed. Do not stop taking medication when you feel better, or when symptoms disappear. Do not save medication.

—Bathe daily and brush teeth regularly. Watch for signs of infection in mouth, anal and vaginal areas.

—Some patients experience brief side effects while taking this medication. If you have any numbness, tingling, rashes or dizziness, report them to your health provider.

—Do not drive or use heavy machinery which requires alertness if you are experiencing any of the side effects.

EVALUATION:

ADVERSE REACTIONS: *CNS:* vertigo, slurred speech, paresthesia, tingling of extremities, formication of extremities. *Gastrointestinal:* gastrointestinal upset. *Hypersensitivity:* pruritus, drug fever, urticaria. *Other:* respiratory arrest following IM administration. *Renal:* nephrotoxicity manifested by decreased urinary output, increased serum creatinine.

OVERDOSAGE: *Signs and symptoms:* renal insufficiency, muscle weakness or apnea may occur.

PARAMETERS TO MONITOR: Monitor therapeutic effect of the drug. Obtain baseline renal studies in the renal impaired and the elderly. Continue renal studies during treatment. Monitor for signs and symptoms of neurologic effects: numbness, tingling, dizziness, slurred speech, generalized weakness.

Joann Sabados-Carolina

COLISTIN SULFATE (POLYMYXIN E)

ACTION OF THE DRUG: Colistin sulfate is a bactericidal drug that alters the lipoprotein cell membrane.

ASSESSMENT:

INDICATIONS: Drug choice is dependent on the identification of the infectious organism by appropriate cultures or smears, or based on the clinical picture. Poor intestinal absorption limits the effectiveness to intestinal tract infections due to *E. coli or Shigella*. Has in vitro bactericidal activity against most gram-negative enteric pathogens.

SUBJECTIVE-OBJECTIVE: The patient in need of antibiotic therapy may present in any number of ways, ranging from asymptomatic to severely ill. Keep in mind common infectious indicators such as fever, inflammation, erythema, edema or pain.

PLAN:

CONTRAINDICATIONS: Hypersensitivity to colistin sulfate.
WARNINGS: In patients with azotemia, or when the recommended dosage is exceeded, the possibility of renal toxicity exists.
PRECAUTIONS: Superinfection may occur with extended therapy. Cross resistance to polymyxin B sulfate occurs.

IMPLEMENTATION:

DRUG INTERACTIONS: Colistin may enhance the activity of surgical neuromuscular blocking agents such as tubocurarine, decamethonium, gallamine triethiodide or succinylcholine. May alter laboratory tests in the following manner: increases serum nitrogen levels, creatinine levels, urine protein and urinary casts.
PRODUCTS (TRADE NAME):
Coly-Mycin S (Available as 25 mg/5 ml powder for oral suspension.)
ADMINISTRATION AND DOSAGE:
Adult and children: 5-15 mg/kg/day po in three divided doses.
IMPLEMENTATION CONSIDERATIONS:
—Obtain a thorough health history: history of renal impairment, hypersensitivity to colistin sulfate, other medications which may cause drug interactions.
—Evaluate client's renal status (BUN, creatinine, and urinalysis) before making the decision to use this drug.

WHAT THE PATIENT NEEDS TO KNOW:
—Medication should be taken exactly as prescribed. Do not stop taking drug once you start feeling better or once symptoms disappear. Do not save medication.
—Bathe daily and brush teeth regularly. Watch mouth, anal and vaginal areas for signs of infection.
—Although side effects related to this drug are uncommon, notify your health provider if you notice any new or discomforting symptoms.

EVALUATION:

PARAMETERS TO MONITOR: Monitor therapeutic effect of the drug. Monitor renal function, especially in patients with renal impairment and in the elderly. Observe for decreased urinary output.

Joann Sabados-Carolina

ERYTHROMYCIN

ACTION OF THE DRUG: Erythromycin is a bacteriostatic or bactericidal macrolide that inhibits ribosomal protein synthesis.

ASSESSMENT:

INDICATIONS: Erythromycin is indicated as the alternative treatment in patients hypersensitive to the penicillins. Effective in the treatment of infections due to the following susceptible organisms: Alpha-hemolytic streptococci, group A beta-hemolytic streptococci, *Entamoeba histolytica, Haemophilus influenzae, Listeria monocytogenes, Mycoplasma pneumoniae, Neisseria gonorrhoeae, Staphylococcus aureus, Streptococcus pneumoniae, Treponema pallidum.* It is effective in the treatment of erythrasma.

SUBJECTIVE-OBJECTIVE: The patient in need of antibiotic therapy may present in any number of ways, ranging from asymptomatic to severely ill. Keep in mind common infectious indicators such as fever, inflammation, erythema, edema or pain.

PLAN:

CONTRAINDICATIONS: Hypersensitivity to any erythromycin.

WARNINGS: Discretion should be used during treatment in pregnant and nursing mothers since the drug crosses the placental border and is secreted in breast milk. Hepatotoxicity has been reported in patients on erythromycin estolate.

PRECAUTIONS: Superinfection may occur with treatment. Use with discretion in patients with tartrazine sensitivity.

IMPLEMENTATION:

DRUG INTERACTIONS: Concurrent use with theophylline derivatives may increase serum theophylline levels. Sulfonamides exert a synergistic effect when used with erythromycins. An antagonistic effect exists with the use of erythromycin and clindamycin or lincomycin. Although concurrent use of penicillin is not indicated, it may exert an antagonistic effect. Erythromycin may cause the following alterations in laboratory values: increased SGPT, increased SGOT, increased alkaline phosphatase, false increase in urinary catecholamines or 17-ketosteroids, decreased serum glucose levels, decreased serum cholesterol, decreased prothrombin.

PRODUCTS (TRADE NAME):
Bristamycin (Available in 250 mg film-coated tablets.) **EES (Erythromycin Ethylsuccinate)** (Available in 200 mg chewable tablets, 400 mg film coated tablets, 200 and 400 mg/5 ml oral suspension, 100 mg/2.5 ml drops.) **Erythromycin** (Available in 250 mg enteric-coated tablets, and 250 and 500 mg film-coated tablets.) **E-Mycin** (Available in 250 mg and 330 mg enteric-coated tablets.) **Erypar** (Available in 250 mg film-coated tablet.) **Erythromycin Base** (Available in 250 and 500 mg film-coated tablets.) **Ethril 250** (Available in 250 mg film-coated tablet.) **Ilosone (Erythromycin Estolate)** (Available in 125 and 250 mg chewable tablets; 125 and 250 mg capsules; 500 mg tablets; 100 mg/ml drops; 125 and 250 mg/5 ml oral suspension.) **Ilotycin** (Available in 250 mg enteric-coated tablet.) **Pediamycin** (Available in 200 mg chewable tablet, 200 and 400 mg/5 ml oral suspension and 100 mg/2.5 ml drops.) **Pfizer-E** (Available in 250 mg film coated tablet.) **RP Mycin**

(Available in 250 mg enteric-coated tablet.) **SKErythromycin** (Available in 250 and 500 mg film-coated tablet). **Wyamycin-S** (Available as 250 and 500 mg enteric-coated tablet.)

ADMINISTRATION AND DOSAGE: Dosage-dependent on the type and severity of the infection. All chewable forms must be fully chewed for complete therapeutic effect. Strength is expressed as erythromycin base equivalence. Due to differences in absorption, 400 mg ethylsuccinate is required to provide the same free erythromycin serum levels as 250 mg erythromycin base, stearate or estolate.

Adults: 250 mg (400 mg ethyl succinate) every 6 hours po; 15-20 mg/kg/day parenterally. Dosage may be increased with the severity of the infection.

Children: 30-50 mg/kg/day po in 3-4 divided doses; 15-20 mg/kg/ day parenterally. Dosage may be increased with the severity of the infection.

IMPLEMENTATION CONSIDERATIONS:

—Obtain a thorough health history: prior history of hepatic impairment or alcoholism; medications which may cause interaction; prior history of hypersensitivity to erythromycin or tartrazine; pregnancy or breast feeding.

—Watch for superinfection.

WHAT THE PATIENT NEEDS TO KNOW:

—Medication should be taken exactly as prescribed. Take all medications even when symptoms have disappeared and you are feeling better. Do not save medication.

—Oral dosage may be taken with meals.

—Bathe daily and brush teeth regularly. Watch mouth, anal and vaginal areas for development of any infection.

—Notify health practitioner if urine or stool color changes, abdominal cramps or diarrhea are experienced, or any new or troublesome symptom develops.

EVALUATION:

ADVERSE REACTIONS: *Gastrointestinal:* nausea, diarrhea, vomiting, abdominal cramps, pseudomembranous colitis, hepatotoxicity (cholestatic hepatitis) have been reported with the use of erythromycin estolate and erythromycin ethylsuccinate (rare). *Hypersensitivity:* rash, urticaria, anaphylaxis. *Other:* sensorineural hearing loss with large doses of erythromycin lactobionate or gluceptate which reverses with discontinuance of drug. *With IV administration:* venous irritation or hepatotoxicity has been reported with erythromycin estolate.

OVERDOSAGE: *Signs and Symptoms:* abdominal cramps, diarrhea, nausea or vomiting occurs.

PARAMETERS TO MONITOR: Obtain baseline laboratory studies for liver if long term therapy is anticipated. Repeat tests periodically to monitor for liver toxicity. Observe for abdominal pain, jaundice, dark urine, pale colored stools or weakness. If large doses are indicated, monitor closely for sensorineural hearing loss. Observe for therapeutic effects and superinfection.

Joann Sabados-Carolina

LINCOMYCIN

ACTION OF THE DRUG: Lincomycin is a bacteriostatic and bactericidal drug that inhibits ribosomal protein synthesis.

ASSESSMENT:

INDICATIONS: Drug choice is dependent on the identification of the infectious organism by appropriate cultures or smears, or based on the clinical picture. Lincomycin is a drug which should be prescribed by physicians. However many practitioners may be responsible for monitoring the progress of the patient on this drug. Lincomycin is only to be used in severe infections due to susceptible strains of streptococci, pneumococci and staphylococci when penicillin or erythromycin is contraindicated. It may produce severe and fatal colitis.

SUBJECTIVE-OBJECTIVE: The patient in need of antibiotic therapy may present in any number of ways ranging from asymptomatic to severely ill. Keep in mind common infectious indicators such as fever, inflammation, erythema, edema or pain.

PLAN:

CONTRAINDICATIONS: Hypersensitivity to lincomycin or clindamycin.

WARNINGS: Lincomycin has been reported to cause severe and fatal colitis characterized by abdominal cramps, diarrhea, rectal passage of blood and mucus. These symptoms may not develop until treatment is completed. Discontinue drug if severe and persistent diarrhea occurs. If drug is not discontinued, follow-up with large bowel endoscopy is indicated. Discretion should be used during therapy in pregnancy and in nursing mothers since the drug crosses the placental barrier and is secreted in breast milk. Safety has not been established for use in newborns.

PRECAUTIONS: Use with caution in patients with gastrointestinal disease, especially colitis due to toxicity. Use with caution in patients with a history of asthma or multiple allergies. Diarrhea associated with drug usage is not tolerated well in patients over 60 years old with severe illness. Discretion should be used in treatment of patients with renal disease. Superinfection may occur with treatment.

IMPLEMENTATION:

DRUG INTERACTIONS: Concurrent use may enhance the effects of neuromuscular blocking agents. Antidiarrheals with kaolin and pectin will decrease the oral absorption about 90%. Use of erythromycin or chloramphenicol may produce antagonistic effects with concurrent use of lincomycin. Antiperistaltic antidiarrheals have the ability to delay removal of the toxins from the colon, thus prolonging diarrhea. IV solution is not compatible with novobiocin, kanamycin, phenytoin sodium, and protein hydrolysates. May alter laboratory values in the following manner: increase serum levels of SGPT, SGOT, alkaline phosphatase, bilirubin, BSP retention and a decreased platelet count.

PRODUCTS (TRADE NAME):

Lincocin (Available as 250 and 500 mg capsules, 250 mg/5 ml syrup, and 300 mg/ml in 2 ml vials and 300 mg/ml in 10 ml vial for injection).

ADMINISTRATION AND DOSAGE:

Adults: 500 mg every 8 hours po, with more severe infections requiring 500 mg every 6 hours po; or 600 mg/day IM as a single dose, more severe infections requiring 500 mg IM every 12 hours; 600 mg-1 gm IV every 8-12 hours. Maximum dose is 8 gm/day.

Children including neonates: (Not recommended in newborns under one month). 30 mg/kg/day po in 3-4 divided doses with more severe infections requiring 60 mg/kg/day in 3-4 divided doses; 10 mg/kg/day IM as a single dose, with more severe infections requiring 10 mg/kg every 12 hours IM; 10-20 mg/kg/day every 8-12 hours IV.

Administer oral dose on an empty stomach. For IV administration: dilute to 1 gm/100 ml. Infuse over 60 minute period to prevent cardiac complications. Administer IM dose deep in large muscle mass.

IMPLEMENTATION CONSIDERATIONS:

—Obtain a thorough health history: history of hypersensitivity to lincomycin or clindamycin, history of asthma or multiple allergies, previous gastrointestinal disorders (especially colitis), renal impairment, other medications which may cause drug interactions, pregnancy or breast-feeding.

—Observe for possibility of superinfection in oral, vaginal or rectal area.

WHAT THE PATIENT NEEDS TO KNOW:

—Medication should be taken exactly as prescribed. Do not stop taking medication once symptoms disappear and do not save any medication.

—Medicine is best absorbed on an empty stomach, one hour before or two hours after meals, with a full glass of water.

—Bathe daily and brush teeth regularly. Watch for signs of infection in mouth, anal and rectal areas.

—Notify practitioner immediately if you have severe and persistent diarrhea, abdominal cramps or blood/mucus in stools. Some people experience side effects from this drug and so you should notify your provider if you have any new or uncomfortable symptoms.

EVALUATION:

ADVERSE REACTIONS: *Cardiovascular:* hypotension and cardiac arrest after rapid IV administration (rare). *CNS:* tinnitus, vertigo. *Gastrointestinal:* abdominal cramps, anorexia, bloating, diarrhea, enterocolitis, flatulence, glossitis, nausea, pruritus ani, stomatitis, vomiting, weight loss. *Hematopoietic:* agranulocytosis, aplastic anemia (rare), leukopenia, neutropenia, pancytopenia, thrombocytopenic purpura. *Hypersensitivity:* angioneurotic edema, anaphylaxis, urticaria, serum sickness, Stevens-Johnson syndrome (rare), erythema multiforme (rare). *Other:* abnormal liver function studies, jaundice. *With IM administration:* pain (occasional), induration (rare), sterile abscess (rare). *With IV administration:* thrombophlebitis.

PARAMETERS TO MONITOR: Observe for indications of colitis: severe diarrhea, abdominal cramps, bloody/mucoid stools. In severe and persistent diarrhea, monitor hydration status: intake and output, skin turgor, condition of mucous membranes, weight. (May need to discontinue drug or follow with large bowel endoscopy.) Monitor therapeutic effect of drug. In extended therapy monitor hepatic, renal and hematologic studies; observe for adverse reactions and superinfection.

Joann Sabados-Carolina

NOVOBIOCIN

ACTION OF THE DRUG: Novobiocin is a bacteriostatic drug that inhibits bacterial cell wall synthesis.

ASSESSMENT:

INDICATIONS: Drug choice is dependent on the identification of the infectious organism by appropriate cultures or smears, or based on the clinical picture. Novobiocin is only to be used in serious infections in which organisms are resistant to other antibiotics. Non-physicians do not usually prescribe this drug; however, they may have responsibility for monitoring the status of patients receiving this medication. It is effective in the treatment of *Staphylococcus aureus infections* and in the treatment of urinary infections due to *Proteus.*

SUBJECTIVE-OBJECTIVE: The patient in need of antibiotic therapy may present in any number of ways, ranging from asymptomatic to severely ill. Keep in mind common infectious indicators such as fever, inflammation, erythema, edema or pain.

PLAN:

CONTRAINDICATIONS: Hypersensitivity to novobiocin.

WARNINGS: Novobiocin should only be used in serious infections because of the common occurrence of rapidly developing resistant strains, and adverse reactions. These include urticaria, maculopapular dermatitis, hepatic dysfunction (rare) or blood dyscrasias (rare).

PRECAUTIONS: Superinfection may occur with treatment. Hypersensitivity reactions may develop with treatment.

PRODUCTS (TRADE NAME):
Albamycin (Available as 250 mg capsules).
ADMINISTRATION AND DOSAGE:
Adults: Usual dose is 250 mg po every 6 hours, or 500 mg every 12 hours.
Continue therapy for 48 hours after temperature returns to normal.
Children: 15-45 mg/kg/day po given in divided doses every 6 to 12 hours.
IMPLEMENTATION CONSIDERATIONS:
—Obtain a thorough health history: prior hepatic impairment, history of hypersensitivity.
—Watch closely for the sudden worsening of a patient who is beginning to get better. Sudden development of resistant strains is common.
—Assess carefully for side effects.

WHAT THE PATIENT NEEDS TO KNOW:
—Medication should be taken exactly as ordered. Do not stop taking medication just because you feel better or the symptoms disappear. Do not save any medication.
—Some patients have side effects from this drug. Notify health practitioner if you have any jaundice, dark urine, pale stools, weakness, skin rashes, or any new or bothersome symptoms.

EVALUATION:

ADVERSE REACTIONS: *Hematopoietic:* leukopenia, eosinophilia, anemia, pancytopenia, agranulocytosis, thrombocytopenia. *Hepatic:* jaundice, increased serum bilirubin, impaired bromosulphalein excretion. *Hypersensitivity:* a high incidence of skin eruptions: urticaria, erythematous rash, maculopapular rash, scarlatiniform rash, Stevens-Johnson syndrome (rare). *Other:* nausea, vomiting, diarrhea, intestinal hemorrhage, alopecia, pain with IM injection.
PARAMETERS TO MONITOR: Monitor therapeutic effect of the drug. Obtain baseline blood and hepatic function studies and continue to monitor during therapy. Resistant strains of organisms may develop suddenly. Observe for signs of superinfection.

Joann Sabados-Carolina

PENICILLINS

ACTION OF THE DRUG: The penicillins interfere with mucopeptide cell wall synthesis.

ASSESSMENT:

INDICATIONS: These are the drugs of choice for broad-spectrum susceptible gram-positive and gram-negative organisms. The choice of drug is dependent on the identification of the infectious organism by appropriate cultures or smears, or based on the clinical picture. Effective in the treatment of the following susceptible organisms: alpha-hemolytic streptococci, group A beta-hemolytic streptococci, streptococci groups C, G, H, L, M, Streptococcus pneumoniae *Spirillum minus* (rat bite fever), *Neisseria gonorrhoeae, Treponema pallidum* (syphilis), *Treponema pertenue* (yaws), *Neisseria meningitidis, Fusobacterium, Bacillus anthracis, Actinomyces israelii, Clostridium perfringens, Clostridium tetani, Corynebacterium diptheriae, Listeria monocytogenes, Staphylococcus, Pasteurella meningitidis.* Also indicated for the prophylaxis against bacterial endocarditis in patients with rheumatic heart disease or congenital heart disease before dental procedures, upper respiratory tract, genitourinary tract, or gastrointestinal tract surgery.

SUBJECTIVE-OBJECTIVE: The patient in need of antibiotic therapy may present in any number of ways ranging from asymptomatic to severely ill. Keep in mind common infectious indicators such as fever, inflammation, erythema, edema or pain.

PLAN:

CONTRAINDICATIONS: Hypersensitivity to penicillin or cephalosporins.

WARNINGS: Anaphylaxis has occurred with oral and parenteral therapy. Use with caution in patients with multiple allergies. Discretion should be used during treatment in pregnant and nursing mothers since the drug crosses the placental barrier and is secreted in breast milk.

PRECAUTIONS: Use with extreme caution in patients with multiple allergies or asthma. Skin testing for allergy may be utilized at the discretion of the practitioner. Use with caution in patients allergic to tartrazine. Prolonged use may lead to hepatic, renal, or hematologic disorders. A minimum of 10 days of therapy is indicated in the treatment of Group A beta-hemolytic streptococci to decrease the risk of rheumatic fever, endocarditis, or glomerulonephritis. In the treatment of gonorrhea, all lesions should be examined for syphilis through a dark-field exam before initiation of therapy. Repeat serologies are necessary once a month for 4 months. Avoid ineffective doses in any therapy to decrease the risk of development of resistant strains.

IMPLEMENTATION:

DRUG INTERACTIONS: Bacteriostatic antibiotics such as tetracyclines and erythromycin may decrease the bactericidal effect of penicillins. Probenecid will prolong blood levels by blocking renal secretion of penicillins. Concurrent use of ampicillin and oral contraceptives has been associated with menstrual irregularities and unplanned pregnancies. Indomethacin, phenylbutazone, or aspirin may increase serum penicillin levels. Concurrent use of antacids may decrease absorption. May interfere with the following laboratory tests: increases SGOT, increases bilirubin, increases serum creatinine, false positive Coombs' test, decreases serum haptoglobin, decreases hemoglobin, decreases hematocrit, decreases platelet count, produces positive lupus erythematosus preparation, false increase in urine glucose and protein, serum uric acid and cerebrospinal protein.

ADMINISTRATION AND DOSAGE: Dosage is dependent on the type and severity of the infection. Table 1-3 lists the various classifications of penicillin. Refer to specific product information for further information.

IMPLEMENTATION CONSIDERATIONS:

—Take a thorough health history: Evaluate the medications that the patient is on for possible interactions with penicillin; determine prior history of penicillin allergy, multiple allergies, asthma, hypersensitivity to procaine or tartrazine; whether patient is pregnant or breast feeding.

—Watch for possible superinfection in the oral, vaginal or rectal areas.

—With IM injections, always aspirate to prevent medicine from entering a blood vessel.

—Observe patients after first dose whenever possible, watching for anaphylactic reactions.

—In treating patients with syphilis or gonorrhea, infected partners must be treated also.

TABLE 1-3. CLASSIFICATION OF PENICILLIN PRODUCTS

Classification	Specific Drugs	Penicillinase-Resistant	Acid-Stable
Acid-Stable Ampicillins	Penicillin V	—	+
	Amoxicillin	—	+
	Ampicillin	—	+
	Bacampicillin	—	+
	Cyclacillin	—	+
	Hetacillin	—	+
Extended-spectrum	Azlocillin	—	NA
	Carbenicillin	—	+
	Mezlocillin	—	NA
	Piperacillin	—	NA
	Ticarcillin	—	NA
Penicillin G	Penicillin G		
Penicillinase-resistant	Cloxacillin	+	+
	Dicloxacillin	+	+
	Methicillin	+	—
	Nafcillin	+	+
	Oxacillin	+	+

+ = yes   − = no   not applicable (NA) if only comes in IM or IV preparation

—If laboratory tests are necessary while patient is on penicillin therapy, remember that penicillin interferes with the accuracy of many values.

WHAT THE PATIENT NEEDS TO KNOW:

—Medication should be taken exactly as prescribed. Do not stop taking medication just because you feel better. Take every dose.

—Be careful to bathe and brush your teeth regularly while using this medication. Watch for any signs of itching, irritation, infection.

—Do not use medication after the date printed on the label.

—Notify practitioner if rash, hives, decreased urination, diarrhea, or other unusual symptoms develop. Penicillin allergies can develop at any time.

—Go to an emergency room quickly if you become short of breath, or have difficulty breathing.

—Always carry a medic alert tag or card if you have any drug allergies.

—If treatment is for a sexually transmitted disease, do not have sexual activity during treatment. All sexual partners should come in for testing and treatment also.

EVALUATION:

ADVERSE REACTIONS: *CNS:* seizures (with high parenteral dosages.) *Dermatologic:* erythema multiforme-like lesions (rare), fixed drug eruptions. *Gastrointestinal:* nausea, vomiting, acute hemorrhagic diarrhea, enterocolitis, pseudomembranous colitis, epigastric distress. *Hematopoietic:* anemia, hemolytic anemia, agranulocytosis, pancytopenia, eosinophilia, leukopenia, transient neutropenia, thrombocytopenia (all are rare and are usually reversible when drug is discontinued.) *Hepatic:* hepatitis (rare.) *Hypersensitivity:* rash, erythema, urticaria, angioedema, laryngeal edema, anaphylaxis, serum sickness syndrome (fever, exanthema, arthritis, lymphadenitis, leukopenia.) *Renal:* interstitial nephritis (rare) *Other: After IM injection:* pain, edema, Jarisch-Herxheimer reactions may occur 2-12 hours after the first dose in the treatment of syphilis (a result of the destruction of treponemas), and may cause severe flu-like illness.

PARAMETERS TO MONITOR: Monitor for therapeutic effect of the drug. Obtain baseline blood, renal and hepatic studies if prolonged treatment is indicated. Obtain baseline blood pressure and pulse before parenteral administration. Advise the patient to wait 30 minutes after oral or IM administration before leaving outpatient setting. Observe for hypersensitivity. Observe for signs of superinfection: yeast overgrowth, thrush, vaginitis, anal pruritus, and vaginal pruritus.

AMOXICILLIN

PRODUCTS (TRADE NAME):

Amoxil (Available as 250 and 500 mg capsules, or powder for oral suspension

which reconstitutes to 125 mg/5 ml, 250 mg/5 ml.) **Amoxicillin, Larotid, Polymox, Sumox, Trimox, Utimox, Wymox** (Available in 250 and 500 mg chewable tablets.)
DRUG SPECIFICS:

This is an extended spectrum penicillin. It is effective against the following susceptible organisms: *E. coli, Haemophilus influenzae, Neisseria gonorrhoeae, Proteus mirabilis, Streptococcus faecalis, Streptococcus pneumoniae*, and non-penicillinase-producing *staphylococcus*.

ADMINISTRATION AND DOSAGE SPECIFICS:

Adults and Children over 20 kg: 250-500 mg po every 8 hours.

Children under 20 kg: 20-40 mg/kg/day po in divided doses every 8 hours.

Continue treatment for a minimum of 48-72 hours after the patient is asymptomatic or cultures are negative.

Uncomplicated gonorrhea: 3 gram po single dose with 1 gm probenecid.

Acute epididymitis or salpingitis: Give 3 grams po with 1 gm po probenecid, followed by tetracycline HCl 500 mg four times daily for 10 days.

Urogeital, anal and pharyngeal gonorrhea in children under 45 kg: Give 50 mg/kg po once, plus probenecid 25 mg/kg once (maximum of 1 gm).

AMPICILLIN

PRODUCTS (TRADE NAME):

Amcill, Omnipen, Polycillin, Principen, SK-Ampicillin, Totacillin (Available as 125, 250, 500 mg capsules; 125 mg tablets, and as a powder for oral suspension that reconstitutes as 125 mg/5 ml, 250 mg/5 ml, 500 mg/5 ml, and pediatric powder which reconstitutes to 100 mg/ml drops.)
DRUG SPECIFICS:

This is an extended-spectrum penicillin. It is effective in susceptible strains of the following organisms: *E. coli, Haemophilus influenzae, Neisseria gonorrhoeae, Neisseria meningitidis, Proteus mirabilis, Salmonella, Shigella*. Give with 1 gm of probenecid for treatment of gonorrhea. Probenecid is not recommended for patients with blood dyscrasias, uric acid kidney stones, or acute gout. An associated non-hypersensitive skin rash has been reported in patients on ampicillin, especially in patients with infectious mononucleosis or with concurrent use of allopurinol.

ADMINISTRATION AND DOSAGE SPECIFICS:

Adults: 250-500 mg po four times a day.

Children under 20 kg: 50-100 mg/kg/day po in divided doses every 6 hours.

Children over 20 kg: 250-500 mg po four times a day.

Uncomplicated gonorrhea: 3.5 gm po with 1 gm of probenecid. In acute epididymitis or salpingitis: continue with 500 mg po four times a day for 10 days. In disseminated gonorrhea: continue with 500 mg po four times a day for one week.

AMPICILLIN SODIUM

PRODUCTS (TRADE NAME):
Omnipen-N, Polycillin-N, Totacillin-N, SK Ampicillin-N (Available in 125, 250, 500 mg, 1 gm, 2 gm vials and 500 mg, 1 gm, 2 gm piggyback units.)
DRUG SPECIFICS:
This is an extended spectrum penicillin. It is effective in susceptible strains of the following organisms: *E. coli, Haemophilus influenzae, Neisseria gonorrhoeae, Neisseria meningitidis, Proteus mirabilis, Salmonella, Shigella.* It is also effective in the treatment of penicillin G sensitive staphylococci, streptococci, or pneumococci.

ADMINISTRATION AND DOSAGE SPECIFICS:
Adults: 250-500 mg IM or IV every 6 hours.
Children: 25-50 mg/kg/day IM or IV in divided doses every 6-8 hours.

AZLOCILLIN SODIUM

PRODUCTS (TRADE NAME):
Azlin (Available in 2, 3, and 4 gm vials for infusion.)
DRUG SPECIFICS:
This is a relatively new product used in the treatment of serious infections and often used concomitantly with an aminoglycoside or a cephalosporin. It is also effective in the treatment of lower respiratory tract infections caused *by E. coli* and *H. influenzae,* and in urinary tract and skin infections caused by *E. coli, P. mirabilis* and *S. faecalis. Give reduced dosage in patients with impaired renal function. Site and severity of the infection, susceptibility of the organism, and defense mechanism of the host all determine dosage for individual patient. Give all medication by IV injection over at least a 5 minute period, or by IV infusion.*

ADMINISTRATION AND DOSAGE SPECIFICS:
Lower respiratory tract infections, skin infections, bone and joint infections: 225 to 300 mg/kg/day. Give IV in divided doses of 3-4 gm every 4-6 hours.
Urinary tract infections: 100 to 200 mg/kg/day. Give IV in divided doses of 2 to 3 gm every 6 hours. Reserve highest dosages for complicated infections.

BACAMPICILLIN HCL

PRODUCTS (TRADE NAME):
Spectrobid (Available in 400 mg film coated tablets and 125/5 ml powder for oral suspension.)

DRUG SPECIFICS:

Used in upper and lower respiratory tract infections, urinary tract infections, skin infections, and acute uncomplicated urogenital infections due to gonorrhea. It is effective against E. coli, P. mirabilis, S. faecalis, N. gonorrhoeae, S. pyrogenes, S. pneumoniae, and H. influenzae as well as non-penicillinase-producing staphylococci. It is more completely absorbed than ampicillin, and so may be administered in lower total daily dosages.

ADMINISTRATION AND DOSAGE SPECIFICS:

Adults: 400 mg every 12-hours. Dose may be doubled in severe infections.

Children or adults weighing less than 25 kg: 25 mg/kg/day in 2 equally divided doses at 12 hour intervals. Dose may be doubled in severe infections.

Gonorrhea: Usual adult dosage for males and females is 1.6 gm bacampicillin plus 1 gm probenecid as a single oral dose.

CARBENICILLIN DISODIUM

PRODUCTS (TRADE NAME):

Geopen, (Available as 1, 2, 5 gm vials, 2, 5, 10, 20 gm piggyback units.)

DRUG SPECIFICS:

This is an extended-spectrum penicillin. It is effective in the treatment of the following susceptible organisms: *E. coli, Proteus, Pseudomonas aeruginosa.* Products vary in the amount of sodium per gram. See hypokalemia and decreased platelet function as signs of toxicity.

ADMINISTRATION AND DOSAGE SPECIFICS:

Urinary Tract Infection:

Adults: Uncomplicated: 1-2 gm IM every 6 hours; Serious: 200 mg/kg/day IV drip.

Children: 50-200 mg/kg/day IM in divided doses every 4-6 hours.

Septicemia, Severe Systemic Respiratory or Soft Tissue Infections:

Adults: Pseudomonas and anaerobes 400-500 mg/kg/day in divided doses or continuous IV. *Proteus* and *E. coli*—300-400 mg/kg/day.

Children: 400-500 mg/kg/day IV divided doses or continuous drip.

CARBENICILLIN INDANYL SODIUM

PRODUCTS (TRADE NAME):

Geocillin (Available as 382 mg film coated tablets.)

DRUG SPECIFICS:

This is an extended-spectrum penicillin. Effective in the following susceptible organisms: *E. coli, Proteus mirabilis, Proteus morgani, Proteus rettgeri, S. faecalis, Enterobacter, Pseudomonas.* Used only in the treatment of urinary tract infections due to *E. coli, Proteus, Enterobacter, Pseudomonas,* or Enterococcus.

ADMINISTRATION AND DOSAGE SPECIFICS:
Adults:
Urinary tract infections: 1-2 tablets po four times a day.
Prostatitis: 2 tablets po four times a day.

CLOXACILLIN SODIUM

PRODUCTS (TRADE NAME):
Cloxacillin Sodium, Cloxapen, Tegopen (Available in 250 and 500 mg capsules, 125 mg/5 ml powder for oral solution.)
DRUG SPECIFICS:
This is a penicillinase-resistant penicillin. It is slightly less resistant to staphylococci than methicillin but more resistant to *B. cereus* penicillinase. Also effective in the treatment of pneumococci or group A beta-hemolytic streptococci.
ADMINISTRATION AND DOSAGE SPECIFICS:
Adults and children over 20 kg: 250-500 mg po every 6 hours.
Children under 20 kg: 50-100 mg/kg po every 6 hours.

CYCLACILLIN

PRODUCTS (TRADE NAME):
Cyclapen-W (Available in 250 and 500 mg tablets, and 125 and 250 mg/5 ml powder for oral suspension.)
DRUG SPECIFICS:
This product has a similar spectrum to ampicillin, but with a lower incidence of diarrhea. It is useful in respiratory tract infections including tonsillitis and pharyngitis caused by group A beta-hemolytic streptococci, as well as infections produced by *H. influenzae.* It is also used in urinary tract infections caused by *E. coli* and *P. mirabilis,* and skin infections caused by group A beta-hemolytic streptococci and staphylococci and non-penicillinase-producing strains. Patients with reduced creatinine clearance require dosage alterations. See manufacturers suggestions for patients in renal failure.
ADMINISTRATION AND DOSAGE SPECIFICS:
Adults: Give 250 mg every 6 hours. 500 mg may be given every 6 hours in GU tract infections.

Children: Give 50 mg/kg/day or 250 mg every 8 hours, depending on severity of infection.

DICLOXACILLIN SODIUM

PRODUCTS (TRADE NAME):
Dicloxacillin Sodium, Dycill (Available in 250 and 500 mg capsules.) **Dynapen** (Available in 125, 250, 500 mg capsules, 62.5 mg/5 ml powder for oral suspension.) **Pathocil** (Available in 250 mg capsules and 62.5 mg/5 ml oral suspension.) **Veracillin** (Available in 250 and 500 mg capsules.)
DRUG SPECIFICS:
This is a penicillinase-resistant penicillin. It is effective in the treatment of penicillinase-producing staphylococci. Also effective in the treatment of pneumococci, group A beta-hemolytic streptococci.
ADMINISTRATION AND DOSAGE SPECIFICS:
Adults and children over 40 kg: 125-250 mg po every 6 hours.
Children under 40 kg: 12.5-25 mg/kg/day po every 6 hours.

HETACILLIN

PRODUCTS (TRADE NAME):
Versapen (Available as 112.5 and 225 mg/5 ml powder for oral suspension.)
Versapen K (Available in 225 mg capsules.)
DRUG SPECIFICS:
This is an extended-spectrum penicillin metabolized to Ampicillin. It is effective in the treatment of the following susceptible organisms: group A beta-hemolytic streptococci, *Streptococcus pneumoniae* (otitis media), non-penicillinase-producing *Staphylococcus aureus, Haemophilus influenzae, E. coli,* Enterococcus, *Proteus mirabilis, Shigella.*
ADMINISTRATION AND DOSAGE SPECIFICS:
Patients over 40 kg: 225-450 mg po four times a day.
Children under 40 kg: 22.5-45 mg/kg/day in divided doses.
Chronic gastrointestinal or urinary tract infection may require prolonged intensive therapy.

METHICILLIN SODIUM

PRODUCTS (TRADE NAME):
Celbenin, Staphcillin (Available in 1, 4, 6 gm vials and 1, 2, 4 gm piggyback units.)

DRUG SPECIFICS:

This is a penicillinase-producing penicillin. Effective in the treatment of infections due to penicillinase-producing staphylococci. Also effective in the treatment of group A beta-hemolytic streptococci. Continue treatment for 48 hours after patient is afebrile or until cultures return to negative. Do not mix with other drugs.

ADMINISTRATION AND DOSAGE SPECIFICS:

Adults: 1 gm IM every 4-6 hours; 1 gm IV every 6 hours in 50 ml sodium chloride.

Children under 20 kg: Usual dose is 25 mg/kg every 6 hours.

MEZLOCILLIN

PRODUCTS (TRADE NAME):

Mezlin (Available in 1, 2, 3 and 4 gm powder for injection.)

DRUG SPECIFICS:

This is a relatively new extended spectrum penicillin which is administered IM or IV. This product is reserved for use in severe or complicated infections. Mezlocillin is effective in the treatment of lower respiratory tract infections, intra-abdominal infections, and urinary tract infections caused by *H. influenzae, K. pneumoniae, P. mirabilis, E. coli, B. fragilis,* and *P. aeruginosa.* It is also used in the treatment of uncomplicated gonorrhea. Mezlocillin may be used in treatment of some mixed infections containing group A beta-hemolytic *Streptococcus.* Used with aminoglycosides, mezlocillin is an effective agent in other serious and life-threatening infections.

ADMINISTRATION AND DOSAGE SPECIFICS:

Urinary tract infections: 1.5 to 3 gm every 6 hours IV or IM.

Lower respiratory tract infections, intra-abdominal infections, skin and gynecological infections: 3 to 4 gm every 4-6 hours IV or IM.

NAFCILLIN SODIUM

PRODUCTS (TRADE NAME):

Nafcil (Available in 500 mg, 1 and 2 gm vials for injection; 1, 2, and 4 gm piggyback units and 250 mg/5 ml powder for oral solution.) **Unipen** (Available in 500 mg tablets; 250 mg capsules; and 500 mg, 1 gm, 2 gm per vial for injection; 1, 2, 4 gm piggyback units and 250 mg/5 ml powder for oral solution.)

DRUG SPECIFICS:

This is a penicillinase-resistant penicillin. Its primary use is in the treatment of infections due to penicillinase-producing staphylococci. Also effective in the treatment of group A beta-hemolytic streptococci and pneumococci. Poorly absorbed orally.

ADMINISTRATION AND DOSAGE SPECIFICS:
   Adults: 250 mg-1 gm po every 4-6 hours; or 500 mg IM every 4-6 hours.
   Children: 250 mg po three times a day or 25-50 mg/kg/day in four divided doses; or 25 mg/kg/day IM in two doses.
   Neonatal: 10 mg/kg po/day in 3-4 doses; or 10 mg/kg/day IM in two doses.
   IV Dosage: 500 mg every 4 hours in 15-30 ml of sodium chloride, injected for 5-10 minutes or slow drip to prevent thrombophlebitis.

OXACILLIN SODIUM

PRODUCTS (TRADE NAME):
   Bactocill, Prostaphlin (Available as 250 mg, 500 mg capsules; 250 mg, 500 mg, 1, 2, 4 gm vials for injection; 1, 2, 4 gm piggyback units and 250 mg/5 ml powder for oral solution.)

DRUG SPECIFICS:
   This is a penicillinase-resistant penicillin. It is used in the treatment of penicillinase-producing staphylococci. Also effective in the treatment of pneumococci or group A beta-hemolytic streptococci. Rare reversible hepatocellular dysfunction has been reported. Monitor liver function. Increased dosages in neonates and infants have produced transient hematuria, albuminuria or azotemia.

ADMINISTRATION AND DOSAGE SPECIFICS:
   Adults: 500-1000 mg po every 4-6 hours for 5 days, or 250 mg-1 gm IM every 4-6 hours.
   Children: 50-100 mg/kg/day po in divided doses every 6 hours for 5 days; or 50-100 mg/kg/day parenterally in 4 divided doses.

PENICILLIN G BENZATHINE

PRODUCTS (TRADE NAME):
   Bicillin (Available in 200,000 U tablets.) **Bicillin L-A** (Available in 300,000 U, 600,000 U, 900,000 U, 1.2 million U, 2.4 million U. for parenteral use.) **Permapen** (Available in 1,200,000 U/dose for injection.)

DRUG SPECIFICS:
   Long-acting IM penicillin. In children administer parenterally in midlateral aspect of thigh. Vary injection site. In adults give IM in gluteal muscle. Aspirate before injection.
   Oral dosage exhibits poor oral absorption and is not recommended for routine use.

ADMINISTRATION AND DOSAGE SPECIFICS:
   Oral dosages: 400,000 to 600,000 units po every 4-6 hours.

Parenteral dosages:
Prophylaxis for Rheumatic Fever: 1.2 million units IM twice a month on a continuous basis.
Streptococcal Upper Respiratory Tract Infection, Skin and Soft Tissue Infection, Scarlet Fever, Erysipelas:
Adults: 2.4 million units IM.
Children 30-60 lbs: 900,000 to 1.2 million units IM.
Children Under 30 lbs: 600,000 units IM.
Yaws, Pinta, Bejel: 1.2 million units IM.
Syphilis: Early: 2.4 million units IM. Latent: 2.4 million units IM once a week for 3 weeks. Congenital: 50,000 units/kg IM.

PENICILLIN G POTASSIUM OR SODIUM (AQUEOUS)

PRODUCTS (TRADE NAME):
Penicillin G Potassium (Available as 200,000 U; 500,000 U; 10,000,000 and 20,000,000 U for injection; 200,000 U, 250,000 U, 400,000 U, 500,000 U. tablets and 250,000 and 400,000 units/5 ml oral suspension.) **Penicillin G Sodium** (Available in 5,000,000 Units for injection.) **Pentids** (Available in 200,000 U, 250,000 U, 400,000 U. and 800,000 U oral tablets; and 200,000 and 400,000 U/5 ml oral suspension.) **Pfizerpen** (Available in 1,000,000 units and 5,000,000 units for injection; and 200,000 U, 250,000 U, 400,000 U, and 800,000 U tablets.)

DRUG SPECIFICS:
Give IM injections deeply, slowly and steadily to prevent needle blockage. Aspiration before injection. Hyperkalemia may develop with large doses. Observe for convulsions, hyperreflexia, or coma. In large doses or extended therapy, monitor renal, cardiovascular and electrolyte function.

ADMINISTRATION AND DOSAGE SPECIFICS:
Adults: 300,000-8 million units/day IM.
Pediatrics: 300,000-1,200,000 units/day IM.
Premature and Infants: 300,000 units/kg/day in two divided doses.

PENICILLIN G PROCAINE OR AQUEOUS (APPG)

PRODUCTS (TRADE NAME):
Crystallicin 300 A.S. (Available in 300,000 and 500,000 U/ml for injection.) **Duracillin A.S.** (Available in 300,000 U/ml for injection.) **Pfizerpen A.S.** (Available in 300,000 and 600,000 U/ml for injection.) **Wycillin** (Available as 300,000, 600,000, and 1,200,000 U/ml for injection.)

DRUG SPECIFICS:

Contains procaine to retard release. Determine if patient is allergic to procaine. Give deep IM in gluteal muscle. Aspirate before injection. Vary injection site.

See latest CDC recommended treatment schedules for disseminated gonorrhea and syphilis dosages. Give with 1 gram probenecid for treatment of gonorrhea. Probenecid not recommended in blood dyscrasia, uric acid kidney stones, or acute gout. This is the drug of choice for gonorrhea. Test cure by repeating smear (gram stain smear for men, endocervical and anal canal cultures for women) approximately 7 to 14 days after therapy. In men, if urethral discharge persists for 3 or more days following initial treatment, follow initial treatment with another 4.8 million units. In women, if cultures remain positive, follow with 4.8 million units daily on 2 successive days.

ADMINISTRATION AND DOSAGE SPECIFICS:

Pneumonia (pneumococcal): 600,000-1,200,000 units/day IM.

Bacterial endocarditis (group A beta-hemolytic streptococci): 600,000-1,200,000 units/day.

Prophylaxis against bacterial endocarditis: 1,000,000 units Penicillin G with 600,000 units APPG IM 30-60 minutes before surgical or dental procedures, then 500 mg Penicillin V every 6 hours for 8 doses.

Sexually Transmitted Diseases:

Acute pelvic inflammatory disease: 4.8 million units IM (in 2 sites), with 1 gm probenecid, followed by 100 mg oral doxycycline, twice a day, for 10 to 14 days.

Uncomplicated gonococcal infections in adults: 4.8 million units IM (in 2 sites), with 1 gm probenecid orally.

Pharyngeal, urethral and anorectal gonococcal infections: 4.8 million units IM, with 1 gm oral probenecid concurrently.

Syphilis: Primary, secondary or tertiary with negative cerebrospinal fluid 600,000 units/day IM for 8 days. Not the drug of choice.

Diphtheria 300,000 to 600-000 units/day IM with antitoxin.

Anthrax: 600,000 to 1,200,000 units/day IM.

Vincent's infection: 600,000 to 1,200,000 units/day IM.

Erysipeloid: 600,000 to 1,200,000 units/day IM.

PENICILLIN V (PHENOXYMETHYL PENICILLIN)

PRODUCTS (TRADE NAME):

Penicillin V (Available in 125, 250 and 500 mg tablets and 125 mg/5 ml and 250 mg/5 ml oral solution.) suspension.) 125 mg = 200,000 units.

DRUG SPECIFICS:

Stable in gastric juices. However, blood levels are higher when administered on an empty stomach. An increased number of penicillin V resistant staphylococcal strains have been reported. Observe for therapeutic effect of the drug.

ADMINISTRATION AND DOSAGE SPECIFICS:
Streptococcal, Scarlet Fever Infection, Erysipelas: 200,000 to 400,000 units po every 6-8 hours for 10 days.

Pneumococcal Infection: 400,000 to 600,000 units every 6 hours until afebrile for 2 days.

Staphylococcal Infection and Fusospirochetosis: 400,000 to 800,000 units po every 6-8 hours.

Prophylaxis for Rheumatic Fever/Chorea: 200,000 to 250,000 units po twice a day continuously.

PENICILLIN V POTASSIUM

PRODUCTS (TRADE NAME):
Beepen-VK, Betapen-VK, Deltapen VK, Detapen-VK, Ledercillin VK, Penapar VK, Pfizerpen VK, Repen-VK, Robicillin VK, SK-Penicillin VK, Uticillin VK, Veetids (Available as 250, 500 mg tablets, and 125 mg/5 ml and 250 mg/5 ml powder for oral suspension.) **Penicillin VK** (Available in 250 and 500 mg tablets; 125 and 250 mg/5 ml oral solution.) **Pen-Vee K, V-Cillin K** (Available in 125 mg tablet and 250 mg/5 ml oral solution).
DRUG SPECIFICS:
Used in the treatment of mild to moderately severe infections when patient can take an oral dosage.
ADMINISTRATION AND DOSAGE SPECIFICS:
Adults: 250-500 mg po 3-4 times a day.
Children: 15-50 mg/kg/day in 3-6 divided doses.

PIPERACILLIN SODIUM

PRODUCTS (TRADE NAME):
Pipracil (Available in 2, 3 and 4 gm powder for injection.)
DRUG SPECIFICS:
Piperacillin is a relatively new extended spectrum product which is effective against a wide number of gram-positive and gram-negative aerobic and anaerobic bacteria. It is often used in the treatment of mixed infections or when treatment is required before the causative organism is identified. It may be possible to use this product alone, when normally two antibiotics might be administered. It has been found useful as concurrent therapy with aminoglycosides although they should not both be mixed in the same syringe. It is used frequently in treatment of gynecological infections including uncomplicated gonococcal urethritis, streptococcal infections,

lower respiratory infections, skin, bone, joint, and urinary tract infections. Preparation may be given IM or IV. Patients with impaired renal function require lower doses.

ADMINISTRATION AND DOSAGE SPECIFICS:
Urinary tract infections, pneumonia: 6 to 16 gm/day IV divided into 4 to 6 doses.
Uncomplicated gonorrhea infections: 2 gm IM single dose.
Complicated or serious infections: 12 to 18 gm/day IV divided into 4 to 6 doses.

TICARCILLIN DISODIUM

PRODUCTS (TRADE NAME):
Ticar (Available as 1, 3, 6 gm vials for injection; 3 gm piggyback units.)
DRUG SPECIFICS:
This is an extended-spectrum penicillin. It is effective against the following susceptible organisms: *E. coli, Enterobacter, Proteus, Pseudomonas aeruginosa, Streptococcus faecalis.*
ADMINISTRATION AND DOSAGE SPECIFICS:
Uncomplicated Urinary Tract Infection:
Adults: 1 gm IM or IV every 6 hours.
Children: 50-100 mg/kg/day IM or IV in divided doses every 6-8 hours.
Complicated Urinary Tract Infections:
150-200 mg/kg/day IV in divided doses every 4-6 hours.
Systemic Septicemia, Respiratory Tract Infection, Soft Tissue Infection:
200-300 mg/kg/day in three, four, or six divided doses.

Joann Sabados-Carolina

POLYMYXIN B SULFATE

ACTION OF THE DRUG: A bactericidal drug that alters the lipoprotein cell membrane.

ASSESSMENT:

INDICATIONS: Drug choice is dependent on the identification of the infectious organism by appropriate cultures or smears, or based on the clinical picture. Ideally, the patient should be hospitalized to monitor the nephrotoxic effects of the drug. This is a drug that is not often prescribed by non-physicians; however, they may frequently have responsibility for monitoring a patient receiving this therapy. Polymyxin B sulfate is effective against all the gram-negative organisms with the exception of *Proteus*. It is also effective in the treatment of acute infections due to susceptible strains of *Pseudomonas aeruginosa, Haemophilus influenzae, E. coli, Enterobacter aerogenes, Klebsiella pneumoniae.* Rarely a first-choice drug.

SUBJECTIVE-OBJECTIVE: The patient in need of antibiotic therapy may present in any number of ways, ranging from asymptomatic to severely ill. Keep in mind common infectious indicators such as fever, inflammation, erythema, edema or pain.

PLAN:

CONTRAINDICATIONS: Hypersensitivity to polymyxins.

WARNINGS: Intramuscular or intrathecal administration should only be given to hospitalized patients. Do not exceed 25,000 units/kg/day. Nephrotoxicity may develop with administration and may be evidenced by proteinuria, cellular urinary casts, azotemia, decreased output, elevated BUN. Neurotoxicity may be evidenced by irritability, weakness, drowsiness, ataxia, perioral paresthesias, numbness of extremities or blurring of vision. Neurotoxicity has resulted in respiratory paralysis. Discretion should be used during treatment in pregnant and nursing mothers since the drug crosses the placental barrier and is secreted in breast milk.

PRECAUTIONS: Renal function should be monitored during treatment. Superinfection may occur.

IMPLEMENTATION:

DRUG INTERACTIONS: Concurrent use with nephrotoxic or neurotoxic drugs may produce additive toxic effects. Avoid concurrent use with anesthetics, neuromuscular blocking agents or drugs with neuromuscular blocking activities since they may produce an additive effect. May alter laboratory values in the following manner: increased serum levels of BUN and creatinine, increased casts and red blood cells in the urine, increased albuminuria.

PRODUCTS (TRADE NAME):

Aerosporin, Polymyxin B Sulfate (Available in 500,000 U/vial for injection, 500,000 U/vial ophthalmic drops and 10,000 U/ml otic drops).

ADMINISTRATION AND DOSAGE: Do not exceed 25,000 units/kg/day. IM administration not recommended because of severe pain at injection site.

Adults and children: 15,000 to 20,000 units/kg/day IV in two divided doses.

Neonates: 40,000 units/kg/day IV.

Intrathecal, adults and children: 50,000 units every day for 3-4 days. Continue with 50,000 units every day for 2 weeks after cerebrospinal cultures are negative.

Intrathecal, under 2 years: 20,000 units every day for 3-4 days, then continue with a dose of 25,000 units every other day for 2 weeks after the cultures are negative.

IMPLEMENTATION CONSIDERATIONS:

—Obtain a thorough health history: renal impairment, hypersensitivity to polymyxin, other medications which may cause drug interactions, pregnancy, breastfeeding.

—Notify anesthesiologist that patient is taking this drug before surgery.

—Force fluids to ensure minimum output is 1,500 cc. This will decrease chances of renal toxicity.

—Drug may alter laboratory tests, including those which may indicate nephrotoxicity.

WHAT THE PATIENT NEEDS TO KNOW:

—Notify your health provider if you notice any decreases in the amount of your urine.

—Some patients taking this drug experience side effects. Be certain to notify your practitioner if you notice any new or discomforting symptoms. Watch especially for dizziness, numbness or tingling.

—Drink at least 2 quarts of water daily while you are taking this medicine.

EVALUATION:

ADVERSE REACTIONS: *CNS:* dizziness, drowsiness, paresthesia, facial flushing, meningeal irritation with intrathecal administration. *Renal:* proteinuria, azotemia, cylindruria, rising blood levels without an increase in drug dose. *Other:* drug fever, urticaria, rash, respiratory arrest, pain at IM injection site, thrombophlebitis at IV infusion site.

PARAMETERS TO MONITOR: Monitor therapeutic effect of drug. Obtain baseline renal function studies and continue to follow throughout therapy. Monitor urinary output. Observe for signs and symptoms of nephrotoxicity or neurotoxicity.

Joann Sabados-Carolina

SPECTINOMYCIN

ACTION OF THE DRUG: Spectinomycin is a bacteriostatic drug that inhibits ribosomal protein synthesis.

ASSESSMENT:

INDICATIONS: Drug choice is dependent on the identification of the infectious organisms by appropriate cultures or smears, or based on the clinical picture. Spectinomycin is a narrow-spectrum drug that is the drug of choice in the treatment of gonorrhea in patients hypersensitive to the penicillins, and in the treatment of penicillinase-producing gonorrhea.

SUBJECTIVE-OBJECTIVE: The patient in need of antibiotic therapy may present in any number of ways, ranging from asymptomatic to severely ill. Keep in mind common infectious indicators such as fever, inflammation, erythema, edema or pain.

PLAN:

CONTRAINDICATIONS: Hypersensitivity to spectinomycin.

WARNINGS: This drug is not effective in the treatment of syphilis. It may also mask the signs of syphilis. Discretion should be used during treatment in pregnant and nursing mothers since the drug crosses the placental barrier and is secreted in breast milk.

PRECAUTIONS: Use with caution in individuals with a history of multiple allergies.

IMPLEMENTATION:

DRUG INTERACTIONS: None reported. May alter laboratory tests in the following manner: increased serum alkaline phosphatase, increased SGOT, and increased BUN with multiple doses. Also a decrease in hemoglobin, hematocrit and creatinine clearance has been reported with multiple doses.

PRODUCTS (TRADE NAME):
Trobicin (Available as 400 mg/ml in 2 and 4 gm vial for injection.)

ADMINISTRATION AND DOSAGE:
Adults: 2 gm as a single dose IM. For antibiotic resistance: 4 gm IM divided between two injection sites. Disseminated gonococcal infections: 2 gm IM twice a day for 3 days.

IMPLEMENTATION CONSIDERATIONS:

—Obtain a complete health history: prior hypersensitivity to spectinomycin; pregnancy or breast feeding.

—Obtain dark-field examination for syphilis of any lesions present before therapy is initiated. Obtain syphilis serology prior to initiation of therapy, and once a month for 3 months. Treat infected partners.

—In treatment of gonorrhea, treat all sexual partners.

—Administer IM deep in the upper outer quadrant of gluteal muscle.

WHAT THE PATIENT NEEDS TO KNOW:

—If therapy is for gonorrhea, do not have sex until treatment is completed. Inform sexual partners of their need for treatment. Repeat blood tests for syphilis are indicated once a month for three months.

EVALUATION:

ADVERSE REACTIONS: *CNS:* dizziness. *Gastrointestinal:* nausea. *Hypersensitivity:* urticaria, fever, chills. *Other:* insomnia, pain at injection site.

PARAMETERS TO MONITOR: Look primarily for evidence of therapeutic effect of drug. Obtain follow-up cultures 1-2 weeks after therapy. Monitor for strains of *Neisseria gonorrhoeae* resistant to spectinomycin.

Joann Sabados-Carolina

TETRACYCLINES

ACTION OF THE DRUG: Tetracyclines are bacteriostatic drugs which inhibit ribosomal protein synthesis.

ASSESSMENT:

INDICATIONS: Tetracyclines are broad-spectrum antibiotics effective in the treatment of a wide variety of organisms. They are the drugs of choice in the following infections: granuloma inguinale, rickettsial diseases, Mycoplasma infections, spirochetal relapsing fever and chlamydia. They are indicated in patients sensitive to penicillin, especially in the treatment of gonorrhea or syphilis. Drug choice is dependent on the identification of the infectious organism by appropriate cultures or smears, or based on the clinical picture.

SUBJECTIVE-OBJECTIVE: The patient in need of antibiotic therapy may present in any number of ways, ranging from asymptomatic to severely ill. Keep in mind common infectious indicators such as fever, inflammation, erythema, edema or pain.

PLAN:

CONTRAINDICATIONS: Hypersensitivity to any of the tetracyclines.

WARNINGS: Discretion should be used during treatment in pregnant and nursing mothers since the drugs cross the placental barrier and are secreted in breast milk. Use of the drugs in pregnancy and in children under 8 years of age may produce tooth discoloration, or inadequate bone or tooth development. Extreme caution should be used in the administration of the drug to patients with impaired renal function. Do not exceed 2 grams in patients with impaired renal function. It may also exacerbate systemic lupus erythematosus. Photosensitivity may occur with treatment. Avoid exposure to the sun or ultraviolet rays.

PRECAUTIONS: Hypersensitivity reactions ranging from mild erythema to anaphylaxis have been reported with use of these drugs. Vertigo may develop with any of the tetracyclines; however, vertigo is more prominent with the use of minocycline. Superinfection may occur with extended therapy. An antianabolic effect has resulted in elevated BUN levels. Use of outdated medicine may lead to damage of the proximal renal tubules. Use with caution in patients with hepatic impairment, since these drugs may cause hepatotoxicity. Determine if the patient is alcoholic.

IMPLEMENTATION:

DRUG INTERACTIONS: Concurrent use of a tetracycline with antacids containing divalent or trivalent cations will impair absorption of the drug. Concurrent use with food, milk, dairy products, or iron preparations may also impair absorption. Concurrent use of oral anticoagulants and a tetracycline may produce an antagonistic effect and downward adjustment of anticoagulant dose may be indicated. Tetracyclines increase the bioavailability of digoxin which could lead to digitalis toxicity. This effect may occur for months after tetracycline is discontinued. Tetracyclines will interfere with the bactericidal action of penicillin. They may alter the following laboratory tests: increased values for SGPT, alkaline phosphatase, SGOT, bilirubin, BUN, creatinine, and proteinuria. May cause a false-positive Coombs' test, may decrease hemoglobin and platelet count, and may alter serum or urine glucose and cerebrospinal fluid protein levels.

ADMINISTRATION AND DOSAGE: May be administered through oral or parenteral route. Avoid topical application to prevent sensitization. Usual doses are as follows:

Oral:
Adults: 1-4 grams/day in 2 or 4 equal doses;
Pediatric: 10-20 mg/day in 4 divided doses.
Parenteral:
Adults: 250-500 mg/day IM or IV.
Pediatric: 15-25 mg/kg/day IM; 12 mg/kg/day IV.

IMPLEMENTATION CONSIDERATIONS:

—Obtain a thorough health history: prior renal damage, hepatic impairment, systemic lupus erythematosus, or alcoholism; medications which may interact with tetracycline; pregnancy or breast-feeding; age; occupation.

—Order baseline hematologic, renal and hepatic laboratory studies if long-term therapy is indicated.

—Be alert to the possibility of superinfection in the oral, vaginal or rectal areas.

—Use with discretion in the elderly.

—Advise patient to use care in driving or using machinery because of the possibility of vertigo.

—Always aspirate before IM injection to prevent medication from entering a blood vessel.

—In the treatment of syphilis, gonorrhea or chlamydial infections, infected partners must be treated also.

WHAT THE PATIENT NEEDS TO KNOW:

—Take medicine on an empty stomach, one hour before or two hours after eating. Follow with a full glass of water.

—If gastrointestinal upset occurs, take a few crackers with the medicine.

—Medicine should be taken exactly as prescribed. Do not stop taking medication when symptoms disappear. Do not save medication. Taking out of date medication may cause rather severe anal irritation.

—Do not use medicine after the date shown on the label.

—Stay out of the sun or ultraviolet light. Sunblockers will not help.

—Use care in bathing and brushing teeth. Watch for signs of infection in mouth, anal or vaginal areas.

—Notify practitioner if diarrhea persists for more than 24 hours.

—Do not take this drug with any iron preparations, antacids, milk or dairy products.

—Watch for dizziness. If it develops it may be severe enough to limit driving or operating machinery.

—Keep medication in light-resistant containers.
—Drug may change the urine glucose test (if you are a diabetic).
—If treatment is for a sexually transmitted disease, do not have sexual activity during the time you take this drug. Your partner needs to be treated also.

EVALUATION:

ADVERSE REACTIONS: *CNS:* ataxia, dizziness, bulging fontanels (infants), increased intracranial pressure, vestibular disturbances. *Dermatologic:* exfolative dermatitis (rare), maculopapular anderythematous rashes, onycholysis and nail discoloration, photosensitivity. *Gastrointestinal:* abdominal discomfort, anorexia, black hairy tongue, epigastric burning, esophageal ulcers, diarrhea with bulky loose stools (if longer than 24 hours must differentiate from superinfection), enterocolitis, fatty liver, glossitis, hepatic toxicity (dose related, increased BUN), nausea, pancreatitis, stomatitis, tooth discoloration, vomiting. *Hematopoietic:* hemolytic anemia, eosinophilia, leukocytosis, leukopenia, neutropenia, thrombocytopenia. *Hypersensitivity:* anaphylaxis, angioedema, fever, pruritus, photosensitivity, serum sickness-like reactions with fever, rash and arthralgia, urticaria. *Other:* benign intracranial edema (vomiting, headache, sixth nerve palsy), diabetes insipidus syndrome, local irritation with IM injection.

OVERDOSAGE: May experience nausea, vomiting, diarrhea, or acute liver damage (rare.)

PARAMETERS TO MONITOR: Obtain baseline blood, renal and hepatic studies if prolonged treatment is indicated, or in patients with renal or hepatic impairment. Continue studies periodically through therapy. In extended therapy, monitor pregnancy status in the reproductive female. Observe for superinfection. Monitor for renal damage: decreased output, proteinuria, increased BUN, increased creatinine. Monitor for hepatic damage: jaundice, abdominal pain, weakness, nausea, vomiting, dark urine, pale stools. Develop a flow sheet to assist in recording therapeutic effects of the drug as well as side effects.

DEMECLOCYCLINE HCL

PRODUCTS (TRADE NAME):
Declomycin (Available in 150 and 300 mg tablets; 150 mg capsules.)
DRUG SPECIFICS:
Most frequently associated with photosensitivity and anaphylactoid reactions. Diabetes insipidus syndrome has been shown with long-term therapy. It is dose dependent and reversible when the drug is discontinued.

ADMINISTRATION AND DOSAGE SPECIFICS:
Adults: 150 mg po four times a day or 300 mg po twice a day.
Children over 8 years: 3-6 mg/lb/day po in 2 or 4 divided doses.

DOXYCYCLINE

PRODUCTS (TRADE NAME):
Doxy-Caps, Doxycycline, Doxycycline Hyclate, Vibramycin (Available as 50, 100 mg capsules, 25 mg/ 5 ml oral suspension; 50 mg/5 ml oral syrup and 100 mg,200 mg/vial for injections.) **Vibra Tabs** (Available in 100 mg tablets.)
DRUG SPECIFICS:
Kidney excretion is not as great as with other tetracyclines. It has been used in the prevention of traveler's diarrhea. It may be taken with food. See latest CDC recommended treatment schedules for sexually transmitted disease dosages.
ADMINISTRATION AND DOSAGE SPECIFICS:
Adult: 200 mg po in two divided doses for the first day. Follow with 100 mg/day in two divided doses or as a single dose.
Children over 8 years: 2 mg/lb/day in two divided doses for the first day. Follow with 1 mg/lb/day in two divided doses or as a single dose.

METHACYCLINE HCL

PRODUCTS (TRADE NAME):
Rondomycin (Available as 150, 300 mg capsules.)
DRUG SPECIFICS:
Derivative of oxytetracycline.
ADMINISTRATION AND DOSAGE SPECIFICS:
Adults: 150 mg po four times a day.
Children over 8 years: 3-6 mg/lb/day in two or four divided doses.

MINOCYCLINE

HCL PRODUCTS (TRADE NAME):
Minocin (Available as 50, 100 mg capsules or tablets; 100 mg/vial for IV injection and 50 mg/5 ml oral suspension.)
DRUG SPECIFICS:
Has delayed kidney excretion compared to other tetracyclines. Half-life is 11-20 hours.

ADMINISTRATION AND DOSAGE SPECIFICS:

Adult: 200 mg po initially. Follow with 100 mg every 12 hours.

Children over 8 years: Initial dose 4 mg/kg. Follow with 2 mg/kg every 12 hours.

OXYTETRACYCLINE

PRODUCTS (TRADE NAME):

E.P. Mycin (Available in 250 mg capsules.) **Oxymycin** (Available in 50 mg/ml injection with lidocaine.) **Oxytetracycline** (Available in 250 mg capsule.) **Terramycin** (Available in 250 mg tablets, 125, 250 mg capsules, 5 mg/gm ophthalmic and otic ointment, 50 and 125 mg/vial for IM injection, 250 and 500 mg/vial for IV injection, 125 mg/5 ml syrup and 100 mg vaginal tablets.) **UriTet** (Available in 250 mg capsule).

DRUG SPECIFICS:

Diarrhea is more common with this preparation than with other tetracyclines. Administer parenteral form deep IM in gluteal muscle mass. Aspirate before injection of medicine to determine needle location. If pain persists after injection, ice may be applied to the area. Avoid rapid IV administration.

ADMINISTRATION AND DOSAGE SPECIFICS:

Adults: 1-2 gram/day po; 100-250 mg IM every 12 hours; 100-250 mg IV every 12 hours. Do not exceed dose of 500 mg every 6 hours.

Children over 8 years: 10-20 mg/lb/day po in four divided doses; 15-25 mg/kg/day in two or three divided doses IM; 10-20 mg/kg/day in two doses IV.

TETRACYCLINE HCL

PRODUCTS (TRADE NAME):

Achromycin V, Cycline, Cyclopar, Deltamycin, Nor-Tet, Panmycin, Re-Tet, Robitet, SK-Tetracycline, Sumycin, Tetrachel, Tetracyn, Tetracycline HCl, Tetralan, Tetram (Available in 250, 500 mg tablets, 100, 250, 500 mg capsules, 125 mg/5 ml syrup, 30 mg/gm ointment, 10 mg/gm ophthalmic ointment, 100 and 250 mg/vial for IM use; 250 or 500 mg/vial for IV use.)

DRUG SPECIFICS:

Shake oral suspension well. Do not use past date on label.

For parenteral form, serum half-life is 6-10 hours. Administer deep into gluteal muscle. Aspirate before injection of medicine to determine location of needle. If pain persists after injection, ice may be applied to the area. Avoid rapid IV administration. Some products contain procaine. Determine hypersensitivity to this, and monitor for adverse reactions.

ADMINISTRATION AND DOSAGE SPECIFICS:
Adults: 1-4 gram/day po; 250-500 mg/day or 300 mg in divided doses every 8-12 hours IV or IM. Do not exceed 500 mg every 6 hours.
Children over 8 years: 10-20 mg/lb/day po; or 12 mg/kg/day in two divided doses IM or IV.

TETRACYCLINE HCL AND AMPHOTERICIN B

PRODUCTS (TRADE NAME):
Mysteclin-F (Available in 250 mg tetracycline HCl and 50 mg amphotericin B capsules, and 125 mg tetracycline HCl and 25 mg amphotericin B/5 ml syrup.)
DRUG SPECIFICS:
This product combines the broad-spectrum antibiotic tetracycline with an antifungal antibiotic. There is no evidence of effectiveness for this product. It is ordered when tetracycline is desired for patients susceptible to candidal superinfections.
ADMINISTRATION AND DOSAGE SPECIFICS:
Adults: Usual dose is 500 mg four times daily.

TETRACYCLINE AND NYSTATIN

PRODUCTS (TRADE NAME):
Achrostatin V (Available in 250 tetracycline HCl and 250,000 units nystatin capsules.) **Declostatin** (Available in 150 mg demeclocycline HCl and 250,000 units nystatin capsules or 300 mg demeclocycline HCl and 500,000 units nystatin tablets.) **Terrastatin** (Available in 250 mg oxytetracycline and 250,000 units nystatin capsules.) **Tetrastatin** (Available in 250 mg tetracycline HCl and 250,000 units nystatin capsules.)
DRUG SPECIFICS:
These products are tetracycline-nystatin combinations which are used to prevent candidal superinfections of the gastrointestinal tract. There is no evidence of effectiveness for these combinations.
ADMINISTRATION AND DOSAGE SPECIFICS:
Adults: Usual dose is 500 mg four times a day.

TETRACYCLINE PHOSPHATE COMPLEX

PRODUCTS (TRADE NAME):
Tetrex (Available in 250 mg capsules.) **Tetrex bidCAPS** (Available in 500 mg capsules.)

NURSING ACTIONS AND SPECIFICS
Store in light-resistant closed container.
ADMINISTRATION AND DOSAGE SPECIFICS:
Adults: 1-4 gram/day po.
Children over 8 years: 10-20 mg/lb/day po.

Joann Sabados-Carolina

VANCOMYCIN

ACTION OF THE DRUG: Vancomycin is a bactericidal drug that inhibits mucopeptide cell wall synthesis.

ASSESSMENT:

INDICATIONS: Drug choice is dependent on the identification of the infectious organism by appropriate cultures or smears, or based on the clinical picture. The drug is often used in severe infections in patients hypersensitive to the penicillins or cephalosporins. It is effective in the treatment of staphylococcal endocarditis, osteomyelitis, pneumonia, soft tissue infections and methicillin-resistant staphylococci. Oral dosage is effective in the treatment of staphylococcal enterocolitis.

SUBJECTIVE-OBJECTIVE: The patient in need of antibiotic therapy may present in any number of ways, ranging from asymptomatic to severely ill. Keep in mind common infectious indicators such as fever, inflammation, erythema, edema or pain.

PLAN:

CONTRAINDICATIONS: Hypersensitivity to vancomycin.
WARNINGS: Nephrotoxicity has been reported with vancomycin, and the toxic effect is increased in high serum levels or prolonged therapy. Avoid use in patients with impaired renal function. Dosage must be altered in the elderly due to the normal decline in renal function. Ototoxicity may occur with renal impairment. Watch for tinnitus which may precede deafness. Avoid use in patients with prior auditory loss. Discretion should be used during treatment in pregnant and nursing mothers since the drug crosses the placental barrier and is secreted in breast milk.
PRECAUTIONS: Vancomycin should be administered by IV, not IM, route. IM injection will cause tissue necrosis. Rapid IV administration may cause hypotension. Dilute solution in 200 ml of glucose or saline solution and infuse over a 30 minute period. IV infusion may cause thrombophlebitis. Rotate infusion sites. Superinfection may occur with treatment.

IMPLEMENTATION:

DRUG INTERACTIONS: Avoid concurrent use with other nephrotoxic or ototoxic drugs such as cephaloridine, colistin, ethacrynic acid, furosemide, gentamicin, kanamycin, paromomycin, polymyxin B, streptomycin, tobramycin, viomycin. Bacteriostatic antibiotics may antagonize the bactericidal effect. Dimehydrinate may mask the ototoxic effect. Vancomycin may enhance the action of oral anticoagulants. Vancomycin may alter laboratory tests in the following manner: increases urine protein or serum urea nitrogen.

PRODUCTS (TRADE NAME):

Vancocin (Available as 500 mg/10 ml vial for injection, 10 gm/powder for oral solution.)

ADMINISTRATION AND DOSAGE: Not to be administered IM.

Adults: 500 mg every 6 hours or 1 gm every 12 hours po or IV. Dose must be altered in renal impairment.

Children: 20 mg/lb/day po in divided doses; 44 mg/kg/day IV in divided doses.

IMPLEMENTATION CONSIDERATIONS:

—Obtain a thorough health history: previous history of renal impairment or auditory damage; drug hypersensitivity; medications which may cause drug interactions; pregnancy or breast-feeding.

—Be alert to possible alterations in laboratory values caused by the medication.

—Obtain baseline kidney function studies. Repeat these periodically with long-term therapy.

—Document hearing function at beginning of therapy. Monitor any changes in hearing closely.

WHAT THE PATIENT NEEDS TO KNOW:

—Take medicine exactly as prescribed. Do not stop medication when you begin to feel better. Do not save medication.

—Notify practitioner if your urine output becomes low or, if you have decreased hearing or ringing in your ears.

—This drug has been associated with side effects in some people so notify your health provider if you experience any new or uncomfortable symptoms.

—Bathe daily and brush teeth regularly. Observe mouth, anal and vaginal areas for any signs of infection.

EVALUATION:

ADVERSE REACTIONS: *Gastrointestinal:* nausea, vomiting. *Hypersensitivity:* chills, fever, eosinophilia, rash, anaphylaxis. *Other:* nephrotoxicity, ototoxicity, superinfection, pain and thrombophlebitis at the infusion site.

PARAMETERS TO MONITOR: Obtain baseline studies of renal and auditory function in patients, particularly those to be on long-term therapy, those who have a previous history of difficulty, or those who are over 60 years old. Perform periodic renal, auditory and vancomycin serum levels. Monitor hematologic, liver and renal function in all patients. Observe patient for signs and symptoms of therapeutic effect, adverse reactions and superinfection.

Joann Sabados-Carolina

ANTIFUNGALS

FLUCYTOSINE

ACTION OF THE DRUG: Flucytosine (5-FC; 5-Fluorocytosine) is a synthetic, fluorinated antifungal agent with fungistatic activity. The antifungal activity is evident when 5-FC is converted to 5-fluorouracil in the fungal cell, thereby competitively inhibiting nucleic acid synthesis. Flucytosine acts as a fungicidal agent when used in high dosages.

ASSESSMENT:

INDICATIONS: Used in the treatment of serious systemic fungal infections caused by susceptible strains of *Candida* and *Cryptococcus*. May cause septicemia, endocarditis, UTI, meningitis, and pulmonary infections.

SUBJECTIVE: History of multiple scaly or blistered red patches on the skin; pruritus, soreness of involved areas. Also, history, temperature, pain, or other symptoms of serious systemic disease.

OBJECTIVE: Multiple scaly or blistered erythematous patches on the skin; brittle nails with yellow discoloration and separation from nail bed; evidence of spores and hyphae with KOH microscopic examination of scrapings from involved areas. May find elevated temperature, murmurs, or pain in specific organ systems suggesting infection.

PLAN:

CONTRAINDICATIONS: Hypersensitivity to flucytosine.

WARNINGS: Administer the drug with extreme caution in those patients with impaired renal function or bone marrow depression. Do not use during pregnancy unless absolutely necessary.

PRECAUTIONS: Adequate serum levels of flucytosine must be maintained to avoid the development of resistant strains of *Candida* and *Cryptococcus*.

IMPLEMENTATION:

DRUG INTERACTIONS: Although therapeutic effect is enhanced by concomitant use of flucytosine and amphotericin B, toxicity is increased. Toxicity can also result from concurrent use of other drugs that depress bone marrow or use during radiation therapy. Avoid concomitant use with hepatotoxic or nephrotoxic drugs. Use of flucytosine can result in increased serum levels of alkaline phosphatase, bilirubin, BUN, creatinine, SGPT, and SGOT. Use also decreases leukocyte and platelet counts and hemoglobin levels.

PRODUCTS (TRADE NAME):
Ancobon (Available in 250 mg, 500 mg capsule.)

ADMINISTRATION AND DOSAGE:
Adults and children: 50-150 mg/kg daily in divided doses at 6-hour intervals.

IMPLEMENTATION CONSIDERATIONS:
—Take a thorough health history. Determine if impaired renal or bone marrow function exists; whether patient is pregnant; previous allergies, especially to flucytosine; and whether patient is taking other drugs that might interact with flucytosine.

—Order baseline renal, hepatic and hematologic studies.

—Inform patient about possible side effects.

—Reduce dosage in patients with decreased renal function.

WHAT THE PATIENT NEEDS TO KNOW:

—If skin rash occurs or if nausea, vomiting or diarrhea become pronounced, notify health provider.

—To avoid or reduce nausea and vomiting, administer the capsules several at a time over a period of 15 minutes.

—If fungal symptoms do not resolve within 2-3 days, notify health provider.

—Take medication as ordered. Do not stop taking medication just because symptoms resolve or you feel better.

EVALUATION:

ADVERSE REACTIONS: *CNS:* headache, drowsiness, confusion, vertigo, hallucinations. *Dermatologic:* macular rash, urticaria. *Gastrointestinal:* nausea, vomiting, diarrhea, ulcerative colitis. *Hematologic:* anemia, neutropenia, leukopenia, eosinophilia, thrombocytopenia, abnormal liver function tests.

PARAMETERS TO MONITOR: Prior to initiating therapy, perform a sensitivity test to determine susceptibility of the organism. Repeat the test periodically to determine if drug resistance has developed. Certain blood tests (complete blood count, hepatic and renal function tests) should be done initially and periodically if patient is on long-term therapy. Observe for signs and symptoms of bone marrow depression, nephrotoxicity, and hepatotoxicity.

Barbara Sommer Wieferich

GRISEOFULVIN

ACTION OF THE DRUG: Griseofulvin is a fungistatic or fungicidal antibiotic derived from *Penicillium griseofulvum*. It acts by being deposited in keratin precursor cells, where it becomes tightly bound, leaving new keratin cells highly resistant to fungal infection as exfoliation occurs.

ASSESSMENT:

INDICATIONS: Used for the treatment of fungal infections involving the hair, skin, and nails due to susceptible species of *Epidermophyton, Microsporum,* and *Trichophyton.*

SUBJECTIVE: History of multiple scaly or blistered red patches on the skin; pruritus, soreness of involved areas.

OBJECTIVE: Multiple scaly or blistered erythematous patches on the skin; brittle nails with yellow discoloration and separation from nail bed; evidence of spores and hyphae with KOH microscopic examination of scrapings from involved areas.

PLAN:

CONTRAINDICATIONS: Hypersensitivity to griseofulvin, history of porphyria or hepatocellular failure.

WARNINGS: Griseofulvin has not been established as safe for use during pregnancy. Avoid using the drug as prophylaxis against fungal infections. Animal studies have raised questions as to tumorigenicity of product which has not yet been resolved.

PRECAUTIONS: Cross-sensitivity is possible, although remote, among individuals allergic to penicillin. Photosensitivity reactions may occur with use. Exacerbation of lupus erythematosus may result from such a reaction. Because of possible adverse reactions, renal, hematologic, and hepatic evaluations should be made periodically.

IMPLEMENTATION:

DRUG INTERACTIONS: Oral warfarin-type anticoagulant activity is decreased when used concomitantly, necessitating dosage adjustment with griseofulvin use. Griseofulvin activity is decreased when used concurrently with barbiturates, requiring dosage adjustments of griseofulvin. Concomitant use of alcohol potentiates the effect of alcohol and produces skin flushing and tachycardia.

ADMINISTRATION AND DOSAGE: Since griseofulvin is absorbed over a long time period, single daily doses are often adequate. The patient must use the medication continuously until the causative organism has been eradicated, as evidenced by both clinical and laboratory examination. This process may require several weeks to many months of therapy, depending upon the causative organism and the site of infection. Concurrent use of topical antifungal agents may be required for the treatment of some fungal infections, primarily tinea pedis.

IMPLEMENTATION CONSIDERATIONS:

—Take a thorough health history: ascertain that patient is not pregnant, allergic to griseofulvin, or taking other drugs that may interact with griseofulvin.

—Absorption rate of griseofulvin is enhanced following a fatty meal.

WHAT THE PATIENT NEEDS TO KNOW:
—Therapy may need to continue for many weeks before laboratory and clinical tests indicate the infection is no longer present.
—Taking the medication with meals which are high in fat causes more of the medication to be absorbed.
—Sometimes people taking this drug develop photosensitivity, or an intolerance to the sun.
—Avoid alcoholic beverages while you are taking this medication.
—Notify provider if you develop sore throat, malaise, fever, skin rash, or other adverse reactions.
—Cleanliness of hair, skin and nails will aid in controlling and limiting the spread of infection.

EVALUATION:

ADVERSE REACTIONS: *CNS:* headache, vertigo, dizziness, syncope, fatigue, insomnia, depression, irritability, memory lapses, impaired judgment, confusion, peripheral neuritis. *Endocrine:* estrogen-type effect in genitals and breasts of children. *Gastrointestinal:* sore throat, nausea, vomiting, epigastric distress, dryness of mouth, oral thrush, black furry tongue, anorexia, diarrhea. *Hematologic:* leukopenia, neutropenia, granulocytopenia. *Hypersensitivity:* photosensitivity, rash, urticaria, angioneurotic edema. *Musculoskeletal:* arthralgia. *Opthalmic:* blurred vision. *Renal:* proteinuria. *Other:* fever, malaise, vaginal discharge, disturbed porphyrin metabolism.
OVERDOSAGE: *Signs and Symptoms:* nausea, vomiting, diarrhea
PARAMETERS TO MONITOR: Observe for therapeutic effect. Periodic renal, hepatic and hematologic laboratory evaluations are necessary, especially for those patients undergoing prolonged therapy. Observe for sore throat, fever, malaise, vaginal discharge, black furry tongue, and diarrhea. Continue medication until laboratory tests indicate infection is no longer present.

GRISEOFULVIN MICROSIZE

PRODUCTS (TRADE NAME):
Fulvicin-U/F (Available in 250 mg, 500 mg tablet). **Grifulvin V** (Available in 500 mg tablet; 125 mg/5ml suspension). **Grisactin** (Available in 125 mg, 250 mg capsule; 500 mg tablet). **Griseofulvin** (Available in 250 mg tablet).
DRUG SPECIFICS:
Divided dosages are recommended for those patients unable to tolerate single dosages.
ADMINISTRATION AND DOSAGE SPECIFICS:
Fungal Infection:
Adults: 500 mg/day/po in single or divided doses following meals.

Children: 13.5 to 23 kg; give 125 to 250 mg po more than 23 kg; give 250 to 500 mg po daily in single or divided doses following meals.

GRISEOFULVIN ULTRAMICROSIZE

PRODUCTS (TRADE NAME):
Fulvicin P/G (Available in 125, 165, 250 and 330 mg tablets.) **Grisactin Ultra** (Available in 125 and 250 mg tablet.) **Gris-PEG** (Available in 125 and 250 mg tablet.)
DRUG SPECIFICS:
Griseofulvin ultramicrosize has approximately 1.5 times the biological activity as griseofulvin microsize, with no advantage in effectiveness or safety.
ADMINISTRATION AND DOSAGE SPECIFICS:
Fungal Infections:
Adults: 250 mg/day in single or divided doses following meals.
Children: 5 mg/kg/day in single or divided doses following meals.

Barbara Sommer Wieferich

KETOCONAZOLE

ACTION OF THE DRUG: Ketoconazole is an imidazole broad-spectrum antibiotic with fungistatic or fungicidal activity. It acts by impairing synthesis of the main sterole of fungi cell membranes (ergosterole), thus producing leakage of cellular components by increased membrane permeability.

ASSESSMENT:

INDICATIONS: Ketoconazole is used in the treatment of systemic fungal infections such as chronic mucocutaneous candidiasis, oral thrush, candiduria, blastomycosis, paracoccidioidomycosis, coccidiodomycosis, histoplasmosis and chromomycosis. It has also been used in the treatment of pityriasis versicolor and vaginal candidiasis.
SUBJECTIVE: Patients may present with a history of fever and chills at onset of infection. Itching is frequently noted but may be associated with more systemic symptoms.
OBJECTIVE: Signs of systemic or vaginal *Candida:* and hypotension at onset of infection are seen. There may be a classic white discharge and erythema associated with thrush. Signs of systemic infections may be more generalized.

PLAN:

CONTRAINDICATIONS: Do not use in the presence of hypersensitivity to this drug. Ketoconazole does not penetrate cerebrospinal fluid adequately, making it ineffective in treating fungal meningitis.

WARNINGS: Although teratogenesis has not been reported, caution is warranted with the use of this drug during pregnancy. Safety during breast-feeding or in children under age 2 has not been carefully evaluated. Usually reversible hepatic toxicity has been reported, as well as a few cases of hepatitis in children. Monitoring of liver function studies is mandatory to detect any liver damage rapidly. Discontinue drug if even minor elevation in liver function studies develops.

PRECAUTIONS: Ketoconazole is a dibasic compound that requires stomach acidity for dissolution and absorption.

IMPLEMENTATION:

DRUG INTERACTIONS: Because of changes in gastrointestinal pH, antacids, anticholinergics or H_2 blockers will inhibit the dissolution and absorption of this drug. At least 2 hours should separate the ingestion of any of these medications and ketoconazole.

PRODUCTS (TRADE NAME):
Nizoral (Available in 200 mg scored tablets.)

ADMINISTRATION AND DOSAGE SPECIFICS:
Adults: Initially give 200 mg/day; may increase up to 400 mg once daily depending upon seriousness of the disease and clinical response.

Children older than 2 years: Give 3.3 to 6.6 mg/kg/day po.

Duration of treatment is not specific and should be based on clinical response. Minimum treatment for candidiasis is 10 days to 2 weeks. Systemic illnesses often require therapy for up to 6 months.

IMPLEMENTATION CONSIDERATIONS:
—Obtain a complete health history: presence of hypersensitivity, concurrent use of other drugs that may produce drug interactions (particularly gastrointestinal drugs), or possibility of pregnancy.

—Do a complete physical examination, noting all sites of infection.

—In patients with achlorhydria, tablets should be dissolved in small amount aqueous 0.2 N HCl solution. Take solution with a straw to avoid discoloring teeth and follow with a full glass of water. Explain to patients how and why this is done.

WHAT THE PATIENT NEEDS TO KNOW:
—Take all medication as ordered. Do not stop treatment when symptoms disappear.

—Notify health care provider if you experience any nausea, vomiting, abdominal pain, diarrhea, fever, dizziness or new or troublesome symptom.

—Take medication with food to decrease stomach upset.

EVALUATION:

ADVERSE REACTIONS: *Gastrointestinal:* abdominal pain, chills, diarrhea, dizziness, fever, headache, gynecomastia, hepatic dysfunction, impotence, nausea, photophobia, pruritus, thrombocytopenia, vomiting. Oligospermia has been reported at excessively high dosages.

OVERDOSAGE: Severe nausea, vomiting and diarrhea occur. Treat supportively, including referral for gastric lavage with sodium bicarbonate.

PARAMETERS TO MONITOR: Observe for therapeutic effects. Watch for shaking chills, fever or other signs of systemic disease to disappear. Watch for signs of gastrointestinal distress. Continue medication until laboratory tests return to normal. Monitor liver function tests and discontinue if even minor elevations occur.

Marilyn W. Edmunds

NYSTATIN

ACTION OF THE DRUG: Nystatin is a polyene antibiotic with fungistatic or fungicidal activity. The drug may allow leakage of intracellular components through the fungal cell membrane by binding to sterols in the cell membrane.

ASSESSMENT:

INDICATIONS: Used in the treatment of intestinal, vaginal and oral fungal infections due to susceptible strains of *Candida albicans* and other *Candida* species.

SUBJECTIVE: History of fever and chills at onset of infection. Frequently has history of recent antibiotic therapy.

OBJECTIVE: Signs of systemic or vaginal Candida: hypotension at onset of infection. May observe classic white discharge and erythema associated with thrush.

PLAN:

CONTRAINDICATIONS: Hypersensitivity to nystatin.

WARNINGS: Although teratogenesis has not been reported, caution is warranted with the use of nystatin during pregnancy.

IMPLEMENTATION:

DRUG INTERACTIONS: Severe superinfection may result with concurrent and prolonged corticosteroid therapy.

PRODUCTS (TRADE NAMES):

Korostatin, Mycostatin, Nilstat (Available in 100,000 units/ml oral suspension, 500,000 unit tablet, 100,000 unit vaginal tablets.) **Nystatin** (Available in 100,000 and 500,000 unit tablets.) **O-V Statin** (Available in 21 oral tablets of 500,000 units each and 14 vaginal tablets of 100,000 units each).

DRUG SPECIFICS:
   This is a systemic antifungal. Shake oral suspension well before use.
ADMINISTRATION AND DOSAGE SPECIFICS:
   Oral Thrush:
   Adults and Children: 400,000 to 600,000 units (4-6 ml), 4 times daily, with one-half the dose being held in each side of mouth a short time before swallowing.
   Older Infants: 200,000 units (2 ml) 4 times daily, with one-half the dose being held in each side of the mouth a short time before swallowing.
   Neonates: 100,000 units (1 ml), 4 times daily, with one-half the dose being held in each side of mouth a short time before swallowing.
   Intestinal Candidiasis:
   Adults: 500,000 to 1,000,000 units, 3 times daily, continued for at least 2 days after absence of symptoms.
   Vaginitis: 1-2 100,000 unit/once daily tablets intravaginally for 2 weeks. Can also be treated with oral doses as in intestinal candidiasis.

   IMPLEMENTATION CONSIDERATIONS:
   —Obtain a complete health history including the presence of hypersensitivity, concurrent use of other drugs which may produce drug interactions (particularly corticosteroids), or possibility of pregnancy.

   —Do a complete physical examination, noting all sites of infection.

WHAT THE PATIENT NEEDS TO KNOW:
   —Take all medication as ordered. Do not stop treatment when symptoms disappear.
   —Notify health care provider if you experience any nausea, vomiting or diarrhea.
   —Shake oral suspension thoroughly before use.

EVALUATION:

   ADVERSE REACTIONS: *Gastrointestinal:* nausea, vomiting, diarrhea.
   OVERDOSAGE: *Signs and symptoms:* severe nausea, vomiting, diarrhea.
   PARAMETERS TO MONITOR: Observe for therapeutic effects. Watch for shaking chills, temperature to disappear. Watch for signs of gastrointestinal distress. Continue medication until results of laboratory tests return to normal.

NYSTATIN-TETRACYCLINE COMBINATIONS

PRODUCTS (TRADE NAME):

Achrostatin V, Tetrastatin (Available in 250,000 units nystatin and 250 mg tetracycline hydrochloride capsule.) **Declostatin** (Available in 500,000 unit nystatin and 300 mg demeclocycine HCl tablets or 250,000 U nystatin and 150 mg demeclocycine HCl capsule.) **Terrastatin** (Available in 250,000 unit nystatin and 250 mg oxytetracycline capsules.)

DRUG SPECIFICS:

A broad spectrum antibiotic used to prevent *Candida* overgrowth during antibiotic therapy, and also for the treatment of existing infections. Provider must consider prescribing information for both nystatin and tetracycline hydrochloride prior to the use of this combination. The medication should be taken one hour before or two hours after meals to enhance absorption. Avoid administration of the medication with milk or other dairy products, antacids, or antidiarrheal suspensions.

ADMINISTRATION AND DOSAGE SPECIFICS:

Adults: 1-2 capsules, 4 times daily.

Barbara Sommer Wieferich and L. Colette Jones

ANTI-INFECTIVES—MISCELLANEOUS

FURAZOLIDONE

ACTION OF THE DRUG: Furazolidone has both antibacterial and antiprotozoal properties. It is bactericidal against gram-positive and gram-negative enteric organisms, including *Salmonella, Shigella, Escherichia coli, Staphylococcus, Aerobacter, Giardia lamblia, Proteus,* and *Vibrio cholerae.* Its mode of action is to interfere with several bacterial enzyme systems and also to minimize the development of resistant organisms.

ASSESSMENT:

INDICATIONS: Furazolidone is indicated in the treatment of bacterial or protozoal diarrhea and enteritis caused by susceptible organisms. It is one of the more potent agents used in the treatment of giardiasis. It is also used as adjunctive therapy in the treatment of cholera.

SUBJECTIVE: The patient may be asymptomatic or present with a history of acute gastroenteritis: acute diarrhea which may contain blood, pus, or mucus; tenesmus; abdominal cramps; nausea; vomiting; anorexia; fever; prostration; and weight loss. The patient may present with a history of chronic diarrhea, steatorrhea, fatigue, and weight loss.

OBJECTIVE: Physical examination may be negative or show signs of gastroenteritis: fever; signs of dehydration and prostration; borborygmi; hyperperistalsis; abdominal distention; diarrheal stools which may contain blood, pus, or mucus. Laboratory: microscopic and culture identification of the causative organism.

PLAN:

CONTRAINDICATIONS: Hypersensitivity to furazolidone; concurrent use of alcohol, sympathomimetics, or tyramine-containing foods. It is also contraindicated in infants under one month of age.

WARNING: Safe use during pregnancy, breast-feeding, and in women of childbearing age has not been established.

PRECAUTIONS: Extreme caution should be used when administering furazolidone to patients with G-6-PD deficiency as acute hemolysis may occur. Orthostatic hypotension and hypoglycemia may also occur.

IMPLEMENTATION:

DRUG INTERACTIONS: Furazolidone may potentiate tyramine sensitivity. Furazolidone in combination with sympathomimetic amines such as nasal decongestants (ephedrine and phenylephrine) or anorectic drugs (amphetamines) is contraindicated, as a hypertensive crisis may occur. Furazolidone may potentiate the effects of other MAO inhibitors. It potentiates CNS depressants such as alcohol, general anesthetics, antihistamines, barbiturates, narcotics, sedatives and tranquilizers. Orthostatic hypotension, CNS depression and hypoglycemia may result. If any of these CNS depressants, except alcohol, must be given with furazolidone, they should be administered with caution and their dosages should be reduced. Furazolidone in combination with alcohol should be avoided as it may cause a disulfiram-like reaction. Furazolidone in combination with tricyclic antidepressants (e.g., Elavil) should be avoided as toxic psychosis may result. Furazolidone also may increase the hypotensive effects of methyldopa, reserpine, and guanethidine. It may potentiate antiparkinsonism drugs, cocaine, insulin and vasopressors. Furazolidone may also cause false positive results in urine tested with Benedict's solution.

PRODUCTS (TRADE NAME):

Furoxone (Available in 100 mg tablets; or 50 mg/15 ml liquid.)

ADMINISTRATION AND DOSAGE: Furazolidone is incompletely absorbed from the gastrointestinal tract. It is well tolerated by patients. The average dose is based on 5 mg/kg/day in four equally divided doses. The maximum dose per day should not exceed 8.8 mg/kg of body weight as this may increase the chance of nausea and vomiting occurring. A positive clinical response should be seen within seven days. If a positive response does not occur, furazolidone should be discontinued and another antibacterial drug prescribed.

Adults: 100 mg four times per day, orally.

Children five to twelve years: 25 to 50 mg po four times per day.

Children one to four years: 17 to 25 mg po four times per day.

Children one month to one year: 8 to 17 mg po four times per day.

IMPLEMENTATION CONSIDERATIONS:

—Obtain a complete health history: history of alcohol abuse, G-6-PD deficiency, hypersensitivity to furazolidone, concurrent use of medications which may interact with furazolidone, possibility of pregnancy, breast-feeding.

—Obtain baseline weight and vital signs.

—Obtain baseline microscopic examination, and culture and sensitivity studies from stool specimen.

—Obtain baseline serum electrolyte studies.

—Hypertensive crises are most likely to occur when large doses have been prescribed or when the drug is continued for more than five days.

—Possible sources for the infection should be investigated, and the patient's family may need to have stool cultures done also.

—Check with the local health department on whether or not the disease is reportable.

WHAT THE PATIENT NEEDS TO KNOW:

—Notify your health provider if you have any side effects, especially fever, rash, abdominal pain, severe nausea, severe vomiting, or headache.

—Avoid cold and hay fever medications, nasal sprays, sedatives, and tranquilizers while on furazolidone, or severe adverse reactions may occur.

—Avoid alcohol and alcohol-containing medications while on this drug, and for four days following your last dose. Failure to eliminate alcohol will cause severe nausea and vomiting.

—If you take furazolidone for more than five days, or are on high doses, the following foods should be avoided: broad beans, cheese, beer, wine, pickled herring, chicken livers, bananas, avocados, chocolate, yeast extracts, and fermented products. Failure to do so will cause severe high blood pressure reactions.

—Furazolidone may color your urine brown.

—Furazolidone may cause a false positive urine glucose result if you are a diabetic and test your urine with Benedict's solution.

—Store your medicine in a dark, light-resistant container.

—Notify your health provider if you have diarrhea which persists for more than one week.

—Bed rest and drinking plenty of fluids are of valuable assistance in addition to drug therapy.

—Keep a record of your weight, the number of bowel movements you have, and how much liquid you are drinking every day.

—Family members may need to have their stools tested also.

—Be certain to wash your hands with soap and water following use of the toilet.

—Avoid handling or preparing food while you are still having loose bowel movements.

—You may be able to infect others as long as you still have loose stools.

EVALUATION:

ADVERSE REACTIONS: *CNS:* headache, malaise; *Gastrointestinal:* nausea, vomiting, abdominal pain, anal pruritus, anorexia, colitis, diarrhea, staphylococcal enteritis. *Hematopoietic:* agranulocytosis, hemolytic anemia in infants under one month of age and in patients with G-6-PD deficiency, hypoglycemia. *Hypersensitivity:* angioedema, arthralgia, fever, hypotension, rash, urticaria, vesicular morbilliform rash.

PARAMETERS TO MONITOR: The health provider should monitor the patient for signs and symptoms of a positive clinical response. Patients with G-6-PD deficiency should be followed closely with hematologic and urine studies. The patient should monitor on a daily basis his weight, the number of stools, and his fluid intake in order to watch for signs of dehydration.

Marna J. Ross

TRIMETHOPRIM-SULFAMETHOXAZOLE (CO-TRIMOXAZOLE)

ACTION OF THE DRUG: Trimethoprim-sulfamethoxazole (TMP-SMX) is a combination of two antimicrobial agents. Their mode of action is to provide sequential and synergistic inhibition of bacterial folate metabolism.

ASSESSMENT:

INDICATIONS: TMP-SMX is indicated for acute and recurrent urinary tract infections caused by susceptible strains of *Escherichia coli, Klebsiella, Enterobacter, Proteus mirabilis, Proteus vulgaris,* and *Proteus morganii.* It is indicated for the treatment of enteritis caused by susceptible strains of *Shigella flexneri* and *Shigella sonnei.* TMP-SMX is indicated for acute otitis media in children, caused by susceptible strains of *Haemophilus influenzae* and *Streptococcus pneumoniae.* It is indicated for acute exacerbations of chronic bronchitis in adults, caused by susceptible strains of *H. influenzae* and *H. pneumoniae.* TMP-SMX is indicated for the treatment of *Pneumocystis carinii* pneumonitis in adults and children. TMP-SMX may have the potential to be useful in a variety of other clinical situations also.

SUBJECTIVE-OBJECTIVE: The patient in need of antibiotic therapy may present in any number of ways, ranging from asymptomatic to severely ill. Keep in mind common infectious indicators such as: fever, inflammation, erythema, edema or pain.

PLAN:

CONTRAINDICATIONS: Do not use with hypersensitivity to trimethoprim or sulfonamides; pregnancy at term; during the nursing period; infants less than two months old; documented megaloblastic anemia secondary to folate deficiency; porphyria; liver disease; and blood dyscrasias. (Refer to trimethoprim, sulfamethoxazole and sulfonamides for more information.)

WARNINGS: TMP-SMX should not be used in the treatment of streptococcal pharyngitis, since patients with infections caused by group A Beta-hemolytic streptacocci may have a greater failure on this drug than they would have on a penicillin. Sulfonamide-associated deaths have been reported due to hypersensitivity reactions, agranulocytosis, aplastic anemia and other blood dyscrasias. Trimethoprim has been reported to interfere with hematopoiesis. Thrombocytopenia with purpura has been reported in elderly patients on diuretics.

PRECAUTIONS: Caution should be exercised when administering TMP-SMX to patients with impaired hepatic or renal function, folate deficiency, severe allergy, bronchial asthma, and G-6-PD deficiency. Dosages should be reduced. The drug should be discontinued immediately if there is any significant reduction in the count of any formed blood element. Benefit compared to risk must be determined before administering TMP-SMX during pregnancy.

IMPLEMENTATION:

DRUG INTERACTIONS: TMP-SMX may increase the effects of oral anticoagulants and prolong the prothrombin time. It may also increase the hypoglycemic response to sulfonylurea oral hypoglycemic agents. Renal excretion of methotrexate may be impaired. Ammonium chloride, ascorbic acid, and paraldehyde may acidify the urine and cause precipitation of sulfonamide and crystalluria. Methenamine when used with TMP-SMX may also cause crystalluria. PABA-containing local anesthetics may inhibit the antibacterial action of TMP-SMX. Leucovorin may also interfere with the antibacterial activity of TMP-SMX, but it may also be used to treat hematologic toxicities induced by the drug. TMP-SMX may cause elevated serum creatinine, bilirubin and alkaline phosphatase levels. (Refer to trimethoprim, sulfamethoxazole and sulfonamides for more information.)

PRODUCTS (TRADE NAME):
Bactrim, Septra (Available with 80 mg trimethoprim/400 mg sulfamethoxazole tablets; double strength: 160 mg trimethoprim/800 mg sulfamethoxazole tablets; 40 mg trimethoprim/200 mg sulfamethoxazole per 5 ml oral suspension.) **SMZ-TMP** (Available in 80 mg trimethoprim/400 mg sulfamethoxazole tablets; double strength: 160 mg trimethoprim/800 mg sulfamethoxazole tablets.)

ADMINISTRATION AND DOSAGE: The combination of sulfamethoxazole and trimethoprim is made to achieve an approximately constant ratio of 20:1 in the blood and tissues. Trimethoprim peaks in the serum in about 2 hours; sulfamethoxazole peaks in approximately 4 hours. Dosages should be reduced in patients with renal insufficiency, and the drug should not be given if the creatinine clearance is less than 15 ml/min. TMP-SMX is not recommended for infants under 2 months of age.

Urinary Tract Infections/Shigellosis:
Adults: 160 mg trimethoprim/800 mg sulfamethoxazole every 12 hours for ten to fourteen days in urinary tract infections, and for five days in shigellosis infections.

Children: 8 mg/kg trimethoprim/40 mg/kg sulfamethoxazole per 24 hours, in two equally divided doses given every 12 hours. Continue for ten days for urinary tract infections, five days for shigellosis.

Otitis Media:

Children: 8 mg/kg trimethoprim/40 mg/kg sulfamethoxazole in 24 hours, given in two equally divided doses every 12 hours for ten days.

Chronic Bronchitis:

Adults: 160 mg trimethoprim/800 mg sulfamethoxazole every 12 hours for fourteen days.

Pneumocystis carinii Pneumonitis:

Adults and children: 20 mg/kg trimethoprim/100 mg/kg sulfamethoxazole per 24 hours; given in equally divided doses every 6 hours for fourteen days.

IMPLEMENTATION CONSIDERATIONS:

—Obtain a thorough health history: hypersensitivities or allergies, history of impaired hepatic or renal function, folate deficiency, bronchial asthma, G-6-PD deficiency, other medications which may cause drug interactions, possibility of pregnancy.

—Obtain baseline laboratory studies for diagnosis.

—Obtain baseline CBC, urinalysis, renal and liver function tests.

—Side effects usually occur within the first two weeks of therapy.

WHAT THE PATIENT NEEDS TO KNOW:

—This medication should be taken exactly as ordered. Do not stop taking the medication once you feel better, or when symptoms are gone.

—Drink one full glass of water with each dose of medication.

—The medicine should be taken one hour before or two hours after meals for best absorption.

—Some patients experience side effects when they take this drug. Any new or uncomfortable symptoms should be reported. Notify the provider immediately if you note any of the following: skin rash, sore throat, fever, mouth sores, or unusual bleeding.

EVALUATION:

ADVERSE REACTIONS: *CNS:* apathy, ataxia, convulsions, fatigue, hallucinations, headache, insomnia, muscle weakness, mental depression, nervousness, peripheral neuritis, tinnitus, vertigo. *Gastrointestinal:* abdominal pain, anorexia, diarrhea, glossitis, hepatitis, jaundice, nausea, pancreatitis, pseudomembranous colitis, stomatitis, vomiting. *Genitourinary:* toxic nephrosis with oliguria or anuria, crystalluria, hematuria. *Hematopoietic:* agranulocytosis, aplastic anemia, hemolytic anemia, hypoprothrombinemia, leukopenia, megaloblastic anemia, methemoglobinemia, purpura, thrombocytopenia. *Hypersensitivity:* arthralgia, anaphylactoid reactions, epidermal necrolysis, erythema multiforme, exfoliative dermatitis, generalized skin eruptions, photosensitization, pruritus, Stevens-Johnson syndrome, urticaria.

Other: drug fever, serum sickness. *With prolonged use:* goiter with or without reduced thyroid function, and superinfections.

OVERDOSAGE: Moderate: nausea, vomiting, abdominal pain, diarrhea. Severe: hematuria, oliguria, anuria.

PARAMETERS TO MONITOR: Monitor for therapeutic effect and for adverse reactions. Clinical response should be carefully monitored due to the increased frequency of organisms resistant to sulfonamides and the possibility of a superinfection developing. A CBC may be obtained weekly for the first eight weeks of therapy and on a periodic basis thereafter. Urinalysis, renal function tests, and microscopic exams should be done periodically throughout therapy, especially for patients with impaired renal function. Liver function tests may be obtained periodically also. The patient should be monitored for signs and symptoms of toxic side effects. Coagulation times should be carefully checked when patients are on anticoagulants.

Marna J. Ross

ANTIMALARIALS

4-AMINOQUINOLINE COMPOUNDS

ACTION OF THE DRUG: These antiprotozoal drugs reduce the ability of DNA to replicate or serve as a template, thereby decreasing protein synthesis in susceptible organisms.

ASSESSMENT:

INDICATIONS: Used in the suppression and treatment of acute malarial attacks due to erythrocytic forms of *Plasmodium ovale, P. malariae, P. vivax* and most strains of *P. falciparum.* It is ineffective against gametocytes of *P. falciparum.* Also used with primaquine to attain radical cure of malaria due to *P. malariae* and *P. vivax.*

SUBJECTIVE: History of malarial symptoms: periodic fever and chills, profound sweating, headache, nausea, body pains and exhaustion. May report being in an area in which malaria is endemic.

OBJECTIVE: Signs of malaria: periodic diaphoresis and remittent fever as high as 104 to 105 degrees Fahrenheit; presence of visual field or retina changes.

PLAN:

CONTRAINDICATIONS: Hypersensitivity to 4-aminoquinoline compounds.
WARNINGS: The drugs should not be used during pregnancy or breast feeding unless absolutely necessary. Since certain strains of *P. falciparum* have developed

resistance to 4-aminoquinoline compounds, treatment with other antimalarial drugs, such as quinine, is recommended for individuals infected with these strains. Use of the drug may precipitate a severe attack of psoriasis or exacerbation of porphyria in those individuals with a history of either disease. Among those individuals on high dosages or prolonged therapy, irreversible retinal damage may occur. Children are highly sensitive to 4-aminoquinoline compounds, primarily chloroquine HCl.

PRECAUTIONS: Use with caution in those patients with glucose-6-phosphate dehydrogenase deficiency, since hemolysis may be precipitated. Use of the drug should be discontinued if any blood dyscrasia develops which is not associated with the disease.

IMPLEMENTATION:

DRUG INTERACTIONS: Concurrent use of phenylbutazone or gold salts may cause severe skin reactions.

ADMINISTRATION AND DOSAGE: Chloroquine phosphate and hydroxychloroquine sulfate are administered orally. For the treatment of malaria, usually an initial loading dose is followed by one half that dose on the succeeding two days. For the suppression of malaria, these drugs are usually initiated two weeks prior to the individual's entrance into a malarious area. The medication is taken once weekly on the same day of the week and is continued for 8 weeks after the individual has left the area. When the absorption of the drug used for acute infection is questionable, when the infection is quite severe, or when nausea and vomiting are present, chloroquine HCl may be given parenterally, usually intramuscularly. Children are highly sensitive to 4-aminoquinoline compounds, primarily chloroquine HCl. Infants and children should never receive more than 5 mg/kg (base) in a single dose.

IMPLEMENTATION CONSIDERATIONS:

—Take a thorough health history: ascertain if the patient is pregnant; has a history of psoriasis, porphyria, or glucose-6-phosphate dehydrogenase deficiency; is allergic to 4-aminoquinoline compounds; or is taking any medications that may interact with 4-aminoquinoline compounds.

—If visual disturbances occur, discontinue the drug immediately and refer patient for evaluation.

WHAT THE PATIENT NEEDS TO KNOW:

—Take all medicatation as ordered. Do not stop medication when symptoms disappear.

—If ringing in the ears, hearing difficulties, or visual disturbances occur, notify health care provider immediately.

—Gastrointestinal upset can be reduced by taking medication with meals. If nausea, vomiting, anorexia, abdominal cramps, or diarrhea become pronounced, notify health care provider.

—Keep this medication out of the reach of children.

EVALUATION:

ADVERSE REACTIONS: *Cardiovascular:* hypotension, electrocardiogram changes. *CNS:* convulsions, mild and transient headaches, neuropathy, psychic stimulation, psychotic episodes. *Dermatologic:* lichen planus-like eruptions, pleomorphic skin eruptions, pruritus, skin and mucosal pigmentation changes. *Gastrointestinal:* abdominal cramps, anorexia, diarrhea, nausea, vomiting. *Hematopoietic:* agranulocytosis, blood dyscrasias. *Ophthalmologic:* accomodation or focusing difficulties, retinal changes, transient corneal edema or opaque deposits, visual blurring, visual halos. *Otologic:* nerve-type deafness, reduced hearing, tinnitus.

OVERDOSAGE: *Signs and symptoms:* Headache, drowsiness, and visual disturbances may occur within 30 minutes of overdose. Cardiovascular collapse, convulsions, respiratory or cardiac arrest are possible. *Treatment:* Immediate production of emesis or for gastric lavage are necessary. Treatment should continue until stomach is completely empty. Following gastric lavage, give activated charcoal via stomach tube within 30 minutes after overdose. Provide symptomatic and supportive therapy as needed.

PARAMETERS TO MONITOR: Initial and periodic ophthalmic examinations should be performed. Make initial determination of glucose-6-phosphate dehydrogenase level in American blacks and in those patients of Mediterranean ancestry. If patient is to undergo prolonged therapy, periodic complete blood counts, urinalysis and observation for signs and symptoms of hemolysis are necessary. Also, if patient is to undergo prolonged therapy, periodically examine knee and ankle reflexes to determine presence of muscular weakness.

CHLOROQUINE HCL

PRODUCTS (TRADE NAME):

Aralen HCl (Available in 50 mg/ml in 5 ml ampules, equivalent to 40 mg/ml—base).

DRUG SPECIFICS:

A parenteral drug of choice for treating acute malarial attacks due to *Plasmodium malariae, P. ovale, P. vivax,* and most strains of *P. falciparum* when oral therapy is ineffective. Intramuscular administration of this drug is necessary when absorption of the oral form is questionable, the infection is quite severe, or nausea and vomiting are present. Children are highly sensitive to chloroquine HCl. Infants and children should never receive greater than 5 mg/kg (base) in a single dose. All patients should resume oral administration of chloroquine phosphate as soon as possible.

ADMINISTRATION AND DOSAGE SPECIFICS:

Adults: 4-5 ml IM initially, and repeated every 6 hours if necessary, with total dose in first 24 hours not to exceed 800 mg (base).

Children: 5 mg/kg (base) initially, repeated in 6 hours if necessary, with total daily dose not to exceed 10 mg/kg (base).

CHLOROQUINE PHOSPHATE

PRODUCTS (TRADE NAME):
   Aralen Phosphate (Available in 500 mg tablet, equivalent to 300 mg base.)
   Chloroquine Phosphate (Available in 250 mg tablet, equivalent to 150 mg base.)
DRUG SPECIFICS:
   Indicated in the suppression and treatment of acute malaria due to *Plasmodium malariae, P. ovale, P. vivax,* and most strains of *P. falciparum.* It is also indicated in the suppression of lupus erythematosus and photosensitivity reactions, and in the treatment of extraintestinal amebiasis, dwarf tapeworms, liver flukes, and rheumatoid arthritis.
ADMINISTRATION AND DOSAGE SPECIFICS:
   Malaria Suppression:
   Adults: 500 mg once weekly on same day of week, beginning 2 weeks prior to entering malarious area and continued for 8 weeks after departure.
   Children: 5 mg/kg (base) once weekly on same day of week, beginning 2 weeks prior to entering malarious area and continuing for 8 weeks after departure.
   Malaria Treatment:
   Adults: 1 gm initially, then 500 mg in 6 hours and 500 mg daily for the next 2 days.
   Children: 10 mg/kg (base) initially, then 5 mg/kg (base) in 6 hours and 5 mg/kg (base) daily for the next 2 days.
   Lupus Suppression:
   Adults: 250 mg twice daily for 2 weeks, then 250 mg daily as maintenance.
Photosensitivity Suppression:
   Adults: 250 mg twice daily for 2 weeks, then 250 mg daily.
   Tapeworm Treatment:
   Adults: 250 mg twice daily for 3 weeks.
   Children: Dosage not established.
   Liver Fluke Treatment:
   Adults: 1.25 gm daily in 3 divided doses for 6 weeks.
   Amebiasis Treatment:
   Adults: 250 mg 4 times daiy for 2 days, then 250 mg twice daily for 2-3 weeks.
   Children: 10 mg/kg (base) twice daily for 2 days, then 5 mg/kg twice daily for 2-3 weeks.
   Arthritis:
   Adults: 250 mg daily with evening meals.

HYDROXOCHLOROQUINE SULFATE

PRODUCTS (TRADE NAME):
   Plaquenil Sulfate (Available in 200 mg tablets, equivalent to 150 mg base.)
DRUG SPECIFICS:
   Indicated in the suppression and treatment of acute malaria attacks due to *Plasmodium malariae, P. ovale, P. vivax,* and susceptible strains of *P. falciparum.* It is also useful in the suppression of discoid and systemic lupus erythematosus and treatment of rheumatoid arthritis.
ADMINISTRATION AND DOSAGE SPECIFICS:
   Adults: 400 mg once weekly on same day of week, beginning 2 weeks prior to entering malarious area and continued for 8 weeks after departure.
   Children: 5 mg/kg (base) once weekly on same day of week, not to exceed adult dosage, beginning 2 weeks prior to entering malarious area and continued for 8 weeks after departure.
   Malaria Treatment:
   Adults: 800 mg initially, then 400 mg in 6 hours and 400 mg daily for the next 2 days.
   Children: 10 mg/kg (base) initially, then 5 mg/kg (base) in 6 hours and 5 mg/ kg (base) daily for the next 2 days.
   Lupus Suppression:
   Adults: 200-400 mg once daily.
   Rheumatoid Arthritis:
   Adults: 400-600 mg once daily until desired effect is obtained, then 200-400 mg daily as maintenance.

Barbara Sommer Wieferich

8-AMINOQUINOLINE DERIVATIVES: PRIMAQUINE PHOSPHATE

ACTION OF THE DRUG: Primaquine phosphate interferes with the metabolism of parasites by causing mitochondrial swelling, thereby inhibiting protein synthesis.

ASSESSMENT:

   INDICATIONS: Used for radical cure (relapse prevented) of *Plasmodium vivax malaria.*
   SUBJECTIVE: History of malarial symptoms: periodic fever and chills, profound sweating, headache, nausea, body pains and exhaustion. May report being in an area in which malaria is endemic.

OBJECTIVE: Signs of malaria: periodic diaphoresis and remittent fever as high as 104 to 105 degrees Fahrenheit.

PLAN:

CONTRAINDICATIONS: Hypersensitivity to 8-aminoquinoline derivatives or primaquine phosphate. Avoid concurrent use of quinacrine HCl, concomitant use of other potential hemolytic agents, and use in those prone to agranulocytopenia due to systemic disease.

WARNINGS: The drug should not be used during pregnancy unless absolutely necessary. Use of primoquine phosphate among those with dark skin, glucose-6-phosphate dehydrogenase deficiency, nicotinamide adenine dinucleotide (NADH) methemoglobin reductase deficiency, or idiosyncratic reactions (leukopenia, hemolytic anemia, or methemoglobinemia), may result in hemolytic reactions. Immediately discontinue the drug if signs or symptoms of hemolysis occur.

PRECAUTIONS: Since anemia, leukopenia, and methemoglobinemia may result from large doses of the drug, recommended doses must not be exceeded.

IMPLEMENTATION:

DRUG INTERACTIONS: Toxicity of antimalarial compounds may result with concurrent use of quinacrine HCl or recent use of quinacrine HCl prior to use of primaquine phosphate.

PRODUCTS (TRADE NAME):

Primaquine Phosphate (Available in 26.3 mg tablet, equivalent to 15 mg base.)

ADMINISTRATION AND DOSAGE: In order to destroy the exoerythrocytic parasitic forms, concomitant administration of primaquine phosphate and chloroquine phosphate is necessary. Initiate primaquine therapy following a course of chloroquine phosphate suppressive treatment or during the last 2 weeks of therapy with chloroquine phosphate.

Malaria Suppression:

Adults: 26.3 mg once daily for 14 days, beginning immediately after leaving malarious area.

Children: 0.3 mg/kg (base) once daily for 14 days, beginning immediately after leaving malarious area.

Radical Cure of Malaria:

Adults: 26.3 mg daily for 14 days or 79 mg once weekly for 8 weeks.

Children: 0.3 mg/kg (base) daily for 14 days or 0.9 mg/kg (base) once weekly for 8 weeks.

IMPLEMENTATION CONSIDERATIONS:

—Obtain a thorough health history: Ascertain if patient is pregnant; if there is a history of glucose-6-phosphate-dehydrogenase deficiency, nicotinamide adenine denucleotide (NADH) methemoglobin reductase deficiency, or idiosyncratic reactions; if there is an allergy to 8-aminoquinoline derivatives or primaquine phosphate, or whether patient is taking any medications that may interact with these drugs.

WHAT THE PATIENT NEEDS TO KNOW:
—Complete the full course of medication therapy, taking medication according to the schedule given you by the health provider.
—Gastrointestinal upset from the medication can be reduced by taking the medication with meals or antacids.
—If nausea, vomiting or abdominal cramps become prolonged, or if the urine becomes dark, notify health provider.

EVALUATION:

ADVERSE REACTIONS: *CNS:* headache, mental depression, confusion. *Dermatologic:* pruritus. *Gastrointestinal:* nausea, vomiting, anorexia, abdominal cramps. *Hematopoietic:* leukopenia, hemolytic anemia in those with glucose-6-phosphate dehydrogenase deficiency, methemoglobinemia in those with methemoglobin reductase deficiency. *Ophthalmic:* difficulty with visual accommodation.

OVERDOSAGE: *Signs and symptoms:* vomiting, burning epigastric discomfort, abdominal cramps, cardiovascular and CNS disturbances, cyanosis, methemoglobinemia, leukocytosis, leukopenia, anemia, granulocytopenia. *Treatment:* Induce emesis and refer for gastric lavage. Provide supportive and symptomatic therapy as needed.

PARAMETERS TO MONITOR: Make initial determination of glucose-6-phosphate dehydrogenase level in American blacks and in those of Mediterranean ancestry. Periodic complete blood counts, urinalysis, and observation for signs and symptoms of hemolysis are necessary.

Barbara Sommer Wieferich

FOLIC ACID ANTAGONISTS

ACTION OF THE DRUG: Pyrimethamine acts as a folic acid antagonist. The therapeutic effect is based on the differential growth requirements and demand for nucleic acid precursors between host and parasite. In sulfonamide products, there is competitive antagonism of para-aminobenzoic acid which is a component in folic acid synthesis.

ASSESSMENT:

INDICATIONS: Used as suppressive therapy of susceptible strains of plasmodia. Susceptibility of plasmodia organisms may vary by locations and time. Used concomitantly with quinine and sulfadiazine in the treatment of chloroquine-resistant strains of *Plasmodium falciparum*. Although ineffective against gametocytes, pyrimethamine arrests sporogony in the mosquito. Also used concomitantly with sulfadiazine or a multiple sulfonamide in the treatment of *Toxoplasma gondii*. These products are compatible with other antimalarial drugs, antibiotics and antidiabetic agents.

SUBJECTIVE: History of malarial symptoms: periodic fever and chills, profound sweating, headache, nausea, body pains, and exhaustion. May report being in an area in which malaria is endemic.

OBJECTIVE: Signs of malaria: periodic diaphoresis and remittent fever as high as 104 and 105 degrees Fahrenheit.

PLAN:

CONTRAINDICATIONS: Hypersensitivity to pyrimethamine, sulfonamides, history of megaloblastic anemia. Do not use in pregancy at term or with nursing mothers. Do not use in infants less than 2 months of age.

WARNINGS: Because large doses of pyrimethamine are required for the treatment of toxoplasmosis, discontinue therapy or reduce the dosage if signs of folic or folinic acid deficiency occur. If necessary, administer leucovorin (folinic acid) 3-9 mg intramuscularly daily for 3 days to return white blood cell and platelet levels to normal. The drug should not be used during pregnancy unless absolutely necessary in the treatment of toxoplasmosis. Such use requires concomitant administration of folinic acid. Parasitic resistance may develop with use of large doses.

PRECAUTIONS: Use with caution in those patients with glucose-6-phosphate dehydrogenase deficiency, since hemolysis may result. For treatment of toxoplasmosis in patients with convulsive disorders, use smaller initial doses.

IMPLEMENTATION:

DRUG INTERACTIONS: Pyrimethamine activity can be inhibited by concurrent use of PABA or folates when treating toxoplasmosis. False increases in urinary alkaloid and barbiturate levels may occur with use of the drug. Anti-folic acid drugs such as sulfonamides or trimethoprim-sulfamethoxazole combinations should not be used concurrently.

ADMINISTRATION AND DOSAGE: These oral preparations may be used either as malaria prophylaxis in patients going into areas where malaria is endemic, or as therapy in acute illness.

IMPLEMENTATION CONSIDERATIONS:

—Obtain a thorough health history: Ascertain whether patient is pregnant; if there is a history of glucose-6-phosphate dehydrogenase deficiency, megaloblastic anemia, or convulsive disorders; allergy to pyrimethamine; or whether patient is taking any medications that may interact with pyrimethamine.

WHAT THE PATIENT NEEDS TO KNOW:

—Complete the full course of medication exactly as instructed by your health provider.

—Gastrointestinal upset can be reduced by taking pyrimethamine with meals.

—Notify health provider if sore throat, fever, unusual bruising or bleeding develops.

EVALUATION:

ADVERSE REACTIONS: *Gastrointestinal:* anorexia, atrophic glossitis, vomiting. *Hematologic:* leukopenia, megaloblastic anemia, pancytopenia, thrombocytopenia.

OVERDOSAGE: *Signs and symptoms:* Acute intoxication is demonstrated by central nervous system stimulation and convulsions. *Treatment:* Refer for administration of parenteral barbiturate. Then give leucovorin (folinic acid).

PARAMETERS TO MONITOR: Make initial determination of glucose-6-phosphate dehydrogenase level in American blacks and in those of Mediterranean ancestry. Semi-weekly complete blood counts, platelet counts, and serum folate levels are necessary, especially in those patients receiving high dosages. Also consider need for repeat sensitivity test when high dosages are given. Observe for signs and symptoms of hemolysis.

PYRIMETHAMINE

PRODUCTS (TRADE NAME):
Daraprim (Available in 25 mg tablet.)
DRUG SPECIFICS:
This is a very inexpensive drug and is used in both prophylaxis and treatment of malaria as well as the treatment of toxoplasmosis. Compliance with therapy over the several weeks necessary is sometimes a problem.
ADMINISTRATION AND DOSAGE SPECIFICS:
Malaria Suppression:
Adults and children over 10 years: 25 mg once weekly.
Children 4-10 years: 12.5 mg once weekly.
Children under 4 years: 6.25 mg once weekly.
Note: Therapy should begin 2 weeks prior to entering malarious area and be continued for 10 weeks after departure.
Chloroquine-Resistant P. falciparum:
Adults:
Pyrimethamine: 25 mg twice daily for 3 days.
Quinine: 600 mg 3 times daily for 14 days.
Sulfadiazine: 2 gm initially, then 500 mg every 6 hours for 6 days.
Children under 15 years: use approximately one-half the adult dosage.
Toxoplasmosis:
Adults:
Pyrimethamine: 50-75 mg for 1-3 weeks, then one-half the dosage for 4-5 weeks.

Sulfonamide: 1-4 gm daily for 1-3 weeks, then one-half the dosage for 4-5 weeks.

Children: 1 mg/kg daily divided into 2 equal doses, then one-half the dosage after 2-4 days and continue therapy for 4 weeks. Use recommended sulfonamide dosage level for children.

PYRIMETHAMINE AND SULFADOXINE

PRODUCTS (TRADE NAME):
Fansidar (Available in 500 mg tablets.)

DRUG SPECIFICS:
Use this preparation considering both the advantages and disadvantages of sulfonamide therapy. This product may produce an acute intoxication syndrome with overdosage which is manifested by CNS stimulation, convulsions, nausea, vomiting, anorexia, and may be followed by megaloblastic anemia, leukopenia, thrombocytopenia, glossitis, and crystalluria. Folinic acid should be administered and renal and hematologic values should be monitored for at least one month following episodes of toxicity.

ADMINISTRATION AND DOSAGE SPECIFICS:
Malaria Prophylaxis:

Adults: Take 500 mg po one or two days prior to entering an endemic area, and continue 500 mg once a week, or 1000 mg every two weeks, for 4 to 6 weeks following return. Follow with a regimen of primaquine.

Children: Take dosage (according to the following scale) one or two days prior to entering an endemic area and once a week for 4 to 6 weeks following return. Follow with a regimen of primaquine.

Children 9 to 14 years: 3/4 tablet weekly or 1 1/2 tablet biweekly.

Children 4 to 8 years: 1/2 tablet weekly or 1 tablet biweekly.

Children under 4 years: 1/2 tablet weekly or 1/2 tablet biweekly.

Malaria Treatment:

Adults: Take 2 to 3 tablets as a single dose, alone or with quinine or primaquine.

Children: Take tablets as a single dose, alone or with quinine or primaquine according to the following schedule:

Children 9 to 14 years: 2 tablets.

Children 4 to 8 years: 1 tablet.

Children under 4 years: 1/2 tablet.

Barbara Sommer Wieferich

QUINACRINE HCL

ACTION OF THE DRUG: Quinacrine HCl reduces the ability of DNA to replicate or serve as a template, thereby decreasing protein synthesis in susceptible organisms.

ASSESSMENT:

INDICATIONS: Used in suppression and treatment of malaria. It is active against the erythrocytic asexual forms of *Plasmodium falciparum, P. malariae,* and *P. vivax,* as well as the sexual forms of *P. malariae* and *P. vivax.* It is ineffective against gametocytes of *P. falciparum* and sporozoites of all forms of malaria. Also useful in the treatment of giardiasis and cestodiasis.

SUBJECTIVE: History of malarial symptoms: periodic fever and chills, profound sweating, headache, nausea, body pains, exhaustion. May report being in an area in which malaria is endemic; previous history of malaria.

OBJECTIVE: Signs of malaria: periodic diaphoresis and fever as high as 104 to 105 degrees Fahrenheit.

PLAN:

CONTRAINDICATIONS: Hypersensitivity to quinacrine HCl.

WARNINGS: The drug should not be used during pregnancy unless absolutely necessary. Since certain strains of *P. falciparum* have developed resistance to synthetic antimalarial compounds, e.g., quinacrine HCl, treatment with other antimalarial drugs, such as quinine, is recommended for individuals infected with these strains. Use of the drug may precipitate a severe attack of psoriasis or exacerbation of porphyria in those individuals with a history of either disease.

PRECAUTIONS: Use with caution in those patients with glucose-6-phosphate dehydrogenase deficiency, since hemolysis may be precipitated. Use of the drug should be discontinued if any blood dyscrasia develops which is not associatd with the malarial disease.

IMPLEMENTATION:

DRUG INTERACTIONS: Concurrent use with primaquine increases the toxicity of primaquine. Quinacrine HCl may inhibit alcohol metabolism, resulting in a minor disulfiram reaction.

PRODUCTS (TRADE NAME):

Atabrine HCl (Available in 100 mg tablet).

ADMINISTRATION AND DOSAGE:

Malaria Treatment:

Adults and Children over 8 years: 200 mg with 1 gm sodium bicarbonate every 6 hours for 5 days, then 100 mg every 8 hours for 6 days.

Children 4-8 years: 200 mg every 8 hours for 24 hours, then 100 mg every 12 hours for 6 days.

Children 1-4 years: 100 mg every 8 hours for 24 hours, then 100 mg once daily for 6 days.

Malaria Suppression:

Adults: 100 mg/day for 1-3 months.

Children: 50 mg/day for 1-3 months.

IMPLEMENTATION CONSIDERATIONS:

—Take a thorough health history: Determine if patient is pregnant; if there is a history of psoriasis, porphyria, or glucose-6-phosphate dehydrogenase deficiency; if there is an allergy to quinacrine HCl; or whether patient is taking any medications that may interact with quinacrine HCl.

WHAT THE PATIENT NEEDS TO KNOW:

—Complete the full course of medication therapy. Take drugs in manner directed by health provider even though all symptoms may have resolved.

—Take this medication with a full glass of water, tea, or fruit juice after meals.

—A yellow discoloration of skin and urine may develop while you are on this drug.

—Onset of any visual disturbances should be immediately brought to the attention of the health provider.

EVALUATION:

ADVERSE REACTIONS: *CNS:* convulsions, dizziness, emotional changes, irritability, mild and transient headaches, nervousness, nightmares, transient psychosis, vertigo. *Dermatologic:* contact dermatitis, exfoliative dermatitis, lichen planus-like eruptions, pleomorphic skin eruptions. *Gastrointestinal:* abdominal cramps, anorexia, diarrhea, hepatitis, nausea, vomiting. *Hematopoietic:* aplastic anemia. *Ophthalmologic:* difficulty focusing, reversible corneal edema or deposits, with visual halos and blurring, retinopathy.

OVERDOSAGE: *Signs and symptoms:* Central nervous system excitation and restlessness, insomnia, convulsions and psychic stimulation, nausea, vomiting, abdominal cramps, diarrhea, vascular collapse, shock, cardiac arrhythmias, cardiac arrest. *Treatment:* Refer and induce emesis or gastric lavage if convulsions are not present. Provide symptomatic and supportive therapy as needed.

PARAMETERS TO MONITOR: Make initial determination of glucose-6-phosphate dehydrogenase level in American blacks and in those of Mediterranean ancestry. If patient is to undergo prolonged therapy, periodic complete blood counts, urinalysis, and observation for signs and symptoms of hemolysis are necessary. Any report of visual disturbances necessitates ophthalmologic examination.

Barbara Sommer Wieferich

QUININE SULFATE

ACTION OF THE DRUG: (1) Quinine reduces the effectiveness of DNA to act as a template in chloroquine-resistant strains of *Plasmodium falciparum*. (2) Parasitic oxygen utilization and carbohydrate metabolism are decreased. (3) Quinine also exerts skeletal muscle relaxant, antipyretic, oxytocic and analgesic effects, as well as cardiovascular effects similar to those of quinidine.

ASSESSMENT:

INDICATIONS: Used in combination with pyrimethamine, and sulfadiazine or tetracycline in the treatment of chloroquine-resistant strains of *P. falciparum*. Used to prevent and treat nocturnal leg cramps, as found in association with diabetes, thrombophlebitis, arteriosclerosis, varicose veins, arthritis, and static foot deformities.

SUBJECTIVE: History of malarial symptoms: periodic fever and chills, profound sweating, headache, nausea, body pains, exhaustion. May report being in an area where malaria is endemic; previous history of malaria.

OBJECTIVE: Signs of malaria: periodic diaphoresis and fever as high as 104 to 105 degrees Fahrenheit.

PLAN:

CONTRAINDICATIONS: Hypersensitivity to quinine; optic neuritis or tinnitus; glucose-6-phosphate dehydrogenase deficiency; pregnancy.

WARNINGS: Use with caution in individuals with cardiac arrhythmias. Caution is necessary with use during lactation, since quinine is excreted in breast milk. Repeated dosages or overdosage may precipitate cinchonism with mild symptoms of headache, nausea, ringing in ears, and slightly disturbed vision.

PRECAUTIONS: Cardiotoxicity may result with quinine use. In very sensitive individuals, reversible thrombocytopenia may occur. Use cautiously in those with myasthenia gravis or asthma.

IMPLEMENTATION:

DRUG INTERACTIONS: Urinary alkalizers may cause renal tubular reabsorption of quinine thereby increasing quinine blood levels. Oral anticoagulant activity may be enhanced when used with quinine. Concomitant use of neuromuscular-blocking agents may be potentiated with quinine use.

PRODUCTS (TRADE NAME):
Quinamm (Available in 260 mg tablet.) **Quine** (Available in 200 and 300 mg capsules.) **Quinine Sulfate** (Available in 130 mg, 195 mg, 200 mg, 300 mg and 325 mg capsules; and 260 and 325 mg tablets.) **Coco-Quinine** (Available in 110 mg/5 ml suspension.)

ADMINISTRATION AND DOSAGE:
Chloroquine-Resistant Malaria:
Adults: 650 mg every 8 hours for 10-14 days.
Children: 25 mg/kg every 8 hours for 10-14 days.
Note: Concurrent use of pyrimethamine 50 mg daily for the first 3 days of quinine therapy plus sulfadiazine 2 gm daily for the first 6 days is recommended.
Nocturnal Leg Cramps: 200-300 mg at bedtime.
Analgesic-Antipyretic: 300-600 mg.

IMPLEMENTATION CONSIDERATIONS:

—Take a thorough health history: ascertain if patient is pregnant or breast-feeding; if glucose-6-phosphate dehydrogenase deficiency, optic neuritis, myasthenia gravis, asthma, or cardiac arrhythmias are present; if client is allergic to quinine; or if client is taking any medications that may interact with quinine.

—Mild side effects are common and client should be counseled regarding them.

WHAT THE PATIENT NEEDS TO KNOW:

—Take all of the drugs ordered, at times and manner prescribed for you.

—Gastrointestinal upset can be reduced by taking quinine with meals.

—Diarrhea, nausea, vomiting, abdominal cramps, or ringing in ears may result. If these things become pronounced, notify your health provider.

—Quinine may cause dizziness and visual blurring. Caution is necessary while driving.

EVALUATION:

ADVERSE REACTIONS: *Cinchonism:* diarrhea, dizziness, headache, nausea, tinnitus, visual blurring. *CNS:* apprehension, confusion, convulsions, delirium, excitement, hypothermia, syncope, severe headache, *Gastrointestinal:* abdominal cramps, diarrhea, nausea, vomiting. *Hematopoietic:* agranulocytosis, hemolytic anemia in glucose-6-phosphate dehydrogenase deficient individuals; thrombocytopenia. *Hypersensitivity:* asthma, flushing, pruritus, rash, urticaria. *Ophthalmologic:* altered color perception, amblyopia, diplopia, mydriasis, night blindness, optic atrophy, photophobia, scotomata, visual blurring.

OVERDOSAGE: *Signs and symptoms:* hypotension, convulsions, paralysis, cardiovascular collapse, coma and death. *Treatment:* Induce emesis and refer for gastric lavage. Provide supportive and symptomatic therapy as needed.

PARAMETERS TO MONITOR: Electrocardiogram may be desirable prior to initiation of therapy if presence of cardiac arrhythmia is questionable. May need to make initial determination of glucose-6-phosphate dehydrogenase level in American blacks and in those patients of Mediterranean ancestry. Periodic complete blood count, urinalysis, and observation for signs and symptoms of hemolysis are necessary.

Barbara Sommer Wieferich

ANTITUBERCULAR DRUGS

ACTION OF THE DRUG: The main action of the antitubercular drugs is their bactericidal or bacteriostatic effect against *Mycobacterium tuberculosis* found intracellularly and/or extracellularly.

ASSESSMENT:

INDICATIONS: *Chemoprophylaxis* is recommended for situations in which there is a high risk of the patient developing active tuberculosis. The duration of prophylactic treatment is currently one year. At present Isoniazid is the only drug recommended for prophylactic therapy. Situations warranting chemoprophylaxis are:

—Close contacts of an individual with an active tuberculosis infection.

—Positive PPD skin reaction in an individual under 35 years of age.

—Positive PPD skin reaction in an individual who is at special risk for developing tuberculosis due to a history of leukemia, Hodgkin's disease, chronic malignancy, prolonged corticosteroid or immunosuppressive therapy, silicosis, gastrectomy, or diabetes mellitus.

—Positive PPD skin reactors with positive, nonprogressive chest x-rays for tuberculosis and negative sputum cultures, who have not received adequate treatment in the past.

—Newly infected persons or those whose skin tests have become positive in the past two years.

Isoniazid prophylaxis is not recommended for healthy individuals over the age of 35 due to their increased risk of developing hepatitis. It is recommended, however, if the patient is at special risk for developing tuberculosis, as indicated above.

Chemotherapy is recommended for patients with active tuberculosis. The nurse practitioner will have the greatest opportunity to monitor clients with pulmonary tuberculosis and this will be emphasized throughout.

It is recognized that non-physician health providers play an important role in tuberculosis case-finding. Although the initial diagnosis and therapy should be coordinated with a qualified physician, long-term management of these patients is frequently carried out by the nurse practitioner. Ability to work with the patient and family, to teach and counsel, is an important part of winning the patient's confidence and aiding compliance.

SUBJECTIVE: In pulmonary tuberculosis the patient may be asymptomatic or exhibit insidious onset of weight loss, fatigue, fevers, night sweats, hemoptysis, and a progressive cough which eventually becomes productive. The patient may present with a history of recent close contact with an infected person, history of past tuberculosis infection, history of recent conversion to a positive tuberculin skin test reaction, or positive chest x-ray for tuberculosis. Other symptoms may be present if the site of tuberculosis is other than in the lungs.

OBJECTIVE: In pulmonary TB, general signs on physical exam may range from no symptoms, to fever, post-tussive apical rales, and cough which may be productive. The patient may have a positive skin test and chest x-ray for tuberculosis. Laboratory data may show a positive smear or culture for tubercle bacilli. For other sites of infection, symptoms would be related to the site.

PLAN:

CONTRAINDICATIONS: *Chemoprophylaxis* is contraindicated during pregnancy; it should be initiated after delivery. It is also contraindicated if the patient has a history of hypersensitivity or severe adverse reactions to isoniazid. *Chemotherapeutic* use of a specific drug is contraindicated when there is a history of hypersensitivity or severe adverse reactions to the drug.

WARNINGS: The provider should never administer only one drug for active tuberculosis as drug resistance is very likely to develop. Two or more drugs should always be given. Drugs which are highly ototoxic should not be given together. Two hepatotoxic drugs should not be given together when clinically active hepatitis is present.

PRECAUTIONS: Caution must be exercised to prevent the development of drug resistance. This may be accomplished by careful monitoring of the following: (1) patient compliance, (2) sputum culture conversions, and (3) selection of appropriate drugs. Due to the long-term nature of the chemotherapeutic regimen, drug toxicity is a special problem. Caution should be exercised in determining dosages for the elderly, unusually small adults, and patients with renal impairment. All patients should be monitored routinely for symptoms of adverse reactions. If toxic effects, adverse reactions, or hypersensitivity reactions should occur, all drugs should be stopped and further evaluation made. Reintroducing drugs after toxic effects or adverse reactions have ceased should be done with caution and under the guidance of a qualified physician. In the event of an unsuccessful treatment regimen, two or more drugs should be added to the therapy, never a single drug.

IMPLEMENTATION:

DRUG INTERACTIONS: See specific drugs for information.

ADMINISTRATION AND DOSAGE: In chemotherapeutic treatment, the concomitant use of two drugs, isoniazid and rifampin, which are bactericidal both intra- and extracellularly, is the treatment of choice for uncomplicated pulmonary tuberculosis. The duration of therapy is usually nine months, or six months after conversion of the sputum to culture negativity with therapy lasting a minimum of nine months. Sputum conversion usually occurs within one to three months after the initiation of isoniazid and rifampin therapy. When necessary, the combination of pyrazinamide and streptomycin may be used to substitute for either one of the bactericidal drugs above. However, there is some controversy over the effectiveness of this shorter, nine-month course of therapy when isoniazid is not used. Currently, intermittent therapy with isoniazid and rifampin is being investigated. The American Thoracic Society recommends that these two drugs be given daily for two to eight weeks, then switched to twice per week for a total of 52 weeks or 39 weeks respectively. The minimum duration of therapy is nine months. Daily dosage recommendations for adults are isoniazid 300 mg and rifampin 600 mg. Twice-weekly dosage recommendations for adults are isoniazid, 15 mg/kg and rifampin, 600 mg. The American Thoracic Society recommends intermittent therapy only for uncomplicated pulmonary tuberculosis.

Whenever a combination of drugs does not exert the effect of two intra- and extracellularly bactericidal drugs, then therapy must continue for the traditional 18 to 24 months. This usually occurs when bacteriostatic drugs are used.

Drug resistance should be suspected if the patient has been treated for tuberculosis in the past. Drugs used in the past regimen may be used again, while waiting for sensitivity studies, if at least two new drugs are also prescribed. Drug resistance is low in United States–acquired infections, but high in tuberculosis infections acquired from Asian, South and Central American and African sources. Drug resistance is less likely to occur when two bactericidal drugs are given rather than when one bactericidal drug is given in combination with bacteriostatic drugs.

Antitubercular drugs should be prescribed in single daily doses unless contraindicated. All drugs, unless stated otherwise, should be taken at the same time each day, preferably in the morning. This is especially important with the combination of isoniazid and rifampin in order to decrease the chance of drug resistance occurring. When poor compliance is suspected, the provider should initiate direct supervision of administration of medications.

Antitubercular drugs have been categorized as first-line (isoniazid, rifampin), second-line (ethambutol, pyrazinamide and streptomycin), and tertiary (P-aminosalicylic acid, ethionamide, cycloserine, capreomycin, and kanamycin.) Of these products, all are bactericidal except ethambutol, P-aminosalicylic acid, ethionamide, and cycloserine, which are bacteriostatic. Streptomycin, capreomycin, and kanamycin require IM administration, while the other products may be given orally.

IMPLEMENTATION CONSIDERATIONS:

—Obtain a thorough health history: previous history of tuberculosis, travel outside the United States, known contacts; history of impairment of liver or kidney; decreased hearing; diabetes mellitus; seizure disorders; alcoholism; malnourishment; pyridoxine deficiency; neurologic disorders; presence of allergies; medications which might produce drug interactions; pregnancy or breast-feeding.

—Obtain thorough baseline physical examination and laboratory tests, including evaluations for ophthalmology and audiometry.

—Remember that potential problems due to the long-term nature of the regimen are most likely to be poor compliance, drug toxicity and drug resistance.

—Patients who are over 60, those who have renal or liver impairment, or those who are of unusually small stature may require decreased dosages.

—The patient should be considered infectious as long as tubercle bacilli are visible microscopically in the sputum. The patient and family need to understand this and how it affects their relationships and activity.

—Report all documented cases to the local health department.

—Establishment of good rapport with the patient and family will be of primary importance in developing an individualized teaching plan, and in obtaining compliance with the therapeutic regimen. Making yourself available to phone calls to discuss progress is helpful.

—Patients should learn to respect the medications they are taking and to keep them out of the reach of small children or others who might take them inadvertently.

WHAT THE PATIENT NEEDS TO KNOW:

—It is very important to take these drugs as ordered. If you forget a dose, take it as soon as you remember, unless it is almost time for the next dose. In that case, the missed dose should not be taken and the regular dosing schedule should be followed. Forgetting to take a dose, or failure to continue with one of the medications may cause the organisms in your body to develop a resistance to the medication. This allows the disease process to continue, with continued risk for you and your close family members and contacts.

—Tuberculosis is a disease that is required to be reported to the local health department. Family members and your close contacts will need to be screened for tuberculosis also.

—This health problem requires long-term treatment. You will need to return for weekly and then monthly visits while you are undergoing therapy.

—You will continue to need periodic sputum examinations, chest x-rays and other laboratory work. This is important in monitoring your recovery progress.

—The medications you take are very powerful, and sometimes produce side effects. Many of these effects are very minor, but they should be evaluated by someone who can make that judgment. Therefore, any new or troublesome symptoms should be reported promptly to your health care provider.

—During the initial period of your illness, you must remember that you are contagious. You must make every effort to cover your mouth when coughing, dispose of sputum and soiled tissues carefully, and act to protect those around you.

—Remember that your whole body is involved in fighting this disease. Your body needs adequate rest, nourishing food, and as restful and quiet a recovery environment as possible.

EVALUATION:

ADVERSE REACTIONS: There are a substantial number of side effects from the various drugs used in antitubercular therapy. Some are mild, while some represent major challenges to the body. Because of the prevalence of adverse reactions, consult this section for each drug involved in the therapeutic regimen.

PARAMETERS TO MONITOR: It is essential for effective treatment that careful monitoring of both bacteriologic studies and toxic side effects of drugs is done regularly. Baseline sputum smears and culture and sensitivity studies, chest x-ray, weight, and renal, hepatic and hematopoietic studies should be obtained. Sputum smears and cultures should be collected every two weeks until three consecutive negative cultures have been obtained. They should then be obtained monthly until therapy is completed. In general, sensitivity studies are required for initial assessment and when bacteriologic response is poor. (Poor bacteriologic response is observed when there is no gradual decrease in the culture size or no conversion to negative cultures.) Sputum conversion usually occurs in one to three months if the patient is on a combination isoniazid and rifampin regimen, or one month longer if he is on another regimen. There is a difference of opinion as to how often to order chest x-rays after the initial one is obtained. It is suggested that they either be obtained when there is a poor bacteriologic response, or on a periodic basis of every two to three months during therapy. Patients are usually seen every one to two weeks for the first two months of treatment, and then on a monthly basis or more often as indicated. *Parameters to monitor each visit:* Follow compliance with total therapeutic regimen, signs and symptoms of toxicity or adverse side effects; sputum smears and cultures; and improvement of clinical syndrome: weight gain, reduced fever, reduced cough, improved sense of well-being and negative bacteriologic studies. *Parameters to monitor after completion of therapy:* Upon completion of therapy, cultures should be obtained every month for six months then every three months for six months.

Marna J. Ross

AMINOSALICYLIC ACID DRUGS

ACTION OF THE DRUG: Aminosalicylic acid (or Para-Amino PASA) and its salts are bacteriostatic for *Mycobacterium tuberculosis.* Aminosalicylic acid competes with the bacterial enzyme systems for PABA and inhibits bacterial folic acid synthesis. It inhibits bacterial resistance to isoniazid and streptomycin.

ASSESSMENT:

INDICATIONS: Aminosalicylic acid and its salts are indicated for use (in conjunction with either streptomycin, isoniazid or both) in the treatment of pulmonary and extrapulmonary tuberculosis. It is used to delay resistance to streptomycin and isoniazid. It should always be used in conjunction with other antitubercular drugs.

SUBJECTIVE-OBJECTIVE: See Antitubercular Drugs introductory section.

PLAN:

CONTRAINDICATIONS: Severe hypersensitivity to aminosalicylic acid and its salts; hypersensitivity to compounds containing *p*-aminophenyl groups such as sulfonamides and certain hair dyes; and hypersensitivity to other salicylates. Potassium aminosalicylate is contraindicated in patients with hyperkalemia or renal impairment; and sodium aminosalicylate is contraindicated in patients on sodium restriction or who have congestive heart failure.

WARNINGS: Safety for use during pregnancy or breast-feeding has not been established.

PRECAUTIONS: Aminosalicylates should be used with extreme caution in individuals with renal impairment, hepatic impairment, gastric ulcer, goiter, G-6-PD deficiency, or blood dyscrasias. Potassium, calcium, and sodium aminosalicylates should be used with extreme caution in individuals with disorders which would be adversely affected by increases in these electrolytes. (For example, potassium aminosalicylate should be used with caution in Addison's disease, acute dehydration, extensive tissue breakdown, concurrent digitalis or diuretic use; calcium aminosalicylate should be used cautiously in patients with carcinoma, hyperparathyroidism, hyperthyroidism, sarcoidosis, nephrocalcinosis; and sodium aminosalicylate should be carefully used in patients with severe liver disease, congestive heart failure, or those on sodium restrictions.) Patients receiving anticoagulant therapy may require dosage adjustments while on aminosalicylates. Aminosalicylic acid and its salts decrease the absorption of rifampin, and should not be used concurrently. If hypersensitivity symptoms develop, all drugs should be stopped and further evaluation made. Hepatic damage, pancreatitis, and nephritis may occur if aminosalicylates are continued in the presence of hypersensitivity reactions. Individuals over sixty are more likely to be susceptible to adverse effects of this drug and may require reduced dosages. They may also be more susceptible to developing anemias.

IMPLEMENTATION:

DRUG INTERACTIONS: Aminosalicylic acid and its salts may increase the effects of oral anticoagulants, anticonvulsants, barbiturates, aminopyrine, and isoniazid. They may decrease the effects of rifampin, pyrazinamide, and sulfa drugs. Aminosalicylic acid and its salts may be inhibited by Benadryl and other anticholinergics. They inhibit the gastrointestinal absorption and urinary excretion of B_{12}. Probenecid and sulfinpyrazone may potentiate the aminosalicylates and thus increase the risk of toxic side effects. PABA may antagonize the bacteriostatic effect of aminosalicylates and should not be given concurrently. Tetracycline should be given at least three hours apart from calcium aminosalicylate. Potassium-sparing diuretics, potassium-containing medications, salt substitutes, potassium supplements, and low salt milk should not be given concurrently with potassium aminosalicylate as hyperkalemia may occur. When aminosalicylic products are taken with aspirin, excess stomach irritation, bleeding and possible ulceration may occur. Acidifying agents such as ascorbic acid and ammonium chloride may increase the probability of crystalluria occurring. Aminosalicylic acid and its salts may also affect laboratory values in the following manner: interfere with urine urobilinogen determinations, may give false-positive to vanillyl/mandelic acid determinations, acetoacetic acid tests, and copper sulfate tests.

ADMINISTRATION AND DOSAGE: Aminosalicylic acid and its salts are readily absorbed from the gastrointestinal tract. Peak serum levels appear in 1.5 to 2 hours after ingestion. The drug is a gastric irritant and should be given in three to four equally divided doses with food. Aminosalicylates are used mainly in re-treatment regimens to prevent bacterial resistance to the more potent antitubercular drugs, and as a second or third drug in antitubercular therapy for children under the age of two. Aminosalicylates should always be administered with either streptomycin, isoniazid, or both of these drugs. Aminosalicylates deteriorate rapidly when in contact with water, sunlight, or heat. In solution, aminosalicylic acid is very unstable. Aminosalicylic acid is administered in doses of ten to twelve grams per day. When aminosalicylic salts are used, dosages must be increased to obtain the equivalent amount of aminosalicylic acid. Sodium and potassium aminosalicylates should be increased 38% and 24% respectively.

IMPLEMENTATION CONSIDERATIONS:

—Obtain a complete health history: history of hypersensitivity to aminosalicylic acid and its salts, compounds containing *p*-aminophenyl groups, aspirin, or other salicylates; history of renal or hepatic impairment, gastric or peptic ulcer disease, G-6-PD deficiency; seizure disorders, congestive heart failure, hyperkalemia, blood dyscrasia, or current sodium restricted diet; taking anticoagulants, potassium-containing medications, digitalis preparations, diuretics, anticonvulsants, probenecid, or other drugs which may produce drug interactions; or possibility of pregnancy.

—High concentrations of the drug are excreted in the urine. This may cause crystalluria and hematuria. High fluid intake and keeping the urine neutral or alkaline with absorbable antacids or fruit juices will decrease the risk of crystalluria.

—Patients receiving anticoagulant therapy will require monitoring of prothrombin times and may need reduced anticoagulant dosages.

—Gastric distress usually disappears after several days; however, if it continues, the drug may need to be discontinued.

—Patient acceptance and tolerance of the drug is poor, usually because of the unpleasant taste in solution, hypersensitivity reactions, and gastric irritation.

WHAT THE PATIENT NEEDS TO KNOW:
—This drug should be taken exactly as ordered.

—To decrease the chance of stomach irritation, or a bitter or sour aftertaste, this drug should be taken with food. If irritation persists, notify your health provider.

—Some people experience side effects from taking this drug. Notify your health provider if you notice any new or troublesome symptoms.

—Stop taking the drug and notify the health provider immediately if any of the following occur: sudden onset of a fever, fatigue, sore throat, joint pain, headache, or itching, as these may be indications of an allergic reaction to the drug.

—Diabetic patients using copper sulfate tests, such as Benedict's solution or Clinitest tablets, may obtain false-positive results while using this drug. Check with your provider on how to monitor urine before changing diet or insulin dosage.

—This drug may color the urine red when it comes into contact with chlorine bleach such as that in toilet bowel cleaners.

—Drink lots of liquid (two quarts a day) while you are taking this medicine.

—Store medicine in a light-resistant, air-tight container. If it turns brownish or purplish, it should be discarded.

—The dry powder form of the medicine should be dissolved in water and stirred immediately before taking.

—Enteric-coated tablets should be swallowed whole to keep the medicine from irritating the stomach.

—This drug and rifampin should be taken at least eight hours apart so that rifampin will be fully absorbed.

EVALUATION:

ADVERSE REACTIONS: *Cardiovascular:* vasculitis. *CNS:* encephalopathy. *Gastrointestinal:* abdominal pain or burning, anorexia, diarrhea, hepatitis, jaundice, nausea, vomiting. *Genitourinary:* albuminuria, crystalluria, glycosuria, hematuria, renal irritation. *Metabolic:* acidosis (with aminosalicylic acid only), goiter (with or without symptoms), hypokalemia. *Hematopoietic:* agranulocytosis, eosinophilia, hemolytic anemia, leukopenia, Loeffler's syndrome, thrombocytopenia. *Hypersensitivity:* fever, infectious mononucleosis-like syndrome, skin eruptions.

OVERDOSAGE: *Symptoms:* severe nausea, vomiting, abdominal pain, diarrhea.

PARAMETERS TO MONITOR: Monitor for therapeutic effect. Periodic monitoring of renal, hepatic, hematopoietic function and serum electrolytes should be done. Patients should be observed for signs and symptoms of hypersensitivity reactions: abrupt onset of high fever which may be intermittent or spiking, or gradual onset of low-grade fever, generalized malaise, joint pains, sore throat, skin rash. Observe for other adverse or toxic reactions including gastrointestinal irritation, goiter, or hypothyroidism. Prothrombin times should be monitored regularly in patients on anticoagulant therapy. During each visit the patient should be questioned closely on pill ingestion to determine compliance.

P-AMINOSALICYLIC ACID (PASA)

PRODUCTS (TRADE NAME):
Aminosalicylic Acid (Available in 500 mg tablets and 500 mg enteric-coated tablets.)
DRUG SPECIFICS:
Aminosalicylic acid should be administered with isoniazid, streptomycin, or both of these drugs.
ADMINISTRATION AND DOSAGE SPECIFICS:
Adults: 10 to 12 grams/day po in two to three equally divided doses.
Children: 200 to 300 mg/kg/day po in three to four equally divided doses.

POTASSIUM AMINOSALICYLATE

PRODUCTS (TRADE NAME):
Teebacin Kalium (Available in 500 mg and 3 gram powder.)
DRUG SPECIFICS:
1.24 grams of potassium aminosalicylate equals 1 gm aminosalicylic acid and contains 6.5 mEq of potassium. Administer with isoniazid and/or streptomycin.
ADMINISTRATION AND DOSAGE SPECIFICS:
Adults: 10/12 gm aminosalicylic acid or equivalent po per day in two to three equally divided doses, up to 20 mg/kg per day.

Children: 200 to 300 mg/kg/day po in three to four equally divided doses.

SODIUM AMINOSALICYLATE

PRODUCTS (TRADE NAME):
  PAS Sodium, Teebacin (Available in 500 mg, one gram tablets; and powder.)
DRUG SPECIFICS:
  1.39 grams of sodium aminosalicylate equals 1 gram aminosalicylic acid, and contains 6.7 mEq of sodium. Administer with isoniazid and/or streptomycin. Sodium aminosalicylate solutions should be prepared within 24 hours of administration. The solution should not be used if its color is darker than when it was first prepared.
  ADMINISTRATION AND DOSAGE SPECIFICS:
  Adults: 10 to 12 gm/day of aminosalicylate or 14 to 16 grams/day po of aminosalicylate sodium in two to three equally divided doses.
  Children: 275 to 420 mg/kg/day po in three to four equally divided doses.

Marna J. Ross

CAPREOMYCIN SULFATE

ACTION OF THE DRUG: Capreomycin is bacteriocidal for *Mycobacterium tuberculosis.* The mode of action is unknown; however, its toxicities are similar to those of the aminoglycosides.

ASSESSMENT:

INDICATIONS: Capreomycin is indicated for use in active pulmonary tuberculosis when the primary drugs of choice cannot be used due to ineffectiveness, drug toxicity, or resistance.
  SUBJECTIVE-OBJECTIVE: See Antitubercular Drugs section

PLAN:

CONTRAINDICATIONS: Do not use with hypersensitivity to capreomycin, concurrent and/or sequential administration of streptomycin, other aminoglycosides, or other ototoxic or nephrotoxic drugs.
  WARNINGS: Safety for use during pregnancy or in infants and children has not been established. Extreme caution should be used when administering capreomycin to patients with renal insufficiency, eighth cranial nerve damage, liver disease, a history of allergies (especially to drugs), myasthenia gravis, or Parkinson's disease.

PRECAUTIONS: Any evidence of decreasing renal function or a BUN above 30 mg/100 ml indicates the need for careful evaluation of the patient and a reduction in the dosage, or withdrawal of the drug. Hypokalemia may occur during therapy without potassium supplementation.

IMPLEMENTATION:

DRUG INTERACTIONS: Concurrent and/or sequential systemic or topical administration of aminoglycosides with capreomycin should be avoided as the risk for ototoxicity and nephrotoxicity is increased. Concurrent administration of anesthetics or neuromuscular blocking agents may increase the risk of neuromuscular blockade occurring. The risk of nephrotoxicity is increased when capreomycin is given concurrently with cephalothin or cephaloridine. Concurrent and/or sequential administration of cisplatin, ethacrynic acid, furosemide, mercaptomerin or vancomycin increases the risk for ototoxicity and nephrotoxicity. Concurrent and/or sequential administration of systemic polymyxins increases the risk for nephrotoxicity and neuromuscular blockade.

PRODUCTS (TRADE NAME):
Capastat Sulfate (Available in 1 gm/5 ml vial for injection.)

ADMINISTRATION AND DOSAGE: Capreomycin is given by deep intramuscular injection. Peak serum levels occur in one to two hours after administration. Capreomycin must be given with at least one other antitubercular agent.

Adult: 1 gm IM daily (not to exceed 20 mg/kg/day) for 60 to 120 days, then 1 gm IM 2 to 3 times per week. The reduced dosage may continue for 18 to 24 months. Reduced dosages may be required in the elderly, unusually small adults, and in individuals with renal impairment.

IMPLEMENTATION CONSIDERATIONS:
—Obtain a thorough health history: history of hypersensitivity to capreomycin, auditory or vestibular impairment, renal insufficiency, liver disease, allergies (especially to drugs), myasthenia gravis and/or Parkinson's disease, drugs taken concurrently which may cause drug interactions, or recent use of any ototoxic or nephrotoxic drugs, possibility of pregnancy.

—Obtain baseline renal, hematopoietic, liver and serum electrolyte studies. Also obtain baseline audiometric measurements and assessment of vestibular function.

—Ascertain if the patient has any disease process or is on any drug which may be affected by hypokalemia.

WHAT THE PATIENT NEEDS TO KNOW:
—This medication should be taken exactly as ordered.
—Some people develop side effects after taking this drug. Some symptoms are mild, and some are more serious. Be certain to notify your health provider if you notice any new or troublesome symptoms.
—Stop taking the drug and notify your health provider immediately if you experience any of the following: hearing loss, ringing or buzzing in the

> ears, a sense of fullness in the ears, dizziness, clumsiness, unsteadiness, or loss of balance.

EVALUATION:

ADVERSE REACTIONS: *CNS:* headache. *EENT:* ototoxicity: hearing loss, tinnitus, vertigo. *Genitourinary:* nephrotoxicity: elevated BUN and nonprotein nitrogen, proteinuria, casts, hematuria, albuminuria, leukocytes, tubular necrosis, decreased creatinine clearance. *Hematopoietic:* eosinophilia, leukocytosis, leukopenia. *Hepatic:* abnormal liver function tests. *Hypersensitivity:* maculopapular rash associated with febrile reaction, urticaria. *Other:* muscle weakness, pain and induration or excessive bleeding at injection site, sterile abscesses.

PARAMETERS TO MONITOR: Audiometric measurement, assessment of vestibular function, and renal, liver, serum electrolytes and urinalysis studies should be done prior to and at regular intervals during therapy. Audiometric testing should be done weekly to detect high-frequency hearing loss. Renal function studies should be monitored weekly throughout therapy. Serum potassium levels should be monitored on a monthly basis. Hypokalemia is less likely to occur when capreomycin is given on a two to three times per week schedule rather than every day.

Marna J. Ross

CYCLOSERINE

ACTION OF THE DRUG: Cycloserine is a bacteriostatic antitubercular agent. It may be bactericidal depending on its concentration at the site of the infection and the susceptibility of the organisms. It inhibits cell wall synthesis in susceptible gram-positive and gram-negative bacteria and in *Mycobacterium tuberculosis*.

ASSESSMENT:

INDICATIONS: Cycloserine is indicated in the treatment of active pulmonary and extrapulmonary tuberculosis when other primary drugs (streptomycin, isoniazid, rifampin, ethambutol) have failed. It is thus considered a third-line drug. It should always be used in conjunction with other antitubercular agents. It is also indicated in the treatment of acute urinary tract infections caused by susceptible gram-positive or gram-negative bacteria, or mycobacteria that have been unresponsive to conventional therapy. However, it is usually less effective than other antimicrobial agents used to treat urinary tract infections caused by bacteria other than mycobacteria.

SUBJECTIVE-OBJECTIVE: See Antitubercular Drugs section.

PLAN:

CONTRAINDICATIONS: Hypersensitivity to cycloserine; epilepsy; depression, severe anxiety, or psychosis; severe renal insufficiency; excessive concurrent use of alcohol.

WARNINGS: Cycloserine should be discontinued or the dosage reduced if the patient develops allergic dermatitis or symptoms of CNS toxicity: convulsions, psychosis, somnolence, depression, confusion, hyperreflexia, headache, tremor, vertigo, paresis, or dysarthria. Cycloserine should be stopped immediately when drug-induced psychotic episodes occur. The patient should be watched closely and suicide precautions taken as necessary until the episode subsides. Recovery usually takes two weeks. Toxicity is related to blood levels above 30 mcg/ml. The ratio of toxic to therapeutic dosage is small.

PRECAUTIONS: Safe use in pregnancy and in children has not been established. Caution should be used when giving cycloserine to individuals with impaired renal function: dosage may need to be reduced. Blood levels should be determined weekly for patients who have impaired renal function, those who are receiving more than 500 mg per day, or those who show symptoms of toxicity.

IMPLEMENTATION:

DRUG INTERACTIONS: Cycloserine taken concurrently with isoniazid may increase the risk of CNS toxicity occurring. This combination should be avoided, or dosage adjustment should be made and the patient monitored closely. Ethionamide potentiates the toxic CNS side effects of cycloserine. Cycloserine potentiates phenytoin action and increases the excretion of Vitamin B12. Taken concurrently with alcohol cycloserine may increase the risk of seizures occurring.

PRODUCTS (TRADE NAME):
Seromycin pulvules (Available in 250 mg capsules.)

ADMINISTRATION AND DOSAGE: Cycloserine is readily absorbed from the gastrointestinal tract with peak serum levels occurring in three to four hours. Large doses are not required in the treatment of urinary tract tuberculosis as the drug is very highly concentrated in the urine.

Adults: 250 mg po every 12 hours for 2 weeks. If no adverse effects occur, this dosage may be maintained or increased to 250 mg two to four times per day. Dosages should not exceed 1 gm per day. Monitor by blood levels.

IMPLEMENTATION CONSIDERATIONS:

—Obtain a thorough health history: previous drug history, other drugs which may cause drug interactions, allergies, epilepsy, renal insufficiency, psychiatric disturbances, alcohol intake, possibility of pregnancy.

—Teaching patient and family is important in obtaining compliance with this long-term therapy.

—Health provider and family should observe patient for any personality changes.

—Concurrent use of alcohol may increase the risk of convulsions and other toxic side effects.

—The elderly, unusually small adults, and patients with renal impairment may require reduced dosages.

—CNS toxicity may occur with blood levels above 30 mcg/ml. Patients receiving more than 500 mg/day should be monitored closely for CNS toxicity.

—The patient may need supplementary Vitamin B12.

WHAT THE PATIENT NEEDS TO KNOW:

—This drug should be taken exactly as ordered.

—Some patients experience side effects after taking this drug. Most of these are mild, but some are more serious. If you notice any new or uncomfortable symptoms, be certain to notify your health provider.

—Stop taking the drug and notify your health provider immediately if any of the following occur: extreme drowsiness, confusion, tremors, dizziness, headache, behavior changes, numbness, and/or skin rash.

—Because this drug often causes drowsiness, do not perform activities which require alertness until the effects of the drug on you personally are known.

—Do not drink alcohol while taking this drug, as it may increase the risk of more severe side effects.

—If you begin to feel uncharacteristically depressed and unhappy, stop taking the drug and notify your health provider at once.

EVALUATION:

ADVERSE REACTIONS: *CNS:* aggression, anxiety, character changes, coma, confusion, convulsions, drowsiness, dysarthria, headache, hyperreflexia, hyperirritability, loss of memory, nervousness, paresis, paresthesias, possible suicidal tendencies and other psychotic symptoms, tremor, vertigo. *Hypersensitivity:* skin rash. *Other:* elevated serum transaminase levels, occasionally Vitamin B12 and/or folic acid deficiency.

OVERDOSAGE: *Signs and symptoms:* CNS toxicity: depression with drowsiness, somnolence, dizziness, hyperreflexia, mental confusion, convulsions, and allergic dermatitis. *Treatment:* Symptomatic and supportive therapy. Pyridoxine [300 mg or more daily] and anticonvulsants may be given to relieve convulsions.

PARAMETERS TO MONITOR: Monitor for therapeutic effect and adverse reactions. Serum blood levels should be obtained periodically, drawn before the first dose of the day. Therapeutic blood levels range from 25 mcg/ml to 30 mcg/ml. In patients with stable but impaired renal function or patients receiving more than 500 mg of cycloserine per day, serum levels should be monitored on a weekly basis. Levels above 30 mcg/ml are associated with increased risk of toxicity and should be avoided. Develop a flow chart of symptoms and question the patient at each visit concerning these symptoms of toxicity.

Marna J. Ross

ETHAMBUTOL HCL

ACTION OF THE DRUG: Ethambutol is bacteriostatic against *Mycobacterium tuberculosis*. It is thought to inhibit the synthesis of RNA in mycobacteria. It is able to reduce the incidence of mycobacterial resistance to isoniazid when the two drugs are used concurrently.

ASSESSMENT:

INDICATIONS: Ethambutol is an effective antimycobacterial agent against *Mycobacterium tuberculosis, M. bovis*, and strains of *M. kansasii*. It is indicated in the initial treatment of tuberculosis when drug resistance or toxicity does not allow the use of a more effective bactericidal drug, and in the re-treatment of tuberculosis. Ethambutol must be used with at least one other antitubercular agent.

SUBJECTIVE-OBJECTIVE: Refer to major discussion under Antitubercular Drugs.

PLAN:

CONTRAINDICATIONS: Do not use in the presence of hypersensitivity to ethambutol; preexisting optic neuritis; children under the age of thirteen; and individuals who cannot cooperate in vision testing.

WARNINGS: Ethambutol may have adverse effects on vision. These effects are generally dose-related.

PRECAUTIONS: Ethambutol should be used in pregnancy only when the potential benefits outweigh the risks to the fetus, as not all the effects of the drug on the fetus are known. Patients with impaired renal function will require reduced dosages, as determined by serum ethambutol levels. Benefits compared to risks should be weighed and caution should be used when administering ethambutol to individuals with impaired vision: cataracts, recurrent inflammatory conditions of the eye, optic neuritis, and diabetic retinopathy. Visual acuity is much more difficult to evaluate in these individuals. Ethambutol may be used in optic neuritis if the clinical judgment of the physician determines that it may be used. Reduced dosages may be required in patients with gout.

IMPLEMENTATION:

DRUG INTERACTIONS: No significant interactions reported.
PRODUCTS (TRADE NAME):
Myambutol (Available in 100 mg and 400 mg tablets.)
ADMINISTRATION AND DOSAGE: Ethambutol is rapidly absorbed and peaks in the serum in two to four hours. It should be given only once every twenty-four hours. Ethambutol must be used in conjunction with at least one other antitubercular drug. When only one bactericidal drug is used in combination with this medication, therapy will generally last 18 to 24 months. It has been used in twice-weekly regimens.

Ethambutol may be taken with food. Dosage must be reduced in patients with renal impairment. Dosages are for adults only.

Initial treatment: 15 mg/kg po in a single daily dose.

Re-treatment: 25 mg/kg po in a single daily dose for 60 days. Dosage is then decreased to 15 mg/kg per day.

IMPLEMENTATION CONSIDERATIONS:

—Obtain a thorough health history: history of hypersensitivity to ethambutol, presence of optic neuritis or other eye disorders, gout, impaired renal function or pregnancy.

—Order baseline ophthalmologic exam (including visual acuity) and renal, hepatic, and hematopoietic studies (including uric acid levels).

—Ethambutol may precipitate an attack of gout in susceptible people.

—Optic neuritis is rare on doses of 15 mg/kg/day. Its incidence increases with higher dosages. It may be unilateral or bilateral. Effects are usually reversible if drug is discontinued immediately.

—Refer to antitubercular drugs section for additional material.

—While the patient is on 25 mg/kg/day dosage, monthly eye exams are advised.

WHAT THE PATIENT NEEDS TO KNOW:

—Take medication exactly as ordered. Establish a routine in taking the medication so you are less likely to forget it.

—Keep medication out of the reach of children, or others for whom it is not prescribed.

—Ethambutol may be taken with food if stomach upset occurs.

—This is a powerful drug, and some people experience side effects from it. Notify your provider immediately if you experience any blurring, loss or fading of vision, eye pain, development of red-green color blindness, or numbness of the extremities. If you notice any new or uncomfortable symptoms, report these promptly to your health provider.

—This drug may cause an attack of gout in people who may have a tendency for this problem. If you having any swelling of joints, tense, hot skin over joints, or joint pain, notify your health provider.

EVALUATION:

ADVERSE REACTIONS: *CNS:* dizziness, disorientation, headache, mental confusion, peripheral neuritis, possible hallucinations. *Dermatologic:* dermatitis, pruritus. *Gastrointestinal:* abdominal pain, anorexia, nausea, vomiting. *Musculo-skeletal:* signs and symptoms of gout, joint pain and swelling. *Ophthalmologic:* optic neuritis: loss of vision and color discrimination, loss of visual acuity, central and peripheral scotoma. *Other:* anaphylactic reactions, bloody sputum, chills, elevated serum uric acid levels, fever, malaise.

PARAMETERS TO MONITOR: Obtain baseline studies for renal, hepatic, hematopoietic and visual functioning. Establish a flow chart to monitor therapeutic effects and adverse reactions. Periodically assess symptoms of gout, changes in visual acuity and subjective eye symptoms. Individuals with renal impairment should have serum levels of ethambutol monitored regularly to determine dosage levels. If the patient receives more than 15 mg/kg of ethambutol/day an ophthalmological exam should be performed on a monthly basis.

Marna J. Ross

ETHIONAMIDE

ACTION OF THE DRUG: Ethionamide is a bacteriostatic antitubercular agent. Its mechanism of action is unknown.

ASSESSMENT:

INDICATIONS: Ethionamide is indicated for the treatment of active pulmonary and extrapulmonary tuberculosis when other primary drugs have failed. It should always be used in conjunction with other antitubercular agents.

SUBJECTIVE-OBJECTIVE: See Antitubercular Drugs section.

PLAN:

CONTRAINDICATIONS: Do not use with severe hypersensitivity to ethionamide or in patients with severe liver damage.

WARNINGS: The use of ethionamide should be avoided during pregnancy and in women of childbearing potential. Teratogenic effects have been reported in animals. Safety during breast-feeding has not been established. Optimum dosage levels for children have not been determined. Patients who are hypersensitive to isoniazid, pyrazinamide, niacin, or other chemically related substances may also be hypersensitive to ethionamide.

PRECAUTIONS: Ethionamide should be used with caution in patients who have diabetes mellitus. Their disease may become more difficult to control and they are more likely to develop hepatitis while on ethionamide. The drug should be stopped if a skin rash appears as it may progress to exfoliative dermatitis.

IMPLEMENTATION:

DRUG INTERACTIONS: Ethionamide may intensify the adverse effects of other antitubercular agents taken concurrently. In combination with cycloserine, toxic CNS side effects, including convulsions, are much more likely to occur. Alcohol may also increase the risk of toxic CNS side effects.

PRODUCTS (TRADE NAME):

Trecator-SC (Available in 250 mg tablets.)

ADMINISTRATION AND DOSAGE: Ethionamide is readily absorbed after it is taken orally, and peak serum levels appear in approximately three hours. It should be given with meals or antacids to reduce gastric irritation. Approximately one third of the patients on ethionamide cannot seem to tolerate its therapeutic dose. Patients may be able to tolerate two thirds to one half the therapeutic dose, but the efficacy of these reduced dosages is uncertain. This is important to note as ethionamide is often used in re-treatment regimens, or in regimens where primary drugs have failed, and thus is often found in combination with marginally effective antitubercular drugs.

Adults: 250 mg po twice daily. Every five days the dose may be increased by 125 mg/po day, until one gram per day is given. Dosages should never exceed one gram per day. The usual adult dose is 0.5 mg to 1 gram po per day. Patients with impaired renal function do not required reduced dosages as only one percent of the dose is excreted in active form.

IMPLEMENTATION CONSIDERATIONS:

—Obtain a complete health history: previous drug history, including any drugs which may cause drug interactions; allergies; or if patient is pregnant.

—Ethionamide should be stopped immediately if a skin rash occurs.

—Ethionamide may cause gastric upset and should be given with meals or antacids.

—Determine if patient has diabetes mellitus.

—Obtain baseline liver function studies.

—Patients may require an antiemetic to control nausea and vomiting.

—The concurrent administration of pyridoxine 50 to 100 mg/day is recommended to prevent neuropathies.

WHAT THE PATIENT NEEDS TO KNOW:

—This drug should be taken exactly as prescribed. If you have any difficulty doing so, notify your health provider promptly.

—This drug sometimes causes gastric upset, including diarrhea, nausea and vomiting. The drug should be taken with meals or with antacids such as Maalox to minimize the upset. Notify your health provider if these side effects continue to increase in severity.

—Many people experience side effects while taking medications. If you notice any new or uncomfortable symptoms these should be reported. Notify the provider immediately if you develop a skin rash, loss of appetite, yellowing of the skin or eyes, general fatigue, depression, or blurred vision.

—Patients with diabetes mellitus may find that their blood sugar is harder to control while on ethionamide.

—Alcohol should be avoided as it increases the risk of side effects.

—Ethionamide may leave a metallic taste in the mouth.

EVALUATION:

ADVERSE REACTIONS: *Cardiovascular:* severe postural hypotension. *CNS:* optic neuritis, peripheral neuritis, psychic disturbances (especially mental depression.) *Dermatologic:* exfoliative dermatitis, rash. *Gastrointestinal:* anorexia, diarrhea, epigastric distress, hepatitis, jaundice, metallic taste, nausea, sialorrhea, stomatitis, vomiting. *Hematopoietic:* thrombocytopenia. *Other:* alopecia, gynecomastia, impotence, pellagra-like syndrome, weight loss.

PARAMETERS TO MONITOR: Monitor for therapeutic effects and adverse reactions. Renal, hepatic and hematologic studies should be monitored periodically throughout therapy. Prior to initiating therapy, and every two to four weeks during therapy, SGOT and SGPT levels should be monitored. However, elevated serum levels may not necessarily be predictive of clinical hepatitis. The levels may return to normal. Compliance may be determined by questioning the patient closely about pill ingestion. Diabetic patients should be followed closely to ensure control of their diabetes, and to determine that they are not developing hepatitis.

Marna J. Ross

ISONIAZID

ACTION OF THE DRUG: Isoniazid is bacteriocidal toward actively growing mycobacteria found both intra- and extracellularly. It is bacteriostatic toward non-actively growing mycobacteria.

ASSESSMENT:

INDICATIONS: *Chemoprophylaxis:* Isoniazid is the drug of choice for prophylactic treatment of tuberculosis in individuals who are at high risk for developing the disease. *Chemotherapeutic:* Isoniazid is one of the major drugs of choice in the treatment of active tuberculosis. It is indicated for use in combination with other antitubercular agents against susceptible mycobacteria.

SUBJECTIVE: In pulmonary tuberculosis the patient may be asymptomatic or exhibit insidious onset of weight loss, fatigue, fevers, night sweats, hemoptysis, and a progressive cough which eventually becomes productive. The patient may present a history of a recent close contact with an infected person, history of past tuberculosis infection, history of recent conversion to a positive tuberculin skin test reaction or positive chest X-ray for tuberculosis. Tuberculosis in non-pulmonary sites will have symptomatology related to the specific site.

OBJECTIVE: General signs of pulmonary tuberculosis on physical examination may range from none to fever, post-tussive apical rales, and cough which may be productive. The patient may have a positive skin test and chest x-ray for tuberculosis. Laboratory data may show a positive smear or culture for tubercle bacilli. Other objective findings may be specific to a non-pulmonary site of infection.

PLAN:

CONTRAINDICATIONS: Isoniazid is contraindicated when there is a history of hypersensitivity to the drug, isoniazid-induced hepatic injury, acute hepatic disease, and/or severe untoward reactions to isoniazid. Prophylactic use of isoniazid is contraindicated in pregnant women and should be deferred until the postpartum period.

WARNINGS: Isoniazid has been associated with hepatitis, severe liver damage, and death. These complications may occur at any time during therapy. Patients who are elderly or who drink alcohol on a daily basis are at greater risk for developing these complications. The drug should be discontinued promptly when signs and symptoms of hepatitis or liver damage appear, and further evaluation made. Breast-fed infants of mothers taking isoniazid should be carefully monitored for adverse side effects.

PRECAUTIONS: Isoniazid should be used with caution in patients with a history of alcoholism, convulsive disorders, hepatic function disorders, and severe renal impairment. There is a possibility that the patient may be hypersensitive to isoniazid if there is a history of hypersensitivity to ethionamide, pyrazinamide, niacin or other chemically related drugs. Isoniazid increases the excretion of pyridoxine (Vitamin B6), therefore anemia and peripheral neuropathies may occur. Patients who are at high risk for developing pyridoxine deficiency are those with a history of diabetes mellitus, malnutrition, or alcoholism. Caution should be used if the patient is currently taking phenytoin, as the dosage of phenytoin may need to be reduced.

IMPLEMENTATION:

DRUG INTERACTIONS: Drugs that increase the chance of side effects from isoniazid are: atropine, disulfiram, meperidine, and sympathomimetics. Hepatotoxicity and increased metabolism of isoniazid may occur with concurrent use of alcohol. Dosage adjustments may be required. Isoniazid may potentiate the effects of the following drugs: coumarin, antihypertensives, antiparkinsonian drugs, narcotics, penicillamine, phenytoin, anticonvulsants, sedatives, sympathomimetics, tricyclic antidepressants, and anesthetics. Isoniazid absorption is decreased by antacids containing aluminum or magnesium. The combination of isoniazid and disulfiram may result in behavioral changes and/or lack of coordination and other neurological symptoms, and should be avoided. Isoniazid combined with rifampin may increase the risk of hepatotoxicity. Isoniazid may also affect laboratory values in the following manner: increased SGOT, SGPT, alkaline phosphatase, bilirubin, potassium and/or isocitric dehydrogenase levels. It may give false positive urine glucose results when copper sulfate tests are used.

PRODUCTS (TRADE NAME):
Isoniazid (Available in 50, 100 and 300 mg tablets and powder.) **Laniazid** (Available in 50 and 100 mg tablets.) **Nydrazid** (Available in 100 mg tablets;100 mg per ml injectable.) **Niconyl, Panazid, Teebaconin** (Available in 50, 100, 300 mg tablets, and 100 gm powder.) **Rifamate** (Available in 300 mg rifampin and 150 mg isoniazid capsules.)

ADMINISTRATION AND DOSAGE:
Isoniazid is well absorbed after oral or intramuscular administration. After oral administration, peak blood levels occur in one to two hours. Single oral doses given daily are the usual mode of administration. Dosage is determined by weight, with the usual adult dose being 5 mg/kg or 300 mg per day. Children's dosages per kg

are usually higher than adults' as they excrete isoniazid more rapidly. Daily administration of pyridoxine is recommended, especially for those patients at high risk for developing peripheral neuropathies.

Isoniazid is the drug of choice in the prophylactic treatment of tuberculosis infections. The usual adult dose is 300 mg per day for one year. Isoniazid is also one of the major drugs of choice in the therapeutic treatment of susceptible strains of tuberculosis. Most tuberculosis infections acquired in the United States and Canada are susceptible to isoniazid. In the therapeutic treatment of tuberculosis, at least two drugs to which the mycobacteria are susceptible should always be used. If tubercle bacilli become resistant to isoniazid, therapy should be changed to another drug to which they are susceptible.

When isoniazid is combined with the bactericidal drug rifampin or the combination of pyrazinamide and streptomycin or capreomycin, therapy is usually required for only nine months. When isoniazid is combined with a bacteriostatic drug such as ethambutol, therapy must continue for the traditional eighteen to twenty-four months. Currently, successful treatment has occurred with isoniazid and rifampin given daily for one month, then on a twice weekly basis for eight months. The twice-weekly doses of isoniazid are higher than the daily doses. They are usually 15 mg per kg body weight or 900 mg of isoniazid twice per week for adults. Rifampin doses remain the same, 600 mg twice a week for adults.

Older adults and individuals with hepatic impairment may require decreased doses of isoniazid. Renal impairment does not usually require a reduction in dosage unless the plasma creatinine level is lower than 6 mg per 100 ml.

Chemoprophylactic:

Adults: 300 mg po per day in single dose; continued for one year.

Children and infants: 10 mg/kg up to 300 mg per day in a single dose; continued for one year.

Chemotherapeutic:

Adults: 5 mg/kg up to 300 mg per day in a single daily dose.

Children and infants: 10-20 mg/kg/day depending on the severity of infection, up to 300-500 mg/day. Give in a single dose.

Rifamate: For adults use two Rifamate capsules, once daily, one hour before or two hours after meals.

IMPLEMENTATION CONSIDERATIONS:

—Obtain a complete health history; hypersensitivity to isoniazid; history of drug-induced hepatitis; acute or chronic liver disease; renal impairment; peripheral neuropathies; convulsive disorders; diabetes mellitus; history of excessive alcohol use; malnourishment; allergic reactions to ethionamide, pyrazinamide, or niacin; other medications which may cause drug interactions; pregnancy or breast-feeding.

—If the patient is taking phenytoin its dosage will probably need to be reduced and phenytoin blood levels monitored.

—Elderly patients are more likely to experience toxic effects.

—Teaching and counseling patient and family about the disease process is important in obtaining compliance with long-term therapy.

—Diabetic conditions are more difficult to control while patient is taking isoniazid. Determine if patient tests his urine with a copper sulfate test, as a different method may need to be substituted.

—Isoniazid in solution may crystallize at low temperatures. It should be allowed to warm to room temperature and crystals should be redissolved before use.

—Patients may experience local transient irritation after an intramuscular injection.

—Patients should be given only a month's supply of the drug at one time.

—Pyridoxine given with isoniazid will help decrease the incidence of peripheral neuropathies.

—Refer to antitubercular drugs section for additional material.

WHAT THE PATIENT NEEDS TO KNOW:

—This drug is of major importance in the treatment of tuberculosis. While it is a valuable treatment aid, like most drugs, it is not without side effects. One of the most serious is that isoniazid may cause hepatitis. If any of the following symptoms occur, you should stop taking the drug and call your health provider immediately: loss of appetite, yellowing of the skin and eyes, dark urine, unusual tiredness or weakness, nausea or vomiting, flu-like symptoms.

—Isoniazid-induced hepatitis is more likely to occur when you drink alcohol regularly. It is best to avoid alcoholic beverages altogether during therapy.

—You should stop taking the drug and call your provider immediately if you experience clumsiness, unsteadiness, numbness, tingling, burning or pain in hands and feet, blurred vision, and/or loss of vision. Also watch for unexplained fever, rash, chills, or arthritic symptoms which may indicate you are becoming overly sensitive to the drug. Any new or troublesome symptom should be reported promptly.

—Isoniazid may increase your need for Vitamin B6 (pyridoxine). You may buy 10-50 mg tablets to take daily.

—Store this medicine in a tight, dark container at room temperature.

—Take isoniazid with other antitubercular drugs you may be taking, before breakfast. If the medicine causes stomach upset, take it with food.

—Antacids such as Maalox should not be taken with isoniazid. They may be taken one hour after your medicine.

—Do not use laxatives more than once a week.

—While you are taking this medicine, some foods such as tuna fish and swiss cheese may cause various symptoms: redness, itching, flushing, rapid or pounding heartbeat, sweating, chills, clamminess, headache, and light-headedness. If you experience any of these symptoms, you need to evaluate what you have eaten, and perhaps exclude it from your diet during the time you are on this medication.

—Keep this drug out of the reach of children or others for whom it is not prescribed. This should be regarded as a dangerous drug and taken care of properly.

—Establish a routine for taking your medicine. Take it every day at the same time. Fit it into your regular routine so that you will not forget it.

EVALUATION:

ADVERSE REACTIONS: *CNS:* convulsions, dizziness, drowsiness, euphoria, hyperreflexia, impaired memory, peripherial neuropathies, visual disturbances, optic neuritis and atrophy, toxic psychosis, changes in affect and behavior, toxic encephalopathy. *Endocrine:* acetonuria, altered thyroid function, glycosuria, gynecomastia, hyperglycemia, hyperkalemia, metabolic acidosis, pellagra, proteinuria, pyridoxine deficiency. *Gastrointestinal:* constipation, dryness of the mouth, epigastric distress, hepatitis, nausea, vomiting. *Hematopoietic:* agranulocytosis, aplastic anemia, eosinophilia, hemolytic anemia, leukopenia, methemoglobinemia, neutropenia, pyridoxine response hypochromic anemia, sideroblastic anemia, thrombocytopenia. *Hypersensitivity:* arthritic symptoms, chills, fever, hematologic reactions, rash (morbilliform, maculopapular, purpuric, urticarial), keratitis, lymphadenitis, vasculitis. *Other:* dyspnea, headache, postural hypotension, rheumatic and systemic lupus erythematosus-like syndrome, tachycardia, urinary retention in males.

OVERDOSAGE: *Signs and symptoms:* Effects may occur from 30 minutes to three hours after isoniazid overdosage. Nausea, vomiting, slurred speech, dizziness, impaired vision and visual hallucinations may be among the early symptoms. Severe overdosage will result in CNS depression, respiratory distress, coma, and severe intractable seizures. *Treatment:* Refer to physician for hospitalization and management.

PARAMETERS TO MONITOR: Initial baseline liver function studies should be obtained, and a physical examination performed which is completely recorded. Because of the number of adverse effects, a good baseline record is important in monitoring future changes. The patient should be seen initially every one to two weeks for the first two months of treatment and then on a monthly basis or more often as indicated. At each visit the patient should be questioned closely about the way he takes his medications, and about his general adjustment to both disease and therapy. Observe for signs and symptoms of therapeutic effect: weight gain, reduced fever, reduced cough, improved sense of well-being and negative bacteriologic studies. Monitor for development of adverse symptoms suggesting toxicity, hepatitis, or progression of disease. Some authorities feel repeat liver function studies should only be obtained if the patient is symptomatic; others feel that they should be obtained on a monthly basis, at least for the first three months. With any reports of suspicious gastrointestinal symptoms, medication should be stopped and liver function studies obtained. If laboratory studies are normal, restart isoniazid at a reduced dosage once the symptoms have disappeared, under the guidance of a physician. If the SGOT, alkaline phosphatase, or serum bilirubin show a threefold increase, isoniazid-induced hepatitis is likely and the drug should be stopped immediately. Thorough ophthalmologic exams should be done periodically. Urine tests may be done for isoniazid to check compliance.

Marna J. Ross

PYRAZINAMIDE

ACTION OF THE DRUG: Pyrazinamide is a bacteriostatic product effective against *Mycobacterium tuberculosis*. It is an analog of nicotinamide, but its mode of action is unknown.

ASSESSMENT:

INDICATIONS: Pyrazinamide is indicated for the treatment of active tuberculosis in any form. It is used when first-line drugs have been tried and found to be ineffective. It should be used only as adjunctive therapy with other antitubercular drugs.

SUBJECTIVE-OBJECTIVE: See Antitubercular Drugs Section.

PLAN:

CONTRAINDICATIONS: Do not use in the presence of hypersensitivity or severe hepatic damage.

WARNINGS: This product should be discontinued if there are any signs of hepatocellular damage or in cases of acute gouty arthritis and hyperuricemia. Because of the potential for development of these problems, the patient should be started on the drug only when he can be closely supervised and when facilities are available for obtaining serum uric acid levels and liver function studies. Because of the relatively recent development of this product, adequate studies on its use in children have not been completed. Therefore, avoid use in children if possible.

PRECAUTIONS: Documentation of organism sensitivity to pyrazinamide should be carried out prior to beginning therapy. The drug should be used cautiously in patients with intermittent porphyria, gout or diabetes because the nature of adverse reactions may make these conditions more difficult to manage.

IMPLEMENTATION:

DRUG INTERACTIONS: This drug has not been on the market long enough for significant drug interactions to have been reported.

PRODUCTS (TRADE NAME):
Pyrazinamide (Available in 500 mg tablets.)

ADMINISTRATION AND DOSAGE: Average adult dose is 20 to 35 mg/kg/day in three or four divided doses. Maximum daily dose is 3 gm. Administer with at least one other effective antitubercular drug.

IMPLEMENTATION CONSIDERATIONS:

—Obtain a complete health history: hypersensitivity, diabetes, intermittent porphyria, gout or hepatic disease.

—Active gouty attacks may be precipitated by this drug.

—The principal adverse reaction is hepatocellular damage, which may be found in as many as 20% of patients placed on pyrazinamide therapy. Early problems may be detectable only by laboratory tests. Early signs of damage may be anorexia, malaise, fever, liver tenderness and hepatomegaly. Splenomegaly may also be seen in some patients. Course may progress to severe hepatic damage and death. Usually, higher dosages of medication are correlated with increased incidence of hepatic damage.

—If hyperuricemia with signs of arthritis develops, or there is any evidence of hepatocellular injury, this drug should be stopped and not resumed.

WHAT THE PATIENT NEEDS TO KNOW:

—Take medication exactly as ordered. Establish a routine in taking the medicine so you are less likely to forget it.

—Keep medication out of the reach of children or others for whom it is not prescribed.

—This is a powerful drug, and some persons experience side effects from it. Notify your health care provider immediately if you experience any loss of appetite, nausea, vomiting, fatigue, dark color to your urine or yellow discoloration of skin and eyes.

—This drug may cause an attack of gout in persons who may have a tendency for this problem. If you have any swelling of joints, tense, hot skin over joints, or joint pain, notify your health care provider.

EVALUATION:

ADVERSE REACTIONS: *Dermatologic:* photosensitivity, rashes. *Gastrointestinal:* diarrhea, hepatocellular damage, nausea, vomiting. *Other:* gout, decreased blood clotting time, sideroblastic anemia.

PARAMETERS TO MONITOR: Obtain baseline studies such as serum uric acid level, SGOT and SGPT prior to beginning therapy. These studies should be repeated every 2 to 4 weeks during the course of therapy. Other liver function studies may be obtained as necessary. Establish a flow chart to monitor therapeutic effects and adverse reactions. Periodically assess for symptoms of gout and hepatocellular damage. Individuals who develop gout or hepatocellular damage should have medication promptly discontinued.

Marilyn W. Edmunds

RIFAMPIN

ACTION OF THE DRUG: Rifampin is an antibiotic with both bactericidal and bacteriostatic action against *Mycobacterium tuberculosis* and *Neisseria meningitidis*. Rifampin exerts its bactericidal action both intra- and extracellularly.

ASSESSMENT:

INDICATIONS: Rifampin is a major antitubercular agent used in the initial treatment and re-treatment of pulmonary tuberculosis. Drug resistance occurs rapidly to rifampin; it should therefore be used in conjunction with at least one other antitubercular agent. Rifampin is also used in short-term therapy for eliminating meningococcal organisms from the nasopharynx of high risk, asymptomatic carriers of *Neisseria meningitidis*.

SUBJECTIVE-OBJECTIVE: See Antitubercular Drugs introductory section.

PLAN:

CONTRAINDICATIONS: Do not use in presence of hypersensitivity to rifamycins, or with active liver disease when the patient is taking another hepatotoxic drug.

WARNINGS: Rifampin has been known to produce liver dysfunction. Fatalities associated with jaundice have occurred in patients who either had liver disease or were taking other hepatotoxic drugs with rifampin. The benefits of using rifampin should be weighed carefully against the risks of further liver damage in these patients. The safety of rifampin during pregnancy and in children under age five has not been established. The risk of possible teratogenic effects should be considered carefully against the benefits in women of childbearing age.

PRECAUTIONS: Caution should be used when administering rifampin to patients with a history of hepatic disease, alcoholism, or who are taking other hepatotoxic drugs. Patients should be cautioned against interrupting their drug regimens as rare renal hypersensitivity reactions have occurred when the drug is restarted. Hypersensitivity reactions such as flu syndrome and rare reactions such as shock, renal failure, and thrombocytopenia may occur when large doses of rifampin have been administered intermittently. These reactions are very uncommon when rifampin is administered in its usual dosage of 600 mg per day at an interval of every 3 to 4 days. Some sources caution against using rifampin in intermittent therapy. Neonates of mothers on rifampin should be observed carefully for evidence of adverse side effects or toxicity.

IMPLEMENTATION:

DRUG INTERACTIONS: Rifampin may increase the requirements for oral anticoagulants such as coumarin, and decrease the effectiveness of oral contraceptives. Rifampin has immunosuppressive properties which may interfere with immunization procedures or immunosuppressive therapy. Corticosteroid metabolism is increased and thus its effectiveness decreased by rifampin. Signs of steroid toxicity may develop in patients taking corticosteroids, once long-term rifampin therapy has stopped. The blood concentrations of oral hypoglycemics, digitalis derivatives, and dapsone are affected by rifampin and dosage adjustments may be required. Rifampin may decrease the effects of methadone and withdrawal symptoms may appear. Probenecid potentiates rifampin. Aminosalicylic acid delays the absorption of rifampin and these drugs should be given at least eight hours apart. Hepatotoxicity may result when rifampin is taken concurrently with alcohol, isoniazid, halothane, or other hepatotoxic drugs. Alcohol may also increase the metabolism of this drug. Rifampin may alter laboratory values in the following manner: increase serum levels of SGPT, SGOT, BUN, uric acid, and bilirubin. It may cause a positive direct and indirect Coomb's test, and interfere with the standard assays for serum folate and B12.

PRODUCTS (TRADE NAME):
Rifadin (Available in 150 and 300 mg capsules). **Rifamate** (Available in 300 mg rifampin and 150 mg isoniazid capsule) **Rimactane** (Available in 300 mg capsules).

ADMINISTRATION AND DOSAGE: Rifampin should always be administered in combination with at least one other antitubercular drug. It is usually given orally, in a single dose, one hour before or two hours after eating. Peak plasma concentrations occur two to four hours after ingestion.

Adult: 600 mg in a single po daily dose. Dosage range is 450-600 mg/day. This is the same whether the therapy is intermittent or daily.

Elderly and debilitated: 10 mg/kg/day. Not to exceed 600 mg/day.

Children 5 years and older: 10-20 mg/kg/day. Not to exceed 600 mg/day.

Rifamate:

Adult: Two rifamate capsules once daily.

IMPLEMENTATION CONSIDERATIONS:
—Obtain a complete health history: history of hypersensitivity, active liver disease or dysfunction, other medications which may cause drug interactions (particularly anti-coagulants, oral contraceptives, other hepatotoxic drugs), daily or excessive alcohol intake, or the possibility of pregnancy.

—Elderly patients are more likely to experience toxic effects from this drug.

—In order to increase compliance with long-term therapy, work to establish rapport with patient. Individualize teaching to patient and family.

WHAT THE PATIENT NEEDS TO KNOW:
—Take medication exactly as ordered. Do not skip doses or double the dosages.

—Do not interrupt or discontinue taking this medication without consulting your health provider. When pills are not taken regularly, the possibility of developing an allergic reaction increases.

—Take this medication with a full glass of water one hour before or two hours after eating. If stomach upset occurs the medicine may be taken with meals.

—This drug may cause drowsiness. Like many other powerful drugs, there may be other side effects associated with it. Notify your health provider immediately if you experience flu-like symptoms, any gastrointestinal problems, bruising or bleeding. Any new or troublesome symptoms should be reported.

—Rifampin may cause a red-orange discoloration of the urine, feces, saliva, sweat, sputum and tears. Soft contact lenses may become permanently discolored and therefore should not be worn.

—Do not drink any alcohol while you are taking this drug as the possibility of developing liver problems is increased.

—Oral contraceptives become less effective while patients are on this drug, and an alternative form of birth control should be used.

—Female patients may develop menstrual irregularities. If this happens, notify your health provider.

—If you are in a methadone maintenance program, notify your methadone clinic that you are taking this medication. Dosage adjustment may be required to prevent withdrawal symptoms.

EVALUATION:

ADVERSE REACTIONS: *CNS:* ataxia, dizziness, drowsiness, fatigue, headache, generalized numbness, inability to concentrate, mental confusion, pain in the extremities, transient low frequency hearing loss, visual disturbances. *Gastrointestinal:* abdominal pain or cramps, anorexia, diarrhea, epigastric distress, flatulence, jaundice, hepatitis, nausea, sore mouth and tongue, transient abnormalities in liver function tests, vomiting. *Genitourinary:* menstrual disturbances. *Hematopoietic:* decreased hemoglobin, eosinophilia, hemolytic anemia, thrombocytopenia, transient leukopenia. *Hypersensitivity:* occurs more frequently with higher dosages, and when there have been interruptions with dosage schedule: eosinophilia, thrombocytopenia, exudative conjunctivitis, fever, flu syndrome, pruritus, renal failure, skin eruptions, sore mouth, sore tongue. *Metabolic:* hyperuricemia.

OVERDOSAGE: *Signs and symptoms:* nausea, vomiting, increasing lethargy, unconsciousness, liver enlargement and tenderness, jaundice. *Treatment:* referral for gastric lavage and activated charcoal administration.

PARAMETERS TO MONITOR: Liver function studies may be obtained periodically or when the patient exhibits symptoms of hepatic toxicity: nausea, vomiting, malaise, fever. Some authorities feel that periodic liver function testing is mandatory in patients with liver disease or who are on other hepatotoxic drugs. Patients who receive rifampin on an intermittent basis should be monitored regularly for symptoms of thrombocytopenia—purpura, petechiae, hematuria. Patients on anticoagulants such as coumarin should have their prothrombin times monitored closely. Compliance may be checked on a periodic basis by observing the color of the urine.

Marna. J. Ross

STREPTOMYCIN SULFATE

ACTION OF THE DRUG: Streptomycin is an aminoglycoside antibiotic and antitubercular agent. It is bactericidal for extracellular tubercle bacilli and bacteriostatic for intracellular bacilli.

ASSESSMENT:

INDICATIONS: Streptomycin is recommended for all forms of susceptible *Mycobacterium tuberculosis*. It must be used in combination with other antitubercular drugs. For other indications for streptomycin see Antiinfective section.

SUBJECTIVE-OBJECTIVE: See Antitubercular introductory section.

PLAN:

CONTRAINDICATIONS: Streptomycin is contraindicated if the patient has a history of hypersensitivity or serious toxic effects from aminoglycosides, especially streptomycin. It is also contraindicated in the presence of labyrinthine disease, myasthenia gravis, concurrent and/or sequential or topical administration of other ototoxic, neurotoxic, nephrotoxic, or neuromuscular blocking agents, and general anesthesia. Streptomycin is contraindicated if the patient is taking capreomycin.

WARNINGS: Usage in pregnancy may cause fetal ototoxicity and deafness. All patients receiving aminoglycosides must be monitored for renal function and eighth cranial nerve function during therapy. The risk of developing toxic side effects is greater in individuals who have impaired renal function, who are are on prolonged therapy, or who receive high doses of aminoglycosides.

PRECAUTIONS: Streptomycin may cause neuromuscular blockade and respiratory depression and paralysis. It should be used with caution in individuals who are at risk for these problems. Caution should be used when administering streptomycin to children, individuals over 60, pregnant women, and to individuals with renal or eighth nerve impairment. Benefit compared to risk should be determined before administering the drug to breast-feeding women.

IMPLEMENTATION:

DRUG INTERACTIONS: The following drugs should not be given concurrently, sequentially, or topically while the patient is on streptomycin as there is a significantly greater risk for neurotoxicity and nephrotoxicity occurring: any neurotoxic, nephrotoxic drug or neuromuscular blocking agent; aminoglycosides, cephaloridine, cephalothin; colistin; capreomycin; cisplatin; ethacrynic acid; furosemide; mercaptomerin; paromomycin; polymomyxins; vancomycin; viomycin; and IV diuretics. Antiemetics may mask ototoxicity signs and symptoms when taken concurrently with streptomycin. Streptomycin in combination with anesthetics may cause neuromuscular paralysis and respiratory depression; they should never be given together. Streptomycin in combination with skeletal muscle relaxants may produce respiratory depression or paralysis. Streptomycin may alter laboratory tests in the following manner: increase serum levels of urea nitrogen, creatinine, and bilirubin, and lower serum haptoglobin levels. False positive Coomb's tests, and elevated urine glucose and proteins have been reported when copper sulfate tests were used.

PRODUCTS (TRADE NAME):
Streptomycin Sulfate (Available in 1 and 5 gm vials for injection.)

ADMINISTRATION AND DOSAGE: In the treatment of tuberculosis, streptomycin should always be given in combination with other antitubercular agents, except capreomycin. Streptomycin should only be given intramuscularly. Peak serum levels occur within 1.5 hours after IM injection. Serum levels above 50 mcg/ml are associated with an increased risk of toxicity. Intramuscular injections should be administered deep into large muscle masses and injection sites should be rotated to decrease irritation. No more than 500 mg/ml should be given per injection site. Injections are painful and sterile inflammatory reactions may occur. Slight dizziness and paresthesias may occur after the injection. Direct contact with the drug should be avoided as sensitization may occur. In the primary treatment of tuberculosis, streptomycin is usually discontinued when the sputum culture becomes negative, usually three to four months after the onset of therapy.

Adults with normal renal function: 1 gm/day IM (may be given five days per week) for two to three months; then two to three times per week for four to six weeks.

Elderly patients, unusually small adults, and individuals with renal impairment: Give reduced dosages, usually 0.5 gm/day IM according to above schedule.

IMPLEMENTATION CONSIDERATIONS:

—Obtain a complete health history: presence of hearing disorders, labyrinthine disease, myasthenia gravis, Parkinson's disease or other neuromuscular disorders, renal impairment; history of hypersensitivity or toxic reactions to aminoglycosides, especially streptomycin; medications which may produce drug interactions; or possibility of pregnancy.

—Order baseline audiogram, caloric stimulation tests, and renal function tests.

—Clients over 60 and individuals with renal impairment will require reduced dosages and careful monitoring for side effects as they are at greater risk for toxic reactions.

—Diabetics who monitor their urine with Clinitest or Benedict's solution may have to use a different urine test as streptomycin may alter the results.

—Adverse effects and toxicity are more likely to occur in individuals receiving high doses of streptomycin, or who are taking other ototoxic, neurotoxic, or nephrotoxic drugs, or who are on prolonged therapy.

—Streptomycin should be stopped immediately if signs and symptoms of ototoxicity develop: Vestibular problems: headache, nausea, vomiting, vertigo in upright position, difficulty reading, positive Romberg test, unsteadiness, ataxia. Auditory problems: usually preceded by vestibular symptoms, highpitched tinnitus, roaring noises, sense of fullness in ears, impaired hearing.

—Observe for signs and symptoms of nephrotoxicity: edema in the extremities, weight gain, or abnormal renal function studies.

—Observe for signs and symptoms of superinfection, especially of the upper respiratory tract.

WHAT THE PATIENT NEEDS TO KNOW:

—Take this medication exactly as ordered.

—Some patients experience side effects while taking this drug. If you notice any new or troublesome symptoms, notify your health provider. Watch especially for dizziness, excessive thirst, blood in urine, clumsiness or unsteadiness, less urine frequency and amount, loss of appetite, loss of hearing, nausea, vomiting, numbness, tingling, burning of face or mouth, ringing or buzzing or feeling of fullness in the ears.

 —To help prevent side effects or renal damage, you should drink at least two quarts of fluid per day.

EVALUATION:

ADVERSE REACTIONS: *CNS:* convulsions, (rare) dizziness, headache, numbness, paresthesias, tingling, vertigo. *Gastrointestinal:* anorexia, nausea, stomatitis, vomiting, weight loss. *Hematopoietic:* altered reticulocyte count, anemia, leukopenia, pancytopenia, thrombocytopenia. *Hepatic:* hepatomegaly, hepatic necrosis. *Other:* arthralgia, hypertension, hypotension, myocarditis, pseudotumor cerebri, splenomegaly, ototoxicity, nephrotoxicity.

PARAMETERS TO MONITOR: Monitor for therapeutic effects and adverse reactions. Audiograms and caloric stimulation tests should be obtained prior to and periodically during long-term or high-dose therapy, and six months after therapy has been completed. Renal function tests should be monitored periodically during therapy to detect nephrotoxicity and to prevent serious neurotoxic reactions. Streptomycin serum levels should be monitored to decrease the risks of toxicity occurring. Individuals with renal impairment should not have peak levels greater than 20 to 25 mcg/ml. If serum levels cannot be monitored, then creatinine clearance rates or serum creatinine levels should be used to monitor the drug and determine when dosage modifications are required. Patients should be asked about symptoms of ototoxicity, neurotoxicity, and nephrotoxicity during each visit. The provider should also observe for signs and symptoms of superinfection, especially upper respiratory infections. Refer to antiinfective section for more details.

Marna J. Ross

ANTIVIRAL DRUGS

ACYCLOVIR

ACTION OF THE DRUG: Acyclovir triphosphate is preferentially accumulated by herpesvirus infected cells where it is incorporated into growing chains of DNA. This action terminates the DNA chain. Thus, inhibitory action may be produced against herpes simplex virus, varicella-zoster virus, cytomegalovirus and Epstein-Barr virus.

ASSESSMENT:

INDICATIONS: This relatively new product is used in the treatment of initial and recurrent mucosal and cutaneous herpes simplex (HSV-1 and HSV-2) infections in immunocompromised adults and children. It has also been utilized for severe initial clinical episodes of herpes genitalis in patients who are not immunocompromised. The relationship between in vitro susceptibility of herpes simplex virus to antiviral drugs and clinical response has not been established.

SUBJECTIVE-OBJECTIVE: Positive history of recent exposure to or previous episodes of herpes simplex or varicella-zoster may be found. Patient may present with signs and symptoms of acute, painful lesions on genitalia, fever and chills. Large multinucleated giant cells may be demonstrated in smears of lesion exudate or scrapings.

PLAN:

CONTRAINDICATIONS: Do not give in the presence of hypersensitivity to acyclovir.

WARNINGS: Because this is a relatively new product, adequate testing of reactions in pregnant or breast-feeding women have not been completed. This product should be used with caution in these individuals. This product is given by IV infusion over at least a one-hour interval to decrease chance of renal tubular damage.

PRECAUTIONS: Dosage should be based upon renal clearance, with lower dosages given for impaired clearance. Maximum urine concentration is reached within the first 2 to 3 hours following infusion, and the patient must be adequately hydrated to prevent precipitation of the product within the renal tubules. Some patients have demonstrated various encephalopathic symptoms following IV infusion of acyclovir. These symptoms vary from mild confusion and lethargy to more serious hallucinations, seizures or coma. As with other products, acyclovir administration may lead to the development of more resistant strains of herpes simplex virus, and prudence should be used in determining the length of therapy.

IMPLEMENTATION:

DRUG INTERACTIONS: Acyclovir half-life may be increased by 18% to 40% when administered with 1 gm probenecid. Because this is a relatively new product, few drug interactions have as yet been reported. Patients receiving concurrent intrathecal methotrexate or interferon should use acyclovir very cautiously.

PRODUCTS (TRADE NAME):
Zovirax (Available in 500 mg powder/10 ml vial for injection.)

ADMINISTRATION AND DOSAGE: (See Topical Antiviral section for topical dosing information.) Initiate therapy as soon as diagnosis has been made. Give medicine by slow IV infusion in concentrations of approximately 7 mg/ml. Consult manufacturer's product information for dosing adjustments in patients with renal impairment.

Mucosal and Cutaneous Herpes Simplex in Immunocompromised Patients:

Adults: 5 mg/kg infused at a constant rate over one hour, every 8 hours for 7 days.

Children 12 years or younger: 250 mg/meter M^2 infused at a constant rate over one hour, every 8 hours for 7 days.

Severe Initial Clinical Episodes of Herpes Genitalis: Same dosage as above, but course lasts only 5 days.

IMPLEMENTATION CONSIDERATIONS:

—Obtain a complete health history, including presence of hypersensitivity of allergies, previous renal disease, and information regarding present course of disease: time of appearance of first symptoms, progression of lesions, home treatment and response.

—For herpes genitalis patients, obtain information regarding sexual contact, and attempt to identify partners who should be warned and treated.

—Approximately 1% of patients receiving this product demonstrate encephalopathic changes. Other major problems occur in patients with reduced renal function. Patients should be observed closely during drug administration and renal and neurologic status monitored.

—Adverse reactions are more likely to arise when drug is infused rapidly. Care must be taken to ensure constant administration of product at the proper concentration.

—Solution should be used within 24 hours after diluted. A precipitate may form in refrigerated solutions which will redissolve at room temperatures.

WHAT THE PATIENT NEEDS TO KNOW:

—This product must be started as soon as your condition is diagnosed. The course of therapy will last several days and will require your cooperation. You will receive the medicine in an IV infusion.

—Notify the nurse promptly if you begin to feel confused, unusually tired, agitated, or note any jerking or trembling of your arms or legs. If you notice any new or troublesome symptoms, discuss these with your health care provider.

—You must keep plenty of water in your body while you are taking this medicine. Try to drink 4 or 5 glasses of water a day, and other liquids if allowed by your diet.

EVALUATION:

ADVERSE REACTIONS: *CNS:* encephalopathic changes such as agitation, coma, confusion, hallucination, lethargy, obtundation, seizures, tremors, and headache. *Other:* diaphoresis, elevated serum creatinine, hematuria, hypotension, nausea, phlebitis at injection site, jitters, and thrombocytosis.

PARAMETERS TO MONITOR: Monitor for therapeutic effect: decrease in pain and clearing of lesions. Evaluate renal function through serum creatinine levels, intake and output recordings, daily weights. Watch for signs of neurologic change or other adverse reaction.

Marilyn W. Edmunds

AMANTADINE HCL

ACTION OF THE DRUG: (1) Amantadine is a virostatic agent with respect to influenza A virus. Its mode of action is not completely understood: however it probably prevents the influenza A virus from entering the host cell. (2) Amantadine is also used in the treatment of Parkinson's disease. The mechanism of action is not known.

ASSESSMENT:

INDICATIONS: Amantadine is used in the prophylactic treatment of respiratory illness caused by influenza A virus when the vaccine is unavailable or contraindicated. It is used in the symptomatic treatment of moderate to severe respiratory illness due to influenza A virus, if therapy is begun promptly after the onset of symptoms. Amantadine is also used in the treatment of idiopathic Parkinson's disease, post-encephalitic Parkinson's disease, drug-induced extrapyramidal reactions, symptomatic Parkinson's disease, and in elderly patients who are thought to develop Parkinson's disease with cerebral arteriosclerosis.

SUBJECTIVE: Positive history of recent exposure to influenza A virus, plus a history of heart disease (rheumatic fever), respiratory disease, metabolic disease (diabetes mellitus) and/or over the age of sixty. Give only when patient has not had inactivated influenza A vaccine. Symptoms of moderate to severe flu syndrome: headache, chills and fever, generalized aches and pains, exhaustion and cold symptoms.

OBJECTIVE: Signs of moderate to severe flu syndrome: temperature of 100-103 degrees Fahrenheit, rhinorrhea, conjunctivitis, cough, injected pharynx, diaphoresis. Patient identified as high risk due to history of underlying disease, close contact with infected person and/or hospital personnel. Influenza A virus identified by sputum culture or serologic test.

PLAN:

CONTRAINDICATIONS: Hypersensitivity to amantadine HCl. Amantadine is contraindicated in nursing mothers.

WARNINGS: The safe use of amantadine during pregnancy and for children under the age of one year has not been established. Use with caution in patients with a history of seizure disorders, congestive heart failure, peripheral edema, hepatic disease, renal impairment, mental illness, eczematoid rash, orthostatic hypotension, and in the elderly, or those receiving CNS stimulants. Dosage reductions or alternative course of treatment may be required. Amantadine should only be given under close medical supervision to patients with cerebral atherosclerosis.

PRECAUTIONS: Toxic levels of amantadine may accumulate in patients with renal impairment or in the elderly due to their decreased glomerular filtration rate. Dosage should be reduced if atropine-like effects occur. Acute parkinsonian crisis may occur in patients with Parkinson's disease if amantadine is stopped suddenly. Patients with a history of seizure disorders may have increased seizure activity.

Patients with a history of congestive failure or peripheral edema may develop congestive heart failure while on amantadine. The potential for abuse exists as amantadine may cause euphoria and hallucinations.

IMPLEMENTATION:

DRUG INTERACTIONS: Amantadine may increase the effects of anticholinergic drugs such as those used in Parkinson's disease. Atropine-like effects, hallucinations, confusion and other signs of excess anticholinergic response may occur. Amantadine dosage should be reduced in these cases. CNS stimulants and psychopharmacologic drugs may increase the effect of amantadine. These agents should be used cautiously in combination, and the patient carefully observed, as CNS and psychic side effects may occur. Amantadine also enhances the therapeutic effects of Levodopa.

PRODUCTS (TRADE NAME):
Symmetrel (Available in 100 mg capsules; 50 mg/5 ml syrup.)

ADMINISTRATION AND DOSAGE: Amantadine is almost completely absorbed after oral administration. It is excreted mainly in the urine. The usual adult dose requires 48 hours to reach maximum tissue saturation.

Prophylactic treatment should begin as soon as possible after exposure to influenza A virus and continue for ten days. It may, if the situation warrants it, be continued up to ninety days. Prophylactic treatment with amantadine is recommended for patients who cannot receive the influenza A virus vaccine. Amantadine may be given with the inactivated influenza A vaccine and continued for two to three weeks while the protection from the vaccine develops.

Therapeutic treatment should be initiated as soon as possible after symptoms appear, and be continued for one to two days after symptoms disappear.

Split dosage regimens may reduce CNS side effects. This drug should be taken after meals for best absorption.

For both prophylactic and therapeutic dosages:

Adult: 200 mg/day po either as a single dose or in two equally divided doses. Do not exceed 400 mg/day.

Children 9-12 years: 100 mg po given twice per day.

Children 1-9 years: 4-8 mg/kg/day or 2-4 mg/lb/day po in two to three equally divided doses. Do not exceed 150 mg/day.

IMPLEMENTATION CONSIDERATIONS:

—Obtain a complete health history: hypersensitivity or allergies, history of epilepsy or seizure disorders, congestive heart failure, peripheral edema, heart disease, orthostatic hypotension, hepatic disease, renal impairment, eczema or recurring eczematoid rash, peptic ulcer disease, enlarged prostate or problem with urinary retention, mental illness, cerebral atherosclerosis, and/or Parkinson's disease; concurrent use of any anti-cholinergic drugs, levodopa, CNS stimulants, or drugs which may induce orthostatic hypotension; possibility of pregnancy.

—Order baseline renal function studies, liver function studies, and hematopoietic studies as indicated by the patient's history.

—Patients over 60 may need to have a lower dosage, especially in the presence of decreased kidney function.

—Order sputum culture and/or serologic tests for influenza A virus to rule out other causative organisms.

WHAT THE PATIENT NEEDS TO KNOW:

—Take this drug exactly as prescribed. Drug must be continued for one or two days even after symptoms disappear.

—Some people experience side effects when taking this medication. Be certain to report any new or uncomfortable symptoms to your health provider. Especially note any swelling of hands or feet; shortness of breath; mood or mental changes such as insomnia, anxiety, confusion or depression; difficult or decreased urination; nausea; or skin rash.

—This drug may cause dizziness, blurred vision, drowsiness and other changes in mental status. Therefore you should avoid tasks which require mental alertness such as driving a car.

—Because this drug sometimes causes insomnia, the last daily dose should be taken several hours before bedtime.

—To aid in the absorption of this medication, take this drug after meals.

—Change positions slowly, especially when moving from lying down. This will avoid lightheadedness. If you do feel dizzy, lie down.

—Do not take any other medications while taking this drug. This includes drugs which you might buy over the counter.

—If you drink alcohol while taking this medication it will increase the action of the drug to produce lightheadedness and to decrease alertness.

—Keep medicine in a closed container and protected from moisture.

—For prophylactic treatment, immunity lasts only while you are taking the drug; it is not a vaccine.

EVALUATION:

ADVERSE REACTIONS: *Cardiovascular:* congestive heart failure, dyspnea, hypotensive episodes, livedo reticularis, peripheral edema. *CNS:* anxiety, ataxia, confusion, convulsions, depression, dizziness or lightheadedness, fatigue, hallucinations, headache, insomnia, irritability, nervous excitement, psychosis, slurred speech, tremor. *Dermatologic:* rash, eczematoid dermatitis (rare). *Gastrointestinal:* anorexia, constipation, dry mouth, nausea, vomiting. *Genitourinary:* impaired urination, urinary retention. *Hematopoietic:* leukopenia and neutropenia (rare), low WBC. *Ophthalmologic:* blurred vision, loss of vision, oculogyric episodes.

OVERDOSAGE: *Signs and symptoms:* CNS changes occur, including hyperactivity, disorientation, confusion, aggressive behavior, tremors, ataxia, blurred vision, visual hallucinations, lethargy, slurred speech, and convulsions. Nausea, vomiting, anorexia, lowered blood pressure, and arrhythmias may also be seen. *Treatment:* Induce vomiting immediately and refer for gastric lavage. Supportive measures include keeping the patient well hydrated, acidifying the urine (to increase excretion of the drug), and monitoring of vital signs, CNS status, electrolytes, urine pH, urinary output and cardiac rhythms.

PARAMETERS TO MONITOR: Monitor for therapeutic effect: either the absence of flu symptoms, or a reduction in the severity of symptoms including temperature. For sustained therapy, the urinalysis, BUN, and serum creatinine should be monitored at each visit in elderly patients and those with renal impairment. History of voiding difficulties and low urinary output should be checked. Patients with cardiovascular disease or those at high risk for congestive heart failure should be observed for signs and symptoms of developing congestive heart failure, peripheral edema, or respiratory disorders. Their electrolytes should be monitored. Patients at risk for orthostatic hypotension or who complain of lightheadedness should have their blood pressure checked lying down, then standing or sitting. All patients should be observed for signs and symptoms of CNS toxicity and other untoward effects. Hepatic and hematopoietic parameters should be monitored as indicated by the patient's history.

Marna J. Ross

SULFONAMIDES

ACTION OF THE DRUG: Sulfonamides exert a bacteriostatic effect against a wide range of gram-positive and gram-negative microorganisms by inhibiting folic acid synthesis by susceptible organisms.

ASSESSMENT:

INDICATIONS: Most often used in the treatment of acute and chronic urinary tract infections, particularly cystitis, pyelitis, and pyelonephritis, when due to *Escherichia coli* or *Nocardia asteroides*. Other indications include trachoma, inclusion conjunctivitis, chancroid, lymphogranuloma venereum, nocardiosis, toxoplasmosis, acute otitis media caused by *Haemophilus influenzae*, and prophylactic therapy against recurrent rheumatic fever. Susceptible organisms include *Streptococcus pyogenes*, *Streptococcus pneumoniae*, some strains of *Bacillus anthracis* and *Corynebacterium diphtheriae*, *Haemophilus ducreyi*, *Brucella*, *Vibrio cholerae*, *Yersinia pestis*, *Nocardia*, *Actinomyces*, *Calymmatobacterium granulomatis*, and *Chlamydia trachomatis*. Several miscellaneous sulfonamides are useful only in the treatment of ulcerative colitis, pre- and postoperative therapy for bowel surgery, or dermatitis herpetiformis.

SUBJECTIVE-OBJECTIVE: The patient in need of antibiotic therapy may present in any number of ways, ranging from asymptomatic to severely ill. Keep in mind common indicators of infection such as fever, inflammation, erythema, edema or pain.

PLAN:

CONTRAINDICATIONS: Hypersensitivity to sulfonamides or chemically similar drugs, such as thiazides and sulfonylureas. Avoid in patients with urinary or intestinal obstruction, pregnant women near term, nursing mothers, infants younger than two months, or porphyria.

WARNINGS: Use with caution in patients with impaired renal or hepatic function. Discontinue drug if urinary output is reduced or if patient develops a rash. Photosensitization can occur with excessive patient exposure to sunlight or ultraviolet light. Sulfonamides are ineffective in the treatment of infections and prevention of sequelae due to group A beta-hemolytic streptococci.

PRECAUTIONS: Adequate fluid intake is necessary to avoid crystalluria or urinary stone formation. In those patients with glucose-6-phosphate dehydrogenase deficiency, hemolytic anemia may occur. Sensitivity reactions to the tartrazine present in some sulfonamides may occur in a few patients, particularly those hypersensitive to aspirin. Discontinue the drug immediately if hypersensitivity reactions or toxicity develop. Use with caution if general anesthesia is necessary. Use lower doses at less frequent intervals when treating the elderly. Use with caution with patients with severe allergy or bronchial asthma.

IMPLEMENTATION:

DRUG INTERACTIONS: Sulfonamides may potentiate the effect of oral anticoagulants, methotrexate, sulfonylureas, thiazide diuretics, phenytoin, and uricosuric agents. Sulfonamides may be displaced from plasma albumin by probenecid, salicylates, phenylbutazone, promethazine, sulfinpyrazone, and indomethacin, resulting in increased effects of sulfonamides. Penicillin use in conjunction with a sulfonamide may reduce the effects of the penicillin. Sulfonamide effect may be antagonized by *p*-aminobenzoic acid (PABA) and possibly PABA derivatives, such as local anesthetics. Concurrent use of methenamine may result in crystalluria. Concomitant administration of sulfonamides with antacids may result in decreased absorption of the sulfonamide. Sulfonamides may alter various laboratory tests: often causes a false-positive urinary glucose test with Benedict's method; infrequently results in positive LE cell test.

ADMINISTRATION AND DOSAGE: Although most sulfonamides are administered orally, several can be given parenterally, primarily intravenously. Other parenteral routes are avoided due to irritation. Some are administered vaginally as creams or suppositories. Sulfonamide dosage is dependent upon the severity of the infection being treated, the sulfonamide used, patient response, and tolerance of the drug. Generally, the short-acting sulfonamides are administered at more frequent intervals than are the intermediate or long-acting sulfonamides. Also, the short-acting sulfonamides usually require an initial loading dose. Taken with food, absorption of sulfonamides tends to be delayed but not reduced.

IMPLEMENTATION CONSIDERATIONS:

—Obtain a complete health history including the presence of allergy to sulfa drugs, aspirin, thiazides or sulfonylureas.

—Take a complete medication history and ascertain whether patient is taking any other drugs that may interact with sulfonamides.

—Ask whether patient is pregnant or breast-feeding.

—Determine if kidney or liver impairment exists. Consider need for laboratory evaluation studies.

—Order baseline urinalysis prior to initiating therapy to determine pH and presence of crystalluria. The urine may need to be alkalinized, depending upon the sulfonamide to be used, if urine volume or pH is exceptionally low.

—Order baseline complete blood count prior to initiating therapy to determine status of blood, especially if patient is to be on long-term therapy.

—For patients over the age of 60, administer lower doses at less frequent intervals.

WHAT THE PATIENT NEEDS TO KNOW:

—Sulfonamides are more fully absorbed when taken on an empty stomach, either one hour before or two hours after meals, along with a full glass of water.

—In order to prevent formation of crystals in the urine, drink large volumes of water while taking this medication.

—Avoid excessive exposure to sunlight or ultraviolet light in order to prevent possible photosensitization.

—Take all medication prescribed. Do not stop taking medication when you feel better and symptoms disappear.

—Inform other health care providers if you must have surgery requiring a general anesthetic while taking this medication.

—Contact your health care provider if there is no improvement of symptoms within a few days following initiation of therapy.

—Notify your health provider promptly if skin rash, blood in urine, bruises, nausea or other adverse effects of therapy develop.

EVALUATION:

ADVERSE REACTIONS: *CNS:* headache, drowsiness, fatigue, dizziness, vertigo, tinnitus, hearing loss, lowered mental acuity, mental depression, convulsions, ataxia, psychoses, insomnia, peripheral neuritis, peripheral neuropathy. *Endocrine:* goiter, hypothyroidism, hypoglycemia. *Gastrointestinal:* anorexia, nausea, vomiting, stomatitis, abdominal pain, hepatitis, jaundice, pancreatitis, diarrhea. *Hematopoietic:* thrombocytopenia, hypoprothrombinemia, petechiae, hemolytic anemia, aplastic anemia, agranulocytosis, purpura, leukopenia, granulocytopenia. *Hypersensitivity:* drug fever, generalized maculopapular or urticarial rash, photosensitization, fever, malaise, pruritus, erythema multiforme, erythema nodosum, exfoliative dermatitis, local irritation, Stevens-Johnson syndrome, scleral and conjunctival injection, periorbital edema, anaphylactic shock. *Renal:* crystalluria, hematuria, proteinuria, renal calculi, toxic nephrosis associated with oliguria and anuria.

OVERDOSAGE: *Signs and symptoms:* Less serious manifestations include anorexia, nausea, vomiting, dizziness, headache, and drowsiness. These minor symptoms disappear within one to two days after the drug is discontinued. Toxic fever may develop prior to serious manifestations, usually occurring one or more days following the end of the infectious fever. Serious manifestations include hemolytic anemia, dermatitis, acidosis, toxic neuritis, hepatic jaundice, and unconsciousness, with one to three weeks necessary for remission of these symptoms. Death is possible. *Treatment:* After immediately discontinuing the medication, administer an emetic and refer for gastric lavage. Alkalinize the urine, and if the kidneys are functioning normally, force fluids.

PARAMETERS TO MONITOR: Blood work consisting of complete blood count, urinalysis, liver and kidney function tests should be done prior to initiating sulfonamide therapy and approximately every month thereafter while patient is on a maintenance dosage. Obtain phenytoin levels on those patients concomitantly on phenytoin; for those concurrently on sulfonylureas, obtain glucose levels. Observe for signs and symptoms of blood dyscrasias: sore throat, fever, pallor, purpura, jaundice. Also observe for signs and symptoms of renal and/or hepatic failure in high-risk patients.

SULFACYTINE

PRODUCTS (TRADE NAME):
Renoquid (Available in 250 mg tablet.)
DRUG SPECIFICS:
A rapidly absorbed, highly soluble sulfonamide. Used primarily in the treatment of acute, non-obstructive urinary tract infections due to susceptible organisms. Due to inadequate clinical experience with this drug, do not administer to children under 14 years.
ADMINISTRATION AND DOSAGE SPECIFICS:
Urinary Tract Infection:
Adults and children over 14: 500 mg orally initially, then 250 mg four times daily for ten days.

SULFADIAZINE

PRODUCTS (TRADE NAME):
Microsulfon, Sulfadiazine (Available in 500 mg tablets.)
DRUG SPECIFICS:
The low solubility of this drug requires a daily urinary output of at least 1500 ml plus alkalinization to prevent crystalluria. The drug is only effective in the treatment of urinary tract infections when used in large doses with alkalinization. An effective prophylactic against rheumatic fever when antibiotics are contraindicated. It is the sulfonamide of choice for treatment of nocardiosis. Useful in the treatment of intraocular infections.
ADMINISTRATION AND DOSAGE SPECIFICS:
Oral:

Urinary Tract Infection, Nocardiosis:
Adult: 2-4 gm initially, then 2-4 gm daily in 3-6 divided dosages.
Children and infants older than 2 months: 75 mg/kg initially, then 150 mg/kg daily in 4-6 divided doses with total daily dose not to exceed 6 gm.
Rheumatic Fever Prophylaxis: 500 mg daily for patients less than 30 kg; 1 gm daily for those over 30 kg.
Intra-ocular Infection: 4 gm initially, then 1 gm every 4 hours.

SULFAMETHIZOLE

PRODUCTS (TRADE NAME):
Microsul (Available in 500 mg and 1 gm tablets.) **Proklar** (Available in 500 mg tablet.) **Thiosulfil** (Available in 250 and 500 mg tablets.) **Urifon** (Available in 500 mg tablet.)

DRUG SPECIFICS:
A short-acting, readily soluble sulfonamide effective in the treatment of urinary tract infections.

ADMINISTRATION AND DOSAGE SPECIFICS:
Adults: 0.5 to 1 gm, 3 or 4 times daily.
Children and infants older than 2 months: 30 to 40 mg/kg/day in 4 divided dosages.

SULFAMETHOXAZOLE

PRODUCTS (TRADE NAME):
Gantanol (Available in 500 mg tablet, 500 mg/5 ml suspension.) **Gantanol-DS** (Available in 1 gm tablet.) **Sulfamethoxazole** (Available in 500 mg and 1 gm tablet.) **Urobak** (Available in 500 mg tablet.)

DRUG SPECIFICS:
An intermediate-acting sulfonamide highly effective against urinary tract infections when used for 7 to 10 days.

ADMINISTRATION AND DOSAGE SPECIFICS:
Urinary Tract Infections:
Adults: 2 gm initially, then 1 gm 2-3 times daily.
Children and infants older than 2 months: 50-60 mg/kg initially, then 25-30 mg/kg every 12 hours.

SULFAPYRIDINE

PRODUCTS (TRADE NAME):
  Sulfapyridine (Available in 500 mg tablets.)
DRUG SPECIFICS:
  The drug of choice for the treatment of dermatitis herpetiformis. Because of its relative insolubility and slow absorption, crystalluria is possible; the patient should be instructed to drink large volumes of fluids.
ADMINISTRATION AND DOSAGE SPECIFICS:
  Dermatitis Herpetiformis:
  Adults: 500 mg orally four times daily until improvement, then decrease dosage by 500 mg at 3-day intervals until symptom-free maintenance is achieved. Dosage increase may be necessary with exacerbation of condition.

SULFASALAZINE

PRODUCTS (TRADE NAME):
  Azulfidine (Available in 500 mg tablet and 250 mg/5 ml oral suspension.) **SAS** (Available in 500 mg tablet.) **Azulfidine En-Tabs** (Available in 500 mg enteric-coated tablet.) **Sulfadyne, Sulfasalazine** (Available in 500 mg tablets.)
DRUG SPECIFICS:
  Indicated in the treatment of mild to moderate ulcerative colitis, adjunctive therapy in severe ulcerative colitis, and as prophylaxis against recurring exacerbation of chronic ulcerative colitis. The drug should be administered after meals. The tendency to develop adverse reactions, primarily anorexia, nausea, and vomiting of gastric mucosal irritation, increases with doses of 4 gm or more daily. If such irritation occurs after initial doses, attempt to more evenly divide the dosage throughout the 24-hour period and consider enteric-coated tablets (although efficacy has not been established.) Also decrease irritation by halving the dosage and then gradually increasing it again. If irritation continues, discontinue the drug for 5-7 days prior to restarting the drug at a lower dose. Caution is necessary when administering the drug to severe asthmatics. After ulcerative colitis is under control, a lower maintenance dosage is often necessary to prevent recurrence of diarrhea.
ADMINISTRATION AND DOSAGE SPECIFICS:
  Ulcerative Colitis:
  Adults: 1-4 gm daily in 4-8 divided doses, then 2 gm daily in 4 divided doses as maintenance.
  Children and infants older than 2 months: 40-60 mg/kg daily in 3-6 divided doses, then 30 mg/kg daily in 4 divided doses as maintenance.

SULFISOXAZOLE

PRODUCTS (TRADE NAME):

Gantrisin (Available in 500 mg tablet, 500 mg/5 ml syrup and pediatric suspension, 400 mg/5 ml injection, 4% opthalmic ointment in 1/8 oz tube, 4% ophthalmic solution in 1/2 oz bottle.) **LipoGastrisin** (Available in 1 gm/5 ml long-acting emulsion.) **SK-Soxazole, Sulfizin** (Available in 500 mg tablets.) **Sulfisoxasole** (Available in 500 mg tablet, 500 mg/5ml suspension, 500 mg/ml syrup, 2 gm/5 ml ampule for injection.) Vaginal creams: **Cantri, Koro-Sulf, Vagilia** (Available as vaginal cream 10% in 3 oz container.)

DRUG SPECIFICS:

A highly soluble sulfonamide, very effective in the treatment of urinary tract infections due to susceptible organisms when used for 7 to 10 days. Also effective against susceptible organisms causing vaginitis; however, topical use may cause sensitization, and the cream may be inactivated by blood and pus.

Use of the ophthalmic ointment or solution for ocular infections requires several precautions: use may cause proliferation of non-susceptible organisms; the drug may slow corneal healing; and its use is incompatible with silver preparations.

LipoGantrisin is a concentrated, time-released drug.

ADMINISTRATION AND DOSAGE SPECIFICS:

Urinary Tract Infection:

Oral:

Adults: 2-4 gm initially, then 4-8 gm daily in 4-6 divided doses.

Children and infants older than 2 months: 75 mg/kg initially, then 150 mg/kg daily in 4-6 divided doses, with total daily dose not to exceed 6 gm.

LipoGantrisin:

Adults: 4-5 gm every 12 hours.

Children and infants older than 2 months: 60-75 mg/kg initially, then 60-75 mg/kg twice daily, with total daily dose not to exceed 6 gm.

Injectable:

Adults and children older than 2 months: 50 mg/kg initially, then 100 mg/kg daily. Subcutaneous: divide into 3 daily doses; Intravenous: divide into 4 daily doses; Intramuscular: divide into 2 or 3 daily doses with no more than 5 ml a day in one site. Note: for subcutaneous and intravenous administration, dilute 5 ml ampule in 35 ml sterile water for injection.

Ophthalmic Infection:

Ophthalmic solution: instill 2-3 drops at least 3 times daily.

Ophthalmic ointment: instill small amount to lower conjunctival sac 1-3 times daily and at bedtime.

Vaginal Infection:

Vaginal cream: insert 2.5-5.0 ml (one half to one applicatorful) cream intravaginally twice daily for 14 days.

SULFONAMIDE COMBINATION PRODUCTS (ORAL)

PRODUCTS (TRADE NAME):
Neotrizine, Sulfaloid, Terfonyl, Triple Sulfa (Available in tablets or 5 ml suspension with 167 mg of each sulfa product.)
DRUG SPECIFICS:
Contains equal amounts of sulfadiazine, sulfamerazine and sulfamethazine, thereby reducing the possibility of crystalluria due to the fact that the solubility of each sulfonamide exists indepedently in solution. Used primarily for urinary tract infections.
ADMINISTRATION AND DOSAGE SPECIFICS:
Urinary Tract Infections:
Adults: 2-4 gm initially, then 2-4 gm daily in 3-6 divided doses.
Children and infants older than 2 months: 75 mg/kg initially, then 150 mg/kg daily in 4-6 divided doses, with total daily dose not to exceed 6 gm.

SULFONAMIDE COMBINATION PRODUCTS—VAGINAL

PRODUCTS (TRADE NAME):
Koro-Sulf, Sultrin (Available as cream or vaginal tablets.) **Triple Sulfa, Trysul** (Available as vaginal cream.)
DRUG SPECIFICS:
Creams contain 3.42% sulfathiazole, 2.86% sulfacetamide, and 3.7% sulfabenzamide. Vaginal tablets contain 172.5 mg sulfathiazole, 143.75 mg sulfacetamide, and 184 mg sulfabenzamide. Full course of therapy is needed in order to be effective. Sex partners should also be treated. Discontinue medication if burning or local irritation occurs. Effective in about 50% of confirmed Haemophilus vaginitis infections.
ADMINISTRATION AND DOSAGE SPECIFICS:
Vaginitis due to hemophilis vaginalis: Use one applicatorful of cream intravaginally twice daily for 4 to 6 days; or one tablet intravaginally twice daily for 10 days. Treatment may be repeated.

SULFAMETHOXAZOLE AND TRIMETHOPRIM

PRODUCTS (TRADE NAME):
Septra, Bactrim (Available in 400 mg sulfamethoxazole and 80 mg trimethoprim tablet, 200 mg sulfamethoxazole and 40 mg trimethoprim/5 ml suspension.)

Septra-DS, Bactrim-DS (Available in 800 mg sulfamethoxazole and 160 mg trimethoprim tablet.)

DRUG SPECIFICS:

This combination is indicated primarily for treatment of acute and chronic urinary tract infections and as prophylaxis for those tending to have recurrent urinary tract infections. Treatment of shigellosis and acute otitis media in children are further indications for use. Its use is contraindicated during pregnancy.

ADMINISTRATION AND DOSAGE SPECIFICS:

Urinary Tract Infection:

Adults: 160/800 mg tablets every 12 hours for 10-14 days.

Children and infants older than 2 months: 40 mg/kg sulfamethoxazole and 8 mg/kg trimethoprim daily in 2 divided doses every 12 hours for 10 days.

Note: For severe urinary tract infections, increase the daily dose by one half and administer in 3 daily doses.

Shigellosis: Follow dosage given for urinary tract infections for 5 days.

Acute Otitis Media: Follow dosage given for children for urinary tract infections.

Note: If creatinine clearance is 15-30 ml/minute, reduce dose by one-half. Avoid the drug if creatinine clearance is less than 15 ml/minute.

Barbara Sommer Wieferich and L. Colette Jones

2

BIOLOGICAL PREPARATIONS

BIOLOGICAL PREPARATIONS

ACTION OF THE DRUG: The biological preparations are composed of a series of vaccines, toxoids and other serologic agents utilized primarily to prevent and/or modify, disease in an otherwise healthy individual. Depending upon the composition of the biological agent, it will be able to provide active or passive immunity to specific disease states.

Types of Agents:

Vaccine: A biological agent made from whole or portions of bacteria or viruses. They may be live attenuated organisms or non-living inactivated organisms.

Toxoid: A vaccine composed of bacterial toxins or endotoxins. Most toxoids are composed of non-living agents, are frequently bacterial, and are in a non-living, inactive state.

AntiSerums: These products are composed of concentrated antibodies (sometimes specific to a given disease) in the gamma globulin portion of serum. Antibodies may be from human or animal sources.

Types of Immunity:

Passive: This type of immunity is produced largely through the transfer of antibodies previously manufactured by animals or humans to a recipient. It provides a very short-lived temporary form of immunity. Natural immunity can be seen in transfer of maternal antibodies to a newborn infant. Artificial immunity is produced through administration of immune serum globulins.

Active: This type of immunity is produced following introduction of an organism into the recipient's system in order to stimulate an antigen-antibody response. This produces a long-acting and, at times, permanent form of immunity. Natural immunity occurs when an individual is exposed and responds to a disease. Artificial immunity is created when there is the introduction of a live vaccine.

ASSESSMENT:

INDICATIONS: Vaccines and toxoids constitute the biological agents utilized in the routine schedule of active immunizations for adults and children. Specific biological agents are reserved for use in individuals in special circumstances where disease is endemic in nature and presents a high risk of infection (i.e., yellow fever, cholera, typhoid).

Other vaccines are recommended for individuals with increased susceptibility to specific disease states (i.e., pneumococcal vaccine, influenza vaccine).

An additional group of biologicals is utilized in screening procedures to identify individuals exposed to a specific state or with a potentially active disease process (i.e., PPD, histoplasmin, coccidioidin).

In special circumstances certain biological agents may be useful to modify a disease process in the previously unimmunized individual (i.e., gamma globulins).

SUBJECTIVE-OBJEJCTIVE: Patient may present a history of exposure to a specific organism, or plans to travel to areas where disease may be endemic.

Presence of individual who is at high risk for infection, as well as children requiring primary immunizations, are also to be assessed.

PLAN:

CONTRAINDICATIONS: Do not give in the presence of active infectious processes, severe febrile illness, or to patients with a history of previous serious side effects. Live attenuated vaccine is usually contraindicated in pregnancy.

WARNINGS: Use with caution all biological agents prepared in media with allergenic properties (i.e., chick embryos) because of the potential for producing allergic reactions. Defer vaccination with live attenuated virus vaccine if there is recent history of acquired passive antibodies (immune serum globulin).

PRECAUTIONS: Screen patients for concurrent or incubating illness. There is an increased risk for use in any individual with compromised immune status (i.e., neonates, the elderly, patients on immunosuppressive therapy, or patients with chronic disease). There is also an increased risk to immunosuppressed individuals if they reside in the household of a recipient of attenuated viral vaccine.

All vaccines should be used with caution in breast-feeding and pregnant individuals.

IMPLEMENTATION:

DRUG INTERACTIONS: Theoretically there is an increase in adverse effects with the simultaneous administration of vaccines with known potent side effects (i.e., cholera, plague, and typhoid). The recent recipient of passive antibodies (maternal, vaccine, or through blood products) may not demonstrate adequate active antibody response to live attenuated vaccine administration.

ADMINISTRATION AND DOSAGE: It is important to follow specific protocols and schedules for administration. There are frequently specialized storage instructions, modes of administration, sites and site preparation techniques. It is important to consult the package insert for each manufacturer's product.

The dosage schedule recommended for primary immunization of infants, children and adults can be found in Table 2-1.

IMPLEMENTATION CONSIDERATIONS:

—Obtain a complete health history, including patient's previous immunization status and reaction to biological agents, history of allergy, especially to eggs or feathers, and results of any known allergy testing. Ask about presence of underlying disease, concurrent infections, use of immunosuppressant drugs, immune serums, blood or blood products, or the possibility of pregnancy.

—Uncomfortable reactions to active vaccines are frequent and generally range from localized irritation and soreness to a systemic response with fever, malaise and anorexia.

—Specific biologicals may predispose the recipient to a variety of hypersensitivity reactions. These range from a localized rash, pruritus or urticaria to an anaphylactic response.

—Keep a record of patient's immunizations, and provide a record patients can take home to update their own personal files.

TABLE 2-1. RECOMMENDED PRIMARY IMMUNIZATION SERIES

Agent	Preferred Ages and Intervals	Dose/ Route	Booster
DPT*	2, 4 and 6 months; 4-6 week intervals	0.5 ml IM	18 months; 4 to 6 years
TOPV**	2, 4 and 6*** months; 6-8 week intervals	Oral drops	18 months; 4 to 6 years
Measles	15 months	0.5 ml SQ	None
Mumps	15 months	0.5 ml SQ	None
Rubella	15 months	0.5 ml SQ	None
Td4****	Used after 7 years of age for primary series; 2 doses at 8 week intervals; 3rd dose 1 year after 2nd dose.	0.5 ml IM	Every 10 years throughout adulthood

*Combined diptheria, tetanus toxoids, and pertussis vaccine.

**Live oral polio vaccine, trivalent

***Sixth month dose optional depending on prevalence and epidemiology of disease in community.

****Combined tetanus and diptheria toxoids, absorbed adult.

—Occasionally titers may be helpful prior to vaccine administration. This is particularly true for rubella.

—Adverse effects may occur immediately or be delayed for some time after preparation has been administered.

WHAT THE PATIENT NEEDS TO KNOW:

—Localized discomfort may often be relieved by symptomatic measures: use of warm compresses to area, acetaminophen, rest and sometimes antihistamines.

—Record this immunization in your own personal health records.

—Notify health care provider immediately if you develop fever, rash, itching, or difficulty breathing.

EVALUATION:

ADVERSE REACTIONS: *CNS:* altered levels of consciousness, headaches, lethargy, seizures. *Dermatologic:* necrosis, rash, subcutaneous nodules, ulceration, urticaria, vesiculation. *Gastrointestinal:* diarrhea. *Hematopoietic:* thrombocytopenia. *Respiratory:* increased respiratory rate, respiratory distress, shortness of breath. *Other:* arthralgia, arthritis, fever, lymphadenopathy, malaise.

PARAMETERS TO MONITOR: In patients receiving immune serums, watch for suppression or modification of disease. In other patients evaluate for adverse effects. On all visits ask patients about whether immunizations are current or not. There has been a decrease in the extent of pediatric immunizations over the past few years, and few adults obtain needed booster immunizations.

Kathy Awalt

ACTIVE IMMUNIZATION—TOXOIDS

DIPHTHERIA TOXOID, ADSORBED

ACTION OF THE DRUG: Diphtheria toxoid provides the individual with an active immune response against the bacteria *Corynebacterium diphtheriae*, the causative agent in diphtheria. The toxoid is composed of the chemically treated toxoid products of the *Corynebacterium* organism.

ASSESSMENT:

INDICATIONS: This toxoid is used as part of the routine schedule of primary immunizations in infancy and childhood. It is recommended as part of the booster (Td) series every ten years from age 12-14 through adulthood.

PLAN:

CONTRAINDICATIONS: Do not give in acute illness, or in states of immunosuppression from medications or disease.

WARNINGS: Hypersensitivity reactions tend to increase with age. The adult form of the toxoid (2 Lf units marked with d) should be utilized in individuals over six years of age. Previous history of the disease does not confer immunity. Immunizations do not confer lifelong immunity but must be continually updated.

PRECAUTIONS: There are two preparations of diphtheria toxoid: adsorbed and plain. In the absorbed form the addition of alum to the toxoid results in an insoluble precipitate, and while it is more likely to cause local reactions, the preparation is more stable than the plain toxoid and adsorbed more gradually. Generally the adsorbed toxoids are recommended over plain forms.

IMPLEMENTATION:

PRODUCTS (TRADE NAME):
Diphtheria Toxoid Adsorbed-Pediatric Combinations: **Diphtheria, Teta-**

nus Toxoid, Plain-Pediatric; Diphtheria, Tetanus Toxoid, Adsorbed-Pediatric; Diphtheria, Tetanus Toxoid, Adsorbed-Adult; Diphtheria, Tetanus, Pertussis Vaccine, Adsorbed-Connaught, Tri-Immunol, Ultrafine Triple Antigen, Triogen, DPT (diphtheria, pertussis, tetanus toxoid, adsorbed-pediatric.) (Available in 5 ml vials.)

ADMINISTRATION AND DOSAGE: Note two strengths, 15 Lf units and 2 LF units and consider appropriate form for client: 15 Lf is used for children 6 years old or younger and 2 Lf is reserved for adults.

The recommended route is deep IM, preferably Z tract method. Usually 0.5 ml of toxoid is used per dose, but this can be reduced while increasing the total number of injections in special circumstances.

Diphtheria toxoid is available in pediatric (D) and adult (d) strength and in a variety of combinations: DT-pediatric diphtheria and tetanus toxoids; dT-adult diphtheria and tetanus toxoids; DTP-pediatric diphtheria, tetanus and pertussis vaccine.

The recommended primary immunization schedule of diphtheria toxoid (as well as pertussis vaccine and tetanus toxoid) in the United States begins at 2 months of life, and is usually in the form of DTP combinations, given three times in the first 6 to 8 months of life, with 4-to-6 week intervals. This is followed by a booster dose one year later (18 months) and a preschool booster dose (4-6 years). Additional booster doses of dT are recommended every ten years throughout adulthood.

IMPLEMENTATION CONSIDERATIONS:
—Determine health history for allergies, previous immunization history.
—Apply skin test (Zoeller-Moloeny) to screen hypersensitivity.
—Assess for any evidence of current illness or immunosuppressed state.
—Determine appropriate strength pediatric D (15 Lf units) or adult d (2 Lf units) and dosage of toxoid.
—Follow manufacturer's directions for storage and preparation, as this may vary from product to product. Shake vial vigorously prior to withdrawing dose.
—Complete immunization record, and counsel patient regarding immunization status and need for boosters.
—Reactions to immunizations may be more severe over six years.

WHAT THE PATIENT NEEDS TO KNOW:
—Obtain and keep a record of immunization status.
—Apply warm compresses to injection site. Relieve general fever and discomfort with analgesics, antipyretics.
—Notify health provider if severe systemic symptoms develop or if no relief is obtained by above measures.

EVALUATION:

ADVERSE REACTIONS: *Hypersensitivity:* May have severe systemic reactions. *Other:* May exacerbate symptoms of current or incubating illness.

PARAMETERS TO MONITOR: Observe for adverse effects.

Kathy Awalt

TETANUS TOXOID

ACTION OF THE DRUG: Tetanus toxoid is a modified form of *Clostridium tetani* toxin which provides active immunization against the disease tetanus.

ASSESSMENT:

INDICATIONS: This vaccine is used as part of the routine schedule of primary immunizations in infancy and childhood. For active immunization against tetanus in adults and children, tetanus toxoid, fluid may be used, although tetanus toxoid, adsorbed is definitely the preferred agent for all primary immunizations, recall immunizations, for people sensitive to horse serum, patients with asthma or other allergies. Tetanus toxoid adsorbed provides a longer lasting immunity compared to the fluid form. It is recommended as part of the booster (Td) series every ten years from age 12-14 through adulthood.

PLAN:

CONTRAINDICATIONS: Do not give in the presence of active infectious disease processes, or active CNS diseases.

WARNINGS: History of natural disease does not confer immunity.

PRECAUTIONS: The possibility exists for development of local vascular necrosis with frequent doses. A higher degree of side effects appears with increasing age.

IMPLEMENTATION:

PRODUCTS (TRADE NAME):
Tetanus Toxoid, Adsorbed Combinations: **Diphtheria and Tetanus Toxoids, Plain-Pediatric; Diphtheria and Tetanus Toxoids, Adsorbed-Pediatric; Diptheria and Tetanus Toxoids, Adsorbed-Adult; Tri-Immunol, Triple Antigen, Triogen, DPT** (diphtheria, pertussis, tetanus adsorbed, pediatric).

ADMINISTRATION AND DOSAGE: Tetanus Toxoid, Adsorbed must be adminstered IM, while Tetanus Toxoid, Fluid may be given IM or SQ. The recommended route is deep intramuscular, preferably Z tract method. Usually 0.5 ml is used per dose, but this can be reduced while increasing the total number of injections in special circumstances. For adsorbed products, 2 doses are given with a 4 to 6 week interval between injections, and a booster one year later. For fluid products, 3 doses are given with a 4 to 8 week interval between injections, and a booster 6 to 12 months later. Boosters of either product should be given every 10 years.

The recommended primary immunization schedule of tetanus in the United

States is usually in the form of DTP combinations starting at 2 months of age, given three times in the first 6 to 8 months of life, with 4- to 6-week intervals. This is followed by a booster dose 1 year later (18 months) and a booster dose pre-school (4-6 years). Additional booster doses of DT are recommended every ten years throughout adulthood. There are two strengths, 7-25 Lf units and 2 Lf units; 7-25 Lf units are used for children 7 years old or younger while 2 Lf units are reserved for adults and children 7 years or older.

In wounds which are tetanus-prone (where anaerobic conditions are present or in which likelihood of exposure to tetanus spores is high) new recommendations for immunization have been released by CDC and the Report of the Committee on Infectious Diseases of the American Academy of Pediatrics. These recommendations are:

Unimmunized or incompletely immunized individual (one or two doses of toxoid): Give one dose of Td or DT followed by completion of immunization in low-risk wound. Give one dose of Td or DT plus 250 to 500 U tetanus immune globulin (TIG) followed by completion of immunization for tetanus-prone wound or wound untreated for more than 24 hours. Give booster every 10 years.

Immunized individual with booster dose within 10 years of primary series: No toxoid is necessary in low-risk wounds. One dose of Td if it has been more than 5 years since immunization in tetanus-prone wounds. If wound is neglected more than 24 hours, give one dose of Td plus 250 to 500 Units tetanus immune globulin (TIG).

Immunized individual with no booster or last booster more than 10 years ago: Give one dose of Td in low-risk wounds and tetanus-prone wounds. Give one dose Td plus 250 to 500 Units tetanus immune globulin (TIG) in wounds neglected for more than 24 hours.

IMPLEMENTATION CONSIDERATIONS:

—Obtain health history, including current immunization status of patient, active CNS disease, previous allergies or adverse reactions to the toxoid.

—Adverse reactions may be more severe in patients over 17 years old.

—Note any evidence of current illness or immunosuppressed state.

—Follow manufacturer's directions for storage and preparation, as this may vary from preparation to preparation.

—Complete immunization record and counsel patient regarding need for boosters.

—Separate syringes and sites should be used if TIG and Td are used together.

WHAT THE PATIENT NEEDS TO KNOW:

—Obtain and keep a record of immunization.

—Apply warm compresses to injection site, relieve general fever and discomfort with analgesics, antipyretics.

—Notify health care provider if severe systemic symptoms develop or if no relief is obtained by above measures.

EVALUATION:

ADVERSE REACTIONS: Vascular necrosis at injection site (rare), localized pain and erythema may occur.
PARAMETERS TO MONITOR: Observe for adverse reactions.

Kathy Awalt

ACTIVE IMMUNIZATION—BACTERIAL VACCINES

CHOLERA VACCINE

ACTION OF THE DRUG: Cholera vaccine provides active immunization against cholera caused by the organism *Vibrio cholerae*.

ASSESSMENT:

INDICATIONS: Cholera vaccine is recommended when traveling or working in an area endemic to cholera. It is required by certain countries prior to entry.

PLAN:

CONTRAINDICATIONS: Do not give if there is a previous history of serious reaction to cholera vaccine, or if the patient is a child under six months of age.
WARNING: Cholera vaccine provides limited protection only, ranging from three to six months. Boosters are needed for continuous protection. Vaccine does not prevent transmission of disease.

IMPLEMENTATION:

PRODUCTS (TRADE NAME):
Cholera Vaccine (Available in 1, 1.5 and 20 ml vials.)
ADMINISTRATION AND DOSAGE: Recommended route is IM. Two initial doses are given at one-month intervals, followed by a booster dose within six months. Dosages are as follows for various age groups:

	#1	*#2*	*Booster*
6 months–5 years:	0.2 ml	0.2 ml	0.2 ml
5–10 years:	0.3 ml	0.3 ml	0.3 ml
Over 10 years:	0.5 ml	0.5 ml	0.5 ml

IMPLEMENTATION CONSIDERATIONS:
—Local pain and induration may develop at site of injection.
—Generalized fever, headaches and gastrointestinal symptoms may occur.

—Symptoms may occur within 24 hours of administration or may be delayed up to three to four days.

WHAT THE PATIENT NEEDS TO KNOW:
—Some patients experience local symptoms, such as mild pain and swelling at injection site, and/or general symptoms of mild fever, headaches or stomach upset.
—Apply warm compresses to injection site to relieve discomfort. Do not apply dressing.
—Take mild analgesic to relieve discomfort and fever.
—Notify health care provider if you develop other symptoms which are not relieved by aspirin.
—Plan to take injection a week or more before traveling abroad as reactions may be delayed a few days in some individuals.

EVALUATION:

ADVERSE REACTIONS: Watch for local induration and pain, mild fever, headaches and gastrointestinal distress.
PARAMETERS TO MONITOR: Observe for adverse effects.

Kathy Awalt

MENINGITIS VACCINE

ACTION OF THE DRUG: Meningococcal polysaccharides induce the formation of human serum bactericidal antibodies which leads to immunity to specific organisms. This product does not provide immunity against all varieties of microorganisms causing meningitis.

ASSESSMENT:

INDICATIONS: These vaccines will stimulate protection against infections caused by *Neisseria meningitidis* Groups A, C, Y, and W-135. Meningitis vaccines should be used in areas where meningitis is endemic or in individuals at high risk. General use is not recommended.

Children over 3 months of age and adults at risk are usually given Group A vaccine. Children over 2 months of age and adults at risk usually receive Group C and Groups A and C vaccine. Groups A, C, Y, and W-135 are reserved for adults over 18 years of age. Health care and laboratory workers with high exposure rates to meningitis may also be considered for vaccination.

PLAN:

CONTRAINDICATIONS: Do not give to patients with immune deficiency conditions, prolonged therapy on corticosteroids, active infections (especially acute respiratory infections), or to women who are pregnant.

PRECAUTIONS: Some patients develop allergic reactions to this preparation, and all patients should therefore be monitored closely following administration of this product. Emergency equipment and medications such as epinephrine 1:1000 should be immediately available for treatment.

IMPLEMENTATION:

ADMINISTRATION AND DOSAGE: All preparations should be given SQ. In children older than 2 years and in adults, one 0.5 ml SQ injection is used. In children 3 to 24 months, two 0.5 ml SQ injections are given one month apart.

IMPLEMENTATION CONSIDERATIONS:

—Obtain a complete health history to establish definite need for this vaccine, and that individual is without immune defect, active infection, and is taking no corticosteroids. Rule out the possibility of pregnancy, since the effects of this product on a fetus are unknown.

—Many reactions to this product are allergic in nature. Occasionally a febrile reaction will develop which is self-limiting.

—This is a new product, and latest information should be obtained based upon further experience with the vaccine.

—Diluent comes with the product for reconstitution. Solution should be shaken until well dissolved. Unused vaccine should be marked with the date, stored between 35-56 degrees F., and discarded within 5 days if not completely used.

WHAT THE PATIENT NEEDS TO KNOW:

—Patients often do not feel well for a short time after taking this vaccine. You may experience a headache and be tired. Localized swelling and a temperature are also produced in some patients as a result of these vaccines. Fever and swelling usually get better within 1 to 2 days.

—Take acetaminophen to reduce swelling and provide greater comfort. Warm compresses may also be applied to injection site to reduce discomfort.

—Notify your health care provider if you develop any other symptoms, or if you do not obtain relief with the above measures.

—This is a medication which should be recorded in your personal immunization record.

EVALUATION:

ADVERSE REACTIONS: *Local:* Injection site may become sore, tender, red and swollen. Lymphadenopathy may also develop in axillary region. Local allergic manifestations at site of injection also sometimes occur. *Systemic:* Febrile reactions may be seen which develop several hours after vaccination and last 24 to 48 hours. More commonly, headaches, chills, cramps, tiredness or malaise are experienced. These are self-limiting. Rarely, a generalized hypersensitivity reaction develops.

PARAMETERS TO MONITOR: Observe patient for at least 15 minutes after giving injection to evaluate for allergic reactions. Monitor for adverse reactions and give supportive therapy as needed.

MENINGOCOCCAL POLYSACCHARIDE VACCINE, GROUP A

PRODUCTS (TRADE NAME):
Menomune-A (Available in 10 and 50 dose vials.)
DRUG SPECIFICS:
This is the only preparation which may be given to children under 2 years of age. It is also a component of several of the other mixtures. Give injections SQ.
ADMINISTRATION AND DOSAGE SPECIFICS:
Adults and children 2 years or older: Give one 0.5 ml SQ injection.
Children 3 to 24 months: Give two 0.5 ml SQ injections at least one month apart.

MENINGOCOCCAL POLYSACCHARIDE VACCINE, GROUP C

PRODUCTS (TRADE NAME):
Menomune-C (Available in 10 and 50 dose vials.)
DRUG SPECIFICS:
Used for children over 2 years of age, and for adults at high risk or in endemic areas.
ADMINISTRATION AND DOSAGE SPECIFICS:
Give one 0.5 ml SQ injection.

MENINGOCOCCAL POLYSACCHARIDE VACCINE, GROUPS A AND C

PRODUCTS (TRADE NAME):
Memomune-A/C, Meningovax-AC (Available in 10 and 50 dose vials.)

DRUG SPECIFICS:
Used for children over 2 years of age, and for adults at high risk or in endemic areas.
ADMINISTRATION AND DOSAGE SPECIFICS:
Give one 0.5 ml SQ injection.

MENINGOCOCCAL POLYSACCHARIDE VACCINE, GROUPS A, C, Y AND W-135

PRODUCTS (TRADE NAME):
Menomune-A/C/Y/W-135 (Available in 10 and 50 dose vials.)
DRUG SPECIFICS:
Used for adults 18 years or older at high risk or in endemic areas.
ADMINISTRATION AND DOSAGE SPECIFICS:
Give one 0.5 ml SQ injection.

Marilyn W. Edmunds

PLAGUE VACCINE

ACTION OF THE DRUG: This vaccine provides active immunization to plague in order to reduce the incidence and severity of disease. The vaccine is a killed preparation of *Yersinia pestis*.

ASSESSMENT:

INDICATIONS: Recommended *only* for individuals in situations with high risk of plague. This includes those traveling or working in geographic areas endemic to plague, or individuals whose work is in contact with the *Yersinia pestis* organism (i.e., with wild rodents and their fleas).

PLAN:

WARNINGS: This vaccine should be administered *only* to those in a high-risk situation. Risk must be weighed against benefit.

IMPLEMENTATION:

PRODUCTS (TRADE NAME):
Plague Vaccine (Available in 20 ml vials.)
ADMINISTRATION AND DOSAGE: Two primary doses are given one month

apart, followed by a third dose 1-3 months later. Boosters are then given at 6-12 month intervals for a total of 5 doses, and 12-24 month intervals as long as exposure exists. An accelerated schedule may be used which provides for 3 doses of 0.5 ml at least 1 week apart. All doses are given IM. Dosage for various age groups is as follows:

Age	Immunization Dose #1	#2–#3	Boosters
Under 1 year:	0.2 ml	0.04 ml	0.02 to 0.04 ml
1–4 years:	0.4 ml	0.08 ml	0.04 to 0.08 ml
5–10 years:	0.6 ml	0.12 ml	0.06 to 0.12 ml
Adults and children over 10 years:	1.0 ml	0.2 ml	0.1 to 0.2 ml

IMPLEMENTATION CONSIDERATIONS:

—There is the possibility of side effects ranging from localized tenderness and erythema to high fever, malaise and headaches.

—Severity of side effects may increase with repeated doses. Use lower doses if severe reactions are anticipated.

WHAT THE PATIENT NEEDS TO KNOW:

—Patients often develop localized swelling and temperature as a result of these injections.

—Apply warm compresses to injection site to reduce discomfort.

—Take antipyretics or mild analgesics as needed.

—Notify your health provider if you develop any other symptoms, or if you do not obtain relief with the above measures.

—This is a medication which should be recorded in your personal immunization record.

EVALUATION:

ADVERSE REACTIONS: Side effects are often unpredictable. There is a wide range of severity and manifestation of symptoms.

PARAMETERS TO MONITOR: Observe for adverse reactions. Give supportive therapy.

Kathy Awalt

PNEUMOCOCCAL VACCINE, POLYVALENT

ACTION OF THE DRUG: Pneumococcal vaccine provides active protection against a variety of pneumococcal infections. The vaccine is composed of purified polysaccharide antigens of the fourteen most common types of pneumococcal organisms.

ASSESSMENT:

INDICATIONS: Pneumococcal vaccine is appropriate for individuals at high risk for compromise of present health status from pneumococcal infection. Specific situations may include: sickle cell disease and/or splenic dysfunction, asplenia, chronic cardiac, respiratory, hepatic, renal or metabolic disease, alcoholic cirrhosis, immunodeficiency via disease or drugs, individuals over age fifty. Also consider individuals at high risk in a living situation that may carry a risk of pneumococcal disease in epidemic or endemic form (i.e., nursing homes). It is also indicated in children 2 years of age or older who are at risk of developing middle ear infections.

SUBJECTIVE OBJECTIVE: History of patient in high risk category for complicated pneumococcal infections. Obtain previous pneumococcal vaccine history and response, and assess present living situation, including close contacts.

PLAN:

CONTRAINDICATIONS: Do not use in children under two years of age, in the presence of acute illness or active infectious process, or with pregnant women.

WARNINGS: Some high risk candidates may not have an effective antibody response to all fourteen strains in the vaccine. Keep epinephrine 1:1000 available for subcutaneous use in immediate allergic reactions.

PRECAUTIONS: In patients who have a history of previous pneumococcal infections, high levels of preexisting pneumococcal antibodies may be present which will result in excessive reactions to this vaccine. Most reactions are local, however, generalized systemic reactions may occur and patients with a previous history of pneumococcal infections should be monitored carefully. Also use care in giving to patients with cardiopulmonary disease in whom a systemic reaction would pose a special threat.

IMPLEMENTATION:

PRODUCTS (TRADE NAME):
Pneumovax 23, Pnu-Imune 23 (Available in 50 mcg/0.5 ml in single and 5 dose vials. Each dose contains 23 polysaccharide isolates per dose.)

ADMINISTRATION AND DOSAGE: Give 0.5 cc IM or SQ. Revaccinations may be necessary in three or more years.

IMPLEMENTATION CONSIDERATIONS:
—Minimal localized soreness and low-grade fever may result.
—Patient may need to be convinced of the usefulness of this injection.
—In patients receiving antibiotic prophylaxis against pneumococcal infection, antibiotics should not be discontinued after vaccination.
—This vaccine may be given simultaneously with whole-virus influenza vaccine or split-virus influenza vaccine without increasing the occurrence of adverse reactions.
—Do not give booster injections of this vaccine to previously vaccinated subjects. Additional doses do not increase antibody titers and may provoke severe local reactions at the site of injection.

> **WHAT THE PATIENT NEEDS TO KNOW:**
> —Sometimes mild soreness at the site of injection develops. This can be relieved through warm compresses on the site.
> —Some patients also develop a mild temperature following this injection. Aspirin or similar antipyretic medication may relieve discomfort and reduce fever.
> —Report any new symptoms you may have to your health provider.

EVALUATION:

ADVERSE REACTIONS: *Hypersensitivity:* Occasionally, anaphylaxis or severe systemic reactions may occur consisting of fever over 104 degrees F (40 degrees C), and leukocytosis. No evidence of permanent sequelae or death has been reported.

PARAMETERS TO MONITOR: Observe for local irritation or development of sensitivity.

Kathy Awalt

TYPHOID VACCINE

ACTION OF THE DRUG: Typhoid vaccine provides active immunization against typhoid fever caused by *Salmonella typhi*. Vaccine is a preparation of the killed typhoid bacilli and provides protection in cases of mild to moderate exposure.

ASSESSMENT:

INDICATIONS: Recommended for use only in individuals exposed to disease or carrier state, and those traveling or working in areas endemic to typhoid fever.

PLAN:

CONTRAINDICATIONS: Do not use in cases of active acute illness or debilitating disease process.

WARNINGS: The level of immunity achieved is variable. The average length of protection is one to two years. The vaccine does not protect in cases of high exposure to typhoid bacilli. Routine use of the vaccine is not indicated in cases of natural disaster (earthquakes, floods, etc.).

IMPLEMENTATION:

PRODUCTS (TRADE NAME):
Typhoid Vaccine (Available in 8 units/ml in 5, 10 and 20 ml vials.)

ADMINISTRATION AND DOSAGE: Preferred route of administration is subcutaneous. Dosages are given twice with a one-month interval. Repeat doses can be administered every three years to patients with continuous exposure. Dosages for various age groups are as follows:

	#1	#2
Under 10 years:	0.25 ml	0.25 ml
Over 10 years:	0.5 ml	0.5 ml

IMPLEMENTATION CONSIDERATIONS:
—There is a wide and variable range of reactions.
—Symptoms may range from localized tenderness to generalized lymphadenopathy and high fever.

WHAT THE PATIENT NEEDS TO KNOW:
—Reactions to this injection are individualized and unpredictable.
—If you develop localized soreness at the injection site, use warm compresses and analgesic for symptomatic relief of mild symptoms.
—Notify your health care provider if symptoms increase in severity or if compresses and aspirin do not relieve symptoms.

EVALUATION:

PARAMETERS TO MONITOR: Watch for localized discomfort.

Kathy Awalt

ACTIVE IMMUNIZATIONS—VIRAL VACCINES

HEPATITIS B VACCINE

ACTION OF THE DRUG: Hepatitis B vaccine induces neutralizing antibody (anti-HBs). This provides protective immunity against the hepatitis B virus.

ASSESSMENT:

INDICATIONS: Used for immunization against infection caused by all known subtypes of hepatitis B virus. It is not effective in preventing infection caused by viruses resposible for hepatitis A, non-A, non-B, or other hepatitis-producing organisms. Its use in preventing infection post exposure has not been studied for sufficient time to determine effectiveness. Because the virus has a long incubation period, it is possible to give the vaccine before the infection is recognized, thus being ineffective in preventing the disease. This vaccine is indicated in individuals who have increased risk of developing hepatitis B such as health and laboratory personnel especially those handling blood and blood products, staff and patients in institutions for the mentally handicapped, persons with high risk such as Alaskan Eskimos, Haitian and Indochinese refugees, military personnel in some overseas areas, morticians and embalmers, prisoners, persons known to use illicit street drugs, persons who repeatedly contract sexually transmitted diseases, homosexual males and female prostitutes.

PLAN:

CONTRAINDICATIONS: Do not give to patients who show any indication of hypersensitivity to the vaccine.

WARNINGS: Immunosuppressed individuals may require larger doses than average in order to build up a supply of circulating antibodies. The use of this product has not been studied in pregnant women, breast-feeding women, or in children under 3 months of age and use in these populations should be avoided.

PRECAUTIONS: Delay using this vaccine in patients with severe active infections, compromised cardiopulmonary status, or severely weakened or debilitated conditions. Be alert for development of anaphylaxis or other generalized allergic reactions.

IMPLEMENTATION:

PRODUCTS (TRADE NAME):
Heptavax-B (Available in 20 mcg antigen/ml for injection.)
ADMINISTRATION AND DOSAGE:
Adults and older children: Give 1.0 ml IM initially and 1 and 6 months later.
Children 3 months to 10 years old: Give 0.5 ml IM initially and 1 and 6 months later.
Dialysis or immunocompromised individuals: Give 2.0 ml IM initially and 1 and 6 months later.
IMPLEMENTATION CONSIDERATIONS:
—Obtain a thorough health history, including allergies, presence of systemic disease, possibility of pregnancy, and documentation of high risk of developing infection from hepatitis B virus.
—Shake medication thoroughly before withdrawing solution. Use sterile needle free of detergents, antiseptics or preservatives in administering medication.
—Do not freeze vaccine or potency will be destroyed.
—This is a new product and updated information will be released as it is obtained. This information should be sought prior to administration of vaccine.
—The length of protection provided by this product has not been established. Probably protection is 5 years, with further immunity maintained by a single booster.
—Product is usually well tolerated and without serious adverse effects.

WHAT THE PATIENT NEEDS TO KNOW:
—Occasionally this vaccine may produce a few side effects. These are usually mild and disappear within a few days. You may note soreness at the site of injection. This may be relieved by warm compresses to the site and use of aspirin or acetaminophen.
—Notify your health care provider if you develop any severe or unusual symptoms such as trouble breathing, itching rash, high temperature.

EVALUATION:

ADVERSE REACTIONS: *Local:* erythema, induration, swelling and warmth at injection site. *Systemic:* Arthralgia, dizziness, headache, fatigue, low grade fever, malaise, myalgia, nausea, and rash have been reported.
PARAMETERS TO MONITOR: Evaluate patient immediately after injection for symptoms of hypersensitivity to vaccine. Monitor adverse reactions.

Marilyn W. Edmunds

INFLUENZA VIRUS VACCINE

ACTION OF THE DRUG: Influenza virus vaccine provides active protection against a variety of influenza viruses. The vaccine consists of inactivated whole or split virus of types A and B. The specific viral strains may vary to protect against the influenza virus prevalent in a specific community.

ASSESSMENT:

INDICATIONS: This vaccine is utilized in individuals who are at high risk for complications following an influenza viral infection. These high-risk categories would include: chronic heart disease, chronic respiratory, renal or metabolic disease, severe anemias, sickle cell disease, immunosuppressed individuals, and individuals over the age of sixty-five.

PLAN:

CONTRAINDICATIONS: Do not give to individuals with history of egg hypersensitivity.
PRECAUTIONS: Two viral preparations are available: whole and split. Whole virus carries a greater incidence of side effects and is recommended for those thirteen years and older. Split virus is recommended for children under thirteen years.

IMPLEMENTATION:

PRODUCTS (TRADE NAME):
Fluogen, Fluzone-Connaught, Influenza Virus [Trivalent] Types A & B
(Available in split virus with 15 mcg A/Brazil/78, 15 mcg A/Philippines/82 and 15 mcg B/Singapore/79 hemagglutinin antigens/0.5 ml). **Fluzone-Connaught** (Available in whole virus with 15 mcg A/Brazil/78, 15 mcg A/Philippines/82 and 15 mcg B/Singapore/79 hemagglutinin antigens/0.5 ml.)

ADMINISTRATION AND DOSAGE: Dosage and administration varies widely depending on vaccine composition and manufacturer. Recommended frequency is one 0.5 ml dose annually for adults and children over 13 years, and two doses (0.5 ml for children 3 to 12 years and 0.25 mg for children 6 to 35 months) separated by a one month interval for children under six years.

IMPLEMENTATION CONSIDERATIONS:
—Obtain health history. Determine presence of allergies.
—Perform skin testing as needed.
—Consider the benefit to patient compared to risk in using whole or split virus preparations.
—Review current recommendations for dosage and administration, as they vary from year to year, type of preparation and manufacturer.
—May increase theophylline blood levels in patients with concurrent therapy.

WHAT THE PATIENT NEEDS TO KNOW:
—Some patients experience side effects to this injection. Fever, malaise and myalgia as systemic side effects are most common in children.
—Report any allergic symptoms to health care provider.
—Report evidence of any new or troublesome symptoms to health care provider.

EVALUATION:

ADVERSE REACTIONS: *Hypersensitivity:* fever, malaise and myalgia, potential anaphylactic response, possible Guillain-Barré syndrome as sequelae.
PARAMETERS TO MONITOR: Watch for adverse effects.

Kathy Awalt

MEASLES VIRUS VACCINE, LIVE ATTENUATED

ACTION OF THE DRUG: Measles vaccine provides active immunity against rubeola virus and its complications.

ASSESSMENT:

INDICATIONS: This vaccine is used in the primary course of immunizations in the young child. Persons susceptible to measles (rubeola) regardless of age may take this vaccine.

PLAN:

CONTRAINDICATIONS: Do not use in immunosuppressed individuals (whether due to therapy or disease), or if patient is pregnant. Do not use in presence of acute febrile illness, recent administration (within three months) of ISG or blood transfusion, or in patients with active tuberculosis.

WARNINGS: Use with caution in patients with a sensitivity to eggs. Vaccine is prepared in a chick embryo culture medium. There are, however, no past reports of allergic response. Vaccine use may potentially exacerbate tuberculosis. Not to be given to patients under 15 months of age due to potential interference with maternal antibodies.

PRECAUTIONS: Atypical, severe local or systemic reactions may occur with a previous history of inactivated vaccine (KMV) immunization.

IMPLEMENTATION:

PRODUCTS (TRADE NAME):
Attenuvax, M-Vac, M R-Vax II (Combined Measles-Rubella.) **M M R II** (Combined Measles, Mumps, Rubella.) (Available in single dose vials.)

ADMINISTRATION AND DOSAGE: A subcutaneous injection of 0.5 cc is given one time. In the United States, the recommended age is approximately 15 months. The vaccine may be given in children 6 to 15 months of age in an epidemic, and the dose must be repeated at 15 months.

See primary immunization schedule in Table 2-1.

IMPLEMENTATION CONSIDERATIONS:
—Obtain a health history, including allergies, other concurrent diseases.
—May need to check results of a tuberculosis screening test.
—May want to check current measles titer in adolescents and young adults immunized at 15 months or younger.
—Immunity to wild rubeola virus is lifelong.
—Review storage and preparation technique of manufacturer (i.e., some products may become inactivated when heated or improper diluent utilized).
—Establish immunization status and record.

WHAT THE PATIENT NEEDS TO KNOW:
—Obtain and keep immunization record and record of titers if drawn.
—Possible mild fever and generalized rash may develop.
—Notify health provider if side effects are not relieved by aspirin.

EVALUATION:

ADVERSE REACTIONS: *CNS:* subacute measles paraencephalitis (rare). May develop tuberculous meningitis with active tuberculosis disease. Possible exacerbation of active tuberculosis. *Dermatologic:* mild fever and generalized rash.
PARAMETERS TO MONITOR: Observe for adverse effects.

Kathy Awalt

MUMPS VIRUS VACCINE, LIVE

ACTION OF THE DRUG: Mumps vaccine provides active immunity against infection by mumps virus and its potential complications. The purpose is to prevent the possible sequelae of wild mumps virus in post pubertal males (orchitis). Also, to prevent mumps meningoencephalitis in children and adults.

ASSESSMENT:

INDICATIONS: This vaccine is used in primary immunization regimen for infants and children. It is also used in individualized cases of prepubertal males with no history of wild mumps virus or immunization.

PLAN:

CONTRAINDICATIONS: Do not use in immunosuppressed individuals (whether from therapy or disease), or in patients with an acute febrile illness. Do not use if patient is pregnant, or has had a recent (within 3 months) administration of ISG or blood products. Do not use in patients hypersensitive to neomycin.
WARNINGS: Not to be given to children under 15 months of age due to potential interference with maternal antibodies.
PRECAUTIONS: Use with care in individuals with a hypersensitivity to eggs, although no allergic reactions have been reported.

IMPLEMENTATION:

PRODUCTS (TRADE NAME):
Mumps Vaccine, Mumpsvax, Biavax II (Combined Rubella-Mumps), **M M R II** (Combined Measles, Mumps, Rubella.) (Available in single dose vials.)
ADMINISTRATION AND DOSAGE: A subcutaneous injection of 0.5 ml is given under normal circumstances. In the United States, 15 months is the recommended age for mumps vaccine. The vaccine can be given separately or in combination with measles (MM), rubella (MR), or measles and rubella (MMR). Individuals not immunized at 15 months can be vaccinated anytime from 15 months to before puberty.

See primary immunization schedule in Table 2-1.

IMPLEMENTATION CONSIDERATIONS:

—Obtain a health history, including allergies.

—Establish and record immunization history.

—If giving mumps vaccine separately from other viral vaccines, allow one month between administration.

—There is no need to establish a mumps titer prior to injection, as no danger to vaccine recipient exists if patient has unknowingly had mumps vaccine or disease.

WHAT THE PATIENT NEEDS TO KNOW:

—Keep a record of this immunization in your personal immunization forms.

EVALUATION:

ADVERSE REACTIONS: *CNS:* febrile seizures, encephalitis, unilateral nerve deafness.

PARAMETERS TO MONITOR: Watch for adverse effects.

Kathy Awalt

PERTUSSIS VACCINE (IN COMBINATION)

ACTION OF THE DRUG: Vaccine provides active immunization against pertussis.

ASSESSMENT:

INDICATIONS: Use as part of the routine schedule of primary immunizations in infancy and childhood.

PLAN:

CONTRAINDICATIONS: Do not use in a generalized acute illness, with an active CNS disorder, or if there is a history of CNS side effects following previous pertussis vaccine administration.

WARNINGS: An episode of pertussis confers lifelong immunity to the disease. This vaccine is not recommended for people over six years of age due to potential serious side effects in older children and adults.

PRECAUTIONS: Controversy exists in cases with a stable CNS disorder and/or seizure disorders. There is a high percentage of side effects with wide variability.

IMPLEMENTATION:

PRODUCTS (TRADE NAME):
Combinations: **Tri-Immunol, Triple Antigen, Triogen, DPT** (diphtheria, pertussis, tetanus toxoid, adsorbed-pediatric).

ADMINISTRATION AND DOSAGE: The recommended route is deep intramuscular, preferably Z tract method. Usually 0.5 ml is given per dose, but this can be reduced while increasing the total number of injections in special circumstances.

The recommended primary immunization schedule of pertussis in the United States is usually in the form of DTP combinations, starting at 2 months of age, and given three times in the first 6 to 8 months, with 4-to-6 week intervals. This is followed by a booster dose 1 year later (18 months) and a preschool booster dose (4-6 years). Routine immunization schedules can be altered in cases of epidemics or increased sensitivity to the vaccine. Pertussis vaccine may be given separately and the dosage decreased.

IMPLEMENTATION CONSIDERATIONS:
—Obtain a health history, especially looking for allergies, CNS disorders, history of seizures, or adverse reations to the vaccine.

—Determine presence of any current illness or immunosuppressed state.

—Follow manufacturer's directions for storage and preparation, as this may vary from preparation to preparation.

—Complete immunization record, and counsel patient regarding need for boosters.

WHAT THE PATIENT NEEDS TO KNOW:
—Obtain and keep a record of this immunization.

—Apply warm compresses to injection site, relieve general fever and discomfort with aspirin.

—Notify health care provider if severe systemic symptoms develop, or if there is no relief from the compresses and aspirin.

—Notify health care provider immediately if convulsions, high fever, screaming, or altered level of consciousness develops.

EVALUATION:

ADVERSE REACTIONS: *CNS:* convulsions, high fever, screaming episodes, altered level of consciousness (rare), encephalitis (rare). *Hypersensitivity:* local erythema, edema, subcutaneous nodule or abscess at injection site, general irritability and gastrointestinal side effects (rare).

PARAMETERS TO MONITOR: Observe for adverse reactions.

Kathy Awalt

POLIOVIRUS VACCINE, LIVE, ORAL, TRIVALENT (TOPV, SALK)

ACTION OF THE DRUG: Poliovirus vaccine provides active immunization against poliomyelitis caused by polioviruses types 1, 2 and 3. It provides both intestinal immunity as well as systemic immunity. This immunity is similar to that produced by natural disease.

ASSESSMENT:

INDICATIONS: This vaccine is used as part of the routine primary immunization schedule in infancy and childhood. Specific monovalent types may be administered in poliomyelitis epidemics (type 1, 2 or 3, depending on viral cause).

PLAN:

CONTRAINDICATIONS: Should not be given in cases of immunosuppression due to disease or therapy. Do not ever give parenterally. Do not give in patients with active infection, diarrhea, vomiting, or in a weakened or debilitated state.

WARNINGS: This vaccine is not routinely recommended in adults over eighteen years unless epidemic risk is present. Use caution in administering to child who is in close contact with an immunosuppressed individual. It is recommended in pregnancy only when the individual is at high risk to polio (i.e., during an epidemic).

PRECAUTIONS: This vaccine is not advised in the presence of a gastrointestinal illness , concurrent enterovirus infection, or immediately after Immune Serum Globulin (ISG) has been administered. This vaccine is not effective in modifying or preventing preexisting or incubating disease.

IMPLEMENTATION:

PRODUCTS (TRADE NAME):
Orimune (Sabin vaccine is available in 0.5 ml single dose dispettes and contains less than 25 mcg each streptomycin and neomycin.)

ADMINISTRATION AND DOSAGE: Two to three primary doses are given in the first six to eight months of life, beginning at 2 months of age. Give 0.5 ml directly or mixed with distilled water, chlorine-free tap water, milk, or on sugar cube, bread or cake. Do not ever give medication parenterally. The first dose of two drops is given po and is usually given with the first DPT. All doses are separated by six-to-eight-week intervals. A booster dose is given at 18 months and again between ages 4 to 6, prior to school entry. Under normal circumstances, dosages are not repeated. See Table 2-1.

IMPLEMENTATION CONSIDERATIONS:
—Obtain health history to check for immunosuppression in patient or close contacts of patient.

—Ascertain absence of gastrointestinal virus or acute illness.

—Establish immunization record and history.

—Check appropriate storage of vaccine. It is usually kept frozen (below O degrees C) and thawed prior to use. Vaccine is active two to seven days after thawing.

—Episodes of wild poliovirus confer lifelong immunity in patient.

—The Salk (inactivated poliovirus) vaccine has limited availability in the United States. Consider use of this vaccine in immunosuppressed individuals or their close contacts or when OPV is indicated.

—In rare cases, vaccine-related paralysis has been produced. Patient, parent or guardian should be advised of this possibility prior to vaccination.

WHAT THE PATIENT NEEDS TO KNOW:
—Establish and keep a record of this immunization.

EVALUATION:

ADVERSE REACTIONS: There is a very low incidence of paralytic poliomyelitis disease from the vaccine. It may occur in a vaccine recipient or very close contacts.

PARAMETERS TO MONITOR: Observe for side effects.

Kathy Awalt

POLIOMYELITIS VACCINE, INACTIVATED (IPV, SALK)

ACTION OF THE DRUG: This vaccine stimulates the production of poliomyelitis antibodies. Four doses are required for adequate immunization. Presence of antibodies may not protect all individuals on exposure.

ASSESSMENT:

INDICATIONS: This product is the treatment of choice in patients who have compromised immune systems and cannot take the Sabin Trivalent Oral Poliovirus Vaccine which would usually be given. In adults who have not been previously vaccinated, the use of IPV vaccine is recommended because the risk of a vaccine-related paralysis following OPV is slightly higher in adults than in children.

Routine immunizations for poliomyelitis is not necessary unless the adult is at increased risk of exposure to wild poliovirus (e.g., country endemic to polio, lab-worker, health care worker).

SUBJECTIVE-OBJECTIVE: Documentation of immune-deficient individual who needs primary immunization to polio.

PLAN:

CONTRAINDICATIONS: Do not give in the presence of active infection, especially of the respiratory system. Do not give if patient has a history of taking corticosteroids or other immunosuppressive agents which would block the action of this drug.

WARNINGS: Examine solution carefully and discard if particulate matter or discoloration is apparent. Have epinephrine available for immediate treatment of severe allergic reactions. Do not give to pregnant women.

PRECAUTIONS: It must be remembered that this drug does not provide immunity against polio to all individuals. This would be especially true if the individual were immune deficient. Allergic reactions to the animal protein, streptomycin, and neomycin present in these products should be assessed.

IMPLEMENTATION:

PRODUCTS (TRADE NAME):

Poliomyelitis Vaccine (Purified)-Connaught (Available in suspensions of 1 ml ampules and 10 ml vials for injection.)

ADMINISTRATION AND DOSAGE: Administer SQ in the deltoid muscle according to the following schedule:

Primary immunization: Give 3 injections, 1 ml SQ each, at four-to-six week intervals. Give a fourth 1 ml dose 6 to 12 months after the third dose. Give 1 ml booster doses every 2 to 3 years. Often given with other primary immunizations.

Supplementary immunization: In all IPV immunized children, a booster dose should be given before starting school. Adults previously immunized with IPV and who are at increased risk of exposure may take a dose of either OPV or IPV. If a primary series of OPV is then completed, necessity for booster IPV every 5 years is avoided.

Unvaccinated or incompletely vaccinated adults: Primary immunization should be completed, or given as an initial series with three doses of 1 ml at one-to-two-month intervals, with a fourth dose six to twelve months after the third.

IMPLEMENTATION CONSIDERATIONS:

—Obtain a complete health history to check for immunosuppression, active infections, corticosteroid use, or possibility of pregnancy. Obtain details of previous vaccinations regarding type and date.

—Vaccine is to be stored in refrigerator between 35 and 46 degrees F.

—Product contains streptomycin, neomycin and protein, which may produce allergies in sensitive individuals.

—Because of rare instances of vaccine-related paralysis, patient, parent or guardian should be advised of this problem before vaccination.

WHAT THE PATIENT NEEDS TO KNOW:

—Observe for any allergic reactions or side effects from this drug and report them to your health care provider.

—This is a vaccination which should be recorded in your personal health records.

EVALUATION:

ADVERSE REACTIONS: Allergic reactions have sometimes been reported due to the presence of protein, streptomycin and neomycin. Rare cases of vaccine-related paralysis have also been reported.

PARAMETERS TO MONITOR: Monitor for adverse effects.

Marilyn W. Edmunds

RUBELLA VIRUS VACCINE, LIVE

ACTION OF THE DRUG: Rubella vaccine provides active immunity to rubella. The purpose of the vaccine is not to protect the recipient, but prevent rubella in pregnant women and potential congenital rubella syndrome in the fetus.

ASSESSMENT:

INDICATIONS: Rubella vaccine is recommended any time from fifteen months of age until puberty, as part of the routine immunization regimen. It is highly recommended in postpubertal females with no history of rubella disease or vaccine after non-pregnant state is ascertained and for health care providers and people in service occupations who come in contact with children and/or pregnant women.

PLAN:

CONTRAINDICATIONS: Do not give in known pregnancy or if possibility of pregnancy within three months of vaccine administration. Do not use with immunosuppressed individuals (either through therapy or disease). Do not use if there is a concurrent acute febrile illness, or recent (within three months) administration of Immune Serum Globulin (ISG) or blood products.

WARNINGS: Do not give routinely to children under 15 months of age due to potential interference with maternal antibodies.

PRECAUTIONS: Utilize serum titers to judge immune status in women of childbearing age prior to vaccine administration. Breast-feeding is not a contraindication to vaccine administration post pregnancy.

IMPLEMENTATION:

PRODUCTS (TRADE NAME):
Biavax II (Combined Rubella, Mumps.) **Meruvax II** (Available in single dose vials.) **M M R II** (Combined Measles, Mumps, Rubella).

ADMINISTRATION AND DOSAGE: A subcutaneous injection of 0.5 ml given one time is the usual protocol. The vaccine can be given alone or in combination with measles (MR), mumps (RM), or measles and mumps (MMR). Allow 4 weeks between doses for separate administration. At present, rubella immunizations in the United States are recommended for all children at approximately 15 months of age.

See primary immunization schedule in Table 2-1.

IMPLEMENTATION CONSIDERATIONS:

—Obtain a thorough health history, including allergies and immunization record.

—Ascertain non-pregnant state of patient.

—Advise strict birth control for women of childbearing age three months post-vaccine administration.

—Carefully review immunization status in female adolescents and young adults. Record a baseline rubella titer at some point in this age group. Revaccination may be necessary.

—Consider use of rubella titer prior to vaccine administration for those with no history of vaccine or disease. Health care provider should weigh cost, availability and accuracy of laboratory testing versus cost, availability and individual need for vaccine.

—Adverse reactions may occur up to several weeks post-vaccination.

WHAT THE PATIENT NEEDS TO KNOW:

—In women of childbearing age, the greatest danger is the damage to the baby if woman should become pregnant within three months after taking this injection. The maximum contraception protection should be provided for three months so this will not happen.

—Keep a record of this immunization, and the rubella titer (if drawn).

—Notify your health provider if you develop any new or uncomfortable symptoms after taking this injection.

EVALUATION:

ADVERSE REACTIONS: *CNS:* transient peripheral paresthesias. *Dermatologic:* A variety of transient symptoms may result: generalized rash, arthralgia, arthritis. *Hematopoietic:* thrombocytopenia. *Other:* lymphadenopathy. Potential danger of congenital rubella syndrome from vaccine virus if it is administered to a pregnant female.

PARAMETERS TO MONITOR: Monitor for adverse reactions.

Kathy Awalt

YELLOW FEVER VACCINE

ACTION OF THE DRUG: Yellow fever vaccine provides active immunization against yellow fever with live attenuated virus vaccine.

ASSESSMENT:

INDICATIONS: This vaccine is recommended for individuals traveling or working in countries endemic to yellow fever.

PLAN:

CONTRAINDICATIONS: Do not use in the presence of acute febrile illnesses, in cases of dysgammaglobulinemia, or if patient is sensitive to eggs. Immunosuppressed individuals via drugs or disease process also should not be given this product.

PRECAUTIONS: This vaccine is administered only at approved World Health Organization Centers.

IMPLEMENTATION:

PRODUCTS (TRADE NAME):
YF Vac (Available in 1, 5, 20 and 100 dose vials.)

ADMINISTRATION AND DOSAGE: Route of administration is subcutaneous. Dosage consists of one injection (0.5 ml) with revaccination in ten years as needed.

IMPLEMENTATION CONSIDERATIONS:
—Obtain health history. Determine if there are any contraindications for use, especially allergies.
—Perform hypersensitivity testing if needed.
—Watch for generalized and mild side effects.

WHAT THE PATIENT NEEDS TO KNOW:
—Some patients experience mild fever and localized discomfort at injection site.
—Take aspirin for fever, and apply warm compresses to injection site to relieve discomfort.
—Notify health care provider if you develop other side effects.

EVALUATION:

ADVERSE REACTIONS: Fever, malaise, headaches. In rare instances encephalitis occurs.

PARAMETERS TO MONITOR: Observe for development of side effects.

Kathy Awalt

AGENTS FOR PASSIVE IMMUNITY—ANTITOXINS AND ANTIVENINS

DIPHTHERIA ANTITOXIN

ACTION OF THE DRUG: Diphtheria antitoxin provides temporary passive immunity from the endotoxin distributed by the bacterium *Corynebacterium diphtheriae.*

ASSESSMENT:

INDICATIONS: Diphtheria antitoxin is used both prophylactically as well as therapeutically for individuals exposed to diphtheria.

SUBJECTIVE: History of exposure to diphtheria, no immunization with diphtheria toxoid. Active clinical symptoms of disease: sore throat, headache, difficulty swallowing.

OBJECTIVE: Presence of cervical adenitis, pharyngitis, laryngitis with characteristic grayish membrane covering pharynx, swelling of throat, fever. Document disease by positive culture of organism.

PLAN:

CONTRAINDICATIONS: Do not use in the presence of immunodeficiency due to medication and/or disease.

WARNINGS: Immunity is temporary, approximately ten to twenty-one days. Follow administration with diphtheria toxoid for active immunity.

PRECAUTIONS: Determine sensitivity to antitoxin prior to administration via skin or conjunctival testing.

IMPLEMENTATION:

PRODUCTS (TRADE NAME):
Diphtheria Antitoxin, Diphtheria Antitoxin-Connaught (Available in 10,000 or 20,000 units/vial.)
ADMINISTRATION AND DOSAGE:
Prophylaxis: 10,000 units in exposed unimmunized individual.
Therapeutic: 20,000 units to 40,000 units if patient has active disease.
IMPLEMENTATION CONSIDERATIONS:
—Obtain complete health history: assess previous immunization status, assess general health status specifically for immunodeficiency problems.
—Determine hypersensitivity via skin or conjunctival testing.
—Follow up prophylactic treatment with throat cultures.
—Administer diphtheria toxoid if needed.

—Consider administration or provision of antihistamines if hypersensitivity develops. Sensitization may not occur for up to ten days.

WHAT THE PATIENT NEEDS TO KNOW:
—Notify health care provider if symptoms of disease develop or become worse.
—Notify health care provider if there is any evidence of localized or systemic allergic reactions: shortness of breath, itching, rash.
—Allergic reactions may be delayed for up to ten days.

EVALUATION:

ADVERSE REACTIONS: *Hypersensitivity:* pruritic rash, shortness of breath, anaphylactic reactions.
PARAMETERS TO MONITOR: Obtain throat culture for positive identification of organism, and repeat throat cultures during therapy. Do hypersensitivity testing prior to giving injection. Observe patient for immediate signs of systemic allergic response. Observe patient for suppression or modification of disease.

Kathy Awalt

TETANUS ANTITOXIN (EQUINE)

ACTION OF THE DRUG: Tetanus antitoxin provides temporary passive immunity against tetanus.

ASSESSMENT:

INDICATIONS: This antitoxin is utilized in individuals requiring temporary immunity against *Clostridium tetani* toxin. It provides tetanus prophylaxis as well as therapy for wounds that are high risk for *Clostridium tetani* infection. Antitoxin is indicated regardless of immunization status if the character of the wound is such that tetanus might occur.

PLAN:

WARNINGS: Since tetanus immune globulin (TIG) is preferred, tetanus antitoxin equine is only utilized in circumstances where TIG is unavailable.

IMPLEMENTATION:

PRODUCTS (TRADE NAME):
Tetanus Antitoxin (Equine) (Available in 1,500 unit vials.)
ADMINISTRATION AND DOSAGE:
Prophylaxis: 3,000 to 10,000 units IM or SQ.
Therapeutic dosage: 40,000 to 100,000 units IV.
IMPLEMENTATION CONSIDERATIONS:
—Conditions that are at high risk for producing *Clostridium tetani* infection:
a. Open wounds without exposure to air and light.
b. Secondary infections of insect bites.
c. Contaminated surgical wounds, specifically related to the gastrointestinal tract.
d. Severe trauma.
—Proper use of aseptic and surgical technique can prevent secondary tetanus infections.
—Prompt and comprehensive treatment of trauma and injuries is important.
—Obtain a complete history of the patient's immunization status.
—Utilize separate syringes and separate injection sites if administration of tetanus toxoid booster is to be given.

WHAT THE PATIENT NEEDS TO KNOW:
—This injection needs to be noted in your personal immunization records.
—Use aseptic and sterile procedures in caring for this wound. These will be demonstrated by your health care provider.
—If wound becomes swollen, inflamed, or has pus, return to your health care provider.

EVALUATION:

ADVERSE REACTIONS: *Hypersensitivity:* localized allergic reactions and/or generalized anaphylactic response. Many people develop flu-like symptoms, local pain and irritation, fever, after receiving equine-based tetanus antitoxin.

PARAMETERS TO MONITOR: Observe for development of symptoms of tetanus, signs of hypersensitivity. Hypersensitivity reactions are a high possibility.

Kathy Awalt

AGENTS FOR PASSIVE IMMUNITY—IMMUNE SERUMS

HEPATITIS B IMMUNE GLOBULIN (HUMAN)

ACTION OF THE DRUG: This is a concentrated human blood plasma preparation with a high degree of hepatitis B antibodies present. Its main purpose is to provide a temporary passive immunity for hepatitis B.

ASSESSMENT:

INDICATIONS: Prophylactic use in individuals at high risk for exposure to hepatitis B. It may attenuate or prevent the disease. Also for possible use in the newborn infant born to a mother with hepatitis B exposure in the third trimester.

PLAN:

CONTRAINDICATIONS: Do not give to known hepatitis B carrier.
WARNINGS: This serum has controversial efficacy in the newborn infant. It provides temporary immunity only. Average half-life is twenty-seven days.

IMPLEMENTATION:

PRODUCTS (TRADE NAME):
H-BIG, Hyper Hep (Available in 1 and 5 ml vials.)
ADMINISTRATION AND DOSAGE: Deep intramuscular route is recommended for administration.
Dosage for maximal exposure (i.e., via blood transfusion): 0.5 ml/kg IM. Repeat in 30 days.
Dosage for minimal exposure: 0.06 ml/kg up to a maximum of 5 ml. Repeat in 30 days.
Dosage for newborn: 0.12 ml/kg.
IMPLEMENTATION CONSIDERATIONS:
—It is preferred to use this specific HBIG to ISG in cases of known hepatitis B exposure.
—Painful injections with localized soreness may result.
—The Z tract method is preferred for maximum deep intramuscular absorption.
—This serum can be administered only IM.
—There is a slight possibility of urticarial rash and/or fever developing.

WHAT THE PATIENT NEEDS TO KNOW:
—Warm compresses may relieve localized soreness.
—Antipyretic agents can be utilized for relief of fever and local discomfort.
—If an itching rash develops, notify your health provider so additional treatment can be prescribed.

EVALUATION:

ADVERSE REACTIONS: *Dermatologic:* rash, urticaria, hematoma at injection site. *Hypersensitivity:* anaphylactic response is possible but extremely rare. *Other:* Degree of protection or modification of disease state may not be achieved. Variables include: initial quality of serum and dosage of administration, individual immune response and specific disease state.
PARAMETERS TO MONITOR: Observe patient for signs and symptoms of

generalized anaphylactic response immediately post administration. Also watch for modification or suppression of disease.

Kathy Awalt

IMMUNE SERUM GLOBULIN, HUMAN (HISG)

ACTION OF THE DRUG: Human immune serum globulin (HISG) is a concentrated preparation of primarily IgG antibodies from human blood plasma. Its main purpose is to provide a temporary passive immunity to specific disease states.

ASSESSMENT:

INDICATIONS: Primarily used to modify and/or prevent hepatitis A and measles (rubeola). Used in cases of hepatitis B when H-BIG (Hepatitis B Immune Globulin) is not available. Possible use in the unprotected pregnant female exposed to varicella and/or rubella.

PLAN:

WARNINGS: Local or systemic reactions cannot be predicted by prior skin testing. Immunity provided is only temporary. Average half-life of HISG is two to three weeks. Individual patient's response to modification or prevention of disease state cannot be guaranteed.

IMPLEMENTATION:

PRODUCTS (TRADE NAME):
Gamastan, Gammar, Immuglobin (Available in 2 and 10 ml vials.)
ADMINISTRATION AND DOSAGE: Route of administration is deep intramuscular. See general administration and dosage parameters on circular packaged with the product. Specifics may vary according to manufacturer.
Hepatitis A: 0.02-0.04 ml/kg IM repeated in four to six months; .06 ml/kg is IM is utilized for cases of continuous exposure.
Rubeola: 0.25 ml/kg IM to prevent disease and 0.05 ml/kg IM to modify the disease.
Hepatitis B: 0.12 ml/kg IM repeated in thirty days.
IMPLEMENTATION CONSIDERATIONS:
—Painful injection with localized soreness may result.
—The Z tract method is preferred for maximum deep intramuscular absorption.
—Administer this product only IM, never IV.
—Slight possibility of urticarial rash and/or fever.

WHAT THE PATIENT NEEDS TO KNOW:
—Warm compresses may relieve localized soreness.
—Active immunization to disease state should eventually be obtained when possible (i.e., rubella, rubeola).
—Antipyretic agents can be utilized for relief of fever and local discomfort.
—Notify the health care provider if an itching rash develops, so additional treatment can be provided.

EVALUATION:

ADVERSE REACTIONS: *Dermatologic:* rash, urticaria, hematoma at injection site. *Hypersensitivity:* anaphylactic response is possible but extremely rare. *Other:* Degree of protection or modification of disease state may not be achieved. Variables include: initial quality of serum and dosage of HISG administered, individual immune response and specific disease state. Transmission of hepatitis B virus via HISG is a remote possibility.

PARAMETERS TO MONITOR: Observe patient for signs and symptoms of generalized anaphylactic respose immediately after HISG administration. Monitor for modification or suppression of disease state.

Kathy Awalt

PERTUSSIS IMMUNE GLOBULIN, HUMAN (HPIG)

ACTION OF THE DRUG: This medication is a preparation of human immune serum globulin with specific pertussis factors. The main purpose of HPIG is to provide temporary passive immunity to pertussis.

ASSESSMENT:

INDICATIONS: The major use for this serum is to provide therapy or prophylaxis to the individual unimmunized against pertussis.

PLAN:

WARNINGS: There is controversial efficacy of this product. Some authorities indicate HPIG is currently inappropriate for use in both therapy and modification of disease.

PRECAUTIONS: Must be used within the first seven days of the disease.

IMPLEMENTATION:

PRODUCTS (TRADE NAME):
Hypertussis (Available in 1.25 ml vials.)
ADMINISTRATION AND DOSAGE: The preferred route of administration is IM.
Prophylaxis: 1.25-2.5 mg IM; repeat as needed in one to two weeks.
Therapy: 1.25 mg IM every 24 to 48 hours.
IMPLEMENTATION CONSIDERATIONS:
—Individual patient response to prevention or modification of disease is extremely variable.
—Controversy exists on the indications for use.
—Local allergic and systemic anaphylactic reactions are possible.

WHAT THE PATIENT NEEDS TO KNOW:
—Active immunity to pertussis should be obtained routinely in children under 7 years of age unless pertussis vaccine is contraindicated. (See pertussis vaccine.)
—Notify your health care provider if signs or symptoms of generalized or localized allergic reactions develop.

EVALUATION:

ADVERSE REACTIONS: *Hypersensitivity:* localized allergic reactions, generalized anaphylactic reaction.
PARAMETERS TO MONITOR: Watch for modification or suppression of disease.

Kathy Awalt

TETANUS IMMUNE GLOBULIN, HUMAN (HTIG)

ACTION OF THE DRUG: This is a preparation of human immune serum globulin with specific tetanus antibody titers. The main purpose is to provide temporary passive immunity against tetanus.

ASSESSMENT:

INDICATIONS: This serum is utilized in individuals requiring temporary immunity against *Clostridium tetani toxin.* It provides tetanus prophylaxis as well as therapy for wounds that are high-risk for *Clostridium tetani* infection. Serum is indicated if wound is tetanus-prone and/or infected and untreated for twenty-four hours regardless of immunization status.

SUBJECTIVE: History of untreated infected wound occurring more than 24 hours previously. Determine history of immunization status with regard to tetanus toxoid. Establish history of injuries with rusty metal; deep penetrating wounds, particularly those that do not bleed: accidents which occur around barnyards or outdoors.

OBJECTIVE: Observe wound for warmth, color, edema, drainage.

PLAN:

WARNINGS: Certain elective surgical procedures as well as injuries by accidents can result in trauma creating a favorable enviroment for the development of tetanus.

IMPLEMENTATION:

PRODUCTS (TRADE NAME):
Homo-Tet, Hu-Tet, Hyper-Tet, Tetanus Immune Globulin (Available in 250 unit vials and disposable syringe.)

ADMINISTRATION AND DOSAGE: Preferred route of administration is IM. Specifics for dosage may vary according to manufacturer.

Prophylaxis: 4 units/kg IM. Maximum dose 250 units IM.

Therapeutic: Exact dosage unknown. Give approximately 140 units/kg IM with a maximum total dose of 3,000 to 6,000 units.

IMPLEMENTATION CONSIDERATIONS:

—Conditions which are high risk for *Clostridium tetani* infection:

a. Open wounds without exposure to air and light.

b. Secondary infections of insect bites.

c. Contaminated surgical wounds, specifically related to the gastrointestinal system.

—Proper use of aseptic and surgical technique can prevent secondary tetanus infections.

—Prompt and comprehensive treatment of trauma and injuries is important.

—Obtain a complete history regarding patient's immunization status.

—Utilize separate syringe and separate injection sites if you are following administration of TIG with a booster of tetanus toxoid.

WHAT THE PATIENT NEEDS TO KNOW:

—This injection needs to be noted in your personal immunization records.

—Use aseptic and sterile procedures in caring for this wound. These will be demonstrated by your health care provider.

—If wound becomes swollen, inflamed, or has pus, return to your health care provider.

EVALUATION:

PARAMETERS TO MONITOR: Watch for symptoms of tetanus or secondary infection of wound.

Kathy Awalt

VARICELLA-ZOSTER IMMUNE GLOBULIN, HUMAN (VZIG)

ACTION OF THE DRUG: VZIG consists primarily of IgG derived from human plasma with specific varicella-zoster antibodies. The main purpose of VZIG is to provide temporary passive immunity to varicella.

ASSESSMENT:

INDICATIONS: Major use is to reduce the morbidity and mortality of individuals at risk of developing progressive varicella. Use is indicated only for "at risk" population with known exposure to varicella in past 96 hours.
SUBJECTIVE-OBJECTIVE: History of recent exposure.

PLAN:

CONTRAINDICATIONS: Not to be given to pregnant women or non-immunodeficient individuals.
WARNINGS: Only administer to individuals meeting specific criteria (e.g., individuals with neoplastic disease, acquired or congenital immunodeficiency, or who are receiving immunosuppressive therapy) plus known varicella exposure.

IMPLEMENTATION:

PRODUCTS (TRADE NAME):
Varicella Immune Globulin 125 units/vial.
ADMINISTRATION AND DOSAGE: Administer by deep intramuscular injection. Dosage follows weight parameters as follows:

Kg weight	Dose/Units
0-10	125 units
10-20	250 units
20-30	375 units
30-40	500 units
40 and over	625 units

IMPLEMENTATION CONSIDERATIONS
—Efficacy is to be expected only if administered within 96 hours of exposure.
—Not known to be effective in prophylactic use for immunosuppressed patients.
—Not known to modify established varicella infections.
—Product is available from local American Red Cross office.

—Product may reduce the number of pox and be helpful in preventing pneumonia and death in treated individuals. Exact dosage to achieve these effects is unknown for each individual.

WHAT THE PATIENT NEEDS TO KNOW:
—This injection is to help in the prevention of chickenpox.
—Following this immunization, report any new or unusual symptoms to your health care provider.

EVALUATION:

PARAMETERS TO MONITOR: Watch for development of fever and characteristic skin lesions of chickenpox. There may be local erythema and swelling at injection site.

Kathy Awalt

RABIES PROPHYLAXIS PRODUCTS

ACTION OF THE DRUG: There are two major modes of prophylaxis for rabies: (1) vaccines which induce active endogenous rabies antibody formation, and (2) globulins which provide rapid passive immune protection but last only a short time. Delays in virus propagation may be produced by passive immunization, allowing more time for rabies vaccine to induce antibodies to the virus. In most cases, adequate treatment requires administration of both vaccine and globulin.

ASSESSMENT:

INDICATIONS: Every year the number of people bitten by animals increases, thus increasing the number of people requiring rabies prophylaxis. The concern over rabies epidemics has reached large scale proportions in some areas of the United States. While the number of actual cases of rabies remains very small, the unpleasant factors associated with the prophylaxis treatment have prompted the development of several new products.

SUBJECTIVE-OBJECTIVE: Although some patients may desire immunization because they work with animals and are hence at greater risk, the major demand for therapy follows animal attack. A thorough history should be obtained about the nature of the injury. Specific treatment decisions may be affected by thorough data collection. Some of the factors to consider are: Type of skin injury, with deep bites which allow inoculation of infectious saliva into the skin being most serious; circumstances of injury, with unprovoked attack by wild animals considered more dangerous; species of animal causing injury, with bats and carnivorous animals such as dogs, cats, raccoons, skunks, foxes, and coyotes more likely being infected; vaccination status of biting animal, with vaccinated pets proving least likely of being rabid; and incidence of rabies in the region, in which there is statistically a greater chance of the animal being rabid if there are other well-documented cases.

The rabies virus enters the body through the skin and travels along the nerve trunk to the brain. The incubation period lasts from 2 weeks to as long as 6 months. Following a bite, the animal must be caught and confined for observation. In cases where the animal changes temperament, either becoming unusually friendly, or viciously biting anything around it, it will be killed and the brain examined to confirm the diagnosis. If the diagnosis is rabies, or if the biting animal cannot be caught, the bitten person should immediately begin antirabies treatment. The disease must be prevented before the virus reaches the brain since the disease is always fatal in humans.

PLAN:

CONTRAINDICATIONS: Repeated doses of Rabies Immune Globulin (RIG) are to be avoided once treatment with vaccine has been started in order to decrease chances of interfering with immunity development. In use of Antirabies Serum, Equine Origin (ARS), use extreme caution in patients with a history of allergy or who have demonstrated any hypersensitivity to horse serum.

WARNINGS: The incidence of rabies is a reportable disease to state health department. Additionally, report any serious reactions to vaccine immediately to the state health department or the Viral Disease Division, Bureau of Epidemiology, Centers for Disease Control in Atlanta, Georgia.

Use of rabies vaccine during pregnancy has produced no fetal abnormalities. Preexposure treatment has also been provided to pregnant women when possibility of rabies exposure is high.

Because of the high incidence of sensitivity reactions to ARS, individuals should have a sensitivity test to the serum. In some cases of positive reaction in which other vaccines are not available, cautious use of a desensitizing regimen may be implemented. Sensitivity reactions vary from immediate shock-like reactions to a serum sickness which develops 6 to 12 days following administration of the medication.

IMPLEMENTATION:

DRUG INTERACTIONS: Corticosteroids and immunosuppressants may block or inhibit the development of active immunity. Thus, the likelihood of the patient developing rabies is much higher in patients who have been receiving these drugs. Adequate antibody titers should be obtained in these individuals if rabies therapy must be implemented.

ADMINISTRATION AND DOSAGE: Following copious flushing and scrubbing of bite site with soap and water, the area should be infiltrated with up to one half the total dose of RIG, if it is to be used. RIG is preferred over ARS because the latter has a higher risk of adverse reactions. Additional treatment with tetanus and antibiotics may also be indicated to control infection.

Postexposure prophylaxis: Therapy should always include both passively administered antibody (preferably TIG) and vaccine (HDCV) unless the patient has been previously immunized with rabies vaccine and has an adequate rabies antibody titer, requiring then only HDCV. Regardless of the interval between exposure and treatment or whether there is a bite or nonbite, this combination therapy of globulin and vaccine is recommended for adequate protection.

For bites caused by wild animals, assume animal is rabid and treat immediately with RIG and vaccine. If further evaluation of the killed animal's brain is negative, discontinue HDCV. In domestic animals in which there is no evidence of untoward behavior, institute no therapy. The treatment regimen of RIG and vaccine may be instituted during the 10-day holding period if the animal becomes rabid. In cases of doubt, institute treatment as if animal were rabid.

In instituting passive immunity, only use ARS if RIG is not available. RIG is given only once, at the beginning of antirabies therapy. Approximately onehalf the dose of either product should be infiltrated around the wound site itself, and the rest injected intramuscularly. Do not exceed recommended doses.

In beginning active immunity, five 1 ml doses of HDCV should be given IM in the deltoid. Doses are given on day of exposure or as soon thereafter as possible and on days 3, 7, 14 and 28 after the first dose.

In individuals warranting preexposure prophylaxis due to the high risk of animal bites, give a 1 ml injection of HDCV IM on days 0, 7, 21 and 28. If a previously immunized person is bitten by a rabid animal, the person should receive two doses of HDCV immediately and one dose three days later.

IMPLEMENTATION CONSIDERATIONS:

—Obtain a complete health history, including a detailed description of the episode where biting occurred, past history of allergies, asthma, hypersensitivity to horse serum or other vaccines, and presence of systemic diseases or long-term drug therapy.

—Begin treatment as soon as possible following biting episode.

—First aid treatment of wound with liberal amounts of soap and continuous flushing of wound with water are an effective way of limiting the chance of rabies development.

—Supervision of therapy by medical personnel is mandatory.

—Consider giving tetanus and antibiotics as necessary to limit other infection at wound site.

—Institute sensitivity testing by intradermal or conjunctival method before using ARS.

Intradermally, give 0.1 ml of 1:100 or 1:1000 normal saline dilution of ARS. Observe area for 10 to 30 minutes. Watch for development of wheal, redness and swelling of the area which document sensitivity to product.

The conjunctival test involves instillation of 0.1 ml of 1:10 normal saline dilution of ARS into the lower conjunctival sac. Dilated vessels, edema, itching and lacrimation with 10 to 15 minutes are considered positive reactions, and can be relieved immediately by washing the eye with epinephrine 1:1000 and normal saline. This test should be used in preference to the intradermal test if there is any possibility of a severe reaction developing.

—Desensitization may be undertaken in individuals in which there are no serums prepared from other animals available. Small amounts of diluted serum are injected SQ every 15 minutes (or longer). The dose is gradually increased as tolerated by the patient. The following schedule has been recommended for desensitization with horse serum:

    a. 0.05 ml of 1:20 dilution SQ
    b. 0.1 ml of 1:10 dilution SQ
    c. 0.3 ml of 1:10 dilution SQ
    d. 0.1 ml undiluted serum SQ
    e. 0.2 ml undiluted serum SQ
    f. 0.5 ml undiluted serum SQ
    g. Inject remaining serum slowly in 0.5 ml doses, reducing the dose by 50% any time that an untoward reaction is noted.

—Watch for allergic reactions, especially in patients receiving ARS. Marked urticaria and severe hypotension may develop within minutes and require epinephrine immediately to prevent development of a shock-like syndrome.

—An additional allergic manifestation may not appear for 6 to 12 days when patient develops a serum sickness. This problem occurs in as many as 40% of all adult patients receiving ARS therapy. See Adverse Reactions section. Large and continuous doses of antihistamines may help alleviate symptoms.

—Assess antibody level following therapy in any patient in whom you have reason to suspect that the level of antibody development is inadequate.

WHAT THE PATIENT NEEDS TO KNOW:

—This medication is very important in protecting you from rabies, a virus which has no treatment once it has developed.

—Follow all instructions given you by your health care provider regarding this treatment. You will be required to make several visits for injections and observation of the wound.

—Notify your health care provider if you note any changes in breathing, begin to itch, or note any new or troublesome symptoms following the administration of any injections.

—You will need to remain under observation for 15 to 30 minutes following each injection to make certain that you have not developed any allergic reactions to the medicine.

—The injections may be stopped if it can be proven that the animal which bit you did not have rabies.

EVALUATION:

ADVERSE REACTIONS: Severe shock-like symptoms or delayed serum sickness may develop following ARS therapy. Watch for any itching, sneezing, coughing, asthma, marked urticaria and severe hypotension. Frequently, patients develop serum sickness which first appears 6 to 12 days following treatment with ARS. Onset may be noted by appearance of headache, itching, skin eruption, lymphadenopathy, and generalized arthralgia. Fever, malaise, chills, and abdominal pain may also be found.

PARAMETERS TO MONITOR: Monitor the general appearance and healing of the wound site. Observe for any adverse reactions, closely monitoring patient following each injection. Question patient carefully about symptoms related to development of serum sickness as therapy progresses. Take time to listen to the concerns and fears of the patient during therapy. Parents in particular may feel guilty if they feel a child has been placed at risk because of their neglect or inattention.

ANTIRABIES SERUM, EQUINE ORIGIN (ARS)

PRODUCTS (TRADE NAME):
Antirabies Serum, Equine Origin (Available in 1000 unit vials for injection.)
DRUG SPECIFICS:
This is a refined, concentrated serum obtained from hyperimmunized horses. This product quickly provides passive immunity to rabies virus although it lasts only about 20 days. It is to be used immediately when it is suspected or documented that rabid animals have bitten individuals and only when Rabies Immune Globulin (RIG) is not available. This product is associated with a high incidence of sensitivity reactions, both immediate and delayed. Sensitivity testing must be carried out prior to using this product. Desensitization is possible in sensitive individuals when use of product is highly desirable. (See Implementation Considerations section.)
ADMINISTRATION AND DOSAGE SPECIFICS:
Give IM one dose of not less than 1000 units/40 lbs (55 u/kg). Half of the dose should be infiltrated into the tissue around the wound whenever possible. When giving with rabies vaccine, do not give in the same syringe or at the same site, as neutralization of the vaccine may take place. Do not repeat dose.

RABIES IMMUNE GLOBULIN, HUMAN (RIG)

PRODUCTS (TRADE NAME):
Hyperab, Imogam (Available in 150 IU per ml for injection.)
DRUG SPECIFICS:
This product is the drug of choice and provides quick, passive protection when given immediately to individuals bitten by animals suspected of being rabid. Protection lasts only about 20 days. Use in all patients, unless a person who has been previously immunized with Rabies Vaccine has an adequate antibody level. Give as soon as possible or up to 8 days after exposure. This product takes approximately one week to stimulate antibody production in the body, so the rapid initiation of

therapy is mandatory. RIG should not be given more than once after therapy has started with vaccine since it may block the production of active immunity. Do not give to individuals allergic to gamma globulin or thimerosal. Unlike ARS, this product has few side effects. Most adverse reactions are found at injection site as tenderness, soreness, or stiffness of muscles. A few cases of angioneurotic edema, nephrotic syndrome and anaphylactic shock have been noted following injection.

ADMINISTRATION AND DOSAGE SPECIFICS:

Give 20 IU/kg (0.133 ml/kg) or 9 IU/lb (0.06 ml/lb) at the time of the first vaccine dose (HDCV). Up to one half the dose should be infiltrated into the wound tissue and the rest administered IM.

RABIES VACCINE, HUMAN DIPLOID CELL CULTURES (HDCV)

PRODUCTS (TRADE NAME):

Imovax Rabies Vaccine (Available in single dose vial of freeze-dried suspension.)

DRUG SPECIFICS:

This vaccine is extremely effective in providing protection from rabies. It takes approximately 7 to 10 days to develop active immune antibody response, but protection lasts up to one year. It may be administered preexposure to individuals working with animals, and to children (who seem to be more vulnerable than adults) traveling to areas of endemic disease. Following local cleansing and treatment of the wound, give RIG for passive immunity, and begin HDCV therapy unless person demonstrates high antibody titer from previous rabies treatment. The sooner treatment is started, the better. This drug has few adverse reactions associated with it, and any serious reactions should be reported to the state health department or the Viral Disease Division, Bureau of Epidemiology, Centers for Disease Control, Atlanta, Georgia. Usual reactions include local swelling, erythema, induration and ache at injection site. A few allergic reactions have been reported, including hives and anaphylaxis. Antihistamines have been effective in alleviating these problems. Aspirin or acetaminophen may also be used for symptomatic therapy. Follow manufacturer's instructions regarding reconstitution of freeze-dried suspension and administration of medication. Do not freeze medication.

ADMINISTRATION AND DOSAGE SPECIFICS:

Preexposure therapy: Give one injection of 1.0 ml IM into deltoid region on day zero, and repeat on day 7 and on either day 21 or 28. Booster doses should be obtained at least every 2 years, depending upon serum level of antibody.

Postexposure therapy: Give 5 doses of HDCV, the first given in conjunction with a dose of RIG. Doses are 1.0 ml and are given IM into the deltoid area on day 0, 3,

7, 14, and 30. World Health Organization recommendations include provision for a sixth dose on day 90, although CDC recommendations do not include this.

Marilyn W. Edmunds

IN VIVO DIAGNOSTIC BIOLOGICALS

COCCIDIODIN

ACTION OF THE DRUG: This is a diagnostic skin test made from cultures of the organism *Coccidioides immitis* and designed to identify through hypersensitivity reactions those individuals with active disease or exposure to the fungal infection coccidioidomycosis.

ASSESSMENT:

INDICATIONS: Use in patient workup when coccidioidomycosis (desert fever or San Joaquin Valley fever) is considered in the differential diagnosis. This is a fungal disease usually affecting the respiratory tract. The spores are carried by the wind and enter the respiratory tract via the nose and mouth. The fungus grows in hot, dry areas, especially in the southwestern United States, Mexico and parts of Central and South America.

SUBJECTIVE: Initial symptoms present like influenza: malaise, fever, productive cough, extreme weakness, loss of energy, poor appetite, loss of weight.

OBJECTIVE: Symptoms predominantly mimic arthritis (pain and swelling of the joints) and tuberculosis (productive cough, consolidation of the chest, decreased breath sounds).

PLAN:

PRECAUTIONS: Utilize the lowest concentration possible. Intense local and systemic reactions may occur with high dosages.

IMPLEMENTATION:

PRODUCTS (TRADE NAME):
Spherulin (Available in strengths of 1:10 and 1:100).
ADMINISTRATION AND DOSAGE SPECIFICS:
Use lowest possible dosage. Administer per intradermal route on the inner aspect of forearm.
IMPLEMENTATION CONSIDERATIONS:
—Obtain health history regarding exposure to people or places where this problem is endemic, previous respiratory problems, arthritis and previous reactions (if any) to skin testing.

—Positive reactions indicate the individual has been in contact with the fungus and does not necessarily have an active infectious process.

—Medication is to be diluted with NaCl only. Once diluted, solution must be refrigerated and used within 24 hours.

—Note evidence of wheal immediately post injection.

—Test is read 24-48 hours post administration.

—If patient is unable to return to have site evaluated by a health professional it may be possible to teach the patient how to interpret the test himself. Draw a circle 5 mm around the injection site and inform the patient to keep this mark and call the health care provider to report the reaction to the test. When the patient calls, ascertain whether there is swelling and/or redness outside the area you have drawn.

WHAT THE PATIENT NEEDS TO KNOW:
—The results of this test should be recorded in your personal records.
—It is important tht the results of the test are communicated to the health care provider and are also recorded in your medical records. You must return to have the test site evaluated, or obtain instructions for checking it yourself.
—Notify your health care provider concerning any unusual skin irritation which develops following this test.

EVALUATION:

ADVERSE REACTIONS: *Dermatologic/Hypersensitivity:* Intense local reactions from severe vesiculation, ulceration and necrosis can occur, as well as systemic allergic response.

PARAMETERS TO MONITOR: 24-48 hours following injection, check site for induration, erythema and size. Positive reactions are areas of induration and erythema 5 mm or greater in size.

Kathy Awalt

HISTOPLASMIN

ACTION OF THE DRUG: This is a preparation of growth products of *Histoplasma capsulatum* designed to identify through hypersensitivity reactions in those individuals with active disease or exposure to the disease histoplasmosis.

ASSESSMENT:

INDICATIONS: Utilized in patient workup when histoplasmosis is suspected or to differentiate histoplasmosis from other sources of infection (e.g., sarcoidosis, coccidioidomycosis). This is a fungal disease caused by inhalation of dust contaminated by *Histoplasma capsulatum* and is found in the rural midwest. It has been seen, however, in most sections of the United States, including urban areas.

SUBJECTIVE: Many asymptomatic infections are believed to occur. The first symptoms resemble those of influenza, including fever and extreme fatigue.

OBJECTIVE: Pulmonary findings both on physical examination and x-ray are similar to tuberculosis.

PLAN:

PRECAUTIONS: Utilize the lowest dosage possible, as severe local and systemic reactions may occur with high dosages. Reactions to skin test may be negative with an acute histoplasmosis infection.

IMPLEMENTATION:

PRODUCTS (TRADE NAME):
Histolyn-CYL, Histoplasmin (Available in 10 dose vials.)
ADMINISTRATION AND DOSAGE: Administer 0.1 ml per intradermal route in precleansed inner aspect of forearm.
IMPLEMENTATION CONSIDERATIONS:
—Obtain health history, including previous exposure to people or places where histoplasmosis is endemic, previous sensitivity testing reaction if any.
—Check for immediate post injection wheal.
—Read reaction at injection site 48-72 hours post administration.
—If patient is unable to return to have injection site evaluated it may be possible to teach the patient how to interpret the test himself. Draw a circle 5 mm around injection site and inform the patient to keep this mark and call the health care provider to report the reaction to the test. When the patient calls, ask whether there is swelling and/or redness outside the area you have drawn.
—TB screening tests should also be performed when considering histoplasmosis as a diagnosis.
—If skin test is positive, follow up with a chest x-ray.
—Baseline antibody titers should be available prior to test as histoplasmin injection may alter titer results.

WHAT THE PATIENT NEEDS TO KNOW:
—The results of this test should be recorded in your personal records.
—It is important that the results of the test are communicated to the health provider also and recorded in your medical records. You must return to have the test site evaluated, or obtain instructions for checking it yourself.
—Notify your health care provider concerning any unusual skin irritation which develops following this test.

EVALUATION:

ADVERSE REACTIONS: *Dermatologic/Hypersensitivity:* Local reactions ranging from vesiculation, ulceration and necrosis may occur, as well as a systemic allergic response.
PARAMETERS TO MONITOR: 48 to 72 hours following injection, check site for induration, erythema and size. Positive reactions are areas of induration and erythema over 5 mm in size.

Kathy Awalt

MUMPS SKIN TEST ANTIGEN

ACTION OF THE DRUG: Mumps skin testing demonstrates cutaneous hypersensitivity to mumps virus.

ASSESSMENT:

INDICATIONS: This product is used to detect the presence of mumps antibodies in individuals so that previous history of mumps may be confirmed or ruled out. When mumps skin test antigen produces a delayed cutaneous reaction in individuals who have had contact or infection with the mumps virus, the immune system is presumed to be intact. This product is undergoing continuing testing to confirm adequacy of action.
SUBJECTIVE-OBJECTIVE: Patient or parent of child may present with questionable history of mumps: febrile reaction, swelling of one or both parotid glands, other incidence of mumps in area. In males, particularly, it may be important to determine that patient has not had mumps, and so would be at risk for the infection.

PLAN:

CONTRAINDICATIONS: Do not give to patients known to be sensitive to eggs, feathers, or chickens as virus is cultivated in chicken embryo. Thimerosal is the preservative used, and some patients may also be sensitive to this chemical.
PRECAUTIONS: Antigen must be injected intradermally, or unreliable or negative reaction will be obtained. Watch for development of allergic reactions due to the nature of this product.

IMPLEMENTATION:

PRODUCTS (TRADE NAME):
Mumps Skin Test Antigen (Available in suspensions of 1 ml vials, which provides enough for 10 tests.)

ADMINISTRATION AND DOSAGE: Inject 0.1 ml antigen on cleansed inner surface of forearm. Take care to inject intradermally. Read reaction in 24 to 48 hours.

IMPLEMENTATION CONSIDERATIONS:

—Obtain a complete health history to detect pattern of allergic reactions or sensitivity to eggs, chickens or feathers. Evaluate carefully previous health and immunization history to determine need for mumps skin testing.

—Accurate testing depends upon intradermal injection. Injecting antigen subcutaneously will invalidate and confuse test results.

—Explain test interpretation to patient if results are to be interpreted by other than the health care provider. Draw area 1.5 cm around injection site. Explain that redness, with or without swelling, which exceeds this line indicates that the person is sensitive to the antigen. A negative reaction, if correctly administered, means nonsensitivity or anergy.

—False-positive reactions may be produced in patients sensitive to egg protein.

WHAT THE PATIENT NEEDS TO KNOW:

—This injection will help us determine if you have previously had mumps.

—A line has been drawn around the injection site. Do not wash this line off. In 24 hours you are to look at this area and see if there is any redness outside of the line. If there is redness, this means you have probably had mumps. If there is no redness, you probably have not had mumps. There may be some swelling present, but the test interpretation depends only upon the amount of redness. Please call your health care provider with the results so that it may be recorded in your medical records.

—If you note any itching, difficulty in breathing or wheezing, contact your health care provider immediately.

EVALUATION:

ADVERSE REACTIONS: Localized itching and swelling may develop, and may persist for several days. Problem is usually mild and self-limiting. More systemic allergic reactions may develop, with possibility of anaphylaxis.

PARAMETERS TO MONITOR: Evaluate patient skin reaction to the antigen. If previous history of mumps is strongly suspected and test is negative, may suspect inaccurate intradermal administration and consider retesting.

Marilyn W. Edmunds

IN VIVO TUBERCULIN TESTS

TUBERCULIN PURIFIED PROTEIN DERIVATIVE (MANTOUX)

ACTION OF THE DRUG: This is a soluble purified derivative product of the tubercle bacilli organism designed to cause a hypersensitivity reaction in those individuals with active tuberculosis, individuals exposed to tuberculosis and those needing further testing.

ASSESSMENT:

INDICATIONS: Utilized in routine TB screening procedures. May be used as a second test to check questionable or positive results of the Tine or Sclavo.

PLAN:

CONTRAINDICATIONS: Not to be given to people with active tuberculosis, or those who have reacted positively to this test before.

WARNINGS: Altered reactivity to the test (suppression) may appear in cases of malnourishment, severe stress and after immunosuppressive medications.

PRECAUTIONS: Questionable reliability of results if given within four weeks of a live viral vaccine (i.e., measles, rubella or mumps). Decreased reactivity may be found in the elderly.

IMPLEMENTATION:

DRUG INTERACTIONS: Steroids and immunosuppressive drugs may alter the reactivity of the TB screening test.

PRODUCTS (TRADE NAME):
Aplisol (Available in 5 TU per 0.1 ml.) **Tubersol-Connaught** (Available in 1 TU, 5 TU and 250 TU per 0.1 ml).

ADMINISTRATION AND DOSAGE: Usual strength is 5 TU (tuberculin units) per 0.1 ml of intermediate strength PPD. Administer 0.1 ml of intermediate strength PPD on inner surface of forearm. If repeat test is indicated, use the other forearm. Route is intradermal only. Under special circumstances dosage can be altered, depending upon history of TB exposure and previous reactivity (i.e., decrease to 1 TU if history of reactivity, increase up to 250 TU with no signs of reactivity and positive history of exposure.)

IMPLEMENTATION CONSIDERATIONS:
—Obtain health history, including previous TB exposure and reactivity to TB screening tests, presence of malnourishment, severe stress, steroids or immunosup-

pressive medications. Determine if patient has received a live viral vaccine within the last four weeks.

—Administer medication on inner surface of cleansed forearm. Avoid hairy areas or areas with little subcutaneous tissue. If this is a repeat test, use a different extremity than the first time.

—Use intradermal route only. Subcutaneous route will yield false negative results.

—Check for immediate post injection wheal.

—Read results in 48-72 hours post administration.

—If patient is unable to return to have injection site evaluated by a health professional, it may be possible to teach the patient how to interpret the test himself. Draw a circle 9 mm around injection site and inform the patient to keep this mark and call the health care provider to report the reaction to the test. When the patient calls, ask about whether there is swelling and/or redness outside the area you have drawn.

—Consider dosage alterations in special circumstances.

—Refrigerate solution and protect from sunlight.

WHAT THE PATIENT NEEDS TO KNOW:
—The results of this test should be recorded in your personal records.
—It is important that the results of the test are communicated to the health provider and also recorded in your medical records. You must return to have the test site evaluated, or obtain instructions for checking it yourself.
—Notify your health provider concerning any unusual skin irritation which develops following this test.

EVALUATION:

ADVERSE REACTIONS: *Dermatologic:* Severe localized reaction may develop if patient is hypersensitive to tubercle bacilli organism (i.e., exposure to tuberculosis or active tuberculosis). Site reactions may range from areas of increased erythema and induration, to vesiculation, ulceration and necrosis.

PARAMETERS TO MONITOR: 48 to 72 hours following injection, check site for induration, erythema and size. Positive reactions are areas of induration and erythema over 9 mm in size. Areas of 5-9 mm are questionable. Areas under 5 mm are negative. Reaction *must* have erythema and induration *plus* increased size.

Kathy Awalt

TUBERCULIN PPD MULTIPLE PUNCTURE DEVICE

ACTION OF THE DRUG: There are several multiple puncture devices contains dried tuberculin purified protein derivative on hidden prongs, concentrated solution, or old tuberculin. These devices are used to identify, through hypersensitivity reactions, individuals with active tuberculosis, individuals exposed to tuberculosis, and those needing further testing.

ASSESSMENT:

INDICATIONS: These devices are utilized as a primary screening device to identify individuals with active tuberculosis, those exposed to tuberculosis, and those needing further evaluation. It may be administered every 1-2 years or more frequently, depending upon the incidence of tuberculosis and epidemiological profile of the community. The PPD (Mantoux) is the most commonly used diagnostic agent. One ml of the concentrated solution for Heaf test contains the equivalent of 100,000 US units of the US Standard Tuberculin PPD. The old tuberculin, Tine test units have been standardized to give reactions equivalent to or more potent than 5 TU of standard old tuberculin administered intradermally in the Mantoux test. All of these multiple puncture devices should be regarded as screening agents, and other appropriate diagnostic procedres utilized for retesting reactors.

PLAN:

CONTRAINDICATIONS: Do not give to patients with active tuberculosis, or to those people who have reacted positively to this test in the past.

WARNINGS: Altered reactivity to this test (suppression) may be found in cases of malnourishment, severe stress and following immunosuppressive medications.

PRECAUTIONS: Questionable reliability of results if this test is given within 4 weeks of receiving a live viral vaccine (i.e., measles, rubella, mumps). Decreased reactivity may be found in the elderly.

IMPLEMENTATION:

DRUG INTERACTIONS: Steroids and immunosuppressive drugs may alter the reactivity of the TB screening test.

PRODUCTS (TRADE NAME):

PPD Multiple Punture Devices: **Aplitest, Sclavo Test PPD, Tuberculin PPD Tine Test** (Available in individual preset puncture devices.)

Tuberculin PPD Concentrated Solution for Heaf Test: **Tuberculin Purified Protein Derivative-Connaught** (Available in concentrated solution with "sterneedle" multipuncture device.)

Old Tuberculin Multiple Puncture Devices: **Tuberculin Mono-Vacc Test** (Available in 5 TU activity per test.) **Tuberculin, Old, Tine Test** (Available in solution containing 7% acacia and 8.5% lactose.)

ADMINISTRATION AND DOSAGE: Apply to a precleansed inner aspect of forearm. Use gentle pressure to allow preset puncture device to properly penetrate skin.

IMPLEMENTATION CONSIDERATIONS:

—Obtain health history, including previous TB exposure and reactivity to TB screening tests, presence of malnourishment, severe stress, steroids or immunosuppressive medications. Determine if patient has received a live viral vaccine within the past four weeks.

—Administer medication on inner surface of cleansed forearm. Avoid hairy areas or areas with little subcutaneous tissue. Press firmly, without twisting, and hold for at least 1 second. All 4 tines should penetrate tissue and a circular depression should be visible. If this is a repeat test, use a different extremity than the first time.

—Check for immediate post injection wheal.

—Read results in 48 hours.

—If patient is unable to return to have injection site evaluated by a health professional it may be possible to teach the patient how to interpret the test himself. Draw a circle 2 mm in size around the injection site and inform the patient to keep this mark and call the health care provider to report the reaction to the test. When the patient calls, ascertain whether there is swelling and induration outside the area you have drawn.

WHAT THE PATIENT NEEDS TO KNOW:

—The results of this test should be recorded in your personal records.

—It is important that the results of the test are communicated to the health care provider and also recorded in your medical records. You must return to have the test site evaluated, or to obtain instructions for checking it yourself.

—Notify your health care provider concerning any unusual skin irritation which develops following this test.

EVALUATION:

ADVERSE REACTIONS: *Dermatologic:* Severe localized reaction may develop if patient is hypersensitive to tubercle bacilli organisms (i.e., exposure to tuberculosis or active tuberculosis.) Site reactions may range from areas of increased erythema and induration, to vesiculation, ulceration and necrosis.

PARAMETERS TO MONITOR: Within 48 hours following injection, check site for induration, erythema and size. Positive reactions are over 2 mm in size around one of the tines, with erythema and induration. Reactions below 2 mm in size are negative.

Kathy Awalt

CARDIOVASCULAR AND DIURETIC DRUGS

ANTIANGINAL AGENTS—
CARDIOVASCULAR SLOW CHANNEL INHIBITORS

DILTIAZEM

ACTION OF THE DRUG: Diltiazem acts through interference with the depolarizing or slow inward current in excitable tissue. In the myocardium this results in excitation-contraction uncoupling of some tissue, although the action potential configuration is not altered. In both ischemic and nonischemic patients, relaxation of both large and small coronary arteries is produced through relaxation of coronary vascular smooth muscle. Little negative inotropic effects are usually seen. Peripherial vascular resistance is reduced as well as systemic blood pressure in a dose-related pattern. Electrophysiologically, diltiazem decreases SA and AV conduction. Functional refractory periods may be prolonged by as much as 20%. Usually no more than first-degree heart block is produced.

ASSESSMENT:

INDICATIONS: Diltiazem is used primarily in the treatment of angina pectoris seconday to coronary artery spasm. It is also used in the management of chronic stable angina in patients who have not responded to therapy with beta-adrenergic blocking agents or nitrates, or who have not been able to use these products.

SUBJECTIVE-OBJECTIVE: Coronary artery spasm should be suspected when the characteristic picture of resting angina with ST segment elevation occurring during attacks is seen (sometimes called Prinzmetal's variant angina). Patient may also present with a well-documented history of angina pectoris unresponsive to other medications.

PLAN:

CONTRAINDICATIONS: Medication should not be used in hypotensive patients, those with second- or third-degree AV block, or in patients with a sick sinus syndrome (unless a functioning ventricular pacemaker is present.)

WARNINGS: Because of the effect on AV conduction, AV node refractory periods may be prolonged without significantly prolonging sinus node recovery time, except in patients with sick sinus syndrome. Thus, very slow heart beats may sometimes be produced, as well as second- and third-degree heart block. If patient has previously taken beta-adrenergic blockers or digitalis, there may be additive effects in decreasing cardiac conduction. Congestive heart failure, hypotension and acute hepatic injury have been reported only rarely in conjunction with this medication.

There are no well-controlled studies using this medication in pregnant women. Laboratory studies suggest that an increased incidence of fetal skeletal damage and death may occur with administration of this drug to pregnant animals. Without further testing, this drug should be given only in the greatest need, to pregnant women. Likewise, no studies have been carried out regarding use of this medication in breast feeding women or in children.

PRECAUTIONS: Because of the metabolism of this drug by the liver and excretion by the kidneys, use this drug with extreme care in patients with impaired renal or hepatic function.

IMPLEMENTATION:

DRUG INTERACTIONS: When used with beta-adrenergic blocking agents or digitalis products, additive effects in prolonging AV conduction may develop. Further studies are warranted to evaluate situations in which this is a particular problem. There seems to be no interference with short- and long-acting nitrates or sublingual nitroglycerin taken concurrently. May increase serum digoxin levels.

PRODUCTS (TRADE NAME):
Cardizem (Available in 30 and 60 mg tablets.)

ADMINISTRATION AND DOSAGE: In all situations the dosage must be individualized. Begin with 30 mg four times daily, before meals and at bedtime. Dose may be increased gradually at 1 to 2 day intervals until 240 mg in divided doses is reached.

IMPLEMENTATION CONSIDERATIONS:

—Obtain a complete health history, including the presence of hypersensitivity, concurrent use of beta-adrenergic drugs or digitalis, underlying systemic disease, and possibility of pregnancy.

—Sublingual, short or long-acting nitrates may be safely taken with this drug, especially to relieve angina during the period of initial titration.

—Adverse reactions are usually mild, and often dosage related.

WHAT THE PATIENT NEEDS TO KNOW:

—Take medication exactly as prescribed. Do not alter dosage or suddenly discontinue medication.

—Some people experience side effects while taking this medication. Notify your health care provider if you develop any new or different symptoms, particularly an irregular heart beat, shortness of breath, nausea, constipation, or if you suddenly develop swelling of hands and feet.

—Carry a Medic-Alert bracelet or other information identifying that you are taking this medication.

—Keep this medication out of the reach of children and all others for whom it is not prescribed.

EVALUATION:

ADVERSE REACTIONS: *Cardiovascular:* arrhythmia (second- and third-degree heart block or asystole), bradycardia, congestive heart failure, edema, flushing, pounding heart, syncope. *CNS:* confusion, depression, dizziness, drowsiness, fatigue, hallucinations, headache, insomnia, lightheadedness, nervousness, weakness. *Dermatologic:* petechiae, rash, urticaria. *Gastrointestinal:* constipation, diarrhea, gastric upset, indigestion, nausea, pyrosis, vomiting. *Other:* nocturia, paresthesia, photosensitivity, polyuria, osteoarticular pain, thirst. Elevations of SGOT, SGPT, LDH, CPK, and alkaline phosphatase may also be transiently found during therapy.

OVERDOSAGE: No toxic response has yet been demonstrated. In patients who have an exaggerated response to the drug, atropine may be given for bradycardia and high-degree AV block, inotropic agents and diuretics given for cardiac failure, and vasopressors given for hypotension.

PARAMETERS TO MONITOR: Observe for therapeutic effect: relief of anginal pain and/or reduction in number of anginal attacks. Also observe for adverse reactions, particularly the development of arrhythmias or congestive heart failure, peripheral edema, and hypotension.

Marilyn W. Edmunds

NIFEDIPINE

ACTION OF THE DRUG: Nifedipine selectively inhibits the passage of extracellular calcium ions through specific ion channels of the cell membrane in cardiac, vascular and smooth muscle cells. Serum calcium concentrations are not altered. The agent causes a decreased peripheral vascular resistance and a fall in systolic and diastolic pressure, with a slight increase in heart rate.

ASSESSMENT:

INDICATIONS: Nifedipine has been used in the relief of vasospastic angina through its action in inhibiting spasm and dilating both normal and ischemic coronary arteries. This helps increase the oxygen available to these areas and may be a factor in reducing Prinzmetal's angina. In patients who have angina at rest with ST segment elevation, in which vasospasm has been documented during angiography, or patients who have effort-associated angina who have been refractory to nitrates or beta-blockers, this agent may be tried. The agent reduces the oxygen utilization of the heart through reducing peripheral vascular resistance, and thus reducing the afterload against which the heart works. In stable angina, medication may be used as adjunctive therapy with beta-blocking agents, although observation for severe hypotension must be conducted.

SUBJECTIVE: Patient may complain of angina, usually of a stable type.

OBJECTIVE: ST segment elevation may be present with complaints of chest pain. ECG changes revert to normal when pain is relieved.

PLAN:

CONTRAINDICATIONS: Do not give in the presence of hypersensitivity to nifedipine.

WARNINGS: Usually reduction in blood pressure of patients receiving this drug is moderate, and well tolerated. Patient taking beta-blockers or other anti-hypertensive medication, as well as selected individuals, may develop severe hypotension upon initial dosage or when dosage is increased. This necessitates careful observation of patients following beginning of therapy. Blood pressure should be monitored in lying, standing, and sitting positions. Patients who have recently stopped taking beta blockers, as well as other selected patients, may experience an increase in severity, duration, and frequency of angina upon beginning therapy or increasing dosage with this drug. Concurrent use of beta blockers may place some patients at greater risk for developing congestive heart failure. This would be particularly true if tight aortic stenosis is also present. Safety for use of this drug during pregnancy has not been established. It has been demonstrated to be teratogenic in laboratory animals.

PRECAUTIONS: May produce mild to moderate peripheral edema, particularly of the lower extremities, in up to 10% of patients. This may present a diagnostic problem in patients prone to develop congestive heart failure.

IMPLEMENTATION:

DRUG INTERACTIONS: Concomitant use with beta blocking agents may increase the likelihood of angina, congestive heart failure, or episodes of severe hypotension. May be administered with nitrates, although there is little clinical information on effects of this combination. May increase serum digoxin levels.

PRODUCTS (TRADE NAME):
Procardia (Available in 10 mg capsules.)

ADMINISTRATION AND DOSAGE: The dosage necessary to achieve the therapeutic objective of pain suppression must be individually determined through careful dosage adjustments.

Initial dose: 10 mg po 3 times/day. Increase both dose and frequency in 7-10 day increments in order to achieve relief of symptoms. Maximum 180 mg/day. If patient can be monitored frequently, dosage could be increased to 20 or 30 mg, 3 times a day over a 3-day period, or even more rapidly if patient is hospitalized. A single dose should rarely exceed 30 mg.

IMPLEMENTATION CONSIDERATIONS:

—Obtain a complete health history, including the presence of hypersensitivity, concurrent use of drugs, underlying systemic disease, and possibility of pregnancy.

—Sublingual or long-acting nitrates may be safely taken with this drug, especially to relieve angina during the period of initial titration.

—A good baseline physical examination may be helpful in determining later changes in peripheral edema or the development of congestive heart failure.

—Adverse reactions are frequent but usually transient and not serious. They are often dosage related.

—Dosages should be gradually tapered when medication is to be discontinued.

WHAT THE PATIENT NEEDS TO KNOW:
—Take medication exactly as prescribed. Do not alter dosage or suddenly discontinue medication.

—Some people experience side effects from taking this medication. Be certain to report any new or troublesome symptoms to your health care provider. The most common symptoms people feel are those related to the vasodilating activity of the drug: dizziness, lightheadedness, giddiness, flushing, heat sensation, headache, nausea, muscle cramps, peripheral edema, nervousness, palpitations, tremor, heartburn, shortness of breath, cough, wheezing, nasal congestion, sore throat.

—Avoid activities which require rapid changes in position. Periods of lightheadedness, especially in the morning when moving from lying to standing position, can usually be relieved by moving slowly.

—Feelings of fainting, developing of excessive fluid, especially in feet, or increases in angina pain should be reported promptly to your health care provider.

—Carry a Medic-Alert bracelet or other information identifying that you are taking this medication.

EVALUATION:

ADVERSE REACTIONS: *Cardiovascular:* angina, dizziness, lightheadedness, myocardial infarction, palpitation, peripheral edema, pulmonary edema, syncope, transient hypotension, ventricular arrhythmias. *CNS:* blurred vision, difficulties with balance, flushing, headache, jitteriness, nervousness, shakiness, sleep disturbances, weakness. *Dermatologic:* dermatitis, pruritus, urticaria. *Gastrointestinal:* constipation, cramps, diarrhea, flatulence, heartburn, nausea. *Respiratory:* cough, dyspnea, nasal congestion, sore throat, wheezing. *Other:* chills, mood changes, muscle cramps, sexual difficulties, tremor. Alteration in laboratory tests (unaccompanied by clinical signs) include: mild to moderate (transient) elevations of alkaline phosphatase, CPK, LDH, SGOT, and SGPT.

OVERDOSAGE: *Signs and symptoms:* Excessive peripheral vascular dilation leading to prolonged systemic hypotension may develop. Significant clinical experience has not been available to determine all symptoms. *Treatment:* Referral to qualified physician for supportive cardiovascular management.

PARAMETERS TO MONITOR: Observe for therapeutic effect: relief of anginal pain and/or reduction in number of anginal attacks. Also observe for adverse reactions, particularly the development of congestive heart failure, peripheral edema, and postural hypotension. Blood pressures and pulses should be taken in lying, sitting, and standing positions. Some of these problems may be brief or may disappear with a slight reduction in dosage.

Marilyn W. Edmunds

ANTIANGINAL AGENTS

NITRATES

ACTION OF THE DRUG: The major action of the nitrate products is the direct relaxation of vascular smooth muscle. This effect is felt in both the arterial and venous circulation. Arterial relaxation decreases systemic vascular resistance and cardiac afterload, while venous relaxation assists in venous pooling of blood, thereby decreasing venous return to the heart and preload. Both of these effects work together to decrease myocardial oxygen consumption. In addition, nitrates increase use of coronary collaterals so that there is better perfusion of the inner layers of the myocardium. Nitrates are readily absorbed sublingually, through the skin, and orally, but those products taken orally are rapidly metabolized in the liver to inactive metabolites and the half-life is only 1 to 4 minutes. Newer transdermal forms of the medication allow it to pass directly into the bloodstream, thus reaching target organs before being inactivated by the hepatic system.

ASSESSMENT:

INDICATIONS: Antianginal agents are used primarily in the relief of pain in acute angina (rapid-acting nitrates such as amyl nitrite, sublingual nitroglycerin and sublingual or chewable isosorbide dinitrate). The long-acting nitrates, topical, transdermal, transmucosal and oral sustained-release nitroglycerin products are also used in the prophylaxis of predictable anginal attacks and to decrease the severity and frequency of anginal attacks. They are also used to reduce the cardiac work load in congestive heart conditions, and for relief of biliary, gastrointestial, urethral and bronchial smooth muscle pain.

SUBJECTIVE: History of angina: crushing, substernal chest pain, brought on usually by exertion or severe emotion and relieved with rest. Angina may be predictable and stable, progressive in nature (Prinzmetal's angina), or occur at rest (decubitus angina).

OBJECTIVE: With chest pain, patient may have tachycardia and blood pressure elevation. Electrocardiogram during pain may indicate T wave elevations, or ST-T wave changes which disappear when angina is relieved.

PLAN:

CONTRAINDICATIONS: Do not use in patients with hypersensitivity to the drug, in patients with severe anemia, increased intracranial pressure, head trauma, cerebral hemorrhage or postural hypotension. Do not give IV nitroglycerin to patients in shock, or those with hypovolemia, hypotension, constrictive pericarditis, pericardial tamponade, or cerebral insufficiency.

WARNINGS: Safety has not been established for the use of nitroglycerin in patients with acute myocardial infarctions (MI). When it is used in patients with recent MIs the transdermal systems are superior and patients must be closely evaluated. IV nitroglycerin administration is particularly hazardous and must be carried out only when patient can be monitored carefully. Safety for use in children, pregnant women and nursing mothers has not been established. No untoward effects on the fetus have been reported but caution should be used.

PRECAUTIONS: Some of these products contain tartrazine which may cause an allergic-type reaction often expressed through symptoms of bronchial asthma. Patients who are allergic to aspirin have a greater tendency to react to tartrazine. IV preparations should be used with care in patients with severe renal or hepatic disease. Tolerance and cross-tolerance may develop to nitrate products that are used for prolonged periods. Excessive dosage may produce violent headaches. All nitrates should be given with care in patients with recent history of cerebrovascular accident (CVA), because of the cerebral vasodilatation which occurs.

IMPLEMENTATION:

DRUG INTERACTIONS: Nitrates increase the effects of atropine-like drugs and tricyclic antidepressants, and decrease the effects of all choline-like drugs. Anticholinergic drugs may be potentiated (especially antihistamines). Do not use concurrently with prazosin because of possibility of interaction. Alcohol, beta-blockers, antihypertensives, narcotics and vasodilators taken with nitrates and nitrites (especially amyl nitrite) may produce severe hypotension and cardiovascular collapse. The pressor actions of sympathomimetic drugs may be antagonized. Cold environment or tobacco reduces the effectiveness of nitroglycerin. Cross-tolerance can develop between all nitrates and nitrites. Nitroglycerin also increases urine VMA and catecholamine levels.

ADMINISTRATION AND DOSAGE: Patient must understand clearly what the uses and limitations are for the nitrate being taken. The patient should understand the dosage schedule and be given instructions about when to seek medical attention during an anginal attack that does not respond to therapy. There are many important considerations in taking this medication by its various routes. Refer to the specific product information sections for details. It is important to note that severe headaches may be produced from excessive dosages. A person using a nitrate for a prolonged period should taper off gradually to avoid precipitating anginal attacks which may be provoked by stopping the drug suddenly.

In choosing the proper preparation for the patient consider the information comparing the action of various products listed in Table 3-1.

IMPLEMENTATION CONSIDERATIONS:

—Obtain a complete health history to determine presence of underlying disease (myocardial infarction, CVA), allergy (especially aspirin), concurrent drug administration which may produce interactions, and possibility of pregnancy. Obtain a complete description of the anginal attacks so that the appropriate therapeutic drug can be selected.

—Tolerance and cross-tolerance with other nitrates may develop over time with repeated use. This may necessitate alternation with other coronary vasodilators.

—Excessive dosage may produce violent headaches which can usually be controlled by lowering the dose and administering analgesics. These headaches will gradually subside.

—Discontinue drug if blurring of vision or dry mouth occurs.

—If patient reports portions of sustained-release medication being passed in the stool, it is likely that GI transit time is too rapid to allow medication to be absorbed. These patients should take oral or sublingual medication.

—Elderly patients may have postural hypotension with these drugs and need to be monitored carefully. They may need to have someone with them when they take the medication.

—Volatile nitrites are sometimes abused to produce sensations of lighthead-

TABLE 3-1. COMPARISON OF NITRATE-NITRITE PRODUCTS

Agents for Acute Angina:

Product	Onset	Duration	Preparation
Amyl nitrite	30 seconds	3-5 minutes	Inhalant
Isosorbide dinitrate	2-5 minutes	1-2 hours	Sublingual/Chewable
Nitroglycerin	3 minutes	10-30 min	Sublingual
	3 minutes	6 hours	Transmucosal
	Immediately	Brief	Intravenous

Agents for Angina Prophylaxis:

Product	Onset	Duration	Preparation
Erythrityl tetranitrate	5 minutes	2 hours	Sublingual/Chewable
	30 minutes	Variable	Oral
Isosorbide dinitrate	15-30 minutes	4-6 hours	Oral
	Slow	12 hours	Sustained Release, Oral
Nitroglycerin	Slow	8-12 hours	Sustained Release, Oral
	30-60 minutes	4-6 hours	Topical Ointment
	30-60 minutes	24 hours	Transdermal
Pentaerythritol tetranitrate	30 minutes	4-5 hours	Oral
	Slow	12 hours	Sustained Release, Oral

edness, dizziness and a feeling of euphoria. Abuse may also produce sexual stimulation.

WHAT THE PATIENT NEEDS TO KNOW:

—For acute anginal attacks, take one tablet sublingually as soon as pain is experienced. Do not chew or swallow medication: let it dissolve under your tongue. Lie down and rest. If pain is not relieved within 1-3 minutes, a second pill may be taken. If pain is not relieved within another 3 minutes, a third pill may be taken. If pain is not relieved you must go to an emergency room immediately for evaluation.

—Nitroglycerin breaks down rapidly. Sunlight will speed up this process. Even under the best storage conditions, these drugs lose their strength in about three months after bottle has been opened. A new prescription should be obtained every three months and old medication discarded. Sublingual medicine which produces burning under the tongue is not always a reliable indicator that drug is still potent. Because some drugs are in a much purer form than others, they do not always produce the characteristic throbbing headache.

—Natural and predictable side effects of nitroglycerin include flushing of the face, brief throbbing headache, increased heart rate, dizziness, and light-headedness when sitting up rapidly. Headache usually lasts no longer than 20 minutes and may be relieved by analgesics. Rest for 10-15 minutes after pain is relieved. Notify your health care provider if blurring of vision, persistent headache or dry mouth occurs.

—Take medication on an empty stomach when possible.

—Do not drink alcoholic beverages while taking nitrate products.

—The active ingredient in nitroglycerin is very easily destroyed. Storage in a plastic or cardboard box allows the nitrate to escape. Cotton plugs in the top of the medicine container or other drugs stored with nitroglycerin will absorb the nitrate. Medication should be stored in the original dark glass container. Remove all cotton wadding and keep container tightly capped and out of sunlight. For topical ointment, keep tube tightly closed.

—For patients using inhalant medication, take it only when lying or sitting down. Because this is a highly flammable product, put out cigarettes and avoid using it around fire or sparks.

—For transmucosal nitroglycerin, do not chew or swallow tablet. Put it inside the cheek, or under your lip, and let it slowly dissolve.

—For topical ointment, spread thin layer on skin, using applicator and ruler. Do not rub or massage the ointment into the skin. Wash off any medication which might have gotten on hands.

—For transdermal application, select a hairless spot (or clip hair) and apply adhesive pad to skin. Washing, bathing or swimming does not affect this system. Do not cut or tear system. If pad should come off, discard it and place a new one on a different site.

—If medication seems not to be as effective after taking it for a while (requiring you to take several pills before getting relief), you may be developing a tolerance to the drug. Discontinuing the drug for several days may be long enough to restore your sensitivity. Take the smallest possible dose in order to minimize the risk of developing tolerance.

—Keep a record of the frequency of your anginal attacks, the number of pills taken, and any side effects. Bring this record with you to each appointment.

—Use nitroglycerin in anticipation of situations in which you can predict anginal attacks will occur. Taking medication before the activity may prevent or reduce the degree of pain.

—This medication is only part of the therapy for angina. Try to avoid situations that precipitate pain (stress, heavy exercise, over eating, smoking). Reduce your calorie intake if you need to lose weight, and develop a program of regular and sensible exercise.

—Avoid excessive intake of foods which stimulate the heart (coffee, tea, caffeinated soft drinks, excessive chocolate).

—Keep this medication out of the reach of children and others for whom it is not prescribed.

EVALUATION:

ADVERSE REACTIONS: *Cardiovascular:* cutaneous vasodilation with flushing, palpitation, postural hypotension, tachycardia. *CNS:* confusion, dizziness, fainting, headache, lightheadedness, signs of cerebral ischemia, transient episodes of vertigo, weakness, palpitation, dizziness, postural hypotension. *Dermatologic:* drug rash, exfoliative dermatitis (rare), topical allergic reactions (localized pruritic eczematous eruptions, vesicular and pruritic lesions, conjunctival and oral mucosal edema). *Gastrointestinal:* local burning in oral cavity, nausea, vomiting. *Hypersensitivity:* Occasional reactions marked by vomiting, profound weakness, restlessness, tachycardia, incontinence, syncope, perspiration, pallor, pronounced hypotension and collapse. *Other:* methemoglobinemia (with high doses of amyl nitrite).

OVERDOSAGE: *Signs and symptoms:* Severe hypotension, reflex tachycardia, and/or paralysis, followed by clonic convulsions and death due to respiratory failure may occur. *Treatment:* Symptoms from IV overdosage will be transient since drug is rapidly degraded. Administer supportive therapy.

PARAMETERS TO MONITOR: Monitor for therapeutic effect and incidence of side effects. Evaluate the number and pattern of anginal attacks. Angina which occurs more frequently and is unresponsive to nitroglycerin therapy, which is precipitated by activity formerly tolerated by patient (crescendo angina) or which occurs when patient is at rest (decubitus angina) are all indications of increasing lack of oxygen to the myocardium. More extensive investigation of cardiac status is warranted. Cardiac monitoring and hospitalization may be indicated. Patient should have periodic ECG evaluations. ECG changes while patient is experiencing angina may document ST-T wave changes which reverse once pain is alleviated. Persistence of ECG changes demonstrates progression of cardiac ischemia and should alert the practitioner to seek medical assistance in evaluating disease status.

AMYL NITRITE

PRODUCTS (TRADE NAME):
Amyl Nitrite Aspirols (Available in 0.18 or 0.3 ml inhalants.) **Amyl Nitrite, Amyl Nitrite Vaporoles** (Available in 0.3 ml inhalants.)

DRUG SPECIFICS:
Inhalant used for immediate relief of angina pectoris. Onset of action is 30 seconds. Crush capsule and wave under patient's nose. May repeat in 3 to 5 minutes as necessary.

ADMINISTRATION AND DOSAGE SPECIFICS:
Use 0.18 or 0.3 ml by inhalation as needed.

ERYTHRITYL TETRANITRATE

PRODUCTS (TRADE NAME):
  Cardilate (Available in 5 and 10 mg SL or oral tablets; 10 mg chewable tablet.)
DRUG SPECIFICS:
  Used as a prophylactic measure for long-term therapy in patients with recurrrent angina or reduced exercise tolerance associated with angina pectoris. Larger doses precipitate more severe headaches.
ADMINISTRATION AND DOSAGE SPECIFICS:
  Sublingual: 5 to 10 mg SL prior to each anticipated incidence of angina.
  Oral: 10 mg three times daily. Up to 100 mg/day may be tolerated.

ISOSORBIDE DINITRATE, CHEWABLE AND SUBLINGUAL

PRODUCTS (TRADE NAME):
  Isogard (Available in 2.5, 5 mg SL tablets.) **Isordil** (Available in 2.5, 5, and 10 mg SL tablets; 10 mg chewable tablet.) **IsosorbideDinitrate** (Available in 2.5 and 5 mg SL tablets.) **Onset** (Available in 5 and 10 mg chewable tablets.) **Sorate** (Available in 2.5 and 5 mg SL tablets; 5 and 10 mg chewable tablets.) **Sorbitrate** (Available in 2.5 and 5 mg SL tablets; 5 and 10 mg chewable tablets.)
DRUG SPECIFICS:
  These chewable and sublingual products are used for the prophylaxis and treatment of anginal attacks. Occasionally, severe hypotensive response may occur to chewable medication, so therapy should be started at low dosage.
ADMINISTRATION AND DOSAGE SPECIFICS:
  Chewable: Take 5 mg initially, and watch for adverse effects. Low dosage may be effective in relieving acute attacks. Increase as needed for relief. Take every 2 to 3 hours for prophylaxis.
  Sublingual: 2.5 to 10 mg for acute attacks. Up to 30 mg may sometimes be warranted. Use every 4 to 6 hours prophylactically.

ISOSORBIDE DINITRATE, ORAL

PRODUCTS (TRADE NAME):
  Dilitrate-SR, Iso-Bid (Available in 40 mg sustained release capsules.) **Isogard** (Available in 5 and 10 mg tablets and 40 mg sustained-release tablets.) **Isordil Tembids** (Available in 40 mg sustained-release tablets or capsules.) **Isordil Titradose** (Available in 5, 10, 20 and 30 mg tablets.) **Isosorbide Dinitrate** (Available

in 5, 10, 20 mg tablets and 20 mg sustained-release capsules and tablets.) **Isotrate Timecelles** (Available in 40 mg sustained-release capsules.) **Sorate** (Available in 10 mg tablets.) **Sorate-40, Sorbide T.D.** (Available in 40 mg sustained-release capsules.) **Sorbitrate** (Available in 5, 10, 20 mg tablets.) **Sorbitrate SA** (Available in 40 mg sustained-release tablets.)

DRUG SPECIFICS:

These oral preparations are used only in the prophylaxis of angina pectoris. Take on an empty stomach unless severe vascular headaches are produced.

ADMINISTRATION AND DOSAGE SPECIFICS:

Tablets: 5 to 30 mg po 4 times daily.

Sustained Release: 40 mg every 6 to 12 hours daily.

NITROGLYCERIN, SUBLINGUAL

PRODUCTS (TRADE NAME):

Nitroglycerin (Available in 0.15, 0.3, 0.4 and 0.6 mg SL tablets.) **Nitrostat** (Available in 0.15, 0.3, 0.4, and 0.6 mg SL stabilized tablets.)

DRUG SPECIFICS:

These sublingual products are used for patients with angina pectoris. Products are very labile, and must be stored carefully in original container, with cotton wadding removed. Stabilized tablets are potent for up to 5 years after manufacturing date, while conventional tablets are stable for only 2 years. Once bottle is opened, tablets are potent for only about 6 months.

ADMINISTRATION AND DOSAGE SPECIFICS:

Prophylaxis: Dissolve one tablet under tongue 5 to 10 minutes before activities causing pain.

Treatment of angina pectoris: Dissolve one tablet under tongue or in buccal pouch at the first sign of an acute anginal attack. Repeat every 3-5 minutes until pain is relieved, or until 3 doses are taken. If no relief after third dose, patient should go to emergency room or clinic.

NITROGLYCERIN, SUSTAINED RELEASE

PRODUCTS (TRADE NAME):

Ang-O-Span (Available in 2.5 mg sustained-release capsules.) **Klavikordal** (Available in 2.6, 6.5 mg sustained-release tablets.) **Nitrocap T.D., Nitroglycerin, Nitrolin, Nitrospan** (Available in 2.6 and 6.5 mg sustained release capsules.) **Nitro-Bid Plateau Caps** (Available in 2.6 mg sustained-release capsules.) **Niong, Nitronet** (Available in 2.5 and 6.5 mg sustained-release tablets.) **Nitroglyn** (Available in 1.3, 2.5, and 6.5 mg sustained-release tablets.) **Nitrong** (Available in 2.5, 6.5

and 9 mg sustained-release tablets.) **N-G-C** (Available in 6.5 mg sustained-release capsules.) **Trates Granucaps** (Available in 2.5 mg sustained-release capsules.)
DRUG SPECIFICS:

"Possibly effective" in the prophylaxis of angina pectoris when used on a regular basis. Monitor systolic blood pressure.
ADMINISTRATION AND DOSAGE SPECIFICS:

One capsule or tablet every 8 to 12 hours. Do not take with food.

NITROGLYCERIN, TOPICAL

PRODUCTS (TRADE NAME):

Nitro-Bid, Nitroglycerin, Nitrol, Nitrong, Nitrostat (Available in 2% ointment.)
DRUG SPECIFICS:

Used for prevention and treatment of angina pectoris. One inch of ointment contains approximately 15 mg nitroglycerin in a lanolin-petrolatum base. The dosage should be adjusted considering both therapeutic and side effects. Monitor especially the blood pressure. Rotate sites of application to avoid skin irritation and sensitization. Discontinue drug by gradually reducing frequency and dosage of application over a 4- to 6-week period, in order to avoid producing withdrawal reactions.
ADMINISTRATION AND DOSAGE SPECIFICS:

Initial dosage: Give 1/2 inch (12.5 mm) every 8 hours, increasing by 1/2 inch with each successive application until desired relief is obtained. Spread ointment onto a 6 x 6 inch skin area (usually chest) in a thin, uniform layer. Cover the area with plastic wrap and hold in place with adhesive tape. Dose depends on surface area covered.

NITROGLYCERIN, TRANSDERMAL SYSTEMS

PRODUCTS (TRADE NAME):

Nitrodisc (Available in 5 mg/24 hr and 10 mg/24 hr transdermal systems.) **Nitro-Dur** (Available in 5 cm^2, 10 cm^2, 15 cm^2, 20 cm^2, and 30 cm^2 transdermal systems.) **Transderm-Nitro** (Available in 2.5, 5, 10, and 15 mg/24 hr transdermal systems.)
DRUG SPECIFICS:

Used for the prophylaxis and treatment of angina pectoris. Transdermal pad applied to skin releases a continuous and well-controlled supply of nitroglycerin beginning in 1 hour and lasting for a minimum of 24 hours.
ADMINISTRATION AND DOSAGE SPECIFICS:

Apply one pad each day to a skin site free of hair on trunk of body. Rotate application site to avoid irritation of skin. Dosage may be increased by applying more systems, or using a higher dosage product. Experiment until the proper therapeutic effect is found, balanced with fewest side effects.

NITROGLYCERIN, TRANSMUCOSAL

PRODUCTS (TRADE NAME):
Susadrin (Available in 1, 2, and 3 mg transmucosal tablets.)
DRUG SPECIFICS:
Transmucosal tablets used for the prophylaxis and treatment of patients with angina pectoris. Tablet is usually placed between lip and gum above upper incisors one time, and the next time in the buccal area between cheek and gum. Tablet adheres to the mucosa and is left to dissolve slowly over a 3- to 5-hour period. If continuous therapy is indicated, take next tablet within one hour of dissolution of the first tablet. Store tablets in original container and avoid exposure to heat.
ADMINISTRATION AND DOSAGE SPECIFICS:
Routine therapy: Take one 1 mg tablet three times daily. If angina occurs while tablet is in place, increase dosage; if angina occurs between tablet administration when no tablet is in place, increase frequency to four times daily.
Prophylaxis: Place 1 tablet in anticipation of pain. Do not exceed 1 tablet every 2 hours.

PENTAERYTHRITOL TETRANITRATE (P.E.T.N.), ORAL AND SUSTAINED RELEASE

PRODUCTS (TRADE NAME):
Duotrate Plateau Caps (Available in 30 and 45 mg sustained-release capsules.) Kaytrate (Available in 30 and 80 mg sustained-release capsules.) Pentraspan (Available in 80 mg sustained-release capsules.) Pentritol (Available in 60 mg sustained-release capsules.) Pentylan (Available in 10 and 20 mg tablets.) Peritrate (Available in 10, 20 and 40 mg tablets, and 80 mg sustained-release tablets.) P.E.T.N (Available in 10 and 20 mg tablets, 30 and 80 mg sustained-release capsules, and 80 mg sustained-release tablets.) Vaso-80 Unicelles (Available in 80 mg sustained-release capsules.)
DRUG SPECIFICS:
Used only for the prophylaxis of angina pectoris. Take on an empty stomach unless severe vascular headaches are provoked.

ADMINISTRATION AND DOSAGE SPECIFICS:

Oral: 10 to 20 mg 3 or 4 times daily initially, increased to 40 mg 4 times daily if needed. Take either 1/2 hour before meals or 1 hour after meals, and at bedtime.

Sustained release: One every 12 hours.

Marilyn W. Edmunds

ANTIARRHYTHMIC AGENTS

ACTION OF THE DRUGS: This category of drugs acts to reduce electrical irregularity of the heart. It does this by acting in one of four major ways:

—Class 1 drugs—quinidine, procainamide, disopyramide—lengthen the effective refractory period of atrial and ventricular myocardium by depressing the fast inward sodium current and decrease the automaticity and excitability of ectopic foci of cardiac muscle.

—Class 2 drugs—beta blockers—reduce sympathetic excitation to the heart.

—Class 3 drugs—amiodarone—lengthen the action potential duration. Class 3 drugs are currently investigational or used only in hospital settings.

—Class 4 drugs—verapamil—selectively block the slow calcium channel in the myocardium and prolongs the effective refractory period in the atrioventricular (AV) node.

ASSESSMENT:

INDICATIONS: The focus for the nurse practitioner is on chronic outpatient prophylaxis of arrhythmias. Emergency or acute care treatment of arrhythmias are not discussed in detail as these are usually viewed as outside this role.

The mechanism of an arrhythmia is important in determining which drug will be effective. The two basic mechanisms within the heart are: (1) increased automaticity resulting in an ectopic focus and (2) reentry through abnormal conduction pathways.

Sinus tachycardia is usually extracardiac in origin. It is usually a physiologic response to stress such as anxiety, exercise, or fever. It is also seen in hypoxia, hypovolemia, pheochromocytoma, hyperthyroidism and congestive heart failure. Rarely is it seen as a chronic abnormality of autonomic regulation. The rate is usually 100 to 200 beats/minute. Therapy consists of correction of the underlying abnormality.

Premature atrial contractions (PAC's) can be caused by either increased automaticity or reentry. They may be seen with anxiety, fatigue, or with alcohol, tobacco, or coffee use. They may be a toxic reaction to drugs such as digitalis, quinidine, or procainamide. They may also be seen in heart disease, especially with distention of the atria as in congestive heart failure. They require therapy if they remain after correction of any underlying problem and the patient is symptomatic (palpitations or syncope).

Evidence suggests that atrial flutter (AFl) is a reentry arrhythmia. It is usually seen in patients with heart disease with distention of the atria, as in congestive heart failure. The rate of flutter is usually 250-450 beats/minute. The AV conduction ratio determines the ventricular rate. A rapid ventricular response can cause cardiovascular decompensation, especially in a diseased heart.

Atrial fibrillation (AF) is due to a total lack of organized activation in the atria. It is usually seen in patients with atrial disease. The ventricular response in untreated AF is 150-220. This rapid rate may be poorly tolerated. Systemic emboli often occur in patients with AF.

Paroxysmal supraventricular tachycardias (PSVT's) are a group of tachyarrhythmias. The most common mechanism is reentry within the AV node. It can also be caused by increased automaticity within the atria or AV node, reentry within the atria, or reentry through an accessory pathway as in Wolff-Parkinson-White (WPW) syndrome. It is characterized by an atrial and ventricular rate of 130-250, 1:1 conduction, and a narrow QRS complex. The PSVT's are not always seen in patients with severe underlying heart disease. The therapy depends on the patient's ability to tolerate the tachycardia as well as the mechanism of the arrhythmia.

Premature ventricular contractions (PVC's) are caused by increased automaticity. They have been classified according to both prevalence and morphological characteristics. Complex PVC's (three or more in a row or early, R on T, PVC's) are associated with increased risk of sudden death. However, underlying heart disease (especially myocardial ischemia or recent myocardial infarction) greatly increases the risk associated with even simple PVC's.

In general, PVC's are treated if any of the following apply: (1) the patient is symptomatic, (2) complex PVC's are present, (3) the patient is one year or less post myocardial infarction, (4) the patient has underlying heart disease, or (5) the patient has angina. PVC's are not treated if all of the following apply: (1) the patient is asymptomatic, (2) the patient has a normal heart, (3) the PVC's are simple, and (4) the PVC's disappear with exercise on a graded exercise test.

The Wolff-Parkinson-White (WPW) syndrome is caused by an accessory conduction pathway in the AV node. It is characterized by a short PR interval, a wide QRS, and delta waves. It is usually seen in otherwise healthy persons. Persons with WPW are susceptible to arrhythmias, usually PSVT, but also atrial flutter and atrial fibrillation.

The Lown-Ganong-Levine (LGL) syndrome's mechanism is not clear, although it is possibly an accessory conduction pathway. It is characterized by short PR interval without delta waves. These persons are also susceptible to PSVT.

Table 3-2 summarizes the suggested treatment of acute and chronic arrhythmias.

SUBJECTIVE: The patient may have no complaints or may complain of palpitations, dizziness, weakness or syncope. The palpitations may be described as fluttering, pounding, skipped beats, heart jumping out of chest. They are often noticed when the patient is sitting quietly or lying in bed. They may be precipitated by anxiety, caffeine, cigarettes, or stimulants such as decongestants, diet pills, or amphetamines.

OBJECTIVE: The patient may have an irregular pulse. A standard 12-lead ECG may show an arrhythmia. However, a 24-hour Holter monitor is usually necessary to document and identify an arrhythmia.

TABLE 3-2. ACUTE TREATMENT AND CHRONIC PROPHYLAXIS OF ARRHYTHMIAS

Arrhythmia	Type of Treatment Indicated*	
	Acute (if indicated)	Chronic Prophylaxis
Sinus tachycardia	Propranolol	Propranolol
Premature atrial contractions	Digoxin	1. Digoxin 2. Quinidine Disopyramide Procainamide 3. Propranolol
Premature ventricular contractions	1. Lidocaine 2. Procainamide	1. Quinidine Disopyramide Procainamide 2. Digoxin 3. Propranolol
Atrial flutter/ atrial fibrillation	1. Cardioversion 2. Digoxin	1. Digoxin 2. Propranolol 3. Quinidine Disopyramide Procainamide 4. Verapamil

*Listed in order of suggested usage.

ANTIARRHYTHMIC AGENTS—CLASS 1

DISOPYRAMIDE

ACTION OF THE DRUG: Disopyramide works to (1) lengthen the effective refractory period of atrial and ventricular myocardium, (2) decrease the automaticity or excitability of ectopic foci of cardiac muscle, and (3) exert an anticholinergic action.

ASSESSMENT:

INDICATIONS: Used in the treatment of premature ventricular contractions.
SUBJECTIVE: Patients may complain of irregular pulse and feeling lightheaded or dizzy. They may or may not have a previous history of cardiac problems. They may also be unaware of any abnormalities.

OBJECTIVE: Pulse may be irregular. Diagnosis is confirmed by 12-lead ECG, with a long lead II demonstrating one or more foci for premature ventricular beats.

PLAN:

CONTRAINDICATIONS: Do not use in the presence of hypersensitivity to disopyramide, second or third degree AV block or cardiogenic shock.

WARNINGS: Disopyramide may cause or worsen congestive heart failure. It may produce hypotension especially in patients with cardiomyopathy. If QRS widening occurs, discontinue the drug. If QT prolongation occurs, worsening of the arrhythmia may occur. Blood glucose levels may be lowered, especially in patients with congestive heart failure, malnutrition, renal or hepatic disease. Reduce dosage if first degree block occurs. Use with caution in patients with glaucoma, myasthenia gravis, or urinary retention because of the drug's anticholinergic effects.

PRECAUTIONS: Treat atrial fibrillation and flutter with digoxin before adding disopyramide or an extremely rapid ventricular rate may result. Use with caution in patients with sick sinus syndrome, Wolff-Parkinson-White syndrome, or bundle branch block.

IMPLEMENTATION:

DRUG INTERACTIONS: Use with other class 1 antiarrythmic drugs may cause severe negative inotropic effects. Disopyramide does not increase serum digoxin levels. Phenytoin or other hepatic enzyme inducers may lower disopyramide plasma levels. Alters laboratory values in the following manner: decreases potassium, elevates cholesterol/triglycerides, elevates liver enzymes, BUN, creatinine, decreases hemoglobin/hematocrit and lowers blood sugar.

PRODUCTS (TRADE NAME):
Norpace CR (Available in 100 and 150 mg capsules).

ADMINISTRATION AND DOSAGE: Reduce dosage in patients with renal or hepatic impairment. Dosage must be individualized; usual dose is 400-800 mg per day in divided doses. 150 mg po every 6 hours for Norspace and 300 mg every 12 hours for Norspace CR.

IMPLEMENTATION CONSIDERATIONS:
—Take a complete health history: history of hypersensitivity, other drugs which may cause drug interactions, other medical problems.

—Look for and treat any underlying factors such as hypoxia, acid-base imbalance, increased or decreased potassium, catecholamines, or drug toxicity.

—This drug often causes or worsens congestive heart failure. Monitor clients with previous history of heart failure carefully.

—If QRS widening occurs, discontinue the drug. If QT prolongation occurs, worsening of the arrhythmia may occur.

—Reduce dosage if first-degree heart block develops.

WHAT THE PATIENT NEEDS TO KNOW:
—Take this medication exactly as ordered. Do not skip doses or double doses.

—Some people have side effects from this drug. Be sure to report any new or uncomfortable symptoms to your health provider. Especially notify them if you note any sudden weight gain, trouble breathing, or increased coughing.

—Be sure to return regularly for visits to your health provider so that your progress on this medication can be followed.

—May cause dizziness or blurred vision, so use caution if driving or performing tasks requiring alertness. Avoid alcoholic beverages since they may increase these symptoms.

EVALUATION:

ADVERSE REACTIONS: *Cardiovascular:* cardiac conduction disturbances, chest pain, congestive heart failure, edema/weight gain, hypotension, shortness of breath, syncope. *CNS:* aches/pains, acute psychosis, depression, dizziness, fatigue/muscle weakness, headache, insomnia, nervousness, numbness/tingling, weakness. *Dermatologic:* dermatoses, itching, generalized rash. *Hematopoietic:* reversible agranulocytosis. *Gastrointestinal:* nausea, pain, bloating, gas, anorexia, diarrhea, vomiting. *Genitourinary:* impotence, urinary frequency and urgency. *Other:* anticholinergic reactions (urinary retention or hesitancy, dry mouth, constipation, blurred vision, nausea).

OVERDOSAGE: *Signs and symptoms:* loss of consciousness, cardiac arrhythmias. *Treatment:* discontinue drug. Treat symptomatically.

PARAMETERS TO MONITOR: Obtain baseline ECG. Monitor for therapeutic effects. Effectiveness may be evaluated by use of a 24 hour Holter monitor. Periodic blood counts and liver and kidney function tests should be collected with patients on long-term therapy. Therapeutic serum level is usually around 2-7 mcg/ml in most laboratories.

PROCAINAMIDE

ACTION OF THE DRUG: Procainamide acts to lengthen the effective refractory period of atrial myocardium considerably more than ventricular myocardium, decreases the automaticity or excitability of ectopic foci of cardiac muscle, and slows conduction in atria, bundle of HIS, and ventricle.

ASSESSMENT:

INDICATIONS: Premature ventricular contractions, paroxysmal supraventricular tachyarrhythmias, atrial flutter, atrial fibrillation, premature atrial contractions.

SUBJECTIVE: Patient may complain of chest pain, irregular pulse, lightheadedness or dizziness. There may or may not be a previous history of cardiac problems.

OBJECTIVE: Rapid regular or irregular pulse may be felt. Diagnosis may be confirmed by 12 lead ECG with a long lead II clearly demonstrating the arrhythmia.

PLAN:

CONTRAINDICATIONS: Hypersensitivity to procainamide, second- and third-degree AV block, or myasthenia gravis.

WARNINGS: A positive ANA test with or without a systemic lupus erythematosus-like syndrome may occur.

PRECAUTIONS: Procainamide may produce untoward responses in an abnormal myocardium. In atrial fibrillation or flutter, procainamide may produce a rapid ventricular response. Use with caution in patients with both liver and kidney disease (because of the danger of excessive drug accumulation) and in bundle branch block.

IMPLEMENTATION:

DRUG INTERACTIONS: Other antiarrhythmic agents exert an additive cardiac depressant effect when administered concomitantly.

PRODUCTS (TRADE NAME):

Procan-SR (Available in 250, 500, and 750 mg tablets). **Pronestyl** (Available in 250, 375, and 500 mg tablets and capsules). **Pronestyl-SR** (Available in 500 mg tablets).

ADMINISTRATION AND DOSAGE: Drug is usually given in order to suppress premature ventricular contractions and to maintain normal sinus rhythm following conversion from atrial fibrillation or atrial flutter. Dose is titrated to achieve maximal therapeutic effect. Prophylaxis dose is calculated only generally on patient weight. The following schedule may be used.

Prophylaxis of PVC's	120 lb	120-200 lb	200+ lb	Frequency
Pronestyl	250 mg	375 mg	500 mg	every 3 hours
Pronestyl-SR	500 mg	500 mg or 1,000 mg	1000 mg	every 6 hours
Procan-SR	500 mg	750 mg	1000 mg	every 6 hours

Maintenance after converting atrial flutter or atrial fibrillation:
Pronestyl: 500-1000 mg every 4-6 hours po.
Procan SR: 1000 mg every 6 hours po.
Pronestyl SR: 1000 mg every 6 hours po.

IMPLEMENTATION CONSIDERATIONS:

—Obtain a thorough health history: hypersensitivity, other antiarrhythmic agents which could cause an additive cardiac depressant effect, other medications which could cause drug interactions, presence of other diseases.

—Procainamide can produce the following changes on an ECG: QRS widening, PR and QT interval prolongation, and QRS and T wave decreased voltage.

—Observe closely for therapeutic effect and check for toxicity.

—Elderly patients may need a decreased dosage.

—With all arrhythmias, look for and treat any underlying factors such as hypoxia, acid-base balance, increased or decreased potassium, catecholamines, or drug toxicity (especially digoxin or quinidine).

WHAT THE PATIENT NEEDS TO KNOW:
—It is very important to take your medicine exactly as prescribed. Do not miss doses or take double doses.

—Some patients experience side effects with this drug. Be certain to report any new or uncomfortable symptoms to your provider, especially: soreness of mouth, throat or gums, unexplained fever or symptoms of upper respiratory infection.

—Take medication with food to avoid upsetting stomach.

EVALUATION:

ADVERSE REACTIONS: *Cardiovascular:* heart block hypotension, ventricular asystole or fibrillation. *CNS:* fever and chills, giddiness, mental depression, psychosis with hallucinations, weakness. *Gastrointestinal:* anorexia, bitter taste, diarrhea, nausea. *Hematopoietic:* agranulocytosis. *Hypersensitivity:* angioneurotic edema, maculopapular rash, pruritus, urticaria. *Other:* lupus erythematosus-like (SLE) syndrome polyarthralgia, arthritis, pleuritic pain, myalgia, skin lesions, pleural effusions, pericarditis. Thrombocytopenia and Coombs-positive hemolytic anemia may be related to this syndrome.

OVERDOSAGE: *Signs and symptoms:* ventricular tachycardia or severe hypotension. *Treatment:* symptomatic.

PARAMETERS TO MONITOR: Obtain baseline ECG. Monitor for therapeutic effects of drug. Effectiveness may be ascertained by 24-hour Holter monitor. Perform baseline blood count, and routine checks for agranulocytosis periodically when patient is on long-term therapy. ANA titer may be done for SLE syndrome. Therapeutic plasma level is usually 3-10 mcg/ml in most laboratories.

QUINIDINE

ACTION OF THE DRUG: Quinidine acts to (1) lengthen the effective refractory period of atrial and ventricular myocardium, (2) decrease the automaticity or excitability of ectopic foci of cardiac muscle, and (3) exert an anticholinergic action.

ASSESSMENT:

INDICATIONS: Premature atrial contractions, premature ventricular contractions, paroxysmal supraventricular tachycardias, atrial flutter and atrial fibrillation. (See preceding discussion).

SUBJECTIVE: Patient may complain of chest pain, irregular pulse, light-headedness or dizziness. There may or may not be a previous history of cardiac problems.

OBJECTIVE: Irregular pulse may be felt. Diagnosis may be confirmed by 12-lead ECG with long lead II demonstrating the arrhythmia.

PLAN:

CONTRAINDICATIONS: Do not use in the presence of hypersensitivity to quinidine, or in patients with second- or third-degree AV block, intraventricular conduction defects, renal failure with significant azotemia, severe congestive heart failure, severe ventricular conduction defects, and abnormal rhythms due to escape mechanisms.

WARNINGS: Treat atrial fibrillation and flutter with digoxin before adding quinidine or an extremely rapid ventricular rate may result.

PRECAUTIONS: Use with caution in patients with severe heart disease (as the drug depresses myocardial contractility), renal disease (because of potential accumulation of quinidine in plasma), hypotension (as it may further reduce blood pressure), digitalis intoxication, myasthenia gravis (because of anticholinergic effects). Give a test dose for hypersensitivity with a short-acting quinidine sulfate. The effect of quinidine is enhanced by potassium and reduced by hypokalemia.

IMPLEMENTATION:

DRUG INTERACTIONS: Quinidine increases digoxin plasma levels. Concurrent administration requires a decrease in digoxin dosage. Quinidine reduces prothrombin levels and causes bleeding in patients on coumarin anticoagulants. Thiazide diuretics prolong the quinidine half-life. The anticholinergic effect of quinidine is additive with other anticholinergic drugs, and antagonistic with cholinergic drugs. Other antiarrhythmic agents exert an additive cardiac depressant effect. Phenobarbital and phenytoin may reduce plasma half-life of quinidine by 50%.

ADMINISTRATION AND DOSAGE: Dosage may vary considerably. Decreasing ectopic activity at the lowest dosage is the therapeutic goal.

IMPLEMENTATION CONSIDERATIONS:

—Take a thorough health history: history of hypersensitivity, drug history of other medications which may cause drug interactions, other medical problems.

—Quinidine may cause the arrhythmia one is trying to suppress. A worsening of an arrhythmia after starting quinidine may be an adverse reaction to the drug.

—Look for and treat any underlying factors which may cause arrhythmias: hypoxia, acid-base imbalance, increased or decreased potassium, catecholamines, or drug toxicity.

—Assess the presence and severity of heart disease. Obtain relevant laboratory studies: chest x-ray, graded exercise test, ECG, echocardiogram, 24-hour Holter monitor.

—Preexisting asthma, muscle weakness and infection with fever may mask quinidine hypersensitivity.

WHAT THE PATIENT NEEDS TO KNOW:
—Take medication exactly as ordered. Do not skip doses or double dosage.
—Some people experience side effects when taking this medication. Report any new or uncomfortable symptoms to your health provider. Note especially any breathing difficulty or dizziness.
—Take quinidine with food to decrease chances of having an upset stomach.

EVALUATION:

ADVERSE REACTIONS: *Cardiovascular:* hypotension, arterial embolism, cardiac asystole, idioventricular rhythms (including fibrillation), paradoxical tachycardia, ventricular ectopic beats, widening of QRS complex. *CNS:* headache, apprehension, confusion, delirium, excitement and syncope, disturbed hearing (tinnitus, decreased auditory acuity), disturbed vision (mydriasis, blurred vision, disturbed color perception, photophobia, diplopia, night blindness, scotomata), optic neuritis. *Dermatologic:* cutaneous flushing with intense pruritus. *Gastrointestinal:* abdominal pain, anorexia, nausea, diarrhea, vomiting. *Hematopoietic:* acute hemolytic anemia, agranulocytosis, hypoprothrombinemia, thrombocytopenic purpura. *Hypersensitivity:* acute asthmatic episodes, angioedema, respiratory arrest, vascular collapse. *Other:* cinchonism (ringing in ears, headache, nausea, disturbed vision).

OVERDOSAGE: *Signs and symptoms:* cardiotoxic effects, hypotension. *Treatment:* Referral for supportive and symptomatic treatment. Sodium lactate, vasoconstrictors and catecholamines may be helpful.

PARAMETERS TO MONITOR: Obtain baseline ECG and monitor for therapeutic effects. A 24 hour Holter monitor may be necessary to confirm effectiveness. Baseline and periodic blood counts and liver and kidney function tests should be obtained. Therapeutic plasma level is around 3-6 mcg/ml in most laboratories.

QUINIDINE GLUCONATE

PRODUCTS (TRADE NAME):
Duraquin (Available in 330 mg sustained-release tablets.) **Quinidine Gluconate** (Available in 324 mg sustained-release tablets and 80 mg/ml [50 mg/ml quinidine] injections.) **Quiniglute Dura-Tabs, Quinatime, Quin-Release** (Available in 324 mg sustained-release tablets.)
DRUG SPECIFICS:
330 mg quinidine gluconate is equivalent to 248 mg quinidine sulfate.

ADMINISTRATION AND DOSAGE SPECIFICS:
Usual dose is 330-660 mg po every 8 hours for Duraquin; 324-648 mg po every 8-12 hours for Quiniglute Dura-Tabs.

QUINIDINE POLYGALACTURONATE

PRODUCTS (TRADE NAME):
Cardioquin (Available in 275 mg tablet).
DRUG SPECIFICS:
275 mg quinidine polygalacturonate is equivalent to 200 mg quinidine sulfate.
ADMINISTRATION AND DOSAGE SPECIFICS:
Usual dose is 275 mg po every 8-12 hours.

QUINIDINE SULFATE

PRODUCTS (TRADE NAME):
Cin-Quin (Available in 100 mg, 200 mg and 300 mg tablets and 200 mg and 300 mg capsules.) **Quinidex Extentabs** (Available in 300 mg sustained-release tablets.) **Quinidine Sulfate** (Available in 200 mg tablets and capsules and 200 mg/ml injections.) **Quinora** (Available in 200 mg and 300 mg tablets.) **SK-Quinidine Sulfate** (Available in 200 mg tablets.)
DRUG SPECIFICS:
Dosage must be individualized depending on patient's symptoms and response to drug.
ADMINISTRATION AND DOSAGE SPECIFICS:
Usual dose is 200-300 mg po every 6-8 hours or 600 mg po every 8-12 hours if the Extentab is used.

Maren Stewart

ANTIARRHYTHMIC AGENTS—CLASS 2

BETA-BLOCKERS

ACTION OF THE DRUG: Beta-blockers compete with beta-adrenergic receptor stimulating agents for available beta-receptor sites, thereby antagonizing the effects of catecholamines released from the adrenergic nerve endings as well as the adrenal medulla. Beta-blocking agents reduce the metabolic (glycogenolytic, lipolytic), myocardial stimulant, vasodilator, and bronchodilator actions of catecholamines. This represents decreases in chronotropic, inotropic, and vasodilator action. Reduction in heart rate and force of contraction, suppression of renin release, and decrease in outflow of sympathetic vasoconstrictor and cardioaccelerator fibers from brain stem vasomotor center are produced.

ASSESSMENT:

INDICATIONS: Propranolol is used for paroxysmal supraventricular tachyarrythmias, especially associated with digitalis or Wolff-Parkinson-White syndrome, sinus tachycardia; tachycardias caused by thyrotoxicosis, atrial flutter, and atrial fibrillation; and premature atrial contractions.

See the beta blocker monograph in the antihypertensive drugs section.

ANTIARRHYTHMIC AGENTS—CLASS 4

VERAPAMIL

ACTION OF THE DRUG: Verapamil (1) inhibits calcium ion influx through slow channels into conductile and contractile myocardial cells and vascular smooth muscle cells, and (2) slows AV conduction and prolongs the effective refractory period within the AV node.

ASSESSMENT:

INDICATIONS: Verapamil is used in supraventricular tachyarrhythmias not controlled by other drugs.

SUBJECTIVE: Patient may complain of chest pain, lightheadedness, dizziness, and irregular pulse. There may or may not a preexisting history of cardiac problems.

OBJECTIVE: Rapid pulse may be felt, and diagnosis confirmed by 12 lead ECG. Long lead II may clearly demonstrate arrhythmia.

PLAN:

CONTRAINDICATIONS: Do not use in the presence of severe hypotension or cardiogenic shock, second- or third-degree AV block, sick sinus syndrome or severe congestive heart failure.

WARNINGS: Verapamil may produce symptomatic hypotension. A rapid ventricular response may occur in patients with atrial flutter/fibrillation. Verapamil may also produce A-V block and bradycardia. It may produce or worsen heart failure due to negative inotropic effects.

PRECAUTIONS: Use with caution in patients with impaired hepatic or renal function.

IMPLEMENTATION:

DRUG INTERACTIONS: Verapamil has an additive effect when used with digitalis, which produces A-V block and bradycardia and can lead to digoxin toxicity by increasing serum digoxin levels. When given with other beta-blockers, there is an additive effect which depresses myocardial contractility and A-V conduction. Administer with caution with other plasma protein-bound drugs since verapamil is highly bound to plasma proteins.

PRODUCTS (TRADE NAME):
Calan, Isoptin (Available in 80 and 120 mg tablets and 5 mg/2 ml injections.)

ADMINISTRATION AND DOSAGE: Dosage must be individualized by titration. Usual dose is 80-120 mg po every 6-8 hours. Total daily dose is from 240 to 480 mg.

IMPLEMENTATION CONSIDERATIONS:

—Obtain a complete health history, including presence of hypersensitivity, concurrent use of other drugs which may produce drug interactions, and underlying systemic problems which may be relevant to the therapy.

—This is a relatively new drug on the market and the health practitioner should watch for new literature about the product as clinical experience is gained.

WHAT THE PATIENT NEEDS TO KNOW:

—Take this medication exactly as ordered. Do not skip doses or double doses.

—Some people have side effects from this medication. Report to your health practitioner any new or uncomfortable symptoms which may develop.

—Keep this medication out of the reach of children and others for whom it is not prescribed.

—Some people experience dizziness and lightheadedness when taking this drug. This is especially seen early in the morning and when changing from lying to standing positions. Move slowly, to allow your body to adjust, when making changes in position.

—Wear a Medic-Alert bracelet and carry a medical identification card specifying that you are taking this drug.

EVALUATION:

ADVERSE REACTIONS: *Cardiovascular:* A-V block, bradycardia, congestive heart failure, hypotension, peripheral edema, severe tachycardia. *CNS:* dizziness, fatigue, headache. *Gastrointestinal:* abdominal discomfort, constipation, nausea, hepatitis.

OVERDOSAGE: *Signs and symptoms:* asystole, A-V block, hypotension. *Treatment:* supportive.

PARAMETERS TO MONITOR: Obtain baseline ECG. Monitor therapeutic effects. May need to evaluate suppression of arrhythmias by having patient use a Holter monitor for 24 hours. Watch for adverse reactions, especially for appearance of congestive heart failure, periodically monitor liver enzymes. Therapeutic plasma level is 100-300 ng/ml in most laboratories.

Maren Stewart

ANTIARRHYTHMIC AGENTS—MISCELLANEOUS

LIDOCAINE HYDROCHLORIDE

ACTION OF THE DRUG: Parenteral lidocaine administration is effective in eliminating many ventricular arrhythmias by increasing the electrical stimulation threshold of the ventricle during diastole. Given as an IV bolus it has an onset of action of 30 to 90 seconds and a short duration of 10 to 20 minutes. With reported IV bolus doses, duration of action may be prolonged to several hours.

ASSESSMENT:

INDICATIONS: This is an emergency drug which is administered in the case of life-threatening arrhythmias frequently following acute myocardial infarction. It may also be required for arrhythmias which develop during surgery or various cardiac evaluation techniques. It is usually given as an IV bolus, followed by a continuous IV infusion to keep ectopic foci suppressed. In all cases it should be given to patients whose cardiac activity can be adequately monitored. In rare cases where monitoring or intravenous infusion equipment is unavailable, but ventricular arrhythmias are strongly suspected, IM injection into deltoid muscle is used. Action of the drug may be observed in 5-15 minutes following IM injection and persist for up to 2 hours. This is a medication which the nurse practitioner should be prepared to give only in emergency situations in which adequate physician personnel are not present. Lidocaine should produce no change in myocardial contractility, absolute refractory period, or in systemic arterial blood pressure in therapeutic doses.

SUBJECTIVE: Patient may complaint of dizziness, lightheadedness, and feeling that "things are fading." Patient may be aware of heart beating faster or irregularly.

OBJECTIVE: Ventricular arrhythmias (VPCs, ventricular tachycardia, ventricular fibrillation) may be documented on monitor or electrocardiogram.

PLAN:

CONTRAINDICATIONS: Do not give to patients with known hypersensitivity to amide local anesthetics, and in patients with advanced degree of sinoatrial, atrioventricular or intraventricular block, Stokes-Adams attacks, or Wolff-Parkinson-White syndrome.

WARNINGS: IV administration should be accompanied by constant cardiac monitoring. ECG should be watched and any development of prolonged P-R interval or QRS complex which indicates depressed myocardial conductivity, or any aggravation of arrhythmias, should signal the practitioner to discontinue this drug. Emergency resuscitation equipment should be available in order to adequately treat patients in whom lidocaine therapy is not effective in suppressing the arrhythmia. Dosage should be lowered and carefully monitored in patients with congestive heart failure, reduced cardiac output, severe liver or renal dysfunction, and the elderly. Electrolytes and acid-base balance should be watched closely in patients receiving long-term infusion therapy. IM injection increases CPK levels and may compromise the use of this test as a diagnostic parameter for acute MI. Safety for use in children and pregnancy has not been established and lidocaine should be used only when potential benefits seem to outweigh possible risks.

PRECAUTIONS: Use lidocaine with caution in patients with hypovolemia, shock, and all types of heart block. The infusion of lidocaine in the presence of bradycardia or heart block may lead to progression of block or promotion of increased ventricular arrhythmias. Other medications should not be added to this infusion. If blood is being infused, do not give lidocaine in dextrose infusions without adding electrolytes at the same time.

IMPLEMENTATION:

DRUG INTERACTIONS: When procainamide is given concomitantly with lidocaine, additive neurological effects may be produced. Concurrent administration with propranolol or cimetidine impairs the clearance of lidocaine and may increase toxic manifestations. Phenytoin and lidocaine together may produce myocardial depression.

PRODUCTS (TRADE NAME):
Lidocaine HCl without Preservatives, Xylocaine HCl without Preservatives(Available in 300 mg in 3 ml automatic injection device for IM administration and 2 mg/ml, 4 mg/ml, 10 mg/ml, 20 mg/ml, 40 mg/ml, 100 mg/ml, 200 mg/ml for IV injections. 10 mg/ml is reserved for IM injections.)

ADMINISTRATION AND DOSAGE:
Intramuscular injection: Give 2 mg/lb; about 300 mg IM (for average patient) in deltoid muscle. LidoPen Auto-Injector comes in 300 mg and is for patients to administer themselves into thigh.

Intravenous: Give 50 to 100 mg (1 mg/kg) bolus over a 2-minute period. One half dose may be repeated in 5-10 minutes. No more than 300 mg lidocaine should be given per hour. Give reduced dosage in elderly patients and those with CHF or reduced cardiac output. Give continuous IV infusion to maintain therapeutic plasma levels. Give 1-4 mg/min (20 to 50 mcg/kg/min or less if patient has CHF or liver disease). Keep patients on this medication until arrhythmia is suppressed, or until patient can be switched to oral medications. Plasma levels should be measured to reduce chances of toxicity. Therapeutic serum levels are 1.5 to 5 mcg/ml. Serum levels of about 7 mcg/ml indicate toxicity. Discontinue therapy if there is any sign of toxicity.

IMPLEMENTATION CONSIDERATIONS:

—Obtain a complete health history from patient or others regarding hypersensitivity, underlying systemic disease, other medications taken concurrently, previous arrhythmias or cardiovascular problems and their treatment, and the possibility of pregnancy.

—Occasionally acceleration of ventricular rate may occur when this medication is given to patients who have atrial fibrillation, and may make arrhythmias worse.

—Administer this drug cautiously in dextrose solutions because of the high number of patients who may have subclinical or overt diabetes mellitus.

—In patients who report a hypersensitivity to procainamide or quinidine, this is a good drug of choice, since there is usually little cross-sensitivity to lidocaine.

—For IM administration, the deltoid muscle is the preferred site of injection since therapeutic blood levels are achieved faster and peak levels are higher from this site. Use only the 10% solution labeled for IM injection and aspirate to avoid possible injection intravascularly. Soreness at injection site may persist for several days.

—For IV injection, use only lidocaine injection without preservatives or catecholamines and clearly labeled for IV use.

—Cardiac monitoring equipment should be available for safe administration of this agent.

—Monitor for toxic effects which may develop suddenly at any time.

WHAT THE PATIENT NEEDS TO KNOW:

—This is a drug which is used to suppress abnormal heart rhythms. It will be used only until the problem is corrected and you can begin taking another oral medicine.

—Some people experience side effects from this drug. Be certain to report any new or troublesome symptoms which you develop.

EVALUATION:

ADVERSE REACTIONS: *Cardiovascular:* bradycardia which may lead to cardiac arrest, cardiovascular collapse, hypotension. *CNS:* apprehension, blurred or double vision, convulsions, dizziness, drowsiness, euphoria, lightheadedness, respiratory depression, respiratory arrest, sensations of heat, cold or numbness, tinnitus, tremors, twitching, unconsciousness. *Hypersensitivity:* allergic reactions (rare): anaphylactic reactions, cutaneous lesions, edema, urticaria. *Other:* febrile response, infection at site of injection, venous thrombosis or phlebitis at injection site, extravasation, and hypervolemia.

OVERDOSAGE: In severe reactions, patient may become unconscious, experience convulsions and respiratory arrest. Medication should be stopped immediately, and the physician and trained personnel should treat the patient symptomatically.

PARAMETERS TO MONITOR: Patient's cardiac activity should be continuously monitored and dosage titrated to suppress arrhythmias; simultaneously observe for toxic symptoms. Fluid and electrolytes should be evaluated through periodic laboratory determination to detect changes in fluid, electrolytes, and acid-base balance. Observe for dilution of serum electrolytes, overhydration provocation of pulmonary edema, and development of hypokalemia after long-term intravenous infusions. Also watch for changes in blood glucose levels in patients who may have subclinical diabetes mellitus. Observe electrocardiogram for signs of depressed myocardial activity: prolongation of P-R interval or QRS. Monitor for CNS changes.

Marilyn W. Edmunds

ANTIHYPERLIPIDEMIC AGENTS

ACTION OF THE DRUG: Lipids are present in the bloodstream, bound tightly to plasma proteins (albumin and globulins). These lipoprotein complexes contain different proportions of high-density and low-density lipids. The four major types of lipoproteins are:

(1) Chylomicrons: largest and lightest of the lipoproteins. These are formed during the absorption of dietary fat in the intestine and are normally in plasma only 1 to 8 hours after the last meal. They impart a cloudiness to plasma and are primarily triglycerides. If a tube of blood from a fasting patient shows this characteristic feature after several hours, the patient may have an inability to handle dietary fat.

(2) Very low-density lipoproteins (VLDL). These are made up of large amounts of triglycerides that were synthesized in the liver and are called pre-beta lipoproteins. This is a carrier state for transferring endogenous triglycerides from the liver to the plasma. Practically all the triglycerides in plasma not in chylomicrons are considered to be VLDL.

(3) Low-density lipoproteins (LDL). When VLDL break down and combine with cholesterol and protein, very little triglyceride is left. This remaining product is then called beta lipoproteins. About 3/4 of cholesterol concentration in plasma is transported in this form. Elevated serum levels of LDL indicate excess cholesterol levels. Patients with high LDL levels are at high risk for developing atherosclerosis.

(4) High-density lipoproteins (HDL). These small, dense lipoproteins are called alpha lipoproteins and contain very small parts of triglycerides. They are mostly protein and cholesterol. They serve as the vacuum cleaners of the tissues, to clear out excess cholesterol. They may inhibit atherosclerotic activity by blocking uptake of LDL cholesterol by vascular smooth muscle cells.

Hyperlipoproteinemia is the term used to indicate an increase in one or more of the classes of lipoproteins and may represent either an excess of cholesterol, triglycerides, or both. Patients with defects in lipid transport or metabolism can be classified on the basis of the types of lipoproteins which are elevated in the plasma. Accurate diagnosis and treatment prescriptions may be formulated through use of these classifications.

Type of hyperlipoproteinemia refers to abnormal lipoprotein patterns, but does not designate specific disease. The classification is made based on overload of a particular lipid transport pathway. Types of hyperlipoproteinemia include:

Type I: loss of enzymatic step in removal of chylomicrons, relatively rare. Seen in infancy and marked by abdominal pain. Does not lead to atherosclerosis. Also called fat-induced or exogenous type.

Type II: excess production or inadequate clearance of LDL. Subgroup (a) has characteristics of high levels of LDL; normal VLDL and slight elevation in triglycerides may be seen. Type II is fairly common and carries with it an increased risk for development of atherosclerosis. Also known as familial hypercholesterolemia. Subgroup (b) has high LDL and VLDL, hypercholesterolemia and hypertriglyceridemia. Xanthomatous lipid deposits are found on knees, feet, elbows, ears.

Type III: block in metabolism of VLDL to LDL, causing an abnormal "intermediate" form of lipoprotein to circulate in plasma. Elevated LDL, VLDL, cholesterol and triglycerides are found. This is a recessively inherited disorder and not as common as some other types. It does carry risk of atherosclerosis with it.

Type IV: excess production or inadequate clearance of VLDL. Triglycerides are increased, but LDL and cholesterol are normal or slightly elevated. This is also called the carbohydrate-induced or endogenous type, and is the most common form. Definite risk for atherosclerosis exists.

Type V: VLDL excess combined with poor chylomicron removal. Elevated VLDL and triglycerides are found, with increases also in chylomicrons. It is not associated with risk of atherosclerosis and is a relatively uncommon type.

Lipids are important in the pathogenesis of atherosclerosis, although their exact mechanism for producing disease is not clear. It appears that there is a metabolic disturbance in the synthesis, transport, and utilization of lipids. In patients in whom there is damage to the vascular endothelial lining (which occurs in most people in the process of aging and may be accelerated by other factors), adherence and eventual buildup of fatty deposits within the lining of the vessel walls of the arterial system may develop, resulting in a gradual occlusion of blood flow. The clinical consequences of this lipid deposition include the development of angina resulting from ischemic heart disease, cerebrovascular disease (including stroke), peripheral ischemia, and renovascular hypertension.

It is still a subject of scientific and clinical controversy whether lowering serum lipids or cholesterol has any positive effect on reducing the risk of atherosclerotic disease. Both diet and drug therapy have proponents and opponents. In patients anxious to reduce elevated levels, behavior modification to reduce other risk factors and dietary methods should always be tried first, as hypolipemic drugs present risks of their own. The use of medication appears to be primarily prophylactic, slowing or preventing the rate of fatty deposition, without dissolving or removing existing fatty plaques.

A summary of usual diet and pharmacologic regimens in the various types of hyperlipoproteinemias is included in Table 3-3:

TABLE 3-3. CLASSIFICATION OF HYPERLIPOPROTEINEMIAS

Type	Diet	Drugs
I	Low fat. No other restrictions.	None are effective.
II a	Low cholesterol, low saturated fats. Increased intake of poly-unsaturated fats.	Cholestyramine Colestipol Probucol Dextrothyroxine Sitosterols
II b	Same as above	Cholestyramine Colestipol Dextrothyroxine Probucol
III	Low cholesterol, low calorie, low saturated fats. High protein.	Clofibrate Dextrothyroxine Nicotinic acid
IV	Low carbohydrate, low alcohol, low cholesterol, low calorie. Maintain protein intake.	Nicotinic acid
V	Low fat, low carbohydrate, low alcohol, high protein.	Nicotinic acid

ANTIHYPERLIPIDEMIC AGENTS— BILE ACID SEQUESTRANTS

ACTION OF THE DRUG: Bile acid sequestrants such as cholestyramine and colestipol work to reduce serum cholesterol levels in the body by forming an insoluble complex with bile salts and thus increasing bile loss through the feces. This loss of bile which is normally recirculated through the enterohepatic cycle causes increased oxidation of cholesterol to form bile, a decrease in low density lipoprotein plasma levels, and a decrease in serum cholesterol levels. Serum triglyceride levels may increase or remain unchanged.

ASSESSMENT:

INDICATIONS: Bile acid sequestrants are used primarily for the treatment of hyperlipoproteinemia, type II. (See introductory section). They may have no effect or moderately increase triglyceride levels. These products are also used to promote increased secretion of bile acids deposited in the skin in patients with partial biliary obstruction, and thereby reduce pruritus. These products are also under investigational use in treating patients with kepone poisoning and pseudomembranous colitis.

SUBJECTIVE: Patient may be asymptomatic.

OBJECTIVE: Xanthomas or lipid deposits may occur on ears, feet, elbows, or knees. In some patients, an arcus senilis, an opaque line partially surrounding the margin of the cornea, may be present. There may be other evidence on ophthalmoscopic or cardiovascular examination of atherosclerotic changes.

PLAN:

CONTRAINDICATIONS: Do not give in the presence of hypersensitivity to these products or with complete biliary obstruction.

WARNINGS: Safety for use in pregnant and breast-feeding women has not been established. Little clinical information is available on the effectiveness of long-term use of these products in children. Potential benefits should be weighed against possible risks in considering bile acid sequestrants in these patients.

This medication must be mixed with water before ingestion. Do not take powder dry. High chloride content may lead to hyperchloremic acidosis.

PRECAUTIONS: Normal absorption of fat-soluble vitamins may be reduced with these products, and patient may be symptomatic of vitamin deficiency if dosage is at high level and/or for prolonged time. Bleeding problems resulting from hypoprothrombinemia from vitamin K deficiency should be anticipated. Normal fat digestion may be impaired. Some patients, especially the very young or small patients, may be more susceptible to development of hyperchloremic acidosis because of the chloride anion exchange. These products may also increase constipation, especially in patients who have a preexisting problem.

IMPLEMENTATION:

DRUG INTERACTIONS: Because these drugs are anion-exchange resins, they may bind with other drugs rather than with bile acid if other medications are taken concurrently. These products will decrease the absorption of cephalexin, clindamycin, chlorothiazide, digitalis preparations, folic acid, iron, penicillin G, phenylbutazone, phenobarbital, thyroid, thyroxine preparations, trimethoprim, and warfarin. If patients have been placed on maintenance levels of any of these drugs and then bile acid sequestrant therapy is discontinued, potential toxic doses may develop once the bile acid resin no longer binds the drug. This would be especially important to consider in digitalis therapy. There may also be malabsorption of fat soluble vitamins if large doses of bile acid sequestrants are taken. Mild elevations of alkaline phosphatase and SGOT and serum phosphorus, and chloride have been seen, with a decrease in serum sodium and potassium levels.

ADMINISTRATION AND DOSAGE: Preparations should be taken 3 times a day before meals. (Although there is no evidence that more than twice daily is therapeutic, patient should get in the habit of having medication with each meal as a part of total dietary modification). These preparations are powders which will rehydrate when added to a liquid. They may be taken with milk, water, juice, carbonated beverages, or made into jello, put into soups, cereals, or fruits with high moisture content such as applesauce, nectars, fruit cocktail, or pineapple. Empty packet or level scoopful into the full glass or bowl. Allow powder to dissolve slowly, without stirring, for at least one minute. (Stirring promotes the formation of lumps.) When dissolved, stir to achieve uniform consistency. Rinse the empty glass or bowl with water in order to ensure taking the full quantity of medicine.

IMPLEMENTATION CONSIDERATIONS:

—Obtain a complete health history, including the presence of hypersensitivity, other medications taken concurrently which may promote drug interactions, dietary therapy, other attempts to reduce cholesterol levels, and possibility of pregnancy.

—Explore dietary management with patient before considering therapy with bile acid sequestrants. Weight reduction should be encouraged, and patient should be in as good health as possible.

—If drug is taken for a long period of time, supplemental doses of vitamins A, D, and K should be given. These should be given orally in a water-miscible form, or through parenteral injection.

—Constipation and hemorrhoids which may be aggravated by constipation may develop. Use of a high bulk diet and a laxative may allow patient to continue with the dosage regimen. Patients should be evaluated to prevent development of impaction.

—Patient must be educated about the long-term nature of this chemical problem and the need for permanent dietary management. The ability of the health care practitioner to establish rapport with the patient, win confidence, and be sensitive to patient reactions will be important in obtaining long-term compliance with diet, medication, and appointment requirements.

WHAT THE PATIENT NEEDS TO KNOW:

—Take this medication as ordered. Do not change dosages or stop taking medication without the knowledge of your health care practitioner.

—The most important thing which you can do in learning to live with this problem is to follow the prescribed diet. Restricting dietary intake of cholesterol and saturated fats, reducing calories, and increasing fluids and fiber content are very helpful. Your health care practitioner will give you a detailed diet explaining the foods which should and should not be eaten.

—This medicine comes in a powder which must be mixed with liquid before you take it. It may be mixed with beverages, soups, fruits, cereals, or jello. It should be added to the liquid and not stirred until it is completely dissolved. Container should be rinsed with water so that you obtain all of the medication in each dose.

—Take other medicine one hour before or 4-6 hours after taking this product. This medicine will delay absorption of other products if taken at the same time.

—Some patients experience side effects from these drugs. Be certain to notify your health care practitioner if you note any new or troublesome symptoms. Especially report persistent stomach upset, constipation, gas, bloating, heartburn, nausea, vomiting, or bleeding of any type.

—Keep this medication out of the reach of children and all others for whom it is not prescribed.

—In order to decrease constipation, eat a high bulk diet (fruit, raw vegetables, bran) and drink at least 2 quarts of fluid per day.

EVALUATION:

ADVERSE REACTIONS: *Cardiovascular:* angina, arteritis, intermittent claudication, myocardial ischemia or infarction, thrombophlebitis. *CNS:* anxiety, arcus juvenilis, dizziness, drowsiness, fatigue, femoral nerve pain, headache, paresthesia, syncope, tinnitus, uveitis, vertigo. *Gastrointestinal:* abdominal discomfort, anorexia, belching, black stools, cholecystitis, cholelithiasis, constipation (most common), diarrhea, diverticulitis, dysphagia, fecal impaction, flatulence, heartburn, hemorrhoids, indigestion, nausea, rectal bleeding, steatorrhea, ulcers, vomiting. *Hypersensitivity:* dermatitis, urticaria. *Musculoskeletal:* arthritis, muscle, joint, and backache. *Renal:* burnt odor to urine, diuresis, dysuria, hematuria. *Other:* bleeding tendencies secondary to hypoprothrombinemia from vitamin K deficiency, vitamin A and D deficiencies, dental bleeding, edema, hyperchloremic acidosis, fatigue, increased libido, osteoporosis, rash and irritation of skin, tongue and perianal area, shortness of breath, weight loss or gain, xanthomas of hands and fingers.

PARAMETERS TO MONITOR: Adequate diagnosis of the type of hyperlipoproteinemia is important in developing precise dietary and therapeutic regimens. If patient is found to have a type II hyperlipoproteinemia, he or she should be started on the specified diet and evaluated clinically. Only when diet modification and weight reduction do not produce significant improvement in cholesterol levels should bile acid sequestrants be used. Baseline serum cholesterol and triglyceride levels should be obtained, and a thorough history and physical should be recorded. Presence of underlying systemic disease may necessitate other laboratory testing at the same time. Patient should be monitored every 3 months for therapeutic effect, i.e., reduction in serum cholesterol and triglyceride levels. If these levels fail to decrease, or if there is a significant rise in triglycerides, medication should be discontinued. If patient continues on medication, observe for development of adverse reactions, especially constipation. Monitor diet for high bulk foods.

CHOLESTYRAMINE

PRODUCTS (TRADE NAME):
    Questran (Available in 4 gm cholestyramine in 9 gm packets of powder.)
DRUG SPECIFICS:
    Used in treating primary type II hyperlipoproteinemia. Also used to obtain partial relief of pruritus from biliary tract obstruction. Experimentally being tested for use in digitalis toxicity. Teach patient drug preparation methods and suggest different ideas for implementing them. Use at least 120 cc liquid for dissolving powder. Adverse reactions more likely with higher dosages. Common side effects

include constipation (severe), abdominal discomfort, flatulence, nausea, and anorexia. Not absorbed from GI tract, but excreted in feces as insoluble bile acid complex.

ADMINISTRATION AND DOSAGE SPECIFICS:

Give 4 gm packet three times daily before meals. Adjust dosage depending upon patient response. Total daily dosage of 14 to 24 gm/day may be necessary to reduce cholesterol level.

COLESTIPOL HYDROCHLORIDE

PRODUCTS (TRADE NAME):

Colestid (Available in 500 gm bottles and 5 gm packets of water insoluble beads.)

DRUG SPECIFICS:

Teach patient drug preparation methods and suggest different ideas for implementing them. Use at least 90 cc of liquid for preparation.

ADMINISTRATION AND DOSAGE SPECIFICS:

Give 15 to 30 gm/day in 2-4 divided doses.

Marilyn W. Edmunds

ANTIHYPERLIPIDEMIC AGENTS—CLOFIBRATE

ACTION OF THE DRUG: Clofibrate acts to lower serum triglycerides and very low density lipoproteins in a number of ways. It (1) inhibits the formation of cholesterol early in the biosynthetic chain. (2) Neutral sterols are excreted in increased amounts. (3) Catabolism of very low density and low density lipoproteins is increased through increased breakdown of free fatty acids in liver, decreased release of VLDL from liver to plasma, and interference with binding of free fatty acids to albumin. (4) Hepatic synthesis of very low density lipoproteins is decreased. Serum cholesterol and low density lipoproteins are also lowered, but in variable amounts. Reduces serum fibrinogen levels and decreases platelet adhesiveness.

ASSESSMENT:

INDICATIONS: Clofibrate is a rather toxic product, reserved for special cases of primary hyperlipidemia, especially in young patients in whom there is a high risk of cardiovascular disease and who have not responded to diet therapy, weight reduction, and other treatment modalities. It is the drug of choice in treatment of primary dysbetalipoproteinemia (type III hyperlipidemia). It is also used with bile-sequestering resins in Type II b where serum triglycerides are elevated. It may be used adjunctively in treatment of patients with xanthoma tuberosum.

SUBJECTIVE: Patient may be asymptomatic.

OBJECTIVE: Patient may have xanthomatous lipid nodules around joints of knee, elbow, and on the ears. Arcus senilis, an opaque line encircling the cornea, may also be present.

PLAN:

CONTRAINDICATIONS: Do not use in severe hepatic or renal impairment, or in primary biliary cirrhosis, as even higher levels of cholesterol may be produced. Safety has not been demonstrated for the use of this product in children, pregnant, or breast-feeding women. It does cross the placental barrier and may provide a hazard to the fetus who is not developed enough to excrete it.

WARNINGS: Clofibrate has been implicated in laboratory animals as a hepatic tumorigen and has been associated with increasing production of cholelithiasis and cholecystitis. There is an increase in cardiac arrhythmias, thromboembolic events, and intermittent claudication. It has been suggested by some studies that there is a substantially increased risk of death from non-cardiac problems with long-term use. Findings are very controversial. No clinical studies have been able to document that use of this product decreases the incidence of fatal myocardial infarction. Medication should be reserved for patients with significant hyperlipoproteinemia not responsive to diet or other medications.

PRECAUTIONS: Use with caution in patients with peptic ulcer disease since activation may be precipitated. Clofibrate may also produce a "flu-like" syndrome of muscular aching, cramping, and soreness which must be distinguished from a viral or bacterial disease. Extreme caution should be used in monitoring liver function, and any indication of hepatic disease should be evaluated thoroughly.

IMPLEMENTATION:

DRUG INTERACTIONS: This product causes potentiation of effect of oral anticoagulants, antidiabetic drugs, cholinesterase inhibitors, and thyroxine. Concurrent use with furosemide may increase effects of both drugs, producing muscular pain, stiffness, and diuresis. Effects of clofibrate may be enhanced by acidifying agents, and neomycin. The product may interfere with the following laboratory tests: SGOT, SGPT, thymol turbidity, CPK, plasma beta lipoproteins (as paradoxical response to decreased LDLP and VLDL). May also decrease plasma fibrogen and increase BSP retention and produce proteinuria.

PRODUCTS (TRADE NAME):
Atromid-S (Available in 500 mg capsules.)

ADMINISTRATION AND DOSAGE: Give 2 gm po daily in divided doses.

IMPLEMENTATION CONSIDERATIONS:

—Use this product with caution in diabetics.

—Usually see a rebound increase in serum lipid levels after 2 to 3 months of therapy and then further decreases may occur.

—Try to control disorder through diet modification, weight reduction and other medications before using this drug.

—Patients concurrently taking oral anticoagulants require frequent prothrombin time determinations while on this product. Some clinicians recommend reduction of oral anticoagulant dose by one half.

WHAT THE PATIENT NEEDS TO KNOW:

—Take this medication as ordered. Do not stop taking medication suddenly.

—Adherence to strict contraceptive measures is essential for women since drug may increase risk of damage to fetus.

—Medication may be taken with food or milk to decrease chance of stomach upset.

—Some people experience side effects from this drug. Be certain to notify your health care provider if you note any new or troublesome symptoms. Especially note and report any chest pain, irregular heart beat, shortness of breath, fever, chills or sore throat, severe stomach pain, nausea, vomiting, blood in the urine, swelling of lower extremities, weight gain, or producing less urine than usual.

—Keep this medication out of the reach of children and all others for whom it is not prescribed.

EVALUATION:

ADVERSE REACTIONS: *Cardiovascular:* angina pectoris, arrhythmias, edema, phlebitis, pulmonary emboli, thrombophlebitis, or xanthoma swelling. *CNS:* blurred vision, dizziness, drowsiness, fatigue, headache, tremor, weakness. *Dermatologic:* allergic reaction (dry skin, dry, brittle hair, pruritus, urticaria), alopecia, skin rash. *Gastrointestinal:* abdominal distress, bloating, dyspepsia, flatulence, gallstones, gastritis, GI bleeding, hepatomegaly, increased appetite, heartburn, loose stools, nausea, stomatitis, vomiting. *Genitourinary:* decreased libido, impotence, renal dysfunction (dysuria, hematuria, proteinuria, decreased urine output). *Hematopoietic:* anemia, eosinophilia, leukopenia. *Musculoskeletal:* arthralgia, muscle cramping, aching and weakness, rheumatoid arthritis (not proven). *Other:* chills, dyspnea, fever, gynecomastia, increased perspiration, lupus erythematosus, polyphagia, weight gain.

PARAMETERS TO MONITOR: Obtain complete history, physical, and laboratory evaluations prior to initiation of therapy. This should include cardiovascular, hepatic, and renal function studies. Observe for reduction in serum triglyceride and very low density lipoprotein levels. These levels should be drawn every 2 weeks within the first few months of therapy and then monthly to detect paradoxical rise in serum cholesterol or triglycerides, as well as to confirm treatment efficacy. If there is no reduction within 3 months, drug should be withdrawn unless used to treat xanthomas. Serum lipid determinations should be obtained to monitor levels of cholesterol and all lipids. Frequent serum transaminase and other liver function tests should also be obtained every month for first 2 months, and then every 2 months until effect is observed, and then every 4 months. If levels continue to rise, or abnormalities become marked, drug should be withdrawn. Periodic evaluations should be made for detecting cholelithiasis in patients with suspicious symptomatology. Complete blood counts with indices should be obtained to monitor for anemia and leukopenia. ECGs should also be obtained periodically to assess for development of abnormal rhythms. Check patients for presence of chest pain, dyspnea, fever, chills, sore throat, irregular heartbeat, weight gain, and signs and symptoms of gallstones, pancreatitis, and renal toxicity.

Marilyn W. Edmunds

ANTIHYPERLIPIDEMIC AGENTS— DEXTROTHYROXINE SODIUM

ACTION OF THE DRUG: Dextrothyroxine sodium acts to (1) increase liver catabolism and excretion of cholesterol and its degradation products through feces and (2) stimulate cholesterol synthesis. Low density lipoprotein levels and cholesterol levels are reduced, but drug has no consistent lowering effect on triglyceride and beta lipoprotein fractions.

ASSESSMENT:

INDICATIONS: In euthyroid patients with no evidence of organic heart disease, dextrothyroxine sodium is used adjunctly in patients with elevated serum cholesterol levels and LDL levels in type II disease. It is also used in the treatment of hypothyroid patients with cardiac disease who cannot tolerate other types of thyroid medication.

SUBJECTIVE: Patients with hyperlipoproteinemia may be asymptomatic. Hypothyroid patient may present with specific complaints. (See section on endocrine drugs.)

OBJECTIVE: Patient may present with xanthomatous lipid deposits on elbows, knees, ears, shoulders, and may have an arcus senilis, a thin opaque line partially encircling the cornea. There may be evidence of hypothyroidism.

PLAN:

CONTRAINDICATIONS: Do not give to euthyroid patients with known organic heart disease (angina pectoris, history of myocardial infarction, history of any cardiac arrhythmias, rheumatic heart disease, congestive heart failure, myocardiopathies, hypertension) liver or kidney diseases, or history of iodism. This product is contraindicated in pregnant women and breast-feeding mothers.

WARNINGS: Use of this preparation in euthyroid patients for the treatment of obesity is dangerous and unwarranted. Dosage necessary to produce weight loss may produce serious toxic manifestations. When used as a thyroid replacement drug in patients with hypothyroidism and concomitant cardiac disease, caution should be used. Angina may be triggered because of increased myocardial demands for oxygen at high doses. If arrhythmias, progressive angina, or ischemia develop, drug may have to be withdrawn. Drug should be discontinued 2 weeks prior to any contemplated surgery in order to reduce the possibility of cardiac arrhythmias during anesthesia. Because of deleterious effects upon both kidney and liver, drug should be used only as a last resort in patients with advanced disease of these organs.

PRECAUTIONS: Increased serum protein bound iodine levels develop which reflect absorption and transport of the drug. Values in the range of 10% to 25% may develop and are normal. Only if signs of iodism develop should medication be discontinued. Medication is not recommended for sustained use in children unless history of familial hypercholesterolemia requires significant reductions in serum cholesterol levels.

IMPLEMENTATION:

DRUG INTERACTIONS: Drug dosage may have to be adjusted if other thyroid drugs are taken concomitantly. Dextrothyroxine sodium may potentiate the effects of digitalis and oral coumarin anticoagulants, and concurrent use requires close supervision. Coumarin dosage should be reduced by one-third when dextrothyroxine is started. Injections of epinephrine in patients with coronary artery disease may precipitate coronary insufficiency, especially if patients are taking additional thyroid products. There is the possibility that insulin or oral hypoglycemic requirements may be increased as dextrothyroxine in diabetic patients may increase blood sugar levels.

PRODUCTS (TRADE NAME):
Choloxin (Available in 1, 2, 4, and 6 mg tablets.)

ADMINISTRATION AND DOSAGE:

Euthyroid Hypercholesterolemic Patients:

Adults: Give 4-8 mg/day po. Start with 1-2 mg and increase in 1-2 mg increments at one-month intervals. Maximum dose is 4-8 mg/day. Monitor effects through serum cholesterol levels.

Children: Give 0.05 mg/kg, and increase in 0.05 mg/kg increments at one month intervals to maximum dose of 4 mg/day.

Hypothyroid Patients with Cardiac Disease: Give 1 mg/day po initially with 1 mg increments at one-month intervals. Maximum dose is 4-8 mg/day. (Maximum dose of patients receiving digitalis is 4 mg/day.)

IMPLEMENTATION CONSIDERATIONS:

—Obtain a complete health history, including the presence of hypersensitivity, cardiovascular (especially angina, infarction, congestive failure and arrhythmias), renal or hepatic disease, and possibility of pregnancy.

—When used as thyroid replacement therapy, closely monitor patients for the development of any arrhythmias, congestive heart failure, or aggravation of angina. If these should develop, reduce dosage or discontinue medication.

—Diabetic patients require special monitoring as dextrothyroxine may affect the dosage of insulin or antidiabetic agents. When dextrothyroxine is started or withdrawn, dosage adjustments of antidiabetic agents must be made.

—Side effects are primarily related to increased metabolism and may be deminished by following restricted dosage schedule.

—Patients least likely to have adverse effects are euthyroid patients with no cardiovascular disease; those most likely to have problems are hypothyroid patients with organic heart disease.

—Monitor closely patients on digitalis since requirements for myocardial oxygen may be dangerously elevated by this drug.

—Drug normally increases PBI to 10-25 mcg%. This indicates routine action of the drug and not a hypermetabolic state.

—Discontinue drug two weeks prior to elective surgery.

WHAT THE PATIENT NEEDS TO KNOW:

—Carefully follow the instructions for taking this medicine given to you by your health care practitioner.

—Women should use secure contraceptive techniques since drug may increase risk of fetal damage and should not be used during pregnancy.

—Tell other health care providers that you are taking this therapy. Arrange with health practitioner to discontinue drug 2 weeks before any elective surgery (including dental).

—Some people experience side effects from this medication. Be certain to report to your health care provider any new or troublesome symptoms. Note especially the presence of chest pain, rapid heartbeat, sweating, headache, diarrhea, or skin rash.

—Keep this medication out of the reach of children and all others for whom it is not prescribed.

—Wear a Medic-Alert bracelet or carry other identifying information stating that you are taking this product.

EVALUATION:

ADVERSE REACTIONS: *Cardiovascular:* angina pectoris, arrhythmias (premature contractions, supraventricular tachycardia), increase in heart size, myocardial ischemia, myocardial infarction (unknown whether drug related), palpitations. *CNS:* dizziness, flushing, headache, hyperthermia, insomnia, lid lag, loss of weight, malaise, muscle pain, nervousness, paresthesias, psychic changes, sweating, tinnitus, tremors, visual disturbances. *Dermatologic:* skin rashes, pruritus. *Gastrointestinal:* anorexia, constipation, diarrhea, dyspepsia, nausea, vomiting. *Other:* altered libido, cholestatic jaundice, diuresis, elevated PBI, exophthalmos, gallstones, hair loss, hoarseness, hyperglycemia, menstrual irregularities, muscle pain, peripheral edema, retinopathy, worsening of peripheral vascular disease.

PARAMETERS TO MONITOR: Obtain baseline history, physical and laboratory evaluations. This should include a thorough cardiac exam and ECG, cardiac enzymes, renal and hepatic function studies, and chest x-ray. Monitor for therapeutic effect by obtaining cholesterol and triglyceride levels monthly throughout therapy. Also monitor for development of adverse reactions. If new arrhythmias are precipitated or patient develops angina or congestive heart failure, dosage should be cut back or discontinued.

Marilyn W. Edmunds

ANTIHYPERLIPIDEMIC AGENTS—GEMFIBROZIL

ACTION OF THE DRUG: Gemfibrozil acts to reduce elevated very low density lipoprotein fractions in serum, thereby reducing serum triglycerides, with some decrease in total serum cholesterol. It is thought to produce this reduction by decreasing the hepatic extraction of free fatty acids, inhibiting peripheral lipolysis. (Hepatic triglyceride production is then reduced.) Synthesis of very low density lipoprotein carriers (apoproteins) is decreased. (This leads to a reduction in levels of very low density lipoproteins.) In addition to these actions, gemfibrozil may also increase high density lipoprotein cholesterol, reduce the breakup of long-chain fatty acids and prevent their incorporation into newly formed triglycerides, accelerate transport of cholesterol from the liver, and increase excretion of cholesterol in the feces.

ASSESSMENT:

INDICATIONS: Gemfibrozil is reserved for the adult patient who has been diagnosed with type V hyperlipidemia, whose serum triglyceride levels are above 750 mg/deciliter, and who has been unresponsive to dietary and weight loss therapy. These patients are at risk for developing abdominal pain and pancreatitis. Laboratory response should be obvious within 3 months, or drug may be discontinued. There is usually no reduction in elevated cholesterol levels although medication may be used in patients with a familial history of hypercholesterolemia as part of a long-term diet and medication regimen.

SUBJECTIVE/OBJECTIVE: Patient may be asymptomatic or may complain of gastric distress. Serum triglyceride levels above 750 mg/deciliters.

PLAN:

CONTRAINDICATIONS: Do not give in the presence of hypersensitivity, severe hepatic or renal dysfunction, preexisting gallbladder disease or primary biliary cirrhosis.

WARNINGS: This medication is pharmacologically similar to clofibrate, and many of the concerns about that drug are probably applicable to gemfibrozil. Because of documented higher incidence of cholelithiasis, non-cardiovascular deaths, cataracts, and (in laboratory animals, decreased fertility and testicular cell tumors), this drug should not be continued if patients demonstrate no substantial reduction in serum lipid levels. There is no conclusive evidence that lowering triglyceride levels decreases the chance of coronary artery disease. Thus, possible benefits must be weighed against possible risks before therapy is instituted. Safety for use has not been established for children, pregnant, or breast-feeding women.

PRECAUTIONS: This medication should be used only as a last resort when diligent efforts to reduce serum levels by other means have failed: dietary elimination of high cholesterol and saturated fatty acids, alcohol restriction, weight loss, exercise increases, and general control of other underlying systemic diseases such as diabetes or hypothyroidism.

Patients on gemfibrozil therapy should be closely monitored: elevated serum lipid levels, CBC and indices, liver function, and ECG. Every attempt for early detection of adverse reactions should be made.

IMPLEMENTATION:

DRUG INTERACTIONS: Concurrent use with anticoagulants necessitates frequent prothrombin times; dosage adjustments may be necessary.

PRODUCTS (TRADE NAME):

Lopid (Available in 300 mg capsules.)

ADMINISTRATION AND DOSAGE: Give 600 mg po 30 minutes before eating in morning and evening. Adjust dosage depending upon serum lipid response. Usual range is 900-1500 mg/day to achieve decrease in lipids.

IMPLEMENTATION CONSIDERATIONS:

—Obtain a complete health history, including the presence of hepatic, renal, or cardiovascular disease, past history of dietary and medication regimens, drugs taken concurrently, and possibility of pregnancy.

—This product may increase the levels of cholesterol excretion, leading to cholelithiasis in susceptible individuals. If there is any suspicious history or symptoms, perform gallbladder x-rays, and discontinue medication if gallstones are found.

—This drug should be used as a last resort. Substantial effort should have been invested in teaching patient about diet, weight loss, alcohol restriction, exercise, and general health habits prior to beginning this product.

—Slight reductions in hemoglobin, hematocrit, and white blood cell count may be observed in the early phases of treatment. These values should stabilize toward normal as therapy continues.

—There may be abnormalities in liver function tests, which develop as a result of therapy. These are generally reversible once therapy is discontinued.

WHAT THE PATIENT NEEDS TO KNOW:

—Take this medication daily 30 minutes before eating in the morning and evening. Medication should not be discontinued or dose changed without the knowledge of your health care provider.

—Some people experience side effects from this product. Be certain to report any new or troublesome symptoms to your health practitioner. Especially note abdominal pain, excess gas, diarrhea, nausea or vomiting which persists.

—It is mandatory that you adhere closely to the special diet in addition to taking this medicine. Work closely with your health care practitioner to design a diet most fitted to your particular needs. Avoid alcoholic beverages, saturated fats, sugar, and cholesterol, and increase amount of daily exercise.

—At times this product may produce dizziness or blurred vision. Do not drive or perform tasks requiring alertness until you are certain of the medication's effects on you.

—Keep this medication out of the reach of children and all others for whom it is not prescribed.

EVALUATION:

ADVERSE REACTIONS: *CNS:* blurred vision, dizziness, headache, insomnia, paresthesia, tinnitus, vertigo. *Dermatologic:* dermatitis, pruritus, rash, urticaria. *Gastrointestinal:* abdominal pain, anorexia, constipation, diarrhea, dyspepsia, dry mouth, epigastric pain, flatulence, gas pains, nausea, vomiting. *Hematopoietic:* anemia, eosinophilia, leukopenia. *Musculoskeletal:* arthralgia, back pain, myalgia, muscle cramps, painful extremities, swollen joints. *Other:* fatigue, increased incidence of cough and urinary tract infections, malaise, syncope. Hypokalemia, increased SGOT, SGPT, LDH, CPK, and alkaline phosphatase may also be seen.

PARAMETERS TO MONITOR: Obtain complete history, physical, and laboratory evaluation prior to initiation of therapy. This should include a number of serum lipid levels to use as baseline. During therapy, periodic serum lipids should be obtained and drug should be withdrawn if substantial response has not been seen in 3 months. Seasonal variation in lipid levels should still be obvious with higher levels in mid winter and late summer. During therapy, patient should have periodic CBC and liver function study evaluations to look for adverse reactions. ECG studies should be obtained if there is any suspicion of development of arrhythmias.

Marilyn W. Edmunds

ANTIHYPERLIPIDEMIC AGENTS—
NICOTINIC ACID (NIACIN)

ACTION OF THE DRUG: Nicotinic acid, a water-soluble vitamin (B3), reduces the levels of serum cholesterol and triglycerides when given in pharmacologic doses. Although the specific mechanism of action is not known, it appears to work by inhibiting the accumulation of cyclic adenosine monophosphate (AMP) in fat cells, thereby reducing lipolysis and release of free fatty acids in adipose tissue. This reduces the amount of fatty acid available to the liver, decreases production of very low density lipoprotein, and causes a reduction in triglyceride synthesis. Since low density lipoprotein is a product of very low density catabolism, less low density lipoprotein is formed as well. Other mechanisms of action possibly include the inhibition of hepatic cholesterol synthesis, increased neutral steroid excretion, and faster removal of chylomicron triglycerides through increased action of lipoprotein lipase. Niacinamide does *not* have this hypolipemic effect.

ASSESSMENT:

INDICATIONS: This product is useful as adjunctive therapy in patients with hypercholesterolemia and hyperbetalipoproteinemia (types II b, III, IV and V) who have not responded substantially to special diets and weight loss regimens. Controversy continues about the effectiveness in reducing coronary artery disease as a result of lowering lipid levels in patients.

SUBJECTIVE-OBJECTIVE: Patient may be asymptomatic.

PLAN:

PRECAUTIONS: Drug should be used only after careful diagnosis, and for patients in which there has been no response to other treatment modalities. Patients should be advised to continue special diets, increase exercise, and work to reduce additional coronary artery disease risk factors: smoking, obesity, etc.

IMPLEMENTATION:

DRUG INTERACTIONS: This product may enhance the effects of antihypertensives, and antagonize effects of antidiabetic drugs by increasing blood glucose levels.

PRODUCTS (TRADE NAME):
Diacin (Available in 200 mg timed release capsules.) **Niac** (Available in 300 mg timed release capsules.) **NICO-400** (Available in 400 mg timed release capsules.) **Nicobid** (Available in 125, 250, and 500 mg timed release capsules.) **Nicolar** (Available in 500 mg tablets.) **Nico-Span** (Available in 400 mg timed release capsules.) **Nicotinex** (Available in 50 mg/5 ml elixir.) **Nicotinic Acid** (Available in 50, 100 mg tablets; 125, 250, 400, and 500 mg timed release capsules; 50 mg/ml and 100 mg/ml injection.) **Span-Niacin-150** (Available in 150 mg timed release capsules.) **Tega-Span** (Available in 400 mg timed release capsules.)

ADMINISTRATION AND DOSAGE: Give 1-2 gm 3 times daily po. Maximum dose 6 gm/day.

IMPLEMENTATION CONSIDERATIONS:
—Obtain a complete health history, including hypersensitivity, presence of underlying systemic disease (especially glaucoma, jaundice, gallbladder disease, diabetes, gout), concurrent medications, and possibility of pregnancy.
—Use this product only in conjunction with other therapeutic regimens.

WHAT THE PATIENT NEEDS TO KNOW:
—Take medication as prescribed. Do not exceed dosage or stop medication without consulting your health practitioner.
—Take with meals to reduce stomach upset.
—Adherence to prescribed diet is important. Restrict dietary intake of saturated fats, sugars, and/or cholesterol. Limit or avoid alcoholic beverages.
—Some patients experience side effects from this product. Be certain to report any new or troublesome symptoms to your health practitioner.
—During the first few months of therapy, some patients note a feeling of warmth and flushing of face, neck, and ears during the first 2 hours after taking the drug. Itching, tingling, and headache may also occur. These symptoms disappear if therapy is continued.
—Avoid changing positions rapidly if you note feeling of lightheadedness. This is especially important in the morning when moving from the lying to standing positions. Avoid activities in which you must move about quickly, or stand without moving for long times.
—Keep this product out of the reach of children and all others for whom it is not prescribed.

EVALUATION:

ADVERSE REACTIONS: *Cardiovascular:* hypotension, palpitations. *CNS:* dizziness, headache, paresthesias, tingling. *Gastrointestinal:* activation of peptic ulcer, diarrhea, epigastric pain, jaundice, impaired liver function. *Other:* decreased glucose tolerance test, dermatoses, gouty arthritis, hyperuricemia, headache, increased sebaceous gland activity, itching, tingling, skin rash, toxic amblyopia, transient flushing.

PARAMETERS TO MONITOR: Obtain history, physical, and laboratory evaluations prior to initiation of therapy. Perform periodic serum lipid level studies in order to monitor therapeutic effects of the medication. Therapeutic plasma concentration of 0.5 to 1.0 mcg/ml is necessary for the effects of nicotinic acid to achieve lipolysis. Plasma levels of triglycerides should fall within hours after institution of therapy, although cholesterol levels do not decrease for several days. Discontinue drug if acceptable results are not seen.

Marilyn W. Edmunds

ANTIHYPERLIPIDEMIC AGENTS—PROBUCOL

ACTION OF THE DRUG: Although the exact mechanism of action is not known, it is theorized that probucol (1) decreases the absorption of dietary cholesterol (2) increases excretion of bile acids in feces, and (3) inhibits the earliest components of cholesterol synthesis.

ASSESSMENT:

INDICATIONS: Probucol is used in adjunctive treatment of high cholesterol levels in patients with diagnosed primary hypercholesterolemia (elevated low density lipoproteins, type II) who have not responded to dietary and weight loss management, or control of underlying diabetes mellitus. It is also used in some patients with combined hypercholesterolemia and hypertriglyceridemia. Response to the drug is variable.

SUBJECTIVE: Patient may be asymptomatic.

OBJECTIVE: Xanthomatous lipid deposits may be found on ears, knees, elbows or shoulders. Arcus senilis, an opaque line partially encircling the cornea, is also sometimes seen. Elevated cholesterol and triglyceride levels are found.

PLAN:

CONTRAINDICATIONS: Do not give in the presence of hypersensitivity.

WARNINGS: Because of the suggestion of cardiotoxicity which has developed in animals, patients with recent myocardial damage, congestive heart failure, multifocal or paired PVCs, prolonged QT interval, or other cardiac arrhythmias should receive the drug with caution or not at all. Safety for use in children, pregnant and breast-feeding mothers has not been established. Because of the long-term effects which persist even when drug has been withdrawn, patients should use birth control for at least 6 months following withdrawal of the drug.

PRECAUTIONS: Probucol should not be continued if hypertriglyceridemia persists several months after therapy.

IMPLEMENTATION:

DRUG INTERACTIONS: None known. Oral anticoagulants and oral hypoglycemic agent dosages are not affected by this product. Although not confirmed, probucol may be responsible for elevations of some laboratory tests: SGOT, SGPT, bilirubin, alkaline phosphatase, creatine phosphokinase, uric acid, blood urea nitrogen, blood glucose.

PRODUCTS (TRADE NAME):
Lorelco (Available in 250 mg tablets.)
ADMINISTRATION AND DOSAGE:
Adults: Take 500 mg twice daily with morning and evening meals. Always take with food.
IMPLEMENTATION CONSIDERATIONS:
—Obtain a complete health history, including the presence of hypersensitivity, recent myocardial damage or arrhythmias, and possibility of pregnancy.
—Perform baseline evaluation studies to document elevated serum cholesterol. Several levels should be obtained during the months prior to initiation of probucol therapy.

—Most adverse reactions are mild and of short duration. Persistent GI problems may require discontinuance of the drug.

—Continue medication as long as a favorable trend is seen in lower cholesterol values. Decreased cholesterol levels should be expected in 2 months. If lowered levels do not develop, discontinue drug.

WHAT THE PATIENT NEEDS TO KNOW:

—Take this medication in morning and evening. Take with meals or food to minimize gastric upset.

—This drug should not be taken by pregnant women. Effective contraceptive measures should be used by women taking this drug, and continued for up to 6 months following discontinuance of the drug.

—The use of the medication is supplemental to your special diet. You should continue to avoid high cholesterol and saturated fatty foods and stay on the diet you have received from your health care practitioner.

—Some patients experience side effects while taking this product. Be certain to notify your health care provider of any new or troublesome symptoms. Especially note the presence of any persistent diarrhea, abdominal pain, flatulence, nausea, or vomiting.

—Keep this medication out of the reach of children and others for whom it is not prescribed.

EVALUATION:

ADVERSE REACTIONS: *CNS:* blurred vision, conjunctivitis, dizziness, diminished sense of taste and smell, headaches, insomnia, paresthesias. *Gastrointestinal:* abdominal pain, anorexia, diarrhea (10% of patients), flatulence, bleeding, heartburn, indigestion, nausea, vomiting. *Dermatologic:* pruritus, rash. *Hematopoietic:* ecchymosis, eosinophilia, low hemoglobin and/or hematocrit, petechiae, thrombocytopenia. *Other:* angioneurotic edema, enlargement of goiter, idiosyncratic reactions including chest pain, dizziness, palpitations, nausea, vomiting and syncope; fetid sweat, hyperhydrosis, nocturia, peripheral neuritis. Abnormal liver function tests, uric acid, BUN, and FBS may also be found.

PARAMETERS TO MONITOR: After accurate diagnosis of hyperlipidemic problem and dietary trial, several baseline cholesterol and triglyceride levels should be obtained. Cholesterol levels should start to decrease within 2 months after initiation of therapy. If no reduction is seen, evaluate patient compliance with diet and medication. Patient should abstain from alcohol, and calories should be restricted in order to increase chances of success. If no reduction is seen within 4 months from initiation of therapy, or if hypertriglyceridemia persists, medication should be discontinued.

Marilyn W. Edmunds

ANTIHYPERTENSIVES

ACTION OF THE DRUG: There are a wide variety of drugs available for the treatment of hypertension. They act at many sites in the body and through numerous mechanisms. These drugs fall roughly into main categories: (1) Diuretics that exert an indirect effect in reducing blood pressure by increasing sodium and water excretion and decreasing vascular tone. (2) Adrenergic inhibiting agents that assist in decreasing cardiac output and/or peripheral resistance; some also inhibit the release of renin. (3) Vasodilators that decrease peripheral resistance.

ASSESSMENT:

INDICATIONS: Drugs are selected and used alone or in combination to decrease elevated diastolic blood pressure. Respected clinical studies support that it is beneficial to use a combination of diet, drug therapy, and reduction of risk factors in treating hypertension. The therapeutic goal in the hypertensive patient is to reduce the blood pressure to normal or near normal with a minimum of untoward effects. Reduction of diastolic pressure below 90 mm Hg has been associated with decreased risk of end organ damage.

SUBJECTIVE: Patient may be asymptomatic, or may complain of not feeling well in general. Headaches, frequently associated with hypertension, are often produced by stress, tension, or other reasons, rather than being related to high blood pressure, unless very severe blood pressure elevations are present. In cases of secondary hypertension, there may be reports of nocturia (if patient is unable to concentrate urine), history of renal trauma (producing renal artery stenosis), or family history of hypertension.

OBJECTIVE: Patient may have elevated blood pressure due to numerous factors: full bladder, anxiety, pain, etc. If the average blood pressure is found to be above 140/90 on three consecutive readings (usually within a 2-4 week period) the patient is assumed to be hypertensive. Blood pressure above 120 diastolic requires immediate medical care. Blood pressure should be obtained in lying, sitting and standing positions in both arms. In cases where coarctation of the aorta is part of the diagnostic differential, blood pressure should also be measured in the lower extremities. Eyes should be examined for the presence of increased arteriovenous (A-V) ratio, nicking, hemorrhages or exudates in the fundus of the eye, and blurring of the disc margins. Chest should be examined for diffuse point of maximum intensity (PMI), displacement of PMI to the left, thrusts, murmurs, and presence of third and fourth heart sounds. (Systolic ejection murmurs and fourth heart sounds commonly develop in hypertensive patients.) Abdomen should be assessed for renal artery bruits. Renal function should be assessed.

PLAN:

PRECAUTIONS: Choice of hypertensive drug depends on many factors: degree of hypertension being treated, presence of other disease states, concurrent use of other drugs, and patient's acceptance of the mild but inescapable side effects which may develop.

IMPLEMENTATION:

DRUG INTERACTIONS: Antihypertensive drugs interact with many other products. Specific product information should be consulted before using other preparations concurrently.

ADMINISTRATION AND DOSAGE: A stepped-care approach to use of drugs has become accepted as the standard for appropriate therapeutic prescription in hypertension. As advocated by the Joint National Committee on Detection, Evaluation, and Treatment of High Blood Pressure, this approach involves a progressive regimen, beginning with use of a single agent with the least toxicity in a category, gradually increasing the dose, and adding drugs sequentially from other drug categories to bring the diastolic blood pressure under control. The pharmacologic effects are balanced in this approach to take advantage of differing mechanisms of action. This stepped-care approach can be summarized in Table 3-4.

Step One Drugs: The drug of choice in beginning antihypertensive therapy is

TABLE 3-4. STEPPED-CARE TREATMENT REGIMEN FOR HYPERTENSION

Level	Drug Action	Suggested Drugs to Use
Step One	Diuretic	Thiazides Indapamide Loop diuretics Potassium-sparing agents
Step Two	Adrenergic Inhibiting Agent	Atenolol Clonidine HCl Guanabenzep Guanadrel Methyldopa Metoprolol Nadolol Pindolol Prazosin HCl Propranolol HCl Rauwolfia alkaloids Timolol
Step Three	Vasodilators	Hydralazine HCl Prazosin
Step Four	Additional Adrenergic Inhibiting Agent	Guanethidine sulfate Captopril Minoxidil

an oral thiazide preparation. Drug is started in a low dosage and increased to maximal level as needed. In many cases one of these preparations used singly will reduce the diastolic blood pressure to an acceptable level. Because these products frequently produce hypokalemia, a potassium supplement may also be used concurrently. Loop diuretics are indicated when hypertension is severe and a prompt response is indicated.

Step Two Drugs: An antiadrenergic agent may be added to the regimen if maximal doses of thiazide diuretics fail to lower the blood pressure to the desired level. These two categories of drugs work synergistically to bring down blood pressure and minimize incidence of side effects, and are superior to use of an antiadrenergic agent alone. There are a variety of drugs within this category, allowing experimentation to find the most advantageous drug combinations for the individual patient. Only after failure to control blood pressure following use of a variety of these preparations should the patient move to the next level.

Step Three Drugs: The third drug to be added to the therapeutic regimen includes a vasodilator. These drugs are most effective when used with a beta-adrenergic blocking agent to control the reflex tachycardia which results from decreased peripheral resistance.

Step Four Drug: Guanethidine, an additional adrenergic inhibiting agent, is saved as the final drug which can be used in refractory hypertension. This drug has marked side effects which make its use as a Step Two drug inappropriate, leaving it for use in more severe cases of hypertension. The initial dose should be small, with dosage increased under supervision.

Some clinicians have suggested that minoxidil and captopril be considered Step Five drugs, and used to augment the armamentarium of medications available for antihypertensive therapy.

IMPLEMENTATION CONSIDERATIONS:

—Obtain a complete health history and physical examination, searching for a secondary cause for hypertension: Cushing's disease, Addison's disease, renal artery stenosis, coarctation of the aorta, pheochromocytoma. Also determine presence of other underlying disease, allergies, or concurrent medications which may affect choice of drug therapy.

—Substantial patient teaching and education will be essential to obtain compliance with therapy. Although taking the medication is important, it is also important to work on decreasing other risk factors and changing dietary habits.

—Collection and recording of a good initial data base: history, physical, and laboratory findings are important in evaluating progress of end-organ damage over the years. The incidence of drug side effects and complications from inadequately treated hypertension are high, and good record keeping is important in evaluating the patient's status.

—Patients should be encouraged to lose weight, restrict sodium intake, avoid stress and emotional pressures, develop regular and realistic exercise patterns, and engage in hobbies or activities which help self-esteem. Taking the medications should be emphasized as only a small part of this total regimen.

—Experimentation should be used in selecting antihypertensive drugs. The lowest possible dosage should be used, and the minimum side effects produced. Patients need to be counseled regarding side effects, and should have a vote in determining therapy when possible. For example, discussing the possibility of impotence is very important with male patients.

—Effectiveness in establishing patient rapport is paramount in obtaining their confidence. This is essential in establishing positive lifetime health modification patterns.

WHAT THE PATIENT NEEDS TO KNOW:

—This medication should be taken exactly as ordered by your health care provider. If you miss a dose, take it as soon as you remember if it is within an hour or two of the scheduled time. If it is close to your next scheduled dose take only the next dose at the regular time. Do not double doses.

—Take medication with a full glass of orange juice (unless not on your diet). Other potassium-rich foods should be used daily. These include: citrus foods (especially oranges and tomatoes), bananas, dried fruits, apricots, cantaloupe, watermelon, nuts, dried beans, beef, and fowl.

—Taking medication is only one part of your treatment regimen. Reduction of other risk factors is also important: lose weight (if overweight), reduce sodium intake, stop smoking, increase exercise, avoid excessive stress and emotional pressures. Avoid use of foods high in sodium: lunch meats, smoked meats, Chinese food, processed cheese, snack foods. Do not salt food when cooking or add salt to your food after it is cooked.

—There are numerous side effects which could develop from use of these preparations. Be certain to notify your health care provider of any new or troublesome symptoms which you may experience. Your medication may need to be changed in order to find the best drugs for you. A close working relationship with your health care provider will be necessary in order to accomplish this. It is therefore very important to keep your appointments for care.

—Keep this medication out of the reach of children and others for whom it is not prescribed. It would be very hazardous for them. Do not leave it lying on night tables or low dressers to present a temptation to young children.

—The goal of therapy is to help you feel as healthy as possible, and to avoid any complications. Generally there is no cure for hypertension, and therapy extends for a lifetime. Taking your medication and reducing other risk factors will help reduce the chance of serious complications. It is important then to keep taking your medicine, even when you feel well, and to keep seeing your health care practitioner regularly.

—Wear a Medic-Alert bracelet and carry a medical identification card specifying that you have hypertension and listing the drugs which you are taking.

EVALUATION:

ADVERSE REACTIONS: There are a variety of side effects seen, depending upon the drugs and the drug combinations used. See sections on individual drugs.

PARAMETERS TO MONITOR: Initial data base should include complete history, physical examination (stressing vital signs, eyes, heart, lungs, abdomen, and peripheral vascular assessment), and laboratory evaluation: complete blood count, uric acid, BUN, glucose, electrolytes, ECG, chest x-ray. Special tests may be done to rule out Addison's disease, pheochromocytoma, Cushing's disease, etc., as indicated. On each visit, the patient should be monitored for therapeutic effect. The goal is reduction of diastolic blood pressure to 90 mm Hg or below in 6 months or less. If blood pressure is not decreased there may be indications of progressive end-organ damage: cardiomegaly, development of third and fourth heart sounds, cardiac murmurs, arrhythmias, rales in the lungs, peripheral edema, weight gain, changes in funduscopic examination of the eye, and development of peripheral neuropathies. Also watch for adverse effects from medications: hypokalemia is the most serious side effect from thiazides; drowsiness, impotence, hypovolemia, and postural hypotension are all seen. Laboratory evaluation of blood and cardiac function should be made periodically through urinalysis, electrolytes, ECG, and other laboratory tests as warranted.

Marilyn W. Edmunds

ANTIHYPERTENSIVES—
ANGIOTENSIN-CONVERTING ENZYME INHIBITOR

CAPTOPRIL

ACTION OF THE DRUG: Through stimulation of the juxtaglomerular apparatus of the kidneys, renin is released into the circulating blood volume to produce angiotensin I. Angiotensin I is then converted by the liver and the lungs to angiotensin II through an angiotensin-converting enzyme (ACE). Angiotensin II is a powerful vasoconstrictor which acts on the adrenal cortex to increase aldosterone secretion. This renin-angiotensin sequence is important in conserving sodium and water as a compensatory mechanism in maintaining blood pressure in the presence of shock, but contributes to increasing pressure found in hypertension. Although the complete mechanism of action of captopril is not yet known, it is thought to prevent the conversion of angiotensin 1 to angiotensin 11 by inhibiting angiotensin converting enzyme (ACE) in the plasma and vascular endothelium. It may interfere with the breakdown of bradykinin, an endogenous peptide that produces vasodilation. There may be other complex actions, since captopril is also effective in low-renin hypertension.

With use of this product, peripheral arterial resistance is reduced in hypertensive patients with usually a mild increase in cardiac output. Renal blood flow increases, but glomerular filtration rate remains unchanged. Plasma renin activity increases due to loss of negative feedback, and serum potassium may increase due to the absence of aldosterone. The maximum antihypertensive effect is noted 60 to

90 minutes following administration, but several weeks of therapy may be required to obtain the gradual decrease of blood pressure to within therapeutic range. Duration of effect seems to be dosage related.

ASSESSMENT:

INDICATIONS: Captopril is not a routine drug to be used in the stepped care treatment of hypertension. Because of its potency, as well as its potential for serious side effects, it is reserved for use in patients who have been unresponsive to multidrug antihypertensive regimens or who have developed side effects to drugs utilized previously. It is prescribed by qualified specialists, although nurse practitioners often have the responsibility of monitoring patient response to therapy. Captopril is effective when used alone; however, it is most frequently combined with a thiazide diuretic since concurrent administration has an additive effect. Captopril has also been found effective for use in patients with heart failure when used adjunctively with diuretics and digitalis. It is reserved for patients who have not responded to conventional therapy.

SUBJECTIVE: Patient presents with a history of known hypertension and therapy with a variety of other antihypertensive drugs. There may be subjective symptoms of hypertension, end-organ damage, or side effects from other medications.

OBJECTIVE: Patient may have cardiomegaly, diffuse PMI, systolic ejection murmur, third or fourth heart sound. There may be evidence of hemorrhage, nicking, or exudates in optic fundus, or blurring of the disc margins if hypertension is severe enough. There may be rales on chest examination and the presence of peripheral edema or paresthesias.

PLAN:

WARNINGS: Membranous glomerulopathy has been found in some patients taking captopril, with the only sign being the development of persistent proteinuria. Many of these patients had preexisting renal disease, and a conclusive link to the medication has not been made. Patients should be screened for prior evidence of disease before contemplating use of this drug.

Use captopril with caution in patients with impaired renal function, who have taken drugs known to depress immune response, or who have serious autoimmune diseases such as lupus. Some patients (especially those with the problems just listed) have developed neutropenia or agranulocytosis 3 to 12 weeks after initiating therapy. In some cases the WBC has fallen slowly over 10 to 30 days. In a small number of cases, myeloid hypoplasia developed, and patients developed either systemic or oral cavity infections. Most patients recovered within 2 weeks after therapy was discontinued.

Safety has not been demonstrated for use of drug in pregnant or breast-feeding women. There is limited experience in using the drug with children, so other therapeutic measures should be explored, leaving this drug as a final alternative.

PRECAUTIONS: In patients with active renal disease or impairment, reduction of blood pressure by captopril may also lead to increased serum BUN and creatinine levels. Discontinuing diuretic therapy may solve this problem, but at times captopril also may have to be stopped to ensure adequate renal perfusion. After undergoing vigorous diuresis, patients also may be more vulnerable to development of hypotensive episodes.

If hypotension occurs during surgery due to general anesthesia, volume expansion may be necessary to override the effects of captopril and normalize blood pressure.

IMPLEMENTATION:

DRUG INTERACTIONS: In patients who have been on severe dietary salt re striction, on dialysis, or who have recently begun diuretic therapy, a drastic reduction in blood pressure is sometimes seen within 3 hours following administration of the first dose of captopril. Other antihypertensive agents which might increase renin levels will enhance the effect of captopril. Potassium-sparing diuretics or potassium supplements should be given cautiously, and only in documented cases of hypokalemia. The administration of captopril reduces aldosterone and leads to increases in serum potassium. Significant increases of potassium may develop even if patient had discontinued spironolactone several months in the past. Ganglionic blocking agents or adrenergic neuron blocking agents may affect sympathetic activity and should be used with caution. Concomitant use of beta-adrenergic blocking agents does not substantially increase the antihypertensive effects of the two products. Captopril may also cause a falsepositive test for urine acetone.

PRODUCTS (TRADE NAME):
Capoten (Available in 25, 50, and 100 mg scored tablets.)

ADMINISTRATION AND DOSAGE: If possible, all other antihypertensive medications should be discontinued at least one week prior to beginning therapy with captopril. For congestive heart failure patients, digitalis and a diuretic should be continued. Consideration should be given to the presence of other underlying disease processes, severity of hypertension, and diet before determining dosage schedule. Medication should be taken one hour before meals. This therapy should be carried out under careful medical supervision.

Initial therapy: Monitor patient closely for at least 3 hours following first dose. Give 25 mg po 3 times daily. If needed, dose may be increased to 50 mg 3 times daily after 1 or 2 weeks. If therapeutic goal has not been achieved in 1-2 weeks, a small dose of a thiazide diuretic may be started and also increased at 1-2 week intervals until blood pressure has reached therapeutic objective. Captopril also may be increased to 100 and then 150 mg 3 times daily. Maximum dose is 450 mg/day of captopril.

Patients with renal impairment: Excretion of drug is reduced, so patients may respond to smaller or less frequent doses. Reduce initial dose and give smaller increments to achieve pressure reduction. Once pressure is within desired range, cut back on daily dose to the minimum amount possible. Furosemide is preferred to use of thiazide diuretic therapy in these patients.

Malignant hypertension: Hospitalize patients and begin therapy with 25 mg 3 times a day, increasing dose every 24 hours until therapeutic objective is reached. Furosemide also may be a necessary component of therapy. Patient must be closely monitored during entire pressure reduction period. Captopril may cause elevation of liver enzymes, transient elevation of creatinine and BUN, and rise in serum potassium concentrations.

Heart failure: Initially 6.25 to 12.5 mg three times daily is given with careful assessment of fluid and salt status because patients have usually been heavily diuresed. Daily dosage is 25 mg three times daily with gradual increase up to 50 mg three times daily. After two week trial, dosage may again be increased. Do not exceed 450 mg/day.

IMPLEMENTATION CONSIDERATIONS:

—Obtain a complete health history, including presence of hypersensitivity, recent use of guanethidine, spironolactone, or other potassium-sparing diuretics, salt restriction, vigorous diuresis, and previous medications taken for control of blood pressure. Assess status of liver, kidney, and cardiovascular function, and the possibility of pregnancy.

—With use of captopril, orthostatic effects and tachycardia do not routinely occur unless patient is severely volume depleted.

—Abrupt withdrawal of medication does not appear to cause a rapid increase in blood pressure.

—Taking medication with food reduces the absorption by 30% to 40%.

—About 95% of drug is excreted in the urine, thus less frequent dosage and smaller amounts are indicated in patients with renal impairment.

—Watch for development of proteinuria and neutropenia or agranulocytosis, especially in patients with previous history of renal disease, autoimmune diseases, or patients who have previously taken drugs which affects the immune response. Whether drug should be discontinued if these signs appears depends upon an evaluation of individual benefits vs. possible risks.

—If patient develops hypotension with initial dose, place patient in supine position and begin IV with 0.9% NACL.

WHAT THE PATIENT NEEDS TO KNOW:

—This is a potent antihypertensive medication which is being utilized to control elevated blood pressure. While you are taking this drug you will need to follow instructions for taking it carefully, and return to your health care provider regularly for evaluation of its effectiveness.

—Take medication exactly as ordered. Do not suddenly stop medication or change dosages without being advised to do so. It may require several weeks of therapy before the full effect of the drug will be known. If you miss a dose, take it as soon as you remember if it is within an hour or two of the time you should have taken it. If it is close to your next scheduled dose, skip it, and take the next dose at the regular time. Do not double doses.

—Keep this medication out of the reach of children and all others for whom it is not prescribed.

—Take this medication one hour before meals. Your body will not absorb all of the medication if you have food present in your stomach when you take the pills.

—Do not take any medications, including cough, cold, or allergy medications which you may buy over the counter without the knowledge of your health care provider.

—Some people experience side effects when taking this drug. Notify your health care provider if you note any new or troublesome symptoms. Report particularly any skin rash, impaired taste perception, dizziness or fainting, excessive perspiration, dehydration, vomiting, diarrhea, mouth sores, sore throat, fever, swelling of hands or feet, chest pains, or irregular heartbeat.

—If you feel lightheaded, particularly in the morning, avoid rapid changes in position. Move slowly, especially from the lying to standing position.

—Take medicine with a full glass of orange juice (unless contraindicated by your diet). Other potassium-rich foods should be used daily. These include: citrus foods (especially oranges and tomatoes), bananas, dried fruits, apricots, cantaloupe, watermelon, nuts, dried beans, beef, and fowl.

—Taking medication is only one part of your treatment regimen. Reduction of other risk factors is also important: lose weight (if overweight), stop smoking, increase exercise, avoid stressful and emotional pressures. Avoid use of foods high in sodium: lunch meats, smoked meats, Chinese food, processed cheese, snack foods. Do not salt food while cooking or add salt to your food after it is cooked.

—The goal of therapy is to help you feel as healthy as possible and to avoid any complications. Generally there is no cure for hypertension, and therapy extends for a lifetime. Taking your medication and reducing other risk factors will help reduce the chance of serious complications. It is important then to keep taking your medicine, even when you feel well, and to keep seeing your health care practitioner regularly.

—Wear a Medic-Alert bracelet, and carry a medical identification card specifying that you have hypertension and the drugs which you are taking.

EVALUATION:

ADVERSE REACTIONS: *Cardiovascular:* angina pectoris, chest pain, congestive heart failure, hypotension (2%), myocardial infarction (rare), palpitations, Raynaud's syndrome, tachycardia. *CNS:* alteration or loss of taste perception (7%), dizziness, fatigue, headache, insomnia, malaise, paresthesias. *Dermatologic:* angioedema of the face, mucous membranes of the mouth, and extremities; flushing, pallor; pruritic maculopapular rash, sometimes with fever and eosinophilia (10% of patients), may develop positive ANA titers; reversible pemphigoid-like lesions; photosensitivity. *Gastrointestinal:* abdominal pain, anorexia, constipation, diarrhea, dry mouth, gastric irritation, nausea, peptic ulcer, vomiting. *Hematopoietic:* agranulocytosis, eosinophilia, hemolytic anemia, neutropenia, pancytopenia. *Renal:* proteinuria, oliguria, polyuria, renal failure, renal insufficiency, urinary frequency. *Other:* dyspnea.

OVERDOSAGE: *Signs and symptoms:* Hypotension may be present. *Treatment:* Volume expansion may be helpful. Place patient in supine position.

PARAMETERS TO MONITOR: Obtain complete baseline studies before initiation of therapy. If patient has been receiving other antihypertensive drugs, discontinue other medications if possible for at least one week. Monitor for therapeutic effect and development of adverse reactions. Several weeks may be required to evaluate the full effect of this drug. Make small dosage adjustments during this period. Blood pressure should be measured in both lying, sitting, and standing positions. Pressure reductions should be about the same in both standing and lying positions. Orthostatic changes or reflex tachycardia should alert health care practitioner to the possibility of volume depletion.

Neutropenia often develops 3-12 weeks after starting medications in patients who are receiving large doses. Smaller doses in patients with only moderate elevations of pressure are less likely to stimulate neutropenia. WBC count and differential should be obtained prior to initiating therapy and should be monitored in patients every two weeks for the first three months of therapy and monthly thereafter. If neutrophils fall to below 1000/mm^2, discontinue drug and monitor patient with differential counts. Neutropenia generally resolves within two weeks, but patient should be evaluated for signs of infection during that time (fever, sore throat, etc.).

Patients also should be closely observed for the development of proteinuria. Dip stick checks for protein (on first morning specimen) or 24-hour quantitative measurements should be performed prior to beginning therapy and once each month for nine months. Most cases of proteinuria occur by the eighth month of therapy. When proteinuria persists or reaches a level exceeding 1 gm/day, use of captopril must be reconsidered. Patient must be watched for other renal symptoms indicating possible development of nephrotic syndrome or membranous glomerulopathy.

Marilyn W. Edmunds

ANTIHYPERTENSIVES—BETA BLOCKERS

ACTION OF THE DRUG: Beta-blockers compete with beta-adrenergic receptor stimulating agents for available beta-receptor sites, thereby antagonizing the effects of catecholamines released from the adrenergic nerve endings as well as the adrenal medulla. Beta-blocking agents reduce the metabolic (glycogenolytic, lipolytic), myocardial stimulant, vasodilator, and bronchodilator actions of catecholamines. This represents decreases in chronotropic, inotropic, and vasodilator action. Reduction in heart rate and force of contraction, suppression of renin release, and decrease in outflow of sympathetic vasoconstrictor and cardioaccelerator fibers from brain stem vasomotor center are produced.

ASSESSMENT:

INDICATIONS: Propranolol is the most widely used of the beta-blocking agents, although it is largely non-specific in its blocking action, and therefore is associated with a wide range of side effects. Newer beta-blocking drugs have more selective blocking action toward the beta-1 receptors in the heart, relative to the beta-2-sites. Because it is impossible to completely disassociate the beta-1 and beta-2-blocking activity, all drugs must be used cautiously in patients with bronchospastic disorders. Beta-blockers are used for the treatment of mild to moderate hypertension as Step

Two drugs. They may be used alone, but are more commonly used with other anti-hypertensive agents. Beta-blockers are used for long-term management of angina pectoris, for long-term prophylaxis in patients with recent myocardial infarction, and for arrhythmias.

SUBJECTIVE-OBJECTIVE: Patient may or may not have preexisting history of cardiac problems. Patient may present with complaints of lightheadedness, and dizziness. History of hypertension unresponsive to diuretic regimen may also be present. Elevated blood pressure may be found.

PLAN:

CONTRAINDICATIONS: Do not use with a history of hypersensitivity to the drug, bronchial asthma, sinus bradycardia, second or third-degree heart block, cardiogenic shock, right ventricular failure secondary to pulmonary hypertension, or congestive heart failure.

WARNINGS: Drug may precipitate or cause congestive heart failure. In Wolff-Parkinson-White syndrome, drug may cause severe bradycardia. Use with caution in patients with chronic bronchitis or emphysema. Drug may mask signs and symptoms of hypoglycemia.

PRECAUTIONS: Use with caution in patients with hepatic impairment.

IMPLEMENTATION:

DRUG INTERACTIONS: Catecholamine-depleting drugs, such as reserpine, given with beta-blockers may produce an excessive reduction of the resting sympathetic nervous activity. Concurrent use with aminophylline or isoproterenol may result in mutual inhibition. Use with digitalis may result in excessive bradycardia. Use with epinephrine, phenylephrine or other sympathomimetics may result in excessive bradycardia and hypertension. Propranolol may either raise or lower blood sugar; it may mask symptoms of hypoglycemia. Dosage of insulin or oral hypoglycemics may need adjustment. Beta-blockers may produce elevated blood urea levels in patients with severe heart disease, elevated serum transaminase, alkaline phosphatase, and lactate dehydrogenase.

IMPLEMENTATION CONSIDERATIONS:

—Obtain a complete health history, including the presence of hypersensitivity, drug history of other medications which may cause drug interactions, and other systemic diseases which may affect therapy.

—Withdrawal of the drug should be done gradually over a period of several weeks.

—Beta-blockers should be withdrawn 48 hours prior to major surgery.

—Watch for signs of asthma, or development of congestive heart failure in patients who cannot adjust to lowered heart rate.

WHAT THE PATIENT NEEDS TO KNOW:

—Take this medication exactly as ordered by your health care provider. Do not skip doses or double doses. If you miss a dose, take it as soon as you remember unless it is close to the time for the next dose.

—Do not discontinue medication without being advised to do so by your health care provider.

—Some people have side effects from this medication. Be sure to report any new or uncomfortable symptoms to your health practitioner. Especially note any sudden weight gain, trouble breathing, or increased coughing.

—This medicine may make you feel dizzy or drowsy. Use caution in driving and in performing tasks requiring alertness.

—Keep this medicine out of the reach of children and all others for whom it is not prescribed.

—Wear a Medic-Alert bracelet and carry a medical identification card specifying that you are taking this product.

EVALUATION:

ADVERSE REACTIONS: *Cardiovascular:* arterial insufficiency usually of Raynaud type, bradycardia, congestive heart failure, intensification of AV block, hypotension, paresthesia of hands. *CNS:* depression, disorientation, dizziness, emotional lability, fatigue, hallucinations, insomnia, lightheadedness, mental confusion (especially in the elderly), reduced alertness, visual disturbances, weakness. *Gastrointestinal:* abdominal cramping, constipation, diarrhea, epigastric distress, ischemic colitis, nausea, mesenteric arterial thrombosis, vomiting. *Hematopoietic:* agranulocytosis, nonthrombocytopenic purpura, thrombocytopenic purpura. *Hypersensitivity:* agranulocytosis, erythematous rash, fever combined with aching and sore throat, laryngospasm and respiratory distress, pharyngitis. *Respiratory:* bronchospasm, dyspnea. *Other:* reversible alopecia.

OVERDOSAGE: *Signs and symptoms:* Bradycardia, cardiac failure, hypotension, and bronchospasm may be seen and should be treated supportively. Atropine, digitalis, diuretics, and vasopressors may be necessary along with isoproterenol and aminophylline.

PARAMETERS TO MONITOR: Obtain complete history, physical, and laboratory work as baseline. This should include complete analysis of vital signs, weight, cardiac and chest assessment. Laboratory work should include CBC, glucose, liver and renal function tests, and ECG. Monitor for therapeutic effect: reduction in blood pressure, relief of angina, stabilization of cardiac rhythm. Also monitor for adverse reactions, especially development of signs or symptoms of congestive heart failure. Check for signs and symptoms of agranulocytosis (sore throat, fever) and thrombocytopenia (bruising). Develop a flow chart of symptoms which you question patient about on each visit so that you may focus consistently on the most important problems for each patient.

ATENOLOL

PRODUCTS (TRADE NAME):
  Tenormin (Available in 50 and 100 mg tablets.)
DRUG SPECIFICS:
  This drug is used primarily in the treatment of hypertension as a step two drug. (It may be used alone but has increased effects when administered in conjunction with thiazide diuretics, and products such as methyldopa, prazosin, and hydralazine.) Atenolol is primarily excreted through the kidneys, and patients with renal impairment (creatinine clearance below 35 ml/min) should have a decreased dose and be closely monitored.
ADMINISTRATION AND DOSAGE SPECIFICS:
  Give 50 mg/day po in the morning, either alone or with other antihypertensive agents and diuretics. If desired effect is not achieved within 2 weeks, may increase dose to 100 mg/day po in the morning. Increasing dosage beyond this is not likely to produce greater effects.

METOPROLOL TARTRATE

PRODUCTS (TRADE NAME):
  Lopressor (Available in 50, 100 mg scored tablets.)
DRUG SPECIFICS:
  This medication is a step two antihypertensive drug which is used in conjunction with other thiazide diuretics and antihypertensive medications. It has significantly reduced blocking activity at beta-2-receptors in the pulmonary system at normal dose levels. Hypotensive effects are potentiated by catecholamine-depleting agents (reserpine). Insulin-induced hypoglycemia may be enhanced. It requires individual evaluation and clinical trials in patients in order to establish optimium dosage. Some patients require dosage three times a day if pressure begins to rise at the end of a 12-hour period. Monitor blood pressure control at end of dosing interval to determine degree of control. Common side effects are diarrhea, dizziness, and fatigue.
ADMINISTRATION AND DOSAGE SPECIFICS:
  Give 100 mg po daily in single or divided doses for at least one week when the medication is sole agent or used in conjunction with other agents. Increase dosage at one week intervals until expected response is obtained. Maximum effective dosage appears to be 100 to 450 mg/day in divided doses.

NADOLOL

PRODUCTS (TRADE NAME):
   Corgard (Available in 40, 80, 120, 160 mg scored tablets.)
DRUG SPECIFICS:
   This is a step two antihypertensive agent which has also been found effective in the long-term treatment of angina pectoris. It has a non-selective beta-adrenergic blocking action. It reduces heart rate, cardiac output, and systolic and diastolic blood pressures, but has no anesthetic-like membrane stabilizing action and little direct myocardial depressant effect. This medication is excreted primarily by the kidneys, and patients with renal impairment require reduced dosage regimens. The long half-life of this medication permits once a day dosing. Do not exceed recommended dosage as accumulation may occur. When medication is to be discontinued, it should be stopped gradually over a period of 2-3 weeks. Bradycardia is a common side effect.
ADMINISTRATION AND DOSAGE SPECIFICS:
   Hypertension: 40 mg po once daily whether used as sole agent or in conjunction with other diuretic and antihypertensive agents. Individualize dosage according to patient response, with increments of 40 to 80 mg until therapeutic response is achieved. Usual dose is 80 to 240 mg once a day. Doses up to 640 mg/day may be given.
   Angina pectoris: Give 40 mg po once daily. Increase dosage in 40- to 80-mg increments at 4-7 day intervals until satisfaction with results is achieved or adverse reactions develop (especially undue slowing of heart). Establish maintenance dose at lowest possible dose to achieve therapeutic results. Usual dose is 80 to 240 mg once daily.

PINDOLOL

PRODUCTS (TRADE NAME):
   Visken (Available in 5 and 10 mg tablets.)
DRUG SPECIFICS:
   This beta-blocker is used primarily for the management of moderate hypertension. It is a step two drug in the antihypertensive stepped-care format. It is comparable in cost with other beta-blocking agents. While this product has been on the market a relatively short time, drug specifics appear to be similar to other beta-blocking agents.
ADMINISTRATION AND DOSAGE SPECIFICS:
   Hypertension: Initially give 5 mg twice daily, alone or with other antihypertensive agents. Patient usually responds with lowered blood pressure within 7 days. If adequate blood pressure response has not developed within 2 to 3 weeks, increase dosage by 10 mg/day increments at 2 to 3 week intervals. Do not exceed 60 mg/day.

PROPRANOLOL HYDROCHLORIDE

PRODUCTS (TRADE NAME):
Inderal (Available in 10, 20, 40, and 80 mg tablets; 1 mg/ml ampules for injection.) **Inderal LA** (Available in 80, 120, and 160 mg capsules).

DRUG SPECIFICS:
This is the beta-adrenergic blocking agent which has been on the market for the longest time and is the best known. It is also used in the widest variety of situations: hypertension (either alone or as a step two drug), cardiac arrhythmias (especially in digitalis overdosage, sinus tachycardia, atrial premature contractions, and tachyarrhythmias due to general anesthesia, and thyroid toxicosis), migraine, angina pectoris secondary to coronary artery disease, idiopathic hypertrophic subaortic stenosis, pheochromocytoma. It is being experimentally tested in treatment of somatic symptoms of anxiety, essential and lithium-induced tremors, and open-angle glaucoma. It provides reversible competitive blocking action at beta-adrenergic receptor sites, resulting primarily in negative chronotropic and inotropic effects on the heart (decreasing rate and force of contraction), slowed atrioventricular conduction, decreased plasma renin levels, bronchoconstriction, hypotension, decreased levels of free fatty acids, and possibly lowers glucose levels. It also has a quinidine-like depressant effect on myocardial function at higher doses. Common side effects include bradycardia, palpitations, hypotension, nausea, cramping, diarrhea, lightheadedness, mild depression, and lethargy.

ADMINISTRATION AND DOSAGE SPECIFICS:
Inderal
Hypertension: Give 40 mg po twice daily, either alone or in combination with other thiazide diuretics and antihypertensive agents. Gradually increase dose to reduce blood pressure to desired level. Up to 640 mg/day may be required, with usual dosage 120 to 240 mg/day. May require large doses or three times daily dosing if blood pressure begins to rise at the end of a 12-hour period.

Arrhythmias: Give 10 to 30 mg 3 or 4 times daily po before meals and at bedtime. Adjust dosage depending upon cardiovascular response of patient. May give 1-3 mg parenterally in emergency situations but do not exceed 1 mg/min. May repeat once in 2 minutes. Monitor carefully. Isoproterenol may be indicated for overdosage.

Angina pectoris: Give 10 to 20 mg 3 or 4 times daily, before meals and at bedtime. Increase dosage every 4 to 7 days until therapeutic effect is satisfactory. Usual dose is 160 mg/day with maximum dose 320 mg/day.

Hypertrophic subaortic stenosis: Give 20 to 40 mg 30 or 4 times daily po, before meals and at bedtime.

Migraine: Give 80 mg/day in divided doses. Increase drug slowly to 240 mg/day to use as migraine prophylaxis. Effectiveness of therapy should be evident in 4-6 weeks or drug may be discontinued. Withdraw medication slowly over 2-3 weeks.

Pheochromocytoma: Give 60 mg/day in divided doses for 3 days prior to surgery.

Use an alpha-adrenergic blocking agent in addition. Patient may be continued on 30 mg/day if surgery is not indicated.

Myocardial infarction: Give 180-240 mg per day in divided doses either in a bid or tid regimen.

Inderal LA

When switching from Inderal to Inderal LA, care should be taken to maintain therapeutic effect. Inderal LA produces lower blood levels.

Hypertension: Give 80 mg once daily, either alone or in combination with thiazide diuretics and other antihypertensive agents. Gradually increase dose to reduce blood pressure to desired level. Up to 640 mg may be required, with usual dosage 120 to 160 mg one a day.

Angina pectoris: Give 80 mg once a day. Increase dosage at 3 to 7 day intervals. Usual dose is 160 mg once a day with maximum dose 320 mg.

Migraine: Give 80 mg once a day. Increase dose gradually. Usual dose is 160 to 240 mg once a day. Effectiveness of therapy should be evident in 4 to 6 weeks or drug may be discontinued. Withdraw medicine slowly over 2 or 3 weeks.

Hypertrophic subaortic stenosis: Give 80 to 160 mg once daily.

TIMOLOL MALEATE

PRODUCTS (TRADE NAME):

Blocadren (Available in 10, 20 mg tablets).

DRUG SPECIFICS

This beta-blocker has little intrinsic sympathomimetic, myocardial depressant or local anesthetic action. It reduces the formation of aqueous humor in the eye without miosis or hyperemia. This is a drug used primarily for the treatment of hypertension, either as the sole therapy or in conjunction with other thiazide diuretics and antihypertensive agents, as a step two drug. It is also useful in patients with recent myocardial infarction as a long-term prophylactic agent. (See ophthalmic drugs for use in open-angle glaucoma. It is contraindicated in patients with a history of bronchial asthma.)

ADMINISTRATION AND DOSAGE SPECIFICS:

Hypertension: Give 10 mg twice daily whether alone or with other agents. After 7-day intervals, may increase to 20-40 mg/day maintenance dose. Total of 60 mg/day in two doses is maximum.

Myocardial infarction: Give 10 mg twice daily after acute period.

Maren Stewart and Marilyn W. Edmunds

ANTIHYPERTENSIVES—CLONIDINE HCL

ACTION OF THE DRUG: Clonidine acts to (1) stimulate peripheral alpha-adrenergic receptors, producing a brief and transient vasoconstriction, and then (2) stimulates the presynaptic alpha-2-adrenergic receptors in cardiovascular integrating centers in the brain stem. As a result of this the bulbar sympathetic cardioaccelerator and sympathetic vasconstrictor center, stimulation is inhibited and total sympathetic outflow from the brain is decreased. Slight reduction in pulse rate and cardiac output occur.

This drug acts to reduce plasma renin levels and promotes excretion of both catecholamines and aldosterone. Renal blood flow and the glomerular filtration rate remain essentially unchanged. Initial stimulation of peripheral alpha-adrenergic receptors may cause a transient vasoconstriction.

ASSESSMENT:

INDICATIONS: Clonidine is a step two drug used in the treatment of mild to moderate hypertension (although it may be used alone or with another antihypertensive drug also). It is indicated for hypertensive patients who have not been controlled on a diuretic alone or who evidence adverse effects from high doses of diuretics required to control diastolic pressure. This product is considered moderately potent and its actions are enhanced when used concomitantly with a diuretic. It has been used investigationally in the treatment of severe migraine headaches, to decrease menopausal flushing, and in detoxification of patients receiving chronic methadone administration. It may be used also as an alternative to methadone in rapid opiate detoxification.

SUBJECTIVE: Patient may be asymptomatic or may complain of not feeling well in general. Headaches, often associated with hypertension, are often produced by stress, tension, or other reasons rather than being related to high blood pressure, unless very severe blood pressure elevations are present. In cases of secondary hypertension, there may be reports of nocturia (if patient is unable to concentrate urine), history of renal trauma (producing renal artery stenosis), or family history of hypertension.

OBJECTIVE: Patient may have elevated blood pressure due to numerous factors: full bladder, anxiety, pain, etc. If the average blood pressure is found to be above 140/90 mm Hg on three consecutive readings, the patient is assumed to be hypertensive. Readings above 120 mm Hg diastolic require immediate medical care. Blood pressure should be obtained in lying, sitting, and standing positions in both arms and, in cases where coarctation of the aorta is part of the diagnostic differential, in the lower extremities. Eyes should be examined for the presence of increased arteriovenous (AV) ratio, nicking, hemorrhages, or exudates in the fundus of the eye and blurring of the disc margins. Chest should be examined for diffuse point of maximum intensity (PMI), displacement of PMI to the left, thrusts, murmurs, and presence of third or fourth sounds. (Systolic ejection murmurs and fourth heart sounds commonly develop in hypertensive patients.) Abdomen should be assessed for renal artery bruits.

PLAN:

CONTRAINDICATIONS: Do not use in the presence of hypersensitivity.
WARNINGS: Use with extreme caution and careful monitoring in patients

with recent myocardial infarction, severe coronary insufficiency, chronic renal failure, or severe cerebrovascular disease. Initial studies suggest teratogenic effects of this drug, and although not conclusive, this drug is not indicated for use in women in whom there is a possibility of pregnancy. Risk must be weighed against possible benefit. Safety for use in children has not been established.

PRECAUTIONS: Patients well controlled on this drug may develop tolerance. This may necessitate periodic evaluations and changes in therapy to keep blood pressure within acceptable limits. Patients on chronic clonidine therapy should be evaluated by an ophthalmologist periodically since retinal degeneration has been suggested from animal studies. Drug should never be stopped suddenly because a rebound hypertension may develop. This may be severe enough to cause hypertensive encephalopathy and death.

IMPLEMENTATION:

DRUG INTERACTIONS: Concomitant administration of a diuretic has been shown to enhance the antihypertensive effects of clonidine. Tolazoline and tricyclic antidepressants (except doxepin) may block the antihypertensive effects. This drug may also increase the CNS depressant effects of barbiturates, alcohol, narcotics, and other sedatives. Excessive bradycardia may occur with concurrent administration with digitalis agents, propranolol, or guanethidine. Discontinuing therapy with concurrent use of propranolol may increase risk of clonidine withdrawal hypertensive crisis, and propranolol should be slowly discontinued first. May produce weakly positive direct antiglobulin Coombs' test.

PRODUCTS (TRADE NAME):
Catapres (Available in 0.1, 0.2 , 0.3 mg scored tablets.)

ADMINISTRATION AND DOSAGE: Dosage must be individualized, based upon patient's blood pressure and therapeutic response to medication.

Adults: Begin dosage with 0.1 mg twice a day. Increase dose 0.1 or 0.2 mg/day until desired response is achieved. Maximum effective dose is 2.4 mg/day, but usual dose is 0.2 to 0.8 mg/day.

IMPLEMENTATION CONSIDERATIONS:

—Obtain a complete health history, including presence of hypersensitivity, other medications taken concurrently, presence of myocardial insufficiency or infarction, cerebral insufficiency, renal dysfunction, history of depression, or possibility of pregnancy.

—Abrupt termination of therapy may produce headache, agitation, and a rapid rise in blood pressure. These can be treated by reinstituting clonidine or using both an alpha and beta-adrenergic blocker. Discontinue therapy over 2 to 4 days by reducing the dosage gradually.

—Patients on long-term care should have periodic ophthalmologic examinations to assess for any retinal deterioration.

—The sedative effects of this medication can be reduced by slowly increasing the daily dosage and giving the largest dose in the evening before going to bed.

—This drug is usually well tolerated, with minimal side effects. Most side effects diminish within 4 to 6 weeks of continuous therapy.

—The ability to establish rapport with the patient, institute diet therapy, and reduce other risk factors, as well as encouraging patient to keep appointments, will be major factors contributing to success in treating patient on a long-term basis.

 —Patient may develop tolerance to clonidine. Reevaluate therapy and consider adding other antihypertensive medications if this should occur.

WHAT THE PATIENT NEEDS TO KNOW:

 —Take this medication exactly as ordered by your health care provider. Do not adjust doses or stop taking medication without being advised to do so. If you miss a dose, take it as soon as you remember if it is within an hour or two of the time you should have taken it. If it is close to your next scheduled dose, skip it, and take the next dose at the regular time. Do not double doses.

 —Therapy for hypertension requires periodic visits to your health care provider and evaluation of your response to medication. There is a wide variety of things which you can do to help reduce your blood pressure, and the health practitioner will assist you in learning the things which will be most helpful for you. This may require taking different drugs at different times, or changing dosages. It is very important for you to return to the health care provider for evaluation of your reaction to therapy.

 —Do not stop taking this medication suddenly. To do so may stimulate very high blood pressure. If you miss taking more than 1 dose in a row, check with your health care provider immediately.

 —Do not take any other medications without the knowledge of your health care provider. This includes over-the-counter drugs which you may buy for colds, cough, or allergy. Use with alcohol should also be discussed with your practitioner.

 —Patients often note an increase in sleepiness after beginning this drug or whenever the dosage is increased. This is felt only briefly and can be minimized by taking the increased or largest dose in the evening before going to bed. Do not attempt to drive or perform any tasks requiring alertness until you know how you will respond to this drug.

 —In order to avoid dizziness, avoid changing positions rapidly, especially when rising from the lying position.

 —Some patients note other side effects from this drug. If you experience any new or uncomfortable symptoms, do not hesitate to report them to your health care provider promptly. Especially note any change in patterns of urination since this drug may produce urinary hesitancy.

 —This medication can cause severe reactions in children or pets who accidently swallow it. It must be kept out of the reach of children or others for whom medication is not prescribed.

 —If you note that your mouth and throat feel dry while taking this medication, dissolving bits of ice in your mouth or chewing sugarless gum may help relieve dryness.

 —You should wear a Medic-Alert bracelet or carry other identifying information about having hypertension and the medications you are taking.

 —Take medication with a full glass of orange juice (unless contraindicated by your diet). Other potassium-rich foods should be used daily. These include:

citrus foods (especially oranges and tomatoes), bananas, dried fruits, apricots, cantaloupe, watermelon, nuts, dried beans, beef, and fowl.

—Taking medication is only part of your treatment regimen. Reduction of other risk factors is also important: lose weight (if overweight), reduce sodium intake, stop smoking, increase exercise, avoid stressful and emotional pressures. Avoid use of foods high in sodium: lunch meats, smoked meats, Chinese food, processed cheese, snack foods. Do not salt food while cooking or add salt to your food after it is cooked.

EVALUATION:

ADVERSE REACTIONS: *Cardiovascular:* cyanosis, congestive heart failure, ECG abnormalities (episodes of second-degree heart block (Wenckebach) and ventricular trigeminy), edema, palpitations, pain in extremities, Raynaud's phenomenon. *CNS:* anxiety, behavioral changes, delirium, depression, dizziness, drowsiness, ear pain, excessive dreaming, fatigue, flushing, headache, insomnia, mental depression, nervousness, nightmares, restlessness, sedation, vivid dreams. *Dermatologic:* angioneurotic edema, hives, rash, pruritus not associated with rash, rash, thinning of the hair, urticaria. *Endocrine:* elevated blood glucose and serum creatinine phosphokinase (transient), gynecomastia, weight gain. *Gastrointestinal:* anorexia, abnormalities in liver function tests (mild and reversible), constipation, dry mouth, malaise, nausea, parotid pain, vomiting. *Genitourinary:* impotence, urinary retention. *Other:* dryness, itching or burning of the eyes, dryness of the nasal mucosa, gynecomastia, hyperglycemia, increased sensitivity to alcohol, pallor, weight gain.

OVERDOSAGE: *Signs and symptoms:* bradycardia, CNS depression, respiratory depression, apnea, hypothermia, miosis, lethargy, agitation, irritability, seizures, diarrhea, and arrhythmias. Profound hypotension, weakness, somnolence, diminished or absent reflexes and vomiting. *Treatment:* Stimulate emesis or refer for gavage and symptomatic treatment. A saline cathartic may increase the GI transit time.

PARAMETERS TO MONITOR: Obtain a complete laboratory data baseline before initiating therapy. This should include electrolytes, cardiac, renal and liver function studies, an electrocardiogram, and a chest x-ray. A urinalysis should also be obtained. These laboratory tests should be repeated at least yearly while patient is taking medication. During therapy, patient should be monitored for therapeutic effect: controlling diastolic blood pressure at a rate of 90 mm Hg or lower with a minimum of side effects. Observe for adverse reactions. Check for postural hypotension and evaluate patient for progressive end-organ damage to heart, lungs, kidneys, and eyes. An ophthalmologic examination should be obtained every 6 months if patient is on long-term therapy.

Marilyn W. Edmunds

ANTIHYPERTENSIVES—GUANABENZ ACETATE

ACTION OF THE DRUG: This alpha-2-adrenergic agonist acts as an antihypertensive medication through stimulation of central alpha-adrenergic receptors. Sympathetic outflow from the brain at the bulbar level to the peripheral circulatory system is thus decreased. Pulse rate is slightly decreased, although no changes in cardiac output are seen during long-term therapy. With prolonged use peripheral vascular resistance is decreased and blood pressure is lowered in both standing and supine positions, although postural hypotension has not been observed. There is no observable change in glomerular filtration rate, renal blood flow, or renal and sodium excretion.

ASSESSMENT:

INDICATIONS: This product is a step-two medication, used in the treatment of hypertension. It has in some cases been used alone rather than with a thiazide diuretic.

SUBJECTIVE: Patient may be asymptomatic or may complain of not feeling well in general. Headaches, often associated with hypertension, are often produced by stress, tension, or other reasons rather than being related to high blood pressure, unless very severe blood pressure elevations are present. In cases of secondary hypertension, there may be reports of nocturia (if patient is unable to concentrate urine), history of renal trauma (producing renal artery stenosis), or family history of hypertension.

OBJECTIVE: Patient may have elevated blood pressure due to numerous factors: full bladder, anxiety, pain, etc. If the average blood pressure is found to be above 140/90 mm Hg on three consecutive readings, the patient is assumed to be hypertensive. Readings above 120 mm Hg diastolic require immdiate medical care. Blood pressure should be obtained in lying, sitting, and standing positions in both arms and, in cases where coarctation of the aorta is part of the diagnostic differential, in the lower extremities. Eyes should be examined for the presence of increased arteriovenous (AV) ratio, nicking, hemorrhages, or exudates in the fundus of the eye and blurring of the disc margins. Chest should be examined for diffuse point of maximum intensity (PMI), displacement of PMI to the left, thrusts, murmurs, and presence of third or fourth sounds. (Systolic ejection murmurs and fourth heart sounds commonly develop in hypertensive patients.) Abdomen should be assessed for renal artery bruits.

PLAN:

CONTRAINDICATIONS: Do not give in the presence of known hypersensitivity to guanabenz.

WARNINGS: Because this is a relatively new product there are no controlled studies documenting safety for usage in pregnancy, breast-feeding women, and in children. Risk to benefit ratio should be examined and product used only when deemed essential.

PRECAUTIONS: This medication should not be stopped suddenly as the possibility of producing a rebound hypertension may develop. Increases in serum catecholamines and symptoms resulting from this may also develop with rapid cessation of therapy. This medication should be used with caution in patients with recent myocardial infarction, cerebrovascular disease, severe coronary insufficiency, or severe hepatic or renal failure. This product causes sedation and drowsiness in many patients.

IMPLEMENTATION:

DRUG INTERACTIONS: Concurrent use with CNS depressants may cause increased sedative effect.

PRODUCTS (TRADE NAME):
Wytensin (Available in 4 and 8 mg tablets.)

ADMINISTRATION AND DOSAGE: Dosage must be individualized, based upon patient's blood pressure and therapeutic response to medication. A starting dose of 4 mg twice a day is recommended, regardless of whether a thiazide diuretic is used or not. Increase medication in increments of 4 to 8 mg per day every 1 to 2 weeks, depending on the patient's response. Do not exceed 32 mg twice daily.

IMPLEMENTATION CONSIDERATIONS:

—Obtain a complete health history, including the presence of hypersensitivity, other medications taken concurrently, presence of myocardial insufficiency or infarction, cerebral insufficiency, renal or hepatic failure, or possibility of pregnancy.

—Abrupt termination of therapy may produce rebound hypertension.

—This drug is usually well tolerated, with minimal side effects. Most side effects are dosage related.

—In patients experiencing drowsiness from this product, give largest dose in evening before going to bed.

—The ability to establish rapport with the patient, as well as encouraging patient to keep appointments, will be major factors contributing to success in treating patient on a long-term basis.

WHAT THE PATIENT NEEDS TO KNOW:

—Take this medication exactly as ordered by your health care provider. Do not adjust doses or stop taking medication without being advised to do so. If you miss a dose, take it as soon as you remember if it is within an hour or two of the time you should have taken it. If it is close to your next scheduled dose, skip it, and take the next dose at the regular time. Do not double doses.

—Therapy for hypertension requires periodic visits to your health care provider and evaluation of your response to medication. There is a wide variety of things which you can do to help reduce your blood pressure, and the health practitioner will assist you in learning the things which will be most helpful for you. This may require taking different drugs at different times, or changing dosages. It is very important for you to return to the health care provider for evaluation of your reaction to therapy.

—Do not stop taking this medication suddenly. To do so may stimulate very high blood pressure. If you miss taking more than 1 dose in a row, check with your health care provider immediately.

—Do not take any other medications without the knowledge of your health care provider. This includes over-the-counter drugs which you may buy for colds, cough, or allergy. You should not drink any alcohol or use other CNS depressant drugs while taking this medication.

—Patients often note an increase in sleepiness after beginning this drug or whenever the dosage is increased. Do not attempt to drive or perform any tasks requiring alertness until you know how you will respond to this drug.

—You should wear a Medic-Alert bracelet or carry other identifying information about having hypertension and the medications you are taking.

—Keep this medication out of the reach of children and others for whom it is not prescribed.

—Taking medication is only part of your treatment regimen. Reduction of other risk factors is also important: lose weight (if overweight), reduce sodium intake, stop smoking, increase exercise, avoid stressful and emotional prssures. Avoid use of foods high in sodium: lunch meats, smoked meats, Chinese food, processed cheese, snack foods. Do not salt food while cooking or add salt to your food after it is cooked.

EVALUATION:

ADVERSE REACTIONS: *Cardiovascular:* arrhythmias, chest pain, edema, palpitations. *CNS:* anxiety, ataxia, blurring of vision, depression, dizziness, drowsinesss, dry mouth, headache, nasal congestion, sleep disturbances, weakness. *Dermatologic:* pruritus, rash. *Gastrointestinal;* abdominal discomfort, constipation diarrhea, epigasotric pain, nausea, vomiting. *Other:* aches in extremities, disturbances in sexual function, dyspnea, gynecomastia, muscle aches, taste disorders, urinary frequency.

OVERDOSAGE: Limited experience shows that hypotension, somnolence, lethargy, irritability, bradycardia and miosis are produced in overdosage. Gastric lavage and symptomatic treatment have been effective.

PARAMETERS TO MONITOR: Obtain a complete laboratory data baseline before initiating therapy. This should include electrolytes, cardiac, renal and liver function studies, an electrocardiogram, and a chest x-ray. A urinalysis should also be obtained. These laboratory tests should be repeated at least yearly while patient is taking medication. During therapy, patient should be monitored for therapeutic effect: controlling diastolic blood pressure at a rate of 90 mm Hg or lower with a minimum of side effects. Observe for adverse reactions. Evaluate for progressive end-organ damage to heart, lungs, kidneys, and eyes.

Marilyn W. Edmunds

ANTIHYPERTENSIVES—GUANADREL SULFATE

ACTION OF THE DRUG: This product is an adrenergic neuron blocking agent which inhibits sympathetic vasoconstriction through inhibition of norepinephrine release from neuronal storage sites and depletion of norepinephrine from nerve endings. Total peripheral resistance is thus decreased through the relaxation of vascular smooth muscle. Venous return is also decreased. Hypotensive effects and reduction in heart rate are both seen. There is no observable change in cardiac output in normal individuals. This medication causes increased sensitivity to circulating norepinephrine, and is thus dangerous in the presence of excess norepinephrine such as that found in pheochromocytoma.

ASSESSMENT:

INDICATIONS: This product is a step-two medication, used in the treatment of hypertension not responding sufficiently to thiazide diuretics alone.

SUBJECTIVE: Patient may be asymptomatic or may complain of not feeling well in general. Headaches, often associated with hypertension, are often produced by stress, tension, or other reasons rather than being related to high blood pressure, unless very severe blood pressure elevations are present. In cases of secondary hypertension, there may be reports of nocturia (if patient is unable to concentrate urine), history of renal trauma (producing renal artery stenosis), or family history of hypertension.

OBJECTIVE: Patient may have elevated blood pressure due to numerous factors: full bladder, anxiety, pain, etc. If the average blood pressure is found to be above 140/90 mm Hg on three consecutive readings, the patient is assumed to be hypertensive. Readings above 120 mm Hg diastolic require immediate medical care. Blood pressure should be obtained in lying, sitting, and standing positions in both arms and, in cases where coarctation of the aorta is part of the diagnostic differential, in the lower extremities. Eyes should be examined for the presence of increased arteriovenous (AV) ratio, nicking, hemorrhages, or exudates in the fundus of the eye and blurring of the disc margins. Chest should be examined for diffuse point of maximum intensity (PMI), displacement of PMI to the left, thrusts, murmurs, and presence of third or fourth sounds. (Systolic ejection murmurs and fourth heart sounds commonly develop in hypertensive patients.) Abdomen should be assessed for renal artery bruits.

PLAN:

CONTRAINDICATIONS: Do not give in the presence of known hypersensitivity to guanadrel sulfate, to patients with known or suspected pheochromocytoma. Do not use concurrently with or within one week of using MAO inhibitors. Do not use in patients with frank congestive heart failure.

WARNINGS: Dizziness, weakness, fainting upon exercise or standing and other problems associated with orthostatic hypotension are common in patients treated with this product. Patients should be carefully instructed to minimize these problems. Bronchial asthma patients may be more difficult to manage because the asthma may be aggravated by catecholamine depletion while sympathomimetic amines may interfere with the antihypertensive effect of guanadrel. Patients should also discontinue this medication 72 hours prior to elective surgery to reduce risk of vascular collapse during surgery. Because this is a relatively new product there are no controlled studies documenting safety for usage in pregnancy, breast-feeding women, and in children. Risk to benefit should be examined and product used only when deemed essential.

PRECAUTIONS: This product often produces salt and water retention which may provoke congestive heart failure. Patients with peptic ulcer should use this medication cautiously as problem could be aggravated by increase in parasympathetic tone. Studies on these problems have not yet been undertaken.

IMPLEMENTATION:

DRUG INTERACTIONS: Guanadrel enhances the activity of direct-acting sympathomimetics like norepinephrine by blocking neuronal uptake. Drugs which can reverse the effects of neuronal blocking agents include tricyclic antidepressants and indirect-acting sympathomimetics such as ephedrine or phenylpropanolamine. Alpha- or beta-adrenergic blocking agents and reserpine may possible potentiate the effects of guanadrel, causing excessive postural hypotension and bradycardia.

PRODUCTS (TRADE NAME):
Hylorel (Available in 10 and 25 mg tablets.)

ADMINISTRATION AND DOSAGE: Dosage must be individualized, based upon patient's blood pressure and therapeutic response to medication. With long-term therapy, some tolerance may develop, necessitating dosage increases. Adjust the dosage weekly or monthly until blood pressure is controlled. A starting dose of 10 mg day is usual. Most patients will require a daily dosage in the range of 20 to 75 mg usually in twice daily doses. If dosage is large, 3 or 4 times daily dosing may be needed.

IMPLEMENTATION CONSIDERATIONS:

—Obtain a complete health history, including the presence of hypersensitivity, other medications taken concurrently, presence of myocardial insufficiency or infarction, cerebral insufficiency, congestive heart failure, bronchial asthma, or possibility of pregnancy.

—The ability to establish rapport with the patient, as well as encouraging patient to keep appointments, will be major factors contributing to success in treating patient on a long-term basis.

—Monitor closely the orthostatic side effects of this preparation and teach patient how to limit problems resulting from this process.

—Side effects from medication appear greatest within the first 8 weeks of therapy and then tend to decrease.

WHAT THE PATIENT NEEDS TO KNOW:
—Take this medication exactly as ordered by your health care provider. Do not adjust doses or stop taking medication without being advised to do so.

If you miss a dose, take it as soon as you remember if it is within an hour or two of the time you should have taken it. If it is close to your next scheduled dose, skip it, and take the next dose at the regular time. Do not double doses.

—Therapy for hypertension requires periodic visits to your health care provider and evaluation of your response to medication. There is a wide variety of things which you can do to help reduce your blood pressure, and the health practitioner will assist you in learning the things which will be most helpful for you. This may require taking different drugs at different times, or changing dosages. It is very important for you to return to the health care provider for evaluation of your reaction to therapy.

—In order to avoid dizziness, avoid changing positions rapidly, especially when rising from the lying position. Sit or lie down immediately if you have any dizziness or weakness. Feelings of lightheadedness may be increased by alcohol, fever, hot weather, prolonged standing, or exercise.

—Do not take any other medications without the knowledge of your health care provider. This includes over-the-counter drugs which you may buy for colds, cough, or allergy.

—You should wear a Medic-Alert bracelet or carry other identifying information about having hypertension and the medications you are taking.

—Keep this medication out of the reach of children and others for whom it is not prescribed.

—Taking medication is only part of your treatment regimen. Reduction of other risk factors is also important: lose weight (if overweight), reduce sodium intake, stop smoking, increase exercise, avoid stressful and emotional pressures. Avoid use of foods high in sodium: lunch meats, smoked meats, Chinese food, processed cheese, snack foods. Do not salt food while cooking or add salt to your food after it is cooked.

EVALUATION:

ADVERSE REACTIONS: *Cardiovascular:* chest pain, palpitations. *CNS:* confusion, depression, dizziness, drowsinesss, faintness, fatigue, headache, paresthesias, psychological problems, sleep disorders, syncope, visual disturbances. *Gastrointestinal:* abdominal discomfort, anorexia, constipation, dry mouth, dry throat, gas pains, increased bowel movements, indigestion, glossitis, nausea, vomiting. *Genitourinary;* ejaculation disturbances, hematuria, impotence, nocturia, peripheral edema, urination urgency or frequency. *Musculoskeletal:* aching limbs, backache or neckache, joint pain or inflammation, leg cramps during the night and day. *Respiratory:* coughing, shortness of breath at rest or on exertion. *Other:* excessive weight gain or loss.

OVERDOSAGE: Limited experience shows that marked dizziness and blurred vision along with postural hypotension may be produced in overdosage. Patient should rest in order to minimize symptoms. Vasoconstrictors such as phenylephrine may be needed in more compromised individuals.

PARAMETERS TO MONITOR: Obtain a complete laboratory data baseline before initiating therapy. This should include electrolytes, cardiac, renal and liver function studies, an electrocardiogram, and a chest x-ray. A urinalysis should also be obtained. These laboratory tests should be repeated at least yearly while patient is taking medication. During therapy, patient should be monitored for therapeutic effect: controlling diastolic blood pressure at a rate of 90 mm Hg or lower with a minimum of side effects. Observe for adverse reactions, especially monitoring extent of orthostatic hypotension through lying, sitting and standing pressures and pulses. Evaluate for progressive end-organ damage to heart, lungs, kidneys, and eyes.

Marilyn W. Edmunds

ANTIHYPERTENSIVES—GUANETHIDINE SULFATE

ACTION OF THE DRUG: Guanethidine accumulates in peripheral adrenergic nerve endings and inhibits norepinephrine release, and therefore adrenergic nerve endings become depleted. Exogenous catecholamines sensitize the effector cells. Intraneuronal stores of norepinephrine are also exhausted, resulting in a prolonged decrease in heart rate and peripheral vascular resistance. Guanethidine is metabolized partially by the liver and excreted by the kidney. Plasma renin activity may be reduced and cardiovascular reflexes may be inhibited, so a high degree of orthostatic hypotension is often produced.

ASSESSMENT:

INDICATIONS: Guanethidine is considered a step-four drug for management of moderate and severe hypertension. It may be used alone, but is more usually used in combination with step one, two and three drugs to more adequately control diastolic blood pressure. It is particularly helpful in renal hypertension, including that caused by renal artery stenosis, pyelonephritis and amyloidosis.

SUBJECTIVE: Patient presents with a history of known hypertension, and therapy with a variety of other antihypertensive drugs. There may be subjective symptoms of hypertension, end-organ damage, or side effects from other medications.

OBJECTIVE: Patient may have cardiomegaly, diffuse PMI, systolic ejection murmurs, third or fourth heart sound. There may be evidence of hemorrhage, nicking, or exudates in optic fundus, or blurring of the disc margins if hypertension is severe enough. There may be rales on chest examination and the presence of peripheral edema or paresthesias.

PLAN:

CONTRAINDICATIONS: Do not give to patients with hypersensitivity to guanetheidine, to patients concurrently using MAO inhibitors, to patients in frank congestive heart failure not due to hypertension, or to patients with hypertension secondary to pheochromocytoma.

WARNINGS: This medication is one of the most potent antihypertensives and it should be reserved for patients uncontrolled by other measures. Its most common side effect is severe orthostatic hypotension, producing dizziness and weakness, which occurs at fairly predictable times. It is most pronounced in the morning after the patient has been recumbent all night. It is also aggravated by alcohol, exercise, and hot weather.

This drug should be administered with caution to patients with decreased renal function, patients with bronchial asthma, and patients with allergies. Drug should be discontinued 1-2 weeks prior to patient undergoing general anesthesia in order to avoid problems with vascular collapse. Safety for use during pregnancy has not been established. Compare risks to possible benefits.

PRECAUTIONS: Use this drug with extreme caution in patients recovering from recent myocardial infarction, patients with myocardial insufficiency, and those suffering from cerebral vascular disease. Because guanethidine slows the heart rate, it should not be given to patients with severe congestive heart failure. Concomitant therapy with a thiazide diuretic may be helpful in reducing sodium and water retention.

Use cautiously in patients with a history of peptic ulcer disease. Also watch for patients with tartrazine sensitivity which may produce an allergic-type reaction. These patients are frequently also hypersensitive to aspirin.

IMPLEMENTATION:

DRUG INTERACTIONS: Guanethidine administered concurrently with digitalis provides an additive effect in slowing of the heart and may produce significant bradycardia. Use of guanethidine with some of the step two drugs, especially the *Rauwolfia* derivatives, may exaggerate postural hypotension, mental depression, and bradycardia. Other drugs which increase the hypotensive effect are alcohol, diuretics, hydralazine, levodopa, methotrimeprazine, propranolol, quinidine, reserpine, and vasodilators. Drugs which may antagonize antihypotensive effect of guanethidine include oral contraceptives, narcotics, antihistamines, cocaine, diethylpropion, ephedrine, methylphenidate, tricyclic antidepressants and other psychopharmacologic agents, amphetamine-like compounds, sympathomimetic agents, and stimulants. Guanethidine increases the responsiveness to norepinephrine and vasopressors which are administered, and the incidence of cardiac arrhythmias may be increased. Guanethidine may impair the hyposecretion effects of anticholinergics. It also may exert an additive hypoglycemic effect with insulin or oral antidiabetic agents. MAO inhibitors should not be given concurrently with guanethidine or within two weeks of their administration.

PRODUCTS (TRADE NAME):
Ismelin Sulfate (Available in 10 and 25 mg scored tablets.)

ADMINISTRATION AND DOSAGE: Average dose is 25 to 50 mg/day po. Dosage should begin at 10 mg/day po and be increased gradually every 5-7 days, depending on patient response. Blood pressure should be evaluated for orthostatic changes and dosage increased only if there is no decrease in normal standing pressure levels. Because of the long half-life (approximately 5 days), the drug accumulates slowly. It may take up to two weeks to adequately evaluate the patient's response to the drug.

Patients who are hospitalized and can be monitored more closely can be given higher doses, usually 25 to 50 mg, which can be repeated every 8 hours as needed until desired response is obtained. Maintenance doses are usually one-seventh of the loading dose.

Guanethidine is usually used in combination with other drugs as part of a hypertensive regimen. The most successful combinations include concurrent use of thiazides and hydralazine. Thiazides used concurrently help in reduction of edema. (If the patient is already on guanethidine, its dosage may need to be reduced when the thiazide is started.) If the patient has been receiving a ganglionic blocking agent, it should be gradually stopped before guanethidine is begun. MAO inhibitors should also be discontinued for at least one week before initiating guanethidine. Once the patient's blood pressure has been brought under control with a combination of drugs, all drug dosages should be reduced to the lowest effective level.

IMPLEMENTATION CONSIDERATIONS:

—Obtain a complete health history, including history of hypersensitivities, bronchial asthma, myocardial infarction, myocardial insufficiency, cerebral vascular disease, peptic ulcer, renal disease, congestive heart failure, use of MAO inhibitors or other drugs which might produce drug interactions, and possibility of pregnancy.

—Up to two weeks may be necessary before it will be possible to adequately evaluate patient's response to this medication. Premature increases in dosage are not warranted. The effects of guanethidine are cumulative, and initial doses should be small with very small increments.

—Dosage requirements may be increased when fever is present.

—Reduced dosages are required in patients with renal impairment. Watch for rising BUN levels. Decreasing blood pressure may further compromise renal blood flow.

—The most frequent and severe side effect of guanethidine is postural hypotension. Patients must be cautioned about living with this medication. Counseling patients about getting out of bed slowly, changing positions carefully, and, in general, staying out of situations that require rapid movements is important in preventing syncopal episodes. On follow-up visits, take blood pressure in lying, sitting, and standing positions. A drop in blood pressure of 10 mm Hg from lying to standing indicates postural hypotension.

—Development of severe diarrhea as a result of unopposed parasympathetic activity may require stopping this drug.

—If possible, withdraw medication 2 weeks before elective surgery, and inform anesthesiologist that patient has been on this medication.

WHAT THE PATIENT NEEDS TO KNOW:

—Take this medication exactly as ordered by your health care provider. Do not increase dosage or stop taking medication suddenly. Take care not to run out of medication. If you miss a dose, take it as soon as you remember if it is within an hour or two of the scheduled time. If it is close to your next scheduled dose, skip it, and take the next dose at the regular time. Do not double doses.

—This is one of the most powerful drugs for controlling your blood pressure. It should be kept out of the hands of children or others for whom it is not prescribed.

—The most frequent side effect from this drug is a feeling of dizziness and lightheadedness when changing positions rapidly. This will be most pronounced in the morning when you attempt to get out of bed. Slowly rise to a sitting position and sit there for a few minutes. Let your body adjust to that position before attempting to stand up. Have something to hold on to if need be. Alcohol, exercise, and hot weather tend to increase this problem. Avoid situations which require you to change positions quickly. Alert your health care provider if you begin fainting or falling, or are having extensive problems with feeling lightheaded.

—Do not take any other medications without the knowledge of your health care provider. This includes cough, cold, or allergy medications which you can buy over the counter.

—Some people experience other side effects from this drug. Notify your health care provider promptly if you have any new or troublesome symptoms. Especially note persistent diarrhea or sudden weight gain or edema, urinary retention, weakness, or slow pulse.

—Take medicine with a full glass of orange juice (unless contraindicated by your diet). Other potassium-rich foods should be used daily. These include: citrus foods (especially oranges and tomatoes), bananas, dried fruits, apricots, cantaloupe, watermelon, nuts, dried beans, beef, and fowl.

—Taking medication is only one part of your treatment regimen. Reduction of other risk factors is also important: lose weight (if overweight), stop smoking, increase exercise, avoid stressful and emotional pressures. Avoid use of foods high in sodium: lunch meats, smoked meats, Chinese food, processed cheese, snack foods. Do not salt food while cooking or add salt to your food after it is cooked.

—The goal of therapy is to help you feel as healthy as possible and to avoid any complications. Generally there is no cure for hypertension, and therapy extends for a lifetime. Taking your medication and reducing other risk factors will help reduce the chance of serious complications. It is important then to keep taking your medicine, even when you feel well, and to keep seeing your health practitioner regularly.

—Wear a Medic-Alert bracelet and carry a medical identification card specifying that you have hypertension and the drugs which you are taking.

EVALUATION:

ADVERSE REACTIONS: *CNS:* Symptoms due to unopposed parasympathetic activity: especially bradycardia, increased bowel movements and diarrhea. Symptoms due to sympathetic blockade: dizziness, lassitude, syncope and weakness. *Other:* anemia, asthma, blurring of vision, cardiac irregularity, chest pain, chest paresthesias, congestive heart failure, depression, dermatitis, diarrhea, dry mouth, dyspnea, fatigue, fluid retention, hair loss, incontinence, increased BUN, inhibition of ejaculation, mental depression, muscle tremor, myalgia, nasal congestion, nausea, nocturia, orthostatic hypotension, parotid tenderness, ptosis of the eye lids, scalp hair loss, skin rash, swelling of feet and lower legs, tremors, vomiting, weight gain (due to fluid retention).

OVERDOSAGE: *Signs and symptoms:* Postural hypotension and syncope, bradycardia, and diarrhea are the main symptoms. *Treatment:* Keep patient supine and treat symptomatically. Patient usually regains adequate blood pressure within 72 hours. If vasopressors are given, monitor closely for development of cardiac arrhythmias.

PARAMETERS TO MONITOR: Obtain a complete physical examination and laboratory data base prior to initiating therapy. This should include CBC, electrolytes, FBS, BUN, liver and renal function studies, a urinalysis, ECG, and chest x-ray. These studies should be repeated periodically while patient is under treatment with this drug. Patient should be monitored for therapeutic effect and development of adverse reactions. Therapeutic goal is to reduce diastolic blood pressure to 90 mm Hg or lower with a minimum of side effects. Dosage adjustments should be made slowly, and allow 3 to 5 days for effects to become obvious. Monitor closely for postural hypotension. Blood pressure should be taken in lying position, after standing for 10 minutes, and soon after exercise if possible. Dosage should be increased only if there has been no decrease in standing blood pressure from previous levels. A drop of 10 mm Hg from lying to standing is considered evidence of postural hypotension.

Marilyn W. Edmunds

ANTIHYPERTENSIVES—HYDRALAZINE HCL

ACTION OF THE DRUG: Hydralazine HCl is a potent peripheral vasodilator whose antihypertensive effect is caused by direct relaxation of arterial smooth muscle. In addition to decreased peripheral vascular pressure, diastolic pressure is reduced, and a reflex increased heart rate, cardiac output, and stroke volume are produced. Renal and cerebral blood flow are increased.

ASSESSMENT:

INDICATIONS: This drug may be used alone but is generally classed as a step three antihypertensive medication, which is used in conjunction with a thiazide diuretic and a drug which inhibits sympathetic activity, such as methyldopa, clonidine, or a beta-blocker. It is used parenterally in severe essential hypertension when rapid reduction of blood pressure is necessary or when patient cannot take drug orally.

SUBJECTIVE: Patient may be asymptomatic or may complain of not feeling well in general. Headaches, often associated with hypertension, are often produced by stress, tension, or other reasons rather than being related to high blood pressure, unless very severe blood pressure elevations are present. In cases of secondary hypertension, there may be reports of nocturia (if patient is unable to concentrate urine), history of renal trauma (producing renal artery stenosis), or family history of hypertension.

OBJECTIVE: Patient may have elevated blood pressure due to numerous factors: full bladder, anxiety, pain, etc. If the average blood pressure is found to be above 140/90 mm Hg on three consecutive readings, the patient is assumed to be hypertensive. Readings above 120 mm Hg diastolic require immediate medical care. Blood pressure should be obtained in lying, sitting, and standing positions in both arms. In cases where coarctation of the aorta is part of the diagnostic differential blood pressure should also be measured in the lower extremities. Eyes should be examined for the presence of increased arteriovenous (AV) ratio, nicking, hemorrhages, or exudates in the fundus of the eye, and blurring of the disc margins. Chest should be examined for diffuse point of maximum intensity (PMI), displacement of PMI to the left, thrusts, murmurs, and presence of third and fourth heart sounds. (Systolic ejection murmurs and fourth heart sounds commonly develop in hypertensive patients.) Abdomen should be assessed for renal artery bruits.

PLAN:

CONTRAINDICATIONS: Do not use with hypersensitivity to hydralazine, in coronary artery disease, or in rheumatic heart disease with mitral valve damage. Also not to be used in patients with systemic lupus erythematosus.

WARNINGS: A clinical picture similar to that for lupus erythematosus has appeared in a few patients. In this case, medication should be discontinued. Drug has not been proven safe in pregnancy, and the question of teratogenesis in humans has not been resolved.

PRECAUTIONS: Drug should be given with caution in patients with rheumatic heart disease or coronary artery disease, because of the possibility of provoking angina and myocardial ischemia as a result of myocardial stimulation. The drug has also been implicated in producing myocardial infarction. Other cardiovascular changes may produce worsening of cerebral ischemia, postural hypotension, and a general decrease in cardiac compensation abilities.

Patients with decreased renal function may have increased renal circulation; however, drug should be used cautiously in patients with advanced renal damage. An antipyridoxine effect may be seen in some patients, producing a worsening of peripheral neuritis which may require pyridoxine therapy if symptoms develop. Some patients may also develop blood dyscrasias, or show hypersensitivity, such as bronchial asthma, to the chemical tartrazine, which many products include. Patients who have an allergy to aspirin may be more likely to react to tartrazine than others in the general population.

IMPLEMENTATION:

DRUG INTERACTIONS: Profound hypotensive episodes may develop through additive effects when hydralazine is used with other anesthetics, antidepressants, quinidine, procainamide, diuretics and other parenteral antihypertensive agents. Hypotensive effects are antagonized by amphetamines, ephedrine, and other sympathomimetic agents, and tachycardia may be provoked by concurrent use. MAO inhibitors also should be used cautiously. May produce positive direct antiglobulin (Coombs') test.

PRODUCTS (TRADE NAME):

Apresoline (Available in 10, 25, 50, 100 mg tablets, and 20 mg/ml injections.) **Dralzine** (Available in 25 mg tablets). **Hydralazine HCl** (Available in 10, 25, 50 mg tablets).

ADMINISTRATION AND DOSAGE:

Adults: Give 10 mg four times daily for the first 2 to 4 days; increase to 25 mg four times daily for the balance of the first week. Then increase dosage to 50 mg four times daily for the following week. Evaluate patient and reduce to lowest dosage which achieves therapeutic effects without adverse reactions. When other medications are used, lower dosages of hydralazine may be effective. Each component of the drug regimen must be individually regulated and evaluated. Some patients seem able to get along on a twice-daily regimen.

After long-term administration, tolerance may develop, requiring increased dosages. Do not give more than 400 mg/day. Adverse reactions seem to be dosage-related.

Parenteral dosage: For emergency use in hospitalized patients who cannot take oral forms, IV or IM medication may be given. Use 20 to 40 mg, repeated as needed. Constant monitoring of blood pressure is mandatory, as pressure may begin to fall within 10 minutes after injection.

IMPLEMENTATION CONSIDERATIONS:

—Obtain a complete health history, including the presence of hypersensitivity (including reactions to tartrazine or aspirin), concurrent use of other medications which might cause drug interactions, presence of underlying systemic disease such as rheumatic or coronary artery disease, renal impairment, and possibility of pregnancy.

—Individual adjustments of this medication dosage, as well as other step one and Step Two antihypertensive drugs, will be important for achieving the therapeutic objectives.

—Teaching, counseling, and establishing rapport with the patient will be important in obtaining patient compliance in taking the medications and keeping clinic appointments.

—Increasing the dosage of hydralazine too rapidly may produce a marked fall in blood pressure if the patient has uremia or very severe hypertension. This may cause certain central nervous system symptoms, ranging from mild anxiety or depression to more severe forms of coma or depression.

—In any situation in which someone whose disorder has been controlled by hydralazine must stop taking the drug, withdraw the medication slowly so as not to precipitate a rapid rise in pressure.

—Pyridoxine may need to be added to the therapeutic regimen if patient develops numbness and tingling or other paresthesias.

—Discontinue therapy if there are indications that patient is developing a blood dyscrasia. Periodic monitoring for blood changes is advised.

—Side effects are usually reversible, especially when dosage is reduced. If symptoms persist, medication should be discontinued.

—Systemic lupus erythematosus (SLE)-like syndrome occurs more frequently in patients receiving doses greater than 200 mg/day, in patients with impaired renal function and in "slow acetylators." (Eskimos, Orientals and American Indians have the lowest incidence of slow acetylators. Egyptians, Israelis, Scandinavians, other Caucasians, and Black populations have the highest incidence of slow acetylators).

—Patients with impaired renal function may require lower doses.

WHAT THE PATIENT NEEDS TO KNOW:

—Take this medication as directed by your health care provider. Changes may need to be made depending upon the response of your blood pressure to the current regimen. Any failure to take medication as directed may make evaluation of the medicine's benefits difficult.

—Do not take other medications, or stop taking this medicine, without the knowledge of your health care provider. Do not take cough, cold, or allergy medications or other over-the-counter medications without the knowledge of your health care practitioner.

—Medicine should be taken with meals or a snack. Taking food at the same time as the medicine helps the body absorb the maximum amount of the drug.

—Some people experience side effects from this drug. Most of these reactions are mild and brief. However, it is important to discuss with your health care provider any new or troublesome symptoms so that they might be properly evaluated. Especially report any unexplained or excessively long periods of feeling tired, periods of fever, chest pain, muscle, or joint aching.

—During the first few days of therapy, medication may cause headaches or a feeling that your heart is pounding. These symptoms should disappear within a few days.

—Change positions slowly to decrease the risk of feeling lightheaded which may accompany this drug. It is most important to move slowly from the lying to standing position, especially first thing in the morning.

—Keep this medication out of the reach of children and all others for whom it is not prescribed.

—If you miss a dose, take it as soon as you remember if it is within an hour or two of the scheduled time. If it is close to your next scheduled dose take only the dose at the regular time. Do not double doses.

—Take medication with a full glass of orange juice (unless not on your diet). Other potassium-rich foods should be used daily. These include: citrus foods (especially oranges and tomatoes), bananas, dried fruits, apricots, cantaloupe, watermelon, nuts, dried beans, beef, and fowl.

—Taking medication is only one part of your treatment regimen. Reduction of other risk factors is also important: lose weight (if overweight), stop smoking, increase exercise, avoid stressful and emotional pressures. Avoid use of foods high in sodium: lunch meats, smoked meats, Chinese food, processed cheese, snack foods. Do not salt food while cooking or add salt to your food after it is cooked.

EVALUATION:

ADVERSE REACTIONS: *Cardiovascular:* angina, edema, postural hypotension, palpitations, paradoxical pressor response, tachycardia. *CNS:* dizziness, headache, mood changes, peripherial neuritis (paresthesias, numbness, tingling), psychotic reactions (anxiety, depression, disorientation), tremors. *Gastrointestinal:* anorexia, constipation, diarrhea, nausea, paralytic ileus, vomiting. *Genitourinary:* difficulty starting stream, impotence (rare). *Hematopoietic:* blood dyscrasias (agranulocytosis, decrease in RBC and hemoglobin, leukopenia, and purpura), lymphadenopathy. *Hypersensitivity:* arthralgia, chills, eosinophilia, fever, hepatitis and obstructive jaundice (rare), pruritus, rash, urticaria. *Ophthalmologic:* conjunctivitis, lacrimation. *Other:* dyspnea, flushing, lymphadenopathy, muscle cramps, nasal congestion, splenomegaly, weight gain.

OVERDOSAGE: *Signs and symptoms:* Headache, hypotension, tachycardia, and generalized skin flushing develop initially. Shock associated with cardiac arrhythmias and myocardial infarction may also develop. *Treatment:* Induce emesis, and refer for gavage and symptomatic treatment. Cardiac functioning must be ensured and treatment for shock should not aggravate tachycardia and arrhythmias which are usually present. General therapy should be overseen by a specialist.

PARAMETERS TO MONITOR: A complete history, physical, and laboratory evaluation should be conducted prior to initiation of therapy. Patient should be seen regularly to evaluate for therapeutic effects and development of adverse reactions. Watch for lupus-like reactions: skin lesions, fever, dermatoses, myalgia, arthralgia, anemia. Discontinue drug if symptoms develop. Most symptoms regress when drug is withdrawn, but some may persist for years. Also watch for chest pain, fever, sore throat, and weakness which may indicate myocardial ischemia or development of blood dyscrasias. Mental acuity changes may result from changes in cerebral blood flow. Edema and weight gain may also be detected. A flow chart should be developed to record individualized parameters in history (such as development of arthralgias, fever, chest pain, continued malaise) physical (such as development of bruising, skin reactions simulating lupus, fever, splenomegaly), and laboratory work which are relevant for each patient. Patient should be seen each week for the first month after being placed on this medication. CBC, LE cell preparations and ANA titers should be drawn periodically. Evaluation of patient's compliance to dosage regimen is important in determining whether dosage prescribed is adequate. Education and teaching should be carried out as needed to reduce other disease risk factors.

Marilyn W. Edmunds

ANTIHYPERTENSIVES—
MECAMYLAMINE HYDROCHLORIDE

ACTION OF THE DRUG: Mecamylamine is a secondary amine which effects the body systemically. This medication acts by competitive antagonism of acetylcholine at autonomic ganglia to reduce the blood pressure in both hypertensive and normotensive patients. It also penetrates the blood-brain barrier and may be responsible for various CNS symptoms.

ASSESSMENT:

INDICATIONS: This drug is rarely used because of the many side effects and profound hypotension produced. It is effective in the treatment of moderate to severe hypertension, and is used in malignant hypertension when there are no complications. It is not routinely used in the stepped-care therapy for hypertension. Nurse practitioners would not prescribe this drug, but may have responsibility for monitoring patient response to it and altering dosages.

SUBJECTIVE: Patient presents with a history of known hypertension and therapy with a variety of other antihypertensive drugs. There may be subjective symptoms of hypertension, end-organ damage, or side effects from other medications.

OBJECTIVE: Patient may have cardiomegaly, diffuse PMI, systolic ejection murmurs, third or fourth heart sounds. There may be evidence of hemorrhage, nicking, or exudates of optic fundus, or blurring of the disc margins if hypertension is severe enough. There may be rales on chest examination, and the presence of peripheral edema or paresthesias.

PLAN:

CONTRAINDICATIONS: Do not give in the presence of hypersensitivity, in uremia, chronic pyelonephritis, glaucoma, organic pyloric stenosis, coronary insufficiency or acute myocardial infarction. Use with caution in patients with renal insufficiency.

WARNINGS: In patients receiving high doses or with renal insufficiency, watch for convulsions, tremors, choreiform movements, and mental changes which may result secondary to the CNS effects of the drug. It is mandatory that patients be withdrawn slowly from this drug (over a period of 3-4 weeks) and other antihypertensive therapy increased. Abruptly stopping the medication may produce rebound hypertension which may precipitate congestive heart failure or cerebrovascular accidents.

PRECAUTIONS: The appropriate selection of this drug for use with patients involves screening patients to eliminate those who might not tolerate decreased blood flow or hypotension. Patients with preexisting compromise to renal, cerebral or cardiovascular blood flow are not candidates for this drug. This drug may produce urinary retention and therefore should be used carefully in patients with urethral strictures, prostatic hypertrophy, or bladder neck obstruction.

The action of this drug may be potentiated by salt depletion. Any situation which may produce fluid and electrolyte changes (diarrhea, vomiting, excessive sweating, high external heat, fever, infection, hemorrhage, surgery, vigorous exercise, pregnancy) may require dosage alterations. Patients who have been on thiazide diuretic therapy may also experience increased sensitivity to this drug.

IMPLEMENTATION:

DRUG INTERACTIONS: Increased hypotension may be precipitated by concurrent use of diuretics, other antihypertensive drugs, alcohol, bethanechol, and general anesthesia. It may potentiate effects of sympathomimetic drugs.

PRODUCTS (TRADE NAME):
Inversine (Available in 2.5, 10 mg scored tablets.)

ADMINISTRATION AND DOSAGE: Medication has a gradual onset of action of about 30 minutes to 2 hours, with duration of up to 12 hours. Give 2.5 mg po twice daily. May increase medication in 2.5 mg increments every 2 days until therapeutic objective is reached. Adjust dose for individual according to response of standing blood pressure and symptoms of hypotension. Usually 25 mg in 3 divided doses is adequate. If used with other agents, reduce the dosage of mecamylamine and other antihypertensive agents by 50% but keep thiazide diuretics at normal level.

IMPLEMENTATION CONSIDERATIONS:
—Obtain a complete health history, including the presence of hypersensitivity, other medications taken concurrently which might produce drug interactions, underlying renal, cerebrovascular or cardiovascular disease, glaucoma, or pyloric stenosis.

—Because of the potency of this drug, it should be reserved for patients with more severe forms of hypertension and not given in mild cases.

—Patients who are not reliable in taking medication, keeping appointments, or accurately reporting response to drug are not good candidates for mecamylamine therapy. It is important for the practitioner to establish rapport with the patient and to provide necessary teaching and counseling in order to obtain maximum compliance.

—While patient is on this medication, do not restrict salt intake. If patient becomes salt depleted, the hypotensive effects of the drug are potentiated. Be alert to other developments in the patient's medical picture which may make him vulnerable to fluid and electrolyte imbalance.

—Partial tolerance may develop to this drug after patient has been maintained for some time. This may require increasing dosages.

—In order to maintain a smooth control of patient's blood pressure, evaluate the pressure in lying, sitting, and standing positions. Therapy adjustments should be based upon the standing pressure. If possible, pressure should be measured at the peak of drug action.

—Because blood pressure may vary throughout the day, smooth control may be more likely if medication is given in 4 or more doses, with the smallest in the morning and the largest in the evening.

—Medication should be taken at the same time every day, preferably following a meal, which enhances absorption.

—Patient should be taught regarding the hypotensive effects of the drug, and warned to withhold a dose if excessive hypotension develops. Patient should notify health care provider if symptoms persist at the time for the second dose. Some patients or family may be taught to take the patient's blood pressure and can be advised to withhold a dose if blood pressure falls below a certain level. Evaluation of patients who can intelligently handle this responsibility should be made.

—Diarrhea, decreased bowel sounds, and abdominal distention are signs of paralytic ileus. Drug should be discontinued at once if these signs develop.

—Constipation may be treated with milk of magnesia.

—Do not stop drug suddenly, but taper off over a period of weeks in order to avoid rebound of hypertension and increase risk of producing cerebrovascular accident.

—Effects of medication may be increased by fever, infection, salt depletion, hemorrhage, and pregnancy.

WHAT THE PATIENT NEEDS TO KNOW:

—Take this medication exactly as prescribed by practitioner. It is important to not alter dosages or skip doses. Abruptly stopping this drug is dangerous.

—This medication frequently produces a feeling of lightheadedness or faintness. This will be especially noted when changing positions rapidly, particularly early in the morning. Time should be allocated to gradually get up in the morning, first to a sitting position, and then standing. Your tolerance for standing in one position may also be decreased.

—Your health care provider will instruct you on how to proceed if you note excessive dizziness, especially when it is time for another dose of medicine.

—Keep this medicine out of the reach of children and all others for whom it is not prescribed.

—This medicine works best when taken right after eating. Often the largest dose is taken in the evening and the smallest dose at lunchtime.

—Do not take any other medication, including cough, cold, or allergy medication which you may buy over the counter, without the knowledge of your health practitioner.

—Do not drink alcoholic beverages while taking this medicine, since it may increase your feelings of dizziness.

—If you note any change in bowel habits, i.e., constipation or the presence of frequent loose stools, notify health care provider.

—The goal of therapy is to help you feel as healthy as possible and to avoid any complications. Generally there is no cure for hypertension and therapy extends for a lifetime. Taking your medication and reducing other risk factors (losing weight, cessation of smoking, increasing exercise, reduction of stress) will help reduce the chance of serious complications. It is important to keep taking your medicine, even when you feel well, and to keep seeing your health practitioner regularly.

—Wear a Medic-Alert bracelet and carry a medical identification card specifying that you have hypertension, and the drugs which you are taking.

EVALUATION:

ADVERSE REACTIONS: *Cardiovascular:* dizziness, lightheadedness, orthostatic hypotension, paresthesias, syncope. *CNS:* blurred vision, convulsions, choreiform movements, dilated pupils, fatigue, mental abnormalities, sedation, tremor. *Gastrointestinal:* abdominal distention, anorexia, constipation, dryness of the mouth and tongue, nausea, paralytic ileus, vomiting. *Other:* decreased libido, impotence, urinary retention.

OVERDOSAGE: If hypotension develops, small doses of pressor amines may be given.

PARAMETERS TO MONITOR: Obtain a complete history, physical and laboratory evaluation prior to initiation of therapy. This should include detailed ophthalmoscopic, heart, chest, and abdominal examination, and laboratory CBC, electrolytes, uric acid, glucose level, urinalysis, ECG, and chest x-ray. Screen patient carefully to determine both physical and mental appropriateness of this candidate for receiving mecamylamine therapy. Monitor for therapeutic effect: decrease in blood pressure when taken in the standing, lying, and sitting positions. Changes in therapy should be based upon standing pressure at peak of medication action and upon patient's subjective complaints of hypotension. Monitor for adverse effects. Follow weights and pulse rate, and evaluate electrolytes periodically to check for imbalance. Check urine for pH as toxicity can be intensified by drugs that increase urinary pH. Watch for urinary retention. Make a flow chart to guide evaluation each visit regarding common signs and symptoms which would indicate target organ damage.

Marilyn W. Edmunds

ANTIHYPERTENSIVES—
METHYLDOPA AND METHYLDOPATE HCL

ACTION OF THE DRUG: Methyldopa is an antiadrenergic agent which is thought to reduce blood pressure through (1) reduction of plasma renin levels (although renal blood flow and cardiac output are not significantly affected); (2) stimulation of brain stem inhibitory alpha-adrenergic receptors to decrease outflow of sympathetic vasoconstrictors and cardioaccelerator impulses, thus producing vasodilation and bradycardia (methyldopa inhibits the enzyme aromatic amino acid decarboxylase through competitive antagonism and chemically converts to a product which functions as an activator of central alpha-2-adrenergic receptors); and (3) false neurotransmission. Tissue concentrations of epinephrine, norepinephrine, serotonin and dopamine are also decreased by methyldopa. Diurnal blood pressure variations rarely occur. Sodium and water are retained, and there is a mild sedative action.

ASSESSMENT:

INDICATIONS: Methyldopa is useful for the treatment of chronic moderate and severe hypertension. It may be used alone, but is more commonly used as a Step Two drug. It is not indicated for the treatment of mild labile hypertension or diastolic elevations caused by pheochromocytoma. Methyldopate HCl is sometimes used parenterally in hypertensive crisis, but other agents which work faster are generally preferred.

SUBJECTIVE: Patient may be asymptomatic, or may complain of not feeling well in general. Headaches, frequently associated with hypertension, are often produced by stress, tension, or other reasons, rather than being related to high blood pressure, unless very severe blood pressure elevations are present. In cases of secondary hypertension, there may be reports of nocturia (if patient is unable to concentrate urine), history of renal trauma (producing renal artery stenosis), or family history of hypertension.

OBJECTIVE: Patient may have elevated blood pressure due to numerous factors: full bladder, anxiety, pain, etc. If the average blood pressure is found to be above 140/90 mm Hg on three consecutive readings (within a 2-4 week interval), the patient is assumed to be hypertensive. Diastolic readings greater than 120 mm Hg indicate need for immediate medical care. Blood pressure should be obtained in lying, sitting, and standing positions in both arms, and in cases where coarctation of the aorta is part of the diagnostic differential, in the lower extremities. Eyes should be examined for the presence of increased arteriovenous (AV) ratio, nicking, hemorrhages, or exudates in the fundus of the eye, and blurring of the disc margins. Chest should be examined for diffuse point of maximum intensity (PMI), displacement of PMI to the left, thrusts, murmurs, and presence of third and fourth heart sounds. (Systolic ejection murmurs and fourth heart sounds commonly develop in hypertensive patients.) Abdomen should be assessed for renal artery bruits.

PLAN:

CONTRAINDICATIONS: Methyldopa should not be used in presence of hypersensitivity, active hepatic disease (hepatitis, cirrhosis), or if previous therapy with methyldopa has caused hepatic dysfunction.

WARNINGS: With prolonged therapy (6-12 months), 10-20% of patients develop a positive direct Coombs' test. In some cases this precedes the development of a hemolytic anemia which may lead to potentially fatal complications. If a positive Coombs' test develops, evaluate patient for possibility of a hemolytic anemia; methyldopa may need to be stopped.

Some patients have also developed hypersensitivity to methyldopa, manifested by severe liver dysfunction. Fever early in the therapy, associated with eosinophilia and abnormalities in one or more liver function tests, may reveal cholestasis. Liver function should therefore be monitored closely, especially in the early phase of treatment.

Occasionally there are hematologic abnormalities which develop as a result of this drug. The most notable is a reduction in the white blood cell count (WBC), affecting primarily the granulocytes. Decrease is reversible once therapy is discontinued.

Methyldopa crosses the placental barrier and can be found in breast milk. Safety during pregnancy and breast-feeding has not been established, and risk should be compared to benefit.

PRECAUTIONS: Use with caution in patients with liver dysfunction and severe cerebrovascular disease. A paradoxical pressor response is seen rarely with use of IV methyldopate HCl and methyldopa. If involuntary choreoathetotic movements are produced by this product, discontinue drug.

IMPLEMENTATION:

DRUG INTERACTIONS: Use with other antihypertensives, alcohol, methotrimeprazine, levodopa, anesthetics, narcotics, quinidine, vasodilators and diuretics potentiates the hypotensive effects. Antagonistic effects may be produced by MAO inhibitors, amphetamines, catecholamines, and tricyclic antidepressants. Methyldopa may potentiate the action of norepinephrine, producing an increased pressor response. Tolbutamide metabolism may be decreased by methyldopa, thereby promoting more hypoglycemic effects. An increased incidence of blood dyscrasia is also noted with tolbutamide administration. Patients may require lower doses of anesthetics. Concurrent use with lithium may produce symptoms of lithium intoxication although lithium blood levels are not elevated. Concomitant use of phenoxybenzamine may lead to total urinary incontinence, which is reversible once therapy is stopped. Use with haloperidol may produce psychiatric symptoms such as aggressiveness, dementia, and irritability. Methyldopa also interferes with the following laboratory tests: BUN, elevated potassium and sodium levels, urinary uric acid, serum creatinine, SGOT (colorimetric method), and falsely high levels of urinary catecholamines.

PRODUCTS (TRADE NAME):
Aldomet (Available in 125, 250, 500 mg tablets and 250 mg/5 ml oral syrup or injections).

ADMINISTRATION AND DOSAGE: Methyldopate HCl is the parenteral form of the drug, which after injection is de-esterified almostly completely to form methyldopa. Peak effect is usually 4-6 hours after administration, with the antihypertensive activity lasting for up to 12 hours following IV dose and up to 24 hours after oral therapy. Approximately 2 days are required for maximal antihypertensive activity, or for hypertension to return after drug has been discontinued.

Oral:

Adults:

Starting dose: 250 mg po 2-3 times/day for 48 hours. Drug may then be increased or decreased, usually at intervals of not less than 2 days until an adequate response.

Maintenance dose: 500 mg-2 gm po given in 2-4 divided doses. (Maximum 3 gm/day.)

Concomitant therapy: 500 mg/day in divided doses when given with other antihypertensive agents (except for thiazides, which require no change). Dosages should be decreased in the elderly or those patients with impaired renal or hepatic function.

Children: 10 mg/kg/day po in 2-4 doses initially; increased to obtain desired therapeutic response (maximum 65 mg/kg or 3 gm daily, whichever is less).

Parenteral:

Adults: 250-500 mg IV in 100 ml 5% dextrose every 6 hours as required. (Maximum 1 gm every 6 hours.)

Children: 20-40 mg/kg in divided doses in 100 ml 5% dextrose every 6 hours (maximum 65 mg/kg or 3 gm/day, whichever is less).

When hypertensive control has been obtained, begin oral therapy with same dosage regimen as being used by parenteral route.

IMPLEMENTATION CONSIDERATIONS:

—Obtain a complete health history and physical examination, searching for a secondary cause for hypertension: Cushing's disease, Addison's disease, renal artery stenosis, coarctation of the aorta, or pheochromocytoma. Also determine presence of other underlying disease, allergies, or concurrent medications which may affect choice of drug therapy. Assess ability of patient to comply with medication and behavior modification necessary for adequate management of hypertension. Evaluate for evidence of end-organ damage and possibility of pregnancy.

—Methyldopa is a step two drug and patient should already have received maximal therapy using a thiazide or loop diuretic. Only when blood pressure cannot be controlled on step one medication, or when side effects require decreasing step one dosage should this product be introduced.

—This drug is usually well tolerated, with few significant adverse effects occurring. Sedation when the medication is started or increased is the most frequent complaint from patients receiving this drug. This problem is usually transient and patients should be advised that it will pass. Headaches and weakness may also be found frequently on initial therapy.

—A significant but rare side effect to watch for is development of a hemolytic anemia. This is often preceded by development of a positive Coombs' test, which occurs in approximately 20% of patients on chronic therapy, is dose-related and may persist for 3 to 18 months after drug is withdrawn. In the absence of other complications, it is usually not clinically significant. If a hemolytic anemia develops, it is often reversed once methyldopa is discontinued or following corticosteroid therapy. Evaluation for other possible causes of hemolytic anemia should also be pursued.

—If a patient has developed both a direct and indirect positive Coombs' test this may interfere with cross-matching of blood.

—Establishing rapport with patients, teaching, and working to obtain patient compliance in taking medication, altering diet, and in keeping future appointments is essential in achieving long-term therapeutic goals.

—To minimize the sedation associated with the dosage increases of this product, suggest that the patient start dosage increases in the evening.

—Occasionally a patient may develop tolerance to this product, usually after 2 or 3 months of therapy. Increasing the dosage of a thiazide diuretic administered concurrently or increasing the dosage of methyldopa may help.

—Collection and recording of a good initial data base (history, physical, and laboratory findings) are important in evaluating progress of end-organ damage over the years. The incidence of drug side effects and complications from inadequately treated hypertension are high, and good record keeping is important in evaluating the patient's status.

—Patients need to be encouraged to lose weight, restrict sodium intake, avoid stress and emotional pressures, develop regular and realistic exercise patterns, and engage in hobbies or activities which help self-esteem. Taking the medications should be emphasized as only a small part of this total regimen.

—Reversible methyldopa hepatotoxicity can occasionally occur, especially during the first few months of therapy. Be alert for chills, fever, headache, pruritus, rash, arthralgia, and enlarged liver. Check liver function tests. Discontinue drug if fever, jaundice, and liver function abnormalities develop.

WHAT THE PATIENT NEEDS TO KNOW:

—Take this medication exactly as ordered by your health care provider. Do not discontinue the medication until told to do so. If you miss a dose, take it as soon as you remember if it is within an hour or two of the scheduled time. If it is close to your next scheduled dose, skip it, and take the next dose at the regular time. Do not double doses.

—It will be important to have regular follow-up visits to evaluate the effectiveness of this medication in decreasing your blood pressure, and to ascertain that adverse effects have not developed.

—Patients often notice feeling sleepy during the initial period of therapy with this drug or when the dosage is increased. If you experience this, it should pass quickly and you should continue to take the medication anyway. Taking the largest dose in the evening is sometimes helpful in handling this problem. Occasionally people note headaches or feelings of weakness upon beginning this drug. If you have feelings of prolonged general fatigue, or if fever or dizziness occur, report them. Be sure to report to your health care provider immediately any symptoms which do not disappear within a week, or which are very troublesome to you.

—Should you see another health care provider, including a dentist, during the time you are taking this drug, you should inform him of this therapy. This would be especially important if he plans to prescribe medication which would interact with the drugs you are already receiving.

—Avoid allergy, cough, or cold medications which you can buy over the counter, unless recommended by your health care provider.

—You should wear a Medic-Alert bracelet or carry other identifying information about your hypertension and treatment.

—Caution is advised in changing positions to avoid dizziness. This is especially true when moving from a lying position to a standing position.

—Keep this medication out of the reach of children and others for whom it is not prescribed.

—The goal of therapy is to help you feel as healthy as possible, and to avoid complications. Generally there is no cure for hypertension, and therapy extends for a lifetime. Taking your medication and reducing other risk factors will help reduce the chance of serious complications. It is important then to keep taking your medicine, even when you feel well, and to keep seeing your health care practitioner regularly.

—Taking medication is only one part of your treatment regimen. Reduction of other risk factors is also important: lose weight (if overweight), reduce sodium intake, stop smoking, increase exercise, avoid stressful and emotional pressures. Avoid use of foods high in sodium: lunch meats, smoked meats, Chinese food, processed cheese, snack foods. Do not salt food while cooking or add salt to your food after it is cooked.

—Take this medication with a full glass of orange juice (unless contraindicated by your diet). Other potassium-rich foods should be used daily. These include: citrus foods (especially oranges and tomatoes), bananas, dried fruits, apricots, cantaloupe, watermelon, nuts, dried beans, beef, and fowl.

—Urine may appear darker because of this drug. This is not harmful.

EVALUATION:

ADVERSE REACTIONS: *Cardiovascular:* angina pectoris, bradycardia, edema, myocarditis (fatal), paradoxical pressor response, orthostatic hypotension. *CNS:* asthenia, decreased mental acuity, depression, dizziness, headache, involuntary choreoathetoid movements, lightheadedness, memory impairment, nightmares, numbness, pain or weakness in hands or feet, parkinsonian-like symptoms, paresthesias, psychic disturbances, psychoses (reversible and mild), sedation, tingling, weakness. *Gastrointestinal:* abdominal distension, abnormal liver function tests, acute colitis (reversible), constipation, diarrhea, flatus, jaundice, liver disorders, mild dryness of mouth, nausea, pancreatitis, sialadenitis, sore or black tongue, vomiting. *Hematopoietic:* eosinophilia, granulocytopenia, hemolytic anemia, leukopenia, thrombocytopenia, positive Coombs' test, positive tests for antinuclear antibody, LE cells and rheumatoid factor, rise in BUN, falsely high urinary catecholamines. *Hypersensitivity:* drug-related fever, lupus-like syndrome. *Other:* arthralgia, breast enlargement, decreased libido, dermatologic reactions including eczema and lichenoid eruptions, skin rash, failure to ejaculate, gynecomastia, impotence, lactation, mild arthralgia, myalgia, nasal stuffiness, tiredness, unexplained fever, weight gain.

PARAMETERS TO MONITOR: At the start of therapy, perform a complete blood count (hematocrit, hemoglobin, WBC, RBC, and differential) to establish a blood data base. Also obtain a baseline Coombs' test and liver function tests. Throughout therapy, monitor for therapeutic effect (i.e., reduction of blood pressure and increase or decrease dosage depending upon clinical results). Patient should achieve therapeutic effect within 48 hours after taking medication or increasing doses. Expect initial complaints of sedation, headache and weakness which should pass with continued therapy. Check for signs and symptoms of edema, fever, anemia, myocarditis, hepatitis, parkinsonism, colitis, pancreatitis, thrombocytopenia. Also monitor for symptoms of end-organ damage (cardiomegaly, cardiac murmurs, development of S3 heart sound, edema, impaired renal function, appearance of nicking, hemorrhages, and exudates in the eye fundus.) Finally, monitor for adverse effects related to drug. Obtain periodic blood counts to check for hemolytic anemia, and repeat Coombs' tests at least at 6 and 12 months of therapy. Liver function studies should be evaluated regularly, especially during the first 4-12 weeks of therapy and if patient develops any unexplained fever. Discontinue medication if involuntary choreoathetotic movement, liver or hematologic disorders appear.

Marilyn W. Edmunds

ANTIHYPERTENSIVES—MINOXIDIL

ACTION OF THE DRUG: Minoxidil acts to reduce systolic and diastolic blood pressure by direct relaxation of vascular smooth muscle, decreasing peripheral vascular resistance. The exact mechanism of action of vascular smooth muscle is not known but it appears to block calcium uptake through the cell membrane.

Reduction in peripheral resistance and the fall in blood pressure stimulate release of renin, increase cardiac output, and lead to conservation of salt and water. Because minoxidil does not interfere with vasomotor reflexes, no orthostatic hypotension is produced and CNS function is not altered. Blood pressure reduction is related to dosage administered, and action is proportional to the extent of hypertension. Renal blood flow and glomerular filtration rate are not altered.

ASSESSMENT:

INDICATIONS: Although minoxidil is a potent vasodilator, it should not be considered a step three drug for routine use in treatment of hypertension. It is a potent drug, reserved for patients who are severely hypertensive, who have target organ damage, and who have not responded to maximal doses of at least two other antihypertensives and a diuretic. It should be prescribed under the direction of a specialist and administered initially in hospitalized patients who can be monitored closely. The nurse practitioner frequently has responsibility for evaluating the patient's response to this medication. Because of the predictable sympathetic, vagal inhibitory and renal homeostatic mechanisms which this medication also stimulates, it is best used concomitantly with graded doses of a beta-adrenergic blocking agent (to prevent tachycardia and increased myocardial workloads), and a diuretic (frequently one acting in the ascending limb of the loop of Henle) to prevent fluid accumulation.

SUBJECTIVE: Patient presents with a history of known hypertension and therapy with a variety of other antihypertensive drugs. There may be subjective symptoms of hypertension, end-organ damage, or side effects of other medications.

OBJECTIVE: Patient may have cardiomegaly, diffuse PMI, systolic ejection murmur, third or fourth heart sound. There may be evidence of hemorrhage, nicking, or exudates in optic fundus, or blurring of the disc margins if hypertension is severe enough. There may be rales on chest examination and the presence of peripheral edema or paresthesias.

PLAN:

CONTRAINDICATIONS: Do not give in the presence of hypersensitivity. In hypertension secondary to pheochromocytoma, minoxidil stimulates increased tumor secretion of catecholamines and therefore should not be used.

WARNINGS: This product has been associated with several severe adverse effects: angina pectoris may be precipitated, and pericardial effusions may develop, occasionally progressing to tamponade. There is also the possibility that this drug may cause a variety of serious cardiac lesions, such as papillary muscle or atrial hemorrhagic lesions, although this has not been documented in humans.

The propensity of the drug to cause fluid and salt retention requires careful monitoring, especially in patients in whom there is a history of preexisting congestive heart failure. Omitting an effective diuretic in the therapeutic regimen may rapidly lead to substantial volume retention and resultant problems.

Because the drug also increases heart rate, angina or congestive failure may worsen or appear for the first time. Sympathetic blockage may prevent this problem and beta-adrenergic blocking agents or other sympathetic nervous system suppressants (clonidine or methyldopa) may be useful.

Intravenous use of minoxidil in patients with malignant hypertension may precipitate myocardial infarction or cerebrovascular accidents if blood pressure is reduced too rapidly. These patients should be hospitalized so that the rate of pressure reduction can be carefully monitored.

Safety for use has not been established in pregnant women, breast-feeding women or in children. Use in these circumstances requires careful evaluation of the risk-benefit ratio.

PRECAUTIONS: Because minoxidil may limit blood flow to the myocardium, its use following myocardial infarction is prudently avoided. While the decreased oxygen demand because of lower blood pressure may have a positive effect on the heart, it is usually possible to achieve that effect with a different medication.

IMPLEMENTATION:

DRUG INTERACTIONS: Concurrent use of minoxidil with guanethidine results in profound orthostatic changes. If at all possible guanethidine should be discontinued prior to use of minoxidil, or patients should be hospitalized and carefully monitored to prevent dangerous orthostasis. Laboratory findings may be altered in the following ways: alkaline phosphatase increases and serum BUN and creatinine levels increase and then decrease to pretreatment levels.

PRODUCTS (TRADE NAME):
Loniten (Available in 2.5 and 10 mg tablets.)

ADMINISTRATION AND DOSAGE:

Adults and children over 12: Give 5 mg/day po in a single dose. Increase to 10, 20 and then to 40 mg in single or divided doses to achieve blood pressure control. Maximum recommended dosage is 100 mg/day.

Children under 12: Give 0.2 mg/kg/day po in a single dose. Increase in 50% to 100% increments until blood pressure is controlled. Maximum recommended dosage is 50 mg/daily.

All dosages should be evaluated against patient blood pressure response. Normally patient should take medication at one level for at least 3 days before evaluation or change in dosage is made. If a patient is closely monitored and the need exists, dosage changes could be made every 6 hours.

Concurrent administration of diuretics is essential and they may be administered in the following amounts: hydrochlorothiazide 50 mg twice daily (or equivalent thiazide dosages), or furosemide 40 mg twice daily, or chlorthalidone 50 to 100 mg once daily. The concurrent use of a adrenergic beta blocker should be the equivalent of propranolol, 80 to 160 mg/day in divided doses.

If beta-blockers are contraindicated, methyldopa 250 to 750 mg twice daily may be given, administered initially at least 24 hours before minoxidil is introduced. Clonidine 0.1 to 0.2 mg twice daily may also be given to suppress the reflex tachycardia.

IMPLEMENTATION CONSIDERATIONS:

—Obtain a complete health history, including presence of hypersensitivity, a thorough history of patient's previous therapeutic regimens for hypertension, concurrent use of guanethidine, presence of target organ damage, or underlying systemic disease such as renal insufficiency, coronary artery or cerebrovascular disease, and concurrent use of other medications. Also assess for the possibility of pregnancy.

—Compliance is often a problem, since a patient placed on this drug is usually receiving a variety of other medications. Your ability to teach, counsel and establish rapport with the patient will be an important factor in obtaining compliance in taking medications and keeping appointments for evaluation.

—Some patients develop hypersensitivity, as manifested primarily through a skin rash. Whether the drug should be discontinued when this appears often depends upon the severity of hypertension and other therapeutic alternatives.

—Patients with renal disease may be more sensitive to this medication, and reduced dosage levels may be indicated to prevent adverse reactions.

—Pericardial effusion may develop in approximately 3% of treated patients. Patients with uremic disease, congestive failure, connective tissue disorders, or marked fluid retention may be more likely to develop pericardial effusion. These patients should be carefully monitored if minoxidil is indicated for treatment of severely elevated pressures. Echocardiography may be indicated if suspicion of pericardial effusion develops. Stopping the drug, along with vigorous diuretic therapy and pericardiocentesis, may be indicated if effusion develops.

—Monitor patient's weight and watch for other evidence of fluid retention.

—Monitor ECG periodically. Watch for development of nonspecific T wave changes. These usually disappear as treatment is continued and are not evidence of myocardial damage.

—If excessive salt and water retention develops and patient gains more than 5 pounds, discontinue thiazide therapy and utilize furosemide. If patient is already on furosemide, increase dosage to control symptoms.

—Evaluate patient's blood pressure in lying, sitting, and standing positions. If lying blood pressure has been reduced less than 30 mm Hg, administer the drug only once a day. If pressure has been reduced more than 30 mm Hg, divide the daily dose into two equal amounts.

—The excessive growth of fine body hair is frequently extremely upsetting to children and women. This develops within 3 to 6 weeks of therapy. Because this happens in approximately 80% of patients, they need to be warned of this reaction and encouraged to keep taking the medication.

—May give medication concomitantly with beta-blockers to prevent reflex tachycardia.

WHAT THE PATIENT NEEDS TO KNOW:

—Minoxidil is a very potent antihypertensive medication, generally taken with a variety of other drugs which are carefully balanced to help reduce your blood pressure. Medications should be taken exactly as indicated by your health care provider. Do not change dosages or discontinue any medications without instructions to do so. If you miss a dose, take it as soon as you remember if it is within an hour or two of the scheduled time. If it is close to your next scheduled dose, skip it, and take the next dose at the regular time. Do not double doses.

—Medication should be taken with a full glass of water or orange juice (unless contraindicated by your diet); food neither enhances nor reduces absorption. Other potassium-rich foods should be used daily. These include: citrus foods (especially oranges and tomatoes), bananas, dried fruits, apricots, cantaloupe, watermelon, nuts, dried beans, beef, and fowl.

—Most patients (80%) experience an increase in growth and darkening of the fine body hair while taking this drug. This usually begins about one month after therapy has started, and may take 2-6 months to return to the normal state after therapy has ended. It is first noted in area of temples, eyebrows, and sideburns, later affecting back, arms and legs.

—Patients may experience some side effects from this drug. Any new or troublesome symptoms should be reported to your health care provider. Especially note the presence of rapid weight gain of more than 5 pounds; unusual swelling of feet, hands, abdomen, or face; difficulty in breathing; awakening in the night coughing and unable to catch breath; dizziness or fainting; increased heart rate of 20 or more beats/minute over normal; new or increasing episodes of chest, left arm, or shoulder pain.

—Keep this and all other medications out of the reach of children or others for whom they are not prescribed.

—Taking medication is only one part of your treatment regimen. Reduction of other risk factors is also important: lose weight (if overweight), stop smoking, increase exercise, avoid stressful and emotional pressures. Avoid use of foods high in sodium: lunch meats, smoked meats, Chinese food, processed cheese, snack foods. Do not salt while cooking or add salt to your food after it is cooked.

—The goal of therapy is to help you feel as healthy as possible, and to avoid any complications. Generally there is no cure for hypertension, and therapy extends for a lifetime. Taking your medication and reducing other risk factors will help reduce the chance of serious complications. It is important then to keep taking your medicine, even when you feel well, and to keep seeing your health practitioner regularly.

—Wear a Medic-Alert bracelet and carry a medical identification card specifying that you have hypertension and the drugs which you are taking.

EVALUATION:

ADVERSE REACTIONS: *Cardiovascular:* ECG changes: changes in direction and magnitude of T waves, pericardial effusion, peripheral edema, rebound hypertension following withdrawl of medication, reflex tachycardia, tamponade. *Hematopoietic:* transient reduction in hematocrit, hemoglobin, and erythrocyte levels, thrombocytopenia. *Other:* breast tenderness, darkening of the skin, fatigue, fluid and electrolyte imbalance, hypersensitivity reactions, hypertrichosis (increase in length, thickness and coloration of fine body hair), increase of alkaline phosphatase and serum creatinine, headache, nausea, rash.

OVERDOSAGE: *Signs and symptoms:* Marked hypotension may develop if large dose is taken concurrently with guanethidine. *Treatment:* Maintain blood pressure, treat symptomatically but avoid sympathomimetic drugs. Angiotensin II, dopamine, phenylephrine, and vasopressin all reverse hypotensive effects of minoxidil but should be reserved for emergency use.

PARAMETERS TO MONITOR: A complete history, physical examination, and laboratory work should be obtained prior to beginning therapy with minoxidil. Patient should be hospitalized for initial doses, and then monitored closely if continued on maintenance therapy. Monitor for extent of blood pressure reduction and for development of adverse reactions. Develop a flow chart of items to evaluate each visit from history (presence of body hair, breast tenderness, dyspnea, chest pain), physical (changes in point of maximum intensity (PMI) or left boarder of cardiac dullness (LBCD) on cardiovascular examination, peripheral edema, rash), and laboratory studies (development of non-specific T wave changes, development of anemias, changes in BUN, creatinine, or alkaline phosphatase levels. Allow at least 3 days between dosage adjustments for full effect of drug to become apparent. Patient should also be monitored for progressive insult to target organs. Evaluate patient compliance and teach and counsel about diet, medications, hypertension, risk factor reduction, or other items as indicated.

Marilyn W. Edmunds

ANTIHYPERTENSIVES—
PARGYLINE HYDROCHLORIDE

ACTION OF THE DRUG: After several weeks of therapy, pargyline HCl exerts antihypertensive effects, although the mechanism of action is unknown. It may form a "false neurotransmitter" in adrenergic nerve endings and may elevate central catecholamine levels, interfering with sympathetic venoconstriction. It may also modify ganglionic transmission. It is a monoamine oxidase (MAO) inhibitor and shares many characteristics with the antidepressant MAO inhibitors.

ASSESSMENT:

INDICATIONS: This medication is not part of the regular stepped care therapy for hypertension and is reserved only for patients with moderate to severe elevations of blood pressure. It may be used alone but is most often used with thiazide diuretics, reserpine, or other antihypertensive agents. It is not prescribed by nurse practitioners; however, they frequently have responsibility for monitoring the patient's response and dosage changes.

SUBJECTIVE: Patient presents with a history of known hypertension and therapy with a variety of other antihypertensive drugs. There may be subjective symptoms of hypertension, end-organ damage, or side effects from other medications.

OBJECTIVE: Patient may have cardiomegaly, diffuse PMI, systolic ejection murmur, third or fourth heart sounds. There may be evidence of hemorrhage, nicking, or exudates in optic fundus, or blurring of the disc margins if hypertension is severe enough. There may be rales on chest examination, and the presence of peripheral edema or paresthesias.

PLAN:

CONTRAINDICATIONS: Do not use in the presence of hypersensitivity, hyperthyroidism, renal failure, pheochromocytoma or paranoid schizophrenia. There is no clinical information available regarding use in children under 12 and in patients with malignant hypertension.

There are many drugs and food whose concurrent use contraindicates administration of pargyline. (See Drug Interactions section.)

WARNINGS: Because pargyline is excreted primarily in the urine, caution should be used in patients with impaired renal function. If BUN begins to increase, drug may have to be withdrawn. Pargyline may induce hypoglycemia, and may precipitate severe hypoglycemia in diabetic patients if not monitored closely. Dosage of antidiabetic agents may need to be reduced to decrease this risk. Patients requiring surgery or who are to receive CNS depressants should have pargyline discontinued at least 2 weeks prior to receiving other CNS drugs. An exaggerated response to anesthetics, antihistamines, hypnotics, sedatives, tranquilizers, and narcotics will be seen if the effect of pargyline is still present. Safety for use in pregnancy and breast feeding has not been established. Risks should be weighed versus potential benefits before this therapy is selected.

PRECAUTIONS: Patients with impaired renal, cardiovascular or cerebrovascular circulation should be closely monitored. They may not be able to tolerate orthostatic hypotension and cerebral or coronary vessel thrombosis may be precipitated. Febrile illnesses increase the hypotensive effect of pargyline and medication should be withheld during periods of temperature elevation. Patients to receive pargyline should be screened for mental stability since previous clinical trials have revealed the development of severe psychotic illnesses in patients with history of emotional problems. Increases of motor activity, restlessness, confusion, disorientation, and agitation may also be precipitated. Because of this, pargyline should also be used with caution in patients with Parkinson's disease. Unlike other MAO inhibitors, no cases of hepatic or optic damage have been noted in conjunction with pargyline therapy. But because they are in the same family, particular evaluation of these systems should be made throughout therapy. The 25 mg tablet contains tartrazine, a substance to which many people, especially those with sensitivity to aspirin, may develop an allergic reaction. Caution should therefore be used in these patients.

IMPLEMENTATION:

DRUG INTERACTIONS: Do not use with centrally or peripherally acting sympathomimetic drugs; parenteral reserpine or guanethidine; methyldopa, levodopa or dopamine; or other MAO inhibitors. (These drugs often augment the effect of pargyline or increase the excitability of the patient.) Caffeine, alcohol, barbiturates, chloral hydrate and other hypnotics, sedatives, tranquilizers, and narcotics, as well as antihistamines, should be used at a reduced dosage to avoid hypotensive effects. Some patients may become refractory to the nerve blocking effects of local anesthetics such as lidocaine. Concomitant use of tricyclic antidepressants may produce vascular collapse and hyperthermia which may be fatal.

While taking this drug, patient should not eat aged or processed cheese, beer, wine, chocolate, yeast extract, avocado, pickled herring, pods of broad beans, ripened bananas, papaya products (including certain meat tenderizers), and chicken livers. These foods often contain pressor amines or tyramine. In some patients, tyramine may precipitate an episode of severe hypertension, headache, chest pain, profuse sweating, palpitation, visual disturbances, tachycardia or bradycardia, coma, and intracranial bleeding.

PRODUCTS (TRADE NAME):

Eutonyl Filmtabs (Available in 10, 25, 50 mg tablets.)

ADMINISTRATION AND DOSAGE: Give 25 mg po once daily, increasing once a week in 10 mg increments until the therapeutic objective is achieved. Maximum dose is 200 mg daily. In patients already receiving antihypertensive medications, in elderly patients, or in patients with sympathectomy, the daily dosage should be 10 to 25 mg. It may take 1-3 weeks before effects of the medication are observed, and medication should not be increased more frequently than once a week. Once pressure is controlled, usually dosage may be reduced to 25 to 50 mg po daily or a level sufficiently low to control pressure and reduce side effects. If pargyline is the sole antihypertensive agent and tolerance develops, addition of another antihypertensive agent may be considered.

IMPLEMENTATION CONSIDERATIONS:

—Obtain a complete health history, including the presence of hypersensitivity (including aspirin), underlying renal, cardiovascular or cerebrovascular disease, concurrent use of medications which may cause drug interactions, emotional status, previous details of hypertensive therapy, and possibility of pregnancy.

—Monitoring the effects of this drug requires evaluation of the patient's blood pressure in lying, sitting, and standing positions. Whether to alter dosage regimens should be based upon the standing pressure at the peak of drug action.

—Effects of this drug may not be exhibited by the patient for up to 3 weeks. Additionally, adverse effects which develop from the drug may also take days to weeks to disappear. If problems develop because of the drug, withhold the medication until all symptoms have disappeared before reinstituting medication.

—Tolerance may develop to this drug, and additional medication may need to be added to the therapy.

—Selecting a patient for use of this drug requires a good understanding of the patient and reassurance of the patient's ability to comply with the dosing regimen. It is important to teach and counsel the patient about the various drugs and foods that should be avoided without being unduly frightening.

WHAT THE PATIENT NEEDS TO KNOW:

—Take this medication exactly as instructed by your health practitioner. Do not skip doses or increase the dosage. This drug must not be stopped suddenly.

—It may take several weeks before your blood pressure begins to respond to this medication. You will need to return for various tests and evaluation to determine your response to the drug.

—Some people experience side effects from this drug. Be certain to notify your health care provider of any new or troublesome symptoms. Especially note headaches or fainting.

—The most common symptom is feeling lightheaded or faint when rapidly changing positions. This is noticed especially in the morning. Time should be planned to sit up slowly, and then rise to a standing position. Avoid activities that require rapid movement or prolonged standing.

—Avoid taking other medications, including cough, cold, or allergy products which may be purchased over the counter, without the consent of your health practitioner. Use of this drug with other medications may be very dangerous.

—Patients who have had heart attacks or angina may note a feeling of increased well-being. This feeling should not be allowed to induce the patient to overwork or engage in strenuous exercise.

—Keep this medication out of the reach of children and all others for whom it is not prescribed.

—If you plan to have dental work done, or any type of surgery, be certain to inform the medical personnel that you have been taking this drug. The medication may make nerve endings insensitive to local anesthetic.

—During the time you take this medication, avoid eating products which require the action of bacteria or molds for their preparation or preservation: processed or aged cheese (cheddar, Camembert, Stilton), beer, and wine. Certain chemicals contained in some foods interact in a negative way with this drug. Because of this, also avoid chocolate, avocado, ripe bananas, papaya products (including some meat tenderizers), chicken livers, yeast extract, pickled herring, and pods of broad beans. Some people have severe and sudden elevations of blood pressure if they continue to eat these foods.

—Wear a Medic-Alert bracelet and carry a medical identification card specifying that you have hypertension and are taking this medication.

EVALUATION:

ADVERSE REACTIONS: *Cardiovascular:* congestive heart failure, fluid retention, orthostatic changes: dizziness, fainting, tachycardia, weakness. *CNS:* blurred vision, headache, hyperexcitability, increased neuromuscular activity, insomnia, nervousness, nightmares. *Gastrointestinal:* constipation, dry mouth, increased appetite, nausea, vomiting. *Hypersensitivity:* drug fever, purpura, rash. *Other:* arthralgia, difficulty voiding, impotence, delayed ejaculation, sweating, weight gain, hypoglycemia.

OVERDOSAGE: *Signs and symptoms:* Agitation, convulsions, hypotension or hypertension, hallucinations, hyperreflexia, and hyperpyrexia may all be seen. *Treatment:* Supportive therapy should be carried out by a specialist. Small doses of norepinephrine might be helpful in controlling hypotension.

PARAMETERS TO MONITOR: Obtain a complete history, physical, and laboratory evaluation prior to initiation of therapy. This should include liver function studies, electrolytes, cardiac enzymes, and renal function studies. An ophthalmologist should also obtain baseline information about the status of the patient's eyes. Then monitor for therapeutic effect: gradual reduction of blood pressure. Watch for development of adverse reactions, particularly postural hypotension, fainting, or syncopal episodes. Repeat hepatic function tests and ophthalmologic exams if there are any symptoms of impairment. Patient's compliance with therapy is important to evaluate in determining whether dosage should be altered.

Marilyn W. Edmunds

ANTIHYPERTENSIVES—PRAZOSIN HCL

ACTION OF THE DRUG: Prazosin produces selective blockage of postsynaptic alpha-adrenergic receptor sites leading to a reduction in peripheral vascular resistance and blood pressure. Blood pressure, especially diastolic pressure, is reduced in both the supine and standing positions. This is due to dilatation of both arterioles and venules caused by direct relaxation of arteriolar and venous smooth muscles. Changes in cardiac output, renal blood flow, and glomerular filtration rate are not significant, and renin release is not increased as it is by the direct-acting vasodilators.

Prazosin is currently under investigational use for treatment of acute congestive heart failure as it tends to decrease both cardiac afterload and preload. Cardiac output and pulmonary congestion are both improved in short-term studies, although tolerance appears to develop in chronic use.

ASSESSMENT:

INDICATIONS: Prazosin is a step two antihypertensive drug useful in the treatment of mild to moderate hypertension. It may be used alone at times. It has been used as adjunctive treatment in congestive heart failure but its tendency to cause sodium and water retention limits its value as the sole therapeutic drug. It is most effective when given with a thiazide diuretic and/or a beta-blocker.

SUBJECTIVE: Patient may be asymptomatic or may complain of not feeling well in general. Headaches, frequently associated with hypertension, are often produced by stress, tension, or other reasons rather than being related to high blood pressure, unless very severe blood pressure elevations are present. In cases of secondary hypertension, there may be reports of nocturia (if patient is unable to concentrate urine), history of renal trauma (producing renal artery stenosis), or family history of hypertension.

OBJECTIVE: Patient may have elevated blood pressure due to numerous factors: full bladder, anxiety, pain, etc. If the average blood pressure is found to be above 140/90 on three consecutive readings, the patient is assumed to be hypertensive. Readings above 120 mm Hg diastolic require immediate medical care. Blood pressure should be obtained in lying, sitting, and standing positions in both arms, and, in cases where coarctation of the aorta is part of the diagnostic differential, in the lower extremities. Eyes should be examined for the presence of increased arteriovenous (AV) ratio, nicking, hemorrhages, or exudates in the fundus of the eye, and blurring of the disc margins. Chest should be examined for diffuse point of maximum intensity (PMI), displacement of PMI to the left, thrusts, murmurs, and presence of third and fourth heart sounds. (Systolic ejection murmurs and fourth heart sounds commonly develop in hypertensive patients.) Abdomen should be assessed for renal artery bruits.

PLAN:

WARNINGS: A sudden and unexplained syncopal episode often develops following the first dose of this medication. Although in some cases the syncope is preceded by a rapid tachycardia, in other cases excessive postural hypotension is responsible for the syncope which may have developed within 30 to 90 minutes of the first dose. The incidence of initial syncope is increased with higher dosages and warrants limiting the initial dose to 0.5 to 1 mg. An increased sensitivity is found in volume-depleted or sodium-restricted patients, and effects are exaggerated after exercise.

Use with caution in patients with history of angina, severe cardiac disease, mental depression or renal function impairment. Safety for use during pregnancy or with children has not been established, and risk should be weighed against possible benefits.

IMPLEMENTATION:

DRUG INTERACTIONS: Concurrent use with diuretics and other antihypertensives, especially propranolol, potentiates the hypotensive effects. Prazosin HCl may interfere with other highly protein-bound drugs. There is a possibility of some interaction also with nitroglycerin, increasing the hypotensive effect.

PRODUCTS (TRADE NAME):

Minipress (Available in 1, 2 and 5 mg capsules.)

ADMINISTRATION AND DOSAGE: Dosage must be titrated to individual blood pressure responsiveness.

Initial dose: Begin with 1 mg capsule, 2 or 3 times daily.

Maintenance dose: Dosage may be slowly increased to 20 mg/day given in divided doses. Give the incremental dosages at bedtime to decrease chances of syncopal episodes. Usual range is 6-15 mg/day. Maximum 40 mg/day in 2 divided doses. When adding a diuretic or other antihypertensive agent, reduce dosages to 1 or 2 mg 3 times a day and retitrate according to blood pressure response.

IMPLEMENTATION CONSIDERATIONS:

—Obtain a complete health history, including hypersensitivities, underlying diseases, other drugs taken concurrently which may promote drug interactions, and possibility of pregnancy.

—In some patients, tolerance to this drug may develop in long-term use. In other patients, tolerance does not develop.

—Observe patient carefully when starting them on this medication if they are currently receiving a beta-blocker, as chances for hypotensive episodes are increased.

—Patients should always be started on the 1 mg capsules since the 2 mg and 5 mg capsules are not indicated for initial therapy.

—After initial dosage adjustments, some patients can be maintained adequately on a twice-daily dosage regimen. Initial doses and increased doses may be given before bedtime to decrease dizziness.

—Peak of action is about 3 hours after administration. Prazosin is excreted mostly in bile and feces, with only a small portion passing out in the urine.

—Consider having patient take initial doses at bedtime to decrease problems with orthostatic hypotension and drowsiness.

WHAT THE PATIENT NEEDS TO KNOW:

—Take this medication exactly as ordered by your health care provider. Do not discontinue taking it unless directed to do so. It may take several weeks before the full effect of the drug is noted. If you miss taking a dose, take it as soon as you remember if it is not long after the scheduled time to take it. If it is close to the next scheduled dose, do not take it, and do not double the dose at the next scheduled period.

—Take medication with a full glass of orange juice (unless contraindicated by your diet). Other potassium-rich foods should be eaten daily. These include: citrus foods (especially oranges and tomatoes), bananas, dried fruits, apricots, cantaloupe, watermelon, nuts, dried beans, beef, and fowl.

—Taking medication is only one part of your treatment regimen. Reduction of other risk factors is also important: lose weight (if overweight), stop smoking, increase exercise, avoid stressful and emotional pressures. Avoid use of foods high in sodium: lunch meats, smoked meats, Chinese food, processed cheese, snack foods. Do not salt food while cooking or add salt after it is cooked.

—Do not take any other medications, including over-the-counter cough, cold, and allergy medications, unless directed to do so by your health care provider.

—Fainting sometimes occurs following the first dosage of this medication. Do not drive or do any tasks requiring alertness for 6 hours following taking this medication.

—Some people experience dizziness, drowsiness, or headache during the first few days of taking this drug. If these symptoms or any other new sensations do not disappear within a few days, notify your health care provider.

—To avoid feelings of lightheadedness, use care in changing positions, especially from the lying to the standing. It may be especially necessary when you wake up in the morning to take time sitting up. This feeling may be more prominent during the first few days of therapy.

—Keep this medication out of the reach of children and others for whom it is not prescribed.

—The goal of therapy is to help you feel as healthy as possible, and to avoid any complications. Generally there is no cure for hypertension, and therapy extends for a lifetime. Taking your medication and reducing other risk factors will help reduce the chance of serious complications. It is important then to keep taking your medication, even when you feel well, and to keep seeing your health practitioner regularly.

—Wear a Medic-Alert bracelet and carry a medical identification card specifying that you have hypertension, and the drugs which you are taking.

EVALUATION:

ADVERSE REACTIONS: *Cardiovascular:* aggravation or development of angina, dizziness, dyspnea, edema, irregular pulse, nausea, orthostatic hypotension, palpitations, peripheral edema, syncope, tachycardia. *CNS:* depression, drowsiness, headache, malaise, nervousness, paresthesias, tinnitus, vertigo, weakness. *Dermatologic:* alopecia, diaphoresis, lichen planus, rash, pruritus. *EENT:* blurred vision, dry mouth, epistaxis, nasal congestion, reddened sclera, tinnitus. *Gastrointestinal:* abdominal discomfort or pain, diarrhea, constipation, vomiting. *Genitourinary:* impotence, incontinence, priapism, urinary frequency. *Ophthalmologic:* possible pigmentary mottling and serious retinopathy. *Other:* arthralgia, diaphoresis, hypothermia, drug-induced lupus erythematosus, leukopenia, weight gain.

OVERDOSAGE: *Signs and symptoms:* depressed reflexes, profound drowsiness, and hypotension. *Treatment:* Support cardiovascular system in cases of hypotension and treat symptomatically.

PARAMETERS TO MONITOR: Monitor for therapeutic effect. Therapeutic objective is to keep diastolic blood pressure below 90 mm Hg with the minimum side effects possible. Obtain baseline history, physical examination and laboratory data including renal, cardiac, and hepatic studies. Repeat urinalysis, ECG, x-ray as needed periodically while patient is on therapy. Monitor blood pressure (sitting, supine and standing) to assess for orthostatic changes, pulse, weight, cardiac and respiratory findings to observe for any adverse reactions.

Marilyn W. Edmunds

ANTIHYPERTENSIVES—RESERPINE

ACTION OF THE DRUG: Reserpine is one of the only *Rauwolfia* alkaloids still being used clinically. Reserpine 0.5 mg is approximately equal to 200 to 300 mg whole root *Rauwolfia*. The antihypertensive action is due to blocking of amine uptake into vesicular storage sites within the nerve endings, thus causing inhibition of catecholamine storage in postganglionic adrenergic nerve endings, and leading to depletion of norepinephrine. Decrease in heart rate and blood pressure is produced; cardiac output and renal blood flow is not markedly altered. Sedative and tranquilizing actions from depletion of amines in the CNS are also produced. These effects may continue even after the drug is discontinued.

ASSESSMENT:

INDICATIONS: Reserpine is a step two antihypertensive drug, useful in the treatment of mild to moderate hypertension after maximal doses of diuretics have either been ineffective or have caused significant side effects. It is occasionally used alone. It was a very popular drug but in recent years has been replaced by more potent medications. It is also used in combination with other antihypertensives to control more severe hypertension. Parenteral administration will reduce blood pressure promptly in emergency situations, although other agents are usually preferred. This medication is also effective in initiating treatment in psychiatric patients with extreme agitation due to psychotic states, primarily in patients intolerant to other antipsychotic drugs or until they can take oral medication.

SUBJECTIVE: Patient may be asymptomatic, or may complain of not feeling well in general. Headaches, often associated with hypertension, are often produced by stress, tension, or other reasons rather than being related to high blood pressure, unless very severe blood pressure elevations are present. In case of secondary hypertension, there may be reports of nocturia (if patient is unable to concentrate urine), history of renal trauma (producing renal artery stenosis), or family history of hypertension.

OBJECTIVE: Patient may have elevated blood pressure due to numerous factors: full bladder, anxiety, pain, etc. If the average blood pressure is found to be above 140/90 on three consecutive readings, the patient is assumed to be hypertensive. Blood pressure readings above 120 mm Hg diastolic require immediate medical care. Blood pressure should be obtained in lying, sitting, and standing positions in both arms and, in cases where coarctation of the aorta is part of the diagnostic differential, in the lower extremities. Eyes should be examined for the presence of increased arteriovenous (AV) ratio, nicking, hemorrhages, or exudates in the fundus of the eye, and blurring of the disc margins. Chest should be examined for diffuse point of maximum intensity (PMI), displacement of PMI to the left, thrusts, murmurs, and presence of third and fourth heart sounds. (Systolic ejection murmurs and fourth heart sounds commonly develop in hypertensive patients.) Abdomen should be assessed for renal artery bruits.

PLAN:

CONTRAINDICATIONS: Do not give in presence of known sensitivity to *Rauwolfia* derivatives, in patients with mental depression, active peptic ulcer, ulcerative colitis, pheochromocytoma, and in patients receiving electroconvulsive therapy or being treated with MAO inhibitors.

WARNINGS: It has been suggested but not conclusively demonstrated in a variety of studies that long-term administration of reserpine to hypertensive women causes a threefold increase in cases of carcinoma of the breast. Because of a tendency to cause drug-induced depression, do not give to patients with past history of depression, and be alert to symptoms of developing depression. Safe and effective use in children has not been established. Safety for use during pregnancy has not been established. Risks must be weighed against possible benefits. Reserpine crosses the placental barrier and is also found in breast milk. Increased respiratory secretions, cyanosis, anorexia, and nasal congestion may occur in infants born to mothers taking reserpine.

PRECAUTIONS: Use with caution in patients with impaired renal or hepatic function. Reserpine causes increased GI motility and secretion; therefore, use with caution in patients with history of ulcerative colitis, gallstones, or peptic ulcer. Discontinuing this medication preoperatively will not ensure cardiovascular stability. The anesthesiologist should be aware that the patient has been taking this drug.

Some of the products may contain tartrazine, a preservative, which may cause allergic-type reactions (including bronchial asthma) in sensitive individuals. These patients may also have aspirin hypersensitivity.

IMPLEMENTATION:

DRUG INTERACTIONS: Enhanced hypotensive effects may be seen when reserpine is given with anesthetics, barbiturates, diuretics, and other antihypertensive drugs, methotrimeprazine, phenothiazines, quinidine, vasodilators, and beta-blocking agents. Cardiac arrhythmias have been precipitated by the use of reserpine concomitantly with quinidine and digitalis. Concurrent use with any other medications should be closely supervised, especially with the thiazides, chlorthalidone, methyldopa, hydralazine, guanethidine, Veratrum alkaloids, and other ganglionic blocking agents. MAO inhibitors should be avoided. The effects of anticholinergics, anticonvulsants, indirect-acting sympathomimetics (ephedrine and amphetamines), levodopa, morphine, salicylates, vasopressors (metaraminol, mephentermine) are decreased.

PRODUCTS (TRADE NAME:)
Lemiserp, Rau-Sed (Available in 0.25 mg tablets.) **Releserp-5** (Available in 0.5 mg timed release capsule.) **Reserpine** (Available in 0.1, 0.25, .5, 1.0 mg tablets.) **Sandril, Serpasil** (Available in 0.1, 0.25 mg tablets and 2.5 mg/ml injections.) **Serpalan, Serpate** (Available in 0.1 mg tablets.) **Reserjen, Reserpoid, Serpanray, SK-Reserpine, Zepine** (Available in 0.25 mg tablets.)

ADMINISTRATION AND DOSAGE: The onset of action for IM dosage is slightly longer than one hour and effects may persist for up to 10 hours. It is metabolized extensively in the liver.

Patients not receiving any other antihypertensive agents: Give 0.5 mg/day. Should be given po for 2-3 weeks and then decreased to 0.1 to 0.25 mg/day.

Patients receiving step one diuretic therapy: In addition to other drugs, add 0.1 mg/day and then increase or decrease depending upon individual response. Reduce dosage for children, elderly, or severely debilitated patients.

Hypertensive crisis: Give 0.5 to 1 mg IM, followed by oral doses of 2 and 4 mg at 3-hour intervals. Titrate dosage depending upon blood pressure. Do not give more than 0.4 mg, but use other agents to help decrease blood pressure.

Psychiatric disorders: Give 0.5 mg/day. Range 0.1 to 1 mg. Adjust according to individual response. May administer 2.5 to 5 mg IM if patient is unable to take orally.

IMPLEMENTATION CONSIDERATIONS:
—Obtain a complete health history, including presence of hypersensitivity, bronchial asthma, cardiac damage or arrhythmias, epilepsy, obesity, renal insufficiency, mental depression, active peptic ulcer, ulcerative colitis, pheochromocytoma, electroconvulsive therapy, concurrent use of drugs which may produce drug interactions, or possibility of pregnancy.

—Discontinue drug at first sign of despondency, early morning insomnia, self-deprecation, or loss of appetite and impotence. Drug-induced depression severe enough to cause suicide may persist for several months following discontinuance of drug.

—People with history of other drug allergy, (particularly to aspirin) or who have bronchial asthma are more likely to be allergic to this drug.

—Exercise caution when treating patients with renal insufficiency since they adjust poorly to lowered blood pressure levels.

—Discontinue drug several weeks prior to elective surgery to avoid hypotension during surgery. Alert anesthesiologist that patient has been on reserpine if surgery is scheduled.

—Patients treated with reserpine plus a beta-blocking agent should be closely observed for evidence of hypotension or excessive bradycardia. Vertigo, syncope or postural hypotension may also accompany these conditions.

—Establishing rapport with patient, using adjunctive diet therapy and medications, working to decrease other risk factors, and continual monitoring of patients response is important in reaching therapeutic objective.

WHAT THE PATIENT NEEDS TO KNOW:

—Take this medication exactly as ordered by your health care provider. If you miss a dose, take it as soon as you remember if it is within an hour or two of the scheduled time. If it is close to your next scheduled dose, skip it, and take the next dose at the regular time. Do not double doses.

—Do not discontinue this medication or change dosages unless advised to do so by your health care provider. Effects of the drug may not be obvious for several weeks and also may last up to one month following end of therapy.

—Some people experience drowsiness, especially the first few days the medication is taken, or when the dosage is increased. This should pass if you continue taking the medication. Do not drive or perform tasks requiring alertness until these symptoms stop.

—If you experience any stomach upset, take this drug with food or milk.

—Do not drink beer, wine, or liquor, or take any other medications without the knowledge of your health care provider. This includes medicines for cough, cold or allergy which you might buy over the counter.

—Some people experience side effects from drugs. If you notice anything new or troublesome, report it promptly to your health provider. Especially note the presence of severe abdominal pain or any change in mood or sleep habits. Weigh regularly and report new or rapid weight gain.

—To avoid dizziness do not change your position quickly, especially when moving from lying to standing.

—Take this medication with a full glass of orange juice (unless it is not on your diet). Other potassium-rich foods should be used daily. These include: citrus foods (especially oranges and tomatoes), bananas, dried fruits, apricots, cantaloupe, watermelon, nuts, dried beans, beef, and fowl.

—Taking medication is only one part of your treatment regimen. Reduction of other risk factors is also important: lose weight (if overweight), stop smoking, increase exercise, avoid stressful and emotional pressure. Avoid use of foods high in sodium: lunch meats, smoked meats, Chinese food, processed chese, snack foods. Do not salt your food while cooking or add salt to your food after it has been cooked.

—Keep this medication out of the reach of children and others for whom it is not prescribed.

—The goal of therapy is to help you feel as healthy as possible, and to avoid any complications. Generally there is no cure for hypertension, and therapy extends for a lifetime. Taking your medication and reducing other risk factors will help reduce the chance of serious complications. It is important then to keep taking your medicine, even when you feel well, and to keep seeing your health care practitioner regularly.

—Wear a Medic-Alert bracelet and carry a medical identification card specifying that you have hypertension, and the drugs which you are taking.

EVALUATION:

ADVERSE REACTIONS: *Cardiovascular:* angina-like symptoms, arrhythmias, bradycardia, fall in blood pressure, orthostatic hypotension, palpitations, syncope. *CNS:* anxiety, blurred vision, CNS sensitization manifested by dull sensorium; cutaneous vasodilation and flushing, deafness, depression, drowsiness, extrapyramidal symptoms (with large doses), nightmares, nervousness, paradoxical anxiety, parkinsonian syndrome (rare), syncope, uveitis. *Dermatologic/Hypersensitivity:* asthma (in asthmatic patients), pruritus, rash. *Gastrointestinal:* abdominal pain, anorexia, diarrhea, dry mouth, GI bleeding, hypersecretion, nausea, vomiting. *Hematopoietic:* thrombocytopenic purpura. *Other:* asthma, breast engorgement, dizziness, dry mouth, dyspnea, dysuria, epistaxis, gynecomastia, headache, impotence or decreased libido, menstrual irregularity, muscular aching, nasal congestion, pseudolactation, weight gain.

OVERDOSAGE: *Signs and symptoms:* Diarrhea, flushing of the skin, conjunctival injection, pupillary constriction, impairment of consciousness (drowsiness progressing to coma), hypotension, hypothermia, central respiratory depression and bradycardia may occur. *Treatment:* Produce emesis and refer for gavage and symptomatic treatment. Observation and treatment may be required for up to 3 days because of long action of the drug. Severe hypotension should be treated with a direct-acting sympathomimetic (levarterenol) rather than an indirect-acting drug (ephedrine).

PARAMETERS TO MONITOR: Obtain a complete data base of physical and laboratory parameters prior to initiating theapy. This should include electrolytes, urine and liver function studies, urinalysis, an electrocardiogram, and chest x-ray. These should be repeated at least yearly while patient is on medication, more frequently if problems are suspected. Monitor for therapeutic effect: reduction of diastolic blood pressure to 90 mm Hg or lower. Monitor for adverse reactions especially development of depression.

Marilyn W. Edmunds

ANTIHYPERTENSIVES—VERATRUM ALKALOIDS

ACTION OF THE DRUG: These products act as antihypertensives through decreasing peripheral resistance. This is accomplished through stimulation of pressor receptors in the baroreceptors of the carotid sinus, aortic arch, and coronary arteries. This stimulation sends signals to the brain indicating that the pressure is higher than its actual level, thus turning on the body's normal compensatory mechanisms in high blood pressure. Sympathetic tone is decreased and vagal tone is increased, thus decreasing both systolic and diastolic blood pressure. The heart is slowed, although cardiac output remains normal. Renal blood flow is not markedly altered.

ASSESSMENT:

INDICATIONS: These preparations, all compounds derived from the Veratrum plants, are not included as part of the step-care therapy for hypertension, but are reserved for use when other antihypertensive therapy has been exhausted. These drugs are effective in mild to moderate hypertension; however, the therapeutic and toxic doses (producing emesis and hypotension) remain so close that it is difficult to give these drugs safely. Dosage recommendations therefore must be general.

SUBJECTIVE: Patient may be asymptomatic, or may complain of not feeling well in general. Headaches, often associated with hypertension, are often produced by stress, tension, or other reasons rather than being related to high blood pressure, unless very severe blood pressure elevations are present. In cases of secondary hypertension, there may be reports of nocturia (if patient is unable to concentrate urine), history of renal trauma (producing renal artery stenosis), or family history of hypertension. Some patients may have been managed initially on other drugs, with hypertension remaining out of control. There may be evidence of end-organ damage or side effects from other drugs.

OBJECTIVE: If the average blood pressure is found to be above 140/90 mm Hg on three consecutive readings, the patient is assumed to be hypertensive. Diastolic readings above 120 mm Hg require immediate medical care. Blood pressure should be obtained in lying, sitting, and standing positions in both arms and in cases where coarctation of the aorta is part of the diagnostic differential, in the lower extremities. Eyes should be examined for the presence of increased arteriovenous (AV) ratio, nicking, hemorrhages, or exudates in the fundus of the eye, and blurring of the disc margins. Chest should be examined for diffuse point of maximum intensity (PMI), displacement of PMI to the left, thrusts, murmurs, and presence of third and fourth heart sounds. (Systolic ejection murmurs and fourth heart sounds commonly develop in hypertensive patients.) Abdomen should be assessed for renal artery bruits.

PLAN:

CONTRAINDICATIONS: Do not give in the presence of hypersensitivity, pheochromocytoma, increased intracranial pressure (not caused by hypertension), Stokes-Adams syndrome, recent cerebrovascular thrombosis or coronary artery occlusion, coarctation of the aorta, or vasovagal syncope.

WARNINGS: Safety for use in pregnant and breast-feeding women has not been established. Weigh possible benefits against potential risks.

PRECAUTIONS: If patients develop a slow heart rate, or have persistent nausea, medication should be discontinued. Use caution when treating patients in whom lowering of blood pressure might create a problem due to underlying pathology: decreased renal function, cerebrovascular disease, angina pectoris, coronary thrombosis. Use care in treating patients with large doses, especially patients with a history of bronchial asthma since medicine may trigger a reflex respiratory depression and direct bronchiolar constriction.

IMPLEMENTATION:

DRUG INTERACTIONS: If using concomitantly with other antihypertensive agents or diuretics, each drug dosage should be reduced by about 50% and patient monitored carefully because of additive effects. MAO inhibitors potentiate the hypotensive action of these drugs, and tricyclic antidepressants, vasopressors, and atropine counteract excessive hypotension. Atropine sulfate also diminishes bradycardia which sometimes develops, while *Veratrum* alkaloids will exaggerate the bradycardia produced by morphine. In patients receiving digitalis and/or quinidine, extreme care must be used to avoid stimulating cardiac arrhythmias arising from increased myocardial irritability. While local anesthetics will abolish the action of *Veratrum* alkaloids on excitable cells, extreme caution should be employed in patients undergoing general anesthesia because of the additive hypotensive effects of both preanesthetic and anesthetic agents.

ADMINISTRATION AND DOSAGE: Gastrointestinal absorption is extremely variable, causing difficulty in developing dosage regimens. A routine should be developed for each individual patient and then evaluations made according to the blood pressure response. It is important to take the medication at the same time daily, while fitting it into the patient's general life style. A suggested routine for the normal individual would be to take medication in three unequal doses: medium size dose immediately following breakfast in the morning, a small dose in the afternoon, and the largest dose at evening. This allows patients to have enough medication to control blood pressure until the next dosing period.

IMPLEMENTATION CONSIDERATIONS:

—Obtain a complete health history, including the presence of hypersensitivity, other medications taken concurrently which may produce drug interactions, underlying cardiovascular, cerebrovascular, renal or respiratory disease, and previous diagnosis and treatment for hypertension. Also inquire about the possibility of pregnancy.

—Hypertensive patients with uremia or chronic renal disease may not tolerate lowered blood pressure, and BUN and creatinine levels may begin to rise.

—Temporary lowering of the medication dose may be necessary during extremely hot weather.

—These medications should be reserved for patients who have demonstrated compliance in therapy and who are reliable in taking medications as ordered and accurately reporting their responses. Because of the potential for toxicity, dangerous conditions could develop if patients do not work closely with the health care provider in evaluation of response to this medication.

—Adverse effects are usually reversible and stop when the drug is withdrawn.

—Many gastrointestinal symptoms may be relieved with the administration of atropine.

—Gastrointestinal absorption is quite variable, and careful dosage titration is necessary.

—Discontinue drug if nausea or excessive bradycardia develop.

WHAT THE PATIENT NEEDS TO KNOW:

—It is very important that this drug be taken exactly as prescribed by your health care practitioner and that you work together to make necessary modifications in your therapy. Taking this medication will require follow up visits and laboratory evaluations to help measure effectiveness of the drug in controlling your blood pressure.

—Keep this medication out of the reach of children and all others for whom it is not prescribed.

—If you experience nausea or vomiting, it make help to take medication 4 hours after eating.

—Do not stop taking this medication suddenly or change doses without consulting with your health care provider.

—Do not take any other medications, including cold, cough, or allergy preparations which you may purchase over the counter, without the knowledge of your health care practitioner.

—There are numerous side effects which could develop from use of this preparation. Be certain to notify your health care provider of any new or troublesome symptoms which you may experience so that they may be adequately evaluated.

—The goal of therapy is to help you feel as healthy as possible and to avoid any complications. Generally there is no cure for hypertension, and therapy extends for a lifetime. Taking your medication and reducing other risk factors (stop smoking, increase exercise, lose weight, avoid high sodium foods, reduce stress) will help reduce the chance of serious complications. It is important to keep taking your medicine, even when you feel well, and to keep seeing your health care provider regularly.

—Wear a Medic-Alert bracelet and carry a medical identification card specifying that you have hypertension, and the drugs which you are taking.

EVALUATION:

ADVERSE REACTIONS: *Cardiovascular:* bradycardia, hypotension. *CNS:* blurring of vision, hiccoughs, mental confusion, paresthesias. *Gastrointestinal:* anorexia, epigastiric and substernal burning (similar to angina), nausea, salivation, unpleasant taste, vomiting. *Respiratory:* bronchiolar constriction, respiratory depression (with large doses), sweating.

OVERDOSAGE: *Signs and symptoms:* Hypotension, bradycardia, nausea, vomiting, and occasional bronchoconstriction may develop. *Treatment:* Usually resolves without treatment in 1-1/2 hours. May give atropine sulfate or vasopressors if indicated for severe reactions.

PARAMETERS TO MONITOR: Obtain a complete history, physical and laboratory examination as baseline prior to initiation of therapy. This should include electrolytes, renal function, and ECG evaluation. Monitor for therapeutic effect: reduction in blood pressure. Also monitor for progression of problem and development of adverse reactions.

CRYPTENAMINE TANNATES

PRODUCTS (TRADE NAME):
Unitensen (Available in 2 mg scored tablets.)

DRUG SPECIFICS:
This 2 mg preparation is equivalent to 260 CSR (carotid sinus reflex) units. Begin therapy at low doses, and increase medication on either a daily or weekly basis, depending upon how closely the patient response can be evaluated.

ADMINISTRATION AND DOSAGE SPECIFICS:
Give 4 to 12 mg po daily in divided doses. Give largest dose in evening before patient retires and the smallest in the afternoon. Evaluate the patient's response in order to determine dosage adjustments.

VERATRUM VIRIDE ALKALOIDS

PRODUCTS (TRADE NAME):
Pro-Amid (Available in 0.2 mg tablets.) **Vera-67** (Available in 2.67 mg tablets.)

DRUG SPECIFICS:
These preparations are made from different *Veratrum* alkaloids. Differences in bioavailability of drugs should preclude switching routinely from one product to another.

ADMINISTRATION AND DOSAGE SPECIFICS:
Pro-Amid: Give 0.2 mg 4 times daily.
Vera-67: Give 1 tablet 3 or 4 times daily.

Marilyn W. Edmunds

CARDIAC GLYCOSIDES

ACTION OF THE DRUG: This group of drugs has an inotropic effect on cardiac cells through enhancement of excitation-contraction coupling triggered by membrane depolarization. It acts through inhibition of sodium and potassium membrane ATPase, the enzyme responsible for breakdown of ATP to supply energy for the sodium-potassium pump. Therefore, electrical properties of the myocardium are altered and intracellular sodium and extracellular potassium concentrations are elevated. Calcium ions move into the cell during depolarization and released from intracellular binding sites on the sarcoplasmic reticulum to mediate the interaction between actin and myosin. The glycosides act to (1) directly increase the force of myocardial contraction; (2) depress the sinoatrial node by stimulating medullary vagal nuclei and increasing sensitivity of the pacemaker cells to acetylcholine; (3) prolong conduction to the atrioventricular node via vagal stimulation; (4) increase the refractory period of the atrioventricular node; and (5) help to increase peripheral resistance. Thus, heart rate is slowed both vagally and extravagally. A diuretic effect may be promoted by increased cardiac output, which increases the glomerular filtration rate, but increased aldosterone may also be released.

Preparations in this drug category differ pharmacokinetically but have the same basic therapeutic action on heart tissue. Some products are absorbed better than others. Because of the variation in purity of some preparations, effects may be variable. Once absorbed, digitalis is bound to plasma albumin in varying degrees and is widely distributed in tissues. Digitoxin is degraded by the liver to inactive products which are excreted by the kidneys. Other digitalis products are excreted by the kidneys in a more active form, thus presenting a danger of toxicity in cases of impaired renal failure.

ASSESSMENT:

INDICATIONS: Cardiac glycosides are used primarily in the treatment of congestive heart failure, arrhythmias, and cardiogenic shock.

In congestive heart failure these drugs increase cardiac output and produce a diuresis which helps relieve symptoms. They are most effective in congestive failure caused by decreased left ventricular function and other low-output syndromes. For arrhythmias, digitalis products are used primarily in the treatment of atrial tachyarrhythmias, fibrillation, flutter, and paroxysmal atrial tachycardia. Rapid rates may also provoke pulmonary edema. Parenteral administration brings a rapid decrease in ventricular response, allowing normal sinus rhythm to reassert itself. Continuing the patient on oral digitalis keeps the tachyarrhythmia suppressed. In shock of·cardiogenic origin, digitalis is used along with a number of other measures designed to strengthen myocardial contractility and decrease pulmonary edema.

SUBJECTIVE: Patients with congestive failure or atrial tachyarrhythmias frequently complain of fatigue, weakness, shortness of breath, dyspnea on exertion, paroxysmal nocturnal dyspnea, and pedal edema. They may also be aware of rapid or irregular heart action, lightheadedness, and dizziness.

OBJECTIVE: In congestive heart failure, patients will have a documented weight gain, and on cardiac examination the PMI may be diffuse and displaced to the left, with the appearance of third heart sound or gallop rhythm. Jugular venous distension may be present. Rales and decreased breath sounds may also be present in the lungs. Pulse may be irregular and/or rapid, producing syncopal episodes. Chest x-ray may indicate cardiac enlargement and sometimes blunting of the costophrenic angles and other symptoms of pulmonary edema. Arrhythmias may be confirmed through use of ECG tracings or 24-hour Holter monitor.

PLAN:

CONTRAINDICATIONS: Do not use this drug in ventricular tachycardia or fibrillation, unless the patient has overwhelming congestive failure which is unrelated to digitalis. Do not give in beriberi heart disease or in patients with hypersensitive carotid sinuses. Allergy to digitalis is rare.

WARNINGS: Digitalis represents a potent cardiac poison and should be respected as such. Treatment for non-cardiovascular problems is unwarranted and dangerous. It should never be used adjunctively in the treatment of obesity. In a patient who has been receiving digitalis, it is frequently a diagnostic dilemma as to whether a patient with arrhythmias and congestive failure needs more digitalis, or whether symptoms represent digitalis toxicity. If there is a question, digitalis products should be withheld temporarily.

Patients with some types of underlying disease or previous treatment are more sensitive to digitalis toxicity and must be monitored closely. Patients with acute myocardial infarction, pulmonary edema, intractable heart failure and rheumatic heart disease, as well as those patients having electrical conversions of arrhythmias, fall into this category. Digitalis may be given to these patients at low doses until the patient's response can be evaluated. Patients with premature ventricular contractions, or who have varying degrees of heart block, may have a worsening of arrhythmias with additional doses of digitalis. Patients with Wolfe-Parkinson-White syndrome and idiopathic hypertrophic subaortic stenosis are prone to lethal arrhythmias, and digitalis should be used only if absolutely necessary.

All digitalis products except digitoxin are delayed in their excretion by renal insufficiency. Thus, dosage adjustments need to be made in this condition. Impaired hepatic function will also require decreased dosage of digitalis since half-life of medication may be prolonged.

Special attention should be paid when using digitalis in the very young and in the elderly, especially those with renal impairment. Small dosage with continuous monitoring of effects is mandatory. Safe use in pregnancy has not been documented. Digitalis does appear in breast milk and may represent a contraindication to use.

PRECAUTIONS: Potassium depletion sensitizes the myocardium to digitalis, and thus digitalis toxicity is more frequent in patients taking diuretics. Corticosteroid therapy, suction, prolonged diarrhea and vomiting, and dialysis may also produce hypokalemia. The usual dosage may need to be lowered in these individuals. It is mandatory to maintain normal serum potassium levels in patients receiving digitalis because hypokalemia may affect the intensity and rate of onset of the action of digitalis. Avoid use of calcium in digitalized patients since serious arrhythmias may be provoked by elevated calcium levels.

Use with caution in patients with thyroid dysfunction since the half-life of digitalis may be altered. Atrial arrhythmias associated with hypermetabolic states are extremely resistant to digitalis, and the underlying problem should be corrected when possible. Some products contain tartrazine, which may cause allergic reactions in susceptible individuals. These persons often are also hypersensitive to aspirin.

IMPLEMENTATION:

DRUG INTERACTIONS: Hypokalemia may increase the effects and toxicity of digitalis. Thiazides and furosemide are most frequently responsible for producing urinary loss of potassium in patients also receiving digitalis. Mineralocorticoids and some antibiotics may also cause increased excretion of potassium. When potassium sparing diuretics such as triamterene, spironolactone and propantheline bromide are used, serum levels of digitalis may rise and eventually reduce the effects of digitalis. Concurrent use of quinidine and digoxin may increase serum digoxin levels and may require reduction in digoxin levels by as much as 50% or use of another digitalis product. Digitalis may decrease the effects of oral anticoagulants and heparin. The effect of these glycosides may be additive with quinidine, procainamide or propranolol. Administer with care in patients receiving thyroid preparations.

Glycosides are also synergistic with, and may produce toxicity when used with, epinephrine, ephedrine, amphotericin, *Rauwolfia* alkaloids, succinylcholine, parenteral calcium salts, corticosteroids, diuretics, glucose, insulin, magnesium, thyroid products, pancuronium and other adrenergic agents. Decreased absorption may occur with concurrent use of antacids, anti-diarrhea adsorbent suspension, anticholinergics, laxatives, neomycin and cholestyramine resins. Microsomal enzymes that metabolize digoxin in the liver and so reduce digitalis effects include antihistamines, anticonvulsants, barbiturates, hypoglycemic agents, rifampin and phenylbutazone. Concurrent use with digitalis products should be avoided because of the problems of developing toxicity. Marked bradycardia may develop if administered in combination with carbamazine, guanethidine, phenytoin, propranolol and reserpine.

ADMINISTRATION AND DOSAGE: Digitalis agents can be roughly divided into three groups based on the rate of action of the drugs (Table 3-5).

Digitalis glycoside mixtures (Gitalin, Acetyldigitoxin, Lantoside C, Deslanoside [Desacetyl-Lantoside C] and Ouabain [G-Strophanthin]) are used only rarely in this country, and then primarily in acute care settings where rapid digitalization is indicated and cardiac monitoring is possible. Therefore, most of these drugs are not discussed more fully in this book.

Digitalization may be accomplished by either a fast dosage schedule (necessitating closer monitoring) or by a slower schedule, which may be instituted on an outpatient basis.

Administer oral digitalis slowly or rapidly, as required by the clinical picture, until the desired therapeutic effect is obtained without symptoms of overdosage. This amount can be predicted approximately from the lean body mass of the patient with allowances made for excretion during the time taken to induce digitalization. Maintenance dosage is also tentatively determined by the amount necessary to sustain the desired therapeutic effect. Recommended dosages are practical average figures that may require considerable modification as dictated by individual sensitivity or associated conditions. Diminished renal function is the most important factor requiring modification of recommended or average dosages. Use parenterally

TABLE 3-5. CLASSIFICATION OF DIGITALIS PREPARATIONS BY ACTION

Category	Drug	Onset of Action	Peak Activity	Elimination
Rapid-acting	Ouabain	5-10 minutes IV	30-60 minutes	1-3 days
	Digoxin	1-2 hours	4-8 hours	12 hours (start)
	Lantoside C	1-2 hours	4-8 hours	2-3 days (end)
Intermediate-acting	Gitalin	2-4 hours	8-12 hours	7-12 days
	Acetyldigitoxin		12-24 hours	2-3 weeks
Long-acting	Digitalis	2-3 hours	8-12 hours	2-3 weeks
	Digitoxin	2-3 hours	6-12 hours	

only when the drug cannot be taken orally or when rapid digitalization is very urgent.

Significant bioavailability differences exist between various products and manufacturers of the same product. It is prudent to write on the prescription the specific product that is to be used to fill the prescription in order to eliminate variability.

IMPLEMENTATION CONSIDERATIONS:

—Obtain a complete health history to determine sensitivities, possible contraindications to drug use, underlying medical problems and concurrent use of other medications that could cause interactions.

—This drug has a very narrow margin of safety and must be used cautiously. The difference between the therapeutic dose and the toxic dose may be small. Watch for arrhythmias or decreases in pulse rate below 60 beats/minute.

—Elderly patients are often more sensitive to the effects of the medication than others. Premature newborns and infants are also vulnerable to the effects of digitalis.

—Patients with hypothyroidism or impaired liver or kidney function will metabolize and excrete digitalis differently, and this must be taken into account both in the initial dosage schedule and in subsequent monitoring.

—If patient is allergic to one cardiac glycoside (which is rare), another may be tried.

—If patient is taking a potassium-wasting diuretic concurrently with digitalis, prescribing a potassium-sparing diuretic in addition may keep the potassium levels within the normal range. Alternatively, prescription of a potassium chloride supplement should be provided to digitalized patients who would be unusually vulnerable to life-threatening arrhythmias from hypokalemia (such as those with severe cases of heart block).

—Once a patient has been treated with digitalis for congestive heart failure, it is advised to keep patient on a maintenance dose even though failure is reversed.

—Patients should be taught precautions to take in administering their medications and when they should report to the health care provider.

—Bioavailability differences between products may be extensive, and it is wise to specify on the prescription exactly the product you want the patient to have. The prescription should not vary from time to time as it is filled.

—Many of the symptoms associated with the need for digitalis (congestive heart failure, arrhythmias) may also indicate digitalis toxicity. Carefully assess patients on return visits, including chest examination, weights, ECGs and x-rays to help determine clinical status and therapy.

—Caution patients to avoid taking an "extra" dose of medication for a missed dose. Accumulation of drugs and chances of toxicity are increased when medication doses are taken too close together.

WHAT THE PATIENT NEEDS TO KNOW:

—Take this drug exactly as ordered by your health care provider. If you forget a dose, take it as soon as you remember. If it is close to the scheduled time for your next dose, do not take the missed dose or double the next dose.

—Taking this drug requires you to be periodically evaluated by your health care provider to see that the drug level is kept within certain specified limits.

—Because the action of the drug is to slow the heart rate as it strengthens contractions, this drug should not be taken if the heart rate is very slow. Your health care provider will teach you or your family members how to take your pulse. You should take your pulse every morning and not take the medicine until checking with your health care provider if the pulse rate is below 60 beats per minute.

—Any new or unusual symptoms that you develop should be reported to your health care provider.

—This drug is a poison and will kill pets and children. Keep it out of the reach of children and others for whom it is not prescribed.

—Men may note sensitivity or enlargement of the breasts due to estrogen-like action of certain digitalis preparations.

—It is advisable to carry a Medic-Alert or other identifying bracelet or card noting that you are taking this drug.

—Reduction of overall salt intake is advised. High sodium foods, including salted snacks, pork, lunch meats, and processed cheese, should be avoided. Do not add salt when cooking or use extra salt when food is cooked.

EVALUATION:

ADVERSE REACTIONS: *Cardiovascular:* arrhythmias (all kinds with ventricular premature contractions and atrial premature contractions being the most common). *CNS:* ambylopia, confusion, delirium, depression, diplopia, disorientation, drowsiness, headache, lethargy, visual disturbances. *Gastrointestinal:* abdominal discomfort, anorexia, diarrhea, nausea, vomiting. *Other:* eosinophilia, facial pain, fever, flashes, halos or white lights around eyes, gynecomastia, joint pain, pruritis, skin rash, thromboembolism, unusual tiredness, urticaria, weakness.

OVERDOSAGE: *Cardiac toxicity:* depression of conductivity, enhancement of automaticity, or a combination: atrioventricular premature beats, increasing atrioventricular block leading to complete heart block, paroxysmal atrial tachycardia, paroxysmal and nonparoxysmal nodal rhythms, ventricular premature beats. (Atrial cardiac arrhythmias are more common in children than other symptoms.) *CNS toxicity:* apathy, aphasia, bad dreams, confusion, delirium, disorientation, drowsiness, hallucinations, headache, lethargy, mental depression, visual disturbances (blurred, yellow or green vision, halo effect, amblyopia, diplopia, scotomas), retrobulbar neuritis (rare), and weakness. *Gastrointestinal toxicity:* abdominal pain, anorexia, diarrhea, nausea, salivation, vomiting. *Other:* severe muscular weakness.

PARAMETERS TO MONITOR: Monitor for therapeutic effect and toxicity. A complete history and physical examination including lying, sitting and standing blood pressure and pulse should be conducted at the time the patient is begun on digitalis therapy. This should include baseline blood studies, electrolytes, hepatic function and renal function studies, a chest x-ray and an ECG. These studies should be repeated periodically while patient is receiving this drug because of usually progressive changes in underlying cardiac status of patients receiving digitalis.

Serum digitalis levels are not a good index of therapeutic levels but are a good indication of toxic ranges. (Digitoxin greater than 35 ng/ml and digoxin greater than 2.0 ng/ml indicates toxicity.) Patients with congestive heart failure should have gradual disappearance of subjective symptoms, and it should be possible to document improvement in cardiac function. Cardiac arrhythmias should also be controlled. The earliest signs of toxicity are often subtle and easy to ignore by both patient and provider: extreme fatigue, tiredness, anorexia, weakness and nausea. These complaints should be noted when volunteered by the patient. Observe for ECG signs of toxicity.

DIGITALIS

PRODUCTS (TRADE NAME):

Digitalis (Available in 32.5 mg, 48.75 mg, 65 mg and 100 mg tablets.) **Digifortis Kapseals, Digitalis Pulvules** (Available in 100 mg capsules.) **Digifortis, Pil-Digis** (Available in 100 mg tablets.)

DRUG SPECIFICS:

This product is made of digitalis leaf and is the least pure and usually the most variable in its effects. The generic preparation is usually the least expensive cardiac glycoside on the market.

ADMINISTRATION AND DOSAGE SPECIFICS:

Digitalizing dose: Give a total average dose of 1.2 gm divided into equal parts administered every 6 hours. Individualize dose to more or less depending upon needs of the patient.

Maintenance dose: 100 to 200 mg/day po. Dose may vary from 30 to 400 mg/day depending upon the needs of the patient.

DIGITOXIN

PRODUCTS (TRADE NAME):

Crystodigin (Available in 0.05 mg, 0.1 mg, 0.15 mg and 0.2 mg tablets and 0.2 mg/ml injection.) **De-tone-1 and De-tone-2** (Available in 0.1 mg and 0.2 mg tablets.) **Digitoxin** (Available in 0.1 mg and 0.2 mg tablets.) **Purodigin** (Available in 0.1 mg, 0.15 mg and 0.2 mg tablets.)

DRUG SPECIFICS:

This is the most potent of the digitalis glycosides. It is the drug of choice for maintenance therapy because it is almost completely absorbed from the gastrointestinal tract. Its slow onset of action makes it undesirable for emergency use. One milligram of digitoxin is therapeutically the equivalent of 1 gm digitalis leaf.

ADMINISTRATION AND DOSAGE SPECIFICS:

Rapid oral digitalizing dose: 0.6 mg initially, followed by 0.4 mg, then 0.2 mg at intervals of 4-6 hours.

Slow oral digitalizing dose: 0.2 mg twice daily for 4 days.

Maintenance dose: 0.05 to 0.3 mg/day. (0.1 mg/day is usual dose.) Elderly patients may require less.

Parenteral digitalizing dose:

Adults: 1.2 to 1.6 mg IV.

Children: Individualized based on response of patient. Usual dose is 0.045 to 0.03 mg/kg, depending on age and weight of child. Premature or immature infants are particularly sensitive to this drug. Therapy should be worked out with physician. Maintenance dose is one tenth of the digitalizing dose.

DIGOXIN

PRODUCTS (TRADE NAME):

Digoxin (Available in 0.25 mg tablets and 0.25 mg/ml injection.) **Lanoxin** (Available in 0.125 mg, 0.25 mg and 0.5 mg tablets, 0.05 mg/ml pediatric elixir and 0.25 mg and 0.1 mg/ml injection.) **SK-Digoxin** (Available in 0.25 mg tablets.)

DRUG SPECIFICS:

Onset of action is faster and of shorter duration than digitoxin. Digoxin may be the drug of choice for use in congestive heart failure because of these features. It can be administered intravenously, intramuscularly or orally.

ADMINISTRATION AND DOSAGE SPECIFICS:

Adults and children 10 years and older:

Rapid oral digitalizing dose: 1 to 1.5 mg po. Loading dose of 0.5 to 0.75 mg usually produces effects in 1-2 hours, becoming maximal in 6-8 hours. Give additional doses of 0.25 to 0.5 mg cautiously every 6-8 hours.

Usual oral maintenance dose: 0.125 to 0.5 mg daily. (Average is 0.25 mg.) In elderly patients, use 0.125 to 0.25 mg.

Slow oral digitalizing dose: In previously undigitalized patients with normal function, maintenance therapy without a loading dose results in a steady blood level in about 7 days.

Infants and children: Digitalizing doses for children with normal renal function range from 40 to 80 mcg/kg depending upon age and weight. Therapy should be decided upon in conjunction with a physician and where continuous cardiac monitoring can take place. Maintenance therapy is 20% to 30% of digitalizing dose daily.

Marilyn W. Edmunds

DIURETICS—
CARBONIC ANHYDRASE INHIBITORS

ACTION OF THE DRUG: These products are nonbacteriostatic sulfonamides which (1) decrease glomerular filtration rate and renal blood flow. They produce increased excretion of potassium, sodium, bicarbonate, and water, resulting in an alkaline diuresis. (2) They also inhibit the action of carbonic anhydrase enzymes, thus blocking the hydration of CO_2 to carbonic acid and ionization to yield hydrogen ions and bicarbonate. This leads to a decreased secretion of aqueous humor in the eye and a decreased intraocular pressure since water is no longer attracted to a hypertonic solution. (See section on antiglaucoma drugs.)

ASSESSMENT:

INDICATIONS: These drugs are used primarily for the treatment of open angle glaucoma; however, several drugs in this category are somewhat useful with other drugs in the control of fluid retention associated with cardiovascular problems. They are also used at times in the treatment of certain seizure disorders such as petit mal epilepsy. The nurse practitioner does not usually prescribe this medication but often assumes responsibility for monitoring the response of a patient to this medication.

SUBJECTIVE: Patient may present with a history of weight gain, fatigue, weakness, paroxysmal nocturnal dyspnea, dyspnea, swollen feet, and high blood pressure.

OBJECTIVE: Patient may present with signs of edema: shortness of breath, jugular venous distention, increased hepatojugular reflux, rales in the lungs, documented weight gain, third heart sound, peripheral edema. When drug is used as an antihypertensive, blood pressure greater than 140/90 mm Hg may be found.

PLAN:

CONTRAINDICATIONS: Do not use in the presence of hypersensitivity to sulfonamides, severe liver or kidney disease, in electrolyte imbalance (especially hyponatremia and hypokalemia), hyperchloremic acidosis, adrenocortical insufficiency, or Addison's disease. Do not use in patients who cannot increase alveolar ventilation (as in severe pulmonary obstruction) as deepening acidosis may be promoted. Do not use for long periods in patients with chronic closed angle glaucoma as closure of the angle may be masked by lowered intraocular pressure in some organic processes. Do not give to patients with demonstrated sensitivity to antibacterial sulfonamides, sulfonamide derivatives, or thiazides as cross-sensitivity has been reported.

WARNINGS: Safety for use in pregnancy has not been demonstrated. Teratogenic effects in rats and mice have been demonstrated at high doses.

PRECAUTIONS: Potassium excretion is increased by carbonic anhydrase inhibitors and is proportional to the extent of diuresis, presenting a substantial risk in rapid diuresis. Patients with low oral potassium intake are also at risk for developing hypokalemia. The risk of hypokalemia may also be increased when used in the presence of severe cirrhosis or with concomitant use of steroids or ACTH. Hepatic coma could also be precipitated. Use with caution in patients with respiratory acidosis.

Increasing the dose does not increase diuresis. However, these drugs, used in combination with other diuretics, may result in decreased fluid retention in some refractory cases.

Hypokalemia produces exaggerated myocardial sensitivity in patients taking digitalis.

IMPLEMENTATION:

DRUG INTERACTIONS: Carbonic anhydrase inhibitors make urine alkaline and thus may enhance the action of amphetamines, catecholamines, procainamide, quinidine, tricyclic antidepressants, and any other basic drug by increasing their reabsorption. They may produce a lowered hypoglycemic response to insulin and oral antiglycemics. Carbonic anhydrase inhibitors can decrease the effects of barbiturates, lithium, salicylates, nitrofurantoin, and other acid substances by reducing their tubular reabsorption. Increased hypokalemic response can result when used concurrently with other diuretics, corticosteroids, and amphotericin B. Hypokalemia may augment digitalis toxicity.

ADMINISTRATION AND DOSAGE: When used for congestive heart failure or edema, increasing the dose does not increase the diuretic effect. Failure of therapy is often due to overdosage or too-frequent dosage. The best diuresis is often produced by administering medication on alternate days, or by giving drug for two days and withholding on the third day.

Drug is available for parenteral use in emergency situations within hospitals. The preferred parenteral route is IV since IM injections are very painful. Drugs vary a great deal in time of onset, peak of action, and duration of effect. See sections on individual drugs for comparisons. Effects are additive when given with other miotics or mydriatics. Dichlorphenamide (used exclusively in the treatment of glaucoma) is 15 times as potent an inhibitor as the other carbonic anhydrase inhibitors and has an onset of action within one hour.

IMPLEMENTATION CONSIDERATIONS:

—Obtain a complete health history, including presence of hypersensitivity to sulfonamides or thiazide diuretics, presence of respiratory acidosis, diabetes, gout, significant liver, renal, or cardiac problems, and possibility of pregnancy.

—There are usually minimal side effects with short-term therapy. Diabetics must be monitored very closely however.

—The side effects which develop are similar to other sulfonamides. The practitioner needs to monitor for adverse effects so that the drug may be discontinued as soon as possible if symptoms develop.

—The most frequent adverse reaction seen even with short-term therapy is the development of paresthesias.

—In long-term therapy, check for metabolic acidosis and hypokalemia. Adjunctive administration of bicarbonate and potassium may be necessary to correct this problem.

—Some patients develop a transient myopia which disappears when drug is discontinued.

—If patient has problems with both edema and glaucoma, the practitioner must work closely with the ophthalmologist in developing a treatment regimen for the patient.

—Do not change brands of carbonic anhydrase inhibitors when patient is stabilized on one product since therapeutic equivalence varies among different products.

WHAT THE PATIENT NEEDS TO KNOW:

—Take medication exactly as instructed by the health care provider. If you miss a dose, take it as soon as you remember. If it is close to the time for the next dose, skip the missed dose and take your regular dose at the proper time. Do not double doses.

—If stomach upset develops from use of the medication, take pills with food.

—Drug may cause drowsiness. Use caution in driving or performing tasks requiring alertness.

—Force fluids while taking this medicine. Drink at least 8 glasses of liquid (preferably water) each day.

—Side effects do occur in some people taking this drug. Notify your health practitioner if you note any new or uncomfortable symptoms. Watch particularly for the development of a sore throat, fever, unusual bleeding or bruising, skin rash, tingling or tremors in hands or feet, or flank or loin pain.

—Take this medication with a full glass of orange juice (unless contraindicated by your diet). Other potassium-rich foods should be used daily. These include: citrus foods (especially oranges and tomatoes), bananas, dried fruits, apricots, cantaloupe, watermelon, nuts, dried beans, beef and fowl.

—Taking medication is only one part of your treatment regimen. Reduction of other risk factors is also important: lose weight (if overweight), stop smoking, increase exercise, avoid stressful and emotional pressures. Avoid use of foods high in sodium: lunch meats, smoked meats, Chinese food, processed cheese, snack foods. Do not salt food while cooking or add salt to your food after it is cooked.

—Keep this medication out of the reach of children and others for whom it is not prescribed.

—The goal of therapy is to help you feel as healthy as possible and to avoid any complications. Taking your medication and reducing other risk factors will help reduce the chance of serious complications. It is important then to keep taking your medicine, even when you feel well, and to keep seeing your health practitioner regularly.

EVALUATION:

ADVERSE REACTIONS: *CNS:* ataxia, confusion, convulsions, depression, disorientation, dizziness, drowsiness, flaccid paralysis, headache, loss of taste and smell, nervousness, paresthesias (particularly tingling in extremities, lips, mouth, and anus), sedation, transient myopia, tinnitus, tremor, vertigo, weakness, xerostomia. *Dermatologic:* pruritus, rash, skin eruptions, urticaria. *Endocrine:* glycosuria. *Gastrointestinal:* anorexia, constipation, diarrhea, dry mouth, hepatic insufficiency, melena, nausea, pancreatitis, vomiting. *Hematopoietic:* agranulocytosis, aplastic anemia, bone marrow depression, hemolytic anemia, leukopenia, pancytopenia, thrombocytopenic purpura. *Hypersensitivity:* photosensitivity. *Renal:* crystalluria, dysuria, glycosuria, hematuria, polyuria, renal calculi, ureteral colic, urinary frequency. *Other:* depression, fever, hypokalemia, hyponatremia, lassitude, malaise, tiredness.

PARAMETERS TO MONITOR: Complete baseline history; physical and laboratory work should be collected prior to initiation of therapy. This should include a thorough evaluation of liver and kidney function. Patient should be monitored for therapeutic effect: weight loss, relief of dyspnea, peripheral edema. Monitor for development of adverse effects through periodic laboratory evaluations.

ACETAZOLAMIDE

PRODUCTS (TRADE NAME):

Acetazolamide (Available in 250 mg tablets, 500 mg sustained release capsules.) **AK-Zol** (Available in 250 mg tablets.) **Diamox** (Available in 125, 250 mg tablets; 500 mg solution for injections.) **Diamox Sequels** (Available in 500 mg sustained release capsules.)

DRUG SPECIFICS:

Used in the treatment of edema secondary to congestive heart failure or drugs. Also used in treating petit mal and unlocalized seizures. (See section on Anti-Glaucoma drugs for use in glaucoma.)

Do not use products interchangeably as bioavailability of different drugs may vary.

Onset of action is 60-90 minutes for tablets, with peak of action from 2 to 4 hours. Action lasts up to 12 hours. Sustained action capsules have onset within 2 hours with their peak between 8 and 12 hours. Duration is between 18 and 24 hours. IV administration will produce results in 2 minutes, peak at 15 minutes, and continue working for 4-5 hours.

ADMINISTRATION AND DOSAGE SPECIFICS:

Congestive heart failure and drug-induced edema: Give 250 to 375 mg po initially in the morning (5 mg/kg.) Then continue taking medication on alternate days, or take for two days and withhold for one day. Sustained release drugs may be used on a twice-daily schedule.

METHAZOLAMIDE

PRODUCTS (TRADE NAME):

Neptazane (Available in 50 mg tablets.)

DRUG SPECIFICS:

This drug is used primarily in the treatment of glaucoma. (See section on Anti-Glaucoma drugs.) Osmotic and miotic drugs may be used with this product. Do not change products as bioavailability of different drugs may vary. Onset of action is 2 to 4 hours, with peak between 6 and 8 hours. Duration of effect is 10 to 18 hours.

ADMINISTRATION AND DOSAGE SPECIFICS:

Give 50 to 100 mg 2 or 3 times daily.

Marilyn W. Edmunds

DIURETICS—LOOP

BUMETANIDE

ACTION OF THE DRUG: Loop diuretics act by inhibiting reabsorption of sodium and chloride in the thick, ascending loop of Henle and in both proximal and distal tubules. This drug is often effective in patients with very low glomerular filtration rates because it is so efficient in inhibiting reabsorption of sodium. The peak diuretic effect is much greater than that observed with other clinically available diuretics. Bumetanide has a fast oral onset but duration of action is shorter than furosemide or ethacrynic acid. Sodium chloride, potassium, hydrogen and other electrolytes plus large volumes of water are excreted in the urine. Bumetanide is more chloruretic than natriuretic and may have maximal effect on the proximal tubule. It may be effective in patients with significant renal insufficiency due to inhibition of the large proportion of filtered sodium.

ASSESSMENT:

INDICATIONS: Loop diuretics are used in the treatment of severe edema in congestive heart failure, cirrhosis of the liver, and renal disease (nephrotic syndrome) where a powerful diuretic is indicated. It may be given parenterally for pulmonary edema when gastrointestinal absorption is reduced and when oral medication is not possible.

SUBJECTIVE: Patient may present with a history of weight gain, fatigue, weakness, paroxysmal nocturnal dyspnea, dyspnea, and swollen feet. History of hypertension may also be present.

OBJECTIVE: Signs of edema and hypertension may be present: shortness of breath, jugular venous distension, hepatojugular reflux, rales in the lungs, documented weight gain, third heart sound (S3), peripheral edema. When drug is used as an antihypertensive, assess level of blood pressure and pulse in standing, sitting and lying positions. Blood pressure in hypertensive patients is greater than 140/90 mm Hg.

PLAN:

CONTRAINDICATIONS: Do not give in the presence of hypersensitivity. Do not give in the presence of anuria, hepatic coma, or dehydration. It has not been proven safe for administration in infants or in the early stages of pregnancy, or to breast-feeding women.

WARNINGS: This drug is a very potent diuretic used in special situations and should usually be given in collaboration with a physician. Excessive diuresis may promote dehydration, volume depletion, and vascular collapse. Elderly patients are particularly vulnerable to these problems, and embolism and vascular thrombosis may also be precipitated.

In patients with hepatic impairment, treatment should be initiated in the hospital under a physician's supervision since hepatic coma may be precipitated. Close monitoring of fluid and electrolytes is mandatory in these patients.

This product may exacerbate or activate systemic lupus erythematosus. Observe for blood dyscrasias, liver damage or idiosyncratic reactions.

PRECAUTIONS: Electrolyte depletion may occur, especially in patients receiving high dosages. In critically ill patients taking these medications, a number of drug-related deaths have occurred. These fall into two main categories: (1) patients with severe myocardial disease who are taking digitalis, who develop hypokalemia and subsequently have fatal arrhythmias, and (2) patients with decompensating hepatic cirrhosis and ascites who develop severe electrolyte deficiencies leading to death. It is also important to note that numerous laboratory tests may be altered by this drug and, therefore, monitoring patient status may be difficult at times.

IMPLEMENTATION:

DRUG INTERACTIONS: The effects of antihypertensive medications may be potentiated, particularly with ganglionic or peripheral adrenergic blocking drugs. Because of reductions in renal clearance, do not use with lithium as lithium toxicity may be precipitated. Concomitant administration with aminoglycoside antibiotics increases the potential for ototoxicity, especially if patient has reduced renal function. When given with alcohol, anesthetics, skeletal muscle relaxants, barbiturates or narcotics, orthostatic hypotension may develop. Hypokalemia is likely in patients concurrently using potassium-depleting steroids, corticosteroids, or ACTH. Patients receiving therapy with digitalis preparations who have excessive loss of potassium may develop digitalis toxicity. Pretreatment with probenecid reduces both the natriuresis and hyperreninemia produced by bumetanide. Indomethacin blunts the increases in urine volume and sodium excretion seen with bumetanide therapy.

PRODUCTS (TRADE NAME):
Bumex (Available in 0.5 and 1.0 mg tablets and 0.25 mg/ml injection.)

ADMINISTRATION AND DOSAGE: Dosage must be adjusted individually for each patient depending upon response. Use lowest dosage possible to avoid profound diuresis and fluid and electrolyte depletion. IV administration should be used only in emergency situations or when patient cannot take medication orally. Change to oral form as soon as patient is able to do so.

Oral: The usual total daily dose is 0.5 to 2.0 mg given as a single dose in the morning. A second or third dose may be given 4 to 5 hours later if diuesis is not adequate. Do not exceed 10 mg/day. In patients with edema, medication may be taken on alternate days or for 3 to 4 days with rest periods of 1 to 2 days in between.

Parenteral: Usually initial dose is 0.5 to 1.0 mg IV or IM. Give IV medication slowly over a 1 to 2 minute period. Dosage may be repeated within 2 to 3 hours if diuresis is inadequate.

IMPLEMENTATION CONSIDERATIONS:

—Obtain a complete health history, including the presence of hypersensitivity (especially to sulfonamide-type drugs); concurrent use of other drugs which may cause drug interactions; underlying systemic disease, especially collagen, cardiovascular, or hepatic; or possibility of pregnancy.

—Renal effects of this drug are primarily dose related.

—Substantial water and electrolyte loss can be avoided by giving small initial doses, weighing patient during therapy, and titrating dose to achieve best effects. Give on intermittent dosage schedule when possible.

—Profound dehydration and electrolyte depletion may develop in patients on this drug. If excessive diuresis occurs, reduce dosage or withdraw drug temporarily.

—Asymptomatic hyperuricemia or gout may be precipitated along with an elevated BUN. This is especially seen in dehydration of patients with renal insufficiency.

—Practitioner may need to instruct the patient to adjust salt intake and use supplementary potassium chloride if patient consistently develops hypokalemia.

—These products may lower serum calcium, and rare cases of tetany have been seen.

—In patients taking more than 80 mg/day, frequent laboratory evaluations should be performed.

—Monitor patients with diabetes or gout very carefully.

—Because cross-sensitivity with furosemide is rare, this product may be substituted at about a 1:40 ratio of bumetanide to furosemide in patients allergic to furosemide.

WHAT THE PATIENT NEEDS TO KNOW:

—Take this medication precisely as ordered by the health care provider. If you miss a dose, take it as soon as you remember if it is within an hour or two of the regular time. If it is close to the time for the next dose, take only the next scheduled dose. Do not double dosage or abruptly stop medication without being advised to do so.

—Some people feel stomach upset after taking this medicine. Taking pills with food or milk may help reduce this feeling.

—Notify your health care provider if muscle weakness, cramps, nausea, diarrhea, blood in urine, impaired hearing, ringing in ears, vertigo, or dizziness develops. If you notice any weight gain, be certain to notify your practitioner.

—Take medication early in the day on either a once- or twice-daily schedule to avoid having to get up at night to void. For twice daily schedules, 8 AM and 2 PM are suggested.

—Keep this medication out of the reach of children and others for whom it is not prescribed.

—Take medication with a full glass of orange juice (unless contraindicated by your diet). Other potassium-rich foods should be used daily. These include: citrus foods (especially oranges and tomatoes), bananas, dried fruits, apricots, cantaloupe, watermelon, nuts, dried beans, beef, and fowl.

—Taking medication is only one part of your treatment regimen. Reduction of weight, increased exercise, and elimination of high-sodium foods are also important. Avoid foods such as lunch meats, smoked meats, Chinese food, processed cheese, and snack foods. Do not salt food while cooking or add salt to your food after it is cooked.

—Wear a Medic-Alert bracelet specifying that you are taking this drug.

—Watch for signs of dizziness, particularly on rising from lying to standing position. Move slowly in order to allow your body time to adjust.

EVALUATION:

ADVERSE REACTIONS: Reactions associated with loop diuretics in general: *CNS:* blurred vision, headache, irreversible hearing loss, tinnitus, vertigo. *Gastrointestinal:* acute pancreatitis, anorexia, diarrhea, dysphagia, jaundice, nausea, vomiting. *Hematopoietic:* agranulocytosis, thrombocytopenia. *Other:* hyperglycemia and hyperuricemia which may precipitate gout, local irritation and pain with parenteral use (occasionally), pruritus, rash, hypocalcemia, hypochloremic alkalosis, hypokalemia, hyponatremia, hypomagnesemia.

Problems associated with bumetanide in particular: *Cardiovascular:* chest pain, ECG changes, hypotension. *CNS:* asterixis. *Gastrointestinal:* abdominal pain, dry mouth, upset stomach. *Genitourinary:* Difficulty maintaining erection, premature ejaculation, renal failure. *Musculoskeletal:* arthritis pain, fatigue, muscle cramps, musculoskeletal pain, weakness. *Other:* dehydration, hives, hyperventilation, nipple tenderness, pruritus, sweating. Most laboratory tests are affected by both hydration and the medication itself.

PARAMETERS TO MONITOR: Obtain complete history, physical and laboratory baseline studies (including CO_2, BUN, WBC, uric acid, glucose, liver function, and electrolytes) prior to initiation of therapy. Monitor for therapeutic effect: reduction in edema which may be evaluated by subjective indications of relief and weight loss, decrease or absence of peripheral edema, no jugular venous distention, reduction in cardiac size, and gradual loss of third (S3) heart sound. Also monitor for progression of edema and development of adverse reactions. Perform periodic evaluation of serum electrolytes. Check for signs and symptoms of fluid and electrolyte imbalance: hyponatremia, hypochloremic acidosis, hypokalemia. Be especially careful in patients concomitantly receiving digitalis. Do serum and urine evaluations in patients complaining of vomiting or having cirrhosis, IV fluids, or severe diuresis. Look for the warning signs of imbalance and dehydration: dry mouth, thirst, weakness, lethargy, drowsiness, restlessness, muscle pains or cramps, muscle fatigue, hypotension, oliguria, tachycardia, arrhythmias, nausea, and vomiting. Also watch for blood dyscrasias, liver damage, or idiosyncratic reactions.

Frequent serum electrolytes, C02, BUN, and calcium levels should be obtained in patients on long-term therapy. FBS, glucose tolerance, and 2-hour postprandial blood sugar evaluations should be obtained in diabetics using bumetanide.

Marilyn W. Edmunds

ETHACRYNIC ACID

ACTION OF THE DRUG: Loop diuretics act by inhibiting reabsorption of sodium and chloride in the thick, ascending loop of Henle and in both proximal and distal tubules. This drug is often effective in patients with very low glomerular filtration rates because it is so efficient in inhibiting reabsorption of sodium. The peak diuretic effect is much greater than that observed with any other clinically available diuretics. Loop diuretics have fast oral onset, work independently of acid-base imbalance, and are effective in patients with impaired renal function. Sodium, chloride, potassium, hydrogen and other electrolytes plus large volumes of water are excreted in the urine. Ethacrynic acid has not been shown to offer an advantage over other loop diuretics and is more ototoxic.

ASSESSMENT:

INDICATIONS: Loop diuretics are used in the treatment of severe edema in congestive heart failure, cirrhosis of the liver, and renal disease (nephrotic syndrome) where a powerful diuretic is indicated. They may be given parenterally for pulmonary edema when gastrointestinal absorption is reduced and when oral medication is not possible. Ethacrynic acid is especially useful in short-term therapy for lymphedema, idiopathic edema and in ascites secondary to malignancy. It is used in patients hospitalized for treatment of nephrotic syndrome or congestive heart failure.

SUBJECTIVE: Patient may present with a history of weight gain, fatigue, weakness, paroxysmal nocturnal dyspnea, dyspnea, and swollen feet. Patient may also have history of high blood pressure.

OBJECTIVE: Signs of edema and hypertension may be present: shortness of breath, jugular venous distention, hepatojugular reflux, rales in the lungs, documented weight gain, third heart sound (S3), peripheral edema. When drug is used as an antihypertensive, assess level of blood pressure and pulse in standing, sitting and lying positions. Blood pressure in hypertensive patients is greater than 140/90 mm Hg.

PLAN:

CONTRAINDICATIONS: Do not give in the presence of hypersensitivity. Patients allergic to sulfonamide-type medications may be allergic to this medication also. Do not give in the presence of anuria, hepatic coma, or dehydration. It has not been proven safe for administration in infants or in the early stages of pregnancy.

WARNINGS: These drugs are very potent diuretics used in special situations and should usually be given in collaboration with a physician. Excessive diuresis may promote dehydration, volume depletion, and vascular collapse. Elderly patients are particularly vulnerable to these problems, and embolism and vascular thrombosis may also be precipitated.

In patients with hepatic impairment, treatment should be initiated in the hospital under a physician's supervision since hepatic coma may be precipitated. Close monitoring of fluid and electrolytes is mandatory in these patients.

Tinnitus may be provoked and hearing loss (usually reversible) may develop with rapid IV injection of high doses or when used in conjunction with other ototoxic drugs.

These products may exacerbate or activate systemic lupus erythematosus. Use with extreme caution in pregnant women, as initial animal research indicates possible hazards to both mother and fetus. Drug appears in breast milk. If use of these drugs is indicated, mother should stop breast-feeding.

PRECAUTIONS: Electrolyte depletion may occur, especially in patients receiving high dosages. In critically ill patients taking this medication, a number of drug-related deaths have occurred. These fall into two main categories: (1) patients with severe myocardial disease who are taking digitalis, who develop hypokalemia and subsequently have fatal arrhythmias, and (2) patients with decompensating hepatic cirrhosis and ascites who develop severe electrolyte deficiencies leading to death. It is also important to note that numerous laboratory tests may be altered by these drugs and, therefore, monitoring patient status may be difficult at times.

IMPLEMENTATION:

DRUG INTERACTIONS: Ethacrynic acid exerts potent effects when used concomitantly with oral anticoagulants and antihypertensive agents, especially ganglionic or peripheral adrenergic blocking agents. When given with alcohol, anesthetics, skeletal muscle relaxants, barbiturates or narcotics, orthostatic hypotension may develop. Hypokalemia is likely in patients concurrently using potassium-depleting steroids, corticosteroids, or ACTH. Patients receiving therapy with digitalis preparations who have excessive loss of potassium may develop digitalis toxicity. Toxicity may also be increased with use of cephalosporins and cardiac glycosides. This diuretic reduces the renal clearance of lithium and so increases the risk of lithium toxicity. Arterial responsiveness to norepinephrine is decreased by this drug. Decrease may not neutralize pressor action, however.

Ethacrynic acid displaces warfarin from plasma protein binding sites, so a reduction in usual anticoagulant dose may be necessary, and extra caution in monitoring clotting time is important.

PRODUCTS (TRADE NAME):

Edecrin (Available in 25 and 50 mg scored tablets). **Sodium Edecrin** (Available in 50 mg vial for reconstitution and injection).

ADMINISTRATION AND DOSAGE: Dosage must be adjusted individually for each patient depending upon response. Use lowest dosage possible to avoid profound diuresis and fluid and electrolyte depletion. IV administration should be used only in emergency situations or when patient cannot take medication orally. Change to oral form as soon as patient is able to do so.

Ethacrynic acid is effective within 30 minutes after oral administration, reaches a peak within 1-2 hours, and is effective for 6-8 hours. For IV administration, it is effective within 5 minutes, reaches a peak within 30 minutes, and duration of action is about 2 hours.

If severe, watery diarrhea develops, discontinue drug and do not readminister.

Adults: Give 50-100 mg/day orally, or a smaller dose if possible to achieve a gradual weight loss (1 to 2 lb/day). Maintenance dose is 50 to 200 mg/day on a continuous or intermittent basis. Adjust dosage upward in increments of 25 to 50 mg and evaluate patients carefully. If patient is taking other diuretics, an additive response has often been seen, and increments should be only 25 mg at a time.

May give IV when unable to take orally. Give 50 mg or 0.5 to 1 mg/kg slowly (over a period of minutes). If second dose is warranted, inject in different site in order to avoid development of thrombophlebitis. Do not give IM or SQ because of extreme pain.

Children: Give 25 mg po with increases of 25 mg to reach desired level of diuresis. Not recommended for IV use in children.

IMPLEMENTATION CONSIDERATIONS:

—Obtain a complete health history, including the presence of hypersensitivity (especially to sulfonamide-type drugs); concurrent use of other drugs which may cause drug interactions; underlying systemic disease, especially collagen, cardiovascular, or hepatic; or possibility of pregnancy.

—Renal effects of this drug are primarily dose related.

—Substantial water and electrolyte loss can be avoided by giving small initial doses, weighing patient during therapy, and titrating dose to achieve best effects. Give on intermittent dosage schedule when possible.

—Profound dehydration and electrolyte depletion may develop in patients on this drug. If excessive diuresis occurs, reduce dosage or withdraw drug temporarily.

—Asymptomatic hyperuricemia or gout may be precipitated along with an elevated BUN. This is especially seen in dehydration of patients with renal insufficiency.

—Practitioner may need to instruct the patient to adjust salt intake and use supplementary potassium chloride if patient consistently develops hypokalemia.

—These products may lower serum calcium, and rare cases of tetany have been seen.

—Liberalization of salt intake may be necessary when taking ethacrynic acid.

—Monitor patients with diabetes or gout very carefully.

WHAT THE PATIENT NEEDS TO KNOW:

—Take this medication precisely as ordered by the health care provider. If you miss a dose, take it as soon as you remember if it is within an hour or two of the regular time. If it is close to the time for the next dose, take only the next scheduled dose. Do not double dosage or abruptly stop medication without being advised to do so.

—Some people feel stomach upset after taking this medicine. Taking pills with food or milk may help reduce this feeling.

—Notify your health care provider if muscle weakness, cramps, nausea, diarrhea, blood in urine, impaired hearing, ringing in ears, vertigo, or dizziness develops. If you notice any weight gain, be certain to notify your practitioner.

—Take medication early in the day on either a once or twice-daily schedule to avoid having to get up at night to void. For twice daily schedules, 8 AM and 2 PM are suggested.

—Keep this medication out of the reach of children and others for whom it is not prescribed.

—Take medication with a full glass of orange juice (unless contraindicated by your diet). Other potassium-rich foods should be used daily. These include: citrus foods (especially oranges and tomatoes), bananas, dried fruits, apricots, cantaloupe, watermelon, nuts, dried beans, beef, and fowl.

—Taking medication is only one part of your treatment regimen. Reduction of weight, increased exercise, and elimination of high-sodium foods are also important. Avoid foods such as lunch meats, smoked meats, Chinese food, processed cheese, and snack foods. Do not salt food while cooking or add salt to your food after it is cooked.

—Wear a Medic-Alert bracelet specifying that you are taking this drug.

—Watch for signs of dizziness, particularly on rising from lying to standing position. Move slowly in order to allow your body time to adjust.

EVALUATION:

ADVERSE REACTIONS: Problems common to loop diuretics in general: *CNS:* blurred vision, headache, irreversible hearing loss, tinnitus, vertigo. *Gastrointestinal:* acute pancreatitis, anorexia, diarrhea, dysphagia, jaundice, nausea, vomiting. *Hematopoietic:* agranulocytosis, thrombocytopenia. *Other:* hyperglycemia and hyperuricemia which may precipitate gout, local irritation and pain with parenteral use (occasionally), pruritus, rash, hypocalcemia, hypochloremic alkalosis, hypokalemia, hyponatremia, hypomagnesemia.

Problems particular to ethacrynic acid: *Endocrine:* acute hypoglycemia with convulsions (rare). *Gastrointestinal:* abdominal discomfort, anorexia, dysphagia, gastrointestinal bleeding, severe and profuse watery diarrhea. *Hematopoietic:* Henoch-Schonlein purpura (rare) in patients with rheumatic heart disease taking other drugs, severe neutropenia (rare). *Other:* abnormal liver function tests in severely ill patients taking many drugs, apprehension, chills, confusion, fatigue, fever, hematuria, hypovolemia, muscle cramps, nystagmus, orthostatic hypotension.

PARAMETERS TO MONITOR: Obtain complete history, physical and laboratory baseline studies (including C02, BUN, WBC, uric acid, glucose, liver function, and electrolytes) prior to initiation of therapy. Monitor for therapeutic effect: reduction in edema which may be evaluated by subjective indications of relief and weight loss, decrease or absence of peripheral edema, no jugular venous distention, reduction in cardiac size, and gradual loss of third (S3) heart sound. Also monitor for progression of edema and development of adverse reactions. Perform periodic evaluation of serum electrolytes. Check for signs and symptoms of fluid and electrolyte imbalance: hyponatremia, hypochloremic acidosis, hypokalemia. Be especially careful in patients concomitantly receiving digitalis. Do serum and urine evaluations in patients complaining of vomiting or having cirrhosis, IV fluids, or severe diuresis. Look for the warning signs of imbalance and dehydration: dry mouth, thirst, weakness, lethargy, drowsiness, restlessness, muscle pains or cramps, muscle fatigue, hypotension, oliguria, tachycardia, arrhythmias, nausea, and vomiting. Also watch for blood dyscrasias, liver damage, or idiosyncratic reactions. Frequent serum electrolytes, C02, BUN, and calcium levels should be obtained in patients on long-term therapy. Monitor for decreased hearing.

Marilyn W. Edmunds

FUROSEMIDE

ACTION OF THE DRUG: Loop diuretics act by inhibiting reabsorption of sodium and chloride in the thick, ascending loop of Henle and in both proximal and distal tubules. This drug is often effective in patients with very low glomerular filtration rates because it is so efficient in inhibiting reabsorption of sodium. The peak diuretic effect is much greater than that observed with any other clinically available diuretics. Furosemide has a fast oral onset, works independently of acid-base imbalance, and is effective in patients with impaired renal function. Sodium, chloride, potassium, hydrogen and other electrolytes plus large volumes of water are excreted in the urine.

ASSESSMENT:

INDICATIONS: Loop diuretics are used in the treatment of severe edema in congestive heart failure, cirrhosis of the liver, and renal disease (nephrotic syndrome) where a powerful diuretic is indicated. It may be given parenterally for pulmonary edema when gastrointestinal absorption is reduced and when oral medication is not possible. Furosemide is used in the treatment of hypertension as a Step One drug, either alone or in combination with other antihypertensive agents.

SUBJECTIVE: Patient may present with a history of weight gain, fatigue, weakness, paroxysmal nocturnal dyspnea, dyspnea, and swollen feet. Patient may also have history of high blood pressure.

OBJECTIVE: Signs of edema and hypertension may be present: shortness of breath, jugular venous distension, hepatojugular reflux, rales in the lungs, documented weight gain, third heart sound (S3), peripheral edema. When drug is used as an antihypertensive, assess level of blood pressure and pulse in standing, sitting and lying positions. Blood pressure in hypertensive patients is greater than 140/90 mm Hg.

PLAN:

CONTRAINDICATIONS: Do not give in the presence of hypersensitivity. Patients allergic to sulfonamide-type medications may be allergic to this medication also. Do not give in the presence of anuria, hepatic coma, or dehydration. It has not been proven safe for administration in infants or in the early stages of pregnancy.

WARNINGS: These drugs are both very potent diuretics used in special situations and should usually be given in collaboration with a physician. Excessive diuresis may promote dehydration, volume depletion, and vascular collapse. Elderly patients are particularly vulnerable to these problems, and embolism and vascular thrombosis may also be precipitated.

In patients with hepatic impairment, treatment should be initiated in the hospital under a physician's supervision since hepatic coma may be precipitated. Close monitoring of fluid and electrolytes is mandatory in these patients.

Tinnitus may be provoked and hearing loss (usually reversible) may develop with rapid IV injection of high doses or when used in conjunction with other ototoxic drugs.

This product may exacerbate or activate systemic lupus erythematosus. Use with extreme caution in pregnant women, as initial animal research indicates possible hazards to both mother and fetus. Furosemide appears in breast milk. If drug is indicated, mother should stop breast-feeding.

PRECAUTIONS: Electrolyte depletion may occur, especially in patients receiving high dosages. In critically ill patients taking these medications, a number of drug-related deaths have occurred. These fall into two main categories: (1) patients with severe myocardial disease who are taking digitalis, who develop hypokalemia and subsequently have fatal arrhythmias, and (2) patients with decompensating hepatic cirrhosis and ascites who develop severe electrolyte deficiencies leading to death. It is also important to note that numerous laboratory tests may be altered by this drug and, therefore, monitoring patient status may be difficult at times.

IMPLEMENTATION:

DRUG INTERACTIONS: Furosemide exerts potent effects when used concomitantly with oral anticoagulants and antihypertensive agents, especially ganglionic or peripheral adrenergic blocking agents. When given with alcohol, anesthetics, skeletal muscle relaxants, barbiturates or narcotics, orthostatic hypotension may develop. Hypokalemia is likely in patients concurrently using potassium-depleting steroids, corticosteroids, or ACTH. Patients receiving therapy with digitalis preparations who have excessive loss of potassium may develop digitalis toxicity. Probenecid prolongs the diuretic action of furosemide by inhibiting its excretion. Toxicity may also be increased with use of cephalosporins and cardiac glycosides. Loop diuretics reduce the renal clearance of lithium and so increase the risk of lithium toxicity. Arterial responsiveness to norepinephrine is decreased by these diuretics. Decrease may not neutralize pressor action, however.

If patient has impaired renal function, avoid use of parenteral furosemide (especially if aminoglycoside antibiotics have been given) since ototoxicity often develops. Furosemide will also enhance the nephrotoxicity of cephaloridine. If patient is receiving high doses of salicylates, concomitant use of furosemide may produce salicylate toxicity at lower doses because of competition with renal excretory sites. Furosemide also antagonizes the skeletal muscle relaxing effect of tubocurarine; it may also potentiate the action of succinylcholine. Concomitant administration of indomethacin may decrease the natriuretic and antihypertensive effect secondary to decreased prostaglandin synthesis. Phenytoin may reduce the absorption of furosemide. Furosemide may increase the fasting blood sugar level and alter glucose tolerance and two-hour postprandial blood sugar levels. BUN, serum uric acid, and urine glucose levels may all be increased. Furosemide may increase the level of blood uric acid and adjustment of antigout medicines may be necessary to control hyperuricemia and gout. It may also raise blood glucose levels or interfere with hypoglycemic effects of antidiabetic agents, requiring alteration of dosages.

PRODUCTS (TRADE NAME):

Furosemide (Available in 20, 40 and 80 mg tablets, and 10 mg/ml oral solution and injections). **Lasix** (Available in 20, 40 and 80 mg tablets, 10 mg/ml oral solution, and 10 mg/ml injection). **SK-Furosemide** (Available in 20 mg tablets.)

ADMINISTRATION AND DOSAGE: Patients with known allergy to sulfonamides may show sensitivity to furosemide. Onset of action following oral administration is 1 hour, with peak effect in 1-2 hours and duration 6-8 hours. Onset of action following IV injection is 5 minutes, with peak effect within 30 minutes and duration about 2 hours.

Tablets should be kept in a dark, closed container, since exposure to light causes discoloration and decomposition. Do not use solution if it is yellow.

Dosage must be adjusted individually for each patient depending upon response. Use lowest dosage possible to avoid profound diuresis and fluid and electrolyte depletion. IV administration should be used only in emergency situations or when patient cannot take medication orally. Change to oral form as soon as patient is able to do so.

Edema: Give 20 to 80 mg/day po in single dose. A second dose may be administered 6-8 hours later if needed to increase diuresis. May increase dosage by 20 or 40 mg at 6-8 hour intervals. Dose which achieves desired amount of diuresis should be used as maintenance dose, which is given once or twice daily. Whenever possible give medication 2 to 4 consecutive days per week, using an intermittent dosing regimen. May also give 20 to 40 mg IM or IV, administered slowly (give over 1-2 minutes if administered IV). Increase dosage by 20-40 mg every 2 hours if needed (80 mg may be needed for patients in acute pulmonary edema). Establish maintenance dose, which should then be given daily. When medication is given by infusion, maximum dosage is 4 mg/min.

Hypertension: Give 40 mg po twice a day. If patient is receiving other antihypertensive medications, reduce their dosage by 50% when furosemide is started. Gradually adjust dosages of all medications depending upon response of patient's blood pressure.

Infants and children: Give 2 mg/kg po or 1 mg/kg IV given slowly and increase by 1 or 2 mg/kg every 6-8 hours (or every 2 hours if giving medication IV) as needed. Maximum 6 mg/kg. For maintenance adjust dose to smallest amount possible to achieve desired results.

IMPLEMENTATION CONSIDERATIONS:

—Obtain a complete health history, including the presence of hypersensitivity (especially to sulfonamide-type drugs), concurrent use of other drugs which may cause drug interactions, underlying systemic disease, especially collagen, cardiovascular or hepatic, or possibility of pregnancy.

—Renal effects of this drug are primarily dose related.

—Substantial water and electrolyte loss can be avoided by giving small initial doses, weighing patient during therapy, and titrating dose to achieve best effects. Give on intermittent dosage schedule when possible.

—Profound dehydration and electrolyte depletion may develop in patients on this drug. If excessive diuresis occurs, reduce dosage or withdraw drug temporarily.

—Asymptomatic hyperuricemia or gout may be precipitated along with an elevated BUN. This is especially seen in dehydration of patients with renal insufficiency.

—Practitioner may need to instruct the patient to adjust salt intake and use supplementary potassium chloride if patient consistently develops hypokalemia.

—These products may lower serum calcium, and rare cases of tetany have been seen.

—In patients taking more than 80 mg/day, frequent laboratory evaluations should be performed.

—Monitor patients with diabetes or gout very carefully.

WHAT THE PATIENT NEEDS TO KNOW:

—Take this medication precisely as ordered by the health care provider. If you miss a dose, take it as soon as you remember if it is within an hour or two of the regular time. If it is close to the time for the next dose, take only the next scheduled dose. Do not double dosage or abruptly stop medication without being advised to do so.

—Some people feel stomach upset after taking this medicine. Taking pills with food or milk may help reduce this feeling.

—Notify your health care provider if muscle weakness, cramps, nausea, diarrhea, blood in urine, impaired hearing, ringing in ears, vertigo, or dizziness develops. If you notice any weight gain, be certain to notify your practitioner.

—Take medication early in the day on either a once- or twice-daily schedule to avoid having to get up at night to void. For twice daily schedules, 8 AM and 2 PM are suggested.

—Keep this medication out of the reach of children and others for whom it is not prescribed.

—Take medication with a full glass of orange juice (unless contraindicated by your diet). Other potassium-rich foods should be used daily. These include: citrus foods (especially oranges and tomatoes), bananas, dried fruits, apricots, cantaloupe, watermelon, nuts, dried beans, beef, and fowl.

—Taking medication is only one part of your treatment regimen. Reduction of weight, increasing exercise, and elimination of high-sodium foods are also important. Avoid foods such as lunch meats, smoked meats, Chinese food, processed cheese, and snack foods. Do not salt food whle cooking or add salt to your food after it is cooked.

—Wear a Medic-Alert bracelet specifying that you are taking this drug.

—Watch for signs of dizziness, particularly on rising from lying to standing position. Move slowly in order to allow your body time to adjust.

EVALUATION:

ADVERSE REACTIONS: Reactions associated with loop diuretics in general: *CNS:* blurred vision, headache, irreversible hearing loss, tinnitus, vertigo. *Gastrointestinal:* acute pancreatitis, anorexia, diarrhea, dysphagia, jaundice, nausea, vomiting. *Hematopoietic:* agranulocytosis, thrombocytopenia. *Other:* hyperglycemia and hyperuricemia which may precipitate gout, local irritation and pain with parenteral use (occasionally), pruritus, rash, hypocalcemia, hypochloremic alkalosis, hypokalemia, hyponatremia, hypomagnesemia.

Problems associated with furosemide in particular: *Cardiovascular:* initial orthostatic hypotension. *CNS:* loss of hearing, paresthesias, xanthopsia. *Dermatologic/ Hypersensitivity:* erythema multiforme, exfoliative dermatitis, necrotizing angitis (with vasculitis, cutaneous vasculitis), photosensitivity, pruritus, purpura, urticaria. *Gastrointestinal:* anorexia, constipation, diarrhea, oral and gastric irritation, hepatic dysfunction. *Other:* fever, glycosuria, muscle spasm, restlessness, sore throat, thrombophlebitis, tiredness, urinary bladder spasm, urinary frequency, weakness. *Hematopoietic:* anemia, aplastic anemia (rare), leukopenia.

PARAMETERS TO MONITOR: Obtain complete history, physical and laboratory baseline studies (including CO_2, BUN, WBC, uric acid, glucose, liver function, and electrolytes) prior to initiation of therapy. Monitor for therapeutic effect: reduction in edema which may be evaluated by subjective indications of relief and weight loss, decrease or absence of peripheral edema, no jugular venous distention, reduction in cardiac size, and gradual loss of third (S3) heart sound. Also monitor for progression of edema and development of adverse reactions. Perform periodic evaluation of serum electrolytes. Check for signs and symptoms of fluid and electrolyte imbalance: hyponatremia, hypochloremic acidosis, hypokalemia. Be especially careful in patients concomitantly receiving digitalis. Do serum and urine evaluations in patients complaining of vomiting or having cirrhosis, IV fluids, or severe diuresis. Look for the warning signs of imbalance and dehydration: dry mouth, thirst, weakness, lethargy, drowsiness, restlessness, muscle pains or cramps, muscle fatigue, hypotension, oliguria, tachycardia, arrhythmias, nausea, and vomiting. Also watch for blood dyscrasias, liver damage, or idiosyncratic reactions. Frequent serum electrolytes, CO_2, BUN, and calcium levels should be obtained in patients on long-term therapy. FBS, glucose tolerance, and 2-hour postprandial blood sugar evaluations should be obtained in diabetics using furosemide.

Marilyn W. Edmunds

DIURETICS—POTASSIUM SPARING

AMILORIDE HYDROCHLORIDE

ACTION OF THE DRUG: Amiloride is a comparatively new potassium sparing drug with relatively weak diuretic, natriuretic and antihypertensive properties. It works in the absence of aldosterone as it is not an aldosterone antagonist.

ASSESSMENT:

INDICATIONS: Amiloride is a weak diuretic compared to the thiazides but may prove helpful as adjunctive therapy in congestive heart failure and hypertension. Use only in patients with documented, persistent hypokalemia or in patients in which hypokalemia would pose a serious risk (i.e., patients with arrhythmias or digitalized patients). If used adjunctly with thiazides, it not only produces an additive effect, but it reduces the risk of hyperkalemia.

SUBJECTIVE: Patient may present with signs of edema: weight gain, fatigue, weakness, paroxysmal nocturnal dyspnea, dyspnea, and swollen feet. Hypertension may also be present.

OBJECTIVE: Practitioner may elicit signs of edema: shortness of breath, jugular venous distention, hepatojugular reflux, rales in the lungs, documented weight gain, third heart sound (S3), peripheral edema. Blood pressure greater than 140/90 mm Hg may also be found.

PLAN:

CONTRAINDICATIONS: Do not use in the presence of hypersensitivity to this product, hyperkalemia (serum potassium above 5.5 mEq/l), concurrently with other potassium-sparing drugs or potassium supplements, or in patients with anuria, chronic or acute renal insufficiency, diabetic nephropathy, or other evidence of impaired renal function.

WARNINGS: Like all potassium-sparing drugs, amiloride may cause hyperkalemia, which may be fatal if untreated. About 10% of the time amiloride produces hyperkalemia if used in therapy as the single agent. Incidence decreases to 1 to 2% when used with a thiazide diuretic. Avoid use in diabetic patients if possible as they seem to be more likely to develop hyperkalemia, even with no evidence of nephropathy. Use with caution in severely ill patients, especially those with cardiopulmonary disease, poorly controlled diabetes, or in patients likely to develop metabolic acidosis. Safety for use in children or in pregnant or breast-feeding women has not been established. Possible benefits must be compared to unknown risks.

PRECAUTIONS: When used with other diuretics and when brisk diuresis is promoted in ill patients who may have cardiac, metabolic, or hepatic dysfunction, a substantial risk of producing hyponatremia, hypochloremia, and elevated BUN levels exists.

IMPLEMENTATION:

DRUG INTERACTIONS: Use with other potassium-sparing drugs such as triamterene or spironolactone can lead to hyperkalemia. Use with oral or IV potassium supplements can also produce hyperkalemia. Do not give with lithium, as toxicity may be provoked due to decreasing the renal clearance of lithium. Amiloride may cause abnormal liver function tests although this is hard to document.

PRODUCTS (TRADE NAME):
Midamor (Available in 5 mg tablets).

ADMINISTRATION AND DOSAGE: Amiloride begins to act in 2 hours after oral administration, with peak action between 6 and 10 hours and duration of action of 24 hours.

Adjunctive or single agent therapy: Give 5 mg/day po, preferably with usual antihypertensive medication or thiazide. May increase to 10 mg/day orally. Further dosage increases are usually ineffective and risky without careful electrolyte monitoring.

IMPLEMENTATION CONSIDERATIONS:

—Obtain a complete health history, including the presence of hypersensitivity, underlying systemic disease, especially of renal insufficiency, diabetes, arrhythmias, cardiopulmonary disease, or other problems likely to produce metabolic acidosis, other medications taken concurrently which may produce drug interactions, and possibility of pregnancy. A documented history of chronic hypokalemia or a condition in which hypokalemia would present a substantial risk to the patient should exist.

—This medication is excreted unchanged by the kidneys and in the feces. It is not metabolized, so it can be given to patients with hepatic dysfunction as long as kidney function is not impaired. Patients with renal impairment retain the drug for extended periods of time and have increased risk of developing hypokalemia.

—This product has little effect on glomerular filtration rate or renal blood flow.

—Use of potassium-sparing drugs are not necessary in patients with essential hypertension who can take a normal diet.

—Amiloride effects on serum electrolytes begin with a single dose, and continue up to doses of 15 mg.

—Because this product is such a weak diuretic, relatively speaking, it is not usually used as one of the step one drugs in treating hypertension. The increased risk of hyperkalemia which exists when it is used as a single agent drug also precludes its use as a step one drug.

—Do not advise a potassium-rich diet or give other potassium-sparing drugs or potassium supplements while patient is on this drug.

—Renal function must be evaluated carefully in patients with elevated BUN and creatinine levels as potassium retention is accentuated in patients with renal impairment.

—Do not give amiloride to diabetics without carefully monitoring serum electrolytes, BUN, and creatinine.

—Discontinue drug at least 3 days before glucose tolerance testing.

—Drug is usually well tolerated, and except for hyperkalemia, few side effects are noted. Adverse reactions are often due to symptoms associated with diuresis or the underlying problem being treated.

> **WHAT THE PATIENT NEEDS TO KNOW:**
> —Take this medication only as ordered. Stopping the medication suddenly or increasing the dosage could be dangerous to your health. If you miss taking a dose, take it as soon as you remember. If it is close to the time for your next dose, skip the missed dose and take the drug on the regular schedule. Do not double doses.
> —This product may be taken with food if it causes stomach upset.
> —Use this medication cautiously if you are driving or performing tasks which require alertness since it may cause visual disturbances, dizziness, or headaches.
> —Contact your health care provider if you develop any illness which causes nausea, vomiting, or diarrhea while you are taking this product.
> —Do not eat excessively potassium-rich foods (bananas, orange juice, dried fruits) or take potassium supplements as you may have been advised to do in the past. This medicine conserves your body's potassium, and you should not add additional quantities to your normal level.
> —Keep this medication out of the reach of children and others for whom it is not prescribed.

EVALUATION:

ADVERSE REACTIONS: Most side effects are rare and occur less than 1% of the time. *Cardiovascular:* angina, arrhythmias, orthostatic hypotension, palpitations. *CNS:* decreased libido, depression, dizziness, encephalopathy, headache, increased intraocular pressure, insomnia, mental confusion, nasal congestion, nervousness, paresthesias, somnolence, tinnitus, tremors, vertigo, visual disturbances. *Dermatologic:* alopecia, dryness of mouth, itching, pruritus, mild skin rash. *Gastrointestinal:* abdominal pain, anorexia, appetite changes, constipation, diarrhea, dyspepsia, flatulence, gastrointestinal bleeding, heartburn, jaundice, nausea, thirst, vomiting. *Genitourinary:* bladder spasms, dysuria, impotence, polyuria, urinary frequency. *Musculoskeletal:* fatigability, muscle cramps, and weakness. *Respiratory:* cough, dyspnea, shortness of breath. *Other:* elevated serum potassium levels (above 5.5 mEq/l), suspected but not confirmed cause of aplastic anemias, abnormal liver function tests, neutropenia, and activation of probable preexisting peptic ulcer.

OVERDOSAGE: *Signs and symptoms:* Not known except for dehydration and signs of hyperkalemia. Watch for bradycardia, ECG abnormalities, fatigue, flaccid paralysis of the extremities, muscular weakness and shock. ECG changes from normal (in mild hyperkalemia) to show tall, peaked T waves or elevations. R wave voltage may drop with increased depth of S wave, widening of P wave (may even disappear), progressive widening of QRS complex, prolongation of PR interval, and ST depression. *Treatment:* Discontinue drug immediately and see that patient receives emergency therapy by qualified physician to reduce serum potassium levels. Monitor electrolyte status. Give symptomatic and supportive therapy. Patient may require dialysis to reduce potassium although it is not known if amiloride itself is dialyzable.

PARAMETERS TO MONITOR: Obtain a complete health history, physical examination and laboratory evaluation prior to initiation of therapy. Monitor for therapeutic effect, i.e., reduction in fluid levels or hypertension of patient. Also evaluate for progression of the problem or development of adverse reactions. Carefully monitor potassium levels, BUN, creatinine and other electrolytes after therapy is initiated, periodically during therapy, and in any illness which could upset the patient's fluid and electrolyte balance. Also check renal function. If BUN goes over 30 mg/100 ml or serum creatinine above 1.5 mg/100 ml, amiloride should be discontinued. Diabetics should be monitored especially carefully and acid-base balance watched in these and other patients likely to develop metabolic acidosis. Mild hyperkalemia is not usually associated with abnormal ECG.

Marilyn W. Edmunds

SPIRONOLACTONE

ACTION OF THE DRUG: Spironolactone acts as both a diuretic and an antihypertensive agent. (1) It increases the excretion of water and sodium while preserving potassium. It acts through competitive binding at aldosterone receptor sites in the distal renal tubular cell nucleus, resulting in changes in nuclear protein synthesis which affects sodium and potassium exchange. Antagonism of aldosterone may also inhibit $H+$ excretion. (2) It may permit an increase in estrogen activity by interfering with testosterone synthesis.

ASSESSMENT:

INDICATIONS: Spironolactone is effective in lowering both systolic and diastolic blood pressure and is used in the treatment of essential hypertension in combination with other drugs. It may be helpful even when aldosterone levels are normal. It is also used in treating hypokalemia in patients or when development of hypokalemia would pose significant risk (i.e., in digitalized patients or patients with arrhythmias). It is most often used as a step two drug. Additionally, it is used to treat edema resulting from cirrhosis of the liver, nephrotic syndrome, and congestive heart failure when other drugs are ineffective or inappropriate. It may also be used for the treatment of primary hyperaldosteronism, where it helps establish diagnosis through a therapeutic trial, or in short-term (preoperative) or long-term therapy when aldosterone level is elevated.

SUBJECTIVE: Patient may present with a history of weight gain, fatigue, weakness, paroxysmal nocturnal dyspnea, dyspnea, swollen feet and in some cases, hypertension.

OBJECTIVE: Signs of edema and hypertension may be present: shortness of breath, jugular venous distention, hepatojugular reflux, rales in the lungs, documented weight gain, third heart sound (S3), peripheral edema. Blood pressure of greater than 140/90 mm Hg may be found in hypertensive patients.

PLAN:

CONTRAINDICATIONS: Do not give in the presence of hypersensitivity, anuria, impaired renal function or insufficiency, or hyperkalemia (serum potassium above 5.5 mEq/l). Do not use with other potassium-sparing drugs or potassium supplements.

WARNINGS: Spironolactone has been shown to be tumorigenic in rats. Chronic toxicity studies show dose-related effects on endocrine organs and liver. Safety for use in pregnant or breast-feeding women has not been established. Spironolactone crosses the placental barrier, and its metabolites are found in breast milk. The hazards of use should be weighed against possible benefits.

PRECAUTIONS: Watch for hyperkalemia, which may promote fatal arrhythmias. Monitor fluid and electrolytes carefully. Spironolactone may also produce hyponatremia and gynecomastia. In patients with impaired renal function, mild acidosis and transient elevations of BUN are often seen.

IMPLEMENTATION:

DRUG INTERACTIONS: Do not use with potassium-rich foods, potassium supplements, or other potassium-sparing products since hyperkalemia may develop. Concomitant use of other antihypertensive agents or diuretics provides additive effects. Ganglionic-blocking drugs especially should be reduced by 50% or added to the drug regimen in decreased dosages. Increases in serum levels of digitalis glycosides may occur with concurrent use of spironolactone. However, the cardiac effect of digitalis products may also be decreased due to the increased potassium levels. Use will reduce the likelihood of digitalis-induced arrhythmias. The effect of oral anticoagulants is decreased due to concentration of clotting factors caused by diuresis. Ammonium chloride and other acidifying agents can induce systemic acidosis when used concurrently. Do not use in patients receiving lithium since renal clearance is altered and the risk of lithium toxicity is increased. Vascular responsiveness to epinephrine is decreased. This is important if the patient is to have general anesthesia. Salicylates may reverse the effects of these products.

PRODUCTS (TRADE NAME):
Aldactone, Spironolactone (Available in 25 mg tablets).

ADMINISTRATION AND DOSAGE: This product is rapidly and extensively metabolized. Peak of action is 2-4 hours after oral administration, and it is excreted in urine and bile over 12-96 hours. May be given in single or divided doses.

In edema, give a large loading dose and then a smaller maintenance dose for at least 5 days. Another more proximally acting diuretic could then be added if diuresis has not been sufficient. Resulting diuresis should then be prompt, but do not decrease dose of spironolactone.

In hypertension, treatment should continue for at least 2 weeks since maximal response may not occur sooner. Individualize dosage carefully for each patient to achieve therapeutic effect at lowest possible dosage.

Edema Associated with Congestive Heart Failure, Hepatic Cirrhosis, or Nephrotic Syndrome:

Adults: Give 100 mg/day po initially. Maintenance dose ranges from 25 to 200 mg/day po for 5 days, and then add another proximally acting diuretic if increased diuresis is indicated.

Children: Give 3.3 mg/kg/day po.

Essential Hypertension: Give 50-100 mg/day po either as a single agent or with other more proximally-acting diuretics for at least 2 weeks.

Hypokalemia: Give 25-100 mg/day po.

Hyperaldosteronism: Refer to physician for therapeutic trial (either short or long term) to confirm diagnosis of primary hyperaldosteronism. For maintenance dose, give 100-400 mg/day po preoperatively or at lowest possible dosage in patients requiring long-term therapy.

IMPLEMENTATION CONSIDERATIONS:

—Obtain a complete health history, including presence of hypersensitivity, other medications taken concurrently which may produce drug interactions, underlying systemic disease. Document case of consistent hypokalemia or situations which would make hypokalemia a serious risk to patient, and ask about possibility of pregnancy.

—Watch for symptoms of hyperkalemia: bradycardia, ECG abnormalities, fatigue, confusion, flaccid paralysis of the extremities, muscular weakness, and shock. Do not give potassium supplementation; advise patient against eating potassium-rich foods.

—Watch for symptoms of hypernatremia: dryness of mouth, thirst, lethargy, drowsiness. Observe for this especially if spironolactone is given with other diuretics.

—Routine use of diuretics in pregnancy is hazardous. Diuretics have not been demonstrated as helpful in preventing or treating toxemia. Indications for using diuretics in pregnancy would be the same as for non-pregnant women. Women should discontinue breast-feeding while using this drug.

—Gynecomastia may develop and is dose and time related. It is normally reversible.

—Because of tumor-producing tendencies in laboratory rats, this drug should be reserved for patients in which other diuretic therapy is either ineffective or inappropriate.

WHAT THE PATIENT NEEDS TO KNOW:

—Take this medication exactly as prescribed. Do not increase dosage or stop taking medication abruptly. If you miss a dose, take it as soon as you remember unless it is close to the time for your next dose. Do not take double doses.

—While taking this medicine do not take potassium supplements or eat foods rich in potassium (i.e., bananas, orange juice, dried fruits) as you may have been advised to do in the past.

—This product may cause staggering, drowsiness or mental confusion when first taken. Do not drive or perform tasks requiring alertness until your response to the medication can be evaluated.

—Report any new or unusual symptoms to your health care provider. Especially note any excessive thirst, dryness of mouth, drowsiness, or lethargy.

—Taking this drug for a very long time may cause breast enlargement. This usually decreases when the drug is stopped.

—Keep this medication out of the reach of children and all others for whom it is not prescribed.

EVALUATION:

ADVERSE REACTIONS: Usually, all problems are reversible when drug is discontinued. *CNS:* ataxia, drowsiness, headache, lethargy, mental confusion. *Endocrine:* amenorrhea, breast tenderness, deepening of voice, gynecomastia, hirsutism, hyperkalemia, impotence, inability to achieve or maintain erection, irregular menses, postmenopausal bleeding, thirst. *Dermatologic/Hypersensitivity:* drug fever, maculopapular or erythematous cutaneous skin eruptions, urticaria. *Gastrointestinal:* cramping, diarrhea, gastrointestinal upset, vomiting. *Other:* fever, fluid and electrolyte disturbance (especially hyperkalemia, hyponatremia, mild acidosis and elevated BUN), suspected but not confirmed relationship to carcinoma of breast.

OVERDOSAGE: *Signs and symptoms:* Unknown except for dehydration and signs of hyperkalemia: bradycardia, ECG abnormalities, fatigue, flaccid paralysis of the extremities, muscular weakness, and shock. ECG changes from normal (in mild hyperkalemia) to show tall, peaked T waves or elevations. R wave voltage may drop with increased depth of S wave, widening of P wave (may even disappear), progressive widening of QRS complex, prolongation of PR interval, and ST depression. *Treatment:* Discontinue drug immediately and see that patient receives emergency therapy by qualified physician to monitor patient. Reduce serum potassium levels. Give symptomatic and supportive therapy. Patient may require dialysis to decrease potassium.

PARAMETERS TO MONITOR: Obtain complete history, physical, and laboratory baseline data prior to initiation of therapy. Monitor for therapeutic effect, i.e., reduction in blood pressure or edema. Also monitor for progression of problem or development of adverse reactions, especially development of hyperkalemia. Perform periodic BUN, creatinine and serum electrolyte evaluations, and if BUN goes over 30 mg/100 ml or serum creatinine over 1.5 mg/100 ml, discontinue drug. Monitor the patient especially closely in any situation in which the patient's fluid and electrolyte balance might be altered. ECG should be obtained if patient is symptomatic or hyperkalemia is suspected.

Marilyn W. Edmunds

TRIAMTERENE

ACTION OF THE DRUG: Triamterene is a potassium-sparing diuretic which acts directly on the distal renal tubule to inhibit reabsorption of sodium ions in exchange for potassium and hydrogen ions in the distal segment of the renal tubule. Its action is not aldosterone dependent. The amount of diuresis produced by this mechanism is limited but can be increased by concurrent use of more proximally acting diuretics.

ASSESSMENT:

INDICATIONS: Triamterene is used in the treatment of edema associated with congestive heart failure, cirrhosis of the liver,and nephrotic syndrome. It is also used in idiopathic edema, steroid-induced edema and in edema due to secondary hyperaldosteronism. It may be used alone or with thiazides to increase effectiveness in refractory cases of hypertension.

SUBJECTIVE: Patient may present with a history of weight gain, fatigue, weakness, paroxysmal nocturnal dyspnea, dyspnea, and swollen feet. Hypertension may also be present.

OBJECTIVE: Signs of edema and hypertension may be seen: shortness of breath, jugular venous distention, hepatojugular reflux, rales in the lungs, documented weight gain, third heart sound (S3), and peripheral edema. When drug is used as an antihypertensive, blood pressure above 140/90 mm Hg is seen.

PLAN:

CONTRAINDICATIONS: Do not use in the presence of hypersensitivity, anuria, severe or progressive liver or kidney disease (except nephrosis), or hyperkalemia (serum potassium above 5.5 mEq/l). Do not use with other potassium-sparing drugs or potassium supplements.

WARNINGS: There are reports of blood dyscrasias, liver damage, and idiosyncratic reactions associated with use of this drug. Use with caution in patients with renal insufficiency. Diabetic patients with nephrotoxicity seem to be more vulnerable to developing hyperkalemia.

Safety has not been demonstrated for pregnant or breast-feeding women. It crosses the placental barrier and may appear in breast milk. Hazards of use must be compared against potential benefits to decide whether this drug should be included in therapy.

PRECAUTIONS: Watch for hyperkalemia which may promote fatal arrhythmias. Monitor fluid and electrolytes carefully. Imbalance occurs infrequently in patients with normal urine output; but if high doses are given for a long period of time, hyperkalemia may develop, thus necessitating discontinuance of the drug. Drug is generally withdrawn gradually to decrease the chance of developing a rebound kaliuresis.

Triamterene may produce mild antihypertensive effects which may be a problem in some patients. Use of full-dose diuretics when salt intake has been kept low (as in congestive heart failure, cirrhosis, or renal disease) may produce a low-salt syndrome. Drug may also cause reversible, mild nitrogen retention, a decreasing nitrogen reserve and the possibility of metabolic acidosis.

IMPLEMENTATION:

DRUG INTERACTIONS: When used with antihypertensive drugs, it may produce an additive effect. As captopril decreases aldosterone production, concurrent administration of triamterene may produce hyperkalemia. Do not use with other potassium sparing drugs or potassium supplements since hyperkalemia may develop. Increases in serum levels of digitalis glycoside may occur with concurrent use of triamterene. However, the cardiac effect of digitalis products may also be decreased due to the increased potassium levels. Do not use in patients receiving lithium since renal clearance is altered and the risk of lithium toxicity is increased. Triamterene will interfere with the fluorescent measurement of quinidine because they have similar spectra for fluoresence. Indomethacin and NSAIDS should be used with caution with patients on triamterene due to possible development of acute renal failure. Serum uric acid levels may also increase in patients predisposed to gouty arthritis. Triamterene may cause a decreasing alkali reserve with the possibility of metabolic acidosis if used with triamterene. Ammonium chloride and other acidifying agents can induce systemic acidosis when used concurrently.

PRODUCTS (TRADE NAME):
Dyrenium (Available in 50 and 100 mg capsules).

ADMINISTRATION AND DOSAGE: Onset of action is 2-4 hours. Most patients respond during the first day of treatment. Maximum effect takes several days and duration depends on renal function but is usually 7-9 hours.

As a single agent give 100 mg po twice daily after meals. When used with another diuretic, total daily dosage of each should be lowered initially and adjusted according to individual response. Maximum dose should be 300 mg/day.

IMPLEMENTATION CONSIDERATIONS:

—Obtain a complete health history, including the presence of hypersensitivity, concurrent use of drugs which may cause drug interactions, underlying cardiovascular, renal, gout, diabetic, or hematopoietic diseases, and possibility of pregnancy.

—Observe for signs of hyperkalemia and other electrolyte imbalance: abdominal cramps, bradycardia, confusion, drowsiness, dry mouth, ECG abnormalities, fatigue, flaccid paralysis of the extremities, muscular weakness, paresthesias, thirst, shock.

—Routine use of diuretics in pregnancy is hazardous. Diuretics have not been demonstrated to be effective in prevention or treatment of toxemia. Indications for use in pregnant women are the same as for non-pregnant women.

—If patient is breast-feeding, this medication should not be used.

—Withdraw drug gradually to prevent excessive rebound of potassium excretion.

WHAT THE PATIENT NEEDS TO KNOW:

—Take this medication exactly as prescribed. Do not change dosage or suddenly discontinue medication. If you miss a dose, take it as soon as you remember. If it is close to the time for the next dose, skip the missed dose and take medication at the regular time. Do not double doses.

—Notify health care provider if you develop dry mouth, headache, weakness, bleeding, bruising, yellowing of skin, cloudy urine, fever, sore throat, sore or bleeding gums, extreme fatigue, or any other new or troublesome symptoms.

—Avoid staying in the sun for a long time since photosensitivity may occur.

—While taking this medicine do not take potassium supplements or eat potassium-rich foods (i.e., bananas, orange juice, dried fruits) as you may have been advised in the past.

—Keep this medication out of the reach of children and others for whom it is not prescribed.

—Wear a Medic-Alert bracelet and carry a medical identification card specifying that you are taking this drug.

EVALUATION:

ADVERSE REACTIONS: Other than hyperkalemia, only occasional problems develop. *CNS:* headache, hypotension, metallic taste, weakness. *Dermatologic/Hypersensitivity:* anaphylaxis, photosensitivity, rash. *Gastrointestinal:* diarrhea, dry mouth, gastrointestinal upset, nausea, vomiting. *Hematopoietic:* blood dyscrasias (rare). *Other:* leg cramps, renal calculi. Elevated BUN and hyperuricemia may also develop.

OVERDOSAGE: *Signs and symptoms:* Problems associated with dehydration and electrolyte imbalance are usually seen. Look for bradycardia, ECG abnormalities, fatigue, flaccid paralysis of the extremities, muscular weakness, and shock. ECG changes from normal (in mild hyperkalemia) to show tall, peaked T waves or elevations. R wave voltage may drop with increased depth of S wave, widening of P wave (may even disappear), progressive widening of QRS complex, prolongation of PR interval, and ST depression. *Treatment:* Discontinue drug immediately, Patient should receive emergency therapy by qualified physician to monitor patient and reduce serum potassium levels. Give symptomatic and supportive therapy.

PARAMETERS TO MONITOR: Obtain a complete history, physical and laboratory baseline prior to initiation of therapy. Monitor for therapeutic effect, i.e., decrease in hypertension or reduction in edema. Also monitor for progression of problem or development of adverse reactions. Follow blood pressure and weight levels. Do periodic BUN, potassium, and kidney function tests, especially in older or diabetic patients. CBC with indices should also be done every 6 months to check for megaloblastosis. Obtain ECG if there is any index of suspicion about presence of hyperkalemia.

Marilyn W. Edmunds

DIURETICS—
THIAZIDES AND RELATED DIURETICS

ACTION OF THE DRUG: Thiazides represent the largest group of orally effective diuretic drugs. The main action of the thiazide diuretic is to inhibit reabsorption of sodium and chloride through direct action on the thick, ascending portion of the loop of Henle in the distal tubule, thus producing diuresis. Carbonate excretion is increased slightly. Thiazides also cause a direct dilation of arteriolar smooth muscles, decreased reactivity of vascular smooth muscles to endogenous pressors and direct reduction of plasma volume and sodium levels, thus providing an antihypertensive effect. They also interfere with insulin release and compete with uric acid for renal tubular excretion sites. They are structurally related to sulfonamide antibacterial drugs but have no antiinfective properties themselves. All of these drugs possess parallel dose-response curves, and there is no difference between them in their clinical efficacy.

ASSESSMENT:

INDICATIONS: Thiazides are used as adjunctive therapy in edema associated with congestive heart failure, hepatic cirrhosis or various forms of renal dysfunction and estrogen or steroid therapy. Thiazides are considered step one drugs used in management of hypertension either as the sole therapeutic agent in mild cases or, in more severe forms, to enhance the effect of other antihypertensive drugs.

SUBJECTIVE: Patients may present with a history of weight gain, fatigue, weakness, paroxysmal nocturnal dyspnea, dyspnea and swollen feet. They may have hypertension.

OBJECTIVE: Signs of edema: shortness of breath, jugular venous distention, increased hepatojugular reflux, rales in the lungs, documented weight gain, third heart sound (S3), peripheral edema. When drug is used as an antihypertensive, assess level of blood pressure and pulse in standing, sitting and lying positions. Blood pressure of 140/90 mm Hg or greater on three consecutive readings indicates hypertension.

PLAN:

CONTRAINDICATIONS: Do not use in the presence of hypersensitivity to thiazides or sulfonamides or in patients with anuria or renal decompensation. Do not give by intravenous route to infants or children. Metolazone should not be used in patients with hepatic coma or pre-coma states.

WARNINGS: Careful consideration should be made concerning the decision to use thiazides in pregnant and nursing mothers since the drugs cross the placental barrier and may be found in breast milk. Cross-sensitivity with sulfonamides may occur. Use with caution in patients with impaired renal function, progressive liver disease or impaired hepatic function. Exacerbation or activation of lupus erythematosus has occasionally been reported.

PRECAUTIONS: Hypokalemia may develop, especially with very aggressive diuresis. Interference with adequate oral electrolyte intake may also produce hypokalemia. This may be avoided or treated by use of liquid potassium supplements or foods with high potassium content. Hyperglycemia may occur, and frank gout may even be precipitated in some patients. Insulin requirements in diabetic patients may be altered (either increased or decreased). Latent diabetes mellitus may become manifest during thiazide therapy. If changes in renal function occur, reduction, withholding or discontinuance of thiazide therapy may be indicated. Discontinue thiazides before carrying out tests for parathyroid and thyroid function. Serum protein-bound iodine levels may be decreased, and calcium excretion is decreased by thiazides. Prolonged therapy may sometimes produce pathologic changes in the parathyroid gland.

IMPLEMENTATION:

DRUG INTERACTIONS: Thiazides may augment or potentiate the effects of other antihypertensive drugs. They may increase the responsiveness to tubocurarine and may decrease arterial responsiveness to norepinephrine. Dosage adjustments of antidiabetic agents are frequently indicated. Thiazides may alter various laboratory test results: all electrolytes, particularly potassium, BUN, uric acid, glucose, and protein-bound iodine. They also raise the level of serum glucose and uric acid, necessitating dosage adjustments of antigout and antidiabetic medications. Potentiation of effects may be seen when administered with alcohol, anesthetic agents, skeletal muscle relaxants, barbiturates, narcotics, and other CNS depressants. Thiazide absorption may be inhibited by cholestyramine. Thiazides antagonize effects of oral anticoagulants and vasopressors. Effectiveness of methenamine may be decreased due to alkalinization of urine. Thiazides also decrease excretion of amphetamines and quinidine. They have a pronounced action in making the myocardium of a patient receiving digitalis more sensitive to toxicity. Hypokalemia may develop with concomitant use of steroids. Concurrent use with amphotericin B, ACTH or corticosteroids may intensify electrolyte imbalance, particularly hypokalemia. Lithium used concomitantly reduces the renal clearance of lithium and adds a higher risk of the development of lithium toxicity. Thiazides interfere with PSP excretion test (which may be decreased) and may produce false-negative phentolamine and tyramine tests. Thiazides may increase blood glucose, serum calcium, uric acid and urine glucose levels and decrease serum magnesium, potassium, sodium and protein-bound iodine levels.

ADMINISTRATION AND DOSAGE: At maximal therapeutic dosage all thiazides are approximately equal in their diuretic potency. Thiazides are often the first line of treatment for hypertensive patients. If a patient is already on another antihypertensive drug, it may eventually be discontinued for a trial of a thiazide alone. Individualize therapy according to patient response. Titration of dosage to gain maximal therapeutic response with the lowest dosage is the objective.

The onset, peak and duration of diuretic action and the approximate equivalent dose for each of the thiazides and related diuretics is given in Table 3-6. The antihypertensive action of these agents requires several days before effects are noted. The diuretic effect is usually more pronounced initially, with the body adjusting after several days. Administration for up to 4 weeks is usually required for evaluation of total therapeutic effects.

IMPLEMENTATION CONSIDERATIONS:
—Obtain a complete health history, including the presence of hypersensitivities (especially to sulfonamides) and underlying systemic diseases (especially diabetes, gout, bronchial asthma, lupus, impaired kidney or liver function). Ascertain if there is a family history of these problems. Although family history or presence of these diseases does not rule out the use of a thiazide preparation, caution must be used

TABLE 3.6. COMPARISON OF THIAZIDE ONSET, PEAK, DURATION AND EQUIVALENT DOSES

	Onset	Peak	Duration	Equivalent Dose
Bendroflumethiazide	1-2 hr	6-12 hr	18-24 hr	5 mg
Benzthiazide	2 hr	4-6 hr	12-18 hr	50 mg
Chlorothiazide	2 hr	4 hr	6-12 hr	500 mg
Chlorothalidone	2 hr	within 2 hr	48-72 hr	50 mg
Cyclothiazide	within 6 hr	7-12 hr	18-24 hr	2 mg
Hydrochlorothiazide	2 hr	4 hr	6-12 hr	50 mg
Hydroflumethiazide	1-2 hr	2-4 hr	6-12 hr	50 mg
Methyclothiazide	2 hr	6 hr	24 hr	5 mg
Metolazone	1 hr	2 hr	12-24 hr	5 mg
Polythiazide	2 hr	6 hr	36 hr	2 mg
Quinethazone	2 hr	6 hr	18-24 hr	50 mg
Trichlormethiazide	2 hr	6 hr	24 hr	2 mg

if such a drug is prescribed, and special monitoring for side effects is indicated. Check for concurrent use of medications and possibility of pregnancy.

—Substantial patient teaching and education will be essential to obtain compliance with therapy. Although taking the medication is important, it is also important to work on decreasing other risk factors and changing dietary habits.

—Discontinue medications 48 hours prior to surgery because they will produce an increased action of muscle relaxants and a decreased effect of pressor amines.

—Discontinue medication before obtaining parathyroid function tests since drugs may decrease calcium excretion.

—Collection and recording of a good initial data base is important. History, physical examination and laboratory findings are important in evaluating progress of end-organ damage over the years. The incidence of drug side effects and complications from inadequately treated hypertension is high, and good record keeping is important in evaluating the patient's status.

—Patients over 60 are often quite sensitive to the effects of standard doses. It is important to begin the patient on a small dose and observe individual patient response before increasing dosage.

—Ascertain what other drugs the patient is taking that may interact with thiazides.

—Poor compliance with multiple daily doses may necessitate switching to a once-daily medication when patient's blood pressure is under control.

WHAT THE PATIENT NEEDS TO KNOW:

—Take medication exactly as ordered. Take medicine with food to decrease gastric irritation. If you miss a dose, take it as soon as you remember if it is within 1 or 2 hours of the scheduled time. If it is close to your next scheduled dose, skip it and take the next dose at the regular time. Do not double doses.

—This drug will make you urinate much more frequently and in greater amounts. It may even cause you to get up at night to go to the bathroom. If you take the last dose 4-6 hours before going to bed at night, this may be reduced. Frequent urination will be greatest when you first take the drug, but it should taper off in a few days as your body loses excess water and adjusts.

—Reduction in circulating blood volume may cause you to feel lightheaded when changing positions rapidly. In order to reduce this feeling, move slowly when changing from the lying position, after standing still for long periods of time, after vigorous exercise and after taking hot baths or showers. Should feeling lightheaded continue to be a problem, using elastic stockings or support hose for legs may decrease this sensation.

—Diuretic use causes the gradual loss of potassium through the urine. You may be advised to eat a potassium-rich diet. Foods that might be included are bananas, citrus fruits (especially tomatoes and oranges), apricots, and dried fruits such as raisins, prunes and dates. Cantaloupe and watermelon in season are also good. Nuts, dried beans, beef and fowl also contain potassium. Usually, dietary potassium intake for the average adult is 50 to 80 meq/day.

—Some thiazide products cause drowsiness when you first begin taking them. This feeling should pass within 1 or 2 weeks.

—Promptly notify your health care provider if you develop any unusual symptoms, especially excessive thirst, hunger or sharp pains in toes or joints.

—Take medication with a full glass of orange juice (unless contraindicated by your diet).

—Taking medication is only one part of your treatment regimen. Reduction of other risk factors is also important: lose weight (if overweight), stop smoking, increase exercise, avoid stressful and emotional pressure. Avoid use of foods high in sodium: lunch meats, smoked meats, Chinese food, processed cheese, snack foods. Do not salt food while cooking or add salt to your food after it is cooked.

—Keep this medication out of the reach of children and others for whom it is not prescribed.

—The goal of therapy is to help you feel as healthy as possible and to avoid any complications. Generally there is no cure for hypertension, and therapy extends for a lifetime. Taking your medication and reducing other risk factors will help reduce the chance of serious complications. It is important then to keep taking your medicine, even when you feel well, and to keep seeing your health care provider regularly.

EVALUATION:

ADVERSE REACTIONS: *Cardiovascular:* orthostatic hypotension, especially aggravated by alcohol, barbiturates, or narcotics. *CNS:* blurred vision, dizziness, fatigue, headaches, lightheadedness, paresthesias, syncope, vertigo. *Gastrointestinal:* anorexia, constipation, cramping, diarrhea, gastric irritation, jaundice, nausea, pancreatitis, vomiting. *Hematopoietic:* agranulocytosis, aplastic anemia, leukopenia, thrombocytopenia. *Hypersensitivity:* purpura, photosensitivity, rash, urticaria, necrotizing angitis, fever, respiratory distress including dyspnea, pneumonitis and anaphylactic reactions, Stevens-Johnson syndrome. *Musculoskeletal:* muscle cramping, spasm, weakness. *Other:* chills, elevated BUN, glycosuria, hypercalcemia, hyperglycemia, hyperuricemia, hypokalemia, impotence, transient blurred vision, restlessness, hematuria, rare idiosyncratic inappropriately increased antidiuretic hormone secretions causing severe fluid and electrolyte derangements after brief therapy.

OVERDOSAGE: *Signs and symptoms:* Lethargy of varying degrees may appear and progress to coma within a few hours. Respiratory and cardiovascular function, state of hydration or serum electrolyte values all show significant changes, although mechanism is unknown. At other times, gastrointestinal irritation, hypermotility and temporary elevation of BUN with other serum electrolyte changes may occur. *Treatment:* Gastric lavage for CNS depression. Gastrointestinal effects are usually short lived but may require symptomatic treatment.

PARAMETERS TO MONITOR: Laboratory evaluation should be done prior to initiating thiazide therapy and once the patient is on a maintenance dose. Usually blood work (complete blood count, electrolytes, BUN, CO_2, glucose, uric acid level, and kidney function tests) and urinalysis are done every 2 months until the patient is stable and then at least every 6 months. On each visit ask questions to detect history compatible with electrolyte imbalance or blood volume depletion: anorexia, weakness, fatigue, thirst, oliguria, vomiting, drowsiness, dizziness or lightheadedness on change of position, muscle cramps. Assess weight, blood pressure, pulse, hydration of mucous membranes. Observe closely for symptoms of renal failure, appearance of hyperglycemia, gout, or digitalis toxicity in patients identified as being at risk for these problems. Evaluate for orthostatic hypotension when patient is on maintenance dose. Difference of more than 10 mg Hg from lying to standing position or increase in pulse when patient rises to standing position may be indicative that patient is volume depleted. Evaluate for signs of therapeutic effect: weight loss, absence of rales in lungs, elimination of third heart sound (S3), decreased peripheral edema, decreased blood pressure.

BENDROFLUMETHIZAIDE

PRODUCTS (TRADE NAME):
   Naturetin (Available in 2.5 mg, 5 mg and 10 mg tablets.)
DRUG SPECIFICS:
   Action lasts for about 24 hours. If administered every other day, or 3-5 days per week, there is relatively little likelihood of causing severe electrolyte disturbances.
ADMINISTRATION AND DOSAGE SPECIFICS:
   Edema: 5 mg each morning; may give in one daily dose if less than 20 mg/day.

Hypertension: Initial dosage is 5 to 20 mg/day. Maintenance dosage is individualized depending upon response but usually ranges from 2.5 to 15 mg/day.

BENZTHIAZIDE

PRODUCTS (TRADE NAME):
Aquatag (Available in 25 mg and 50 mg tablets.) **Benzthiazide, Exna, Hydrex, Marazide, Omuretic, Proaqua, Urazide** (Available in 50 mg tablet.)
DRUG SPECIFICS:
Action begins within 2 hours, lasts 12-18 hours and peaks within 4-6 hours.
ADMINISTRATION AND DOSAGE SPECIFICS:
Edema: 50 to 200 mg/day should be used for several days or until dry weight is attained. Titrate dosage to obtain therapeutic response.
Hypertension: Initial: 50 to 200 mg/day. Titrate dosage to obtain therapeutic response. Maximum dosage is 50 mg four times daily.

CHLOROTHIAZIDE

PRODUCTS (TRADE NAME):
Chlorothiazide (Available in 250 mg and 500 mg tablets.) **Diuril** (Available in 250 mg and 500 mg tablets, 250 mg/5 ml oral suspension and 500 mg/20 ml powder for injection.) **SK-Chlorothiazide** (Available in 250 mg and 500 mg tablets.)
DRUG SPECIFICS:
Administration with meals will help reduce gastric upset. Shake oral suspension well before using. Store in tight, well-closed containers. Intravenous therapy is used primarily in emergency situations. Doses of 250 mg given two to three times a day produces a greater diuresis than larger doses given once a day. Current studies suggest that doses greater than 250 mg do not produce an increased effect due to bioavailability. Manufacturers have not revised dosage to reflect these early reports.
ADMINISTRATION AND DOSAGE SPECIFICS:
Edema: Usual adult dosage is 0.5 to 1 gm once or twice a day (po or IV). It may be administered 3-5 days per week in some patients.
Hypertension: Usual adult starting dose is 0.5 to 1 gm/day. Maximum dose is 2 gm/day. Titrate dosage to obtain therapeutic effects.
Infants and children: Intravenous route is not recommended. Usual pediatric oral dose based on 10 mg/lb/day in two doses.
Infants under 6 months: up to 15 mg/lb/day in two doses.
Infants up to 2 years: 125 to 375 mg/day in two doses.
Children 2 to 12 years: up to 375 mg to 1 gm/day in two doses.

CHLORTHALIDONE

PRODUCTS (TRADE NAME):
    Chlorthalidone, Hygroton (Available in 25 mg, 50 mg and 100 mg tablets.)
Thalitone (Available in 25 mg tablets.)
DRUG SPECIFICS:
    Give in the morning with food. Chlorthalidone has a more prolonged action than most thiazides (up to 72 hours.) It is often used to potentiate action of other agents and is often more expensive. Increases in serum uric acid and decreases in potassium are dose related.
ADMINISTRATION AND DOSAGE SPECIFICS:
    Edema: 50 to 100 mg/day or 100 mg on alternate days or three times weekly. Maximum dose is 200 mg/day.
    Hypertension: 25 to 50 mg initially daily. Dosage above 100 mg usually does not increase effectiveness. Titrate dosage to obtain therapeutic effects. Maintenance dose may often be lower than initial dose.

CYCLOTHIAZIDE

PRODUCTS (TRADE NAME):
    Anhydron, Fluidil (Available in 2 mg tablet.)
DRUG SPECIFICS:
    Duration of action is prolonged. Give in one dose in morning.
ADMINISTRATION AND DOSAGE SPECIFICS:
    Edema: Usual adult dosage is 1 or 2 mg/day. Reduce dosage once edema is eliminated. One or 2 mg on alternate days or two to three times per week is often sufficient for maintenance.
    Hypertension: Usual dosage is 2 mg/day; 2 mg three times daily is maximum dose. Titrate dosage to obtain therapeutic effects.

HYDROCHLOROTHIAZIDE

PRODUCTS (TRADE NAME):
    Chlorzide, Diaqua, Diu-Scrip (Available in 50 mg tablets.) **Esidrix, Hydrochlorothiazide, Hydro-DIURIL** (Available in 25 mg, 50 mg and 100 mg tab-

lets.) **Hydromal, Hydro-Z-50, Hyperetic, Lexor** (Available in 50 mg tablets.) **Oretic, SK-Hydrochlorothiazide, Thianal** (Available in 25 mg and 50 mg tablets.) **Zide** (Available in 50 mg tablets.)

DRUG SPECIFICS:
Hydrochlorothiazide is usually one of the least expensive drugs.

ADMINISTRATION AND DOSAGE SPECIFICS:
Edema: 25 to 200 mg until dry weight is attained; 25 to 100 mg/day or intermittently for maintenance. Maximum dosage is 200 mg/day.

Hypertension: Usual starting dose is 50 to 100 mg/day; 200 mg/day in divided doses is maximum.

Infants and children: Dosage is based on 1 mg/lb/day, given in two doses.

Infants under 6 months: Up to 1.5 mg/lb/day in two doses may be required.

HYDROFLUMETHIAZIDE

PRODUCTS (TRADE NAME):
Diucardin, Saluron (Available in 50 mg tablets.)

DRUG SPECIFICS:
Hydroflumethiazide is a long-acting drug.

ADMINISTRATION AND DOSAGE SPECIFICS:
Edema: Initial adult dose is 50 mg once or twice daily. Maintenance dose may be 25 to 200 mg. Give in divided doses when dosages exceed 100 mg or more daily. Intermittent therapy may be used three to five times a week.

Hypertension: Usual starting dose is 50 mg twice daily. Titrate dosage based on therapeutic effect. Usual maintenance dose is 50 to 100 mg/day. Maximum dose is 200 mg/day.

METHYCLOTHIAZIDE

PRODUCTS (TRADE NAME):
Aquatensen (Available in 5 mg tablets.) **Enduron** (Available in 2.5 and 5 mg tablets.)

DRUG SPECIFICS:
Methyclothiazide is a long-acting drug. Some products are fairly expensive.

ADMINISTRATION AND DOSAGE SPECIFICS:
Edema and hypertension: Usual adult dose ranges from 2.5 to 10 mg once daily for both starting and maintenance doses. Maximum dose is 10 mg.

METOLAZONE

PRODUCTS (TRADE NAME):
Diulo, Zaroxolyn (Available in 2.5 mg, 5 mg and 10 mg tablets.)
DRUG SPECIFICS:
Metolazone is a long-acting thiazide. It does not affect glomerular filtration rate. It should not be used in children or in patients with prehepatic coma. Particular adverse effects noted with this drug are chest pain, chills and rapid heart beat. Highest doses are indicated for patients with paroxysmal nocturnal dyspnea.
ADMINISTRATION AND DOSAGE SPECIFICS:
Edema: 5 to 20 gm once daily. Titrate dosage to obtain therapeutic effects.

POLYTHIAZIDE

PRODUCTS (TRADE NAME):
Renese (Available in 1 mg, 2 mg and 4 mg tablets.)
DRUG SPECIFICS:
Polythiazide is very long acting and often expensive.
ADMINISTRATION AND DOSAGE SPECIFICS:
Edema: 1 to 4 mg daily. Initially, doses up to 12 mg daily in divided doses may be required.

QUINETHAZONE

PRODUCTS (TRADE NAME):
Hydromox (Available in 50 mg tablets.)
DRUG SPECIFICS:
Quinethazone is a sulfonamide with the same effects as the thiazides. It is used for edema associated with premenstrual tension. It may precipitate gout and is often expensive.
ADMINISTRATION AND DOSAGE SPECIFICS:
Give in 50 to 100 mg daily dose; 150 to 200 mg doses are occasionally needed.

TRICHLORMETHIAZIDE

PRODUCTS (TRADE NAME):
Aquazide, Diurese (Available in 4 mg tablets.) **Metahydrin, Naqua, Tri-**

chlormethiazide (Available in 2 mg and 4 mg tablets.) **Trichlorex** (Available in 4 mg tablets.)
DRUG SPECIFICS:
 Trichlormethiazide is inexpensive and long-acting.
ADMINISTRATION AND DOSAGE SPECIFICS:
 Edema: 1 to 4 mg/day.
 Hypertension: 2 to 4 mg/day.

Marilyn W. Edmunds

DIURETICS—THIAZIDE-POTASSIUM-SPARING COMBINATION DRUGS

PRODUCTS (TRADE NAME):
 Alazide, Aldactazide, Spiractazide, Spironazide, Spirozide (Available as 25 mg spironolactone with 25 mg hydrochlorothiazide tablets). **Dyazide** (Available as 50 mg triamterene and 25 mg hydrochlorothiazide tablets). **Moduretic** (Available in 5 mg amiloride hydrochloride and 50 mg hydrochlorothiazide tablets).
DRUG SPECIFICS:
 If a stable dose of a combination of diuretic products is eventually established for a patient needing therapy for edema or hypertension, one of these products might be considered. The advantages of this type of combination drug include providing additive effects of diuretics and antihypertensive medications through different mechanisms of action and minimization of hypokalemia. Taking a smaller number of pills per day may help increase patient compliance with the therapeutic regimen. Disadvantages include inflexibility in dosage adjustment of individual medications as clinical picture changes, and the greater expense of combination drugs as opposed to individual drugs. See specific prescribing information for each product.
ADMINISTRATION AND DOSAGE SPECIFICS:
 Alazide, Aldactazide, Spiractazide, Spironazide, Spirozide: Give 2-4 tablets po daily.
 Dyazide: Give 1-2 tablets twice daily after meals.
 Moduretic: Give 1-2 tablets daily with meals.

Marilyn W. Edmunds

INDAPAMIDE

ACTION OF THE DRUG: Indapamide represents the first of a new class of antihypertensive diuretics called indolines. The drug acts by decreasing peripheral resistance and altering transmembrane calcium currents to produce its antihypertensive effect. Cardiac output, rate and rhythm, glomerular filtration rate and renal plasma flow are not affected. In conjunction with other antihypertensive drugs, indapamide appears to have an additive effect typical of thiazide-type diuretics.

ASSESSMENT:

INDICATIONS: This produce is a step one medication used in the treatment of hypertension. It is a new drug, used in place of a thiazide diuretic, alone or in combination with other antihypertensive drugs. It is also used to reduce the salt and fluid retention associated with congestive heart failure.

SUBJECTIVE: Patients may be asymptomatic or may complain of not feeling well in general. Headaches, often associated with hypertension, are often produced by stress, tension or other reasons rather than being related to high blood pressure, unless very severe blood pressure elevations are present. In cases of secondary hypertension there may be reports of nocturia (if patient is unable to concentrate urine), history of renal trauma (producing renal artery stenosis) or family history of hypertension.

OBJECTIVE: Patients may have elevated blood pressure due to numerous factors (e.g., full bladder, anxiety, pain). If the average blood pressure is found to be above 140/90 mm Hg on three consecutive readings, the patient is assumed to be hypertensive. Readings above 120 mm Hg diastolic require immediate medical care. Blood pressure should be obtained in lying, sitting and standing positions in both arms and, in cases where coarctation of the aorta is part of the diagnostic differential, in the lower extremities. Eyes should be examined for the presence of increased arteriovenous (AV) ratio, nicking, hemorrhages or exudates in the fundus of the eye and blurring of the disc margins. Chest should be examined for diffuse point of maximum intensity (PMI), displacement of PMI to the left, thrusts, murmurs and presence of third or fourth heart sound. (Systolic ejection murmurs and fourth heart sounds commonly develop in hypertensive patients.) Abdomen should be assessed for renal artery bruits.

PLAN:

CONTRAINDICATIONS: Do not give in the presence of known hypersensitivity to indapamide or other sulfonamide-derived drugs. Do not give to patients with anuria.

WARNINGS: Because this is a relatively new product there are no controlled studies documenting safety for use in pregnant or breast-feeding women and in children. The risk to benefit ratio should be examined and the product used only when deemed essential. There is no evidence that use of diuretics prevents toxemia of pregnancy or is useful in its management. Hypokalemia occurs commonly with diuretics and should be monitored for during therapy.

PRECAUTIONS: Hypokalemia may develop, especially with very aggressive diuresis. Interference with adequate oral electrolyte intake may also produce hypokalemia. This may be avoided or treated by use of liquid potassium supplements or food with high potassium content. Hyperglycemia may occur and frank gout may even be precipitated in some patients. Insulin requirements in diabetic patients by be altered (either increased or decreased). Latent diabetes mellitus may become manifest during diuretic therapy. If changes in renal function occur, reduction, withholding or discontinuance of diuretic therapy may be indicated. Use indapamide with caution in patients with impaired hepatic function or progressive liver disease, since minor changes in fluid and electrolyte status may precipitate hepatic coma. Prolonged therapy may produce changes in the parathyroid gland, producing hypercalcemia and hypophosphatemia. Discontinue medication before tests for parathyroid function are performed. Indapamide may decrease serum protein-bound iodine levels without signs of thyroid disturbance. There is also the possibility that this product, like thiazides, may exacerbate or activate systemic lupus erythematosus.

IMPLEMENTATION:

DRUG INTERACTIONS: Do not use indapamide concomitantly with lithium because of the risk of producing lithium toxicity as renal clearance is reduced. Indapamide may also reduce the arterial responsiveness to norepinephrine slightly.

PRODUCTS (TRADE NAME):

Lozol (Available in 2.5 mg tablets.)

ADMINISTRATION AND DOSAGE SPECIFICS: Dosage must be individualized, based upon patient's blood pressure and therapeutic response to medication. A starting dose of 2.5 mg once a day in the morning is recommended. When used for edema of congestive heart failure, increase dosage to 5 mg once daily after 1 week, or after 4 weeks when treating for hypertension. If the response is insufficient, combine indapamide with other antihypertensive medications, reducing the usual dose of other agents by 50% during the initial period of therapy. There is little experience with doses above 5 mg daily.

IMPLEMENTATION CONSIDERATIONS:

—Obtain a complete health history, including the presence of hypersensitivity especially to sulfonamides and underlying systemic diseases (especially diabetes, gout, lupus, impaired kidney or liver function), other medications taken concurrently or possibility of pregnancy. Although family history or presence of these diseases does not rule out the use of this product, caution must be used if such a drug is prescribed, and special monitoring for side effects is indicated.

—Substantial patient teaching and education will be essential to obtain compliance with therapy. Although taking the medication is important, it is also important to work on decreasing other risk factors and changing dietary habits.

—This drug is usually well tolerated, with minimal side effects. Most side effects are transient. Patients usually require potassium supplementation to prevent hypokalemia.

—In patients experiencing drowsiness from this product, give largest dose in evening before going to bed.

—The ability to establish rapport with the patient, as well as encouraging patient to keep appointments, will be major factors contributing to success in treating patient on a long-term basis.

WHAT THE PATIENT NEEDS TO KNOW:

—Take this medication exactly as ordered by your health care provider. Do not adjust doses or stop taking medication without being advised to do so. If you miss a dose, take it as soon as you remember if it is within 1 or 2 hours of the time you should have taken it. If it is close to your next scheduled dose, skip it, and take the next dose at the regular time. Do not double doses.

—Therapy for hypertension requires periodic visits to your health care provider and evaluation of your response to mediation. There is a wide variety of things that you can do to help reduce your blood pressure, and the health care provider will assist you in learning what will be most helpful for you. This may require taking different drugs at different times or changing dosages. It is very important for you to return to the health care provider for evaluation of your reaction to therapy.

—This product will make you urinate more frequently. Take early in the day to avoid having to get up at night.

—Do not take any other medications without the knowledge of your health care provider. This includes over-the-counter drugs that you may buy for colds, cough or allergy. You should not drink any alcohol or use other CNS depressant drugs while taking this medication.

—Patients often note an increase in sleepiness after beginning this drug or whenever the dosage is increased. Do not attempt to drive or perform any tasks requiring alertness until you know how you will respond to this drug. Report any episodes of muscle weakness or cramps, nausea, vomiting or dizziness to your health care provider.

—You should wear a Medic-Alert bracelet or carry other identifying information about having hypertension and the medications you are taking.

—Keep this medication out of the reach of children and others for whom it is not prescribed.

—Taking medications is only part of your treatment regimen. Reduction of other risk factors is also important: lose weight (if overweight), reduce sodium intake, stop smoking, increase exercise, avoid stressful and emotional pressures. Avoid use of foods high in sodium: lunch meats, smoked meats, Chinese food, processed cheese, snack foods. Do not salt food while cooking or add salt to your food after it is cooked.

—Diuretic use causes the gradual loss of potassium through the urine. You may be advised to eat a potassium-rich diet. Foods that might be included are bananas, citrus fruits (especially tomatoes and oranges), apricots, and dried fruits such as raisins, prunes and dates. Cantaloupe and watermelon in season are also good. Nuts, dried beans, beef and fowl also contain potassium. Usually dietary potassium intake for the average adult is 50 to 80 mEq/day.

EVALUATION:

ADVERSE REACTIONS: *Cardiovascular:* irregular heart beat, orthostatic hypotension, palpitations, premature ventricular contractions. *CNS:* anxiety, agitation, blurred vision, blurring of vision, depression, dizziness, drowsiness, head-ache, insomnia, irritability, loss of energy, lethargy, malaise, muscle cramps or spasm, numbness of the extremities, nervousness, tension, vertigo. *Dermatologic:* hives, pruritus, rash, vasculitis. *Gastrointestinal:* abdominal discomfort, anorexia, constipation, diarrhea, gastric irritation, nausea, vomiting. *Genitourinary:* fre-quency of urination, nocturia, polyuria. *Other:* dry mouth, flushing, glycosuria, hyperuricemia, hyperglycemia, hyponatremia, hypochloremia, hypokalemia, in-crease in serum urea nitrogen or creatinine, impotence or reduced libido, rhinorrhea, tingling of extremities, weight loss.

OVERDOSAGE: *Symptoms:* Disturbances of electrolyte balance occur, accom-panied by nausea, vomiting, weakness and gastrointestinal distress. Hypotension and depressed respiration may also be noted in some patients. *Treatment:* Produce emesis or perform gastric lavage. Monitor fluid and electrolyte status and treat symptomatically.

PARAMETERS TO MONITOR: Obtain a complete history, physical exam-ination and laboratory evaluation for baseline values before initiating therapy. This should include electrolytes, cardiac, renal and liver function studies, an ECG and a chest x-ray. A urinalysis should also be obtained. These laboratory tests should be repeated at least yearly while patient is taking medication, more frequently for electrolytes. During therapy, patient should be monitored for therapeutic effect: controlling diastolic blood pressure at a rate of 90 mm Hg or lower with a minimum of side effects and reduction in edema. Observe for adverse reactions, particularly hypokalemia. Evaluate for progressive end-organ damage to heart, lungs, kidneys and eyes.

Marilyn W. Edmunds

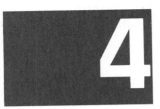

CENTRAL NERVOUS SYSTEM DRUGS

ANALGESICS—ANTIGOUT PREPARATIONS

ALLOPURINOL

ACTION OF THE DRUG: Allopurinol inhibits the production of uric acid by decreasing the production of xanthine oxidase, an enzyme that metabolizes purine hypoxanthine to xanthine and xanthine to uric acid. This drug has no analgesic or anti-inflammatory properties and is therefore not beneficial in the treatment of acute gout, but rather is used in prophylactic therapy for recurrent or chronic gout, and in patients with renal failure significant enough to increase their uric acid levels to a point where they may develop gouty attacks.

ASSESSMENT:

INDICATIONS: Gout is a form of arthritis caused by overproduction or under-excretion of uric acid. The drugs used in the treatment of gout vary in their method of action. Some are used in the treatment of the acute attack primarily to relieve pain and inflammation; others act to alter the body's response to, production of, or distribution of uric acid. The use of allopurinol should be decided on the basis of objective findings demonstrating any of the following conditions. (1) On a general diet, patient is an over-producer of uric acid (24-hour urine shows uric acid excretion greater then 700 mg/day). (2) A uric acid nephropathy with impaired renal function (creatinine clearance less than 80 ml/min). (3) Tophi. (4) Documentation of kidney stones by x-ray of the abdomen. (5) Primary or secondary hyperuricemia associated with blood dyscrasias and their treatment. (6) Gout not controlled by uricosuric drugs alone, due to patient intolerance of drug, or ineffectiveness of drug. (7) Drug is for prophylactic therapy in patients with lymphomas, leukemias, or other malignancies requiring chemotherapy or radiation therapy which results in an increase in the serum uric acid.

SUBJECTIVE: The patient complains of an initial or recurrent attack of inflammation, erythema, swelling, or extreme tenderness and pain, usually in a single or asymmetric joint pattern. At least 50% of initial attacks occur in the great toe at the metatarsal phalangeal joint (podagra). This disease manifests itself usually in the lower extremities. Joints affected may be in the instep, ankles, heels, or knees, although some patients are also bothered in wrists, fingers and elbows. In patients with a severe or progressive form of the disease, additional joints may be involved. These symptoms are sudden in onset and patients complain of being unable to tolerate clothing, shoes, or even bed coverings on the area. There may be a historical association of minor trauma to the involved joint, alcohol ingestion, use of a new drug such as hydrochlorothiazide, or low-dose aspirin consumption.

OBJECTIVE: Recurrent presentation of podagra or other joint involvement with erythema, heat, swelling and tenderness is seen. Hyperuricemia (serum uric acid greater than 7.0 mg/100 ml) is also found. Diagnosis is made on the basis of monosodium urate crystals found in the white cells of synovial fluid aspirated from the inflamed joint and examined under a compensated polarized light microscope. Patients should also be examined for tophi (monosodium urate crystals) deposited along bony surfaces, the pinna of the ear, on tendons, or in cartilagenous areas.

PLAN:

CONTRAINDICATIONS: Do not give in presence of hypersensitivity to the drug, especially with skin manifestation. Do not use in children, with the exception of those with hyperuricemia secondary to neoplastic diseases and their therapy. This drug is excreted in breast milk and should not be used in breast-feeding women.

WARNINGS: Discontinue drug at first sign of skin rash which is erythematous, maculopapular, and pruritic, as continued use could lead to erythema multiforme and/or general vasculitis. This can occur even several months or a year after therapy has begun. Clinical cases of hepatotoxicity have been described and allopurinol can increase serum alkaline phosphatase or serum transaminase levels, so liver function studies should be performed in the first months of therapy, particularly in patients with known hepatic problems. Drowsiness may occur so drug should be started when patient is not going to be operating dangerous equipment or driving. This drug should be used in pregnant women only if benefits outweigh the potential unknown hazards. Animal studies show no adverse effects, but the effects of xanthine oxidase inhibition in humans is not known.

PRECAUTIONS: Allopurinol may precipitate a gouty attack during the initial treatment phase. This is easily preventable by oral prophylactic use of colchicine 0.5 mg twice daily for 2 weeks to 1 month. Good fluid intake and neutral or alkaline pH of urine are important to prevent the possibility of xanthine calculi. Patients with impaired renal function require decreased dosage, and renal function should be carefully monitored. Nausea, vomiting, anorexia, intermittent abdominal pain, and diarrhea have been reported.

IMPLEMENTATION:

DRUG INTERACTIONS: Hypersensitivity may occur in patients with renal compromise taking thiazides and allopurinol concurrently. Concomitant use with ampicillin may increase the chance for skin rashes. Mercaptopurine and azathioprine will have increased effects if used with allopurinol, so their dosage must be decreased. An increase in hepatic iron concentration is seen if used with iron preparations. Serum half-life of theophylline are also increased with administration of allopurinol. Allopurinol will increase the half-life of anticoagulants; the therapeutic significance of this has not been established, but coagulation studies should be followed. Concomitant use with uricosuric agents may decrease the excretion of oxypurinol, the active metabolite of allopurinol. Decreased dosage may be needed.

PRODUCTS (TRADE NAME):
Allopurinol, Lopurin, Zyloprim (Available in 100 and 300 mg tablets.)

ADMINISTRATION AND DOSAGE: Gastrointestinal side effects are usually reduced if medication is taken with meals. The dosage to control gout and hyperuricemia is variable. The average is 200-300 mg for patients with mild gout; 400-600 mg for those with moderately severe or tophaceous gout. Dosages over 300 mg should be given in divided doses; less than that can be given once daily. Allopurinol has a short half-life but its active metabolite oxypurinol is also active, allowing for decreased dose frequency. To reduce the chance of precipitating gout, begin with 100 mg daily dose, and increase weekly until the serum uric acid level is less than 6.0 mg/100 ml and then maintain that dose.

A creatinine clearance of 20 ml/min requires only 200 mg/day, and a clearance of less than 10 ml/min requires no more than 100 mg/day. In patients receiving neoplastic therapy, 600-800 mg in divided doses with a large amount of fluid intake for 2-3 days is recommended.

In transferring patients from uricosuric agents, a gradual increase of allopurinol with a gradual decrease of the other agent should be made, over a period of several weeks, monitoring to maintain a normal serum uric acid level.

In pediatric cases associated with neoplastic therapy, give 100 mg three times daily in children 6-10 years, and adjust dose according to response. Give only 50 mg three times daily to children under 6 years of age.

IMPLEMENTATION CONSIDERATIONS:

—Obtain a complete health history, including the presence of hypersensitivity, concurrent drug administration which could cause drug interactions, history of renal impairment, and possibility of pregnancy.

—Obtain 24-hour urine for uric acid level and creatinine clearance.

—Look for evidence of renal impairment or stones. Obtain serum BUN, and x-ray of abdomen if necessary.

—Teach patient about the need for good fluid intake while on this medication.

—Document gouty attacks by joint aspiration which demonstrates urate crystals, or make a diagnosis through the triad of gout symptoms, hyperuricemia and a rapid response to colchicine.

—If patient develops a maculopapular rash anytime during therapy, stop the drug immediately. It should not be restarted.

—Check specific gravity of urine to determine if patient is drinking enough fluid. Monitor for alkaline or neutral pH, which is desirable for patients on this therapy.

—Obtain baseline blood work of uric acid, liver function studies, renal function studies, and complete blood count to rule out blood dyscrasias.

WHAT THE PATIENT NEEDS TO KNOW:

—This drug helps to control gouty attacks, but does not cure them. There is a possibility of recurrent gout attacks, but frequency and severity will decrease if drug is taken regularly.

—Take this medication as outlined by your health care provider. Many patients are able to use one dose a day unless they find it causes stomach distress. Do not take more than the prescribed amount or take extra tablets if a gout attack occurs.

—Medication should be taken with food in order to decrease chances of stomach upset.

—Drink at least 8 glasses of fluid (especially water) every day while on this medication in order to prevent the development of kidney stones.

—Taking this drug will require periodic visits to your health care provider and laboratory tests to determine liver and kidney function, and to determine the proper dosage.

—Do not take any new medications without the knowledge of your health care provider. Some medications may be affected by this drug.

—Keep a record of all gouty attacks so that these can be analyzed on your office visits.

—Contact your health care provider immediately for any kind of skin rash that develops while taking this medicine.

—This medication causes drowsiness in some people. Do not drive or do tasks requiring alertness until you know how this drug affects you.

—Keep this prescription out of the reach of children or others for whom the drug is not prescribed.

EVALUATION:

ADVERSE REACTIONS: *CNS:* drowsiness, neuritis. *Dermatologic:* alopecia, erythematous maculopapular pruritic rash, even up to several months after therapy started, exfoliative, urticarialor purpuric lesions, and Stevens-Johnson Syndrome. *Gastrointestinal:* diarrhea, intermittent abdominal pain, nausea, vomiting. *Hematopoietic:* agranulocytosis, anemia, aplastic anemia, bone marrow deprssion, leukopenia, pancytopenia, thrombocytopenia. (Most often seen in patients on medications causing similar adverse reactions). *Other:* drug idiosyncrasies with fever, chills, arthralgias, skin rash, pruritus, nausea, vomiting, and interstitial nephritis may be seen, occasional development of cataracts (exact association unknown), vasculitis leading to hepatotoxicity and death.

PARAMETERS TO MONITOR: Evaluate for therapeutic effects: decrease in frequency and severity of gouty attacks, resolution of tophi. Uric acid level should be obtained when therapy is initiated and then again in two weeks. Potential effect of the drug is seen in 5-10 days after therapy is started. Dosage should be adjusted to maintain a serum uric acid level of less than 7 mg/100 ml. Levels as low as 2-3 mg/100 ml are not harmful. Monitor for adverse reactions. Look for rash, appearance of tophi, or change in joint deformities. Obtain history of frequency, duration and severity of gout attacks, symptoms compatible with the development of renal calculi, or cataracts. Ask about GI distress and drowsiness. Periodic determination of liver and renal function, creatinine clearance, BUN, and complete blood counts should be done, particularly in the first months of therapy. Specific gravity of urine may be checked to make sure patient is getting adequate fluid intake.

Carole Hill

COLCHICINE

ACTION OF THE DRUG: The mechanism of action of colchicine in relieving gouty attacks is not completely known. It is believed to be involved in the inhibition of leukocyte migration and phagocytosis that causes the inflammatory response in gout. It also decreases uric acid deposition by reducing lactic acid production of leukocytes, and interferes with kenin formation. Colchicine is not an anti-inflammatory, an analgesic, or a uricosuric agent. It is used in the treatment of acute gouty attacks, or prophylactically with allopurinol or other uricosuric agents to prevent an acute attack when initiating therapy with these agents. Long-term, it is used to prevent acute attacks and as a diagnostic tool to confirm the diagnosis of gout when joint aspiration is not possible.

ASSESSMENT:

INDICATIONS: Used when the diagnosis of gout is either confirmed or suspected by patient history and physical exam. It is effective in relieving the pain of acute attacks. It is also used in conjunction with allopurinol or other uricosuric agents in order to avoid precipitating a gouty attack until the serum uric acid level is reduced to normal and stabilized. It has no effect on uric acid levels itself. It may be used prophylactically to prevent recurrent attacks, but only in combination with a uricosuric agent.

SUBJECTIVE: Patient complains of an initial or recurrent attack of inflammation, erythema, swelling, extreme tenderness, and pain in a single or asymmetric joint pattern. It is most often seen in the first metatarsal phalangeal joint (podagra). The disease of gout usually manifests itself in the lower extremities: instep, ankles, heels, knees (in decreasing frequency), followed by wrists, fingers and elbows. Other joints are also involved but are usually seen in patients with a progressive or severe form of the disease. The symptoms may be sudden in onset, and may be precipitated by minor trauma, obesity, alcohol ingestion, and use of drugs such as hydrochlorothiazide or low doses of aspirin, allopurinol or uricosurics. Renal failure may also cause hyperuricemia leading to acute attacks. Patients will complain of being unable to tolerate clothing, shoes, or even bed covers on the site or inflammation, and cannot obtain relief by any of the usual methods of heat, elevation or aspirin.

OBJECTIVE: The initial or recurrent presentation of podagra or a similar inflammatory joint. Uric acid level is found to be greater than 7 mg/100 ml. A documented diagnosis is made from monosodium urate crystals found in the white cells of synovial fluid aspirated from an inflamed joint, and examined under a compensated polarized light microscope.

PLAN:

CONTRAINDICATIONS: Do not use in the presence of hypersensitivity to the drug, in patients with severe renal, hepatic, or cardiac disorders, or in patients with blood dyscrasias. Do not use in pregnancy because of the possibility of fetal harm.

WARNINGS: Use with caution in debilitated and elderly patients, especially in those with renal or gastrointestinal problems, or heart disease. Reduction of dosage is indicated if weakness, anorexia, nausea, vomiting, or diarrhea appears. This drug may adversely affect spermatogenesis in humans and has been found to arrest cell division in other animals. It is not known if this drug is excreted in human milk. Use and efficacy have not been established for pediatric use.

PRECAUTIONS: Prolonged therapy may cause bone marrow depression, thrombocytopenia, and aplastic anemia. Blood work should be monitored periodically to assess for these complications. This agent is shown to produce reversible malabsorption of vitamin B_{12} by altering ileal mucosa function.

IMPLEMENTATION:

DRUG INTERACTIONS: Colchicine is inhibited by acidifying agents and potentiated by alkalinizing agents. Patients on this agent may have an increased sensitivity to CNS depressants. It also decreases gut absorption of vitamin B_{12} Sympathomimetics are enhanced by colchicine. It may increase serum levels of SGOT and alkaline phosphatase. It may also decrease thrombocyte values during therapy. Colchicine may give false-positive results when testing urine for blood or hemoglobin.

PRODUCTS (TRADE NAME):

Colchicine (Available in 0.5 or 0.6 mg tablet, in 1 mg/2 ml injection; and in 0.5 mg granules.) **Colsalide** (Available in 0.432 mg.) Also available in colchicine and probenecid combinations. (See probenecid.)

ADMINISTRATION AND DOSAGE:

Acute attack of gout: Begin therapy at first warning of an acute attack. The delay of only a few hours greatly reduces the therapeutic effectiveness. Oral route: 1 to 1.2 mg initially, followed by 1 tablet every one to two hours until pain is relieved, or nausea, vomiting or diarrhea develop. Do not exceed total dose of 4-8 mg. Pain is usually relieved in 12 hours and gone in 24 to 48 hours.

IV route: Give 1-2 mg initially, then 0.5 mg every 3 to 6 hours until pain is relieved. Total dose is 4 mg.

Prophylactic therapy: Give 0.5 to 1 mg/day in daily or divided doses, usually in combination with a uricosuric agent.

In patients with less than one yearly attack the usual dose is 0.5 or 0.6 mg three or four days per week. In patients with more than one yearly attack, the dose is 0.5 or 0.6 mg taken every day. Severe cases may require as much as 1 or 1.8 mg daily. Prophylactic therapy may be used for patients to be treated with allopurinol or uricosuric agents. In this case, use 0.5 or 0.6 mg po daily for about one month when other agents are first started.

Prophylactic therapy in patients undergoing surgery: Give 0.5 or 0.6 mg three times daily for three days before surgery and three days after surgery. To be used in patients known to have more than one attack per year.

IMPLEMENTATION CONSIDERATIONS:

—Obtain a complete health history including the presence of hypersensitivity, concurrent drug administration which would cause drug interactions, history of renal or hepatic failure, or other systemic diseases, and possibility of pregnancy.

—Diagnose gout through presence of symptoms of hyperuricemia, response to colchicine within 12 hours, or uric acid crystals from joint aspiration under polarized light microscope.

—See patient frequently to check for weakness, anorexia, nausea, vomiting or diarrhea as these are the first indications of toxicity and dosage should be reduced.

—Injectable dose is not to be given IM or SQ, but must be given IV only.

—Watch for symptoms of vitamin B_{12} deficiency.

—Obtain baseline blood uric acid level, hepatic and renal function studies.

WHAT THE PATIENT NEEDS TO KNOW:

—This is a medicine which you should keep on hand in case you develop an attack of gout. At the first sign of difficulty, take 2 tablets, and then 1 tablet every hour or every two hours until symptoms are relieved, or until you develop nausea, diarrhea or vomiting. Do not take more than 12 tablets.

—If you are taking this medication regularly with other drugs, take it with meals in order to reduce gastrointestinal upset.

—Medicine must be taken regularly as ordered if it is to help prevent gouty attacks.

—While you are taking the drug on a daily basis, stop drug if you notice symptoms of nausea, vomiting or diarrhea, and notify your health care provider. Also report any skin rash, fever, sore throat, unusual bleeding or bruising.

—Do not take any other medications without the knowledge of your health care provider. Some drugs interact adversely with this product.

EVALUATION:

ADVERSE REACTIONS: *Gastrointestinal:* abdominal pain, diarrhea (may be severe, requiring paregoric or opiate derivatives), nausea, vomiting. (These are worse in patients with peptic ulcer or spastic colon.) *Hematopoietic:* Prolonged use may cause bone marrow depression with agranulocytosis, aplastic anemia, and thrombocytopenia. *Other:* azoospermia, peripheral neuritis, purpura, myopathy, and hair loss.

OVERDOSAGE: *Signs and symptoms:* There is usually a latent period between overdosage and onset of symptoms. Deaths have been reported with as little as 7 mg. The first symptoms are gastrointestinal as described above. Bloody diarrhea is known to occur secondary to hemorrhagic gastroenteritis. Burning sensations of throat, stomach, and skin may also occur. Extensive vascular damage or severe dehydration with hypovolemia may result in shock. Kidney damage with hematuria or oliguria may occur. Muscular weakness leading to paralysis may also develop. The patient, though conscious, may experience delirium or seizure activity. Death usually results from hypovolemia or respiratory depression. *Treatment:* Use gastric lavage, and symptomatic treatment of shock, respiratory depression. Use of atropine or morphine may help abdominal pain. Recently the use of peritoneal dialysis or hemodialysis has been recommended.

PARAMETERS TO MONITOR: Monitor for therapeutic effects: decrease in frequency and severity of gouty attacks. Patients treating acute attacks with a loading dose can usually reach a maximum dose level before the onset of GI side effects. Monitor adverse reactions. Uric acid levels and renal, hepatic and complete blood counts should be obtained prior to therapy and repeated periodically, especially in the first months of therapy. Watch especially for signs of gastrointestinal distress and blood dyscrasias: sore throat, fever, bleeding tendencies or weakness. When colchicine is used in conjunction with allopurinol or uricosuric agents, uric acid levels should be obtained so drug can be withdrawn when normal levels are reached.

Carole Hill

URICOSURIC AGENTS

ACTION OF THE DRUG: Uricosuric agents increase the elimination of urate salts by blocking renal tubular reabsorption. They also decrease the miscible urate pool, urate deposition, and promote reabsorption of urate deposits. Sulfinpyrazone also has platelet inhibitory and anti-thrombotic effects. These drugs do not have significant anti-inflammatory or analgesic properties and therefore are of little help during an acute episode of gout.

Probenecid inhibits tubular secretion of penicillin and can therefore increase plasma levels 2-4 times normal irrespective of the route of administration of the drug.

ASSESSMENT:

INDICATIONS: Probenecid is often used as conjunctive therapy in the treatment of venereal diseases with penicillin preparations, because of its ability to increase the plasma level of penicillin. Uricosuric agents are primarily used to reduce uric acid levels in patients who are underexcreters. Confirm diagnosis of gout through serum uric acid levels greater than 7 mg/100 ml and a 24-hour urine test for uric acid of less than 800 mg/day. Patients have usually had more than one acute episode before being started on these agents.

The patient should not be started on these agents during an acute episode of gout as these agents may induce an attack or worsen the severity of an existing attack. Colchicine is often given concurrently when initiating treatment with these agents to prevent the precipitation of an acute episode of gout brought on by a shift in the miscible urate pool. Sulfinpyrazone is used only in patients refractory to all other modalities.

SUBJECTIVE: The patient complains of an initial or recurrent attack of inflammation, erythema, swelling, extreme tenderness and pain, usually in a single or asymmetric joint pattern. At least 50% of initial attacks occur in the great toe at the metatarsal phalangeal joint (podagra). This disease manifests itself usually in the lower extremities. Joints affected may be in the instep, ankles, heels, or knees, although some patients are also bothered in wrists, fingers and elbows. In patients with a severe or progressive form of the disease, additional joints may be involved. These symptoms are sudden in onset and patients complain of being unable to tolerate clothing, shoes, or even bed coverings on the site of inflammation. There may be a historical association of minor trauma to the involved joint, obesity, alcohol ingestion, use of a new drug such as hydrochlorothiazide, or low-dose aspirin consumption.

OBJECTIVE: Recurrent presentation of podagra or other joint involvement with erythema, heat, swelling and tenderness is seen. Hyperuricemia (serum uric acid greater than 7.0 mg/100 ml) is also found. Documented diagnosis is made on the basis of monosodium urate crystals found in the white cells of synovial fluid aspirated from the inflamed joint and examined under a compensated polarized light microscope. Patients should also be examined for tophi (monosodium urate crystals) deposited along bony surfaces, the pinna of the ear, on tendons, or in cartilagenous areas. A 24-hour urine test for uric acid of less than 800 mg/day demonstrates that the patient is an underexcreter. The acute attack must have resolved before these agents can be used; they have no effect on the acute episode.

PLAN:

CONTRAINDICATIONS: Do not use in people hypersensitive to the drug, in children under the age of two, or those with blood dyscrasias or uric acid kidney stones. Therapy should not be instituted until the acute episode has resolved. Sulfinpyrazone is contraindicated in active peptic ulcer disease or symptoms of gastrointestinal ulceration. There is a cross-sensitivity to phenylbutazone and other pyrazoles so drug should not be given to patients sensitive to these agents.

WARNINGS: Initiation of therapy with these agents may precipitate an acute attack of gout, and concomitant use of colchicine is often given to prevent such an attack. Use in pregnancy is recommended only when benefits outweigh potential effects to fetus. Probenecid is known to cross the placental barrier, but exact effects on fetus are not known. The use of salicylates in small or large doses is contraindicated in patients on probenecid because they antagonize the uricosuric action of this drug. Patients needing mild analgesia should be instructed to use only acetaminophen products.

PRECAUTIONS: The urine should be alkalinized to prevent hematuria or formation of urate stones, especially during the initial stages of therapy. Use caution in prescribing for patients with a history of peptic ulcer disease, acute or intermittent porphyria, or G-6-PD deficiency. For patients receiving sulfinpyrazone, this agent sometimes contains tartrazine, which may cause hypersensitivity (bronchial asthma) in some patients, particularly if they are salicylate sensitive. Alternate forms of therapy should be considered in these patients.

IMPLEMENTATION:

DRUG INTERACTIONS: Salicylates antagonize the uricosuric action of these drugs. Uricosurics potentiate the effects of the following drugs by decreasing renal tubular excretion: sulfonamides, sulfonylureas, naproxen, indomethacin, rifampin, dapsone, pantothenic acid, aminosalicylic acid, and methotrexate. Additionally, sulfinpyrazone affects anticoagulants by potentiating their platelet aggregation effects.

ADMINISTRATION AND DOSAGE: These agents are to be started only after the acute attack has subsided. Recommend this treatment in patients having more than one acute attack per year. If less than that, try to control attacks by having colchicine on hand.

IMPLEMENTATION CONSIDERATIONS:

—Obtain a complete health history, including the presence of hypersensitivity, concurrent drug administration which could cause drug interactions, history of active peptic ulcer disease, GI ulceration, renal insufficiency, kidney stones, or in patients with blood dyscrasias, G-6-PD deficiency, hypersensitivity to aspirin, tartrazine, phenylbutazone or other pyrazoles, or the possibility of pregnancy.

—Obtain a 24-hour urine test for uric acid level and creatinine clearance.

—Assess frequency and severity of attacks to decide if concomitant therapy with colchicine is indicated.

—Teach the patient about the need for good fluid intake while on this medication.

—This medication may give false urine tests in diabetics using Clinitest.

—Obtain baseline creatinine, BUN, uric acid level, and urine pH.

WHAT THE PATIENT NEEDS TO KNOW:

—This drug will not alter acute gouty attacks, but does help prevent attacks if taken regularly. During the initial dosage, an acute attack may be precipitated, but this will decrease future chances of severe attacks. Drug does not cure gout, but should help control it.

—Take this medication as outlined by your health care provider. Taking it with meals may help to decrease gastrointestinal side effects.

—Drink at least 8 glasses of fluid (especially water or citrus juices) every day while on this medication in order to prevent the development of kidney stones.

—Observe stools and urine for blood.

—Contact your health care provider if you develop any rash, stomach problems, or any new or troublesome symptoms.

—Keep this medication out of the reach of children and all others for whom it is not prescribed.

EVALUATION:

ADVERSE REACTIONS: *Dermatologic:* drug fever, flushing with dizziness (sulfinpyrazone), pruritus, rashes. *Gastrointestinal:* anorexia, constipation, diarrhea, nausea, vomiting. *Hematopoietic:* hemolytic anemia in patients with G-6-PD deficiency. *Other:* exacerbations of acute attacks of gout. Rarely anaphylaxis, nephrotic syndrome, hepatic necrosis, and aplastic anemia.

OVERDOSAGE: *Signs and symptoms for sulfinpyrazone:* nausea, vomiting, diarrhea, epigastric pain, ataxia, respiratory distress, seizure activity, and coma. *Treatment:* No specific antidote is known. Therapy involves emesis, gastric lavage, and supportive therapy.

PARAMETERS TO MONITOR: Evaluate for therapeutic effects: decrease in frequency and severity of gouty attacks. Monitor for progression of arthritis process: joint deformity, destruction, or tophi formation. Monitor for adverse reactions. Monitor alkalinity of urine, specific gravity of urine (to make sure patient is properly hydrated), periodic blood work for blood counts, uric acid levels and renal function. Once uric acid is normal, maintain drug for 6 months and then gradually decrease dosage every 6 months until uric acid level is within normal range and not increasing.

PROBENECID

PRODUCTS (TRADE NAME):

Benemid, Probalan, Probenecid, Probenimead, SK-Probenecid (Available in 500 mg tablets.) Combination products: **ColBENEMID, Proben-C, Probenecid with Colchicine** (Available in 0.5 mg colchicine and 500 mg probenecid.)

DRUG SPECIFICS:

Because probenecid can increase the serum level of penicillin, it is often used with penicillin in the treatment of venereal disease. There is cross-sensitivity to phenylbutazone and other pyrazoles so do not use this product in sensitive patients. Patients needing mild analgesia should be instructed to us acetaminophen products and not aspirin.

ADMINISTRATION AND DOSAGE SPECIFICS:

Initial: Give 250 mg two times daily for one week.

Maintenance: Give 500 mg two times daily. Therapy may be increased by 500 mg/day every 4 weeks with a maximum dose of 2 grams or until urine urate excretion is less than 700 mg/day. If an acute attack occurs, continue regimen and add colchicine .25 mg two times daily for 1 week, then 0.5 mg two times daily until uric acid levels are within normal range. Colchicine can then be discontinued until there is another attack. If attacks occur frequently, then the two agents should be used together indefinitely. Once normal uric acid levels have been maintained for 6 months, daily dosage may be decreased by 500 mg every 6 months until there is a slight rise in the uric acid level. Drug is maintained at that level.

Children 2 years or older: Initially give 25 mg/kg, then 40 mg/kg every 6 hours.

Concurrent use with penicillins or cephalosporins: (Only in patients without renal impairment).

Adults and children more than 50 kg: Give 2 gm/day in divided doses.

Children: Give 25 mg/kg initially, then 40 mg/kg/day in divided doses.

Treatment of gonorrhea: Use 1 gm plus other therapy.

SULFINPYRAZONE

PRODUCTS (TRADE NAME):

Anturane (100 mg tablets, 200 mg capsules.)

DRUG SPECIFICS:

Anturane capsules contain tartrazine, to which some people (especially those sensitive to aspirin) may show hypersensitivity. Sulfinpyrazine has platelet inhibitory and antithrombotic effects and so potentiates the effects of anticoagulants. This drug is usually only used in patients refractory to all other modalities of therapy. Its use is contraindicated in patients with active peptic ulcer disease.

ADMINISTRATION AND DOSAGE SPECIFICS:

Initial dose: Give 200-400 mg/day in two divided doses. Take with meals.

Maintenance dose: Give 400 mg/day in divided doses; may be increased to 800 mg/day or as low as 200 mg/day as long as serum uric acid remains normal. Therapy should be continued even during acute episodes and patient may be switched from other uricosuric agents to this drug at full maintenance dose.

Carole Hill

ANALGESICS—ANTIMIGRAINE AGENTS

ACTION OF THE DRUG: The main action of the antimigraine agents is (1) to block nerve impulses in the alpha or beta receptors of the sympathetic nervous system. (2) The ergot alkaloids used in the prophylaxis and treatment of vascular headaches are alpha adrenergic blocking agents. (The exception is propranolol hydrochloride, not an ergot derivative, but rather a beta adrenergic blocking agent discussed under the cardiovascular drugs.) (3) The alpha adrenergic blocking agents vasodilate smooth muscle tissue in the peripheral vascular system and uterus. The result is a reduction in cerebral blood flow and arterial pulsation. (4) Other actions include an oxytoxic effect on the myometrium and a decrease in blood pressure.

ASSESSMENT:

INDICATIONS: These drugs are used in the prophylaxis and treatment of vascular headaches. They relieve pain associated with vascular headaches by constricting dilated cerebral arteries. They are also used less frequently for oxytoxic and other smooth muscle spasmogenic effects.

SUBJECTIVE: History of migraines, vascular headaches, headache pain of a periodic, throbbing, severe nature; may be unilateral and often over one eye; photophobia and sensitivity to sound may be present; nausea and vomiting; family history of vascular headaches or history of motion sickness as a child; series of headaches in clusters, history of hypertension, food allergy or birth control pills. Headache may be improved by sleep or vomiting.

OBJECTIVE: Signs of sweaty hands and feet, scalp tenderness, autonomic dysfunction such as miotic pupil, red eye and unilateral nasal congestion.

PLAN:

CONTRAINDICATIONS: These drugs are contraindicated in coronary artery disease and conditions in which a sudden change in blood pressure may be detrimental or dangerous. Ergot preparations are also contraindicated for patients with infections, peripheral vascular disease, hepatic or renal dysfunction, pregnancy, pruritus, in young children and in cases of severe hypertension.

WARNINGS: The ergot alkaloids stimulate uterine contraction and are particularly harmful to the pregnant uterus. These migraine agents are slowly and incompletely absorbed from the gastrointestinal tract. Ergotamine is sequestered in various tissues, accounting for its long-lasting and toxic actions. Elderly patients and nursing mothers should be monitored closely when using this drug.

IMPLEMENTATION:

DRUG INTERACTIONS: When used with other vasoconstrictors, vasoconstriction may be increased.

ADMINISTRATION AND DOSAGE: These products are available in oral, sublingual, parenteral and rectal forms, and as a solution for inhalation. Prescription requires consideration of many factors, including whether the purpose of the agent is to prevent or to treat migraine. Oral and rectal preparations are slowly and incompletely absorbed from the gastrointestinal tract. To speed up this absorption, caffeine is combined with oral and rectal preparations of the ergot alkaloids. Persons who cannot tolerate oral preparations are given rectal forms of the agent. Sublingual tablets are more quickly absorbed than either rectal or oral preparations. Intramuscular and subcutaneous preparations are commonly used, but absorption is often incomplete and slow.

Ergotamine is metabolized and eliminated most slowly of all the ergot alkaloids, followed by dihydroergotamine, dehydroergotoxine mesylate, ergonovine and methylergonavine.

IMPLEMENTATION CONSIDERATIONS:

—Obtain a complete health history to identify etiology of headache, e.g., tension, migraine, or cluster, and to rule out contraindications for use of this drug: renal or liver disease, pregnancy.

—Be alert for peripheral vascular signs of acute poisoning or chronic toxicity.

—In addition to the migraine agents, digital pressure on one side of the carotids approximately half way between the sternum and maxillary bones may reduce extracranial and intracranial blood flow, thereby relieving migraine pain.

—Prolonged antimigraine agent use can lead to acute overdosage or chronic toxicity because of the wide variability in its absorption, metabolism, and excretion.

—Diagnosis of vascular headaches can be confirmed by relief of pain following IM injection of 1 ml (0.5 mg) ergotamine.

—Abrupt discontinuation of antimigraine agents after prolonged use can result in rebound migraine headaches; therefore they should be discontinued slowly.

—Early use of antimigraine agents at the onset of an attack increases the efficacy of these drugs in relieving migraine pain and symptoms.

—If more than 8 mg of oral ergotamine is needed to relieve migraine pain, the patient risks acute poisoning.

—Rebound migraine headaches may occur when a patient discontinues excessive use of ergots.

WHAT THE PATIENT NEEDS TO KNOW:

—Take medication precisely as ordered. Do not increase dosage without consulting health care provider as acute poisoning or overdosage may be produced.

—Avoid exposure of arms and legs to cold temperatures after taking this medication.

—Contact your health care provider immediately if numbness, coldness of the extremities, or pain in legs during walking occurs.

—Oral drugs may produce stomach upset. Take medicine with milk or meals if possible to decrease these effects.

—Common side effects of these antimigraine agents include: headache, nausea, vomiting, diarrhea, dizziness, and lightheadedness when changing positions rapidly.

—After taking this drug, lie down immediately in a quiet, dark room to help obtain relief of symptoms. Relaxation techniques may also assist in making you feel better.

—If more than 8 mg of oral ergotamine is needed to relieve migraine pain, contact your health care provider immediately.

—Do not use this drug if you suspect you are pregnant.

EVALUATION:

ADVERSE REACTIONS: *Cardiovascular:* anginal pain, bradycardia, coronary fibrosis, murmurs, precordial distress and pain, transient tachycardia. *CNS:* confusion, depression, dizziness, drowsiness, fixed miosis, hallucination, muscle pain in extremities, numbness and tingling in toes, weakness, especially in legs. *Gastrointestinal:* nausea and vomiting. *Renal:* retroperitoneal fibrosis. *Respiratory:* pleural and pulmonary inflammation, pleuropulmonary fibrosis. *Other:* coldness, eosinophilia, leg cramps, localized itching and edema, neutropenia, numbness and tingling, peripheral vascular effects, vascular insufficiency.

OVERDOSAGE: *Signs and symptoms:* Numb, cold, pale extremities, muscle pain at work and rest, decreased or absent arterial pulses, drowsiness, confusion, depression, convulsions, hemiplegia, tabetic manifestations and fixed miosis. *Treatment:* Withdraw the causative agent, and refer to maintain adequate circulation to extremities through vasodilators, anticoagulants, and low molecular weight dextran.

PARAMETERS TO MONITOR: The severity and chronicity of the migraine attacks dictates which parameters to monitor. Initial baseline data should include a complete neurological, respiratory and cardiovascular assessment, including a detailed health history. Parameters to monitor each visit: Monitor for therapeutic effect: decrease in number and severity of migraine headaches. To determine whether overdosage, toxicity or adverse reactions are developing, monitor patients every three months for blood pressure measurements in standing, sitting and lying positions, peripheral vascular assessment, pulse assessment, respiratory, cardiovascular assessment and auscultation for bruits. A urinalysis is also indicated in methysergide maleate therapy.

CAFERGOT

PRODUCTS (TRADE NAME):

Cafergot, Ercaf, Ergo-Caff (Available as suppositories equivalent to 2 mg ergotamine tartrate and 100 mg caffeine; or as oral tablets equivalent to 1 mg ergotamine tartrate and 100 mg caffeine.) **Migral** (Available in 1 mg ergotamine tartrate, 50 mg caffeine, 25 mg cyclizine HCl tablets.) **Wigraine** (Available in 1 mg ergotamine tartrate, 100 mg caffeine, 0.1 mg belladonna alkaloids, 130 mg phenacetin tablets or suppository.)

DRUG SPECIFICS:

Cafergot is a combination of ergotamine tartrate and caffeine used for the treatment of migraine and vascular headaches. Ergotamine tartrate is an alpha adrenergic blocking agent useful in vasoconstriction of cerebral vessels. The caffeine is combined with this drug to expedite the absorption of the ergot alkaloid. In addition to the warning noted for the ergot alkaloids, patients should be advised that chronic use may potentiate habituation and exacerbate peptic ulcers. Insomnia, restlessness, and nervousness are the most common side effects. Xanthines can enhance the cardiac effects of this drug. Also false elevation in serum urate levels, VMA urinary levels, and catecholamines may be noted by health care provider.

ADMINISTRATION AND DOSAGE SPECIFICS:

Migraine treatment: Administer 2 tablets orally at the start of an attack, followed by one tablet every half hour to a maximum of 6 tablets per attack, 10 per week. Or, administer 1 suppository at the start of an attack. This dose may be repeated 1 hour later if needed. Do not exceed 2 suppositories per attack, 5 per week.

DIHYDROERGOTAMINE MESYLATE

PRODUCTS (TRADE NAME):

D.H.E. 45 (Available in injectable solution equivalent to 1 mg of dihydroergotamine mesylate per ml).

DRUG SPECIFICS:

Dihydroergotamine mesylate is an alpha adrenergic blocking agent possessing pharmacologic and toxic properties similar to ergotamine. The drug causes cerebral vasculature to constrict, but it does not have an oxytoxic effect. Therefore, this product can be used during pregnancy. The side effects of this drug are milder than those of ergotamine. The drug should be taken at the onset of migraine headache to offset the associated cerebral vascular dilatation.

ADMINISTRATION AND DOSAGE SPECIFICS:
Migraine treatment: Administer 1 mg IM to be repeated at hourly intervals, not to exceed a total of 3 mg; or administer 1 mg IV to be repeated once. The total weekly dose should not exceed 6 mg.

ERGOTAMINE TARTRATE

PRODUCTS (TRADE NAME):
Ergomar, Ergostat (Available in 2 mg sublingual tablets). **Gynergen** (Available in 1 mg tablets). **Medihaler Ergotamine** (Available as an aerosol spray in a 2.5 ml vial, equivalent to 0.36 mg/spray or 9 mg/ml).

DRUG SPECIFICS:
Ergotamine tartrate is used for the treatment of migraine and vascular headaches. It is an alpha adrenergic blocking agent which exerts direct vasoconstriction on cranial blood vessels, relieving pulsations thought to be responsible for vasoconstriction. It should not be used for migraine prophylaxis in the prodromal stage, since it can precipitate an attack. Patients should be advised to contact health care provider if signs of ergotism (overdosage) or cardiovascular irregularities occur. These drugs are contraindicated in pregnancy because of their oxytoxic effects. Prolonged use or dosage above the recommended levels is hazardous. Propranolol interacts with the ergot alkaloids, blocking their effects. The ergot products may cause increases in serum urea, nitrogen, urine proteins, and prophyrins. Dependence on ergotamine may develop, necessitating gradual withdrawal from these products.

ADMINISTRATION AND DOSAGE SPECIFICS:
Migraine treatment: Administer 2 mg orally or sublingually at the start of an attack, followed by 1 mg every half hour as needed for full relief, up to 6 mg per migraine attack or 10 mg per week. The total amount is then used for subsequent attacks. For intramuscular or subcutaneous injection, administer 0.25 mg, repeated in 40 minutes, if needed, for full relief. The total amount needed is then used at the first sign of subsequent attacks. For inhalation dosage, administer 0.36 mg (1 metered spray) at the beginning of an attack, then repeat every 5 minutes as needed, up to 2.16 mg (6 metered sprays) per 24 hours, or 12 mg per week. The total amount required may be used at the first sign of subsequent attacks.

METHYSERGIDE MALEATE

PRODUCTS (TRADE NAME):
Sansert (Available in 2 mg tablets.)

DRUG SPECIFICS:
Methysergide maleate is used as a migraine prophylaxis for patients suffering

from one or more severe vascular headaches per week. Its exact mode of action is unknown, but it is thought to block serotonin activity in the CNS which may be related to vascular headaches. This drug can produce highly toxic effects. Therefore, continuous administration should not exceed 6 months. After each 6-month course of therapy 3 to 4 weeks should be drug free, followed by another 6-month course of medicine. Advise patients to administer the drug with meals to avoid gastric irritation. Health care providers should monitor weight, and watch for signs of edema, toxicity, and fibrosis at regular 3-month intervals.

ADMINISTRATION AND DOSAGE SPECIFICS:

Migraine prophylaxis: Administer 4 to 8 mg daily in divided doses with meals or milk.

Doreen C. Harper

ANALGESICS—ANTIPYRETIC AGENTS

ACETAMINOPHEN

ACTION OF THE DRUG: Acetaminophen is an analgesic and antipyretic agent. It produces analgesia by an elevation in the pain threshold, and produces antipyresis by directly acting on the temperature regulating centers of the hypothalamus, increasing body dissipation of heat by vasodilation. The exact mechanism of the analgesic effect is not known though it is known to inhibit prostaglandin synthesis of the central nervous system. It does not, however, affect prostaglandin synthesis peripherally, therefore having no anti-inflammatory activity. Acetaminophen does not inhibit platelet aggregation, prothrombin response, or produce gastrointestinal ulcerations.

ASSESSMENT:

INDICATIONS: Use in minor to moderate musculoskeletal pain, headache, toothache, myalgias, neuralgias, and fever believed to be of no serious origin.

SUBJECTIVE: Acetaminophen provides temporary relief for a wide range of types of pain, especially of a musculoskeletal origin, as well as headache, dental pain, myalgia, neuralgias, minor soft tissue trauma, or minor surgical procedures. It also aids in the reduction of fever secondary to viral, flu-like syndromes, or immunizations. It can be used to treat fever associated with bacterial illnesses, but the causative agent and appropriate antibacterial agent must still be determined and treated. It is the drug of choice for fever in children or during pregnancy, though the health care provider should be contacted prior to using drug. It is also used in patients with aspirin allergy, bleeding problems, or gout.

OBJECTIVE: Physical findings will be compatible with any of the above complaints and represent a minor variation from normal, i.e., minimal to moderate heat, swelling, tenderness, and inability to carry out normal activities. Temperature elevation may be present. Any physical finding that demonstrates serious pathogenesis needs further exploration, i.e., fever with lethargy, disorientation, pain with clinical signs of infection, fracture or malignancy.

PLAN:

CONTRAINDICATIONS: Do not use in the presence of hypersensitivity to the drug or G-6-PD deficiency. Patients with severe renal insufficiency, anemia, cardiac or pulmonary disease should not be given this drug as they are more susceptible to toxic effects.

WARNINGS: Do not exceed recommended dosage or use for longer than ten days.

PRECAUTIONS: Monitor patient for failure to improve, or worsening of symptoms. Prolonged use may result in symptoms of restlessness, or excitation upon withdrawal of the agent. This drug is metabolized by the liver so patients with hepatic problems should be carefully watched. Monitor use in alcoholics or seizure patients on phenobarbital, as hepatotoxic problems may develop.

IMPLEMENTATION:

DRUG INTERACTIONS: Alcohol or phenobarbital may increase the conversion of acetaminophen to its toxic metabolite, thereby increasing hepatic necrosis. There is only minimal interaction with anticoagulants.

PRODUCTS (TRADE NAME):

Products are manufactured by a number of different companies, and come in a variety of dosages and forms. See Table 4-1 for summary.

ADMINISTRATION AND DOSAGE: Acetaminophen comes in a variety of forms: tablets, liquid, drops and suppositories. Because this preparation is widely used in children, choose the format which is most appropriate for the patient age.

Adult: 325-650 mg po every 4 hours. Long term, maximum 2.6 Gm/day. Short term not to exceed 4gm/day.

The following doses for children not to exceed 5 doses in 24 hours.

Children 0-3 months: 40 mg.
Children 4-11 months: 80 mg.
Children 1-2 years: 120 mg.
Children 2-3 years: 160 mg.
Children 4-5 years: 240 mg.
Children 6-8 years: 320 mg.
Children 9-10 years: 400 mg.
Children 11-12 years: 480 mg.

IMPLEMENTATION CONSIDERATIONS:

—Obtain a complete health history including presence of allergies, liver impairment, excessive alcohol intake, kidney problems, or possibility of pregnancy.

—Rule out the possibility of serious pathology for the underlying pain or fever.

—If the patient is pregnant, the frequent use of this drug should be discouraged.

TABLE 4-1. ACETAMINOPHEN PRODUCTS, DOSAGE, AND FORMS

| *Product* | *Tablet* | Form and Amount of Agent Present | | | |
		Capsule	*Elixir*	*Drops*	*Suppository*
A'cenol	325 mg	500 mg			
Aceta	325 mg				300 mg
Acetaminophen	325 mg		120 mg/5ml	100 mg/0.6 ml	120, 125,
	500 mg				325, 600,
	650 mg				650 mg
Actamin	325 mg				
Anuphen					120, 650 mg
Dapa	325				
Datril	325 mg				
Datril 500	500 mg				
Febrigesic		500 mg			
G-1	325 mg				
G-lixir			120 mg/5 ml		
Liquiprin				120 mg/2.5 ml	
Panex	300 mg				
Pedric wafers	120 mg		120 mg/5 ml		
Phenaphen		325 mg			
SK-APAP	325 mg		120 mg/5 ml	60 mg/0.6 ml	
Tapar	325 mg		120 mg/5 ml		
Tempra			120 mg/5 ml	100 mg/ml	
Tylenol	325 mg	325 mg	120 mg/5 ml		
			100 mg/ml		
Chewable	80 mg				
Extra strength	500 mg	500 mg	165 mg/5 ml		

If patient is determined to take a pain reliever, this is the drug of choice over aspirin.

—Chronic use of this drug should be avoided as it can lead to nephrotic or hepatic problems if taken in large doses over a long period of time.

WHAT THE PATIENT NEEDS TO KNOW:

—This is a medication to be used for pain or fever, but is not to be taken over a long period of time.

—This drug should not be used for arthritis, as it has no effect on inflammation.

—Mothers should review with the health care provider the proper dose of the drug for their child. Dosage is figured according to age and weight of child. Be accurate to avoid over- or underdosage.

—Suppository form of this drug should be inserted rectally and patient should not move bowels, but allow the medication to be absorbed.

—Sometimes this medication can cause adverse effects. If you notice any new or troublesome symptoms, notify your health care provider. Especially note any sore throat, easy bruising, bleeding or yellow color to skin.

—Keep this medication out of the reach of children and all others for whom it is not prescribed.

EVALUATION:

ADVERSE REACTIONS: Problems usually occur only with long-term usage. *Hematopoietic:* cyanosis, hemolytic anemias, leukopenia, methemoglobinemia, neutropenia, pancytopenia, sulfhemoglobinemia. *Hypersensitivity:* skin eruption, urticaria. *Other:* drowsiness, excitation, hypoglycemia, jaundice.

OVERDOSAGE: Excessive medication results in hepatotoxicity manifested by anemias, cyanosis, tachycardia, excitation progressing to delirium, coma, shock, seizures and death. Early signs of overdosage may be nausea, vomiting or abdominal pains. Toxic doses range from 5.8 gm to 10 gm or 70 to 140 mg/kg. Lethal dose is 15 gm or 200 mg/kg. It is very important to administer the antidote, acetylcysterne, shortly after the overdose is discovered. Children appear to be more resistant to toxicities than adults. Hepatic damage may not be evident for up to two weeks, so liver enzymes should be analyzed at regular intervals.

PARAMETERS TO MONITOR: Monitor for symptomatic relief of pain and reduction of temperature. Observe for adverse reactions, especially symptoms of hepatic or renal toxicity in patients on long-term use. Acetaminophen is a fairly safe drug if used properly and in short duration.

Carole Hill

ANALGESICS—
SLOW-ACTING ANTIRHEUMATIC DRUGS (SAARDS)

GOLD COMPOUNDS (CHRYSOTHERAPY)

ACTION OF THE DRUG: The exact mechanism of action of gold is not known. Gold is a heavy metal that interferes with a wide range of biochemical reactions on a cellular level. It is felt it may inhibit lysosomal enzyme activity in macrophages and decrease their phagocytic activity. It is also believed that it in some way affects the antigen formation in the autoimmune response of patients with rheumatoid arthritis. It appears to suppress the synovitis of active rheumatoid disease and therefore reduce the amount of damage done.

ASSESSMENT:

INDICATIONS: Use in documented rheumatoid arthritis that has been progressive or without remission despite other methods of therapy, including high doses of non-steroidal anti-inflammatory drugs. None of these agents are without significant risk and toxic effects. Patients on these drugs need constant follow up and regular evaluation. This medication would be prescribed by a specialist, with the nurse practitioner frequently responsible for monitoring the progress of the patient receiving the drug. Both patient attitude and compliance history and drug action and side effects must be understood before beginning therapy. Gold compounds are indicated in the treatment of active rheumatoid disease in both juvenile and adult patients. It is most successfully used in continually active, progressive disease early in the course of treatment, and will have little effect once joint destruction has already occurred. It may be of use in limiting further destruction and should therefore be instituted in patients with acute and widespread synovitis.

SUBJECTIVE: Patient complains of a long history of severe or recently progressive pain, stiffness, or weakness in his/her joints. They may tire quickly, or complain of inability to carry out activities of normal living. They also complain of swelling, heat, and redness of joints (usually of the hands, but it may involve most other joints). By the time a patient is a candidate for use of gold compounds, he/she has undergone extensive testing and has been diagnosed as having rheumatoid arthritis. They have taken other medications with no relief or a gradual worsening of symptoms.

OBJECTIVE: Confirmed diagnosis of rheumatoid arthritis may be demonstrated on the basis of joint aspiration; x-ray findings showing joint space narrowing, juxta-articular erosion, osteoporosis, and even subluxation; abnormal laboratory values, with an anemia of chronic disease, elevated sedimentation rate and platelet count, positive L.E. prep, L.E. latex, and a positive rheumatoid factor. Physical findings include obvious or beginning joint deformities, with periarticular swelling or other abnormalities, particularly of the PIP and MCP joints. Subcutaneous nodules may also be found over bony prominences or around involved joints or extensor surfaces of long bones.

PLAN:

CONTRAINDICATIONS: Gold is contraindicated in combination with other slowacting antirheumatoid drugs; severe diabetes; liver failure or in patients with a past history of hepatitis. Additionally it is contraindicated in patients with impaired renal function or other severely debilitated people with problems such as heart failure. Patients with systemic lupus erythematosus should not receive gold, as it greatly increases their skin manifestations.

There is some disagreement about whether gold is contraindicated in Sjögren's syndrome: some authorities feel it is, and other rheumatologists state they have had improvement both of the rheumatoid arthritis as well as the Sjögren's syndrome when using gold in these patients.

Gold is also contraindicated in patients with agranulocytosis, abnormal hemorrhagic tendencies, or other blood abnormalities. It should not be used in patients with past history of toxic reactions to other heavy metals or gold. It should not be used in patients with severe dermatologic problems such as eczema, or those with colitis. Pregnant or breast-feeding women should not receive gold nor should any patient having induced or acquired bone marrow depression.

WARNINGS: This drug has many toxic effects and only 30-35% of patients gain benefit from its use. Patients should be warned of this before being started on this agent.

Initial baseline evaluation of any patient to be started on this drug is essential. This evaluation should include a complete blood count with differential, and platelet count. Urine should also be analyzed for protein and blood. An exact protocol should be followed for laboratory work to be repeated, looking at various indicators for problems. Elderly patients do not tolerate this drug well, and patients with diabetes or congestive failure must be under good control before initiating therapy.

A number of patients experience what is known as the "nitritoid reaction with the use of Myochrysine. This is a benign reaction caused by the aqueous medium the gold is in. It results in the patient feeling flushed and lightheaded, and occasionally leads to fainting. These symptoms occur immediately after the injection, and for this reason it is advised that patients receiving Myochrysine should be lying down and remain recumbent for 10 to 15 minutes after the injection. This problem is self-limited and requires no other intervention.

PRECAUTIONS: Do not use with penicillamine or cytotoxic drugs. Use with caution in patients with a history of blood dyscrasias, allergies to medications, skin rashes, marked hypertension, or compromised vascular profusion of cerebral or cardiac tissues. Renal adenomas have been shown in rats on long-term therapy, but these findings have not been demonstrated in humans. Possibility of carcinogenesis, mutagenesis and impairment of fertility have been raised and are under study.

IMPLEMENTATION:

DRUG INTERACTIONS: Gold compounds may be used concurrently with systemic corticosteroids, salicylates and other slow-acting antirheumatic drugs. Gold compounds are not to be used with immunosuppressants or pyrazoline derivatives such as phenylbutazone and oxyphenbutazone because of the potential for blood dyscrasias.

ADMINISTRATION AND DOSAGE: The empirical regimen includes three phases in the administration and use of gold: (1) a 2 or 3 week period of injections that increase gradually to test for severe reactions or unusual problems; (2) a loading period" of weekly injections, until a total dose of 1 gm of injected gold is reached, and (3) a decreasing frequency of dosage sequencing until a maintenance dose is achieved.

Gold is a heavy metal and comes in two solution forms for injection: one in an oil medium and the other in an aqueous medium. They are both painful injections and should be given only in the gluteus muscle. There is an oral form of gold that looks promising for future use, but it is only being used in the United States in controlled studies at the present time.

Use the following dosage regimen for prescribing both aqueous and oil medication in adults:

Gold sodium thiomalate for juvenile arthritis: Based on child's weight after initial 10 mg dose. The recommended dose is 1 mg/kg, not to exceed 50 mg. Give in the dosage schedule shown in Table 4-2.

TABLE 4-2. DOSAGE REGIMEN FOR AQUEOUS AND OIL MEDICATIONS

Phase	Week	Dosage	Blood work	Urine Dip-stick
One	1	10 mg	Baseline before medication	Baseline
	2	25 mg		
	3	25 mg	CBC	Yes
			no	Yes
Two	4-22	50 mg/week until total of 1 gm cumulative reached	Every other week	Every week
Three	23-36	50 mg every other week	Yes with results before medication	Yes
	37-54	50 mg every third week	Yes with results before medication	Yes
	55+	50 mg every fourth week	Yes with results before medication	Yes

Aurothioglucose for children 6-12: Give 1/4 of adult dose, governed by body weight in the same schedule as above.

IMPLEMENTATION CONSIDERATIONS:

—Obtain a complete health history, including the complete diagnostic and therapeutic history of the patient's arthritis, presence of drug sensitivities, underlying diseases such as renal, liver, cardiovascular, or hematopoietic diseases which would contraindicate using gold compounds, possibility of pregnancy, or other drugs taken concurrently which might cause drug interactions.

—Obtain complete baseline physical and laboratory examinations.

—Remember that only 30-35% of patients may benefit from this drug and the patient should be counseled so as not to develop unrealistic hopes.

—This is a painful injection and must be given in the gluteus muscle.

—Patients receiving Myochrysine injections should remain lying down for 15 minutes following the injection, and then be helped carefully to their feet. They should be monitored for any symptoms of nitritoid reaction.

—Shake vial well before administering the injection, and check to ensure proper concentration of medication.

—Check color of medication. Do not use if darker color than pale yellow.

WHAT THE PATIENT NEEDS TO KNOW:

—This drug is a very potent, slow-acting drug which may be helpful in some patients in actually halting joint destruction caused by arthritis. It does not help all patients, and a thorough trial will take 12 to 20 weeks before response to the drug can be determined.

—There are possibly serious toxic side effects that can occur with this drug. You must work closely with your health care providers in keeping appointments, getting laboratory work drawn, and reporting any new or troublesome symptoms which develop.

—You and the health care provider should especially watch for problems which may develop in the kidneys, your skin, or in your blood.

—This medication requires weekly injections for at least 26 weeks, and then monthly injections on a long-term basis.

—Some people experience a brief increase in pain and joint achiness for 1-2 days after receiving the injection, which then disappears. You should contact your health care provider if you are still having great discomfort after 2 days.

—The most common toxic effects are skin rashes, ulcers or sores in the mouth.

—Notify your health care provider if you note a metallic taste in your mouth, purple blotches, bruising, or problems with bleeding.

EVALUATION:

ADVERSE REACTIONS: *Dermatologic:* The most common side effects are mucocutaneous, which occur in about 15% of all patients. Gold dermatitis has a variety of appearances but is always pruritic. (Often this pruritus occurs before the rash presents itself, and is seen most commonly periorbitally and on the palms and dorsum of the hands.) Stomatitis may be demonstrated with painful ulcers on the buccal mucosa, tongue, palate or pharynx. These may be preceded by a metallic taste. *Gastrointestinal:* cholestatic jaundice (rare), and colitis. *Hematopoietic* (occur in about 1% of patients): aplastic anemia, granulocytopenia, thrombocytopenia. *Renal:* 5-8% of patients may have asymptomatic proteinuria or microscopic hematuria (only seen with use of urine dipsticks), which may progress to nephrotic syndrome or glomerulitis if therapy is not discontinued.

PARAMETERS TO MONITOR: Obtain a complete history, physical examination and laboratory evaluation for baseline data prior to initiating therapy. These should include complete blood count, indices, platelet, liver and renal function studies, and evaluation studies of cardiac status if indicated. X-rays of joints should also be obtained so progression of disease can be followed.

This drug should be given according to a protocol established by therapist. Each week patient should be monitored for: (1) History: complaints of itching, sores in mouth, metallic taste. Ask about symptomatic improvement of joint pain or limitation after 20 weeks of therapy. (2) Physical: signs of itching, ulcers in mouth, limitation of joint movement, resolution of subcutaneous nodules. (3) Laboratory: WBC greater than 5000; urine protein-free or only trace; RBC and indices.

Gold dermatitis may appear in a variety of ways, but is always pruritic and itching often precedes development of the rash itself. Check for this especially between 400-800 mg cumulative dose as this is when it is most likely to occur. If there is any sign of gold dermatitis, drug must be stopped as soon as possible or it can led to exfoliative dermatitis. When symptoms resolve one can resume therapy at 25 mg weekly, usually without problems. Topical steroids may be used in mild cases of the dermatitis until it clears, or low-dose oral steroids may be indicated for more severe dermatitis.

The metallic taste in the mouth is often a warning sign which precedes the painful oral ulcers. If this sign should develop, the dosage should be cut in half and the patient carefully monitored.

If asymptomatic proteinuria or microscopic hematuria are found through use of urine dipsticks, therapy may continue if there is less than 50 mg/100 ml of protein. If higher than this, the gold should be stopped. If the urine returns to normal in one to two weeks, therapy can be resumed at half the previous dosage. If the proteinuria reappears immediately, the gold must be discontinued. If treatment is continued, nephrotic syndrome or glomerulitis may develop.

If there is an exacerbation of the arthritis during maintenance management therapy, go back to weekly injections for 6-8 weeks until the symptoms are suppressed.

If there is no patient improvement after phase two (see Table 4-2) is completed and a total of 1 gm of gold has been given, several choices for continued therapy exist: (1) discontinue the medication as the patient is not responsive to this drug; (2) continue phase 2 for 10 more weeks; or (3) increase the injection dosage by 10 mg every 1 to 4 weeks until improvement occurs. Do not exceed total injection doses of 100 mg.

AURANOFIN

PRODUCTS (TRADE NAME):
   Ridaura (Available in 3 mg tablet.)
DRUG SPECIFICS:
   Product has just come on the market. Seek current information for this drug.
ADMINISTRATION AND DOSAGE SPECIFICS:
   No information yet. Seek current information from manufacturer.

AUROTHIOGLUCOSE

PRODUCTS (TRADE NAME):
   Solganal (Available in oil preparation for IM injection in 50 mg/ml in 10 ml vial.)
DRUG SPECIFICS:
   There appear to be fewer skin eruptions, and a greater incidence of stomatitis and albuminuria with this preparation. Oil and aqueous preparations may be alternated. This injection is painful and should be given deep into the gluteus muscle.

ADMINISTRATION AND DOSAGE SPECIFICS:
Refer back to Administration and Dosage in general. See parameters to monitor for dosage procedure if exacerbation develops, or if there is no improvement in patient's condition after phase two is completed.

GOLD SODIUM THIOMALATE

PRODUCTS (TRADE NAME):
Myochrysine (Available as an aqueous preparation for injection in 10, 25, 50 mg/ml ampules.)
DRUG SPECIFICS:
There appear to be more skin eruptions, and a greater incidence of stomatitis and albuminuria with the aqueous solution than the oil preparation, so a number of authorities recommend alternating oil and aqueous preparations.

This injection is painful and should be given only in gluteus muscle. This preparation is also responsible for producing a "nitritoid-like response" in some patients (see Warnings), and patients must remain lying down for 10-15 minutes following injection to decrease possibility of fainting.

Shake vial well prior to injection, and make certain proper concentration of medication is used.
ADMINISTRATION AND DOSAGE SPECIFICS:
Refer back to Administration and Dosage in general section. See Parameters to Monitor for dosage procedure if exacerbation develops, or if there is no improvement in patient's condition at the conclusion of phase two.

Carole Hill

HYDROXYCHLOROQUINE SULFATE

ACTION OF THE DRUG: The mechanism of action of this drug is not understood. It is believed that the antimalarial drugs, of which this is one, in some way suppress the formation of antigens in the body. These antigens produce the hypersensitivity reactions leading to the physiologic changes of rheumatoid arthritis and systemic lupus erythematosus.

ASSESSMENT:

INDICATIONS: Use in documented rheumatoid arthritis that has been progressive or without remission despite other methods of therapy, including high doses of non-steroidal anti-inflammatory drugs. This agent is not without significant risk and toxic effects. Patients on this drug need constant follow up and regular evaluation. This medication would be prescribed by a specialist, with the nurse practitioner frequently responsible for monitoring the progress of the patient receiving the drug. Both patient attitude and compliance history and drug action and side effects must be understood before beginning therapy. This drug is a second line agent for long-term use in the treatment of rheumatoid arthritis.

In addition to rheumatoid arthritis, medication may be used in confirmed diagnosis of systemic or discoid lupus erythematosus. This drug is also used in the treatment of malaria. (See Antimalarials).

SUBJECTIVE: Patients complain of a long history of severe or recently progressive pain, stiffness, or weakness in their joints. They may tire quickly, or complain of inability to carry out activities of normal living. They also complain of swelling, heat, and redness of joints (usually of the hands, but it may involve most other joints). By the time patients are candidates for use of this drug, they have undergone extensive testing and have been diagnosed as having rheumatoid arthritis. They have taken other medications with no relief or a gradual worsening of symptoms.

OBJECTIVE: Confirmed diagnosis of rheumatoid arthritis may be demonstrated on the basis of joint aspiration; x-ray findings showing joint space narrowing, juxta-articular erosion, osteoporosis, and even subluxation; abnormal laboratory values, with an anemia of chronic disease, elevated sedimentation rate and platelet count, positive L.E. prep, L.E. latex, and a positive rheumatoid factor. Physical findings include obvious or beginning joint deformities, with periarticular swelling or other abnormalities, particularly of the PIP and MCP joints. Subcutaneous nodules may also be found over bony prominences or around involved joints or extensor surfaces of long bones.

PLAN:

CONTRAINDICATIONS: Do not give in the presence of hypersensitivity to this and other aminoquinoline compounds. Any retinal or visual field changes that have occurred in relation to use of any 4-aminoquinoline compounds should preclude the use of this drug for treatment of arthritis, as changes are significant and non-reversible. Do not use these drugs concomitantly with other slow-acting antirheumatic drugs.

WARNINGS: Children are especially sensitive to this agent, and deaths have been reported with children on this medication.

The most serious side effect of this drug is damage to the eyes, which usually appears in two forms: (1) retinopathy with irreversible visual loss, and (2) corneal infiltration (which may be somewhat reversible when the medication is stopped). The retinopathy does appear to be dose-related, so patients should have an expert ophthalmologic evaluation prior to initiation of the drug, and periodically every 3 to 6 months throughout therapy. The drug should be discontinued with any visual complaints, or symptoms such as seeing flashing lights or light streaks, as the retinal damage may progress even after the drug is discontinued.

Patient's reflexes and motor strength should also be regularly evaluated to look for muscle weakness. Decreased muscle strength is an indication for stopping the drug.

This drug should not be used to treat arthritis during pregnancy.

PRECAUTIONS: Use with caution in patients with G-6-PD deficiency anemia, or patients with hepatic disease or alcoholism. The chance for dermatologic reactions will be increased if used in conjunction with other drugs that commonly cause skin reactions.

IMPLEMENTATION:

DRUG INTERACTIONS: Do not use this product with other slow-acting antirheumatic drugs, especially gold, as concurrent use will greatly increase the chance of dermatologic reactions. Acidifying agents decrease the effectiveness of chloroquine by increasing urinary excretion. Alkalinizing agents such as bicarbonate decrease urinary excretion and potentiate the effects of the drug. MAO inhibitors affect the liver and therefore increase the effect of chloroquine by decreasing hepatic metabolism of the drug.

PRODUCTS (TRADE NAME):
Plaquenil Sulfate (Available in 200 mg tablets.)
ADMINISTRATION AND DOSAGE:
Rheumatoid arthritis: Use 400-600 mg po daily with meals or food to prevent GI upset. If patient experiences side effects, try a reduced dosage for 5-10 days, and then resume full dose.

Maintenance dose: Continue 400-600 mg po daily for 4-12 weeks, until patient has symptomatic improvement. Then reduce dosage by 50% to 200-400 mg po daily, and maintain that dosage.

This medication requires 4-12 weeks of therapy before improvement is seen. If there is no improvement after 6 months, discontinue the drug.

If the drug is stopped while the patient is feeling relief from symptoms, the agent can be reintroduced with exacerbation of the disease. Corticosteroids or nonsteroidal anti-inflammatory drugs may be used with this drug until the effects of this slow-acting drug become apparent.

Lupus erythematosus: Give 400 mg po 1 to 2 times daily initially. This may be continued for several weeks to months. Then a 200-400 mg po daily dose may be used for prolonged maintenance. This drug is beneficial in skin and rheumatic-like symptoms, but will have little effect on lupus symptoms of other body organs.

IMPLEMENTATION CONSIDERATIONS:
—Obtain a complete health history, including drug sensitivities, other drugs taken concurrently which might produce drug interactions, presence of underlying systemic disease, G-6-PD deficiency, previous history of retinal or visual problems, liver disease or high alcohol intake, past treatment history for arthritis or lupus erythematosus, and possibility of pregnancy.

—A thorough physical examination, paying particular attention to evaluation of muscle strength and reflexes, should be performed prior to initiation of therapy and relevant laboratory data collected. This will serve as a baseline against which further evaluations can be compared.

—The most common side effects are visual or dermatologic problems and these must be watched for on every visit. A complete evaluation by an ophthalmologist should be conducted prior to beginning therapy.

—This drug may turn patient's urine a yellow or brown color.

—Potential for reducing pain and deformity in arthritic patients, as well as reducing skin and joint manifestations of lupus erythematosus, must be explained to patients. They must be educated about what the reasonably expected therapeutic results include.

—This drug may cause alopecia or bleaching of hair and patients should be warned about this.

WHAT THE PATIENT NEEDS TO KNOW:

—There will be no immediate relief from pain with this drug, as benefits are not usually seen for up to 12 weeks. This medication is a slow-acting drug which may help to prevent some of the damage of rheumatoid arthritis, not just to relieve the pain. Because it is such a powerful drug you will need to be carefully supervised while you take this medication. This will require return visits to your health care provider, and additional laboratory work.

—This drug may cause your urine to turn a yellow or brown color. This is a normal and expected reaction.

—This medication may cause stomach upset which can be reduced by taking it with food or milk.

—Keep this medicine in the amber-colored bottle it comes in. The medicine will be decomposed by light.

—The most common side effects from this drug are skin rashes or itching. Report these immediately to your health care provider.

—Report any difficulties with your vision: decreased vision, seeing halos around lights, light flashes, light streaks, or blurred vision.

—Also report any muscle weakness, hair loss or bleaching of color (without use of hair products), fever, sore throats, unusual bleeding, bruising, or black and blue spots on your body or in your mouth that seem to appear without injury to the area.

—Take medication exactly as ordered. Do not take any other medications, including those which you may buy over-the-counter, without the knowledge of your health care provider.

—Keep this medication out of the reach of children and all others for whom it is not prescribed. This drug is powerful enough to kill children, even if only small doses are taken.

EVALUATION:

ADVERSE REACTIONS: *CNS:* ataxia, convulsions, dizziness, headache, insomnia, irritability, nerve conductive hearing loss, nervousness, vertigo. *Dermatologic:* alopecia, bleaching of hair, mucosal discoloration, pruritus with skin rash of just about any variety, including severe exfoliative dermatitis. *Gastrointestinal:* anorexia, diarrhea, gastrointestinal distress, nausea (up to 15% of all patients), vomiting. *Hematopoietic:* agranulocytosis, aplastic anemia, hemolytic anemia (in patients with G-6-PD deficiency), leukopenia, thrombocytopenia. *Neuromuscular:*

decreased or lost reflexes, decreased muscle strength. *Ophthalmologic:* atrophy, "bull's eye" pigmentation changes, corneal edema with linear opacities (usually reversible), decreased ability to recover from photo-stress test, retinal edema, visual field defects. These serious retinopathies are not reversible when the drug is stopped and may progress in severity despite discontinuation.

OVERDOSAGE: *Signs and symptoms:* The overdose effects of this drug can occur within 30 minutes of ingestion. Visual disturbances, headache and drowsiness may progress to convulsions. This drug also affects the cardiovascular system, producing collapse and arrest with ECG changes that progress from atrial standstill to ventricular fibrillation. *Treatment:* Due to the rapid onset of lethal symptoms, treatment must be immediate with emesis and referral for gavage and supportive treatment. This condition represents a medical emergency and top priority should be given to caring for the patient.

PARAMETERS TO MONITOR: In using this drug it is extremely important to collect accurate and comprehensive baseline information: history, physical exam (including muscle strength and reflexes, and a thorough ophthalmologic evaluation), and laboratory studies including CBC, L.E. prep, L.E. latex, rheumatoid factor and sedimentation rate. Blood count and sedimentation rate should be repeated at regular intervals to monitor for hemolytic problems as well as disease activity. Routine liver and renal studies should also be obtained. Ophthalmologic exam (including visual fields, acuity, funduscopic, and slit lamp evaluations) should be repeated every 3 months until the maintenance dose is reached, and then every 6 months. Monitor for therapeutic effect and development of adverse reactions. Develop a flow chart, and record after each visit the presence or absence of various common symptoms such as bruising, visual complaints, alopecia, pain, tiredness, stiffness, joint inflammation, subcutaneous nodules, gastrointestinal distress, etc.

Carole Hill

PENICILLAMINE-D

ACTION OF THE DRUG: This drug is a degradation of penicillin. It is a chelating agent used as a heavy metal antagonist and is useful in such things as lead and copper poisoning. Its mode of action in the treatment of rheumatoid arthritis is not understood. It is known to be effective in relieving the symptoms of arthritis and in some way suppressing the disease progression.

ASSESSMENT:

INDICATIONS: Use in documented rheumatoid arthritis that has been progressive or without remission despite other methods of therapy, including high doses of non-steroidal anti-inflammatory drugs. This agent is not without significant risk and toxic effect. Patients on this drug need constant follow up and regular evaluation. This medication is prescribed by a specialist, with the nurse practitioner frequently responsible for monitoring the progress of the patient receiving the drug. Both patient attitude and compliance history and drug action and side effects must be understood before beginning therapy.

In addition, it is also indicated in two other completely unrelated illnesses: Wilson's disease, because of its ability to remove copper through the kidney; and in the treatment of cystinuria because of its ability to exchange with cystine to form a more soluble product.

SUBJECTIVE: Patients complain of a long history of severe or recently progressive pain, stiffness, or weakness in the joints. They may tire quickly, or complain of inability to carry out activities of normal living. They also complain of swelling, heat, and redness of joints (usually of the hands, but it may involve most other joints). By the time patients are candidates for the use of penicillamine, they have undergone extensive testing and have been diagnosed as having rheumatoid arthritis. They have taken other medications with no relief or a gradual worsening of symptoms.

OBJECTIVE: Confirmed diagnosis of rheumatoid arthritis may be demonstrated on the basis of joint aspiration; x-ray findings showing joint space narrowing, juxta-articular erosion, osteoporosis, and even subluxation; abnormal laboratory values, with an anemia of chronic disease, elevated sedimentation rate and platelet count, positive L.E. prep, L.E. latex, and a positive rheumatoid factor. Physical findings include obvious or beginning joint deformities, with periarticular swelling or other abnormalities, particularly of the PIP and MCP joints. Subcutaneous nodules may also be found over bony prominences or around involved joints or extensor surfaces of long bones.

PLAN:

CONTRAINDICATIONS: Penicillamine is contraindicated for use in pregnancy; patients with aplastic anemia or agranulocytosis; or those hypersensitive to penicillamine. Patients with a history of or active renal impairment should not receive this drug, due to possible toxic effects on the kidney. It is contraindicated in combination with other drugs that could potentiate blood dyscrasias such as gold compounds, cytotoxic drugs, or pyrazoline derivatives such as phenylbutazone or oxyphenbutazone.

WARNINGS: About 50% of patients taking this drug have untoward reactions, some of which are fatal. Medical supervision through administration course is mandatory. This drug has many toxic side effects and as with gold, only about 30% of patients put on this agent obtain benefit from its use. Patients should be warned of this before starting the agent. This drug requires patient compliance, as it is an oral preparation which they must administer themselves.

Initial baseline evaluations of patients to be started on this drug are essential. This should include a complete blood count with differential and platelet count and should be repeated on a regular basis. Renal function must also be determined, with particular attention to proteinuria or hematuria, which are common side effects of this drug.

PRECAUTIONS: Patients who have been on gold therapy in the past with adverse reactions which caused it to be discontinued also seem to have problems with penicillamine. They should be monitored especially carefully when placed on penicillamine therapy.

IMPLEMENTATION:

DRUG INTERACTIONS: This drug increases the effect of isoniazid. It reacts with iron preparations if taken at the same time and this will decrease the effect of penicillamine. Do not use concurrently with other drugs known to produce blood dyscrasias because of the possibility of potentiation of adverse effects. This product may cause the patient's ANA titer to become positive. May produce increased serum alkaline phosphatase and LDH and positive cephalin flocculation and thymol turbidity tests.

PRODUCTS (TRADE NAME):

Cuprimine (Available in 125 and 250 mg capsules.) **Depen** (Available in 250 mg tablets.)

ADMINISTRATION AND DOSAGE: These dosage schedules are well known and recommended by the research done by Jaffe in the late 1970s for the treatment of rheumatoid arthritis. Recommendations can be summarized in Table 4-3.

Maintenance dose is that dose at which clinical improvement begins to occur. When a maintenance dose is reached, the blood and urine follow-up should continue

TABLE 4-3. DOSAGE SCHEDULE FOR PENICILLAMINE-D

Time	Dosage	Blood work	Urine Studies
Initial	125-250 mg daily for 3 months	Complete baseline evaluation before starting, then every 2 weeks.	Renal function then dip-stick tests for blood and protein every 2-4 weeks.
3 months	Increase by 125-250 mg daily to total dose of 250-500 mg daily	Complete blood count and platelets every 2 weeks	Dipstick tests for blood and protein every 2 weeks.
6 months	Increase by 125-250 mg to total of 375-750 mg daily	Complete blood count and platelets every 2 weeks.	Dipstick tests for blood and protein
9 months	If no improvement, increase 250 mg every 3 months to total 1,000 mg.	Continue blood work every 3 weeks.	Continue urine testing every 2 weeks.
12 months on 1,000 mg.	If no improvement after 3-4 months of 1,000 mg dosage, discontinue drug.		

every 2 weeks for 6 months and then monthly thereafter for as long as the patient receives the medicine. If an exacerbation occurs during therapy, the use of non-steroidal anti-inflammatory drugs is indicated rather than a rapid increase in the penicillamine dosage.

If remission occurs, continue maintenance dose for 3 months, then attempt to decrease the dose by 125 mg steps every 3 months. Previous experience shows a relapse often occurs within a few weeks, requiring a return to the previous maintenance dose.

Doses up to 500 mg daily may be taken at one time. Doses greater than 500 mg should be divided. This medication should be taken on an empty stomach 1 hour before meals or 2 hours after meals, and should not be taken with other medications.

No therapeutic effect may be seen for 3 to 6 months.

Children: The starting dose for children is 50 mg daily. Increase the dose by 50 mg in no less than 4-week time periods. Maximum dose is 450 mg daily in children less than 20 kg, and 600 mg in other children. The average maintenance dose is 375 mg daily.

IMPLEMENTATION CONSIDERATIONS:

—Obtain a complete health history, including hypersensitivity, other medications taken concurrently which may cause drug interactions, history of kidney or renal problems, skin problems, mouth sores, autoimmune diseases or positive ANA tests, blood dyscrasias, liver impairment, and possibility of pregnancy.

—There is a high incidence of cross-sensitivity in patients who are allergic to penicillin.

—The nurse's ability to teach, counsel and establish rapport with this patient will be important in obtaining compliance with dosage regimen and testing, as well as keeping appointments. Patients must be taught the things they should communicate to the practitioner, and to be realistic about the expectations of results.

—Only 30% of all patients benefit from this agent. Whether the patient will benefit or not cannot be determined for 3-6 months.

—If patient's ANA titers become positive, this does not mean the drug must be stopped. The patient must be very carefully observed for the development of any autoimmune problems.

—The most common side effects from penicillamine are skin eruptions. These can range from a mild form to a severe exfoliative or pemphigoid-like reaction. Most are mild and quickly clear up once the drug is stopped.

—About 10-25% of patients develop an alteration or decrease in the ability to taste. It usually occurs within the first 8 weeks of therapy and then disappears with no intervention.

WHAT THE PATIENT NEEDS TO KNOW:

—This medication is a very potent, slow-acting drug which may be helpful in some patients in actually halting joint destruction caused by arthritis. It does not help all patients, and a thorough trial will take 3-6 weeks before response to the drug can be determined.

—There are possibly serious toxic side effects that can occur with this drug. You must work closely with your health care providers in keeping appointments, getting laboratory work drawn, and reporting any new or troublesome symptoms which develop.

—You and your health care provider should watch especially for the development of cloudy, dark or bloody urine, skin rashes, sores in the mouth, purple blotches, bruising, or bleeding problems.

—You may experience a change in your sense of taste. This usually returns to normal after you have been on the medicine for a few months.

—Do not take any medications, including drugs which you can purchase over the counter, without the knowledge of your health care provider.

—This medicine should be taken on an empty stomach 1 hour before meals or 2 hours after meals. Do not take other medicines at the same time.

—Do not take this drug if there is any possibility that you are pregnant.

EVALUATION:

ADVERSE REACTIONS: High incidence (over 50%) of adverse reactions in patients on this drug. Many reactions are potentially fatal. *CNS:* alteration or decrease in ability to taste (10-25%), optic neuritis (reversible), pyridoxine-responsive motor neuropathy, tinnitus. *Dermatologic:* generalized pruritus, lupus erythematosus-like reactions, migratory polyarthralgias, mild skin eruptions to severe exfoliative or pemphigoid-like reactions, rashes (early or late in therapy), stomatitis, thyroiditis, urticaria. *Gastrointestinal:* altered taste perception, anorexia, cheilosis, colitis, diarrhea, epigastric pain, gingivostomatitis, glossitis, hepatic dysfunction, intrahepatic cholestasis, nausea, oral ulcerations, reactivation of previous peptic ulcer disease, stomatitis, vomiting. *Hematopoietic:* agranulocytosis, aplastic anemia, bone marrow depression, eosinophilia, hemolytic anemia, leukocytosis, leukopenia (2%), monocytosis, red cell aplasia, thrombocytopenia (4%). *Renal:* hematuria, nephrotic syndrome (if drug is not stopped), proteinuria. *Other:* alopecia, bronchial asthma, dermatomyositis, drug-induced autoimmune syndromes: systemic lupus erythematosus, myasthenia gravis, Goodpasture-like syndromes; hyperpyrexia, lichen planus, mammary hyperplasia, polymyositis.

PARAMETERS TO MONITOR: Obtain a complete history, physical examination and laboratory data prior to initiating therapy. These should include complete blood count, indices, platelets, liver and renal function studies. X-rays of joints should also be obtained so progression of disease can be followed.

This drug should be given according to a protocol established by the therapist. Both therapeutic effects and adverse effects should be checked. Each week the patient should be monitored for: (1) History: complaints of itching, alterations in taste, sore mouth, changes in color or character of urine, bruising, bleeding, fever. After 3-6 months of therapy ask about symptomatic improvement of joint pain or limitation of movement. (2) Physical: signs of itching, ulcers in mouth, limitation of joint movement, resolution of subcutaneous nodules. (3) Laboratory: WBC greater than 5000; urine protein and blood free, RBC with indices and platelets. Also obtain sedimentation rate, rheumatoid factor. Liver function studies should be monitored every 3 months for the first year, then every 6 months. ANA titers should be evaluated to detect autoimmune problems.

Carole Hill

ANALGESICS—NARCOTIC-AGONISTS

ACTION OF THE DRUG: (1) Narcotic analgesics are thought to inhibit painful stimuli in the substantia gelatinosa of the spinal cord, brain stem, reticular formation, thalamus and the limbic system. (2) Opiate receptors in each of these areas interact with neurotransmitters of the autonomic nervous system, producing alterations in reaction to painful stimuli. (3) The narcotic action of the drug is manifested by pain relief, sedation, euphoria, mental clouding, respiratory depression, miosis, decreased peristaltic motility, depression of the cough reflex, and orthostatic hypotension.

ASSESSMENT:

INDICATIONS: Narcotic analgesics are used for symptomatic treatment of moderate to severe pain of an acute nature. May be used to relieve pain from acute coronary, pulmonary, hepatic, renal or peripheral vascular origin; for preoperative medications; in severe diarrhea and cramping; detoxification of narcotic addictions (methadone only); persistent cough (codeine); dyspnea related to left ventricular failure or pulmonary edema, post-surgical trauma and labor and the chronic, severe, intractable pain of terminal illness. The use of narcotic analgesics on an ambulatory basis must be justified by the health care provider; particularly since neither the nurse practitioner nor the physician's assistant have legal sanction to prescribe these drugs. In primary care situations the synthetic narcotic analgesics are often used.

SUBJECTIVE: Assess the patient's perception of pain, elicit history of pain including its onset, location, quality and quantity, aggravating and relieving factors.

OBJECTIVE: Alterations in many of the following may be observed: tensed muscles; observable autonomic reactions such as alterations in respirations, blood pressure, pulse, perspiration, pupillary reaction; restlessness; affective responses (crying, moaning); changes in baseline blood pressure and pulse rates.

PLAN:

CONTRAINDICATIONS: These drugs should be withheld from persons with seizure disorders, severe respiratory depression, asthmatic conditions, chronic obstructive pulmonary disease, increased intracranial pressure, emphysema, kyphoscoliosis, undiagnosed acute abdominal conditions, colitis, Addison's disease, myxedema, hepatic cirrhosis, chronic cor pulmonale, and women of childbearing age.

WARNINGS: The main drawback of using the opioids particularly on a primary care basis, is the associated risk of physical and psychological dependence for the patient. Extreme caution should be exercised when prescribing opioids for the elderly, pregnant women, debilitated persons and patients in shock, in acute stages of alcohol intoxication, in children or newborns. Patients with reduced blood volume have been shown to be more susceptible to the hypotensive effects of the opioids. Exacerbation of urinary retention in patients with benign prostatic hypertrophy have also been reported. Finally, narcotic analgesics, as well as any CNS depressants are contraindicated in persons with increased intraocular pressure, head injury or loss of consciousness.

PRECAUTIONS: Once the narcotic analgesic is metabolized, the patient may experience an increased sensitivity to pain. The drugs should be administered two hours before delivery or surgery to prevent associated respiratory depression in the neonate or patient. Although there may be no significant respiratory depression of the mother when morphine is administered prior to delivery, the neonate may exhibit respiratory depression due to an immature blood-brain barrier. The opioids cross the placental barrier and are excreted in breast milk. Serum amylase levels may be elevated significantly by the opioids and their cogeners, while serum lactate levels may be significantly decreased.

Pain is often a key symptom necessary for diagnosing acute conditions. The use of narcotic analgesics can mask this symptom, obscuring progress of the disease, particularly in abdominal conditions. The use of narcotic analgesics is not recommended in these situations. The cough reflex is suppressed by these products and this may be a problem in patients with pulmonary problems. Caution should be used in elderly and debilitated patients. Increased ventricular response rate may be provoked in patients with supraventricular arrhythmias. These products may also aggravate preexisting convulsive states. Some products contain tartrazine which produces asthma-like symptoms in sensitive individuals. The analgesic effect of morphine is potentiated by methocarbamol and chlorpromazine. Use with cimetidine may lead to episodes of apnea, confusion, and muscle twitching.

IMPLEMENTATION:

DRUG INTERACTIONS: The CNS depressant effects may be potentiated by the concomitant use of other narcotic analgesics, alcohol, antianxiety agents, barbiturates, anesthetics, non-barbiturate sedative hypnotics, phenothiazines, sedative-hypnotics, skeletal muscle relaxants, and tricyclic antidepressants. (Respiratory depression, hypotension, profound sedation and coma may also result.) Narcotic use with furosemide or ethacrynic acid may aggravate or produce orthostatic hypotension. Death resulting from acute narcotic overdosage with the use of meperidine within 14 days of an MAO inhibitor have been reported. The effectiveness of diuretics given to patients with congestive heart failure may be decreased by narcotic analgesics. Concurrent use of opioids with anticholinergics may produce paralytic ileus. The phenothiazines enhance the sedative effects but antagonize the narcotic analgesics. The effects of poisonous venom from the scorpions *Centruroides sculpturatus ewing and C. gertschi stahnke* are potentiated by the narcotic analgesics. Narcotic analgesics should be withheld from patients stung by these insects. Morphine increased the anticoagulant activity of coumarin and other anticoagulants.

The blood concentration of methadone may be decreased sufficiently by concurrent administration of rifampin or phenytoin that withdrawal symptoms may be seen. Plasma amylase or lipase levels may be unreliable for 24 hours following administration of narcotics.

ADMINISTRATION AND DOSAGE: The amount of pain experienced by the patient will determine the dosage of narcotic and the route of administration. The route of administration for this category includes: oral, rectal, intramuscular, subcutaneous and intravenous routes.

Generally, the onset of action for opioids administered orally is between 15 and 30 minutes. The absorption of opioids in subcutaneous administration may vary considerably due to variation in drug solubility. The effect of a dose of opioids is considerably less after oral than after parenteral administration. Likewise, the time-effect curve is prolonged with the oral route, lengthening the duration of action.

The dosage of narcotic analgesic is dependent on the severity of pain experienced by the patient, his response to the pain and the medication, and the nature of the illness.

The narcotic analgesics are metabolized by the liver and excreted through the kidney in a conjugated form; 90% of the drug is excreted during the first 24 hours.

A summary of drugs which may be found in the narcotic analgesic category may be found in Table 4-4.

IMPLEMENTATION CONSIDERATIONS:

—Obtain a complete health history including the presence of or plans for pregnancy, or breast feeding, age (young or old); history or presence of brain injury; respiratory, prostatic, renal, gallbladder, liver, thyroid or Addison's disease. Also determine if patient has history of allergic or adverse reaction to morphine and its cogeners. If any of these conditions are present, withhold the drug.

—Assess the patient's pain tolerance and if narcotic analgesics are indicated, begin treatment with the smallest effective dose possible.

—Recheck patient at regular frequent intervals.

—Whenever possible, begin pain treatment with non-narcotic analgesics and supportive pain measures.

TABLE 4-4. NARCOTIC ANALGESIC DRUGS

Drug Name	Onset	Duration
Fentanyl	5-15 min	1-2 hours
Meperidine	10-15 min	2-5 hours
Codeine	15-30 min	4-6 hours
Hydromorphone	15-30 min	4-5 hours
Levorphanol	60 min	4-8 hours
Methadone	10-15 min	4-6 hours
Morphine	20 min	6-7 hours
Oxycodone	30 min	4-5 hours
Oxymorphone	5-10 min	4-5 hours

—Remember that pain relief is maximized if the drug is given prior to the patient's perception of intense pain.

—Assess dependency behaviors among patients. For example: inability to wean from drug; frequent requests for drug; and utilization of numerous health providers and/or health care facilities.

—Avoid use of alcohol or other CNS depressant medications concurrently.

—Be familiar with regulations concerning the use and dispensation of narcotic analgesics.

—Narcotic analgesics may depress the cough and sigh reflexes. In postoperative patients, particularly long-term smokers, atelectasis and pneumonia may result.

—The narcotic analgesics are classified according to abusive potential as mandated by the Controlled Substances Act of 1970.

WHAT THE PATIENT NEEDS TO KNOW:

—Take this medication as advised by your health provider. Do not alter dosages. Although this product has the potential for addiction, it is most effective when taken before you experience severe pain.

—If you are not experiencing substantial pain, use other methods for relieving pain whenever possible.

—Do not take any other medications without the knowledge of your health provider. This applies to cough, cold, or allergy products which you may purchase over the counter as well as to cholinergic drugs, antihistamines, allergy, cold remedies, barbiturates, non-narcotic analgesics, tricyclic antidepressants, other narcotics, or anticonvulsants which may be prescribed for you. If you drink alcoholic beverages it produces an additive effect with these drugs which could have an adverse effect upon you.

—Some patients experience side effects from this drug. Be certain to report to your health care provider any new or troublesome symptoms. Common side effects include suppression of cough reflex, dizziness, lightheadedness, nausea, drowsiness, sweating and flushing.

—Avoid operating heavy machinery, driving or performing tasks requiring alertness after taking this medication.

—Urinate frequently and monitor bowel habits daily. Report any problems with constipation to health care practitioner.

—Rise from lying or sitting positions slowly to minimize feelings of lightheadedness. Avoid standing in one position for long periods.

—During initial doses of opioids, lie down for short periods to avoid developing nausea.

—Take medications exactly as prescribed and work to taper doses down if taken over a long time. It may be important to jot down times when medication was last taken to prevent overdosing.

—Family members should alert the health care practitioner if any of the following develop in the patient: presence of shallow, slow respirations; shortness of breath; pupil constriction; deep sleep; vomiting; abdominal pain; palpitations; and skin rash.

—Keep this medication out of the reach of children and all others for whom it is not prescribed. Dispose of all extra medication when there is no longer any need for it. Do not keep it for another time.

EVALUATION:

ADVERSE REACTIONS: *Cardiovascular:* bradycardia, decreased blood pressure, palpitations. *CNS:* anorexia, biliary tract spasm, constipation, disorientation, dry mouth, euphoria, headache, paralytic ileus, stupor, syncope, transient hallucinations, vomiting. *Hypersensitivity:* itching, skin rash, sneezing, urticaria. *Respiratory:* respiratory distress, shortness of breath.

OVERDOSAGE: *Signs and symptoms:* Acute: profound respiratory depression, respiratory rate less than 12 breaths/minute; irregular shallow respirations, deep sleep, stupor or coma, miosis, cyanosis, gradually decreasing BP, oliguria, clammy skin, hypothermia. *Chronic:* constricted pupils, constipation, skin infections, mood changes, depressed level of consciousness, skin infections, itching, needle scars, abscesses. *Treatment:* Induce emesis and refer for gastric lavage and supportive treatment, especially to prevent respiratory depression. Artificial respiration and narcotic antagonists (preferably naloxone) are used to combat overdosage.

PARAMETERS TO MONITOR: The severity of pain experienced by the patient determines which parameters need to be monitored. The initial data base should include diagnostic tests necessary for establishing a diagnosis of the predisposing condition. In the initial visit, the health provider should check vital signs, respiratory, cardiovascular, and abdominal status. The patient taking narcotic analgesics to combat pain should be seen at least weekly and perhaps more frequently, depending on the nature of the condition. Regular visits to monitor pain relief and frequency of narcotic analgesic administration should be advised. Assess common side effects, adverse reactions, and drug's interference in activities of daily living or life style patterns. Acute or chronic toxicity signs and symptoms should be monitored as well as withdrawal symptoms including yawning, sneezing, tremors and diaphoresis. Specific signs and symptoms to be assessed include: respirations, blood pressure in lying, sitting and standing positions, breath, heart and abdominal sounds, bowel and urinary functions.

CODEINE

PRODUCTS (TRADE NAME):

Codeine Phosphate (Available in 15, 30, and 60 mg tablets; 15, 30 and 60 mg/ml tablet for parenteral dosage and 30 and 60 mg/ml Tubex.) **Codeine Sulfate** (Available in 15, 30, and 60 mg tablets, and 15, 30 and 60 mg tablets for parenteral use.)

DRUG SPECIFICS:

Codeine has two primary therapeutic effects: analgesic and antitussive. Codeine is relatively less strong than morphine and does not have the drug abuse potential of morphine. Codeine is often combined with non-narcotic analgesics, centrally acting muscle relaxants, and cough medications. Non-combination forms of codeine are classified as a Schedule II controlled substance.

ADMINISTRATION AND DOSAGE SPECIFICS:
   Pain Relief:
   Adults: 15 to 60 mg po, IM or SQ every 4 hours as needed.
   Infants and children: Give 0.5 mg/kg every 4 hours, po, IM or SQ as needed.
   Antitussive:
   Adults: Give 5-10 mg po 4-6 times a day.
   Infants and children: Give 0.175 0.25 mg/kg po 4-6 times a day.

FENTANYL

PRODUCTS (TRADE NAME):
   Sublimaze (Available in .05 mg/ml injection.)

DRUG SPECIFICS:
   Fentanyl is a very potent short-acting narcotic used for relief of moderate to severe pain and preoperative sedation and operative and postoperative analgesia. 0.1 mg dose of fentanyl is equivalent to 10 mg of morphine. Fentanyl may produce bradycardia. The respiratory depressant effects of fentanyl are particularly dangerous and mandate that the provider have resuscitative measures and narcotic antagonists present. Intravenous medication should be administered slowly to prevent muscle rigidity of the accessory muscles. Further narcotic administration in the postoperative state should be reduced to 1/4 or 1/2 the usual recommended dose. It is classified as a Schedule II controlled substance.

ADMINISTRATION AND DOSAGE SPECIFICS:
   Preoperative:
   Adults: Give O.05 mg to 0.1 mg IM.
   General Anesthetic Adjunct:
   Adult: At induction give O.05 mg to 0.1 mg IV; repeat at 2- 3- minute intervals. Maintenance O.025 mg IV or IM as needed.
   Postoperative:
   Adults: O.05 to 0.1 mg IM every 1 to 2 hours IM for pain.
   Children 2 to 12 years: 0.02 to O.03 mg/20 to 25 lb.

HYDROMORPHONE HYDROCHLORIDE

PRODUCTS (TRADE NAME):
   Dilaudid (Available in 1, 2, 3, and 4 mg tablets; 1, 2, 3 and 4 mg/ml injection;

and 5 mg rectal suppositories.) **Hydromorphone** (Available in 1, 2, 3, and 4 mg/ml Tubex injections.)

DRUG SPECIFICS:

A very potent synthetic compound which maximizes analgesic effects, and minimizes some of the common side effects of morphine, Dilaudid has 7-10 times the analgesic action of morphine. Dilaudid produces less sedation, nausea, vomiting and constipation than its counterpart. Incidence of respiratory depression is marked, requiring close observation. Use the lowest dose possible to prevent this adverse reaction. Rectal suppositories are particularly useful for producing a prolonged effect. This drug is contraindicated for use in patients with migraine headaches.

ADMINISTRATION AND DOSAGE SPECIFICS:

Severe Pain:

Adults: 2 to 4 mg every 4-6 hours IM or SQ; 2 mg po every 4-6 hours; 1 suppository twice a day.

Children: Safety and effectiveness in children have not been established.

LEVORPHANOL TARTRATE

PRODUCTS (TRADE NAME):

Levo-Dromoran (Available in 2 mg/ml injections and 2 mg tablets.)

DRUG SPECIFICS:

This preparation is used for the relief of moderate to severe pain. It is often used preoperatively to reduce apprehension and to prolong analgesia. It has a relatively longer onset of action than other narcotic agonist analgesics.

ADMINISTRATION AND DOSAGE SPECIFICS:

Adults: 2 to 3 mg po, or SQ. May also be given by slow IV injection.

MEPERIDINE HYDROCHLORIDE

PRODUCTS (TRADE NAME):

Demerol Hydrochloride (Available in 25, 50, 75 and 100 mg injectable solution; 50 and 100 mg tablets; and 50 mg/5 ml bottles of 16 fluid ounce syrup).

Meperidine Hydrochloride (Available in 25, 50, 75 and 100 ml injectable solution and Tubex.)

DRUG SPECIFICS:

This is a synthetic narcotic analgesic with less potency than morphine (60 to 80 mg doses are approximately equivalent to 10 mg morphine) for the relief of moderate to severe pain, preoperative sedation, postoperative analgesia, obstetrical anesthesia and IV administration for supportive anesthesia. The duration of action is slightly shorter than morphine (2-4 hours). The major metabolite, normeperidine, can accumulate and cause tremors and convulsions. When administering merperidine HCl with phenothiazine and many other tranquilizers, reduce the dosage of Demerol by 25 to 50% since they potentiate the action of Demerol. Each dose of syrup should be taken in one-half glass of water since, if undiluted, it can exert a topical anesthetic effect on mucous membranes. This is classified as a Schedule II controlled substance.

ADMINISTRATION AND DOSAGE SPECIFICS:

Pain Relief:

Adults: 50 mg to 150 mg every 3-4 hours IM, SQ or po.

Children: 0.5 to 0.8 mg/lb every 3-4 hours, IM, SQ or po.

METHADONE HYDROCHLORIDE

PRODUCTS (TRADE NAME):

Dolophine, Methadone HCl (Available in 10 mg/ml ampules; in 5 and 10 mg tablets; and 40 mg diskets of water soluble crystalline material, and 1 mg/ml oral solution.)

DRUG SPECIFICS:

Methadone hydrochloride is a synthetic narcotic analgesic used primarily in the detoxification, treatment and maintenance of heroin addicts or for severe pain. When the drug is used for severe pain, it is administered intramuscularly. The dosages are specific to the desired therapeutic effects. The drug is highly addictive. It is longer acting (36 to 48 hours) and less sedating and euphoric than morphine. When used for heroin addicts for more than 3 weeks methadone moves from a treatment phase to a maintenance phase. The side effects of this drug diminish after long-term use, except for constipation and sweating. Respiratory depression and arrest remain one of its serious adverse reactions. It is classified as a Schedule II controlled substance.

ADMINISTRATION AND DOSAGE SPECIFICS:

Pain Relief:

Adults: 2.5 to 10 mg every 3-4 hours IM, SQ or po.

Childen: Not recommended.

Narcotic Detoxification:

Adults: Specific to severity of withdrawal symptoms: 15 to 40 mg po once daily for 21 days with the dose gradually reduced every few days.

Narcotic Maintenance: 40 to 120 mg or higher once daily po.

MORPHINE

PRODUCTS (TRADE NAME)

Morphine Sulfate (Available in 10, 15, 30 mg soluble tablets; 3, 10, 15 mg/ml solution for IM or SQ injection; 2 to 15 mg/ml solution for injection, 15 and 30

mg oral tablets, 10 mg/5 ml oral solution.) **RMS Uniserts** (Available in 5, 10 and 20 mg rectal suppositories.) **Roxanol** (Available in 20 mg/ml oral solution.)
DRUG SPECIFICS:

Morphine is the primary narcotic analgesic used for relief of severe pain. It is the narcotic analgesic against which all others are compared. It also produces sedation and euphoria when pain is present. Traditionally, morphine sulfate is used for preoperative sedation and postoperative analgesia. Morphine is more effective against dull continuous pain than sharp spasmotic pain. Its use is contraindicated with papaverine for relief of biliary tract spasm. Oral use is not recommended because it is poorly absorbed in the GI tract. IV medication should be given slowly over a 4 to 5 minute period. Monitor carefully for respiratory depression. Protect drug from light and freezing. This is classified as a Schedule II controlled substance.

ADMINISTRATION AND DOSAGE SPECIFICS:

Severe Pain:

Adults: Administer 5 mg to 20 mg every 4 hours as indicated SQ or IM; IV administration doses range from 2 to 15 mg/5 ml injected over a 5 minute period. Oral administration 5 mg to 15 mg every 4 hours.

Children: Administer subcutaneously 0.1 to 0.2 mg/kg per dose. Use minimum effective dose; maximum dose not to exceed 15 mg.

OPIUM

PRODUCTS (TRADE NAME):

Pantopon (Available in 20 mg/ml (1/3 grain) hydrochloride of opium alkaloids in injectable solution.)

DRUG SPECIFICS:

Pantopon is a highly purified form of opium exhibiting the actions of both morphine and codeine without the side effects. Its use has been replaced primarily by morphine. It is equivalent to 15 mg of morphine. This is a controlled substance and requires a narcotic number to prescribe. It is recommended for relief of severe pain in place of morphine and as a preoperative medication.

ADMINISTRATION AND DOSAGE SPECIFICS:

Severe Pain:

Adults: 5 mg to 20 mg every 4-6 hours as needed. Administer only by IM or SQ injection.

OPIUM COMBINATIONS

PRODUCTS (TRADE NAME):

Brown Mixture (Available as 12% paregoric in glycyrrhiza fluid extract, antimony potassium tartrate and alcohol.) **Paregoric** (Available as liquid of opium tincture equivalent to 2 mg/5 ml morphine.) **Opium Tincture** (Available in tincture 10% opium in 18% alcohol.)

DRUG SPECIFICS:

Paregoric is equivalent to 0.04% morphine. Opium Tincture is equivalent to 1% morphine. Avoid confusing these two medications. Paregoric is used for cramps, diarrhea, and teething pain in infants (as a topical application to gums). Its use in teething and colic for infants is not preferred because of its opium derivatives. Its absorption in the gut is improved if administered in water, which turns it a milky color. It can be taken with food if GI upset occurs. These products are classified as Schedule II controlled substances.

ADMINISTRATION AND DOSAGE SPECIFICS:

Diarrhea:
Adults: Tinctures 0.6 ml to 1.5 ml po; Camphorated Tincture: 5-10 ml four times daily po.
Children: Camphorated tincture 0.25 to .5 ml/kg. Tincture of Opium: dosage not yet established.

OXYCODONE HCL AND HYDROCODONE BITARTRATE

PRODUCTS (TRADE NAME):

Dicodid (Available in 5 mg tablets of Hydrocodone.) **Oxycodone HCl** (Available in 5mg/5 ml solution.)
Combinations Products: **Anexsia-D** (Available in 7 mg hydrocodone bitartrate, 325 mg ASA and 30 mg caffeine tablets.) **Anadynos-DHC, Christodyne-DHC, Duradyne-DHC** (Available in 5 mg hydrocodone bitarbrate, 224 mg ASA and 32 mg caffeine tablets.) **Norcet** (Available in 7.5 mg hydrocodone bitartrate and 650 mg acetaminophen tablet.) **Percocet-5** (Available in 5 mg oxycodone and 325 mg acetaminophen tablet). **Percodan, Tylox** (Available in 4.5 mg oxycodone hydrochloride and 0.38 mg oxycodone terephthalate tablets.) **Vicodin** (Available in 5 mg oxycodone bitartrate and 500 mg acetaminophen tablet).

DRUG SPECIFICS:

These agents are similar in their action and structure but are not identical. They may be given alone but are usually combined with other analgesics. (See narcotic analgesic combinations for complete information). They are opium alkaloids and morphine-like in their actions. They are semisynthetic narcotics with primary actions that affect the central nervous system and organs composed of smooth muscle. Their principal actions are those of analgesia and sedation. They are similar to codeine in that they retain at least one half of their analgesic activity in the oral form. They are used to treat moderate to severe pain of an acute nature. They produce drug dependence similar to morphine. They should not be used in patients hypersensitive to any of the combination tablet ingredients. They potentiate the effects of other narcotics, sedatives or CNS depressants such as alcohol if taken concomitantly. The side effects are similar to those with morphine, most commonly dizziness, lightheadedness, sedation, or GI distress with nausea or vomiting.

Overdosage and treatment are as with morphine. Naloxone may be used as a narcotic antagonist.

ADMINISTRATION AND DOSAGE SPECIFICS:
Adults: 1-2 tablets every 4-6 hours as needed for pain.

Doreen C. Harper

ANALGESICS—NARCOTIC AGONIST-ANTAGONIST

ACTION OF THE DRUGS: These products are potent analgesic agents which act through the central nervous system, possibly at the limbic system. They also antagonize the action of narcotics. Thus, they may produce withdrawal symptoms in patients with narcotic dependency, but are also less likely to be abused than pure narcotic agonists.

ASSESSMENT:

INDICATIONS: These products are used primarily for the relief of moderate to severe pain. They are also used for preoperative analgesia and for mothers during active labor, in the parenteral form. These products may be preferred over narcotics for use in ambulatory patients because their potential for abuse is less.

SUBJECTIVE: Assess the patient's perception of pain. Elicit history of pain including its onset, location, quality and quantity, aggravating and relieving factors.

OBJECTIVE: Alterations in many of the following may be observed: Tensed muscles; observable autonomic reactions such as alterations in respirations, blood pressure, pulse, perspiration, pupillary reaction; restlessness; affective responses (crying, moaning); changes in baseline blood pressure and pulse rates.

PLAN:

CONTRAINDICATIONS: Do not give in the presence of hypersensitivity.

WARNINGS: Use with extreme caution in patients who are emotionally unstable and in those patients with a previous history of drug abuse. As both psychological and physiological dependence may occur, this drug should be given under careful supervision and prescribed only in limited amounts. Do not give to patients with head injury, as clinical course must be observed without the confusing effects of medication. Safe use in children and in women during pregnancy (other than during labor) has not been established. If patients receiving therapeutic doses demonstrate any evidence of hallucinations, confusion or disorientation, medication should be discontinued.

PRECAUTIONS: Because of the tendency for respiratory depression caused by these products, use cautiously in patients with respiratory impairment, especially asthma, obstructive respiratory conditions and cyanosis. Use cautiously in patients with impaired renal and hepatic function, since drug is metabolized in the liver and excreted by the kidneys. Greater side effects tend to occur in patients with extensive liver disease. In patients who have demonstrated dependence to narcotics, these products may produce withdrawal symptoms. These products have been known to provoke seizures, especially in those patients with known seizure disorders. These products may be used preoperatively, except in patients having biliary surgery, since spasm of the sphincter of Oddi may be produced by these products. These products also should not be used in patients with myocardial infarction, since they may produce increased work for the heart.

IMPLEMENTATION:

DRUG INTERACTIONS: Phenothiazines, droperidol and other tranquilizers may potentiate the action of butorphanol. Alcohol should be used cautiously with these products due to the potential for increased CNS depression. Concomitant administration of pancuronium with butorphanol may cause an increase in conjunctival changes. Narcotic analgesics, general anesthetics, sedatives, phenothiazines, other tranquilizers, hypnotics, or other CNS depressants may all potentiate nalbuphine.

ADMINISTRATION AND DOSAGE: All of these products are available in parenteral form, while only pentazocine is available orally. Preparations should not be given to children less than 12 years of age since there is little experience with these medications in this age group. Medications should be given by intramuscular injection, as subcutaneous injection may produce damage to tissues. When frequent injections are needed, each dose should be given in a different site, with rotation of sites important to avoid producing tissue injury.

IMPLEMENTATION CONSIDERATIONS:

—Obtain a complete health history, including the presence of respiratory, hepatic or kidney disease, pregnancy or breast-feeding, recent myocardial infarction, or evidence of previous emotional instability, drug dependency, or drug misuse.

—Assess the patient's pain tolerance, and if these products are indicated, begin treatment with the smallest effective dose possible.

—Recheck patient at regular and frequent intervals to assess action of medication.

—Assess dependency behaviors among patients. For example: inability to wean from drug; frequent requests for drug; and utilization of numerous health providers and/or health care facilities.

WHAT THE PATIENT NEEDS TO KNOW:

—Take this medication as advised by your health care provider. Do not alter dosages. Although this product has the potential for addiction, it is most effective when taken before you experience severe pain.

—As you begin to feel better, use other methods for relieving pain whenever possible.

—Some patients experience side effects from this drug. Be certain to report to your health care provider any new or troublesome symptoms. Common side effects include: feeling sleepy, nausea, vomiting, dizziness, blurred vision, sweating, feeling tired, dry mouth, headache, and confusion.

—Avoid operating heavy machinery, driving, or performing tasks requiring alertness after taking this medication.

—Keep this medication out of the reach of children and others for whom it is not prescribed.

EVALUATION:

ADVERSE REACTIONS: *Cardiovascular:* bradycardia, circulatory depression, hypertension, hypotension, palpitations, shock, tachycardia. *CNS:* agitation, alteration of mood, blurred vision, clammy feeling, confusion, crying, depression, diplopia, disorientation, dizziness, dysphoria, euphoria, faintness, floating feeling, hallucinations, headache, hostility, insomnia, lethargy, lightheadedness, nervousness, nystagmus, numbness, paresthesias, syncope, tingling, tinnitus, tremor, unreality, unusual dreams, vertigo. *Dermatologic:* burning, edema of face, hives, itching, nodules, pruritus, rash, severe sclerosis, soft tissue induration, sting on injection, ulceration, urticaria. *Gastrointestinal:* abdominal distress, anorexia, bitter taste, cramps, constipation, diarrhea, dry mouth, dyspepsia, nausea, vomiting. *Hematopoietic:* depression of white blood cells, transient eosinophilia. *Respiratory:* asthma, depression, dyspnea, shallow breathing. *Other:* alterations of uterine contractions during labor, blurred vision, flushing, speech difficulty, urinary retention or urgency, warmth.

OVERDOSAGE: *Signs and symptoms:* Sleepiness, dysphoria and respiratory depression are usually seen. *Treatment:* Give parenteral naloxone, and treat symptomatically.

PARAMETERS TO MONITOR: The severity of pain experienced by the patient determines which parameters the nurse needs to monitor. The initial data base should include diagnostic tests necessary for establishing a diagnosis of the predisposing condition. The patient taking this medication should be seen at least weekly, perhaps more frequently depending on the nature of the condition. Assess patient for therapeutic effect and for the presence of common side effects, dependency, and interference in activities of daily living or life style patterns. Specific signs and symptoms to assess include: respiratory rate, blood pressure in lying, sitting and standing positions, breath and heart sounds, and bowel and urinary functions.

BUTORPHANOL TARTRATE

PRODUCTS (TRADE NAME):
  Stadol (Available in 1 mg/ml and 2 mg/ml injections.)

DRUG SPECIFICS:
This product has 30 times the narcotic antagonist activity of pentazocine and 1/40 the activity of naloxone. Many patients taking this product experience sedation, and many also have nausea, and cold and clammy feelings. There are very few reported cases of overdosage, although this drug is a potent analgesic. Onset of action is 10 minutes following IM injection, and almost immediately following IV injection. Peak activity is 30 to 60 minutes following IM injection. The respiratory depression effect of 4 mg of butorphanol is similar to that of 10 mg of morphine, and is easily reversed with naloxone. Do not give to children under 18 years.

ADMINISTRATION AND DOSAGE SPECIFICS:
Intramuscular: 1 to 4 mg, repeated every 3 to 4 hours as necessary. Do not give doses greater than 4 mg.
Intravenous: 0.5 to 2 mg, repeated every 3 to 4 hours as necessary.

NALBUPHINE HCL

PRODUCTS (TRADE NAME):
Nubain (Available in 10 mg/ml injection.)

DRUG SPECIFICS:
This drug is a potent analgesic equivalent to morphine, and has about three times the potency of pentazocine on a milligram basis. This product does not increase pulmonary artery pressure or systemic vascular resistance, reactions produced by other agonist-antagonists. This medication frequently produces sedation in patients, and may also produce sweaty, clammy feelings, nausea, vomiting, dizziness and vertigo. Product tends to be more expensive than other agonist-antagonist products.

ADMINISTRATION AND DOSAGE SPECIFICS:
Adults: 10 mg SQ, IM or IV, repeated every 3 to 6 hours as necessary. Do not give more than 20 mg in one dose, or more than 160 mg/day.

PENTAZOCINE

PRODUCTS (TRADE NAME):
Talwin (Available in 30 mg/ml injections.) **Talwin NX** (Available in 50 mg scored tablets.)

DRUG SPECIFICS:
Pentazocine is a synthetic opioid with weak narcotic antagonist properties. It is used primarily for the relief of moderate to severe pain or as a preoperative or preanesthetic medication. Drug is not recommended for individuals with history of psychiatric illness or drug dependence. Although the drug is not technically classified as a narcotic, there have been documented instances of psychological and physical dependence. This product is not recommended for pain relief of acute my-

ocardial infarction with hypertension or left ventricular pressure since it is known to increase systemic and pulmonary pressure and peripheral resistance. It should be given intramuscularly whenever possible since subcutaneous injection may produce severe tissue damage at injection site. Do not mix this product with other chemicals during injection.

ADMINISTRATION AND DOSAGE SPECIFICS:

Pain relief in adults: Administer 30 mg IM, SQ or IV every 3-4 hours. Do not exceed doses of 60 mg IM or 30 mg IV. Total daily dose should not exceed 360 mg. Deep intramuscular injection rather than subcutaneous injection is strongly recommended due to tissue damage which can occur at injection sites. Constant rotation of sites is essential. For chronic administration, 50 mg oral tablets are recommended every 3-4 hours.

Labor: Administer a single 30 mg IM dose once contractions become regular. A 20 mg IV dose will also give adequate pain relief. This dose may be repeated at 2-3 hour intervals up to a maximum of three doses as needed.

Doreen C. Harper and Marilyn W. Edmunds

ANALGESICS—NARCOTIC COMBINATIONS

PRODUCTS (TRADE NAME):

See Table 4-5.

TABLE 4-5. CONTENTS OF NARCOTIC ANALGESIC COMBINATION PRODUCTS

Product	Narcotic	ASA	Acetaminophen	Phenacetin	Other Agents
Acetaminophen with Codeine					
Elixir	12 mg codeine		300 mg		
#2	15 mg codeine		300 mg		
#3	30 mg codeine		300 mg		
#4	60 mg codeine		300 mg		
A.P.C. with Codeine					
1/4 gr	15 mg codeine	227 mg		162 mg	32 mg caffeine
1/2 gr	30 mg codeine	227 mg		162 mg	32 mg caffeine
1 gr	60 mg codeine	227 mg		162 mg	32 mg caffeine
A.S.A. with Codeine Compound					
Cap #2	15 mg codeine	230 mg		150 mg	30 mg caffeine
Cap #3	30 mg codeine	230 mg		150 mg	30 mg caffeine
Cap #4	60 mg codeine	230 mg		150 mg	30 mg caffeine
Duradyne DHC Tablets	5 mg hydrocodone bitartrate	230 mg	150 mg		30 mg caffeine

TABLE 4-5. *(Continued)*

Product	Narcotic	ASA	Acetaminophen	Phenacetin	Other Agents
Empirin with Codeine					
No. 2	15 mg codeine	325 mg			
No. 3	30 mg codeine	325 mg			
No. 4	60 mg codeine	325 mg			
Fiorinal with Codeine					
No. 1	7.5 mg codeine	200 mg		130 mg	40 mg caffeine & 50 mg butalbital
No. 2	15 mg codeine	200 mg		130 mg	40 mg caffeine & 50 mg butalbital
No. 3	30 mg codeine	200 mg		130 mg	40 mg caffeine & mg butalbital
Papa-deine					
#3	30 mg codeine	210 mg		150 mg	30 mg caffeine
#4	60 mg codeine	210 mg		150 mg	30 mg caffeine
Percobarb	4.5 mg oxycodone & 0.38 oxycodone terephthalate	224 mg		160 mg	32 mg caffeine & 100 mg hexabarbital
Percocet-5 mg oxycodone tablets				325 mg	
Percodan	4.5 mg oxycodone & 0.38 mg oxycodone terephthalate	325 mg			
Proval #3	30 mg codeine		325 mg		
Tylenol with Codeine					
Elixir	12 mg codeine		120 mg		
Tab #1	7.5 mg codeine		300 mg		
Tab #2	15 mg codeine		300 mg		
Tab #3	30 mg codeine		300 mg		
Tab #4	60 mg codeine		300 mg		
Tylox	4.5 mg oxycodone & 0.38 mg oxycodone terephthalate		500 mg		
Vicodin	5 mg hydrocodone bitartrate		500 mg		

DRUG SPECIFICS:

Narcotic analgesic combination drugs are used as analgesics for moderate to severe pain. They produce their effects by working on the pain centers of the central nervous system. They are combinations of acetaminophen, aspirin, phenacetin and caffeine. They contain narcotics such as codeine, and oxycodone or hydrocodone.

Some agents also contain a form of barbiturate which is added for its sedative effects. Prescriptions must be written by physicians, as these drugs are controlled substances. These agents are used in moderate to severe pain of an acute origin, in postsurgical or postextractional pain. These drugs are addicting and should only be used for a brief period of time.

See individual drug sections regarding contraindications, dosage, adverse reactions, etc.

ADMINISTRATION AND DOSAGE:

Generally 1 to 2 tablets or capsules are taken every 4 to 6 hours for acute pain. Not recommended for children.

Carole Hill

ANALGESICS—NONNARCOTIC

ACTION OF THE DRUGS: These products act centrally, producing analgesia. Propoxyphene and ethoheptazine are chemically related to narcotic analgesics but are not comparable in analgesic potency or abuse potential. Methotrimeprazine has potent CNS depressant activity and is a phenothiazine derivative.

ASSESSMENT:

INDICATIONS: These products are used primarily for the relief of mild to moderate pain. They are also used in combination with other products for pain alone or when pain and fever are both present.

SUBJECTIVE: Assess the patient's perception of pain. Elicit history of pain, including its onset, location, quality and quantity and aggravating and relieving factors.

OBJECTIVE: Alterations in many of the following may be observed: tensed muscles, observable autonomic reactions such as alterations in respirations, blood pressure, pulse, perspiration and pupillary reaction, restlessness, affective responses (crying, moaning), changes in baseline blood pressure and pulse rates.

PLAN:

CONTRAINDICATIONS: Do not give in the presence of hypersensitivity to the products involved, including phenothiazines. For methotrimeprazine, do not give concurrently with antihypertensive agents, including MAO inhibitors, or in the presence of CNS depressant overdosage, comatose states, myocardial infarction, renal or hepatic disease or severe hypotension. These products are usually not given to children under 12 years of age.

WARNINGS: Following administration of methotrimeprazine, orthostatic hypotension, fainting, dizziness or sedation may occur. Patients should be carefully supervised while taking this product, especially for the first 6 hours after the initial dose. Depression of spermatogenesis and a possible antifertility effect has been suggested in animals, and methotrimeprazine should be used cautiously in men and in women of childbearing years. Propoxyphene products in overdoses, especially when used with other CNS depressants, are a major cause of drug-related deaths. Fatalities from overdosage often occur within the first hour. Thus, careful monitoring of patients is required, with the restriction of medication in patients who are emotionally unstable, have abused drugs in the past or who may be considered unreliable in medication dosage. When propoxyphene products are taken in high doses over a long time, dependence may develop. Prescribe with the same degree of caution as used with narcotics. Safety for use during pregnancy, lactation and for children has not been established.

PRECAUTIONS: Methotrimeprazine should not be administered for longer than 30 days unless narcotics are contraindicated and periodic blood counts and liver function studies can be carried out. Elderly and debilitated patients may be more sensitive to the effects of methotrimeprazine, and dosage should be decreased and vital signs closely monitored during initiation of therapy. Tasks requiring alertness should not be performed while patient is on this drug, since medication may increase response time.

IMPLEMENTATION:

DRUG INTERACTIONS: These medications have CNS depressant effects additive with those of other depressants, including alcohol. Concomitant administration of carbamazepine and propoxyphene may increase carbamazepine levels and produce fatigue, ataxia, nausea, dizziness and headaches. Cigarette smoke may induce liver enzymes responsible for metabolizing propoxyphene and thus, dosages may be subtherapeutic in smokers. Methotrimeprazine should not be used with antihypertensive drugs, especially MAO inhibitors. Use methotrimeprazine cautiously with atropine, scopolamine and succinylcholine. Methotrimeprazine has additive effects with narcotics, barbiturates, general anesthetics, meprobamate, reserpine and aspirin.

ADMINISTRATION AND DOSAGE: All of the propoxyphene products are available in oral form, while methotrimeprazine comes as an injection. Many propoxyphene products are available in combination with other drugs. There is no conclusive evidence that propoxyphene combined with other analgesics is more effective than propoxyphene or other analgesics alone.

IMPLEMENTATION CONSIDERATIONS:

—Obtain a complete health history, including the presence of respiratory or hepatic disease, pregnancy or breast-feeding, or evidence of previous emotional instability, drug dependency or drug misuse.

—Assess the patient's pain tolerance and if these products are indicated, begin treatment with the smallest effective dose possible.

—Recheck patient at regular and frequent intervals to assess action of medication.

—Assess dependency behaviors among patients. For example: inability to wean from drug, frequent requests for drug, and use of numerous health care providers and/or health care facilities.

WHAT THE PATIENT NEEDS TO KNOW:
—Take this medication as advised by your health care provider. Do not alter dosages. Although this product has the potential for addiction, it is most effective when taken before you experience severe pain.
—As you begin to feel better, use other methods for relieving pain whenever possible.
—Some patients experience side effects from this drug. Be certain to report to your health care provider any new or troublesome symptoms. Common side effects include dizziness, sedation, nausea and vomiting. You may also note a feeling of lightheadedness, especially when arising from a lying position. Move slowly in order to decrease this feeling.
—Avoid operating heavy machinery, driving or performing tasks requiring alertness after taking this medication.
—Keep this medication out of the reach of children and all others for whom it is not prescribed.

EVALUATION:

ADVERSE REACTIONS: *Cardiovascular:* orthostatic hypotension. *CNS:* disorientation, dizziness, euphoria, headache, lightheadedness, minor visual disturbances, sedation, slurring of speech, weakness. *Dermatologic:* rashes. *Gastrointestinal:* abdominal pain, constipation, dry mouth, epigastric distress, jaundice, liver dysfunction, nausea, vomiting. *Genitourinary:* difficulty urinating, uterine inertia. *Hematopoietic:* agranulocytosis. *Other:* chills, nasal congestion, pain at injection site. Other reactions for methotrimeprazine may be noted by consulting section on phenothiazines.

OVERDOSAGE: *Signs and symptoms:* Sedation is the usual problem, although patient may have respiratory depression and be comatose. Cyanosis and hypoxia are also present due to decreased ventilatory rate. Hypotension and deterioration of cardiac performance may follow. *Treatment:* Refer for management of CNS effects and resuscitative measures. Give naloxone to counteract effect of medication.

PARAMETERS TO MONITOR: The severity of pain experienced by the patient determines which parameters the nurse needs to monitor. The initial data base should include diagnostic tests necessary for establishing a diagnosis of the predisposing condition. The patient taking this medication should be seen at least weekly, and perhaps more frequently depending on the nature of the condition. Assess for therapeutic effect. Assess patient for presence of common side effects, dependency and interference with activities of daily living or life style patterns. Specific signs and symptoms to assess include respiratory rate, blood pressure in lying, sitting and standing positions, breath and heart sounds and bowel and urinary functions.

METHOTRIMEPRAZINE

PRODUCTS (TRADE NAME):
Levoprone (Available in 20 mg/ml injection.)
DRUG SPECIFICS:
This product is a phenothiazine derivative with potent CNS depressant activity. It reduces motor activity and produces sedation and tranquilization. It also raises the pain threshold and produces amnesia. It is often used in obstetric analgesia, where it is important to avoid respiratory depression. It should be used with the same precautions as other phenothiazine products. It should be administered by deep intramuscular injection into large muscles, with rotation of injection sites. Do not give intravenously. It may be mixed in the same syringe with atropine sulfate or scopolamine but no other drugs.
ADMINISTRATION AND DOSAGE SPECIFICS:
Pain: 10 to 20 mg deep IM every 4-6 hours as required. Although up to 40 mg may be given, start with 10 mg doses until individual patient response is assessed. Reduce dosage in elderly patients to 5 mg.
Obstetric analgesia: 15 to 20 mg IM initially, with subsequent adjustment of doses as needed.
Preanesthesia medication: 2 to 20 mg IM 45 minutes to 3 hours prior to surgery. The usual dose is 10 mg, with 20 mg given if greater sedation is desired. Small doses of atropine sulfate or scopolamine may be given at the same time.
Postoperative analgesia: 2.5 to 7.5 mg IM may be given immediately, while effects from general anesthesia are still present. Additional doses may then be given in 4 to 6 hours.

PROPOXYPHENE HCL

PRODUCTS (TRADE NAME):
Darvon (Available in 32 mg and 65 mg capsules/pulvules.) **Dolene, Pargesic 65, SK-65** (Available in 65 mg capsules.) **SK-65 APAP, Wygesic** (Available in 65 mg tablets.) **Propoxyphene HCl** (Available in 32 mg and 65 mg capsules.)
DRUG SPECIFICS:
Propoxyphene HCl is a centrally acting opioid, structurally related to methadone. It is used primarily as a weak analgesic but contains physical and psychological addictive properties. To improve its overall effect, the drug is often combined with non-narcotic analgesics. Propoxyphene produces respiratory and CNS depressant effects similar to those produced by the narcotic analgesics. It is classified as a Schedule IV controlled substance.
ADMINISTRATION AND DOSAGE SPECIFICS:
Prolonged pain relief:

Adults: 65 to 100 mg orally every 4 hours as needed.
Children: No recommended dose established at this time.

PROPOXYPHENE HCL COMPOUNDS

PRODUCTS (TRADE NAME):

Bexophene, Darvon Compound-65, Dolene Compound-65, Elder 65 Compound, Margesic Compound No. 65, Pargesic Compound 65, Proxagesic Compound-65, SK-65 Compound (Available in 65 mg capsules with 227 mg aspirin, 162 mg phenacetin and 32.4 mg caffeine.) **Darvon Compound** (Available in 32 mg capsules with 227 mg aspirin, 162 mg phenacetin and 32.4 mg caffeine.) **Darvon with A.S.A.** (Available in 65 mg capsules with 325 mg aspirin.)

DRUG SPECIFICS:

These combination products may or may not produce a greater analgesic effect than the same analgesic products administered alone.

ADMINISTRATION AND DOSAGE SPECIFICS:

Pain: 65 mg po every 4 hours as needed. Do not exceed 390 mg/day.

PROPOXYPHENE NAPSYLATE

PRODUCTS (TRADE NAME):

Darvon-N (Available in 100 mg tablets and 10 mg/ml oral suspension.)

DRUG SPECIFICS:

This preparation differs only slightly from propoxyphene HCl in that it can be produced as a stable liquid and tablet. A dose of 100 mg propoxyphene napsylate is required to equal 65 mg of propoxyphene HCl due to differences in molecular weight.

ADMINISTRATION AND DOSAGE SPECIFICS:

Give 100 mg every 4 hours as needed for pain. Do not exceed 600 mg/day.

PROPOXYPHENE NAPSYLATE COMBINATIONS

PRODUCTS (TRADE NAME):

Darvocet-N 50 (Available in 50 mg tablets with 325 mg acetaminophen.) **Darvocet-N 100** (Available in 100 mg tablets with 650 mg acetaminophen.) **Darvon w/A.S.A.** (Available in 65 mg capsules with 325 mg aspirin.) **Darvon-N w/A.S.A.**

(Available in 100 mg tablets with 325 mg aspirin.)

DRUG SPECIFICS:

These combination products may or may not be more effective in producing analgesia than the analgesic products administered alone.

ADMINISTRATION AND DOSAGE SPECIFICS:

Pain: 100 mg every 4 hours as needed. Do not exceed 600 mg/day.

Doreen C. Harper and Marilyn W. Edmunds

ANALGESICS—NONNARCOTIC COMBINATIONS

PRODUCTS (TRADE NAMES):

(See Table 4-6 on page 422.)

DRUG SPECIFICS:

Non-narcotic analgesics are combination drugs used mainly for their analgesic properties. They represent combinations of acetaminophen, aspirin, caffeine, phenacetin, antacids, ethoheptazine, or propoxyphene in different combinations. (Refer to individual Product listings for detailed information on their normal usage, contraindications, precautions, drug interactions, and adverse reactions).

Caffeine is a plant extract, with mild cerebral, respiratory and cardiac stimulant effects, as well as some diuretic activity. It has no analgesic property, but is useful in vascular headaches.

Phenacetin is an analgesic from the same family as acetaminophen, being a *p*-aminophenol derivative with similar actions and side effects. There have been some hepatic and renal problems with this drug, and many companies have voluntarily withdrawn this preparation from their combination products.

These combination products are used for mild to moderate pain. If an antipyretic effect is sought, a non-combination agent should be prescribed. Do not give in the presence of hypersensitivity to these agents.

For each combination drug, check the individual Product listings for implementation, and evaluation material.

ADMINISTRATION AND DOSAGE: Usual adult dosage is one to two tablets or capsules every 4-6 hours for pain.

Carole Hill

ANALGESICS—NON-STEROIDAL ANTI-INFLAMMATORY DRUGS (NSAIDS)

ACTION OF THE DRUG: Non-steroidal anti-inflammatory drugs (NSAIDS) are a group of drugs with analgesic, anti-inflammatory and antipyretic effects that are

TABLE 4-6. NONNARCOTIC—ANALGESIC COMBINATIONS

Product	Ingredients and Their Amounts				
	Aspirin	Acetaminophen	Phenacetin	Caffeine	Other
A.S.A. Compound	227 mg		160 mg	32.5 mg	
Anacin tablets	400 mg			32 mg	
Anacin-3		500 mg		32 mg	
Anacin Arthritis Formula	300 mg				20 mg alum OH; 60 mg Mg OH
Bromo Seltzer		325 mg		32 mg	sodium bicarb, citric acid and 2.8 gm na citrate
Capron	227 mg	65 mg		32 mg	
Darvocet-N 50		325 mg			50 mg propoxyphene napsylate
Darvocet-N 100		650 mg			100 mg propoxyphene napsylate
Darvon w/A.S.A.	325 mg				100 mg propoxyphene naphsylate
Dolor	230 mg	230 mg		30 mg	100 mg calcium carbon and 50 mg dry milk
Empirin Compound	227 mg			32 mg	
Excedrin				65 mg	
Excedrin PM		500 mg			25 mg pyrilamine maleate
Fiorinal	200 mg			40 mg	50 mg butalbital
Gemnisyn	325 mg	325 mg			
P-A-C Compound	227 mg		163 mg	32 mg	
Pargesic Compound	227 mg			32 mg	65 mg propoxyphene hydrochloride
Propoxyphene HCl Compound	227 mg			32.4 mg	12.5 mg propoxyphene hydrochloride
S-A-C Tablets		150 mg		30 mg	230 mg salicylamide
Sal-Fayne	227 mg		162 mg	32 mg	
Trigesic	230 mg	125 mg		30 mg	
Trilisate	500-750 mg				293-440 mg choline trisalicylate, 362-546 mg magnesium trisalicylate
Vanquish	227 mg	149 mg		33 mg	25 mg aluminum hydroxide gel and 50 mg magnesium hydroxide

used in the treatment of rheumatic diseases, degenerative joint disease, osteoarthritis, and acute musculoskeletal problems. The exact mode of action of NSAIDS is not known though it is felt that they work through inhibition of the synthesis of prostaglandins. These agents are also associated with inhibition of platelet aggregation, but this effect appears to be dose-related. Ibuprofen has also been approved for use in dysmenorrhea because of its prostaglandin inhibition.

ASSESSMENT:

INDICATIONS: When history and physical have documented a disease process that significantly affects a person's normal pattern of living due to changes in mobility and/or pain, the use of NSAIDS is indicated. They are specifically indicated in the treatment of moderate to severe musculoskeletal pain, rheumatoid arthritis, osteoarthritis, ankylosing spondylitis, degenerative joint disease, and acute or chronic problems involving the bursa, or tendons of the body.

SUBJECTIVE: The patient complains of musculoskeletal pain or tenderness of involved areas, inflammation, stiffness, and an alteration in normal activities of life. The onset may be insidious, with the patient showing only tiredness; sudden; or following a change in activity or minor trauma, depending on the particular type of arthritic problem. Specific history of onset, duration, and location are important in determining which arthritic condition exists.

OBJECTIVE: Evaluate for signs of inflammation: tenderness, erythema, increased warmth, swelling. Joint stiffness, decreased range of motion, or crepitus may also be present. Distribution, location, as well as pattern (i.e. monoarticular, asymmetrical, symmetrical) and number of involved joints must be determined. Radiographic studies may show changes of degeneration or destruction within the joints, synovial thickening, and/or spur formation. Laboratory findings from examination of synovial fluid help establish a specific diagnosis and document the indications for these therapeutic agents.

PLAN:

CONTRAINDICATIONS: NSAIDS are not to be used in patients who have shown sensitivity to the specific drug in the past. They are also not to be used in patients displaying hypersensitivity to aspirin, as all of the specific agents are closely related to aspirin and there is potential for cross-sensitivity. Do not give alternate agents in this category to patients who have manifested symptoms of bronchospasm, asthma, rhinitis, urticaria, nasal polyps, or angioedema following use of any agents within this group.

WARNINGS: These drugs should be used with caution and under close observation in patients prone to or with previous history of upper gastrointestinal diseases. Other methods of treatment should be attempted in patients with active peptic ulcer disease. The safe use and efficacy of most of these agents (except aspirin and tolmetin sodium) for children under 14 years of age has not been established. The safety and efficacy has also not been established in pregnancy because of the relationship of prostaglandins to uterine activity. Some of these products are known to be excreted in breast milk, and safety has not been established for use in breast-feeding women.

PRECAUTIONS: These agents should be used with caution in patients with impaired renal function or history of upper GI problems. Because of the actions on platelets, patients should be carefully monitored if shown to have bleeding time abnormalities or be on anticoagulant therapy.

IMPLEMENTATION:

DRUG INTERACTIONS: Since the agents under this class are structurally somewhat different, their specific drug interactions vary; therefore check specific generic agents for drug interactions which should be monitored.

ADMINISTRATION AND DOSAGE: NSAIDS are first line drugs in the treatment and control of the various forms of arthritis and in many of the uni-articular inflammatory processes. The chemical structure of these agents varies somewhat, and therefore failure to symptomatically improve with the use of one agents does not mean there will be no improvement with a second agent. Salicylates are the most commonly used anti-inflammatory agents. Because of the low cost, efficacy, and low toxicity, all the other NSAIDS are compared to salicylates in terms of their therapeutic benefits and side effects. (See Table 4-7 and specific product information.)

The full therapeutic effect of the agents may not be seen in many chronic problems for 1-2 weeks, and therefore this time period should be considered before changing therapy.

IMPLEMENTATION CONSIDERATIONS:

—Obtain a complete health history, including presence of sensitivity to aspirin or any of the products within this group, gastrointestinal problems, renal dysfunction, history of asthma or allergic respiratory problems, anticoagulant therapy, bleeding problems, other drugs taken concurrently which may cause drug interactions, and possibility of pregnancy or breast-feeding.

—Since the chemical structure of these agents differ, the specific agent should be checked before prescribing the drug.

—Some agents should be used only for short-term therapy because of their toxic side effects. The duration of therapy should be considered when selecting a particular agent for chronic arthritic problems.

—In uniarticular problems, be certain that any infective process is ruled out. NSAIDS may relieve symptoms but not affect the invasive agent, allowing more extensive damage to take place if used inappropriately.

WHAT THE PATIENT NEEDS TO KNOW:

—Take these medications exactly as ordered. Do not increase or decrease dosages without changes being recommended by your health care provider. Evaluation of the action of these drugs will require returning to your health care provider periodically for checkups.

—Gastrointestinal upset is the most common complication and should be reported to the health care provider. Bowel movements should also be observed for the presence of blood or tarry stools which result from excessive irritation.

—Take these medications with meals or with milk in order to minimize gastric irritation. Use of an antacid with the medicine may also be helpful.

—Patients who have chronic arthritic problems may need to take medicine for 1 to 2 weeks before noting any improvement. Medicine should be taken regularly during this time in order to evaluate fairly whether it will be effective or not.

—Keeping a certain level of medicine within the body at all times is important in maintaining the anti-inflammatory effect of the drug. If you do not take your medicine regularly, the drug level may be too low to be effective.

—If a dose is missed, take it as soon as possible after the missed dose was due. If the next dose is due shortly do not take the missed dose, but instead resume the regular dosage schedule. Do not take an increased amount of medicine to make up for a missed dose.

—Blurred vision, or any other eye problems, ringing in the ears, and rashes should immediately be reported to the health provider.

—Some patients experience drowsiness, lightheadedness, or decreased alertness from this medicine. Do not drive or perform tasks requiring alertness until you evaluate your reaction to this drug.

—Do not use two anti-inflammatory (NSAIDS) at the same time.

EVALUATION:

ADVERSE REACTIONS: (See individual product listings for specifics.) *Cardiovascular:* asthma, congestive failure, fluid retention, hypertension, pulmonary edema. *CNS:* confusion or inability to concentrate, depression, dizziness, blurred or decreased vision, corneal or ophthalmologic problems (varies with agents), lightheadedness, malaise, somnolence, tinnitus, vertigo. *Dermatologic:* erythema multiforme, pruritus, rash, skin irritation or rash related to sun exposure, Stevens-Johnson syndrome. *Gastrointestinal:* abdominal pain, anorexia, bloating, constipation, diarrhea, dyspepsia, flatulence, GI bleeding (upper or lower), heartburn, indigestion, nausea, vomiting, *Genitourinary:* hematuria (with some agents or worsened renal failure.) *Hematopoietic:* agranulocytosis, anemia, aplastic anemia, increased prothrombin time, hemolytic anemia, leukopenia, thrombocytopenia.

OVERDOSAGE: *Signs and symptoms:* See any of the adverse effects, especially tinnitus, gastrointestinal symptoms and somnolence. *Treatment:* Induce emesis or refer for gastric lavage followed by activated charcoal. Treat shock symptomatically. Dialysis is of little use with most of these agents. Contact the poison control center for information regarding specific drugs.

PARAMETERS TO MONITOR: Monitor therapeutic effects: reduction of symptoms allowing patient to return to previous activities without pain. Patient should be evaluated 3-4 weeks after starting medication to look for first signs of improvement. If there is no reduction in symptoms, or if patient develops side effects, an alternate agent in this same group can be tried.

Patients should be monitored for adverse effects, particularly for GI and CNS symptoms. Periodic laboratory analysis should also be carried out while patient is on this medicine. Stool specimens should be obtained to check for occult bleeding;

TABLE 4-7. COMPARATIVE DOSAGE REGIMEN FOR NON-STEROIDAL ANTI-INFLAMMATORY DRUGS*

Drug	Adult Dosage	Dosage Regimen
Fenamates		
Meclofenamate sodium	200-400 mg** 400 + mg not approved	50-100 mg every 6-8 hours
Mefenamic acid	1000 mg	500 mg then 250 mg every 6 hours
Indole derivatives		
Indomethacin	50-200 mg/day**	25-50 mg every 6, 8, or 12 hours
Sulindac	300 mg (acute)	150 mg every 12 hours
	400 mg (chronic)	200 mg every 12 hours
Tolmetin sodium	800-2000 mg***	200-500 mg every 6 hours
Oxicams		
Piroxicam	10-20 mg	20 mg every 24 hours
Propionic acid derivatives		
Ibuprofen	1200-1600 mg 2000 + mg anti-inflammatory	300-600 mg every 6 hours
Fenoprofen	1200-2400 mg	200-600 mg every 6 hours
Naproxen	500-750 mg	250-375 mg every 12 hours
Pyrazoles and derivatives		
Phenylbutazone	100-600 mg	100 to 600 mg
Oxyphenbutazone	100-400 mg	400 mg then 100 mg every 6 hours for one week
Salicylates		
Aspirin	3-6 Gm po***	2, 3 or 4 tablets every 4 hours

*See non-narcotic analgesic section for other drugs in this category. None of the products have established dosages for children (although 65 mg/kg/day in divided doses is usually given) with the following exceptions:

**Not recommended for children.

***Children: Tolmetin Sodium: Give 15-30 mg/kg in divided doses every 6-8 hours. More than 30 mg/kg/day not approved. Aspirin: 65 mg/kg/day in divided doses. Sulindac is being studied for pediatric use and may soon be approved for use.

CBCs with indices to evaluate for anemia , hematologic problems, or reduced ability to fight infection. These evaluations should be performed at least biannually. In patients who have underlying cardiovascular disease, watch for development of congestive heart failure.

FENEMATES:
MECLOFENAMATE SODIUM

PRODUCTS (TRADE NAME):
　Meclomen (Available in 50, 100 mg tablets.)
DRUG SPECIFICS :
　One of the fenemate derivatives, this drug has the ability to block the action of prostaglandins as well as inhibit their synthesis, as opposed to the other NSAIDS that only inhibit prostaglandin synthesis.

　This drug is recommended for the treatment of acute and chronic rheumatoid and osteoarthritis, but not for other acute musculoskeletal problems. It has less tinnitus-like side effects than aspirin but significantly more diarrhea problems (10 to 33% of all patients) and nausea (10%), so it is not recommended as one of the initial NSAIDS to use in the treatment of these diseases. Other side effects that are seen in less than 10% of the patients include headaches, dizziness and skin rashes. Patients should be told to notify their health care provider if medication causes nausea, vomiting, abdominal pain or diarrhea. This drug may be taken with antacids, which may reduce some of the symptoms.

　It is not recommended in the treatment of pregnant or breast-feeding women, or in the treatment of children under 14 years of age.

　Drug Interaction: Meclofenamate Sodium increases the prothrombin time in patients receiving anticoagulants.

　　ADMINISTRATION AND DOSAGE SPECIFICS:
　Adult: 200-400 mg po daily in 3-4 divided doses. Maximum dose 400 mg/day.

　Titrate dosage to achieve symptomatic relief with smallest possible dosage. Results should be apparent in 1-2 weeks. Administer with milk, meals or antacids.

MEFENAMIC ACID

PRODUCTS (TRADE NAME):
　Ponstel (Available in 250 mg tablets.)
DRUG SPECIFICS:
　A fenemate derivative, mefenamic acid is recommended for the treatment of dysmenorrhea. (See section on gynecologic drugs.) For acute pain in both adults and children (7 to 14 years of age), give 500 mg initially then 250 mg q 6 hours for short-term therapy—no greater than 1 week.

INDOLE DERIVATIVE:
INDOMETHACIN

PRODUCTS (TRADE NAME):

Indocin (Available in 25 and 50 mg capsules and 75 mg sustained-release capsule, soon to be released in suppository form.)

DRUG SPECIFICS :

Indomethacin is a potent prostaglandin synthesis inhibitor with significant toxic side effects. Therefore,this drug should be used in short-course therapy for acute musculoskeletal disorders such as tendonitis, bursitis, trauma, or other inflammatory arthropathies such as acute gouty arthritis, Reiter's syndrome, or psoriatic arthritis. It should only be used in chronic therapy for patients with moderate to severe rheumatoid arthritis who do not respond to other less toxic NSAIDS or other forms of therapy. There is an increased possibility of adverse reactions when used in the elderly.

Use with salicylates is not recommended. Less than 10% of patients on this medication experience gastrointestinal side effects such as nausea, dyspepsia, or changes in bowel habits. Over 10% of the patients experience headache and slightly less experience vertigo, somnolence, depression or fatigue. These symptoms do appear to be dose-related, though many experience the side effects after 1 or 2 doses. Patients should be warned against these side effects and initial doses should be taken at home and when tasks requiring alertness are not required.

Other adverse reactions specific to this agent include: *Cardiovascular:* edema, hypertension. *Dermatologic:* ecchymosis, exfoliative dermatitis, petechiae, pruritus. *EENT:* blurred vision, corneal deposits, hearing loss, retinal disturbances, tinnitus. *Genitourinary:* hematuria, renal failure. *Hematopoietic:* agranulocytosis, aplastic anemia, hemolytic anemia, leukopenia, thrombocytopenic purpura.

Drug Interactions: Indomethacin increases anticoagulant effects. In combination with corticosteroids it increases the chances of gastrointestinal ulcer formation. It decreases the diuretic and antihypertensive effects of furosemide. Probenecid increases the effect of indomethacin by decreasing kidney excretion and can therefore lead to toxic side effects at lower doses. This agent also leads to increased blood sulfonamide levels in combination with those drugs. Indomethacin in large doses increases the serum level of lithium and can lead to toxic side effects in psychiatric patients on this drug.

ADMINISTRATION AND DOSAGE SPECIFICS:

Acute gouty arthritis: Use 50 mg three times daily for 3-5 days, then reduce to 25 mg three times daily. Gradually wean patient off medication as soon as possible.

Recurrent gout: Use 25 mg 2 times daily in patients who do not tolerate colchicine.

Moderate to severe rheumatoid or osteoarthritis or severe ankylosing spondylitis: Use 25 mg two to three times daily. If this is tolerated, increase dose by 25 or 50 mg/day on a weekly basis, monitoring symptoms until satisfactory response or total daily dose of 150 mg to 200 mg is reached. Patients with severe morning stiffness may respond to 50 to 100 mg doses at night or bedtime and other NSAIDS during the day.

Acute shoulder: 75 to 150 mg in 3 to 4 divided doses no longer than 7—14 days. Sustained release 75 mg q 12 hours.

INDOLE DERIVATIVE: SULINDAC

PRODUCTS (TRADE NAME):
   Clinoril (Available in 150 and 200 mg tablets.)
DRUG SPECIFICS:
   Sulindac is used in acute or prolonged therapy of patients with osteoarthritis, rheumatoid arthritis, ankylosing spondylitis, acute subacromial bursitis, or supraspinatus tendonitis (acute painful shoulder), and acute gouty arthritis. This drug is excreted by the kidneys, and patients with renal failure should be carefully monitored. It is not recommended for use in pregnant or breast-feeding women. Studies are presently underway evaluating its use in children.
   The most common adverse reactions (greater than 1%) are: *CNS:* dizziness, headache, nervousness, tinnitus. *Dermatologic:* rashes. *Gastrointestinal:* constipation, dyspepsia, nausea, pain. Reactions are less common than similar side effects with the use of indomethacin.
   Drug interactions: Sulindac can potentiate the anticoagulant effect of warfarin products by increasing the prothrombin time. It can decrease the effect of the uricosuric action of probenecid. It has no interaction with the sulfonylureas or oral hypoglycemic agents, as opposed to most of the other NSAIDS. Aspirin interferes with the action of sulindac.
ADMINISTRATION AND DOSAGE SPECIFICS:
   Arthritis and ankylosing spondylitis: Use 150-200 mg two times daily with food. Maximum dose 400 mg/day.
   Acute painful shoulder or gout: Use 200 mg two times daily with food. Use for 7 days in gout, 7-14 days for painful shoulder. Safety in children not established.

INDOLE DERIVATIVE: TOLMETIN

PRODUCTS (TRADE NAME):
   Tolectin (Available in 200 mg tablets.) **Tolectin DS** (Available in 400 mg capsule.)
DRUG SPECIFICS:
   This drug is used in the treatment of acute exacerbations and prolonged man-

agement of rheumatoid arthritis and osteoarthritis. It is one of the few NSAIDS approved for the treatment of juvenile rheumatoid arthritis in children over the age of two. It has comparable effects to aspirin in controlling disease, with fewer of the side effects and decreased interference with liver function tests.

Most common side effects include: *Cardiovascular:* sodium and water retention leading to edema in some patients with underlying cardiovascular problems. *CNS:* dizziness, headache, tinnitus. *Dermatologic:* skin rash. *Gastrointestinal:* GI upset.

Drug interactions: Tolmetin can increase the prothrombin time if used with anticoagulants. Aspirin interferes with tolmetin blood levels. Phenobarbital decreases the effect of this drug. Tolmetin increases the effect of phenytoin, the sulfonamides and the oral hypoglycemia agents, as do many of the other NSAIDS.

ADMINISTRATION AND DOSAGE SPECIFICS:
Adult:
Osteoarthritis: Give 400 mg po three times daily with meals.
Rheumatoid arthritis: Give 600 to 1800 mg/day in 3-4 doses with meals. Maximum of 2 grams/day po.
Children over 2 years: 1-20 mg/kg/day in 3-4 doses with meals. Doses higher than 30 mg/kg/day not recommended.

OXICAMS: PIROXICAM

PRODUCTS (TRADE NAME):
Feldene (Available in 10 and 20 mg capsules.)
DRUG SPECIFICS:
This drug is a member of the oxicam family. It is indicated in the treatment of acute exacerbations and long-term management of rheumatoid and osteoarthritis. Its biggest advantage is in increasing patient compliance because it can be administered in a one-time daily dose.

It should not be administered in patients with hypersensitivity to oxicams or patients who develop allergic manifestations (such as nasal polyps, bronchospasm, or asthma) to aspirin or other NSAIDS. Not recommended for use in pregnant or breast-feeding women, or for use in children.

Patient should be evaluated for signs of renal disease, as an elevated BUN may develop (which usually reverses with discontinuation of the drug.) The drug is renally cleared, and should be used with caution in patients with renal disease.

There appear to be fewer side effects with this agent than with aspirin, with gastrointestinal problems the most common. Other side effects are: *Cardiovascular:* edema. *CNS:* dizziness, headache. It is unclear whether oxicams cause any adverse reactions within the eye, but because many of the NSAIDS cause adverse eye reactions, patients with eye complaints should be seen by an ophthalmologist. *Dermatologic:* rashes. *Other:* hematologic changes.

Drug interactions: Piroxicam may potentiate anticoagulants. Concurrent administration of aspirin interferes with piroxicam absorption. No other interactions have been established, but since it is protein-bound, it may affect other protein-bound drugs.

ADMINISTRATION AND DOSAGE SPECIFICS:

Use 20 mg one time daily. No therapeutic effects may be seen for 2 weeks. After that time, evaluate patient to see whether product should be continued or discontinued.

PROPIONIC ACID DERIVATIVE: FENOPROFEN CALCIUM

PRODUCTS (TRADE NAME):

Nalfon (Available in 200, 300 mg capsules, and 600 mg tablets.)

DRUG SPECIFICS:

Fenoprofen is used in the treatment of acute exacerbations and chronic therapy of rheumatoid arthritis and osteoarthritis.

Administer medication 30 minutes before meals or 2 hours after meals as food interferes with absorption. In cases where patient has substantial gastrointestinal disturbance, medication may be taken with meals.

Drug interactions: Patients receiving hydantoins, sulfonamides, or sulfonylureas should be observed for toxicity as these agents compete for albumin-binding sites. This agent also increases the effect of phenytoin and will increase the prothrombin time in patients receiving anticoagulant therapy.

ADMINISTRATION AND DOSAGE SPECIFICS:

Mild to moderate pain: Give 200 mg po every 4-6 hours on empty stomach.

Chronic pain: Give 300-600 mg every 6-8 hours on empty stomach. Maximum dose 3200 mg/24 hours.

PROPIONIC ACID DERIVATIVE: IBUPROFEN

PRODUCTS (TRADE NAME):

Motrin (Comes in 300, 400 and 600 mg coated tablets.) **Rufen** (Available in 400 mg tablets and 600 mg tablets.) New OTC drug—**Advil** (coated 200 mg tablets) and **Nuprin** (200 mg tablets.)

DRUG SPECIFICS:

Ibuprofen is used for relief of signs and symptoms of both chronic and acute arthritis. It is also used for relief of mild to moderate pain and has been approved for use in the treatment of dysmenorrhea. OTC drugs for temporary relief of headache, toothache, musculoskeletal pain and to reduce fever. Advil and Nuprin are available as over-the-counter preparations.

Drug interactions: Use in conjunction with aspirin is not recommended. Ibuprofen can potentiate the effect of phenytoin, and can effect coagulation studies (prothrombin time.) Phenobarbital can decrease the effect of ibuprofen by increasing hepatic breakdown. Patients receiving hydantoins, sulfonylureas, or sulfonamides should be observed for toxicity of these agents as they compete for albumin binding sites.

ADMINISTRATION AND DOSAGE SPECIFICS:

Mild to moderate pain: Give 400 mg po every 4-6 hours.

Chronic pain and acute exacerbations: 300-600 mg po every 6-8 hours. (Anti-inflammatory and rheumatoid arthritis patients generally require the higher doses.)

Primary dysmenorrhea: 400 mg every 4 hours.

Children: Safety not established.

PROPIONIC ACID DERIVATIVE: NAPROXEN

PRODUCTS (TRADE NAME):

Anaprox (Available in 275 mg naproxen sodium tablets.) **Naprosyn** (Available in 250, 375 and 500 mg tablets.)

DRUG SPECIFICS:

This product is used for the relief of mild to moderate pain. Naproxen has been found to be especially successful in the treatment of ankylosing spondylitis, rheumatoid arthritis, osteoarthritis, tendinitis, and bursitis. It is used for the treatment of acute gout and for the relief of dysmenorrhea. The advantage of this drug is that it can be given two times daily, or in some patients once daily, thus increasing compliance.

Drug interactions: This agent can affect anticoagulants by increasing the prothrombin time. Phenobarbital can decrease the effect of naproxen, and this agent can increase the effect of phenytoin. Patients receiving hydantoins, sulfonamides, or sulfonylureas should be observed for toxicity of these agents, as they compete for albumin binding sites. Probenecid is reported to retard plasma clearance of naproxen, leading to increased serum levels. Increased urinary levels of 17-ketogenic steroids is produced by naproxen, so withdrawal of the drug for 72 hours before testing patients for adrenal function is indicated. This drug may interfere with urinary assay of 5-hydroxyindoleacetic acid (5-HIAA) studies also. Do not exceed 1250 mg (1375 mg naproxen sodium) per day.

ADMINISTRATION AND DOSAGE SPECIFICS:

Mild to moderate pain, dysmenorrhea, acute tendinitis, bursitis: Give 500 mg initially, followed by 250 mg every 6 to 8 hours, or 550 mg naproxen sodium followed by 275 mg naproxen sodium every 6 to 8 hours.

Rheumatoid arthritis, osteoarthritis, spondylitis: Give 250 mg to 375 mg po every 12 hours. Doses do not have to be equal. Long-term therapy may require the higher dosage range. If there is no symptomatic effect in 2 weeks, continue trial for 2 more weeks before discontinuing the agent.

Acute gout: 750 mg (825 mg naproxen sodium) followed by 250 mg (275 mg naproxen sodium) every 8 hours until attack ends. Do not exceed 1250 mg per day.

PYRAZOLES AND DERIVATIVES: PHENYLBUTAZONE AND OXYPHENBUTAZONE

PRODUCTS (TRADE NAME):

Phenylbutazone: **Azolid, Butazolidin** (Available in 100 mg tablets and capsules.) **Phenylbutazone** (Available in 100 mg tablets.) Oxyphenbutazone: **Oxalid, Tandearil** (Available in 100 mg tablets.)

DRUG SPECIFICS:

These drugs have significant side effects and should only be used in short-course therapy and for exacerbations of acute gouty arthritis, ankylosing spondylitis, active rheumatoid arthritis, psoriatic arthritis, osteoarthritis (if unresponsive to other NSAIDS), traumatic inflammation, and painful shoulder (tendonitis, bursitis, capsulitis.) These drugs do not stop the progression of the underlying disease.

A complete history and physical examination plus complete hematologic and urine testing should be performed on patients who are to receive this drug. Patients should be followed frequently and hematologic evaluations done at one to two week intervals during therapy.

Blood dyscrasias are the most serious toxic reactions, and are related to hypersensitivity rather than dosage. They can develop in patients who have taken the drug in the past without problems. Patients over 60 years of age should not be on this drug longer than 1 week, and there appears to be an increase in adverse reactions in people over 40 years of age. It is contraindicated in children less than 14, senile patients, and pregnant or breast-feeding females as well as in other situations in which NSAIDS should not be given. It should also not be used in patients with a history of congestive heart failure, hypertension, parotitis, stomatitis, severe renal or hepatic disease, history of peptic ulcer disease, or active ulcer disease.

The most serious side effects are agranulocytosis, leukopenia, thrombocytopenia, and aplastic anemia which has caused fatalities in some older patients. Other adverse reactions frequently seen are: *Cardiovascular:* congestive failure, hypertension, myocarditis, pericarditis. *CNS:* agitation, confusion, headache. *EENT:* blurred vision, hearing loss, optic neuritis, retinal detachment, tinnitus. *Endocrine:* hyperglycemia, pancreatitis, thyroid hyperplasia, toxic and nontoxic goiter. *Gastrointestinal:* abdominal distention, diarrhea, esophagitis, gastritis, salivary gland enlargement, stomatitis, ulcer formation or activation, vomiting. *Renal:* glomerulonephritis, hematuria, nephrotic syndrome, proteinuria, renal failure or necrosis.

As is evidenced by the list of adverse reactions, phenylbutazone and oxyphen-

تتت
تتث

butazone therapy are not without risk. Therefore, patients should be warned to discontinue therapy and immediately contact their health care provider if there is any sign of fever, epigastric pain, sore throat, mouth lesions, unusual bleeding or bruising, tarry stools, skin rash, weight gain or edema, weakness or tiredness. The need for frequent visits to the health care provider, and for laboratory tests, should be emphasized.

Drug interactions: Phenylbutazone and oxyphenbutazone effects are increased by certain androgen hormones. They increase the effect of anticoagulants and phenytoin. Tricyclic antidepressants decrease the effect of these agents as well. They also potentiate the effect of diabetic hypoglycemic agents and insulin, so these patients should be carefully monitored. They decrease the effect of digitalis glycosides and therefore could increase the chance of congestive failure in some patients. They may also alter liver function tests and give a false-positive Coombs' test.

ADMINISTRATION AND DOSAGE SPECIFICS:

Take medication with meals or milk, or use products which include antacids.

Acute gout: Give initial dose of 400 mg followed by 100 mg four times daily for 7 days.

Other problems: Give 300-600 mg in equal divided doses. Symptomatic improvement should occur in one week. If there is no improvement, discontinue agent. If improvement occurs, decrease dose to the smallest possible level which still produces a therapeutic effect. This may be as little as 100 mg/day.

Carole Hill

ANALGESICS—SALICYLATES
ANTI-INFLAMMATORY

ACTION OF THE DRUG: Salicylates are used in the treatment of mild to moderate pain, and in the reduction of fever. They have analgesic, antipyretic, and anti-inflammatory effects. The exact mechanism of action for these agents is not understood. It is known they reduce fever partially through vasodilation; they also inhibit prostaglandin synthesis which affects the pain stimulation and inflammatory process. They have a depressant effect on the central and peripheral pain receptors. They also interfere with Factor III of the clotting mechanism. Aspirin is the most potent prostaglandin inhibitor of this group and therefore has the greatest anti-inflammatory effect of the salicylates.

ASSESSMENT:

INDICATIONS: Salicylates are used in the treatment of various forms of arthritis (i.e., rheumatoid arthritis osteoarthritis, degenerative joint disease, etc..) It is used in the treatment of systemic fever produced by viral illnesses, or in therapy for pain arising from trauma to soft tissue or muscle. Myalgias, neuralgias, arthralgias, headache and dysmenorrhea are also indications for salicylates. The anti-inflammatory effects are useful in treating systemic lupus erythematosus, acute rheumatic fever and other similar conditions.

SUBJECTIVE: This drug is effective in patients complaining of mild to moderate pain of a musculoskeletal nature, and in conditions causing mild fever. It is useful for many of the same conditions in which non-steroidal anti-inflammatory drugs are used.

OBJECTIVE: Signs of inflammation such as tenderness, erythema, increased warmth, and swelling may be present. Joint stiffness, decreased range of motion, or crepitus may also be found. The distribution, location, as well as pattern of involvement (i.e., monoarticular, asymmetrical, symmetrical) and number of joints involved should be determined. Systemic fever or muscular tenderness may be observed also.

PLAN:

CONTRAINDICATIONS: Do not use in the presence of hypersensitivity to salicylates or other non-steroidal anti-inflammatory drugs, as cross-sensitivity may appear (except with sodium salicylate, salicylamides or choline salicylate.) Drugs should also be used cautiously in patients who have hypersensitivity to some drugs, asthma and nasal polyps, as this triad may predispose patients to sensitivity to these drugs. This medication should not be used in patients with bleeding, active gastric ulcers, hemophilia or vitamin deficiency. Magnesium salicylate is contraindicated in patients with severe renal disease.

WARNINGS: Avoid use in patients with hepatic disease. There should be careful use in patients on anticoagulant therapy or patients with abnormalities of clotting. Avoid use prior to surgery, due to platelet effect; or before labor, as bleeding may increase. Use with caution in patients with symptoms suggesting transient ischemic attacks, who should have a complete neurologic evaluation prior to initiation of therapy. In pain which persists for more than 10 days, further evaluation is needed. Discontinue or reduce dosage if tinnitus develops. Magnesium salicylates or salsalate is not recommended in children under twelve. Use during pregnancy, especially during the third trimester, should be avoided due to adverse effects on fetus. Salicylates are found in breast milk.

PRECAUTIONS: Use cautiously to determine presence of gastric irritation, especially in patients with past history of upper gastrointestinal problems. Also use with caution in patients with blood dyscrasias, or impaired renal function. Salsalate and choline salicylate have been reported to cause less gastrointestinal irritation and should be considered if patient does not tolerate aspirin well. Hydration should be monitored carefully in children as they seem to be more prone to salicylate intoxication. Any children with recurrent upper respiratory infection symptoms within a short time span or disorientation should not be given salicylates due to positive association with Reye's syndrome. This acute, life-threatening problem is characterized by vomiting and lethargy which may procede to delirium and coma with permanent brain damage and possible death. Use of aspirin following influenza or chickenpox also seems more highly correlated with development of Reye's syndrome.

IMPLEMENTATION:

DRUG INTERACTIONS: These products increase the chance of gastrointestinal bleeding when used with alcohol. Increased R-aminosalicylic acid (PAS) effect may be caused by decreased excretion by the kidneys or decreased protein binding. There is an increased effect on anticoagulants, sulfonylureas and sulfonamides if used concomitantly with salicylates. Ascorbic acid increases the effect of salicylates by increasing renal tubular reabsorption. They interact with nonsteroidal antiinflammatory drugs (NSAIDS) to increase effects, side effects, and toxicities. They also increase the effect of methotrexate. Phenylbutazone inhibits any uricosuric activities of the salicylates, and salicylates in turn inhibit uricosuric activities of probenecid and sulfinpyrazone. Salicylates also potentiate the effects of phenytoin, and inhibit hyperuricemia produced by pyrazinamide. Salicylates can affect the following lab studies by increasing the results or giving false positive findings: amylase, SGOT, SGPT, uric acid, catecholamines, and urinary glucose using Benedict's clinitest. False negative results may be found in serum carbon dioxide, glucose, potassium and thrombocyte values.

ADMINISTRATION AND DOSAGE: The administration and dosage varies for each of the salicylate products, so each individual product must be checked before prescribing. All forms of the medication exist for these agents, again depending on the individual product. There are tablets, capsules, drops, chewable preparations, suppositories and injectable forms. Aspirin is the most active agent and has the greatest amount of salicylate per unit. Check individual agents for specifics.

IMPLEMENTATION CONSIDERATIONS:

—Obtain a complete health history to check for presence of hypersensitivity to aspirin or other non-steroidal anti-inflammatory preparations, history of asthma and nasal polyps, gastrointestinal problems or ulcer disease, concurrent use of other drugs which may cause interactions, or other underlying hepatic or renal disease.

—Check for occult blood in stool prior to beginning medication. This will help you evaluate whether positive studies in the future are a chance event or not.

—Rule out any infective process as the causative factor in uniarticular joint problems, or systemic fever, as salicylates will reduce the inflammation or fever, but will not treat the causative agent.

—Patients with diabetes who are testing their urine with Benedict's clinitest may get incorrect readings. They may need to switch to another form of urine testing while using salicylate products. Salicylates also potentiate oral hypoglycemic agents, and diabetics should be alert to signs of hypoglycemia.

—Check for signs of bleeding in patients who are on anticoagulants or have bleeding problems.

—Many salicylate products are not recommended for use in children under 12 years of age. Be certain to check the individual agent when prescribing for children.

—Patients with high fevers should be monitored closely to see that they respond to aspirin within one hour. Further treatment is required if they do not respond.

WHAT THE PATIENT NEEDS TO KNOW:

—This drug may cause gastric upset because it is so strong. These symptoms may be reduced by taking medicine with food, milk, or a full glass of water.

—Notify your health care provider if you notice any ringing in your ears, any abnormal bleeding, bruising, or bloody or black tarry stools.

—Arthritis or rheumatic fever may require extra-large doses of medicine.

—Chronic problems may require taking the medicine for more than a week before you notice any decrease in symptoms.

—Take medicine regularly in order to reduce inflammation. If medicine is taken irregularly, a high level of medicine in the blood is not maintained, and it cannot help reduce symptoms as successfully as with regular use.

—Do not begin taking any other medications without the knowledge of your health care provider. This includes drugs you may purchase over the counter.

—Contact your health provider if fever does not decrease in 24-48 hours, or if patient becomes lethargic or hard to awaken.

—Keep this medicine out of the reach of children and all others for whom it is not prescribed.

—If you are unable to take medicine in the form prescribed, call your health practitioner so that another form may be ordered. Medicine is available in chewable tablets, and suppositories to aid in administration.

EVALUATION:

ADVERSE REACTIONS: *CNS:* tinnitus, visual disturbances. *Dermatologic:* edema, hives, rashes, redness. *Gastrointestinal:* anorexia, epigastric discomfort, heartburn, nausea.

OVERDOSAGE: Symptoms may progress from mild to severe with hyperventilation, sweating, thirst, headache, drowsiness, skin eruptions, and electrolyte imbalance progressing to CNS depression, stupor, convulsions and coma, tachycardia, and respiratory insufficiency. Respiratory and metabolic acidosis are most often seen in children. *Treatment:* Induce emesis, and refer for gastric lavage and symptomatic treatment as indicated. Increased hydration with systemic bicarbonate will speed excretion. Short-acting barbiturates may be needed to control convulsions. Dialysis may be helpful in severe overdose cases. Toxic levels are above systemic salicylate levels of 35 mg/100 ml.

PARAMETERS TO MONITOR: Patients should be monitored for therapeutic effect: subjective relief of pain, reduction in temperature to 101° or below. Also observe for temperature that does not resolve, and progression of disease. For arthritis, the higher doses are usually needed to control symptoms. Medicine should be gradually increased while monitoring for subjective improvement, increased strength of grip, increased mobility, and improved ability to carry on normal activities. Check patient for signs of occult bleeding through use of regular blood counts and stool checks. Check for signs of toxicity, especially tinnitus. Periodic salicylate levels may be beneficial if dosage is approaching maximum levels, or if there is a question of patient compliance. For rheumatic fever, follow recommended doses and monitor symptoms and physical signs for any sign of improvement. Here again serum salicylate levels may be helpful in preventing toxicity.

ACETYLSALICYLIC ACID (ASPIRIN)

PRODUCTS (TRADE NAME):
   Aspergum (Available with 210 mg acetylsalicylic acid in a gum base.) **Aspirin, A.S.A.** (Available in 5 gr [325 mg] oral tablet, 65 to 75 mg chewable tablets, 75 to 650 mg suppository.) **Bayer Timed-Release** (Available in 650 mg timed-release tablet.) **Children's Aspirin** (Available with 65 to 81 mg acetylsalicylic acid.) **Ecotrin** (Available in 325 mg enteric-coated tablet.) **Easprin** (Available in 975 mg enteric-coated tablets.) **Hipirin** (Available in 487.5 mg tablet.) **Measurin** (Available in 650 mg tablet.)

DRUG SPECIFICS:
   Aspirin is the most commonly used anti-inflammatory agent. It represents the standard against which all other agents are compared. Hypersensitivity often exists in asthmatics with rhinitis. Prolonged use may cause decreased serum levels which requires an increased or titrated dosage. Patients on long-term therapy should have serum salicylate levels drawn periodically to evaluate therapy. Gastric side effects are the most common adverse reactions.

ADMINISTRATION AND DOSAGE SPECIFICS:
   Mild to moderate pain: Give 325 to 650 mg po initially, then repeat every 4 hours.
   Arthritis: 2.6 to 5.2 gm/day po in divided doses.
   Juvenile rheumatoid arthritis: 90 to 130 mg/kg/24 hours in 4 to 6 divided doses.
   Acute rheumatic fever: Give up to 7.8 gm/day in divided doses.
   Children: 65 mg/kg/day in 4 to 6 divided doses.
   TIA's in men: 1300 mg in divided doses 2 to 4 times daily.

ACETYLSALICYLIC ACID (ASPIRIN), BUFFERED

PRODUCTS (TRADE NAME):
   These products contain various amounts of aspirin in combination with antacids for the purpose of reducing gastrointestinal distress. Patients should be cautioned about taking these medications for gastrointestinal distress, as the aspirin may only increase that symptom. A summary of products and their components can be found in Table 4-8.

DRUG SPECIFICS:
   Aspirin-antacid combinations are used with patients who experience gastrointestinal distress from plain aspirin products. This combination is also claimed to increase the dissolution of the agent so that it reaches the bloodstream faster. Dosage and administration are the same as for plain aspirin (above.)

Table 4-8. CONTENTS OF VARIOUS BUFFERED ASPIRIN TABLETS

Products	Amount Aspirin	Amount and Type Antacid
Alka-Seltzer	324 mg effervescent tab	1.9 mg sodium bicarbonate 1 Gm citric acid
Ascriptin	325 mg/tablet	150 mg aluminum OH and MG OH
Ascriptin A/D	325 mg/tablet	300 mg aluminum OH and MG OH
Asperbuf	325 mg/tablet	130 mg aluminum OH
Buffered Aspirin	325 mg/tablet	Varies with manufacturer
Bufferin	324 mg/tablet	97.2 mg magnesium carbonate and 48.6 mg aluminum glycinate
Bufferin Arthritis Strength	486 mg/tablet	145.8 mg magnesium carbonate and 72.9 mg aluminum glycina

CHOLINE SALICYLATE

PRODUCTS (TRADE NAME):
   Arthropan (Available in 870 mg/5 ml liquid.)
DRUG SPECIFICS:
   This is a liquid form of salicylate with fewer gastrointestinal side effects than aspirin. It may be the drug of choice over sodium salicylate if a sodium restriction is necessary. It has a nasty aftertaste which may be reduced by giving it in water. Do not give with antacids.
ADMINISTRATION AND DOSAGE SPECIFICS:
   Adults and children over 12 years: Give 870 mg po initially; repeat every 3-4 hours. Give no more than 6 times daily.
   Rheumatoid arthritis: Start with 0.87 to 1.74 gm po up to four times daily. If antacids are required, give this agent before meals, and antacids at least 2 hours after meals.

DIFLUNISAL

PRODUCTS (TRADE NAME): Dolobid (250 and 500 mg capsulets).
DRUG SPECIFICS:
   This preparation is a derivative of salicylic acid, but is chemically different than aspirin and is not metabolized to salicylic acid. Its exact mechanism of action is not known, but it is known to be a prostaglandin synthetase inhibitor. This drug is recommended for the treatment of mild to moderate pain of musculosketal dis-

orders and following surgery. The advantage of this drug is its long half life requiring dosing only every twelve hours. It produces significant analgesia in one hour with maximum analgesia in two to three hours. It is compared to Tylenol with codiene or Darvocet with its effectiveness of pain relief. It is not recommended for use as an antipyretic agent. It does have uricosuric effects and some platelet inhibitory function but these are reversible. Peptic ulceration and GI bleeding have been reported with this product so it should be used with caution in those with a positive history of GI problems.

ADMINISTRATION AND DOSAGE SPECIFICS:

Mild to moderate pain: Initial dose of 1000 mg followed by 500 mg every 12 hours. If pain is not severe this may be reduced to 250 mg every 8 to 12 hours.

Osteoarthritis: 500 to 1000 mg daily in 2 divided doses. Dosage may be increased or decreased according to patient response. Maintenance doses higher than 1500 mg daily are not recommended.

This drug is not recommended in pregnancy and is excreted in human milk. The safety of this drug in children under 12 has not been established.

MAGNESIUM SALICYLATE

PRODUCTS (TRADE NAME):

Doan's Pills (Available in 325 mg tablets.) **Durasal** (Available in 480 mg tablets.) **Efficin** (Available in 500 mg tablets.) **Magan** (Available in 545 mg tablets.) **Mobidin** (Available in 600 mg.) **MS-650** (Available in 650 mg tablets.)

DRUG SPECIFICS:

This is a sodium-free salicylate with a lower incidence of gastrointestinal problems than aspirin. It is not recommended for use in children under 12 years of age.

ADMINISTRATION AND DOSAGE SPECIFICS:

Adults and children over 12 years: Give 600 mg po 3-4 times daily. May be increased to 3.6 or 4.8 gm po daily at 3 to 6 hour intervals.

Rheumatic Fever: Give up to 9.6 gm po.

SALICYLAMIDE

PRODUCTS (TRADE NAME):

Salicylamide (Available in 325 mg tablets.) **Uromide** (Available in 667 mg tablets.)

DRUG SPECIFICS:

This compound is less effective than aspirin because it is metabolized to a much greater degree before it gets into the circulation. It is to be used for temporary relief of pain but if pain persists more than 10 days, the patient should be evaluated further.

ADMINISTRATION AND DOSAGE SPECIFICS:

Adult: Give 325 to 650 mg po 3-4 times daily. Can be used as a uricosuric agent with 1.8 gm po daily. Not recommended for long-term use.

SODIUM SALICYLATE

PRODUCTS (TRADE NAME):

Sodium Salicylate (Available in 1 and 1.5 gm injections; 325, 650 mg enteric-coated tablets; 325, 650 mg tablets.) **Uracel 5** (Available in 324 mg enteric-coated tablet.)

DRUG SPECIFICS:

This preparation is less effective than an equal dose of aspirin. It should not be used in patients on a low sodium diet. Some physicians recommend giving 1 gm vitamin K with each gram of this drug. Some also give 1/2 gm sodium bicarbonate per gram of this agent to decrease excretion of the drug. The advantage of this agent is that it comes in an IV injectable form and is sometimes used on an in-patient basis for patients with acute exacerbations of rheumatoid arthritis, or in patients with acute rheumatic fever.

ADMINISTRATION AND DOSAGE SPECIFICS:

Give 325-650 mg po or IV every 4-6 hours.

Rheumatic fever: Give 10-15 gm in divided doses every 4-5 hours.

SODIUM THIOSALICYLATE

PRODUCTS (TRADE NAME):

Arthrolate, Asproject, Nalate, Rexolate, Sodium Thiosalicylate, Thiocyl, Thiodyne, Thiosol, Thiosul, Tusal (Available in 50 mg/ml injection.)

DRUG SPECIFICS:

This is another salicylate with the advantage of an injectable form. This agent has no oral form. It can be used for the treatment of acute gout, musculoskeletal pain and rheumatic fever.

ADMINISTRATION AND DOSAGE SPECIFICS:

Musculoskeletal pain: Give 50 to 100 mg IM daily or on alternate days.

Acute gout: Give 100 mg every 3-4 hours IM for 2 days, then 100 mg daily.

Rheumatic fever: Give 100 to 150 mg IM every 4-6 hours for 3 days, then 100 mg 2 times daily until patient is without symptoms.

Carole Hill

ANTICONVULSANTS

There is a wide variety of drugs which control convulsive behavior through depression of abnormal neuronal discharges in the central nervous system. These products work in a variety of ways. Products are usually most effective in one type of seizure activity, and the best drug for the problem should be prescribed. Frequently patients are started on parenteral therapy, and when seizure activity has come under control, oral therapy is initiated.

Because of the variety of medications and the high incidence of side effects associated with each, the selection of an anticonvulsant medication tends to be a therapeutic experiment for each patient. When control is not maintained with one product, another may be added, or another product substituted.

Recent data suggests that although the majority of epileptic mothers receiving anticonvulsive therapy deliver normal infants, there is an association between the use of anticonvulsant drugs and an elevated incidence of birth defects in children born to these women. This relationship seems to be especially pronounced in women taking phenobarbital or phenytoin, although other anticonvulsants may also be implicated. Women under therapy who contemplate pregnancy, therefore, present a special dilemma in selection of therapeutics.

A summary of the types of anticonvulsants and the types of seizure activity for which they are most appropriate may be found in Table 4-9.

Marilyn W. Edmunds

ANTICONVULSANTS— ACETAZOLAMIDE

ACTION OF THE DRUG: Acetazolamide is a carbonic anhydrase inhibitor which acts to decrease abnormal paroxysmal or excessive discharge from central nervous system neurons. Although the action is not completely understood, the production of acidosis may also contribute to the therapeutic action.

ASSESSMENT:

INDICATIONS: Although nurses do not usually prescribe this medication, they frequently have responsibility for monitoring the patient taking this product. This product is used in the treatment of grand mal, petite mal, myoclonic jerk seizures, and mixed seizure disorder patterns. The best results have been found in controlling petite mal seizures in children. This product is also used in non-convulsive therapy in the treatment of chronic open angle glaucoma and edema. (See ophthalmic and diuretic sections of this book for additional information.)

SUBJECTIVE: Patient may present with a history of grand mal, petite mal,

TABLE 4-9. ANTICONVULSANT DRUGS AND THEIR PRIMARY USES

Drugs	Primary Uses
Barbiturates	
Amobarbital sodium	All forms of epilepsy, status epilepticus, eclampsia, tetanus, drug reactions
Mephobarbital	Grand mal and petite mal seizures
Metharbital	Grand mal, petite mal, myoclonic, mixed seizures
Pentobarbital sodium	Status epilepticus, drug reactions, tetanus
Phenobarbital	All forms of epilepsy, status epilepticus, severe recurrent seizures, eclampsia
Secobarbital sodium	Status epilepticus, drug reactions, tetanus
Thiopental sodium	Status epilepticus
Benzodiazepines	
Clonazepam	Petite mal, myoclonic seizures
Clorazepate	Focal seizures
Diazepam	All forms of epilepsy, status epilepticus, severe recurrent seizures, tetanus
Hydantoins	
Ethotoin	Grand mal and psychomotor seizures
Mephenytoin	Gran mal, psychomotor, focal, Jacksonian seizures
Phenytoin	Grand mal, psychomotor seizures, status epilepticus
Oxazolidinediones	
Paramethadione	Petite mal seizures
Trimethadione	Petite mal seizures
Succinimides	
Ethosuximide	Petite mal seizures
Methsuximide	Petite mal seizures
Phensuximide	Petite mal seizures
Other drugs	
Acetazolamide	Grand mal, petite mal, myocolonic, mixed seizures
Carbamazepine	Grand mal, mixed, psychomotor seizures
Magnesium sulfate	Eclampsia
Paraldehyde	Status epilepticus, eclampsia, drug reactions
Phenacemide	Psychomotor seizures
Primidone	Grand mal, psychomotor, focal seizures
Valproic acid	Petite mal seizures

or mixed seizure disorders. In the absence of a positive history, patient may present with complaints of "blackouts," awakening to find signs of incontinence, bitten tongue, soft tissue injuries, or fractures.

OBJECTIVE: Family or other reliable sources may be able to describe seizures. There may be evidence of physical injury following a "blackout." Positive studies such as skull x-rays, serum glucose, magnesium, or calcium evaluations; cerebrospinal fluid studies; CT scan of the head; pneumograms; brain scans; or cerebral angiograms may show etiology of convulsion. EEG may be normal or positive in a patient with epilepsy.

PLAN:

CONTRAINDICATIONS: Do not give in the presence of known hypersensitivity to sulfonamides. Should also not be given if there is marked kidney and liver disease or dysfunction, adrenal insufficiency, hyperchloremic acidosis, or if there are depressed serum sodium or potassium levels.

WARNINGS: Do not use in the first trimester of pregnancy unless the potential benefits outweigh possible risks. There is a suggestion that teratogenic and embryocidal effects may be present in pregnant animals taking this drug.

PRECAUTIONS: Because acetazolamide may precipitate or aggravate acidosis, use with extreme caution in patients with emphysema or pulmonary obstruction.

IMPLEMENTATION:

DRUG INTERACTIONS: This product may induce hypokalemia, which may make patient more vulnerable to digitalis toxicity. Use with corticosteroids or ACTH will accelerate potassium depletion. Use with quinidine may potentiate and prolong the action of quinidine.

PRODUCTS (TRADE NAME):
Acetazolamide, AK-Zol (Available in 250 mg tablets.) **Diamox** (Available in 125 and 250 mg tablets, and 500 mg injection.)

ADMINISTRATION AND DOSAGE: Because of bioequivalence variance between manufacturers, brand interchange is not recommended. The parenteral solution should be given IV, since IM injections are painful due to the alkaline pH of the solution.

Epilepsy: 8 to 30 mg/kg/day in divided doses. The optimum range appears to be 375 to 1000 mg/day.

Adjunctive anticonvulsant therapy: In addition to other medications, give 250 mg/day. Increase dosage slowly as needed to obtain greater seizure control.

IMPLEMENTATION CONSIDERATIONS:

—Obtain a complete health history, including the presence of hypersensitivity to sulfonamides, underlying systemic disease (especially cardiac, renal, or hepatic), concurrent use of medications, and possibility of pregnancy.

—Document rationale for therapy, and ascertain that the patient's condition is being closely followed by a physician.

—Obtain baseline complete blood count, liver function tests, kidney function tests, ECG, EEG, or other tests as indicated by choice of drug.

—Investigate all legal ramifications with the diagnosis of epilepsy (e.g., driver's license revocation).

—Do not abruptly discontinue anticonvulsant therapy.

—If parenteral form of medication is used, reconstituted solutions should be used within 24 hours. IM injections are to be avoided whenever possible due to the painful nature of the solution.

—Cases of myopia have been reported. This will disappear upon lowering dose or discontinuing the drug.

—Side effects are usually minimal in short-term therapy. Paresthesias are often seen.

WHAT THE PATIENT NEEDS TO KNOW:

—This medication must be taken every day as prescribed. It should not be stopped even though you may have no seizures and may be feeling well.

—If a dose of medicine is missed, take it as soon as possible. If it is nearly time for the next dose, take the next dose only. Continue with regular medication schedule.

—If a dose of medicine is being missed frequently, contact your health care provider and discuss this.

—This medicine may decrease your alertness. Do not drive, operate machinery, or do other activities that require alertness, until you know how you react to this medicine.

—You will need to have health checkups on a systematic basis while taking this drug. Checkups will be more frequent for the first few months of drug therapy.

—Do not stop this medicine without consulting with your health care provider. This is very important.

—Notify your health care provider if unusual bleeding or bruising, sore throat, fever, or other new and troublesome symptoms develop.

—Wear a Medic-Alert necklace or bracelet and carry a medical identification card with your diagnosis and the anticonvulsant medication you are taking.

—Keep this medication out of the reach of children and all others for whom it is not prescribed.

EVALUATION:

ADVERSE REACTIONS: *CNS:* confusion, convulsions, drowsiness, flaccid paralysis, paresthesias, transient myopia. *Dermatologic:* rash, urticaria. *Hematopoietic:* agranulocytosis, bone marrow depression, hemolytic anemia, leukopenia, pancytopenia, thrombocytopenic purpura. *Other:* acidosis, anorexia, crystalluria, fever, glycosuria, hematuria, hepatic insufficiency, melena, renal calculus.

PARAMETERS TO MONITOR: Prior to initiating therapy, a complete blood count, liver function tests and a urinalysis should be obtained. Complete blood count should be repeated every month while taking medication. Watch for reduction in incidence of seizures, and monitor for adverse effects. Reduce dosage or discontinue drug if myopia develops.

Marilyn W. Edmunds

ANTICONVULSANTS—
BENZODIAZEPINES

ACTION OF THE DRUG: Benzodiazepines are capable of suppressing the spike and wave discharge in seizures and of decreasing the frequency, amplitude, duration and spread of the discharge in minor motor seizures.

ASSESSMENT:

INDICATIONS: Used in minor motor seizures and also in the treatment of Lennox-Gastaut syndrome (petit mal variance) and patients who have failed to respond to succinimides. The nurse practitioner does not usually initiate drug therapy with this product, however, they may often be given responsibility for long-term monitoring of patients taking this medication.

SUBJECTIVE: History of infantile spasms, seizures started by photosensitivity, staring into space for several seconds without a response and myoclonic jerks.

OBJECTIVE: Observation of a seizure.

PLAN:

CONTRAINDICATIONS: Do not use with hypersensitivity to benzodiazepines, narrow-angle glaucoma, clinical or biochemical evidence of liver disease. Also avoid use in patients with open-angle glaucoma, unless receiving treatment.

WARNINGS: Has a depressant effect on the central nervous system; therefore, avoid undertaking activities that require alertness, and physical coordination. Use of alcohol and its effects may be addictive. Use may constitute a risk factor if patient is a pregnant woman or even of childbearing age. Because effects are not known, avoid use if patient is breast-feeding. Withdrawal symptoms can occur if the drug is stopped too abruptly. Whether physical and mental development will be adversely affected following long-term use in pediatric patients is not known. Addictive-prone individuals need to be closely monitored.

PRECAUTIONS: When used with patients who have a mixed type of seizure activity, the drug may increase or precipitate the onset of generalized tonic-clonic seizures. Also use with precaution in patients with impaired renal function. Abrupt withdrawal can produce status epilepticus. May cause difficulty in patients with some types of respiratory problems because of increased secretions.

IMPLEMENTATION:

DRUG INTERACTIONS: Carbamazepine may increase the metabolism of clonazepam, thereby increasing the amount of drug available to the patient. Clonazepam may reduce phenytoin and primidone plasma concentrations. Multiple anticonvulsants together may result in an antidepressant effect. Valproic acid in conjunction with clonazepam may produce petit mal seizures.

ADMINISTRATION AND DOSAGE: Adding clonazepam to multiple anticonvulsants may result in an increase of depressant effects. Maintenance dosage must be individualized for each person.

IMPLEMENTATION CONSIDERATIONS:

—Obtain a complete health history, including the presence of hypersensitivity, concurrent drug therapy or the presence of renal or respiratory disease, or the possibility of pregnancy.

—Explain to the family and the patient possible side effects of the drug.

—Counsel patient and family about the transient drowsiness, ataxia and behavior disorders (aggression, hyperactivity, irritability and difficulty in concentration) which may occur with initial therapy, but which subside with continued medication.

WHAT THE PATIENT NEEDS TO KNOW:

—Take dose only as prescribed. Do not double medication doses if you miss one dose. Do not stop taking medication without being instructed to do so.

—Drug will often produce drowsiness, especially when beginning therapy. It is suggested that you do not drive or operate heavy machinery because of this.

—Report difficulty with excessive secretions and coughing, or any changes in your behavior, to your health care provider immediately.

—Wear a Medic-Alert or some type of identifying bracelet or chain which states your seizure problem and your medication.

—Do not drink alcohol while using this medication.

—Do not take this drug if you plan to become pregnant, if you are pregnant, or if you are breast-feeding a baby.

—Do not stop taking the drug suddenly.

—Keep a record of any seizures you have: duration, type, and time of day. Bring this record with you on all visits for health care.

—Taking the drug as ordered and regular follow-up care with your health provider are important.

EVALUATION:

ADVERSE REACTIONS: The most common side effects occurring are: drowsiness (50% of patients), ataxia (approximately 30% of patients) and behavior problems (approximately 23% of patients). However, these problems subside with continued medication. Other adverse effects include: *Cardiovascular:* palpitations. *Central Nervous System:* ataxia, abnormal eye movements, aphonia, choreiform movements, dysarthria, "glassy-eyed" appearance, headache, hemiparesis, hypotonia, nystagmus, respiratory depression, slurred speech, tremor and vertigo. *Dermatologic:* hair loss, hirsutism, ankle and facial edema and skin rash. *Gastrointestinal:* anorexia, increased appetite, nausea, sore gums, dry mouth, gastritis, hepatomegaly. constipation, diarrhea, encopresis. *Genitourinary:* dysuria, enuresis, nocturia, urinary retention. *Hematopoietic:* anemia, leukopenia, thrombocytopenia, eosinophilia. *Re-

spiratory: chest congestion, rhinorrhea, shortness of breath, hypersecretion in upper respiratory passage. *Other:* muscle weakness and incoordination, dehydration, fever, lymphadenopathy, weight loss or weight gain. Increased salivary and bronchial secretions may cause difficulties for children. Also, behavior disturbances can occur in the manner of aggression, hyperactivity, irritability and difficulty in concentration.

OVERDOSAGE: *Signs and Symptoms:* Somnolence, confusion, coma and decreased reflexes may occur. *Treatment:* Monitoring of respirations, pulse rate, blood pressure, along with general supportive measures and immediate gastric lavage should be provided.

PARAMETERS TO MONITOR: As baseline studies obtain: complete blood count, liver function tests, convulsant levels, tonometry reading to check for glaucoma, and urinalysis. If patient is a child, also obtain baseline height and weight. On subsequent visits periodically repeat complete blood count, urinalysis and convulsant levels. Eyes should be checked by tonometry yearly for glaucoma. If patient is a child, keep a running log on height and weight of child, as well as checking with parents about the child's progress in school once a maintenance dose is achieved. On all clients evaluate compliance in taking medication and determine presence of continued seizures.

CLONAZEPAM

PRODUCTS (TRADE NAME:)
    Clonopin (Available in 0.5 mg and 1 and 2 mg tablets.)
DRUG SPECIFICS:
    Whenever possible the daily dose should be divided into three equal doses. If impossible to do this, give the largest dose before bedtime.
ADMINISTRATION AND DOSAGE SPECIFICS:
    Adults: Initial dose is 1.5 mg po divided into three doses per day. After four to nine days, dosage may be increased by 0.5 mg 1.5 mg/day every three days until the seizures stop or until the side effects preclude any further increase. Maximum recommended daily dose is 20 mg.
    Infants and children up to 10 years or 30 kg: initial dosage between O.01 to O.03 mg/kg/day po, however not to exceed O.05 mg/kg/day, given in two or three divided doses. Dosage should be increased by not more than 0.25 to 0.5 mg every third day until a daily maintenance rate of 0.1 to 0.2 mg is reached.

CLORAZEPATE DIPOTASSIUM

PRODUCTS (TRADE NAME):
    Tranxene (Available in 3.75, 7.5 and 15 mg capsules, 3.75, 7.5 11.25, 15 and

22.5 mg tablets; SD half strength tablets 11.25 mg and SD tablets 22.5 mg).

DRUG SPECIFICS:

Medication is used as adjunctive therapy in the management of partial seizures and for the symptomatic relief of anxiety. It may cause drowsiness and alcohol and other CNS depressants should not be taken concurrently. Begin medication at lowest dosages and increase gradually. Do not abruptly stop medication or change doses radically.

ADMINISTRATION AND DOSAGE SPECIFICS:

Adults and children over 12 years: Initial dose is 7.5 mg three times daily. Increase by no more than 7.5 mg every week. Maximum dose not to exceed 90 mg/day.

Children 9 to 12 years: Initial dose is 7.5 mg twice daily. Increase by no more than 7.5 mg every week. Maximum dose not to exceed 60 mg/day.

DIAZEPAM

PRODUCTS (TRADE NAME):

Valium (Available in 2, 5, and 10 mg tablets, and 5 mg/ml injection.) **Valrelease** (Available in 15 mg sustained-release capsules.)

DRUG SPECIFICS:

Used as adjunctive therapy in treatment of seizures. Not found to be effective as sole therapy. Parenteral form is used in treating status epilepticus and severe recurrent seizure disorders. It may cause drowsiness and alcohol and other CNS depressants should not be taken concurrently. Begin medication at lowest dosages and increase gradually. Do not abruptly stop medication or change doses radically.

Parenteral usage should be reserved for emergencies, and given under the direction of a physician. Administer slowly to prevent cardiac arrest and/or apnea. Use care to avoid local irritation, swelling, phlebitis, and other vascular impairment during injection.

This product is also used as a muscle relaxant and for anxiety. (See other sections for more information.)

ADMINISTRATION AND DOSAGE SPECIFICS:

Dosage must be individualized, with elderly and debilitated patients receiving lower doses. In some cases patients may require larger doses. Increments in medication should be cautiously added to the recommended doses.

Adults: 2 to 10 mg po 2 to 4 times daily. Give sustained-release capsules 15 to 30 mg once daily.

Geriatric or debilitated patients: 2 to 2.5 mg po once or twice daily. Gradually increase dose as needed.

Children older than 6 months: 1 to 2.5 mg po three or four times daily initially. Gradually increase dose as needed.

Parenteral therapy: Inject IV medication slowly only into large veins, 1 minute for each 5 mg. This is very important.

Adults: Give 5 to 10 mg IV initially, repeated as necessary at 10 to 15 minute intervals. Maximum IV dose is 30 mg. Therapy may be repeated in 2 to 4 hours as needed.

Children 5 years and older: Give 1 mg every 2 to 5 minutes. Maximum IV dose is 10 mg. Repeat in 2 to 4 hours as needed.

Children 30 days to 5 years: Give 0.2 to 0.5 mg slowly every 2 to 5 minutes. Maximum IV dose is 5 mg.

Linda Ross

ANTICONVULSANTS— CARBAMAZEPINE

ACTION OF THE DRUG: Anticonvulsants may act directly on the motor cortex to inhibit the spread of seizure activity, or cause central nervous system depression. Sometimes the exact mechanism of action is not known. (See also the sections on sedatives, barbiturates and hydantoins).

ASSESSMENT:

INDICATIONS: A nurse practitioner does not usually initiate anticonvulsant therapy. However, it is often their responsibility to monitor the patient on anticonvulsant therapy, make dosage changes, and initiate appropriate referrals. Carbamazepine is used in refractory temporal lobe, psychomotor, grand mal epilepsy and mixed seizure patterns. Petit mal seizures do not appear to be controlled by carbamazepine. This product is also used in the treatment of trigeminal neuralgia and glossopharyngeal neuralgia.

SUBJECTIVE: Patient may present with a history of grand mal, petit mal, Jacksonian, or psychomotor epilepsy. In the absence of a positive history, patient may present with complaints of "blackouts," awakening to find signs of incontinence, bitten tongue, soft tissue injuries, or fractures. There may also be a history of chronic alcohol abuse. Family or other reliable sources may be able to describe seizures.

OBJECTIVE: There may be evidence of physical injury following a "blackout." Positive studies such as skull X-rays, serum glucose, magnesium, or calcium; cerebrospinal fluid studies; CT scan of the head; pneumograms; brain scans; or cerebral angiograms may show etiology of convulsion. EEG may be normal, or positive in a patient with epilepsy.

PLAN:

CONTRAINDICATIONS: Carbamazepine should not be used in patients with AV heart block; history of bone marrow depression; blood disorders associated with serious abnormalities in blood count, platelets or serum iron; hypersensitivity to tricyclic antidepressants; pregnancy; nursing mothers; or MAO inhibitor therapy within the past 14 days.

WARNINGS: All patients on anticonvulsants should be told to avoid activities that require alertness and good psychomotor coordination until central nervous system response to the drug has been evaluated. Never stop anticonvulsant therapy abruptly as this could precipitate a seizure. An increased incidence of birth defects may be related to the use of anticonvulsants during pregnancy. Nursing mothers should stop nursing if placed on anticonvulsant medication.

PRECAUTIONS: Carbamazepine should be used cautiously in patients with cardiac, renal or hepatic damage, increased intraocular pressure, or a history of drug-induced hematologic reactions. Serious blood dyscrasias may develop and could be fatal.

IMPLEMENTATION:

DRUG INTERACTIONS: Use of this product with anticoagulants, coumarin or indandione derivatives may produce decreased serum anticoagulant levels. Concurrent use with barbiturates, benzodiazepines, hydantoins, succinimides or valproic acid produces decreased serum levels of these drugs. Use with oral contraceptives may reduce the reliability of contraceptive action and produce breakthrough bleeding. Erythromycin, propoxyphene, isoniazid, or troleandomycin produces increased plasma levels of carbamazepine, possibly leading to toxicity. Cimetidine may also alter serum carbamazepine levels. Tricyclic antidepressants produce increased central nervous system depression and decreased effects of anticonvulsant. This drug may increase BUN, SGPT, SGOT, bilirubin, and serum alkaline tests. Urine sugar and urine protein levels may be increased. Thyroid function test values may be decreased.

PRODUCTS (TRADE NAME):
Tegretol (Available in 100 and 200 mg chewable tablets).

ADMINISTRATION AND DOSAGE: Initiating therapy with low doses and gradually increasing drug until an adequate response is achieved may minimize side effects. If adding a drug to existing anticonvulsant therapy, the new drug should be added gradually while the other anticonvulsant is gradually decreased. Never abruptly discontinue anticonvulsant therapy. Gradual withdrawal is suggested. Taking drug with food may decrease gastric irritation.

When it is possible, total daily dosage should be given in 3 to 4 divided doses. This product may be used alone or added to other anticonvulsant therapy.

Adults and children over 12 years: Initially give one tablet twice daily on first day. Gradually increase by up to 200 mg daily using a 3 or 4 times daily regimen until the optimum response is obtained. Maximum dose is 1000 mg daily for ages 12 to 15 years. Above 15 years, maximum dose is 1200 mg daily. Maintenance dose is usually 800 to 1200 mg daily.

Children 6 to 12 years: Initially give 1/2 tablet twice daily on first day. Gradually increase by adding 100 mg daily, using a 3 to 4 times daily regimen until optimum response is obtained. Do not exceed 1000 mg daily. Maintenance dose is usually 400 to 800 mg daily.

IMPLEMENTATION CONSIDERATIONS:

—Obtain a complete health history, including the presence of hypersensitivity, underlying systemic disease (especially cardiac, renal, hepatic, hematologic, or optic dysfunctions), concurrent use of medications, and possibility of pregnancy.

—Document rationale for therapy, and ascertain that the patient's condition is being closely followed by a physician.

—Obtain baseline complete blood count, liver function tests, kidney function tests, ECG, EEG, or other tests as indicated by choice of drug.

—Elderly patients may be more sensitive to standard drug dosages.

—Investigate all legal ramifications with the diagnosis of epilepsy (e.g. driver's license revocation, etc.).

—Do not abruptly discontinue anticonvulsant therapy.

WHAT THE PATIENT NEEDS TO KNOW:

—This medicine must be taken every day as prescribed. It should not be stopped even though you have no seizures and are feeling well.

—If a dose of medicine is missed, take it as soon as possible. If it is nearly time for the next dose, take the next dose only. Continue with regular medication schedule.

—If a dose of medicine is being missed frequently, contact your health provider and discuss this.

—This medicine may decrease your alertness. Do not drive, operate machinery, or do other activities that require alertness, until you know how you react to this medicine.

—You will need to have regular health checkups on a systematic basis while taking this drug. Checkups will be more frequent for the first few months of drug therapy.

—Do not stop this medicine without consulting with your health provider. This is very important.

—Taking this drug with food may decrease gastric irritation.

—Notify your health provider if unusual bleeding or bruising, sore throat or fever, or other new and troublesome symptoms develop.

—Wear a Medic-Alert necklace or bracelet and carry a medical identification card stating your diagnosis and the anticonvulsant medication you are taking.

—Keep this medication out of the reach of children and all others for whom it is not prescribed.

EVALUATION:

ADVERSE REACTIONS: *Cardiovascular:* adenopathy, aggravation of coronary artery disease or hypertension, arrhythmias, AV block, congestive heart failure, hypotension, edema, myocardial infarction, syncope, thrombophlebitis. *CNS:* blurred vision, confusion, dizziness, disturbances of coordination, drowsiness, fatigue, headache, nystagmus, paresthesias, peripheral neuritis, tinnitus, unsteadiness. *Dermatologic:* aggravation of disseminated lupus erythematosus, alopecia, altered pigmentation, erythema multiforme and nodosum, exfoliative dermatitis, photosensitivity reactions, pruritic and erythematous rashes, Stevens-Johnson syndrome, urticaria. *EENT:* conjunctivitis, dry mouth and throat, hallucinations, nystagmus, transient diplopia, visual hallucinations. *Gastrointestinal:* abdominal pain, anorexia, constipation, diarrhea, glossitis, nausea, stomatitis, vomiting. *Genitourinary:* acute urinary retention, azotemia, elevated BUN, glycosuria, impotence, oliguria with hypertension, proteinuria, renal failure, urinary frequency. *Hematopoietic:* agranulocytosis, aplastic anemia, eosinophilia, leukocytosis, leukopenia, purpura, thrombocytopenia. *Hepatic:* abnormal liver function tests, hepatitis, hepatic cellular necrosis, jaundice. *Metabolic:* alterations of thyroid function, chills, diaphoresis, fever, hypocalcemia, inappropriate antidiuretic hormone syndrome. *Other:* scattered punctate cortical lens opacities, osteomalacia, aching joints and muscles, leg cramps.

OVERDOSAGE: *Signs and symptoms:* Dizziness, ataxia, drowsiness, stupor, nausea, vomiting, restlessness, agitation, disorientation, tremor, slowed or hyperactive abnormal reflexes, flushing, cyanosis, increased or decreased blood pressure, urinary retention and coma may develop. *Treatment:* Referral for gastric evacuation through emesis or lavage. Treat symptomatically and monitor vital signs and ECG. There is no specific antidote. Treat shock with IV fluids, oxygen, corticosteroids and other supportive measures.

PARAMETERS TO MONITOR: Prior to initiating therapy, complete blood counts (including platelets, reticulocytes and serum iron) should be obtained. Significant abnormalities rule out the use of this drug. These tests should be repeated frequently (possibly even weekly) during the first three months of therapy and monthly thereafter for at least 2 to 3 years. If aplastic anemia develops, this will require appropriate, intensive monitoring and therapy for which specialized consultation should be sought.

Obtain urinalysis, kidney function and liver function tests every three months. Periodic eye examinations are recommended. Assess for decrease in seizures and monitor anticonvulsant blood levels as indicated. Therapeutic level is 3 to 14 mcg/ml (in adults).

Mary Ann Bolter

ANTICONVULSANTS— HYDANTOINS

ACTION OF THE DRUG: Hydantoins work as an anticonvulsant. Primary site of action is the motor cortex, where the spread of seizure activity is inhibited by either increasing or decreasing the sodium ions across the motor cortex during the generation of nerve impulses.

ASSESSMENT:

INDICATIONS: Treatment of grand mal and psychomotor seizures. Used rarely in Parkinson's syndrome, Meniere's syndrome. Sometimes used to treat status epilepticus as well as migraine and trigeminal neuralgia. Although not FDA approved for this purpose, it is sometimes used to treat digitalis-induced arrhythmias. Also used in some disturbed nonepileptic psychotic patients. Useful in treatment of ventricular arrhythmias after open-heart surgery and acute myocardial infarction; however this is not the drug of choice.

SUBJECTIVE: Patient may present with a history of grand mal, petit mal, Jacksonian, or psychomotor epilepsy. In the absence of a positive history, patient may present with a history of "blackouts," awakening to find signs of incontinence, bitten tongue, soft tissue injuries, or fractures. There is often a history of chronic alcohol abuse.

OBJECTIVE: Family or other reliable sources may be able to describe seizures. There may be evidence of physical injury following a "blackout." Possible studies such as skull x-rays, serum glucose, magnesium, or calcium evaluations; cerebrospinal fluid studies; CT scan of the head; pneumograms; brain scans; or cerebral angiograms may show etiology of convulsion. EEG may be normal, or positive in a patient with epilepsy.

PLAN:

CONTRAINDICATIONS: Do not use with exfoliative dermatitis, hematologic or hepatic disorders, known hypersensitivity to drug, or if breast-feeding. It should not be given parenterally in Adams-Stokes syndrome, sino-atrial block, sinus bradycardia, second and third degree atrio-ventricular block.

WARNINGS: Abrupt withdrawal of this drug may precipitate status epilepticus. Usage in pregnancy increases the risk of teratogenic effects. It has been associated with neonatal hemorrhage. Its use is not indicated in seizures due to hypoglycemia. Subcutaneous or perivascular injection should be avoided because of the highly alkaline nature of the solution. It should be administered intravenously very slowly.

PRECAUTIONS: A small percentage of the population metabolize this drug slowly. Therefore, it is necessary to watch carefully for toxic effects. Alcohol should be avoided while patients are on this drug. Avoid in patients with hypotension, impaired liver function, osteomalacia, who are gravely ill, or the elderly. Lymph node hyperplasia has been reported which in rare cases procedes to malignant lymphoma. Hydantoins may inhibit insulin release, or elevate blood sugar levels in patients with hyperglycemia.

IMPLEMENTATION:

DRUG INTERACTIONS: Hydantoin drug interactions are frequent and often extensive. It is wise to monitor carefully the administration of this drug with concomitant use of any other medication, or vitamins. It may also cause changes in various laboratory tests. The most important interactions are summarized here.

Phenytoins decrease the anticoagulant effects of dicumarol, decrease the action of oral contraceptives (thus leading to higher incidence of contraceptive failure especially in low estrogen contraceptives), reduces the antiarrhythmic properties of disopyramide and quinidine, impair the absorption of furosemide, and speed up the metabolism of digitoxin, thus promoting need for higher digitalis doses. Phenytoins have also been reported to inhibit the action of corticosteroids, particularly dexamethasone and prednisolone. Drugs which increase the effects of phenytoin are coumarin and dicumarol anticoagulants, disulfiram, phenylbutazone, chloramphenicol, cimetidine, sulfonamides, isoniazid, and salicylates. Medications which decrease the effects of phenytoin and thus may produce need for higher dosages are: barbiturates, carbamazepine, antacids, calcium gluconate, oxacillin, antineoplastic drugs, increased dietary calcium, folic acid, CNS depressants and alcohol. Use with tricyclic antidepressants in high doses may precipitate seizures. Hydantoins increase the effects of antihypertensive drugs, sedative and sleep-inducing drugs. It also antagonize the effects of vitamin D. Hydantoins increase the effect of griseofulvin, methotrexate, propranolol. Phenobarbital and valproic acid either increase or decrease level of hydantoins. This drug may interfere with the metyrapone and the 1-mg dexamethasone tests. Glucose and alkaline phosphatase blood levels may be increased. PBI blood levels may be decreased.

ADMINISTRATION AND DOSAGE: All doses must be individualized. Dosage for children is usually larger on a weight basis than for adults. The client should be given a single dose within the therapeutic range and then the amount should gradually be increased until seizures are controlled, or until symptoms of overdosage or toxicity make further increases inadvisable. Medicine should not be stopped abruptly as it may precipitate status epilepticus. Drug compliance is mandatory for the client to maintain a therapeutic level. Avoid changing products once patient is controlled on a particular drug. Accurate dosage of oral suspension is often difficult to administer.

IMPLEMENTATION CONSIDERATIONS:

—Obtain a complete health history, including the presence of hypersensitivity, concurrent use of other medications, hepatic or cardiac problems and the possibility of pregnancy.

—Drugs that control grand mal seizures are not effective for petite mal seizures. If both types of seizures are present a combination of drugs is essential to achieve control.

—Client should keep a record of seizures and bring this to each visit so improvement in control can be monitored. Number of seizures, duration, progression characteristics, time of day, and reaction to seizure should be noted.

—The importance of good oral hygiene, especially of gingivae, should be emphasized in client teaching.

—Provide nutritional counseling regarding the foods rich in vitamin D, particularly if client is an institutionalized or nutritionally deprived child.

—Observe elderly patients for signs of confusion or agitation. The health care provider should be notified regarding these symptoms.

—Adverse effects are frequently found in long-term therapy. The client and family must be educated about their appearance and treatment.

—Prescriptions should be written for a particular brand of medication, and the prescription should note "No substitutions." Once a client is controlled on a brand, he should remain on that brand.

—Drug should be discontinued if patient develops skin rash. Medication may be reinstituted after rash completely disappears only if rash is mild.

—If lymph node enlargement develops, substitute other anticonvulsants whenever possible.

WHAT THE PATIENT NEEDS TO KNOW:

—Take the medicine with food or milk to decrease stomach upset.

—When taking or giving the liquid form of medication, shake the medication well before measuring dose.

—Take only the amount prescribed.

—Maintain good oral hygiene: brush teeth and gums with soft toothbrush twice daily. Rinse mouth well. See a dentist every six months.

—Wear Medic-Alert identification or other bracelet or chain which states your medical problem and the medication you are taking.

—The medication may make your urine appear pink, red, or red-brown.

—Chewable tablets must be chewed or crushed before they are swallowed.

—Do not change brands or dosage forms unless ordered by the health care provider.

—When undergoing any kind of surgery, including dental work, alert the physician or dentist that you are on an anticonvulsant medication.

—Notify health provider immediately if you develop a rash, fever or sore throat. Medication may need to be stopped.

—Avoid alcoholic beverages while on this drug.

—Accurate measuring of oral suspension is important.

EVALUATION:

ADVERSE REACTIONS: *CNS:* apathy, ataxia (not to be confused with unsteadiness in a toddler), confusion, diplopia, dizziness, drowsiness, dysarthria, extrapyramidal reactions, fatigue, fever, hallucinations and delusions, headache, inattentiveness, insomnia, lethargy, muscle twitching, nystagmus, ocular disturbances, postural disturbances, poor memory, slurred speech. *Dermatologic:* acne-like eruptions, bullous, exfoliative or purpuric dermatitis, lupus erythematosus, morbilliform rash, Stevens-Johnson syndrome. *Endocrine:* hirsutism. *Gastrointestinal:* diarrhea, constipation, gingival hyperplasia, nausea, vomiting. *Hematopoietic:* agranulocytosis, anemia, aplastic anemia, bleeding tendency, bruising, epistaxis, granulocytopenia, hemolytic anemia, leukopenia, pancytopenia, petechiae, thrombocytopenia. *Others:* alopecia, chest pain, edema, fever, hepatitis with jaundice, Hodgkin's disease, lymph node hyperplasia, multiple myeloma, nephropathology, numbness, periarteritis, photophobia, polyarthropathy, weight gain.

OVERDOSAGE: *Signs and symptoms:* Ataxia, coma, dysarthria, hypotension, nystagmus, unresponsive pupils may be seen. *Treatment:* There is no specific antidote. Refer to physician. Give general supportive care: lavage, maintenance of airway and blood pressure are indicated. Hemodialysis is utilized, especially with drug toxicity in children.

PARAMETERS TO MONITOR: As baseline, obtain complete blood count and differential, liver function tests, calcium level, and urinalysis. Repeat periodically. Obtain an anticonvulsant blood level at two weeks after medication is initiated, and regularly with visits. Electroencephalogram (EEG) should be obtained initially, and then yearly while client is on drug. At each visit assess for: compliance in taking drug (drug blood level will help do this), adequacy of dental hygiene, adequacy of vitamin D and folic acid intake. Develop a flow chart to use in following number of seizures and appearance and progression of specific side effects. If used for digitalis-induced arrhythmias, obtain continuous ECG monitoring and watch for depression of SA node and prolongation of PR interval.

ETHOTOIN

PRODUCTS (TRADE NAME):
   Perganone (Available as 250 and 500 mg tablets.)
DRUG SPECIFICS:

Has fewer side effects than many other preparations. Diarrhea, drowsiness and sedation are the most commonly found untoward effects. Gum hyperplasia is less than with other preparations. Drug should be taken after food. When used with phenacemide, paranoia may sometimes develop. Caution patients against using heavy machinery and driving if drug has a sedative effect on them. Stress the importance of taking drug regularly and properly.

ADMINISTRATION AND DOSAGE SPECIFICS:

Adults: 500 mg to 1 gram orally the first day with dosage gradually increasing over a period of several days until seizure control is obtained, or daily dose reaches 5 grams. Usually amount is divided into 4 6 doses.

Children Up to 750 mg a day orally initially. Usual maintenance dose in children ranges from 500 mg to 1 gram daily. Administer in 4 6 divided doses daily.

MEPHENYTOIN

PRODUCTS (TRADE NAME):
   Mesantoin (Available as 100 mg tablets.)
DRUG SPECIFICS:

Used in focal and Jacksonian seizures. Less incidence of gum hyperplasia with this preparation. Drug has more sedative effect, and drowsiness frequently occurs. Clients should be warned against driving and operating heavy machinery because of this. Mephenytoin is more likely than some other drugs to cause skin rashes and blood dyscrasia, and therefore is used less with children. If given to children, blood counts should be taken before therapy, two weeks after, and at monthly intervals.

ADMINISTRATION AND DOSAGE SPECIFICS:

Adults: 50-100 mg orally once a day. Can be increased by an additional 50-100 mg in three or four divided doses at one-week intervals. Maximum dosage is 800 mg.

Children: Dosage is the same as for adults. However, maximum dosage is 400 mg.

PHENYTOIN SODIUM

PRODUCTS (TRADE NAME):

Dilantin (Available as 30 mg/5 ml or 125 mg/5 ml suspension, or 50 mg chewable tablets, 30 and 100 mg capsules, and 50 mg/ml injection.) **Ditan** (Available in 100 mg capsules.) **Diphenylan Sodium** (Available in 30 and 100 mg capsules.) **Phenytoin Sodium** (Available as 100 mg capsules, and 50 mg/ml injection.) Combination Products: **Dilantin with Phenobarbital Kapseals** (Available in 100 mg capsules with 16 or 32 mg phenobarbital.)

DRUG SPECIFICS:

Dosage should be individualized to provide maximum benefit. With recommended dosage, a period of seven to ten days may be required to achieve therapeutic blood levels. Check with your own laboratory for therapeutic range of values. Use with caution in hypotensive and severe myocardial insufficiency patients. Phenobarbitals and bromides, if previously administered, should be withdrawn gradually. Do not change from one phenytoin drug to another because of differences in bioavailability. In using the oral suspension, shake well and protect from freezing. There are two types of therapy: "prompt" and "extended" capsules. Capsules labeled "extended" may be used once daily in some patients. Capsules labeled "prompt" should always be given two or three times a day. Do not use chewable tablets for once-a-day treatment. Drug is excreted in breast milk.

ADMINISTRATION AND DOSAGE SPECIFICS:

Adults: 100 mg orally three times a day initially. Gradually increase to achieve level desired. Maintenance dose is 300 400 mg, but it may reach 600 mg.

Children: Initially 5 mg/kg/day orally in 2 or 3 equally divided doses. Gradually increase to achieve level desired up to 300 mg. Maintenance dosage 4-8 mg/kg/day.

Children six years of age and older: May require the minimal adult dosage of 300 mg/day.

Alternative dosage format for adults: Single oral dose of 300 mg extended capsule may be given at one time if patient has been maintained on a regular schedule. It is very important on this regimen not to skip a dose.

Linda Ross

ANTI-CONVULSANTS—
MAGNESIUM SULFATE (PARENTERAL)

ACTION OF THE DRUG: Anticonvulsants may act directly on the motor cortex to inhibit the spread of seizure activity, or cause central nervous system depression. Sometimes the exact mechanism of action is not known. (See also the sections on sedatives, barbiturates and hydantoins.)

ASSESSMENT:

INDICATIONS: Nurse practitioners do not usually initiate anticonvulsant therapy. However, it is often their responsibility to monitor the patient on anticonvulsant therapy, make dosage changes, and initiate appropriate referrals. Magnesium sulfate (parenteral) is used in hypomagnesemic seizures, and for prevention and control of seizures in preeclampsia or eclampsia.

SUBJECTIVE: Patient may present with a history of grand mal, petit mal, Jacksonian, or psychomotor epilepsy. In the absence of a positive history, patient may present with complaints of "blackouts," awakening to find signs of incontinence, bitten tongue, soft tissue injuries, or fractures. A history of chronic alcohol abuse may also be found. Famiily or other releiable sources may be able to describe seizures.

OBJECTIVE: There may be evidence of physical injury following a "blackout." Positive studies such as skull X-rays, serum glucose, magnesium, or calcium; cerebrospinal fluid studies; CT scan of the head; pneumograms; brain scans; or cerebral angiograms may show etiology of convulsion. EEG may be normal, or positive in a patient with epilepsy.

PLAN:

CONTRAINDICATIONS: Magnesium sulfate (parenterally) should not be used in digitalized patients, individuals with decreased respiration, or urinary output less than 100 ml in 4 hours prior to giving medication.

PRECAUTIONS: Magnesium sulfate (parenteral) should be used cautiously in patients with heart block, myocardial damage, severe renal dysfunction, and respiratory disease. Use with caution with women in labor as it crosses the placental barrier.

IMPLEMENTATION:

DRUG INTERACTIONS: Magnesium sulfate (parenteral) used with anesthetics, barbiturates, hypnotics, or narcotics increases central nervous system depression. Used with neuromuscular blocking agents, the blockage is also increased.

PRODUCTS (TRADE NAME):
Magnesium Sulfate (Available in 10, 12.5and 50% with volume equivalent to 1, 1.25, 2.5 and 5 gm/10 ml or 8, 10 and 40 mEq magnesium/10 ml.)

ADMINISTRATION AND DOSAGE: Intramuscular administration of magnesium sulfate provides an effect in about 1 hour and lasts for 3 to 4 hours. The intravenous route produces effects immediately and lasts about 30 minutes. Monitor carefully for toxicity.

Adults: 1-5 gm IM (8-40 mEq) as a 25-50% solution, up to six times daily in alternate buttocks. Or may give 1 to 4 gm IV (8-32 mEq) as a 10 to 20% solution at a rate no greater than 1.5 ml of a 10% solution (or equivalent) per minute. May also be given as an IV infusion: Give 4 gm (32 mEq) in 250 ml of 5% dextrose injection at a rate no greater than 4 ml per minute. Usual adult limits are up to 40 gm (320 mEq) daily.

Children: Give 100 mg IM (0.8 mEq) per kg of body weight as a 50% solution.

IMPLEMENTATION CONSIDERATIONS:

—Obtain a complete health history, including the presence of hypersensitivity, underlying systemic disease (especially cardiac, renal, hepatic, hematologic, or optic dysfunctions), concurrent use of medications, and possibility of pregnancy.

—Document rationale for therapy, and ascertain that the patient's condition is being closely followed by a physician.

—Obtain baseline complete blood count, liver function tests, kidney function tests, ECG, EEG, or other tests as indicated by choice of drug.

—Elderly patients may be more sensitive to standard drug dosages.

—Investigate all legal ramifications with the diagnosis of epilepsy (e.g. driver's license revocation, etc.).

—Do not abruptly discontinue anticonvulsant therapy.

WHAT THE PATIENT NEEDS TO KNOW:

—Notify your health provider if unusual bleeding or bruising, sore throat or fever, or other new and troublesome symptoms develop.

EVALUATION:

ADVERSE REACTIONS: *Cardiovascular:* circulatory collapse, depressed cardiac function, flushing, heart block, hypotension. *CNS:* depressed reflexes, drowsiness, flaccid paralysis, hypothermia. *Other:* hypocalcemia, respiratory depression leading to respiratory paralysis.

OVERDOSAGE: *Signs and symptoms:* Early signs of toxicity include profound thirst, feeling of warmth, sedation, confusion, depressed deep tendon reflexes, and muscle weakness. Signs indicating need for immediate treatment include flushing, circulatory collapse, hypotension, hypothermia, hypotonia, reduced heart rate and reduced respiratory rate. *Treatment:* Supportive measures to restore neuromuscular, respiratory and circulatory function must be utilized. Calcium gluconate given intravenously will reverse magnesium intoxication, but do not give to a digitalized patient as arrhythmias may develop.

PARAMETERS TO MONITOR: Magnesium sulfate (parenteral): Prior to initiating therapy, cardiac function (including ECG), renal function, serum magnesium level, patellar reflex determination and respiratory status (rate should be at least 16 per minute before each injection) should be obtained. Monitor vital signs every 15 minutes if the drug is being given intravenously. Maximum infusion rate is 150 mg per minute.

Observe for respiratory depression and signs of heart block. Monitor intake and output. Urinary output should be 100 ml or greater in the 4-hour period prior to each dose.

Check magnesium blood levels after repeated doses. Levels of greater than 2.5 mEq per liter may demonstrate effective anticonvulsant levels; levels of approximately 4 mEq per liter begin to produce symptoms of overdosage; levels of approximately 10 mEq per liter may cause loss of deep tendon reflexes; levels of 12 to 15 mEq per liter may cause respiratory paralysis. Normal average serum magnesium levels are 1.5 to 2.5 mEq per liter (1.8 to 3 mg per 100 ml).

Mary Ann Bolter

ANTICONVULSANTS— OXAZOLIDINEDIONES

ACTION OF THE DRUG: These dione-type drugs raise the threshold for cortical seizures, but do not modify seizure pattern.

ASSESSMENT:

INDICATIONS: Used in petit mal seizures refractory to treatment with other drugs. Can be used in myoclonic and akinetic epilepsy after other drugs have been used and found to be ineffective.

SUBJECTIVE: Patient may present with a history of grand mal, petit mal, Jacksonian, or psychomotor epilepsy. In the absence of a positive history, patient may present with complaints of "blackouts," awakening to find signs of incontinence, bitten tongue, soft tissue injuries, or fractures. A history of chronic alcohol abuse is often obtained.

OBJECTIVE: Family or other reliable sources may be able to describe seizures. There may be evidence of physical injury following a "blackout." Positive studies such as skull X-rays, serum glucose, magnesium, or calcium; cerebrospinal fluid studies, CT scan of the head, pneumograms; brain scans; or cerebral angiograms may show etiology of convulsion. EEG may be normal, or positive in a patient with epilepsy.

PLAN:

CONTRAINDICATIONS: Do not use if there is any indication of hypersensitivity to the drug itself; blood dyscrasias, severe hepatic or renal dysfunction.

WARNINGS: Serious side effects may occur; therefore it is imperative that the patient be supervised carefully during the first year of therapy. These drugs should only be used when other drugs for petit mal epilepsy have been ineffective.

PRECAUTIONS: Use during pregnancy may cause congenital abnormalities. Neonatal hemorrhage may occur because of lowered vitamin K-dependent clotting factors. Abrupt withdrawal of this drug may precipitate petit mal status.

IMPLEMENTATION:

DRUG INTERACTIONS: High doses of tricyclic antidepressants and antipsychotics may provoke seizures. Mephenytoin or phenacemide used with dione-type anticonvulsants, increases the risk of toxicity. Both aminosalicylic acid (PAS) and oral anticoagulants raise the central nervous system depressant effects of this category.

ADMINISTRATION AND DOSAGE: Begin with smallest dose and increase gradually until symptoms are controlled. Take with food or milk to lessen gastric irritation. When replacing this medication with another anticonvulsant medication, start the other medication, and reduce the oxazolidinedione slowly. If discontinuing medication, reduce it gradually so as to avoid petit mal status. Taking drug with food may decrease gastric irritation.

IMPLEMENTATION CONSIDERATIONS:

—Take a complete patient history, including presence of hypersensitivity, underlying systemic diseases (especially renal or liver dysfunction, eye problems or eye diseases), other medications taken concurrently, and possibility of pregnancy. Also look for history of alcohol abuse, particularly if patient will be taking paramethadione solution.

—Perform a complete physical examination, noting particularly the condition of the eyes and mouth in order to evaluate any future changes.

—Document rationale for therapy, and ascertain that the patient's condition is being closely followed by a physician.

—Petit mal seizures are less likely to occur in women of reproductive age, but it may be necessary to discuss whether patient is pregnant or planning on becoming pregnant.

—Discuss with the family and patient common side effects of the medication which should be reported to the health care provider: edema, urinary frequency, burning or clouding of urine.

—Mild sedation may occur with these medications and the patient should be cautioned about driving or use of machinery in which this might be a problem.

—Elderly patients may be more sensitive to standard drug dosages.

—Obtain baseline complete blood count, liver function tests, kidney function tests, EEG, ECG, or other tests as indicated by patient problems.

—Investigate all legal ramifications with the diagnosis of epilepsy (e.g. driver's license revocation, etc.)

WHAT THE PATIENT NEEDS TO KNOW:

—Take this medication exactly as ordered. Do not stop taking it even if you have no seizures and are feeling well. This medication should be taken with food or milk to avoid upsetting your stomach. If a dose of medicine is missed, take it as soon as possible. If it is nearly time for the next dose, take only the next dose. Do not take the missed dose and do not double the next dose. Continue with regular medication schedule.

—The medicine may make you drowsy, so caution must be exercised in driving, operating heavy machinery, or performing tasks which require alertness.

—Any signs or symptoms of urinary frequency, burning, cloudiness of urine, or any unexplained swelling should be reported to your health care provider.

—Sometimes this medicine may make your eyes unusually sensitive to the sun. Wearing dark glasses may help relieve this.

—If you continue to have seizures while taking this medication, the record of the number of seizures and a description of them should be kept, and brought with you when you see your health care provider.

—Taking medication regularly, as ordered, and keeping visits to your health provider are essential while you take this drug.

—Wear a Medic-Alert or other bracelet identifying your medical problem and the medicine you are taking.

—Yearly evaluations by dentist and eye doctor while you on this medication will help detect any problems you may be having with the drug.

—Keep this medication out of the reach of children and all others for whom it is not prescribed.

EVALUATION:

ADVERSE REACTIONS: *Cardiovascular:* changes in blood pressure. CNS: drowsiness, fatigue, headache, increased irritability, insomnia, malaise, myasthenia gravis-like syndrome, paresthesias, personality changes, vertigo. *Dermatologic:* acneiform or morbilliform rash, alopecia, erythema multiforme, exfoliative dermatitis, petechiae. *EENT:* diplopia, epistaxis, photophobia, retinal hemorrhage. *Gastrointestinal:* abdominal pain, anorexia, bleeding gums, gastric distress, hiccoughs, nausea, vomiting, weight loss. *Genitourinary:* albuminuria, fatal nephrosis, vaginal bleeding. *Hematopoietic:* agranulocytosis, aplastic anemia, eosinophilia, hypoplastic anemia, leukopenia, pancytopenia, thrombocytopenia, retinal and petechial hemorrhages, *Hepatic:* abnormal liver function tests. *Other:* alopecia, proteinuria, sore throat and fever.

PARAMETERS TO MONITOR: Prior to initiating therapy, a complete blood count, liver function studies, and urinalysis should be obtained. If significant abnormalities exist, use another type of drug. The CBC should be repeated monthly for 12 months. If no abnormalities have appeared, the interval between studies may be increased. Repeat other tests periodically while patient is taking drug.

Some degree of neutropenia with or without a corresponding decrease in leukocytes is not uncommon. Therapy should be stopped if the neutrophil count is 2,500 cu mm or less. More frequent examinations are necessary when the count is less than 3,000 cu mm.

Liver function tests and urinalysis should be done monthly. Obtain baseline blood pressure, eye examination, gynecological examination; repeat at least yearly.

Therapeutic level for Paramethadione is 60 to 71 mcg/ml. Therapeutic level for Trimethadione is 20 to 40 mcg/ml.

Ask on each visit about prominent side effects, and evaluate patient for extent of compliance in taking the drug.

PARAMETHADIONE

PRODUCTS (TRADE NAME):
Paradione (Comes as both 150 mg capsules and 300 mg/ml oral solutions.)
DRUG SPECIFICS:
Paramethadione has a slightly greater sedative effect than trimethadione. Paramethadione capsules should not be broken or chewed; and the oral solution has a high alcoholic content (65%) and should be diluted with 1/2 glass of water. Use the calibrated dropper to measure the solution, dilute with juice, milk or water before taking. 300 mg tablet contains tartrazine which may cause some allergic-type reactions.

Phenytoin is often administered with this agent in the treatment of mixed types of seizures. This drug has more of a sedative effect than trimethadione. It is known to have the potential for producing fetal malformations and serious side effects.
ADMINISTRATION AND DOSAGE SPECIFICS:
Adults: Initially 300 mg orally three times a day for one week and then begin to increase on a weekly basis, 300 mg per day until seizures are controlled. Total daily dose should not exceed 2.4 grams.

Children 6 years and older: 300 mg three times a day. Readjust dosages by response.

Children ages 2 to 6 years: 200 mg three times a day.

Children up to age 2 years: 100 mg orally three times a day.

TRIMETHADIONE

PRODUCTS (TRADE NAME):
Tridione (Available in 150 mg chewable tablets; 300 mg capsules and 40 mg/ml solution.)
DRUG SPECIFICS:
Trimethadione chewable tablets may be crushed in a small amount of water before administration. Store below 40 degrees centigrade and in a tight container.

Trimethadione has less of a sedative effect than paramethadione. It is known to have the potential for producing fetal malformations and serious side effects.

ADMINISTRATION AND DOSAGE SPECIFICS:

Adults: Initial dose is 300 mg orally, three or four times a day for 1 week. Then begin to increase weekly by 300 mg until desired effect is obtained. Total daily dose is 2.4 grams.

Children 12 years and older: 400 mg three times a day. Dose maintenance can be 40 mg/kg/24 hours.

Children 6 to 12 years: 300 mg three times a day.

Children 2 to 6 years: 200 mg three times a day.

Children up to age 2 years: 100 mg three times a day.

Linda Ross

ANTICONVULSANTS— PHENACEMIDE

ACTION OF THE DRUG: Anticonvulsants may act directly on the motor cortex to inhibit the spread of seizure activity, or cause central nervous system depression. Sometimes the exact mechanism of action is not known. (See also the sections on sedatives, barbiturates and hydantoins.)

ASSESSMENT:

INDICATIONS: Nurse practitioners do not usually initiate anticonvulsant therapy. However, it is often their responsibility to monitor the patient on anticonvulsant therapy, make dosage changes, and initiate appropriate referrals. Phenacemide is used only for severe refractory epilepsy.

SUBJECTIVE: Patient may present with a history of grand mal, petit mal, Jacksonian, or psychomotor epilepsy. In the absence of a positive history, patient may present with complaints of "blackouts," awakening to find signs of incontinence, bitten tongue, soft tissue injuries, or fractures. There may also be a history of chronic alcohol abuse. Family or other reliable sources may be able to describe seizures.

OBJECTIVE: There may be evidence of physical injury following a "blackout." Positive studies such as skull x-rays, serum glucose, magnesium, or calcium; cerebrospinal fluid studies; CT scan of the head; pneumograms; brain scans; or cerebral angiograms may show etiology of convulsion. EEG may be normal, or positive in a patient with epilepsy.

PLAN:

PRECAUTIONS: Phenacemide should be used cautiously in patients with severe hepatic dysfunction, history of allergy (especially to other anticonvulsants), or history of personality disturbances. This drug is extremely toxic. Use only when other anticonvulsants are ineffective.

IMPLEMENTATION:

DRUG INTERACTIONS: Phenacemide has no significant drug interactions.
PRODUCTS (TRADE NAME):
Phenurone (Available in 500 mg tablets.)

ADMINISTRATION AND DOSAGE: Duration of action is approximately five hours. Phenacemide can produce serious side effects and direct organ toxicity. It is usually administered when other anticonvulsants are ineffective. Initiating therapy with low doses and gradually increasing drug until an adequate response is achieved may minimize side effects. If adding a drug to existing anticonvulsant therapy, the new drug should be added gradually while the other anticonvulsant is gradually decreased. Never abruptly discontinue anticonvulsant therapy. Gradual withdrawal is suggested. Taking drug with food may decrease gastric irritation.

Adults: 500 mg three times daily. May increase by 500 mg each week. The effective total daily dose usually ranges from 2 to 3 gm.

Children ages 5 to 10 years: 250 mg three times daily. May increase by 250 mg each week. Maximum is 1.5 gm daily.

IMPLEMENTATION CONSIDERATIONS:

—Obtain a complete health history, including the presence of hypersensitivity, underlying systemic disease (especially cardiac, renal, hepatic, hematologic, or optic dysfunctions), concurrent use of medications, and possibility of pregnancy.

—Document rationale for therapy, and ascertain that the patient's condition is being closely followed by a physician.

—Obtain baseline complete blood count, liver function tests, kidney function tests, ECG, EEG, or other tests as indicated by choice of drug.

—Elderly patients may be more sensitive to standard drug dosages.

—Investigate all legal ramifications with the diagnosis of epilepsy (e.g., driver's license revocation, etc.).

—Do not abruptly discontinue anticonvulsant therapy.

WHAT THE PATIENT NEEDS TO KNOW:

—This medicine must be taken every day as prescribed. It should not be stopped even though you may have no seizures and may be feeling well.

—If a dose of medicine is missed, take it as soon as possible. If it is nearly time for the next dose, take the next dose only. Continue with regular medication schedule.

—If a dose of medicine is being missed frequently, contact your health care provider and discuss this.

—This medicine may decrease your alertness. Do not drive, operate machinery, or do other activities that require alertness, until you know how you react to this medicine.

—You will need to have regular health checkups on a systematic basis while taking this drug. Checkups will be more frequent for the first few months of drug therapy.

—Do not stop this medicine without consulting with your health practitioner This is very important.

—Taking this drug with food may decrease gastric irritation.

—Notify your health care provider if unusual bleeding or bruising, sore throat or fever, or other new and troublesome symptoms develop.

—Wear a Medic-Alert necklace or bracelet and carry a medical identification card identifying your diagnosis and the anticonvulsant medication you are taking.

—Keep this medication out of the reach of children and all others for whom it is not prescribed.

EVALUATION:

ADVERSE REACTIONS: *CNS:* aggressiveness, depression, dizziness, drowsiness, headache, insomnia, paresthesias, suicidal tendencies. *Dermatologic:* rashes. *Gastrointestinal:* anorexia, weight loss. *Genitourinary:* nephritis. *Hematopoietic:* agranulocytosis, aplastic anemia, leukopenia. *Hepatic:* hepatitis, jaundice.

OVERDOSAGE: *Signs and symptoms:* Excitement or mania, followed by drowsiness, ataxia and coma, are symptoms of acute overdosage. *Treatment:* Refer for gastric evacuation either by inducing emesis or lavage. General supportive measures are needed. After recovery, a careful evaluation of liver and kidney function, mental status and blood-forming organs should be obtained.

PARAMETERS TO MONITOR: Prior to initiating therapy, a complete blood count, liver function tests and a urinalysis should be obtained. Significant abnormalities of these tests could rule out the use of phenacemide. Complete blood count should be repeated every month for one year. If no abnormality has developed, the interval may be lengthened. Marked depression of the blood count is indicative of need for withdrawal of the drug.

Urinalysis and liver function studies should be monitored monthly throughout therapy. Discontinue drug if signs and symptoms of dysfunction develop.

Mary Ann Bolter

ANTICONVULSANTS— PRIMIDONE

ACTION OF THE DRUG: Primidone is an anticonvulsive drug which alters seizure patterns and raises the seizure threshold. The mode of action is not known. Phenobarbital and phenylethylmalonamide (PEMA) are metabolites of primidone.

ASSESSMENT:

INDICATIONS: Although nurses would not usually prescribe this medication, they are often given responsibility for monitoring the patient on primidone therapy. Primidone is used for the control of grand mal, focal or psychomotor epileptic seizures. It is often used with other drugs in the therapy of refractory seizures. It has also been used experimentally in the treatment of benign familiar or essential tremors.

SUBJECTIVE: Patient may present with a history of grand mal, focal or psychomotor seizure disorders. In the absence of a positive history, patient may present with complaints of "blackouts," awakening to find signs of incontinence, bitten tongue, soft tissue injuries or fractures.

OBJECTIVE: Family or other reliable sources may be able to describe seizures. There may be evidence of physical injury following a "blackout." Positive studies such as skull x-rays, serum glucose, magnesium, or calcium; cerebrospinal fluid studies; CT scan of the head; pneumograms; brain scans; or cerebral angiograms may show etiology of convulsion. EEG may be normal or positive in a patient with epilepsy.

PLAN:

CONTRAINDICATIONS: Do not give in the presence of hypersensitivity to phenobarbital, or if the patient is known to have porphyria.

WARNINGS: Safety for use in pregnant women has not been established. There appears to be an association between the use of this drug and an elevated incidence of birth defects in children born to these women. The drug is usually not given to breast-feeding women since it is excreted in large quantities in breast milk, producing drowsiness or somnolence in children. Patients should understand that it may take several weeks for the appropriate therapeutic level of medication to be determined, and that regulation to control seizure activity may take some time. Patients or providers should never abruptly stop this medication, since there would be high risk of provoking status epilepticus.

PRECAUTIONS: Total daily dosage should not exceed 2 grams. Adequate baseline general blood studies should be obtained, and repeated at least every 6 months while patient is taking this medication.

IMPLEMENTATION:

DRUG INTERACTIONS: Although there are no reported drug interactions with primidone, it must be remembered that this drug is rapidly metabolized to phenobarbital and PEMA, and that all drug interactions reported for the barbiturates might be relevant in the individual receiving primidone.

PRODUCTS (TRADE NAME):
Myidone (Available in 250 mg tablet.) **Mysoline** (Available in 50 and 250 mg tablets, and in 250 mg/5 ml oral suspension.) **Primidone** (Available in 250 mg tablets.) **Primoline** (Available in 250 mg tablets.)

ADMINISTRATION AND DOSAGE: Dosage must be individualized, based upon patient response. Medication is absorbed from GI tract and is found in peak levels in about 3 hours. It is rapidly metabolized to PEMA and phenobarbital, with PEMA appearing in a few hours, while levels of phenobarbital may take several days to detect. The amount of primidone metabolism and the levels of the metabolites found vary among individuals. Serum blood levels of both primidone and phenobarbital should be obtained in order to determine therapeutic levels. The clinically effective serum level for primidone is between 5 and 12 mcg/ml, and 15 to 45 mcg/ml for phenobarbital. Begin at low dose and increase slowly to avoid over-sedation.

Adults and children over 8 years of age with no previous therapy: Use the following schedule:

Days 1-3: 100 to 125 mg at bedtime; Days 4-6: 100 to 125 mg twice daily; Days 7-9: 100 to 125 mg three times daily; Day 10 and thereafter: 250 mg three times daily. Increase by 50 mg doses as needed. Do not exceed doses of 500 mg four times daiy.

Children under 8 years of age with no previous therapy: Use the following schedule:

Days 1-3: 50 mg at bedtime; Days 4-6: 50 mg twice daily; Days 7-9: 100 mg twice daily; Day 10 and thereafter: 125 to 250 mg three times daily.

Adjunctive anticonvulsant therapy: Start primidone at 100 to 125 mg at bedtime and gradually increase primidone as other medications are decreased. If goal is to continue with primidone alone, wean other drug over a two to three week interval.

IMPLEMENTATION CONSIDERATIONS:

—Obtain a complete health history, including the presence of hypersensitivity to phenobarbital, underlying systemic disease, concurrent use of medications, and possibility of pregnancy.

—Document rationale for therapy, and ascertain that the patient's condition is being closely followed by a physician.

—Obtain baseline complete blood count, and SMA-12 screening blood studies, EEG, or other tests as indicated by the problem.

—Investigate all legal ramifications with the diagnosis of epilepsy (e.g., driver's license revocation).

—Do not abruptly discontinue anticonvulsant therapy.

—Obtain serum phenobarbital and primidone levels to determine if dosing regimen keeps patient within therapeutic level.

—Rarely, megaloblastic anemia develops as a result of primidone therapy. This may be treated with folic acid supplements without discontinuing medication.

—Ataxia and vertigo commonly develop. Patient needs to be encouraged to continue taking the medication, since these symptoms will disappear within a few days if therapy is continued. In situations where symptoms persist, decrease dosage of primidone until problems disappear.

—Follow mood changes in patients, since severe irritability or personality deterioration as a result of the drug may necessitate its discontinuance.

WHAT THE PATIENT NEEDS TO KNOW:

—This medication must be taken every day as prescribed. If should not be stopped even though you may have no seizures and may be feeling well.

—This medication may be taken with food if it causes stomach upset.

—If a dose of medicine is missed, take it as soon as possible. If it is nearly time for the next dose, take the next dose only. Continue with regular medication schedule. If a dose of medicine is being missed frequently, contact your health care provider and discuss this.

—This medicine may decrease your alertness. Do not drive, operate machinery, or do other activities that require alertness, until you know how you react to this medicine. Sedation will decrease with continued use.

—You will need to have health checkups on a regular basis while taking this drug. Checkups will be more frequent for the first few months of drug therapy.

—Do not stop this medicine without consulting with your health care provider. This is very important.

—Notify your health care provider if unusual bleeding, skin rash, joint pain, fever, or other new or troublesome symptoms develop. Often patients initially have a little staggering when they walk, or experience feelings of dizziness. These usually disappear after taking the drug for a few days.

—Wear a Medic-Alert bracelet or necklace and carry a medical identification card with your diagnosis and the anticonvulsant medication you are taking.

—Keep this medication out of the reach of children and all others for whom it is not prescribed.

EVALUATION:

ADVERSE REACTIONS: *CNS:* ataxia, diplopia, drowsiness, emotional disturbances, fatigue, hyperirritability, mood changes, nystagmus, paranoia, vertigo. *Dermatologic:* morbilliform skin eruptions. *Gastrointestinal:* anorexia, nausea, vomiting. *Hematopoietic:* megaloblastic anemia.

PARAMETERS TO MONITOR: Prior to initiating therapy, a complete blood count, SMA-12 blood screening, and EEG should be obtained. Complete blood count and SMA-12 should be obtained every 6 months during therapy. Watch for reduction in number and severity of seizures, and monitor serum primidone and phenobarbital levels to establish and maintain therapeutic dosage regimen. Monitor for adverse effects, particularly megaloblastic anemia, mood and personality disorders.

Marilyn W. Edmunds

ANTICONVULSANTS— SUCCINIMIDE-TYPE

ACTION OF THE DRUG: Succinimide-type anticonvulsants elevates seizure threshold in the cortex and basal ganglia and reduces synaptic response to low frequency repetitive stimulation. These products also suppress the wave pattern of the EEG.

ASSESSMENT:

INDICATIONS: Control of petit mal seizures. Methsuximide is used for refractory petit mal cases.

SUBJECTIVE: Patient may present with a history of grand mal, petit mal, Jacksonian, or psychomotor epilepsy. In the absence of a positive history, patient may present with complaints of "blackouts," awakening to find signs of incontinence, bitten tongue, soft tissue injuries, or fractures. A history of chronic alcohol abuse is often obtained.

OBJECTIVE: Family or other reliable sources may be able to describe seizures. There may be evidence of physical injury following a "blackout." Positive studies such as skull X-rays, serum glucose, magnesium, or calcium; cerebrospinal fluid studies; CT scan of the head; pneumograms; brain scans; or cerebral angiograms may show etiology of convulsion. EEG may be normal, or positive in a patient with epilepsy.

PLAN:

CONTRAINDICATIONS: Do not give in the presence of hypersensitivity to drugs in this category.

WARNINGS: Do not use in patients with liver or renal disease. There is also the possibility of inducing blood dyscrasias or systemic lupus erythematosus. Safety during pregnancy is not established, and risk must be weighed against benefit if patient is breast-feeding.

PRECAUTIONS: It is important to gradually increase or decrease dosage. Sometimes this drug will increase the frequency of grand mal attacks. It may also impair the patient's ability to operate heavy machinery because of significant drowsiness.

IMPLEMENTATION:

DRUG INTERACTIONS: Succinimides will decrease the effect of amphetamines. Concomitant administration with other anticonvulsants can result in increased libido or frequency of grand mal seizures. Chloramphenicol or other bone-depressing drugs should not be used in conjunction with this medication. Tricyclic antidepressants and antipsychotics in high doses may also provoke additional seizures.

ADMINISTRATION AND DOSAGE: The initial doses of succinimides should be small, and dosage increases should be gradual and guided by drug levels in the blood. Seven to ten days are required for drug level to reach therapeutic range. When drug is to be discontinued, or replaced with another anticonvulsant, it should be reduced slowly, while at the same time increasing the other drug.

IMPLEMENTATION CONSIDERATIONS:

—Obtain a complete health history, including presence of hypersensitivity, underlying systemic disease (especially renal, hepatic, or blood disorders), concurrent use of medications, and possibility of pregnancy.

—Baseline laboratory studies including complete blood counts, liver function studies, kidney function studies, EEG, ECG, or other tests as indicated by choice of drug.

—Patient should keep a record regarding occurrence of uncontrolled seizures: time, duration, characteristics and reaction.

—Counsel the patient and family regarding the possibility of transient personality changes. These should be reported back to the health provider.

—Document rationale for therapy, and ascertain that the patient's condition is being closely followed by a physician.

—Elderly patients may be more sensitive to standard drug dosages.

—Investigate all legal ramifications with the diagnosis of epilepsy (e.g. driver's license revocation.)

WHAT THE PATIENT NEEDS TO KNOW:

—Take this medication exactly as prescribed. It should not be stopped even though you may have no seizures and may be feeling well. If a dose of medicine is missed, take it as soon as possible. If it is nearly time for the next dose, take only the next dose. Do not double dose. Continue with the regular medication schedule. Avoid alcoholic drinks while on this drug.

—If medication upsets stomach, take it with food or milk.

—Wear a Medic-Alert or other bracelet or chain identifying your health problem, and the medication you are taking.

—Do not discontinue this drug abruptly. Do not change the dosage of medication except as advised by your health provider.

—This drug depresses alertness and may affect your ability to drive or operate heavy machinery.

—Notify your primary provider if you have any unusual reactions to the drug: skin rash, joint pain, unexplained fever, sore throat, unusual bleeding or bruising, drowsiness, dizziness, or blurred vision.

—The use of this drug is not advised in pregnancy. Advise your health provider if you intend to become pregnant.

—It is crucial that medication be taken in the amount specified, and at the times indicated by the provider if seizures are to be avoided.

—Regular follow-up appointments with your health provider are mandatory to evaluate your reactions to this drug.

—Keep this medication out of the reach of children and all others for whom it is not prescribed.

EVALUATION:

ADVERSE REACTIONS: *CNS:* ataxia, dizziness, drowsiness, dyskinesias, euphoria, fatigue, headaches, hiccoughs, irritability, hyperactivity, lethargy, and mood or mental changes. *Dermatologic:* pruritic, erythematous rashes; Stevens-

Johnson syndrome, urticaria. *EENT:* blurred vision, periorbital edema, photophobia. *Gastrointestinal:* anorexia, abdominal pain, cramps, diarrhea, nausea, vomiting, weight loss. *Genitourinary:* urinary frequency, vaginal bleeding. *Hematopoietic:* eosinophilia, leukopenia, monocytosis, pancytopenia. *Other:* alopecia, muscular weakness, systemic lupus erythematosus. *Psychiatric or psychological:* aggressiveness, confusion, depression, disturbances of sleep, hypochondriacal behavior, inability to concentrate, instability, mental slowness, and night terrors.

OVERDOSAGE: *Signs and symptoms:* Same as adverse reactions. *Treatment:* Referral for gastric evacuation. Treat symptomatically and use supportive measures as needed.

PARAMETERS TO MONITOR: Prior to initiating therapy, obtain liver and kidney function tests and complete blood count. If any abnormalities exist, use drug with extreme caution. These tests should be repeated at routine intervals throughout therapy. Serum levels should be periodically obtained to monitor for therapeutic levels of anticoagulants. On each visit ask about possible side effects, psychological status. Evaluate seizure activity carefully to determine if drug dosage is adequate.

ETHOSUXIMIDE

PRODUCTS (TRADE NAME):
Zarontin (Available as 250 mg capsules or 250 mg/5 ml syrup.)
DRUG SPECIFICS:
Used in combination therapy when other forms of epilepsy coexist with the petit mal form. This drug does not significantly alter blood serum or urinary laboratory values when taken at therapeutic levels. Therapeutic levels of ethosuximide are 40 to 100 mcg/ml. Store medication in well-closed, light-resistant containers. Take drug with meals to decrease gastric discomfort.
ADMINISTRATION AND DOSAGE SPECIFICS:
Adults and children above 6 years: 250 mg twice daily initially, increase by 250 mg every 4 to 7 days until seizures are controlled or total daily dose reaches 1.5 gm. The optimal dosage for most children is 20 mg/kg daily.
Children 3 to 6 years: 250 mg per day orally initially, increase by 250 mg every 4 to 7 days until seizures are controlled or total daily dose reaches 1 gm.

METHSUXIMIDE

PRODUCTS (TRADE NAME):
Celontin Kapseals (Available in 150 and 300 mg capsules.)
DRUG SPECIFICS:
Used in combination therapy when other forms of epilepsy coexist with the

petit mal form. Store in well-closed, light resistant container in a cool place. Contains FD&C Yellow # 5, tartrazine, which can cause an allergic type reaction in some susceptible populations. This drug can also change some laboratory values: It may causea positive albumin in the urine and a positive BUN. Therapeutic levels for methsuximide are 10 to 40 mcg/ml.

ADMINISTRATION AND DOSAGE SPECIFICS:

Adults: 300 mg once a day initially; increase by 300 mg at weekly intervals until seizures are controlled or total daily dose reaches 1.2 gm.

Children: Usual adult dosage. Small children may require adjustment using 150 mg capsule.

PHENSUXIMIDE

PRODUCTS (TRADE NAME):

Milontin Kapseals (Available as 500 mg capsules.)

DRUG SPECIFICS:

Used in combination therapy when other forms of epilepsy coexist with the petit mal form. Shake suspension well before pouring. Take drug with meals to decrease gastric discomfort. May be administered in combination with other anticonvulsants when mixed forms of seizures exist. Can change urine to pink, red or red-brown colors. With prolonged use, efficacy of the drug decreases. Also it is the least toxic but the least effective of this group. Drowsiness and dizziness may be relieved by decreasing dosage.

ADMINISTRATION AND DOSAGE SPECIFICS:

Adults and children: 500 mg twice daily initially, increased by 500 mg at weekly intervals until seizure control or total daily dose reaches 3 gm.

Linda Ross and Mary Ann Bolter

VALPROIC ACID

ACTION OF THE DRUG: Anticonvulsants may act directly on the motor cortex to inhibit the spread of seizure activity, or cause central nervous system depression. Sometimes the exact mechanism of action is not known. (See also the sections on sedatives, barbiturates and hydantoins).

ASSESSMENT:

INDICATIONS: A nurse practitioner does not usually initiate anticonvulsant therapy. However, it is often their responsibility to monitor the patient on anticonvulsant therapy, make dosage changes, and initiate appropriate referrals. Valproic acid is used in treatment of simple (petit mal) seizures, complex absence seizures, and multiple seizure types. It has also been used prophylactically to prevent recurrent febrile seizures in children.

SUBJECTIVE: Patient may present with a history of grand mal, petit mal, Jacksonian, or psychomotor epilepsy. In the absence of a positive history, patient may present with complaints of "blackouts" awakening to find signs of incontinence, bitten tongue, soft tissue injuries, or fractures. There may also be a history of chronic alcohol abuse. Family or other reliable sources may be able to describe seizures.

OBJECTIVE: There may be evidence of physical injury following a "blackout." Positive studies such as skull x-rays, serum glucose, magnesium, or calcium; cerebrospinal fluid studies; CT scan of the head; pneumograms; brain scans; or cerebral angiograms may show etiology of convulsion. EEG may be normal, or positive in a patient with epilepsy.

CONTRAINDICATIONS: Valproic acid should not be given to patients hypersensitive to the drug, and to patients with hepatic dysfunction.

PRECAUTIONS: Valproic acid should be used with caution in patients with blood dyscrasias, renal or hepatic dysfunction. Animals taking valproic acid show reduced fertility, however, this action has not been demonstrated in humans.

WARNINGS: Hepatic failure, often fatal, has occurred in patients receiving valproic acid, most often within the first six months of therapy. Teratogenicity is produced in human offspring when this drug is taken by pregnant women. The drug is also excreted in breast milk.

IMPLEMENTATION:

DRUG INTERACTIONS: Alcohol, anesthetics, antidepressants, MAO inhibitors or central nervous system depressants used with this product increase central nervous system depression. This is seen especially with phenobarbital. Anticoagulants, aspirin, dipyridamole or sulfinpyrazone and valproic acid may prolong the bleeding time. Used with phenytoin and clonazepam, breakhrough seizures and other unpredictable therapeutic effects may develop. Urine ketone tests and thyroid function studies may also be altered by these products.

PRODUCTS (TRADE NAME):
Depakene (Available in 250 mg capsules, 250 mg/5 ml syrup as sodium valproate.) **Depakote** (Available in 250 and 500 mg enteric-coated tablets as divalproex sodium.)

ADMINISTRATION AND DOSAGE: Initiating therapy with low doses and gradually increasing drug until an adequate response is achieved may minimize side effects. If adding a drug to existing anticonvulsant therapy, the new drug should be added gradually while the other anticonvulsant is gradually decreased. Never abruptly discontinue anticonvulsant therapy. Gradual withdrawal is suggested. Taking drug with food may decrease gastric irritation. The capsules should be swallowed without chewing or breaking to avoid local irritation of the mouth and throat. Mixing the syrup with carbonated beverages may cause local irritation. The average well-tolerated serum concentration is 40 to 100 mcg/ml.

Adults and children: 15 mg/kg daily, increase by 5 to 10 mg/kg at one week intervals until seizure control is obtained. If total daily dose exceeds 250 mg, give in divided doses. Usual limit is 30 mg/kg daily.

IMPLEMENTATION CONSIDERATIONS:

—Obtain a complete health history, including the presence of hypersensitivity, underlying systemic disease (especially cardiac, renal, hepatic, hematologic, or optic dysfunctions), concurrent use of medications, and possibility of pregnancy.

—Document rationale for therapy, and ascertain that the patient's condition is being closely followed by a physician.

—Obtain baseline complete blood count, liver function tests, kidney function tests, ECG, EEG, or other tests as indicated by choice of drug.

—Elderly patients may be more sensitive to standard drug dosages.

—Investigate all legal ramifications with the diagnosis of epilepsy (e.g. driver's license revocation, etc.).

—Do not abruptly discontinue anticonvulsant therapy.

—Watch for signs of hepatotoxicity such as malaise, weakness, lethargy, anorexia, vomiting and loss of seizure control.

—Urine ketone tests may be altered and diabetic control may be more difficult to monitor.

WHAT THE PATIENT NEEDS TO KNOW:

—This medicine must be taken every day as prescribed. It should not be stopped even though you may have no seizures and may be feeling well.

—If a dose of medicine is missed, take it as soon as possible. If it is nearly time for the next dose, take the next dose only. Continue with regular medication schedule.

—If a dose of medicine is being missed frequently, contact your health care provider and discuss this.

—This medicine may decrease your alertness. Do not drive, operate machinery, or do other activities that require alertness, until you know how you react to this medicine.

—You will need to have regular health checkups on a systematic basis while taking this drug. Checkups will be more frequent for the first few months of drug therapy.

—Do not stop this medicine without consulting with your health practitioner. This is very important.

—Taking this drug with food may decrease gastric irritation.

—Notify your health provider if unusual bleeding or bruising, sore throat or fever, or other new and troublesome symptoms develop.

—Wear a Medic-Alert necklace or bracelet and carry a medical identification card identifying your diagnosis and the anticonvulsant medication you are taking.

—Keep this medicine out of the reach of children and all others for whom it is not prescribed.

EVALUATION:

ADVERSE REACTIONS: *CNS:* aggression, ataxia, coma, depression, diplopia, dizziness, emotional upset, headache, hyperactivity, incoordination, insomnia, nystagmus, psychosis, sedation, weakness. *Dermatologic:* petechiae, skin rash, transient increases in hair loss. *Endocrine:* abnormal thyroid tests, irregular menses, secondary amenorrhea. *Gastrointestinal:* abdominal cramps, acute pancreatitis, anorexia, constipation, diarrhea, increased appetite and weight gain, indigestion, nausea, pancreatitis, vomiting. *Hematopoietic:* anemia, bone marrow suppression, bruising, frank hemorrhage, increased bleeding time, inhibited platelet aggregation, leukopenia, thrombocytopenia. *Hepatic:* hepatitis, severe hepatotoxicity and death, transient SGPT, SGOT enzyme elevations.

OVERDOSAGE: *Signs and symptoms:* Deep coma is produced. *Treatment:* Referral for gastric lavage is of limited value as the drug is rapidly absorbed. Use general supportive measures and maintain an adequate urinary output. Naloxone has been reported to reverse the CNS depressant effects of valproic acid. Use with caution, as it can also reverse the antiepileptic effects of the drug.

PARAMETERS TO MONITOR: Prior to initiating therapy, obtain liver function studies, platelet counts and prothrombin time. If abnormalities exist, use this drug with caution. Repeat tests at least every 2 months. Discontinue drug if significant dysfunction appears.

Monitor for therapeutic level of anticonvulsant. Therapeutic serum levels for most patients will be 50 to 100 mcg/ml.

Mary Ann Bolter

ANTIEMETIC AND ANTIVERTIGO AGENTS

ACTION OF THE DRUG: Drugs are helpful as antiemetic or antivertigo products when they act to reduce indirect stimulation of the vomiting center (as do anticholinergic agents) or when they reduce dopamine, which acts as a mediator to induce vomiting. There are also several drugs effective in controlling vomiting for which the mechanism of action is not known.

ASSESSMENT:

INDICATIONS: Vomiting may be produced by direct action on the vomiting center of the brain, by indirect action through stimulation of the chemoreceptor trigger zone and by increased activity of chemical neurotransmitters. Thus, drugs, metabolic disorders, radiation, motion sickness, gastric irritation, vestibular neuritis or increases in central trigger zone dopamine or vomiting center acetylcholine may all provoke vomiting. Drugs act by one or more mechanisms to inhibit this response. Antiemetic or antivertigo preparations are used most frequently to prevent and treat motion sickness and to prevent and control nausea and vomiting that occurs with anesthesia and surgery. Antidopaminergic preparations (primarily the phenothiazines: chlorpromazine, perphenazine, prochlorperazine, promethazine, and triflupromazine) and other antiemetic medications (benzquinamide, diphenidol, hydroxyzine HCl and some of the corticosteroids) are used almost exclusively for controlling nausea and vomiting. Anticholinergic medications (antihistamines such as buclizine, cyclizine, dimenhydrinate, diphenhydramine and meclizine and scopolamine and trimethobenzamide) are also used for controlling motion sickness. Of all the products, meclizine, dimenhydrinate and diphenidol are the only products used to control vertigo.

SUBJECTIVE: The health care provider may elicit a history of motion sickness or extrapyramidal reactions due to antipsychotic therapy, labyrinthitis, vertigo, Meniere's syndrome, radiation therapy or diabetes. Nausea and vomiting is one of the most common adverse reactions to drug therapy and may occur after taking almost any drug.

OBJECTIVE: Patients may be without objective findings unless vomiting is ongoing. With some cases of vomiting, other CNS findings may be present, such as nystagmus, sensory hearing deficit, and a positive Romberg's sign.

PLAN:

WARNINGS: These medications should be used with extreme caution in patients performing work that requires mental alertness, since some products produce drowsiness in selected individuals. These preparations are not recommended for use in children because in combination with some illnesses, they may contribute to the development, the misdiagnosis or the severity of symptoms in Reye's syndrome, an encephalopathy often fatal in children.

PRECAUTIONS: Vomiting is often an important diagnostic clue and may point to serious underlying problems. The cause of the vomiting or nausea should be determined, and appropriate treatment undertaken to eliminate the problem. These products should not be the only form of therapy in cases of nausea or vomiting. Attempts to maintain hydration, restore electrolyte balance and reduce accompanying symptoms should be made. Use of antiemetic drugs without adequate diagnostic exploration may prohibit the diagnosis of other, more serious problems.

IMPLEMENTATION:

DRUG INTERACTIONS: The sedative effect of some antiemetic medications is potentiated by concurrent use of other CNS depressants. They also have an additive effect with anticholinergic drugs. Anticholinergic antiemetics can intensify the anticholinergic side effects of the MAO inhibitors as well as the tricyclic antidepressants. The drug interactions may vary, depending upon the type of antiemetic or antivertigo drug but would be similar to other anticholinergic or antidopaminergic products.

ADMINISTRATION AND DOSAGE: These products generally come in tablets, sustained action capsules and concentrates for oral use. For patients who are vomiting or so nauseated that they are unable to take oral medications, injection or suppository forms are usually available. When medications are given for motion sickness, they should be administered 30-60 minutes before the estimated travel time.

IMPLEMENTATION CONSIDERATIONS:

—Obtain a complete health history to rule out hypersensitivity, concurrent use of drugs that would cause drug interactions (especially MAO inhibitors) and possibility of pregnancy.

—In all cases, search for the underlying cause of vomiting, nausea, or vertigo.

—In women of childbearing years, always investigate the possibility of pregnancy. These drugs should not be used for treatment of morning sickness since safety in pregnancy has not been demonstrated.

—Dosage should be as low as possible, and therapy should be terminated as quickly as possible. Intravenous preparations should be reserved for severe cases in hospitalized patients.

WHAT THE PATIENT NEEDS TO KNOW:

—Take this medication as instructed by your health care provider. Do not double dose or alter medication schedule.

—If the drug is taken for motion sickness, it should be administered 30-60 minutes before departure and 30 minutes before meals thereafter.

—Do not drive, operate hazardous machinery or engage in tasks that require alertness while taking these drugs.

—Do not take any other medications without the knowledge of your health care provider. It is especially important to avoid other CNS depressants, including alcohol, because of the sedative effect.

—While some patients experience drowsiness while taking this medication, this is usually transient and will disappear with continued use of the drug.

—Keep this medication out of the reach of children and all others for whom it is not prescribed. Overdosages of this medicine may be very toxic.

EVALUATION:

ADVERSE REACTIONS: See sections on individual drugs for specific information.

PARAMETERS TO MONITOR: During the initial visit, a complete history should be obtained in addition to vital signs and cardiovascular and neurologic assessment. A previous history of similar problems, exposure to drugs, radiation, toxins or other persons with similar symptoms should be investigated. The possibility of pregnancy should be investigated. Once treatment has started, monitor for therapeutic effects. Medication may be started with injection or suppository and when switched to oral form when control has been established. Monitor for adverse effects.

ANTICHOLINERGIC/ANTIEMETIC AGENTS

BUCLIZINE HCl

PRODUCTS (TRADE NAME):
Bucaldin-S Softabs (Available in 50 mg tablets.)
DRUG SPECIFICS:
Buclizine HCl is an antiemetic with central anticholinergic activity. It is also used for nausea and vomiting associated with motion sickness and may be useful for the symptoms associated with labyrinthitis. The softab may be swallowed, chewed or dissolved in the mouth. These tablets contain tartrazine, which may precipitate allergic reactions, particularly in persons sensitive to aspirin. The drug is contraindicated in pregnant women or in persons with known buclizine hypersensitivity.
ADMINISTRATION AND DOSAGE SPECIFICS:
Antiemetic:
Adults: 50 mg three times a day with a maintenance dose of 50 mg twice a day.

CYCLIZINE

PRODUCT (TRADE NAME):
Marezine (Available in 50 mg tablets and 50 mg/ml injectable solution.)
DRUG SPECIFICS:
Cyclizine is an antiemetic, anticholinergic and antihistaminic agent that also reduces the sensitivity of the labyrinthine apparatus. The drug is used primarily in the treatment of nausea and vomiting of motion sickness. Persons who take this drug are often predisposed to the CNS depressant effects of the antihistamine agents. The injectable solution is a sterile solution appropriate for intramuscular injection only. The drug is contraindicated in pregnancy and in children. The drug has been used in postoperative nausea and vomiting, but this use is no longer recommended because of its dangerous hypotensive effects.
ADMINISTRATION AND DOSAGE SPECIFICS:
Antiemetic:
Adults: 50 mg tablets po 30 minutes before travel; repeat every 4-6 hours; maximum 300 mg/day. Administer 50 mg IM every 4-6 hours.

DIPHENHYDRAMINE HCL

PRODUCTS (TRADE NAME):
Benadryl (Available in 25 mg and 50 mg capsules, 12.5 mg/5 ml elixir with

14% alcohol, lotion or ointment and 10 mg or 50 mg/ml injection.) **Bendylate** (Available in 25 mg and 50 mg capsules; and 10 mg/ml or 50 mg/ml injection.) **Caladryl** (Available in 12.5 mg/5 ml elixir and in 1% cream or lotion.) **Diphenhydramine HCl** (Available in 25 mg and 50 mg capsules and 10 mg and 50 mg/ml injection.) **Fenylhist** (Available in 25 mg and 50 mg capsules.) **Nordryl** (Available in 10 mg or 50 mg/ml injection.) **SK-Diphenhydramine** (Available in 25 mg and 50 mg capsules.) **Surfadil** (Available in 1% cream or lotion.) **Valdrene** (Available in 50 mg tablets.) **Zalydryl** (Available in lotion form equivalent to 2% diphenhydramine, 2% zinc oxide and 2% alcohol.)

DRUG SPECIFICS:

Diphenhydramine is an antihistamine that blocks histamine receptors on peripheral effector cells. Diphenhydramine has anticholinergic, antitussive, antiemetic and sedative properties. It is used often in allergic conjunctivitis, allergic reactions to blood or plasma, allergic rhinitis, uncomplicated angioedema, pruritus and urticaria, insomnia, motion sickness, vasomotor rhinitis and anaphylactic reactions and adjunctively to epinephrine and antiparkinsonian therapy. The drug is not indicated for treatment of lower respiratory disease, in newborn or premature infants, and in pregnant or nursing mothers. It has a high incidence of CNS depressant effects associated with its use. Use of these agents in the elderly or debilitated is more likely to produce CNS depressant effects. The most frequent adverse reactions occurring with diphenhydramine are sedation, dizziness, disturbed coordination, epigastric distress and thickening of bronchial secretions.

Pediatric fatalities have resulted from doses of 100 mg of diphenhydramine. Topical preparations can cause a high degree of hypersensitivity. With intravenous use, blood pressure should be carefully monitored.

ADMINISTRATION AND DOSAGE SPECIFICS:

Adults: 50 mg three to four times daily po or 10 to 50 mg IM or IV; maximum daily dosage is 400 mg.

Children over 20 lbs: 12.5 to 25 mg po three to four times daily or 5 mg/kg daily either po or parenterally.

SCOPOLAMINE

PRODUCTS (TRADE NAME):

Scopolamine HSr (Available in 0.4 mg and 0.6 mg soluble tablets.) **Transderm-Scop** (Available in 1.5 mg transdermal therapeutic system that delivers 0.5 mg scopolamine over 3 days.) **Triptone** (Available in 0.25 mg capsules.)

DRUG SPECIFICS:

These products come in oral form as well as in a new transdermal package that is placed postauricularly and releases medication at a constant rate over a 3-day interval. The transdermal mechanism allows for lower dosage and produces fewer adverse anticholinergic effects than the oral forms. Scopolamine is used to control motion sickness in adults. Its use is contraindicated in patients with narrow angle glaucoma, prostatic hypertrophy and pyloric obstruction. It also should be used with caution in patients with renal or hepatic dysfunction, intestinal obstruction or cardiac disease or in the elderly. Potentially fatal idiosyncratic reactions have occurred with therapeutic doses. Safety has not been demonstrated for use in children or in pregnant or breast-feeding women. Common adverse effects include drowsiness, dryness of mouth, blurred vision, dilation of the pupils and impairment of eye accommodation. More infrequently, dizziness, restlessness, disorientation, confusion, memory disturbances, urinary retention, rashes, erythema, and dry and itchy eyes may occur. Excessive dosages may lead to delirium, fever, stupor progressing to coma, respiratory failure and eventually death. Antidote for overdosage is physostigmine. The transdermal system should be applied behind the ear and will dispense a uniform amount of medication (0.5 mg) over 3 days.

ADMINISTRATION AND DOSAGE SPECIFICS:

Motion sickness: 0.25 to 0.8 mg po 1 hour before anticipated travel.

Prolonged therapy: Apply one patch postauricularly at least 4 hours before the antiemetic effect is desired. Replace every 3 days for continued therapy.

TRIMETHOBENZAMIDE HCL

PRODUCTS (TRADE NAME):

Spengan (Available in 100 mg/ml injection.) **Tigan** (Available in 100 mg and 250 mg capsules, 200 mg suppositories, 100 mg pediatric suppositories and 100 mg/ml injection.) **Trimethobenzamide HCl** (Available in 100 mg/ml injection.)

DRUG SPECIFICS:

Trimethobenzamide HCl is an antiemetic that inhibits the chemoreceptor trigger zone in the medulla. It is used for the control of nausea and vomiting. Extreme caution should be exercised in using this agent with children since the drug has been linked to the development of Reye's syndrome. Also the drug can cause extrapyramidal symptoms that can be confused with Reye's syndrome or encephalopathy in children or elderly adults. The drug should only be used in children with prolonged vomiting of known etiology. The drug is contraindicated in patients with a known hypersensitivity to trimethobenzamide. Suppositories are contraindicated for persons with a known hypersensitivity to benzocaine; the suppository form is also contraindicated in newborns and premature infants, while the injectable form is contraindicated in children. The adverse effects of this drug include parkinsonian-like symptoms, blood dyscrasias, blurred vision, coma, convulsions, disorientation, depression, dizziness, drowsiness, headache, diarrhea, jaundice, muscle cramps, and opisthotonos. Persons who are currently receiving or have received other CNS agents (phenothiazines, barbiturates, and belladonna derivatives) should not receive this product. Antiemetics should not be used in acute abdominal conditions since they may obscure the diagnosis. The injectable form of the drug is intended only for intramuscular use, since the injectable solution is highly irritating to the tissues, causing pain, stinging, burning, redness and swelling at the injection site. To minimize these effects, inject deeply into the upper outer quadrant of the gluteal region and avoid the escape of solution along the route.

ADMINISTRATION AND DOSAGE SPECIFICS:

Adult: 250 mg po three to four times daily, 200 mg three to four times daily via the IM route or 200 mg three to four times daily via rectal suppositories.

Children between 30 and 90 lbs: 100 mg po three to four times daily or 100 to 200 mg three to four times daily via rectal suppositories.

Children under 30 lbs: 100 mg rectal suppositories three to four times daily.

ANTICHOLINERGIC, ANTIEMETIC AND ANTIVERTIGO AGENTS

DIMENHYDRINATE

PRODUCTS (TRADE NAME):

Dimentabs (Available in 50 mg tablets.) **Dimenhydrinate** (Available in 50 mg tablets, 12.5 mg/4 ml and 50 mg/1 ml solution for injection.) **Dramamine** (Available as 50 mg tablets, 100 mg suppositories, 12.5 mg/4 ml, and 50 mg/1 ml solution for injection.) **Eldodram, Marmine** (Available in 50 mg tablets.) **Motion-Aid Elixir** (Available in 12.5 mg/4 ml elixir.) **Trav-Arex, Vertiban** (Available in 50 mg tablets.)

DRUG SPECIFICS:

Dimenhydrinate is an antiemetic, antivertigo agent used in motion sickness or radiation sickness or following anesthesia. Its exact pharmacologic mechanism is unknown, but it appears to depress motion-induced stimulation of the labyrinthine structures. Its CNS sedative effects are more pronounced than other antiemetics, especially with high doses.

The drug is contraindicated in pregnancy, in children under age 3, in patients using ototoxic drugs and in persons with known hypersensitivity to dimenhydrinate, diphenhydramine or theophylline. Dimenhydrinate may interfere with anticoagulation therapy, so patients should be advised to contact health care provider if neurologic or vascular problems occur. These agents can decrease erythrocytes, leukocytes, and platelet counts and can reduce the uptake of radioactive iodine 131. For prevention of motion sickness, administer 30-60 minutes before departure.

ADMINISTRATION AND DOSAGE SPECIFICS:

Adults: 50 to 600 mg/day po in divided doses: 100 mg rectally one to two times daily as needed; or 50 mg as needed IV. (Dilute parenteral form in 10 ml sodium chloride injection.)

Children over 3 years: 1.25 mg/kg three to four times a day with a maximum dosage of 300 mg/day in po or IV form.

MECLIZINE HCl

PRODUCTS (TRADE NAME):

Antivert (Available as 12.5 mg and 25 mg tablets and 25 mg chewable tablets.) **Bonine, Dizmiss** (Available as 25 mg chewable tablets). **Meclizine Hydrochloride** (Available in 12.5 mg and 25 mg tablets and 25 mg chewable tablets). **Motion Cure** (Available in 25 mg chewable capsule.) **Wehvert** (Available in 25 mg tablets.)

DRUG SPECIFICS:

Meclizine HCl is an antiemetic, anti-motion sickness and antivertigo agent with anticholinergic properties. Its use is contraindicated in pregnant women and children because it has been associated with teratogenicity in rats. Due to its antihistaminic characteristics, the drug has CNS depressant effects. Therefore, providers need to caution patients from taking other CNS depressants when taking this product. The injectable solution should be stored in a cold place to prevent discoloration.

ADMINISTRATION AND DOSAGE SPECIFICS:

Motion sickness: 50 mg 1 hour prior to departure; repeat every 24 hours as needed.

Vertigo: 25 to 100 mg/day as needed in divided doses.

ANTIDOPAMINERGIC ANTIEMETIC AGENTS

CHLORPROMAZINE HCL

PRODUCTS (TRADE NAME):

Chlorpromazine HCl (Available in 10 mg, 25 mg, 50 mg, 100 mg and 200 mg tablets, 100 mg/ml concentrate and 25 mg/ml injection.) **Chloramead, Promapar** (Available in 10 mg, 25 mg, 50 mg, 100 mg and 200 mg tablets.) **Thorazine** (Available in 10 mg, 25 mg, 50 mg, 100 mg and 200 mg tablets, 10 mg/5 ml syrup, 30 mg/ml and 100 mg/ml concentrate, 25 mg and 100 mg suppositories, 25 mg/ml injection, and 30 mg, 75 mg, 150 mg, 200 mg and 300 mg timed-release Spansules.)

DRUG SPECIFICS:

This product is a phenothiazine derivative used for control of nausea and vomiting and for the therapy of intractable hiccoughs. Patients should be warned not to use alcohol or CNS depressant drugs concurrently and that the medication might cause drowsiness. Patients should not be involved in activities requiring alertness. Medication may also discolor urine pink or reddish brown. Photosensitivity may occur, and patient should avoid prolonged exposure to sunlight. This drug is also used as an antianxiety agent, and more information may be obtained in that section of this book. For severe vomiting, intramuscular medication is generally indicated and is started at a low dose. Hypotension must be watched for, and larger doses may be given depending upon patient response. Medication is switched to oral form as soon as patient can tolerate it.

ADMINISTRATION AND DOSAGE SPECIFICS:

Nausea and vomiting:

Adults: 10 to 25 mg po every 4-6 hours as needed, 50 to 100 mg rectally every 6-8 hours as needed or 25 mg IM. If no hypotension develops, IM dose may be increased to 50 mg every 3-4 hours.

Children over 6 months: 0.25 mg/lb po every 4-6 hours, 0.5 mg/lb rectally every 6-8 hours or 0.25 mg/lb IM every 6-8 hours as needed. Children up to 5 years should not receive more than 40 mg/day. Children 5 to 12 years should not receive more than 75 mg/day unless severely vomiting.

PERPHENAZINE

PRODUCTS (TRADE NAME):

Trilafon (Available in 2 mg, 4 mg, 8 mg and 16 mg tablets, 8 mg Repetabs, 16 mg/5 ml concentrate and 5 mg/ml injection.)

DRUG SPECIFICS:

This product is a phenothiazine derivative used for control of severe nausea and vomiting and for therapy of intractable hiccoughs in adults. Patients should be warned not to use alcohol or other CNS depressant drugs concurrently and that the medication might cause drowsiness. Patients should not be involved in activities requiring alertness. Medication may also discolor urine pink or reddish brown. Photosensitivity may occur, and patient should avoid prolonged exposure to sunlight. This drug is also used as an antianxiety agent and more information may be obtained in that section of this book. For severe vomiting, intravenous or intramuscular medication is generally indicated and is started at a low dose. Intravenous use should be reserved for hospitalized patients and given in a slow drip infusion. Hypotension and extrapyramidal side effects may develop, and medication should be discontinued if they occur. Medication should be switched to oral form as soon as patient can tolerate it.

ADMINISTRATION AND DOSAGE SPECIFICS:

Nausea, vomiting or hiccoughs: 8 to 16 mg po daily in divided doses. Occasionally, as much as 24 mg may be needed. For rapid control of vomiting, 5 mg IM may be given. Higher doses and intravenous therapy should be reserved for hospitalized patients.

PROCHLORPERAZINE

PRODUCTS (TRADE NAME):

Compazine (Available in 5 mg, 10 mg and 25 mg tablets, 10 mg, 15 mg, 30 mg and 75 mg sustained-release Spansules, 5 mg/5 ml syrup, 10 mg/ml concentrate, 2.5 mg, 5 mg and 25 mg suppositories and 5 mg/ml injection.) **Prochlorperazine** (Available in 5 mg, 10 mg and 25 mg tablets and 5 mg/ml injection.)

DRUG SPECIFICS:

This product is a phenothiazine derivative used in the treatment of nausea and vomiting as well as for therapy in anxiety states. It may cause drowsiness and discolor the urine pink or reddish brown. Photosensitivity may develop, and the patient should be warned against excessive exposure to sunlight. Action of intramuscularly administered medication may last for up to 12 hours. In children, therapy lasting longer than 1 day is generally not needed.

ADMINISTRATION AND DOSAGE SPECIFICS:

Nausea and vomiting in adults: 5 to 10 mg po three or four times daily or 15 mg sustained-release tablet may be ordered every morning or a 10 mg sustained-release tablet given every 12 hours. Medication may be given rectally, 25 mg twice daily, or 5 to 10 mg IM, repeated in 3-4 hours as necessary. Do not exceed 40 mg/day IM.

Adjunct to anesthesia: 5 to 10 mg IM or IV 1-2 hours before induction of anesthesia. IM dose may be repeated once after 30 minutes or for control of acute symptoms during and after surgery.

Nausea and vomiting in children over 20 pounds: In children 40 to 85 lbs, give 2.5 mg three times daily or 5 mg twice daily. Do not exceed 15 mg/day. In children 30 to 39 lbs, give 2.5 mg two or three times daily orally or rectally. Do not exceed 10 mg/day. In children 20 to 29 lbs, give 2.5 mg one or two times daily orally or rectally. Do not exceed 7.5 mg/day. If intramuscular medication is indicated, give 0.06 mg/lb.

THIETHYLPERAZINE MALEATE

PRODUCTS (TRADE NAME):

Torecan (Available in 10 mg tablets and suppositories and 5 mg/ml injection.)

DRUG SPECIFICS:

This phenothiazine derivative probably acts directly on the chemoreceptor trigger zone and the vomiting center itself to reduce nausea and vomiting. It should not be given in the presence of hypersensitivity to the phenothiazines or if patient has reduced level of consciousness. It must not be given during pregnancy. There are many drug interactions for phenothiazines (see phenothiazine antipsychotic drug section). Alcohol and other CNS depressants should not be taken concurrently. Intravenous use of this drug is to be avoided since it will produce severe hypotension. Intramuscular use should be limited to deep injection at or shortly before the termination of anesthesia. Dosage has not been determined for children.

ADMINISTRATION AND DOSAGE SPECIFICS:

Nausea and vomiting: 10 to 30 mg/day in divided doses.

TRIFLUPROMAZINE HCL

PRODUCTS (TRADE NAME):
Vesprin (available in 50 mg/5 ml oral suspension and 10 or 20 mg/ml injection.)
DRUG SPECIFICS:
This phenothiazine derivative is used for the control of severe nausea and vomiting. Patients should be warned not to use alcohol or other CNS depressant drugs concurrently and that the medication might cause drowsiness. Patients should not be involved in activities requiring alertness. Medication may also discolor urine pink or reddish brown. Photosensitivity may occur, and patients should avoid prolonged exposure to sunlight. Activity of drug may last for up to 12 hours following intramuscular administration in children.
ADMINISTRATION AND DOSAGE SPECIFICS:
Adults: 20 to 30 mg po total daily dose for prophylaxis; 5 to 15 mg IM for vomiting, repeated every 4 hours as needed up to 60 mg, or 1 mg IV, up to 3 mg total daily dosage.
Children over 2.5 years: 0.2 mg/kg po, not to exceed 10 mg/day in three divided doses: 0.2 to 0.25 mg/kg IM may be given, not to exceed 10 mg/day.

ANTIDOPAMINERGIC ANTIEMETIC AND ANTIVERTIGO AGENTS

PROMETHAZINE HCL

PRODUCTS (TRADE NAME):
Phenergan, Promethazine HCl (Available in 12.5 mg, 25 mg and 50 mg tablets, 6.25 mg and 25 mg/5 ml syrup, 12.5 mg, 25 mg and 50 mg suppositories and 25 mg and 50 mg/ml IM injection.) **Promethacon** (Available in 25 and 50 mg suppositories.) **Remsed** (Available in 50 mg tablets.)
DRUG SPECIFICS:
Promethazine, a phenothiazine derivative, is effective in the treatment of motion sickness and in the prevention and control of nausea and vomiting associated with surgery and anesthesia. Promethazine potentiates the action of barbiturates and narcotics. Dosage of barbiturates should be reduced by at least one half and narcotic dosage reduced by one fourth to one half when given in combination with promethazine. Alcohol and other CNS depressants should not be used concurrently. This product causes drowsiness, and patients should be cautioned not to perform tasks requiring alertness. Medication may discolor urine pink or reddish brown. Patients should be warned that this product may produce photosensitivity. Do not

use in premature or newborn infants. Subcutaneous injection may result in tissue necrosis; intra-arterial injection may produce gangrene of the extremity.

ADMINISTRATION AND DOSAGE SPECIFICS:

Motion Sickness:

Adults: 25 mg 30 minutes to 1 hour before travel; repeat 8-12 hours later if needed. On succeeding days, take 25 mg on arising and again before the evening meal.

Children: 12.5 to 25 mg twice daily.

Nausea and Vomiting:

Adults: 12.5 to 25 mg po, IM or rectally every 4-6 hours as needed. If parenteral medication is indicated, give 25 mg deep IM. Intravenous medication should be given to hospitalized patients only.

Children: 0.25 to 0.5 mg/kg IM or rectally every 4-6 hours as needed. For parenteral medication, do not give more than one half of the adult dose. Preoperatively, equal doses of promethazine and a barbiturate or narcotic and an atropine-like drug may be given.

ANTIEMETICS, MISCELLANEOUS AGENTS

BENZQUINAMIDE HCL

PRODUCTS (TRADE NAME):

Emete-Con (Available in 50 mg injection.)

DRUG SPECIFICS:

This drug has an antiemetic, antihistaminic, sedative, and mild anticholinergic effect, although the exact mode of action is not known. Effects are usually demonstrated within 15 minutes. It is used in the prophylaxis and treatment of nausea and vomiting due to anesthesia and surgery. It should be used judiciously in only those patients in whom emesis would bring harm. Atrial and ventricular arrhythmias and sudden increases in blood pressure have been associated with the intravenous use of this product. It may mask overdosage of toxic drugs or confuse the diagnosis of some diseases that produce nausea. Safety has not been demonstrated in children. This product may potentiate the effect of other pressor agents or epinephrine-like drugs if given concurrently. Drowsiness and dry mouth seem to be the most common adverse reactions; however, muscular twitching, shaking and weakness may be found, as well as anorexia, nausea, insomnia, fatigue, restlessness, headache, excitement, nervousness and widespread autonomic nervous system reactions. Hives, rashes and allergic reactions may also be demonstrated.

ADMINISTRATION AND DOSAGE SPECIFICS:

Prophylaxis with anesthesia: 50 mg (0.5 to 1 mg/kg) IM at least 15 minutes before terminating anesthesia. Repeat in 1 hour, then every 3-4 hours as necessary.

Intravenously, 25 mg (0.2 to 0.4 mg/kg) may be given as a single dose slowly (1 ml/ minute), with the following doses given intramuscularly.

ANTIEMETICS, MISCELLANEOUS AGENTS

HYDROXYZINE

PRODUCTS (TRADE NAME):
Atarax (Available in 10 mg, 25 mg, 50 mg and 100 mg hydroxyzine HCl tablets and 10 mg/5 ml syrup.) **Hydroxyzine HCl** (Available in 10 mg, 25 mg, 50 mg and 100 mg tablets, and 25 mg, 50 mg, 75 mg and 100 mg/ml injection.) **Hydroxyzine Pamoate** (Available in 25 mg, 50 mg and 100 mg capsules.) **Vistaril** (Available in 25 mg, 50 mg and 100 mg capsules, 25 mg, 50 mg, 75 mg and 100 mg/ml injection and 25 mg/5 ml oral suspension.)

DRUG SPECIFICS:
This drug has antiemetic and antihistamine properties but is primarily used in patients with anxiety. (See Antianxiety Agents for more information.)

ADMINISTRATION AND DOSAGE SPECIFICS:
Nausea and vomiting: 25 to 100 mg IM for adults and 1.1 mg/kg (0.5 mg/lb) IM for children.

Preoperative and postoperative adjunctive medication: 25 to 100 mg IM for adults and 1.1 mg/kg (0.5 mg/lb) IM for children.

Preoperative and postpartum adjunctive therapy: 25 to 100 mg IM.

Doreen C. Harper and Marilyn W. Edmunds

ANTIEMETICS AND ANTIVERTIGO AGENTS, MISCELLANEOUS AGENTS

DIPHENIDOL

PRODUCT (TRADE NAME):
Vontrol (Available in 25 mg tablets.)

DRUG SPECIFICS:
This very potent drug is used for treatment of vertigo through action on the vestibular apparatus and for inhibition of the chemoreceptor trigger zone in controlling nausea and vomiting. Because it may cause hallucinations, disorientation and confusion, its use should be confined to hospitalized patients unresponsive to other therapy. These symptoms, although occurring in only about 0.5% of patients,

may begin after 3 days of therapy at recommended doses. More usual side effects are drowsiness, depression, sleep disturbance, dry mouth, gastrointestinal irritation and blurred vision. Rash, headache, heartburn and malaise may also develop. These side effects usually subside spontaneously within 3 days of discontinuing therapy. Treatment should be given by a physician who carefully examines both potential risks and benefits. It has been helpful in Meniere's disease, middle and inner ear surgery and labyrinthine vertigo, which produces nausea and vomiting. It has also been used for nausea and vomiting due to anesthesia and malignant neoplasms. Because the drug is excreted through the kidneys, it should not be given in the presence of anuria. Safety for use has not been established for pregnant and breast-feeding women. Because of the anticholinergic effects, it should be used cautiously in patients with glaucoma, peptic ulcer, prostatis hypertrophy, pyloric and duodenal obstruction and organic cardiospasm. Because the product contains tartrazine, sensitive individuals may develop an asthma-like reaction. Overdosage may produce hypotension and respiratory depression.

ADMINISTRATION AND DOSAGE SPECIFICS:

Adults: 25 to 50 mg every 4 hours for nausea or vertigo.

Children over 25 lbs: 0.4 mg/lb for nausea or vomiting; may repeat in 4 hours as needed. Do not exceed 2.5 mg/lb in 24 hours.

ANTIPARKINSONIAN AGENTS

ACTION OF THE DRUG: The two main actions of the antiparkinsonian agents are either to (1) block the uptake of acetylcholine at postsynaptic muscarinic cholinergic receptor sites or (2) elevate the functional levels of dopamine in motor regulatory centers. These drugs exert a wide range of effects on the organs affected by the autonomic nervous system, including the eye, respiratory tract, heart, gastrointestinal tract, urinary bladder, nonvascular smooth muscle, exocrine glands and the CNS. The antiparkinsonian agents reduce muscle tremors and rigidity, improving mobility, muscular coordination and performance.

ASSESSMENT:

INDICATIONS: These drugs are used as antiparkinsonian agents and to reduce the extrapyramidal side effects of antipsychotic agents.

SUBJECTIVE: Practitioner may elicit a history of Parkinson's disease, concurrent antipsychotic drug therapy, drooling, and/or difficulty with coordination and walking. Patient may be in the middle-aged or elderly category, and have tremors at rest made worse by emotional stress. There may be failure of arms to move when walking, rigidity first occurring in the proximal musculature, inability to perform activities of daily living, and a history of manganese poisoning, hypoxia, carbon monoxide poisoning, iron intoxication, or a family member with Parkinson's disease.

OBJECTIVE: The practitioner may find frozen muscles, resting tremors of hands, arms, lips and eyelids, pillrolling movement of hands, cogwheel rigidity of the limbs, stooped posture, a monotonous weak voice, flat, labile affect, mask-like expression and unilateral weakness, festinating gait, athetosis, chorea, tics and bradykinesia.

PLAN:

CONTRAINDICATIONS: These drugs are contraindicted for persons with known hypersensitivity, acute narrow angle glaucoma, asthma, history of epilepsy, peptic ulcer disease, skin lesions, acute psychoses, history of melanoma, those exposed to rubella, or patients on CNS stimulants and MAO inhibitors.

WARNINGS: Caution should be exercised in using the dopaminergic drugs in patients with severe cardiovascular, pulmonary, renal, hepatic or endocrine disease, peptic ulcer, chronic wide angle glaucoma, diabetes, and psychiatric illnesses. They should be administered cautiously to children, pregnant or breast-feeding women and to the elderly since their safety has not been established in these groups. These preparations are known to aggravate preexisting arrhythmias secondary to myocardial infarction. Excessive doses are associated with toxicity. Early signs of toxicity include muscle twitching, intermittent winking and sudden extreme weakness and bradykinesia. The anticholinergic agents should be used with caution in patients with glaucoma, pyloric, duodenal or bladder neck obstruction; prostatic hypertrophy, myasthenia gravis, peptic ulcer, cardiac, liver, or kidney dysfunction, in children, the elderly, chronically ill or alcoholic patients and in pregnant or breast-feeding women. Early signs of toxicity include: agitation, restlessness and insomnia, or sudden increase in parkinsonian symptoms.

PRECAUTIONS: The anticholinergics and some dopaminergics must be withdrawn slowly because many of these drugs have long half-lives. When withdrawing a preparation and beginning a new preparation, the new drug should be started in small doses and the old drug should be withdrawn gradually. These agents are usually initiated at the lowest dose possible and increased gradually until the maximum therapeutic effect has been obtained. The numerous adverse effects of these drugs can be controlled by decreasing the dosage. Common side effects include dry mouth, blurred vision, dizziness, nausea and vomiting, drowsiness, nervousness and urinary hesitancy. In addition, patients taking levodopa may experience ataxia, mild depression, peripheral edema, and skin mottling.

IMPLEMENTATION:

DRUG INTERACTIONS: Common drug interactions differ according to whether the preparation is an anticholinergic or a dopaminergic agent. Among the drugs which interact with the anticholinergic agents, several interactions are noted. The anticholinergics combine additively with amantidine, procainamide, quinidine, phenothiazines, the MAO inhibitors, and the antidepressants, increasing their toxicity. They also potentiate the sedative actions of the CNS depressants. The concurrent use of anticholinergics and antipsychotic agents may precipitate a psychotic episode. The dopaminergic agents interact with relatively few drugs. The additive effects of amantadine and the anticholinergics were previously noted and excessive CNS stimulation may occur when dopaminergic drugs are given concurrently with other CNS stimulants. These drugs may elevate BUN, SGOT, SGPT, LDH, bilirubin, ad alkaline phosphatase. WBC, hemoglobin and hematocrit may be reduced. Levodopa may cause false-negative readings with Clinistix and false-positive readings with Clinitest. Urine catecholamines may show false-positive results, whereas urinary VMA may show false negative results.

ADMINISTRATION AND DOSAGE: These drugs fall into two major categories: anticholinergics (benztropine, biperiden, diphenhydramine, ethopropazine, procyclidine, orphenadrine, and trihexphenidyl), and dopaminergic agents (amantadine, bromocriptine, carbidopa, and levodopa). These drugs are available in tablets, sustained-release capsules, syrups, elixirs, and IV and IM injections. These drugs are generally well absorbed from the gastrointestinal tract. Peak blood levels are achieved from 1-6 hours depending on the route of administration and the type of drug administered, except for the sustained-release capsules which reach peak plasma blood levels in 8 to 12 hours. Sustained-release capsules are not recommended for initial therapy because they do not allow enough flexibility in dosage regulation. Also, IV injection of the anticholinergics can cause hypotension and incoordination. Often carbidopa and levodopa are administered concurrently in the preparation. Carbidopa/levodopa acts to retard the peripheral breakdown of l-dopa. If this combination drug is administered following levodopa, then levodopa should be discontinued at least 8 hours prior to initiating therapy with carbidopa-levodopa. The combination should be substituted at a dosage level which provides 25% of the previous levodopa dose. Occasionally, when these combination doses are excessive, both drugs can be titrated individually.

IMPLEMENTATION CONSIDERATIONS:

—Obtain a complete health history, including the presence of hypersensitivity, concurrent use of medications which may produce drug interactions, presence of asthma, renal, liver, cardiovascular disease, epilepsy, other contraindications for the drug, or the possibility of pregnancy.

—Long-term use of the dopaminergic and the anticholinergic agents often leads to akinesia, tardive dyskinesia and dystonia. Reduce the dosage to the minimum effective level to counteract these effects and taper doses as necessary to avoid excessive medication.

—Multiple vitamin preparations containing pyridoxine (B6) will reduce the effects of levodopa by increasing its peripheral conversion to dopamine. However, levodopa-carbidopa combinations seem unaffected by B_6 administration.

—Gastrointestinal side effects are common for the antiparkinsonian agents, and health care providers need to identify methods for decreasing these side effects.

—The dopaminergic agents can interfere with urinary glucose tests in diabetic patients. Check blood glucose levels frequently. Keep in mind levodopa may cause false negative readings with Clinistix and false positive readings with Clinitest.

—The anticholinergic agents may impair sweating ability, interfering with the body's heat regulatory mechanism.

—Paralytic ileus has been reported as a significant adverse reaction of the anticholinergic agents.

—Numerous laboratory tests may be altered by these medications and this should be taken into account while monitoring patient status.

WHAT THE PATIENT NEEDS TO KNOW:
—Take this medication exactly as ordered by your health care provider. Clinical improvement may take 2-3 weeks so do not stop taking medication unless advised to do so by your provider.
—Take antiparkinsonian agents after meals to avoid stomach upset.
—Avoid taking vitamin preparations with Vitamin B6 (pyridoxine.)
—Contact your health provider immediately if parkinsonian symptoms become suddenly worse, if intermittent winking or muscle twitching occurs, if abdominal pain, constipation, distention, or urinary problems occur.
—Some patients experience drowsiness, dizziness, or lightheadedness, especially as they move from lying to standing positions. It is best to avoid driving or tasks requiring alertness, or tasks requiring rapid changes of movement when possible.
—Urine, sweat and saliva may darken after exposure to air.
—Avoid overexertion during hot weather.
—Periodic ophthalmologic examinations are necessary when taking anticholinergic drugs.
—Common side effects include dry mouth, dizziness, drowsiness, and gastrointestinal symptoms.

EVALUATION:

ADVERSE REACTIONS:
Dopamine agents: *Cardiovascular:* arrhythmias, palpitations, phlebitis, tachycardia. *CNS:* bradykinesia, depression, muscle twitching, psychotic reactions, rigidity. *Gastrointestinal:* diarrhea, epigastric distress, GI bleeding, nausea, vomiting. *Ocular:* blepharospasm, blurred vision, diplopia. *Other:* alopecia, bitter taste, edema, hemolytic anemia, hot flashes, leukopenia, skin rash, urinary retention.

Anticholinergic agents: *Cardiovascular:* orthostatic hypotension, palpitation, tachycardia. *CNS:* agitation, confusion, delirium, depression, hallucinations, headache, memory loss, muscle cramping, numbness, paresthesias. *Gastrointestinal:* constipation, dilatation of the colon, paralytic ileus, vomiting. *Ocular:* diplopia, increased intraocular pressure, mydriasis. *Other:* decreased sweating, flushing, skin rash.

OVERDOSAGE: Early signs of toxicity in the dopaminergic agents are muscle twitching and blepharospasm. Overdosage is a common phenomenon, particularly with long-term drug therapy. It is recognizable because the patient experiences a sudden onset of progressively worsening parkinsonian symptoms. These drugs should be tapered gradually.

PARAMETERS TO MONITOR: Health providers should perform a complete health assessment, including a complete blood count, electrolytes, enzymes, blood glucose and a urinalysis, prior to initiating therapy with the antiparkinsonian agents. Persons who are concurrently taking MAO inhibitors or with preexisting arrhythmias are not candidates for this drug. Parameters to monitor at each visit: During each visit the provider should assess blood pressure in lying, sitting and standing positions, pulse, temperature, cardiovascular, gastrointestinal, and neurological function. Periodic tonometry examinations should be included as well as tests for hepatic and renal function. Blood glucose should be checked frequently in diabetics.

AMANTADINE HYDROCHLORIDE

PRODUCTS (TRADE NAME):
Symmetrel (Available in 100 mg capsules and 50 mg/5 ml syrup.)
DRUG SPECIFICS:
Amantadine HCl is an antiparkinsonian agent which enhances the release of dopamine from the presynaptic nerve endings. The drug has no anticholinergic activity. It is indicated for the relief of parkinsonian and drug-induced extrapyramidal symptoms. It also exerts an antiviral action, inhibiting the release of viral nucleic acid into host cells. Its use is also indicated for the prophylaxis against the Asian (A) strain of influenza. (See Antiinfective section.) It is especially effective in relieving akinesia and rigidity of Parkinson's disease. It is usually more effective when used in combination with levodopa. The common side effects of this drug include irritability, anxiety, nausea, dizziness, ataxia, confusion, constipation, urinary retention, peripheral edema and skin mottling. The most frequently occurring adverse drug reactions are depression, congestive heart failure, orthostatic hypotensive episodes, and psychosis. Rare cases of leukopenia and neutropenia have been reported. This drug should be withdrawn slowly. The provider should use caution in persons with heart, renal or liver disease or in patients with a history of psychosis or seizure disorders. Advise the patient not to administer the last dose of medication at bedtime, because insomnia can develop. Caution the patient about orthostatic hypotensive changes and how to compensate for these changes.
ADMINISTRATION AND DOSAGE SPECIFICS:
Parkinsonism: Administer 100 mg 1 to 2 times a day up to a maximum of 400 mg per day.
Drug-induced extrapyramidal reactions: Administer 100 mg twice a day up to a maximum of 300 mg per day.

BELLADONNA ALKALOIDS

PRODUCT (TRADE NAME):
Bellafoline (Available in 0.25 mg tablets and 0.5 mg/ml injection.)
DRUG SPECIFICS:
Belladonna alkaloids are anticholinergic agents which compete with acetylcholine for muscarinic receptors at the postganglionic fibers of the parasympathetic

nervous system. This drug is used to treat paralysis agitans, postencephalitic parkinsonism, and spastic and rigid states due to CNS injury. This drug is often used in combination with antacids or phenobarbital to control gastrointestinal disturbances. There are also other drugs which may be used listed in the gastrointestinal anticholinergics-antispasmodics sections.

ADMINISTRATION AND DOSAGE SPECIFICS:

Parkinsonian symptoms: 0.25 to 0.5 mg po 3 times daily; 0.5 to 1 ml 1-2 times daily parenterally.

BENZTROPINE MESYLATE

PRODUCT (TRADE NAME):

Cogentin (Available in 0.5, 1.0, and 2.0 mg tablets and 1 mg/ml injectable solution for IV or IM use.)

DRUG SPECIFICS:

Benztropine mesylate contains anticholinergic and antihistaminic properties. It is a synthetic anticholinergic compound of atropine and diphenhydramine. Pharmacologically, the drug inhibits excessive cholinergic activity in the striatal fibers. The drug is used as an adjunct to parkinsonism treatment and for the management of extrapyramidal symptoms (except tardive dyskinesia) induced by the antipsychotic agents. Intramuscular injection is used to provide rapid (15 minutes) relief from acute dystonic reactions. Oral doses of the drug are cumulative; therefore, therapy should begin with a low dose which is increased gradually at five to six-day intervals as necessary. The drug is contraindicated for persons with known hypersensitivity, in pregnant or breast-feeding women, in persons with glaucoma, and in children. Excessive doses of this medication can produce muscle weakness and exaggerated anticholinergic effects. Supervise closely at the beginning of treatment or with dosage increases. Advise the patient to contact the health care provider immediately upon the occurrence of eye pain or gastrointestinal complaints. Also counsel the patient to refrain from alcohol, driving, or using precision machinery due to the drug's CNS depressant effects; or from taking concurrent over-the-counter cough, cold or allergy medications. Taking the drug with meals will help reduce the GI side effects.

ADMINISTRATION AND DOSAGE SPECIFICS:

Parkinsonian symptoms: Administer 1.0 to 2.0 mg po or parenterally; range is 5 to 6 mg.

Drug-induced extrapyramidal side effects: Administer 1 to 4 mg twice daily.

BIPERIDEN

PRODUCTS (TRADE NAME):

Akineton (Available in 2 mg tablets and 5 mg/ml ampules for IM or IV administration.)

DRUG SPECIFICS:

Biperiden is an anticholinergic which blocks central cholinergic receptors restoring the balance between cholinergic and dopaminergic activity in the basal ganglia. Biperiden is used for the relief of parkinsonian and drug-induced extrapyramidal side effects. Biperiden is contraindicated in persons with known hypersensitivity to this drug, in pregnant or breast-feeding women, and in children. Concomitant administration of anticholinergics, narcotic analgesics, antipsychotic agents, phenothiazines, antidepressants, or certain antiarrhythmics is not recommended. Health care providers should be alert to checking periodic intraocular pressure determinations. Advise patients that frequent dose adjustments are usually required to stabilize symptoms, that the drug can be taken with or after meals to lessen gastric irritation, that high environmental temperatures, including hot baths or saunas, may result in hyperthermia or anhydrosis. When biperiden is used in conjunction with the antipsychotics, concomitant therapy is not recommended for more than three months. Intravenous or intramuscular administration may produce incoordination.

ADMINISTRATION AND DOSAGE SPECIFICS:

Parkinsonism symptoms: Administer 1-2 mg 3 to 4 times a day orally with meals.

Drug-induced extrapyramidal symptoms: Administer 2 mg 1 to 3 times a day orally. Administer 2 mg IM or IV for acute symptoms; repeat every half hour to a maximum of four doses a day.

BROMOCRIPTINE MESYLATE

PRODUCTS (TRADE NAME):

Parlodel (Available in 2.5 mg tablets and 5 mg capsules.)

DRUG SPECIFICS:

Bromocriptine directly stimulates the dopamine receptors in the corpus striatum. Product is used as adjunctive treatment to levodopa for idiopathic or postencephalitic Parkinson's disease. This medication is especially helpful in patients who are beginning to deteriorate or develop tolerance to levodopa. Concomitant use allows levodopa dosage to be decreased, often reducing adverse effects from levodopa. This is a relatively new drug, so long term outcome of patients on this medication has not been evaluated. Start patients on low dosage, evaluate every two weeks to achieve maximum therapeutic response. Dosage may be increased every 2 to 4 weks by 2.5 mg/day with meals. Medication should also be slowly reduced by 2.5 mg/day increments if adverse reactions develop.

ADMINISTRATION AND DOSAGE SPECIFICS:

Parkinson's disease: Initiate therapy with 1.25 mg tablet, twice daily with meals. Increase after 2 to 4 weeks as needed by 2.5 mg/day. Do not exceed 100 mg/day.

CARBIDOPA-LEVODOPA

PRODUCTS (TRADE NAME):
Lodosyn (Available in 25 mg tablets.) **Sinemet-10/100** (Available in tablet form equivalent to 10 mg carbidopa and 100 mg levodopa.) **Sinemet-25/100** (Available in tablet form equivalent to 25 mg carbidopa and 100 mg levodopa.) **Sinemet-25/250** (Available in tablet form, equivalent to 25 mg carbidopa and 250 mg levodopa.)

DRUG SPECIFICS:
Carbidopa-levodopa is a fixed combination antiparkinsonian agent used in all types of parkinsonian treatment, and is composed of both carbidopa and levodopa. Carbidopa competes for the enzymes dopa decarboxylase, retarding the peripheral breakdown of levodopa. This action increases the amount of circulating levodopa in central motor regulating centers. This combination of drugs decreases the dosage requirement by 75%, which decreases the side effects associated with levodopa. Carbidopa can lower the blood levels of creatinine and uric acid. When a provider plans to change a patient from levodopa to carbidopa-levodopa, levodopa must be discontinued at least 8 hours prior to initiating therapy with this product.

ADMINISTRATION AND DOSAGE SPECIFICS:
Relief of parkinsonian symptoms: For patients not receiving levodopa: administer 1 tablet (10/100 or 25/100) 3 times a day initially. Increase by one tablet daily until a maximum of 8 tablets is given. Patients receiving levodopa: discontinue L-dopa at least 8 hours prior to initiating therapy with this product. Administer one tablet (25/250) 3 to 4 times a day in patients previously requiring 1500 mg or more of levodopa each day. If less than 1500 mg of levodopa was used, 1 tablet (10/100) 3 to 4 times a day is administered and adjusted accordingly.

CHLORPHENOXAMINE HCL

PRODUCTS (TRADE NAME):
Phenoxene (Available in 50 mg tablets.)

DRUG SPECIFICS:
Chlorphenoxamine is an antihistamine which may depress motor nerve centers in the brain and spinal cord. It is used primarily as an adjunct in antiparkinsonian therapy. It is most effective in improving muscle strength, endurance and reducing rigidity. It has minimal effect on tremors. This drug is often combined with other anticholinergics of levodopa. A high incidence of drowsiness, dry mouth and sedation occurs when using this drug. It is contraindicated in asthma, narrow angle glaucoma, peptic ulcer, elderly persons, pregnant and breast-feeding women or persons on MAO inhibitor therapy.

ADMINISTRATION AND DOSAGE SPECIFICS:
Parkinsonism: Administer 50 mg po three times a day initially, gradually increasing the dosage up to 400 mg/day.

CYCRIMINE HYDROCHLORIDE

PRODUCTS (TRADE NAME):
Pagitane HCl (Available in 1.25 and 2.5 mg tablets.)
DRUG SPECIFICS:
Cycrimine is an anticholinergic agent that inhibits hyperactive cholinergic activity in striatal fibers. It is used as an adjunct in the treatment of all forms of Parkinson's disease (postencephalitic, arteriosclerotic, or idiopathic.) The drug is contraindicated for persons with known hypersensitivity, in pregnant or breast-feeding women, in persons with glaucoma, and in children. Excessive doses of this medication can produce muscle weakness and exaggerated anticholinergic effects. Supervise closely at the beginning of treatment or with dosage increases. Advise the patient to contact the health provider immediately upon the occurrence of eye pain or gastrointestinal complaints. Also counsel the patient to refrain from drinking alcohol, driving or using precision machinery due to the drug's CNS depressant effects. Do not take concurrently with over-the-counter cough, cold or allergy medications. Taking the drug with meals may help reduce the gastrointestinal side effects.
ADMINISTRATION AND DOSAGE SPECIFICS:
Postencephalitic parkinsonism: 0.5 mg po 2 times a day.
Idiopathic parkinsonism: 1.25 mg po 3 times a day.
Arteriosclerotic parkinsonism: 1.25 mg po 3 times a day. The maximum recommended dose is 20 mg po daily.

ETHOPROPAZINE HYDROCHLORIDE

PRODUCT (TRADE NAME):
Parsidol (Available in 10 and 50 mg tablets.)
DRUG SPECIFICS:
Parsidol is a phenothiazine derivative antiparkinsonian agent with anticholinergic properties. It is used as an adjunct in parkinsonian therapy. Parsidol is effective in the relief of most symptoms including tremors. It does not potentiate other CNS depressants. A high incidence of side effects is associated with this drug and it is poorly tolerated by older patients. The drug is contraindicated in persons with known hypersensitivity to phenothiazines, with glaucoma and in children.

This drug may also be used in the control of extrapyramidal disorders due to CNS drugs such as reserpine and the phenothiazines.

ADMINISTRATION AND DOSAGE SPECIFICS:

Parkinsonism: Administer initial dose of 10 mg 4 times daily; may be increased in 10-mg increments every 2 to 3 days until the desired response is achieved. Moderate symptoms require 100-400 mg daily; severe symptoms may require 500-600 mg daily.

LEVODOPA

PRODUCTS (TRADE NAME):

Dopar (Available in 100, 250, and 500 mg capsules.) **Larodopa** (Available in 100, 125, 250 and 500 mg capsules and 100, 250 and 500 mg tablets.)

DRUG SPECIFICS:

Levodopa is an antiparkinsonian agent which is a metabolic precursor of dopamine. It enters the CNS by crossing the blood brain barrier and is converted to dopamine. The available level of dopamine is elevated, and the symptoms of Parkinson's disease are reduced. The drug is usually administered with food to reduce its common gastrointestinal side effects. The drug is contraindicated in patients with a known hypersensitivity, and in persons with a history of melanoma, skin lesions, narrow angle glaucoma, and patients on MAO inhibitor therapy. Two weeks are required after discontinuation of the MAO inhibitors before levodopa can be administered. Concurrent use of levodopa and vitamin B_6 (pyridoxine) will reverse the effects of L-dopa. The drug acts additively with the antihypertensive agents, producing hypotensive effects. Phenothiazines, sympathomimetics, sedatives, and methyldopa counteract the effects of L-dopa and should be discontinued prior to initiating L-dopa therapy. Providers should monitor patients for signs of depression, hallucinations, and mental status to determine if compliance is a problem. If a compliance problem is suspected, then plasma levodopa levels should be obtained. Levodopa can produce increases in serum levels of alkaline phosphatase, SGOT, SGPT, BUN, bilirubin, and LDH. It can also cause false positive Coombs' tests and false glucose urine determinations. CBCs, urinalysis, hemoccult stool testing and tonometry should be done every 6 months due to the adverse effects of this drug. Baseline ECGs should be obtained prior to instituting therapy with L-dopa and repeated if arrhythmias occur during therapy.

ADMINISTRATION AND DOSAGE SPECIFICS:

Relief of antiparkinsonian symptoms: Administer 0.5 1 gm po daily in two or more doses. Dosage may be increased gradually in increments of 0.75 mg every 3 to 7 days as tolerated. The usual optimum dose should not exceed 8 gm.

ORPHENADRINE HYDROCHLORIDE

PRODUCTS (TRADE NAME):
Disipal (Available in 50 mg tablets.)
DRUG SPECIFICS:
This product is an antiparkinsonian agent with antihistamine and centrally acting skeletal muscle relaxant properties. It is effective in the relief of rigidity and the control of autonomic symptoms. Its use with chlorpromazine is contraindicated since it has resulted in hypoglycemic coma. It may also interact with barbiturates, phenylbutazone, and griseofulvin, reducing their phamacological effects. The drug is contraindicated in patients with known hypersensitivity to orphenadrine, bladder neck obstruction, cardiospasm, glaucoma, myasthenia gravis, prostatic hypertrophy, pyloric or duodenal obstruction or stenosing peptic ulcer. The drug should be used with caution in cardiac patients. If used for long-term therapy, periodic blood, liver and urine evaluations are recommended. The anticholinergic side effects, usually the most bothersome to patients, include dryness of the mouth, tachycardia, urinary retention, blurred vision, increased ocular tension, and constipation. These drugs are additive with CNS depressants and anticholinergics. Advise the patient to take precautions against drowsiness and to observe for urinary hesitancy or retention.

ADMINISTRATION AND DOSAGE SPECIFICS:
Parkinsonism: Administer 50 mg po three times a day.

PROCYCLIDINE HCL

PRODUCT (TRADE NAME):
Kemadrin (Available in 5 mg tablets.)
DRUG SPECIFICS:
Procyclidine HCl is a synthetic antiparkinsonian agent which inhibits hyperactive cholinergic activity in the striatal fibers. It is used primarily as an adjunct in the treatment of all forms of parkinsonism and in the management of the drug-induced extrapyramidal symptoms. It is more effective in the relief of rigidity than tremor and is effective in the relief of excessive salivation. It is contraindicated in angle closure glaucoma, in children and in persons with known hypersensitivity to the drug. This drug produces the commonly known side effects and warrants precautions and warnings similar to other antiparkinsonian agents. Additionally, hypotensive patients who receive this drug should be monitored closely. This drug should be withheld from persons who have urinary retention or tachycardia.

ADMINISTRATION AND DOSAGE SPECIFICS:
Parkinsonism: Administer 8-10 mg po in 3 to 4 divided doses daily. Dosage may range from 6 to 15 mg daily.
Extrapyramidal symptoms: Administer 10-20 mg in 3 divided doses daily.

TRIHEXYPHENIDYL HCL

PRODUCT (TRADE NAME):
   Artane (Available in 2 and 5 mg tablets; in elixir containing 2 mg/5 ml; and in 5 mg sustained-release capsules.) **Aphen** (Available in 2 and 5 mg tablets.) **Trihexane, Trihexidyl, Trihexy-2, Trihexy-5, Trihexyphenidyl Hydrochloride, Tremin** (Available in 2 and 5 mg tablets.)

DRUG SPECIFICS:
   Trihexyphenidyl HCl exerts a direct inhibitory effect upon the parasympathetic nervous system. It also has a relaxing effect on smooth musculature, exerted directly on the muscle tissue and indirectly through an inhibitory effect on the parasympathetic nervous system. These drugs are used as adjuncts in the treatment of Parkinsonism and for the control of drug-induced extrapyramidal side effects. The major effect of the drug is on rigidity, although most symptoms improve to some degree. The sequel dosage form should only be used for maintenance therapy after patients have been stabilized on tablets or elixir. Intraocular pressures should be monitored regularly by health care providers for persons on antiparkinsonian agents. Geriatric patients taking this drug frequently develop increased sensitivity to this drug and require strict dosage control. Its side effects, contraindications, and clinical nursing implications are those commonly identified for the antiparkinsonian agents.

ADMINISTRATION AND DOSAGE SPECIFICS:
   Idiopathic parkinsonism: Administer 6-10 mg po per day in 3 to 4 divided doses; initial dose begins as 1 mg first day and is increased in 2 mg increments at intervals of 3 to 5 days until a total dosage of 6-10 mg is reached. Once maintenance dose is reached, sustained release capsule may by used; 5 mg 1 to 2 times per day.
   Drug-induced parkinsonism: Give 5-15 mg po per day; begin therapy at 1 mg and continue to raise it until therapeutic level is achieved.

                                                              Doreen C. Harper

---

CNS STIMULANTS

AMPHETAMINES

ACTION OF THE DRUG: (1) Amphetamines are central nervous system stimulants acting on the cerebral cortex and on the reticular activating system. They stimulate the medullary respiratory center, raise both systolic and diastolic blood pressure, contract urinary bladder sphincter muscle, facilitate monosynaptic and polysynatic transmission in the spinal cord and exert a pressor effect on the vascular system. (2) Also may produce a calming effect on the hyperactive child.

ASSESSMENT:

INDICATIONS: Used in the treatment of narcolepsy, as an adjunct to other Parkinson drugs, psychogenic disorders or adjunct to phenobarbital in grand mal epilepsy. Useful in petit mal seizures to counteract the sedative effect of trimethadione. An adjunct in the treatment of orthostatic hypotension and alcoholism, urinary incontinence and nocturnal enuresis. In children it is used for hyperactivity in conjunction with other remedial therapies. It is used in obesity and weight reduction when other therapy has been ineffective. However, the FDA is being asked to delete this use from the pharmacological preparations.

SUBJECTIVE: Patient may present with a history of petit mal seizures, chronic alcohol abuse, or urinary incontinence and nocturnal enuresis. Children may have history of reduced attention span, hyperactivity, inability for task completion, and irritable behavior.

OBJECTIVE: Family or reliable sources should be able to describe occurrence of petite mal seizures, other central nervous system diseases, or hyperactivity in children.

PLAN:

CONTRAINDICATIONS: Drug should not be used in the presence of overwhelming drowsiness, increasing energy and alertness, advanced arteriosclerosis, agitated hyperthyroidism, hypersensitivity to drug, nephritis, and history of drug abuse or psychosis in children.

WARNINGS: Drug tolerance may occur quite quickly, often within three to four weeks. If this happens, discontinue drug. Amphetamines mask extreme fatigue and this presents a potential for drug abuse. Chronic intoxication may be marked by severe dermatoses, hyperactivity, marked insomnia, personality changes and irritability. Psychosis may also develop, plus visual hallucinations, compulsive, stereotyped behavior and poor concentration may also be found. Long-term administration may inhibit growth in children in some cases. It may also exacerbate behavioral disturbances and thought disorders in children. It is not recommended for children under three for behavioral disorders, or children under twelve for weight reduction.

PRECAUTIONS: Use only under direction of health care provider. The smallest quantity feasible should be prescribed at one time, to minimize the possibility of overdosage. Avoid during pregnancy, or in sexually active women without birth control, because of risk of congenital abnormalities. Do not use in breast-feeding mothers.

IMPLEMENTATION:

DRUG INTERACTIONS: Use with general anesthesia may produce cardiac arrhythmias. Guanethidine action will be decreased. MAO inhibitors potentiate the effects of amphetamines, which may result in a hypertensive crisis; therefore amphetamines should not be administered during or within fourteen days following the administration of MAO inhibitors. Insulin requirements in diabetes mellitus may be altered with the use of amphetamines or changes in dietary regimen. Thiazide diuretics and sodium bicarbonate can increase effects of amphetamines by increased renal tubular reabsorption, whereas ascorbic acid can decrease the effect of renal tubular reabsorption. Haldol decreases the effect by decreasing the uptake of drugs at its site of action. Phenothiazines decrease effect of amphetamines by decreasing uptake of drugs into its site of action.

ADMINISTRATION AND DOSAGE: The smallest quantity feasible should be prescribed or dispensed at one time to minimize the possibility of overdosage. To decrease insomnia, administer six hours before bedtime, or if using the extended release tablet, 12-14 hours before bedtime. With children who are on the drug for behavioral syndromes, it may be possible to discontinue therapy during summer months or for other times when child is under less stress. Store capsules at temperatures between 15 and 30 degrees Centigrade in a well-closed container. Extended-release capsules should not be used for initiation of dosage, or until the conventional titrated daily dose is equal to or greater than the dosage provided in the extended-release dosage form. Discontinue drug slowly after prolonged treatment, since abrupt withdrawal may precipitate extreme fatigue and mental depression.

IMPLEMENTATION CONSIDERATIONS:

—Obtain a complete health history, including the presence of hypersensitivity, concurrent medications taken, hypertension, diabetes, convulsions, thyroid disease and possibility of pregnancy.

—Evaluate history for any evidence of substance abuse.

—Obtain baseline studies which might be affected by drug: height and weight in children, blood pressure, complete blood count and urinalysis.

—In children it is important to monitor reports from both parents and school on performance and behavior.

—Parents should be cautioned to observe child for dizziness or euphoria.

—It may be difficult to evaluate the therapeutic effects of this drug in some patients. In children it may be necessary to interrupt therapy to see if the medication is responsible for the desired therapeutic effect.

—Evaluate any other health problems which may be related to behavior.

WHAT THE PATIENT NEEDS TO KNOW:

—Your dosage of medicine and when you take it must be especially determined for your situation. Please take all medication exactly as you are instructed.

—Do not chew or crush sustained-release or long-acting tablets.

—Prescription is not renewable. You will need to see your health provider for each prescription you need.

—This prescription is only for you. Other members of your family should not take it, even if they may feel they share the same problems.

—If you note any uncomfortable changes be certain to report them to your health provider. Especially watch for changes in appetite, blurred vision, inability to sleep, feeling of restlessness, heart pounding, changes in bowel habits, skin rashes, or headache.

—Dryness of the mouth can be relieved by sucking on hard sugarless candy, ice chips, or sugarless gum.

—If you are planning on becoming pregnant, or are breast-feeding, make certain provider knows this.

—Before driving, operating heavy machinery, or doing work which requires alertness, evaluate your reaction to this drug. Your ability to do these tasks may be impaired.

—You may feel a change in attitude about sexual activity, or changes in your sexual performance.

EVALUATION:

ADVERSE REACTIONS: *Cardiovascular:* increase in blood pressure, palpitations, tachycardia. *CNS:* blurred vision, dysphoria, euphoria, headache, insomnia, overstimulation, restlessness, sweating. *Gastro-intestinal:* anorexia, constipation, diarrhea, dryness of mouth, unpleasant taste, weight loss. *Integumentary:* urticaria. *Other:* change in libido, impotence.

OVERDOSAGE: *Signs and Symptoms:* Because of slow excretion of amphetamines (5-7 days), a cumulative effect may occur with continued administration. Watch for arrhythmias, dizziness, excoriation of the skin, hallucinations, hypertension, paranoid ideation and hyperpyrexia which can lead to death from cardiovascular collapse or convulsions. *Treatment:* Referral for immediate gastric lavage, maintenance of adequate circulatory and respiratory exchange.

PARAMETERS TO MONITOR: For children taking medication for hyperactivity: Obtain height and weight in children before starting medication, and every 3-4 months thereafter. Also obtain baseline evaluation of child's school and home behavior, including periodic teacher ratings. For all patients taking the medication: obtain baseline complete blood count, blood chemistries, urinalysis, weight and blood pressure. Do repeat evaluation of these studies at least yearly. Evaluate compliance of the individual in taking the drug, and observe for drug abuse or drug tolerance. Designate specific symptoms to follow which will be indicative of therapeutic effect: decrease in Parkinsonian tremors, relief of sedative effects of other drugs, less orthostatic hypertension, urinary incontinence, or nocturnal enuresis, etc.

AMPHETAMINE COMPLEX

PRODUCTS (TRADE NAME):

Biphetamine 12 1/2 and 20 (Available in 6.25 mg dextroamphetamine and 6.25 mg amphetamine or 10 mg dextroamphetamine and 10 mg amphetamine capsules.)

DRUG SPECIFICS:

This is a combination product used primarily for treatment of hyperactivity in children and obesity.

ADMINISTRATION AND DOSAGE SPECIFICS:

Abnormal behavioral disorder in children: Establish control with dextroamphetamine. Then switch to once daily therapy with this product.

Obesity: 1 capsule daily early in morning.

AMPHETAMINE SULFATE

PRODUCTS (TRADE NAME):

Amphetamine Sulfate (Available in 5 and 10 mg tablets.)

DRUG SPECIFICS:

As anorexic: take 30-60 minutes before meals. Last dose 6 hours before bedtime. *Exogenous obesity:* not recommended for use in children under 12 years of age. In general: not recommended for children under three years of age. High potential for abuse. Swallow capsules whole.

ADMINISTRATION AND DOSAGE SPECIFICS:

Narcolepsy:

Adults: 5-60 mg orally two to three times a day depending on the individual response.

Children 6-12 years of age: oral 2.5 mg two times a day, with the dosage being increased by 5 mg at one-week intervals until the desired response is obtained, or with capsule 15 mg once a day.

Children 12 years and older: Oral, 5 mg two times a day, the dosage increasing by 10 mg at one-week intervals until desired response is obtained, or with capsule 15 mg once a day.

Behavioral Syndrome:

Children 3-6 years: oral 2.5 mg once a day, the dosage increasing by 2.5 mg at one-week intervals until desired response is obtained.

Children 6 years and older: 5 mg po one or two times a day, the dosage increasing by 5 mg at one-week intervals until the desired response is obtained.

Anorexia:

Adults: 5-10 mg orally three times a day.

Exogenous Obesity: Usually dosage is one or two 15-mg Spansule daily, taken in the morning; or up to 30 mg tablet daily, taken in divided doses of 5-10 mg 30-60 minutes before meals.

DEXTROAMPHETAMINE SULFATE

PRODUCTS (TRADE NAME):

Dexampex (Available in 5 and 10 mg tablets and 15 mg capsule.) **Dexedrine**

(Available in 5 and 10 mg tablets, 5 mg/5 ml elixir, 5, 10, and 15 mg sustained-release capsule.) **Dextroamphetamine** (Available in 5, 10 mg tablet and 15 mg sustained-release capsule.) **Ferndex** (Available in 5 mg tablet.) **Span Cap No.1** (Available in 15 mg sustained-release capsule.)

DRUG SPECIFICS:

Has stronger central action and weaker peripheral action than amphetamine, therefore fewer undesirable cardiovascular effects.

ADMINISTRATION AND DOSAGE SPECIFICS:

Narcolepsy:

Adult: Oral 5-20 mg one to three times a day, or with extended release capsule, 5-30 mg once a day.

Children 6-12 years: Oral 2.5 mg twice a day. Dosage can be increased by 5 mg at one-week intervals until therapeutic level. Extended release capsule: 5-15 mg orally once a day.

12 years and older: 5 mg twice a day. Dosage increased by 10 mg at oneweek intervals until therapeutic effect is obtained. Extended-release capsules: 10 or 15 mg orally once a day.

Behavioral Syndrome:

Children 3 to 6 years: 2.5 mg po once a day, increasing by 2.5 mg at one week intervals until therapeutic effect is obtained. Range 2.5 to 40 mg.

Children 6 years and older: 5 mg po once or twice a day, increasing by 5 mg at one week intervals until therapeutic effect is obtained. Range 2.5 -40 mg. Extended release capsule: 5 to 15 mg po once a day.

METHAMPHETAMINE HCL

PRODUCTS (TRADE NAME):

Desoxyn (Available in 5 mg tablets, 5, 10 and 15 mg long-acting tablets.) **Methampex** (Available in 10 mg tablets.)

DRUG SPECIFICS:

Keep container tightly closed. 15 mg dosage strength contains FD&C Yellow 5 which may cause allergic-type reactions in certain susceptible individuals, particularly those with aspirin sensitivity.

ADMINISTRATION AND DOSAGE SPECIFICS:

Behavioral Syndrome:

Children 6 years and older: 2.5 mg to 5 mg orally one or two times a day. Usual daily amount 20-25 mg per day. Extended release capsule: 5-15 mg orally once a day.

Obesity: 1 Gradumet tablet 10 or 15 mg in morning. Tablet: 2.5 mg or 5 mg 30 minutes before meal. Treatment should not exceed a few weeks in duration.

AMPHETAMINES—COMBINATION PRODUCTS

PRODUCTS (TRADE NAME):
(See Table 4-10.)

Linda Ross

TABLE 4-10. CONTENTS OF AMPHETAMINE COMBINATION PRODUCTS

| | Dextroamphetamine | | Amphetamine | | | |
	Sulfate	Saccharate	Aspartate	Sulfate	Adipate	How Supplied
Amphaplex-10	2.5 mg	2.5 mg	2.5 mg	2.5 mg		tablets
Amphaplex-20	5 mg	5 mg	5 mg	5 mg		tablets
Delcobese-5	1.25 mg	1.25 mg		1.25 mg	1.25 mg	tab or cap
Delcobese-10	2.5 mg	2.5 mg	2.5 mg	2.5 mg	tab or cap	
Delcobese-15	3.75 mg	3.75 mg		3.75 mg	3.75 mg	tab or cap
Delcobese-20	5 mg	5 mg		5 mg	5 mg	tab or cap
Obetrol-10	2.5 mg	2.5 mg	2.5 mg	2.5 mg		tablet
Obetrol-20	5 mg	5 mg	5 mg	5 mg		tablet

MUSCLE RELAXANTS

ACTION OF THE DRUG: The main action of the skeletal muscle relaxants is (1) to decrease muscle tone and involuntary movement without loss of voluntary motor function. (2) These drugs inhibit transmission of impulses in the motor pathways at the level of the spinal cord, the brain stem (centrally acting) or interferes with the contractile mechanism of the skeletal muscle fibers (direct myotrophic blocking). (3) Other actions include mild sedation, reduction of anxiety and tension, and alteration of pain perception.

ASSESSMENT:

INDICATIONS: Used for relief of pain in musculoskeletal and neurological disorders involving peripheral injury and inflammation, such as: muscle strain or sprain, arthritis, bursitis, low back syndrome, cervical neck syndrome, tension headaches, cerebral palsy and multiple sclerosis.

SUBJECTIVE: Practitioner may find history of pain due to acute muscular trauma or inflammation (sprains or strains); tetanus, low back syndrome, arthritis, multiple sclerosis, spinal cord disease, or cerebral palsy; muscular tension with or without intermittent relief, headache, muscle rigidity.

OBJECTIVE: Practitioner may find signs of muscle spasm, hyperreflexia, hypertonia, edema, inflammation, decreased range of motion in affected joints, muscle atrophy, wasting, or asymmetry.

PLAN:

CONTRAINDICATIONS: The agents should not be used with persons with glaucoma, myasthenia gravis, tachycardia, prostatic hypertrophy, urinary retention, duodenal obstruction and ulcer disease. They are also contraindicated for children and in pregnant or breast-feeding women.

WARNINGS: Caution should be exercised when administering these drugs to the elderly or debilitated, persons with compromised respiratory function, hepatic or renal dysfunction, arrhythmia or coronary insufficiency. Hypersensitivity reactions are common in persons allergic to other carbamate derivatives such as meprobamate. Rarely the first dose of skeletal muscle relaxants will produce an idiosyncratic reaction within minutes or hours. Symptoms include: extreme weakness, transient quadriplegia, dizziness, ataxia, temporary loss of vision, diplopia, mydriasis, dysarthria, agitation, euphoria, confusion, and disorientation.

PRECAUTIONS: Reported incidences of hepatotoxicity, nephrotoxicity and blood dyscrasias have occurred with the use of skeletal muscle relaxants. Signs of hepatotoxicity include abdominal pain, high fever, nausea and diarrhea. Signs of blood dyscrasias include fever, sore throat, mucosal irritation, malaise and petechiae. Concomitant use of other CNS drugs, including alcohol, will potentiate the sedative actions of this drug. Therefore, these drugs are not recommended for persons with alcoholism.

IMPLEMENTATION:

DRUG INTERACTIONS: The skeletal muscle relaxants are known to interact additively with CNS depressants, including sedatives, narcotic analgesics, antianxiety agents, hypnotics, and alcohol, general anesthetics, MAO inhibitors, tricyclic antidepressants, and anticholinergic drugs including cyclobenzaprine and orphenadrine. Cyclobenzaprine may interfere with the antihypertensive activity of the alpha-adrenergic blockers.

ADMINISTRATION AND DOSAGE: These products are available in a tablet and injectable form. When given orally, these drugs are purported to be of questionable benefit. The oral dose would have to be 5-10 times greater than the parenteral dose to obtain true muscle relaxation. For this reason, the parenteral form of these drugs is recommended rather than the oral form. The parenteral form of the drug can cause local tissue irritation.

Skeletal muscle relaxants, like other CNS depressants, can become habit-forming. Their long-term use is not recommended. The efficacy and safe usage of these drugs has not been established in children.

IMPLEMENTATION CONSIDERATIONS:

—Obtain a complete health history, including the presence of hypersensitivity, concurrent drug use which would produce drug interactions, history of respiratory, renal, hepatic, or cardiac dysfunction. These drugs also should not be dispensed to women who are pregnant or breast-feeding, or to persons with a history of drug dependency.

—Side effects which occur most frequently include drowsiness, diplopia, dizziness, weakness, mild muscular incoordination, anorexia, nausea, vomiting, syncope and hypotension.

—Discontinue the drug if no improvement occurs after 45 days, since the risk of hepatotoxicity increases with long-term use of these drugs.

—Use the lowest dosage possible, monitoring for signs and symptoms of hepatotoxicity, blood dyscrasias and dependency.

—Abrupt termination of these drugs can cause withdrawal symptoms after long-term use, so gradually reduce the dosage of the drug before termination.

—Combine the drug regimen with additional programs to build up muscles and restore function, including exercise, diet, and physiotherapy if indicated.

—Do not use these medications with persons having a history of alcoholism or suspected alcohol abuse.

WHAT THE PATIENT NEEDS TO KNOW:

—Take this medication as advised. Do not stop taking medicine suddenly, or increase dosage without supervision.

—Avoid driving, operating heavy machinery or doing tasks requiring alertness while taking this drug.

—Avoid using medicine that depress central nervous system functioning. For example, antihistamines, allergy or cold medications, sedatives, tranquilizers, sleeping medications, anticonvulsants, narcotic analgesics, or tricyclic antidepressants.

—If a dose of medication is missed, it may be taken within the hour it was scheduled. If it is close to the next scheduled dose, take regular dose only and omit missed dose.

—Contact your provider immediately if the following side effects occur: dizziness or fainting, mental depression, unusual fast heartbeat, wheezing, shortness of breath, difficult breathing, abdominal pain, high fever, nausea, diarrhea, sore throat, malaise, mucosal ulceration or petechiae.

—Take the last dose at bedtime so that drowsiness will assist in producing sleep.

—Keep this medicine out of the reach of children and all others for whom it is not prescribed.

EVALUATION:

ADVERSE REACTIONS: *Cardiovascular:* chest pain, flushing, hypotension, petechiae, palpitations, syncope, tachycardia, thrombophlebitis. *CNS:* ataxia, blurred vision, confusion, headache, insomnia, irritability, paresthesias. *Gastrointestinal:* abdominal pain, anorexia, bleeding, diarrhea, hiccoughs, nausea. *Hematopoietic:*

agranulocytosis, hemolytic anemia, leukopenia, pancytopenia, thrombocytopenia. *Hypersensitivity:* anaphylactic reactions, angioedema, asthma-like reaction, dermatoses, erythema, fever, pruritus, rash. *Renal:* dysuria, enuresis, urinary retention. *Respiratory:* dyspnea, nasal congestion, shortness of breath, wheezing. *Other:* dyspepsia, dysrhythmia, euphoria, metallic taste, pain or sloughing at injection site, tremors.

OVERDOSAGE: Overdosage of carisprodol has resulted in shock, coma, respiratory depression and death. Other CNS depressants and psychotropic drugs can be additive, even when taken in the usual recommended doses. In cases of overdosage, the drug should be removed from the stomach and, if necessary, respiratory assistance, CNS stimulants and pressor agents should be administered by a qualified physician.

PARAMETERS TO MONITOR: The acuteness of the musculoskeletal disorder or type of neurological impairment dictates the duration of drug use. Based on the duration of use, the health care practitioner should monitor specific clinical parameters. The initial data base should include a neurological, musculoskeletal and cardiovascular assessment, a urinalysis, and complete blood count. If liver dysfunction or associated abdominal conditions are suspected, then liver function tests should be conducted. Parameters to monitor each visit: pulse, heart sounds, breath sounds, respiratory rate. Observe for signs and symptoms of therapeutic effect, such as increased range of motion, relief from muscle spasm, and pain relief. Be alert to signs and symptoms of adverse drug reactions, and drug dependence.

BACLOFEN

PRODUCTS (TRADE NAME):
   Lioresal (Available in 10 and 20 mg tablets.)
DRUG SPECIFICS:
   Baclofen acts primarily as a skeletal muscle relaxant. It is a derivative of gamma-aminobutyric acid (GABA). Its action is related to inhibition of monosynaptic and polysynaptic reflexes in the spinal cord. It is used chiefly for treatment of spasticity resulting from multiple sclerosis, especially for flexor spasm. The drug is also indicated for spinal cord disease or injury. The drug is not recommended for stroke, cerebral palsy or Parkinson's disease. This medication can cause withdrawal symptoms and hallucinations; therefore, therapy should be discontinued slowly. The drug causes CNS depressant side effects and patient should be advised accordingly. Advise diabetic patients that baclofen may cause an increase in urine glucose and that they should notify provider immediately if any changes occur. Baclofen should be used with caution in renal patients, where spasticity sustains upright posture and balance in locomotion and in epileptic patients. The drug may increase serum levels of alkaline phosphatase, aspartate, SGOT and blood sugar.
ADMINISTRATION AND DOSAGE SPECIFICS:
   Muscle relaxant, antispastic: Begin dosage regimen with 5 mg 3 times a day

for 3 days. Thereafter, increase the dose in increments of 5 mg per dose every 3 days until the desired response is obtained. The dosage is adjusted according to the reversal of spasticity symptoms. The maximum daily dose is 80 mg.

CARISOPRODOL

PRODUCT (TRADE NAME):
    Carisoprodol, Rela, Soma, Soprodol (Available in 350 mg tablets.)
DRUG SPECIFICS:
    Carisoprodol is a centrally acting muscle relaxant which blocks polysynaptic neuronal activity in the descending reticular formation and the spinal cord. This drug is used in the treatment of acute painful musculoskeletal conditions. The exact mechanism for muscle relaxation is unknown, but it may be related to this drug's sedative properties. The tricyclic antidepressants may enhance the CNS effects of carisoprodol, especially drowsiness. Carisoprodol can also decrease total leukocyte count and increase eosinophil count.
ADMINISTRATION AND DOSAGE SPECIFICS:
    Muscle relaxant: 350 mg po 3 times a day and at bedtime. Administration with meals will help reduce gastric distress.

CHLORPHENESIN CARBAMATE

PRODUCTS (TRADE NAME):
    Maolate (Available in 400 mg tablets).
DRUG SPECIFICS:
    Chlorphenesin carbamate is a central muscle relaxant; its mechanism of skeletal muscle relaxation is not known, but it is structurally related to methocarbamol. This product contains tartrazine which may produce asthma-like reactions in patients sensitive to the chemical. Chlorphenesin carbamate is used for muscle spasms and muscle pain secondary to sprains, trauma, or inflammation. This drug has caused rare cases of leukopenia, thrombocytopenia, agranulocytosis, and pancytopenia. On occasion, persons may experience paradoxical stimulation instead of sedation. This occurrence is usually controlled by decreasing the dosage. If allergic reactions occur, discontinue the drug.
ADMINISTRATION AND DOSAGE SPECIFICS:
    Muscle relaxation: 800 mg 3 times daily until a therapeutic effect is achieved; then give maintenance dose of 400 mg 3 times daily. Treatment should not exceed 8 weeks because safety in long-term usage of this medication has not been determined.

CHLORZOXAZONE

PRODUCT (TRADE NAME):

Chlorzoxazone, Paraflex (Available in 250 mg tablets.)

DRUG SPECIFICS:

Chlorzoxazone is a centrally acting skeletal muscle relaxant. The drug acts on the spinal cord and subcortical levels of the brain where it inhibits polysynaptic reflex arcs responsible for maintaining skeletal muscle spasm associated with musculoskeletal disorders. The drug may cause urine to appear orange or red when it is exposed to air, but it is not nephrotoxic. Chlorzoxazone can increase SGPT, SGOT, alkaline phosphatase and bilirubin.

ADMINISTRATION AND DOSAGE SPECIFICS:

Adults: Give 250 to 750 mg 3 times daily. Initial dose for painful musculoskeletal conditions should be 500 mg 3 times daily. If adequate response is not obtained, the dosage may be increased to 750 mg 3 to 4 times daily and then gradually reduced to a maintenance dose of 250 mg 3 times daily once the therapeutic effect is achieved. Administration with meals may help avoid GI irritation.

Children: Give 20 mg/kg not to exceed 125 mg to 500 mg 3 times daily. The tablets may be crushed and mixed with food.

CYCLOBENZAPRINE HCL

PRODUCTS (TRADE NAME):

Flexeril (Available in 10 mg tablets).

DRUG SPECIFICS:

Cyclobenzaprine HCl relieves acute skeletal muscle spasm of local origin without interfering with muscle function. These drugs are ineffective in muscle spasm of CNS origin. Cyclobenzaprine HCl is structurally related to the tricyclic antidepressants with sedative and anticholinergic effects. Its use is contraindicated with concurrent use of the tricyclic antidepressants or MAO inhibitors or within 14 days after their discontinuation. Do not give in hyperthyroidism, arrhythmias, congestive heart failure, myocardial infarction and known hypersensitivity to the tricyclic antidepressants. Advise the patient that the drug can cause drowsiness and dry mouth.

ADMINISTRATION AND DOSAGE SPECIFICS:

Local muscle spasm: 80 mg 3 to 4 times daily. Do not administer for longer than 2 to 3 weeks.

DANTROLENE SODIUM

PRODUCTS (TRADE NAME):

Dantrium (Available in 25, 50 and 100 mg capsules; .32 mg/ml powder for IV use.)

DRUG SPECIFICS:

Dantrolene sodium is a direct-acting skeletal muscle relaxant which affects the contractile response of the skeletal muscle. This drug is used to control spasticity resulting from upper motor neuron disorders of spinal cord injury, stroke, cerebral palsy or multiple sclerosis. The drug must be taken for one week before beneficial effects become apparent. It has a potential for hepatotoxicity, particularly in women, persons over 35, and in persons taking other medications. Hepatic function should be monitored with frequent SGOT and SGPT determinations, alkaline phosphatase and bilirubin tests. Therapy should be discontinued in 45 days if no observable benefit is derived. The drug is contraindicated in hepatic dysfunction, where spasticity maintains upright posture and balance in locomotion, or where spasticity maintains increased function. There is a questionable drug interaction between Dantrium and estrogen. Patients should be cautioned about the CNS depressant effects and photosensitivity reaction evoked by this drug. The dosage should be titrated and individualized for maximum effect. The lowest dose compatible with optimal response is recommended.

ADMINISTRATION AND DOSAGE:

Spasticity:

Adults: Begin therapy with 25 mg once daily; increase to 25 mg 2-4 times daily; and then by increments up to as high as 100 mg 2-4 times daily if necessary. Doses of higher than 400 mg per day are not recommended. Each dosage should be maintained for 4 to 7 days to determine the patient's response.

Children: Begin with 1 mg/kg daily and increase by 0.5 mg/kg increments to a maximum of 3 mg/kg 2-4 times daily.

DIAZEPAM

PRODUCT (TRADE NAME):

Valium (Available in 2, 5, and 10 mg tablets, and 5 mg/ml injectable solution.)

Valrelease (Available in 15 mg sustained-release tablets.)

DRUG SPECIFICS:

Diazepam acts at the spinal level to inhance presynaptic activity, and at supraspinal sites, the brain stem reticular system and the reticular facilitatory system. Calming effects are produced. There may be direct muscle depression through action at neuromuscular synapses. It acts to relief skeletal muscle spasm due to local pathology producing reflex spasms. It is also helpful in reducing spasticity, athetosis, stiff-man syndrome and other upper motor neuron disorders. It is also used an an antianxiety agent and an anticonvulsant. (See other sections for more information.)

ADMINISTRATION AND DOSAGE SPECIFICS:

Dosage must be individualized, with elderly and debilitated patients receiving lower doses. In some cases patients may require larger doses than those suggested. Increments in medication should be cautiously added to the recommended doses.

Adults: 2 to 10 mg po 2 to 4 times daily. Give sustained release capsules 15 to 30 mg once daily.

Geriatric or debilitated patients: 2 to 2.5 mg po once or twice daily. Gradually increase dose as needed.

Children older than 6 months: 1 to 2.5 mg po three or four times daily initially. Gradually increase dose as needed.

Parenteral therapy: Inject IV medication slowly only into large veins, 1 minute for each 5 mg. This is very important.

Adults: Give 5 to 10 mg IV initially, repeated as necessary at 10 to 15 minute intervals. Maximum IV dose is 30 mg. Therapy may be repeated in 2 to 4 hours as needed.

Children 5 years and older: Give 1 mg every 2 to 5 minutes. Maximum IV doses is 10 mg. Repeat in 2 to 4 hours as needed.

Children 30 days to 5 years: Give 0.2 to 0.5 mg slowly every 2 to 5 minutes. Maximum IV dose is 5 mg.

METAXALONE

PRODUCTS (TRADE NAME):

Skelaxin (Available in 400 mg tablets.)

DRUG SPECIFICS:

Metaxalone is a centrally acting muscle relaxant. Its mode of action has not been specifically determined, but may be due to its sedative effects. It does not directly relax skeletal muscle in man. The drug is contraindicated in persons with known tendency toward drug-induced hemolytic or other anemia, with preexisting liver or renal dysfunction, with known sensitivity to metaxalone, or who are pregnant or breast-feeding. Advise patients that metaxalone causes drowsiness, and to avoid other CNS depressants. Since the drug is known to produce false positives for urine glucose with Benedict's solution, Clinitest and Fehling's solution, advise diabetic patients to test their urine with Clinistix, Diastix or Tes-Tape.

ADMINISTRATION AND DOSAGE SPECIFICS:

Muscle Relaxation:
Adults: 800 mg 3-4 times daily.
Children: Not recommended for children under age 12.

METHOCARBAMOL

PRODUCTS (TRADE NAME):

Delaxin (Available in 500 mg tablets.) **Marbaxin 750** (Available in 750 mg tablets.) **Methocarbamol** (Available in 500 and 700 mg tablets and 100 mg/ml injection.) **Metho-500** (Available in 500 mg tablets.) **Robaxin** (Available in)500 and 750 mg tablets; injectable solution of 100 mg/ml.) **SK-Methocarbamol** (Available in 500 and 700 mg tablets.)

DRUG SPECIFICS:

Methocarbamol is a centrally acting skeletal muscle relaxant that is a derivative of guaifenesin (glyceryl guaiacolate). Its action is related to blocking of polysynaptic activity in the CNS, producing relief of discomfort from acute musculoskeletal conditions or tetanus. Intramuscular and intravenous administration must be carefully executed because the injectable form of the drug causes vascular extravasation. The parenteral form of the drug is contraindicated in renal dysfunction, as it has been implicated in causing acidosis and urea retention. The drug increases the level of hemoglobin in urine and false elevations in urinary VMA and 5-HIAA determinations. Advise the patient about drowsiness and CNS depressant precautions. Also advise the patient that the drug may change the color of standing urine to green or black.

ADMINISTRATION AND DOSAGE SPECIFICS:

Relief of muscle spasm: 1.5 gm orally 4 times per day as initial loading dose for the first 3-4 days of treatment. The maintenance dose is 750-1000 mg per day in 4 divided doses. Intravenous and intramuscular dosage should not exceed 30 mg (3 vials) per day for more than 3 days, except in the treatment of tetanus. Specifically for intravenous dosage, do not exceed a rate of 3 ml (300 mg) per minute. Methocarbamol injection for IV infusion may be mixed with sodium chloride injection or 5% dextrose solution. Avoid vascular extravasation which may lead to thrombophlebitis. For IM administration, do not administer more than 5 ml into each gluteal region. The parenteral form of this drug is not recommended for subcutaneous injection.

ORPHENADRINE CITRATE

PRODUCTS (TRADE NAME):

Marflex (Available in 100 mg tablets.) **Norflex** (Available in 100 mg sustained release tablet and 30 mg/ml for injection.) **Orpheradrine Citrate** (Available in 100 mg tablets, 100 mg sustained release tablets, and 30 mg/ml injection.) **O'Flex, X-Otag** (Available in 30 mg/ml.)

DRUG SPECIFICS:

Orphenadrine citrate is a centrally acting skeletal muscle relaxant which exhibits anticholinergic properties. The drug's exact mode of action remains to be determined, but it may be related to its analgesic characteristics, since it does not directly relax skeletal muscle. Its use is indicated for the relief of acute painful musculoskeletal conditions, particularly discogenic disease, tension, and past trauma. It also exerts a major effect on parkinsonian rigidity. The drug is contraindicated in patients with known hypersensitivity to orphenadrine, bladder neck obstruction, cardiospasm, glaucoma, myasthenia gravis, prostatic hypertrophy, pyloric or duodenal obstruction or stenosing peptic ulcer. The drug should be used with caution in cardiac patients. If used for long-term therapy, periodic blood, liver and urine evaluations are recommended. The anticholinergic side effects, usually the most bothersome to patients, include dryness of the mouth, tachycardia, urinary retention, blurred vision, increased ocular tension, and constipation. These drugs are additive with CNS depressants and anticholinergics. Advise the patient to take precautions against drowsiness and to observe for urinary hesitancy or retention.

ADMINISTRATION AND DOSAGE SPECIFICS:

Muscle spasm: Administer 100 mg tablet in the morning and evening. Or administer 60 mg intramuscularly or intravenously every 12 hours.

QUININE SULFATE

PRODUCT (TRADE NAME):

Quinamm (Available in 260 mg tablets).

DRUG SPECIFICS:

Quinine sulfate acts directly on skeletal muscle by increasing the refractory period in the muscle fiber and by decreasing the excitability of the motor end plate. The drug is used for the prevention and treatment of nocturnal recumbency leg muscle cramps associated with arthritis, diabetes, varicose veins, thrombophlebitis, arteriosclerosis and static foot deformities. This drug is contraindicated in children, in women of childbearing potential, in pregnant or breast-feeding women, in persons with known quinine hypersensitivity, and in patients with glucose-6-phosphate dehydrogenase deficiency. The administration of Quinamm has been associated with thrombocytopenic purpura and G-6-PD deficiency and interacts additively with warfarin and other oral anticoagulants. Side effects include tinnitus, dizziness, and gastrointestinal disturbances. Discontinue the drug if ringing in the ears, deafness, skin rash, or visual disturbances occur.

ADMINISTRATION AND DOSAGE SPECIFICS:

Relief of leg muscle cramps: Administer one tablet at bedtime; increase the dose to one tablet at the evening meal when necessary.

Doreen C. Harper

MUSCLE RELAXANTS
—COMBINATION DRUGS

PRODUCTS (TRADE NAME):
  Chlorofon-F, Chlorzone Forte, Chlorzoxazone with A.P.A.P., Parafon Forte, Tuzon, Zoxaphem (Available in tablet form with 250 mg chlorzoxazone and 300 mg acetaminophen.)
DRUG SPECIFICS:
  These products are combination, centrally acting, skeletal muscle relaxants containing chlorzoxazone and acetaminophen. Use is indicated in acute musculo-skeletal conditions that require symptomatic relief from muscle spasms and pain. The drug is contraindicated in persons sensitive to either component, in pregnant or nursing mothers and in children. Precaution should be exercised in using these drugs with persons who have hepatic dysfunction or history of allergic reactions to drugs. Drugs may cause urine to discolor orange or purple.
ADMINISTRATION AND DOSAGE SPECIFICS:
  Relief of muscle spasm and pain: Administer two tablets four times a day.

PRODUCTS (TRADE NAME):
  Methocarbamol with A.S.A., Robaxisal (Available in tablet form with each tablet containing 400 mg methocarbamol and 325 mg aspirin.)
DRUG SPECIFICS:
  These products are centrally acting skeletal muscle relaxants. The mechanism of action is due to the CNS depressant effects of methocarbamol and the anti-inflammatory analgesic effects of aspirin. They are indicated for relief of acute musculoskeletal conditions. The drugs are contraindicated in persons with known hypersensitivity to methocarbamol or aspirin, in pregnant or breast-feeding mothers and in children under 12 years. The most frequent side effects noted are drowsiness, dizziness and nausea. These drugs should be administered cautiously in persons on anticoagulant therapy or with gastritis or peptic ulcer. Advise the patient to contact the health care provider immediately if abdominal bleeding occurs and to administer the drug with food or meals to avoid gastric distress. Caution patient about the drug's CNS depressant effects.
ADMINISTRATION AND DOSAGE SPECIFICS:
  Relief of muscle spasm and for analgesia: Administer two tablets three to four times daily, or in severe conditions, use three tablets three to four times daily for 1-3 days.

PRODUCTS (TRADE NAME):
  Carisoprodol Compound, Soma Compound, Soprodol Compound (Available in tablet form with 200 mg carisoprodol, 160 mg phenacetin and 32 mg caffeine.)
DRUG SPECIFICS:
  These products are combination, centrally acting, skeletal muscle relaxants

containing carisoprodol, phenacetin and caffeine. They are used for treatment of acute muscle spasms and for relief of pain associated with musculoskeletal conditions. Their use is contraindicated in acute intermittent porphyria, in persons sensitive to any of its components or related compounds such as meprobamate, in children under 5 years and in pregnant or breast-feeding mothers. Phenacetin has been associated with severe kidney disease and cancer of the kidney when taken over long periods of time. Advise the patient of the drug's CNS depressant effects, the physical and psychological addictive effects and the withdrawal effects due to abrupt cessation of the drug. Health care providers should exercise caution when administering this drug to persons with anemia, cardiac, renal, pulmonary, or hepatic disease or known hypersensitivity to CNS stimulation. The common side effects noted are drowsiness, dizziness, nervousness and palpitations.

ADMINISTRATION AND DOSAGE SPECIFICS:

Relief of muscle spasm and pain: One to two tablets three to four times a day.

PRODUCTS (TRADE NAME):

Soma Compound with Codeine (Available in tablet form with 200 mg carisoprodol, 160 mg phenacetin, 32 mg caffeine and 16 mg codeine phosphate.)

DRUG SPECIFICS:

Soma Compound with Codeine is a combination, centrally acting, skeletal muscle relaxant containing carisoprodol, phenacetin, caffeine and codeine phosphate that has narcotic analgesic properties. It is used for treatment of acute muscle spasms and relief of pain associated with musculoskeletal conditions. Its use is contraindicated in acute intermittent porphyria, in persons sensitive to any of its components or related compounds such as meprobamate, in children under 5 years and in pregnant or breast-feeding women. Phenacetin has been associated with severe kidney disease and cancer of the kidney when taken over long periods of time. Advise the patient of the drug's CNS depressant effects, the physical and psychological addictive effects and the withdrawal effects due to abrupt cessation of the drug. Health care providers should exercise caution when administering this drug to persons with anemia, cardiac, renal, pulmonary or hepatic disease or known hypersensitivity to CNS stimulants. The common side effects noted are drowsiness, dizziness, nervousness and palpitations. Other side effects secondary to the codeine phosphate include nausea, vomiting, constipation, miosis and sedation.

PRODUCTS (TRADE NAME):

Norgesic (Available in tablet form with 25 mg orephenadrine citrate, 385 mg aspirin and 30 mg caffeine). **Norgesic Forte** (Available in tablet form with 50 mg orephenadrine citrate, 770 mg aspirin and 60 mg caffeine.)

DRUG SPECIFICS:

Norgesic and Norgesic Forte are combination, centrally acting, skeletal muscle relaxants indicated for the relief of mild to moderate pain and muscle spasms of acute musculoskeletal conditions. The drug is contraindicated in persons with glaucoma, pyloric or duodenal obstruction, achalasia, prostatic hypertrophy, obstructions at the bladder neck, myasthenia gravis or known hypersensitivity to aspirin or caffeine and in pregnant or breast-feeding women and children under 12 years of age. Advise the patient about the CNS depressant effects and the gastric irritation potential. Safe long-term use of this drug has not been established. Common side effects include anticholinergic characteristics such as dry mouth, constipation, tachycardia, urinary hesitancy or urgency, nausea and vomiting.

ADMINISTRATION AND DOSAGE SPECIFICS:

Relief from pain and muscle spasms: One to two tablets three to four times daily.

PRODUCTS (TRADE NAME):

Quinite (Available in 260 mg quinine sulfate and 195 mg aminophylline tablets.)

DRUG SPECIFICS:

This combination tablet uses the ability of quinine to decrease the excitability of the motor endplate and also to increase the refractory period by direct action on the muscle fiber. The physiologic action of aminophylline is not proven, but it may act to depolarize muscle membrane, increase metabolic rate of muscle or increase blood flow through the muscle itself. Because of these actions, this medication is used primarily as prophylaxis of muscle cramps occurring at night that are associated with diseases affecting peripherial circulation (diabetes, arthritis, varicose veins, arteriosclerosis, and thrombophlebitis.) It is contraindicated in patients with quinine sensitivity and G-6-PD deficiency and in pregnant women or women of childbearing potential. The action of warfarin and other oral anticoagulants may be potentiated with concurrent administration of this product. Thrombocytopenic purpura and hemolysis may develop following administration of this medication to sensitive individuals. Other adverse reactions are usually mild and self-limiting, including gastrointestinal and visual disturbances, rash, tinnitus and dizziness. Occasional deafness may be provoked. (Consult sections on Aminophylline and Quinine Sulfate for specifics.)

ADMINISTRATION AND DOSAGE SPECIFICS:

Adults: One tablet at bedtime. If necessary, a tablet may also be taken after evening meal.

Doreen C. Harper

PSYCHOTHERAPEUTIC DRUGS— ANTIANXIETY AGENTS

BENZODIAZEPINES

ACTION OF THE DRUG: These drugs (1) apparently act at the limbic, thalamic and hypothalamic levels of the central nervous system producing a calming effect.

(2) These agents also have anticonvulsant, skeletal muscle relaxant, sedative, and hypnotic actions in varying degrees. (3) Appetite-stimulating and weak analgesic effects have also been described.

ASSESSMENT:

INDICATIONS: Used for the relief of anxiety, tension, and fears that occur alone or as the result of illness. Other indications include management of delirium tremens after alcohol withdrawal; premedication for surgical and endoscopic procedures, or electric cardioversion; treatment of convulsive disorders (diazepam only); and relief of muscle spasm.

SUBJECTIVE: The provider may elicit a history of feelings of apprehension, uncertainty, fear, an unpleasant state of tension, a sense of impending doom, insomnia, irritability, hypersensitivity to stress, difficulty with concentration, or nightmares. There may be complaints of easy fatigability, headaches, malaise, weakness, restlessness, or nervousness. Anxiety could also be manifested as gastrointestinal disturbances such as anorexia, indigestion, flatulence, frequent bowel movements, diarrhea, or nervous stomach. Episodes of chest pain, palpitations, tachycardia, shortness of breath, tightness in the chest, and increased respiratory rate can be symptomatic of anxiety. Additionally, urinary frequency, urgency, decreased sex drive, and menstrual irregularities may be present.

OBJECTIVE: Alterations in the mental status exam such as inability to concentrate, slow speech or rapid speech may be noted. Other signs could include weight loss or weight gain, tremors, nail biting, restlessness, agitation, hyperventilation, diaphoresis, hand-wringing, tachycardia, premature atrial or ventricular contractions, or brisk deep tendon reflexes.

PLAN:

CONTRAINDICATIONS: Do not give in the presence of hypersensitivity to benzodiazepines, acute narrow angle glaucoma, untreated open angle glaucoma, or for the management of chronic pain.

WARNINGS: Thoroughly investigate the causes of organic disease that may be manifested as anxiety. The effectiveness of benzodiazepines in treatment that exceeds four months has not been studied. Minor tranquilizers have been associated with an increased risk of congenital malformations when given during the first trimester of pregnancy. Benzodiazepines are excreted in breast milk and have been shown to cause nursing infants to lose weight and become lethargic. Benzodiazepines should not be used with alcohol. Habituation, withdrawal symptoms, and development of tolerance to these agents have occurred, but are usually related to high dosages over long periods of time. The drugs generally have long half-lives and can have cumulative effects. Alterations of liver and renal function tests, blood counts, and bilirubin values are sometimes found with extended use. These drugs are not intended for use in the treatment of psychotic patients. Clients with a history of seizures or epilepsy should be tapered slowly from benzodiazepines.

PRECAUTIONS: Since depression commonly accompanies anxiety, patients must be questioned and observed for suicidal tendencies. Use with caution and in decreased dosages in the presence of hepatic or renal dysfunction to prevent excessive accumulation and subsequent increased effect. Administer drugs cautiously to patients with treated open angle glaucoma. Treatment with these drugs should proceed slowly in the elderly (over age 60), the debilitated, those with limited pulmonary reserve, and those in whom a hypotensive episode might precipitate cardiac dysfunction. Mental alertness, cognitive functions, and physical abilities may be impaired with use. Administer these drugs in conjunction with counseling or psychotherapy for maximum benefit.

IMPLEMENTATION:

DRUG INTERACTIONS: Simultaneous administration of the benzodiazepines with any of the following substances may increase either agent's effect: alcohol, anesthetics, monoamine oxidase (MAO) inhibitors, or central nervous system depressants such as antihistamines, barbiturates, phenothiazines, narcotics, sedatives, tranquilizers, hypnotics, anticonvulsants, or tricyclic antidepressants. Concomitant use of cimetidine or disulfiram with the benzodiazepines may slow their elimination from the body. Caffeinated products and excessive cigarette smoking can antagonize the anxiolytic effect of these drugs.

ADMINISTRATION AND DOSAGE: Psychic or physical dependence may result with prolonged use of benzodiazepines. No clinical studies have provided data to determine the efficacy of therapy continued longer than four months. These drugs should be discontinued gradually after prolonged use. Initial doses in the elderly and debilitated should be decreased, since these patients are more susceptible to drowsiness, ataxia, mental confusion, and oversedation. Dosages should be individualized for each patient, with adjustments required for persistent drowsiness, ataxia or visual disturbances.

Give prescriptions for the smallest amount possible to reduce the opportunity for overdose, particularly in those patients with a history of drug addiction or dependence. Withdrawal symptoms are often delayed for as long as one week after abrupt cessation of therapy. Administering the benzodiazepines during or immediately after meals decreases the incidence of gastrointestinal side effects. Refer to specific products for usage recommendations in children.

IMPLEMENTATION CONSIDERATIONS:

—Obtain a complete health history including hypersensitivities, underlying systemic disease (especially pulmonary, cardiac, liver or renal disease, epilepsy or seizures, myasthenia gravis, mental illness and drug abuse or dependence), possibility of pregnancy, lactation, or concurrent use of medications (both prescribed and over the counter) which may present drug interactions.

—Question the patient about a personal or family history of glaucoma. If there is a positive family history, tonometry may be advisable prior to initiating therapy.

—Elderly patients (over age 60) and those with chronic illnesses may require a decreased initial dosage and need careful monitoring of individual response before alterations in dosage are made.

—Abrupt termination of these agents may cause delayed withdrawal symptoms of abdominal or muscle cramps, vomiting, diaphoresis, tremor or convulsions. Tapering the dosage for those clients on prolonged therapy helps prevent this occurrence.

—Take lying, sitting and standing blood pressures.

—Obtain baseline studies and physical examination prior to initiating therapy.

—Observe patient for signs and symptoms of depression or suicidal tendencies.

—Explore alternatives for coping with stress and change with the patient, for example, increased regular physical activity, muscle relaxation exercises, and hobbies.

—Specific precautions and diluting directions accompany various injectable preparations. Consult the most recent manufacturer publications for this information.

WHAT THE PATIENT NEEDS TO KNOW:

—Take this medication exactly as ordered. Do not stop medication unless advised to do so by your health care provider. If you forget a dose, take it as soon as you remember it if within one to two hours of the regular dosage time. If it is later than two hours, skip the dose, and take the next dose at the regular time. Do not double the dosage.

—It is essential that you keep regular appointments with your medical care provider so that your progress can be checked and side effects of the drug can be monitored.

—This drug can cause dizziness, lightheadedness, drowsiness and unsteadiness. It may decrease your ability to think or react clearly and quickly. You should not drive, operate hazardous machinery, or perform activities requiring alertness, until you know how your body responds to the drug. These symptoms will often stop after you have taken the medicine for several weeks. Additionally, sit up and change to standing positions slowly to minimize these symptoms and prevent falls.

—If you have any new or troublesome symptoms while taking this medication, be certain to let your health provider know promptly. Notify your provider immediately if you notice any of the following side effects: ulcers or sores in the mouth, hallucinations, feelings of confusion, difficulty sleeping, skin rash, yellowing of eyes or skin, slow pulse, difficulty with breathing, sore throat and fever, unusual nervousness, excitement, irritability, depression or eye pain.

—Keep this medication out of the reach of children and all others for whom it is not prescribed.

—Inform your health care provider if you begin taking any new prescriptions or nonprescription drugs. Many different medications can change the way this drug will affect you. Therefore your provider may want to increase or decrease the dosage.

—You should not drink beer, wine, or liquor while you are taking this medicine.

—Cigarette smoking and the use of caffeinated beverages (coffee, tea, cola) can decrease the effect of the medicine.

—This medication is not intended for pregnant women. If you are pregnant, breast feeding, or if you should become pregnant while taking this medicine, you should inform your health care provider immediately.

—This drug may be habit-forming. Use it for the least time possible.

EVALUATION:

ADVERSE REACTIONS: *Cardiovascular:* bradycardia, edema, hypotension, palpitations, tachycardia. *CNS:* apathy, ataxia, clumsiness, confusion, depression, disorientation, drowsiness, dysarthria, euphoria, excitement, extrapyramidal symptoms, fatigue, headache, insomnia, lightheadedness, paradoxical reactions (excitement, hallucinations, agitation, hostility or rage), syncope, unsteadiness, visual disturbances, weakness. *Gastrointestinal:* anorexia, constipation, difficulty swallowing, dry mouth, hiccoughs, jaundice, nausea, vomiting. *Genitourinary:* changes in libido, incontinence, menstrual irregularities, urinary retention. *Hematopoietic:* agranulocytosis, leukopenia, neutropenia. *Hypersensitivity:* pruritus, skin rash, urticaria. *Other:* abuse, dependence, increase or decrease in body weight and joint pain, overdose, tolerance, and unexplained sore throat and fever. Phlebitis and thrombosis at site of intravenous therapy may also develop.

OVERDOSAGE: *Signs and symptoms:* Somnolence, confusion, coma, diminished reflexes and hypotension may develop. *Treatment:* Refer for gastric lavage to empty the stomach. Monitor vital signs. Render supportive mechanisms as required, i.e., IV fluids, maintenance of adequate airway, administration of levarterenol or metaraminol for hypotension. Always consider the possibility of the ingestion of more than one agent.

PARAMETERS TO MONITOR: Obtain baseline physical examination and complete blood count, differential, serum blood urea nitrogen (BUN), creatinine, glucose, bilirubin, aspartate aminotransferase (SGOT), alanine aminotransferase (SGPT), alkaline phosphatase, albumin, total protein, prothrombin time, and urinalysis. The effectiveness of prolonged use (more than four months) has not been studied. Therefore, careful consideration must be given to continuing therapy beyond that time. Some important factors to consider in determining necessity for return visits include: alterations in laboratory tests, the possibility of developing dependence on the drugs, and the occurrence of withdrawal symptoms after prolonged use in high dosages. In those clients with impaired renal or hepatic function, or in those receiving higher dosages than recommended, a repeat of baseline tests is advisable after three months and periodically thereafter. Patient response to these agents will vary greatly. The timing of return visits will be determined by the therapeutic response of the patient as measured by changes in signs and symptoms of anxiety and depression, and performance of mental status and neurologic exams. Additionally, assess for evidence of jaundice, monitor vital signs of blood pressure and pulse, and inspect the skin and mucous membranes for evidence of adverse reactions. Use of alcohol and other medications concurrently with the benzodiazepines should be closely questioned. Interviews with the patient should be conducted in a manner that will allow therapeutic listening, and counseling to aid the patient in long-term relief of anxiety and development of coping mechanisms once medication is withdrawn.

ALPRAZOLAM

PRODUCTS (TRADE NAME):
   Xanax (Available in 0.25 mg, 0.5 mg and 1 mg tablets.)
DRUG SPECIFICS:
   Action peaks in one to two hours; half-life 12-15 hours. Effectiveness and safety in children less than age 18 has not been determined.
ADMINISTRATION AND DOSAGE SPECIFICS:
   Adults: Initial dose 0.25 to 0.5 mg po three times each day; titrate to maximum dose of 4 mg po each day in divided doses.
   Elderly, debilitated: Initial dose is 0.25 mg po two or three times each day. Increase as tolerated.

CHLORAZEPATE DIPOTASSIUM

PRODUCTS (TRADE NAME):
   Tranxene (Available in 3.75 mg, 7.5 mg, and 15 mg tablets and capsules.) **Tranxene-SD** (Available in 22.5 mg tablets.) **Tranxene-SD Half Strength** (Available in 11.25 mg tablets.)
DRUG SPECIFICS:
   Peak effect is in 60 minutes; half-life is two days. Some reports indicate a fall in hematocrit with prolonged usage. Also used as an adjunctive medication for partial seizures. Can be given once each day. Tablets of 22.5 mg are not for initial therapy but may be used once daily for those patients stabilized on 7.5 mg three times day. For children less than 9 years drug is not recommended.
ADMINISTRATION AND DOSAGE SPECIFICS:
   Anxiety:
   Adults: Usual dose is 30 mg each day. May be given in 3 divided doses. May also be given as single bedtime dose of 15 mg. Adjust gradually with a range of 15-60 mg each day.
   Elderly, debilitated: First dose is 7.5 to 15 mg each day. Maximum daily dose is 90 mg.
   Partial Seizures Adjunct:
   Adults: Maximum initial dosage for over age 12 is 7.5 mg three times each day. Increase subsequent dosage by no more than 7.5 mg each week. Maximum dosage is 90 mg each day.

Children ages 9-12: Maximum initial dose is 7.5 mg two times each day. Increase not to exceed 7.5 mg each week. Maximum dosage 60 mg each day.

Acute alcohol withdrawal:

Consult latest manufacturers guide for recommended dosing schedule.

CHLORDIAZEPOXIDE

PRODUCTS (TRADE NAME):

A-poxide (Available in 5, 10 and 25 mg capsules.) **Chlordiazepoxide HCl** (Available in 5 mg, 10 mg, and 25 mg capsules.) **Libritabs** (Available in 5, 10 and 25 mg tablets.) **Librium** (Available in 5 mg, 10 mg, 25 mg tablets and capsules; and 100 mg/2 l injection.) **Lipoxide** (available in 5, 10, and 25 mg capsules). **Murcil** (Available in 5, and 10 mg capsules.) **Reprosans-10** (Available in 10 mg capsule.) **Sereen** (Available in 10 mg capsules.) **SK-Lygen** (Available in 5, 10 and 25 mg capsules.) **Tenax, Zetran** (Available in 10 mg capsules.)

DRUG SPECIFICS:

Peak levels attained in one to four hours with the half-life at 5-30 hours. The ingestion of antacids or food slows absorption. Use with caution in patients with porphyria since this condition may be exacerbated. Concurrent usage with oral anticoagulants may affect blood coagulation. This drug is also used as an antidyskinetic. IV injection must be carried out slowly to avoid producing respiratory arrest. Injection not advised for children younger than age

Not recommended for children less than 6 years.

ADMINISTRATION AND DOSAGE SPECIFICS:

Anxiety: Usual adult dose is 5 to 25 mg three or four times each day; 5 to 10 mg three to four times each day may be given several days preoperatively to allay anxiety.

Elderly, debilitated: Usual dose is 5 mg two to four times per day.

Alcohol withdrawal: Injection used initially if severe. If oral is used, give 50 to 100 mg as needed up to 300 mg each day, then taper to maintenance dose.

Children over age 6: 5 mg two to four times each day.

DIAZEPAM

PRODUCTS (TRADE NAME):

Valium (Available in 2 mg, 5 mg and 10 mg tablets, and 5 mg/ml injection.) **Valrelease** (Available in 15 mg sustained-release capsules.)

DRUG SPECIFICS:

Peak blood levels are reached within one to two hours with a half-life of 20 to 50 hours. Not recommended for use in children less than 6 months. Injectable form is used as an anticonvulsant in status epilepticus. If used concurrently with rifampin, the half-life is shortened; with isoniazid (INH) it is prolonged. Ingestion of food or antacids decreases the rate of absorption of diazepam. Some studies have hypothesized that diazepam may be implicated as a tumor promoter. When this effect is noted, it may work in combination with prolactin. Therefore, existing tumors of the kidney, breast or prostate, which are prolactin sensitive, could be more susceptible to such an effect. Reports are inconclusive. However, use in patients with a known carcinoma should be carefully weighed from a risk-benefit perspective.

IM use is not recommended since absorption is slow and erratic. For specifics regarding IV dosages, refer to the latest manufacturers' information.

ADMINISTRATION AND DOSAGE SPECIFICS:

Anxiety and management of convulsive disorders: 2 to 10 mg two to four times each day. Sustained release capsules 15 to 30 mg each day.

Skeletal muscle spasm: 2 to 10 mg three to four times each day. Sustained release capsules 15 to 30 mg each day.

Acute alcoholic withdrawal: First 24 hours give 10 mg three or four times, then decrease to 5 mg three or four times each day.

Elderly or debilitated: 2 to 2.5 mg once or two times each day, then gradually increase as tolerated and needed.

Children: Usual dose is 1 to 2.5 mg three or four times each day initially, then gradually increase.

HALAZEPAM

PRODUCTS (TRADE NAME):
Paxipam (Available in 20 and 40 mg tablets.)
DRUG SPECIFICS:
Action peaks in 1 to 3 hours; half-life is 14 hours. Individualize dosages as needed and tolerated. No recommendations for children established.
ADMINISTRATION AND DOSAGE SPECIFICS:
Adults: 20 to 40 mg po three or four times each day. Optimal range is 80 to 160 mg po each day.
Elderly, debilitated: 20 mg po one or two times each day.

LORAZEPAM

PRODUCTS (TRADE NAME):
Ativan (Available in 0.5 mg, 1 mg and 2 mg tablets; and 2 and 4 mg/ml injection.)
DRUG SPECIFICS:
Action peaks in 2.5 hours; half-life is 10 to 15 hours. In elderly patients, or

those on prolonged treatment, symptoms of upper gastrointestinal disease must be monitored. Patients may experience withdrawal manifested as insomnia two or three nights after cessation of therapy. Not recommended for children less than age 18. IM injection is used as a preanesthetic agent for adults only. It is also given IV for sedation and relief of anxiety. Consult the latest manufacturer information for specifics of injectable dosing.

ADMINISTRATION AND DOSAGE SPECIFICS:

Anxiety: Initial dose is 2 to 3 mg po two or three times each day. Usual range is 2 to 6 mg each day in divided doses with the largest dose before sleep.

Insomnia: Single bedtime dose of 2 to 4 mg po.

Elderly, debilitated: Initial dose is 1 to 2 mg po in divided doses each day.

OXAZEPAM

PRODUCTS (TRADE NAME):

Serax (Available in 10, 15, 30 mg capsules and 15 mg tablets.)

DRUG SPECIFICS:

Peak blood levels at two to four hours. Half-life is 5 to 20 hours. The incidence of cumulative toxicity is low. Tartrazine is contained in the 15 mg tablet, which may cause an allergic-type reaction, especially in patients with aspirin allergy. (Symptoms of bronchial asthma develop.) Medication is often used in treating elderly (over age 60) clients. Dosages not established in children under 12. Contraindicated for use in children under 6 years. It has been implicated as an agent which may cause systemic lupus erythematosus.

ADMINISTRATION AND DOSAGE SPECIFICS:

Anxiety: Usual adult dose is 10 to 30 mg po three or four times each day.

Elderly or debilitated: Start with 10 mg po three times each day, then increase gradually to 15 mg three or four times each day.

Alcohol withdrawal: 15 to 30 mg three or four times each day.

PRAZEPAM

PRODUCTS (TRADE NAME):

Centrax (Available in 5 and 10 mg capsules and 10 mg tablets.)

DRUG SPECIFICS:

This drug is not recommended for patients less than 18 years. Peak blood levels at six hours after administration.

ADMINISTRATION AND DOSAGE SPECIFICS:

Adults: Usual dosage is 30 mg po each day with dosages gradually adjusted within range of 20 to 60 mg each day.

Elderly, debilitated: Initial dose is 10 to 15 mg po each day in divided doses. This drug may be given in a single bedtime dose. Recommended to start with 20 mg, with optimum dosage from 20 to 40 mg.

Carol Ann Vittek

ANTIANXIETY AGENTS— CARBAMATE DERIVATIVES

ACTION OF THE DRUG: Meprobamate and tybamate are carbamate derivatives that appear to act at several sites of the central nervous system, including the thalamus, the limbic system, and polysynaptic reflex arcs in the spinal cord. The drugs function as anxiolytis, skeletal muscle relaxants, anticonvulsants, hypnotic, and produce effects of sedation and alteration of emotional states. A related product, chlormezanone, acts to allay mild anxiety without interfering with clarity of mind or consciousness.

ASSESSMENT:

INDICATIONS: Carbamates are used in the treatment of anxiety and tension, as skeletal muscle relaxants, in relief of insomnia, and as anticonvulsants in the treatment of petit mal epilepsy.

SUBJECTIVE: The provider may elicit a history of feelings of apprehension, uncertainty, fear, an unpleasant state of tension, a sense of impending doom, insomnia, irritability, hypersensitivity to stress, difficulty with concentration or nightmares. There may be complaints of easy fatigability, headaches, malaise, weakness, restlessness, or nervousness.

Anxiety could also be manifested as gastrointestinal disturbances such as anorexia, indigestion, flatulence, frequent bowel movements, diarrhea, or nervous stomach. Episodes of chest pain, palpitations, tachycardia, shortness of breath, tightness in the chest, and increased respiratory rate can be symptomatic of anxiety. Additionally, urinary frequency, urgency, decreased sex drive, and menstrual irregularities may be present.

OBJECTIVE: Alterations in the mental status exam such as inability to concentrate, slow speech or rapid speech may be seen. Other signs could include weight loss or weight gain, tremors, nail biting, restlessness, agitation, hyperventilation, diaphoresis, hand wringing, tachycardia, premature atrial or ventricular contractions, or brisk deep tendon reflexes.

PLAN:

CONTRAINDICATIONS: Do not give in the presence of hypersensitivity to meprobamate or related agents such as carisoprodol, mebutamate, tybamate, or carbromal. Do not give to patients with acute intermittent porphyria.

WARNINGS: Thoroughly investigate the causes of organic disease that may be manifested as anxiety. The effectiveness of carbamates in treatment that exceeds four months has not been studied. These drugs may cause seizures in epileptics. The use of minor tranquilizers has been associated with an increased risk of congenital malformations when given during the first trimester of pregnancy. Meprobamate is present in breast milk, so use with caution in nursing mothers. Drug dependence and withdrawal symptoms after prolonged use have been reported. Serum levels of aspartate aminotransferase (SGOT), alanine aminotransferase (SGPT), alkaline phosphatase, bilirubin and cholesterol can be increased with extended use of high dosages. Additionally, platelet counts can decrease, and urine porphyria and aminolevulinic acid levels can rise.

PRECAUTIONS: Since depression commonly accompanies anxiety, patients must be questioned and observed for suicidal tendencies. Use with caution and in decreased dosages in hepatic or renal dysfunction, and in the elderly (over age 60) or debilitated individuals. Mental alertness, cognitive functions, and physical abilities may be impaired with use. The presence of tartrazine (FD&C Yellow No. 5) in some of these products may produce hypersensitivity reactions in some patients, most notably those with aspirin allergy in which a bronchial asthma-like attack may be provoked. Administer in conjunction with counseling or psychotherapy for maximum therapeutic effect.

IMPLEMENTATION:

DRUG INTERACTIONS: Simultaneous administration of meprobamate and other central nervous system depressants produces an additive effect. Taken in conjunction with other anticonvulsants, meprobamate can change the seizure pattern. This drug can diminish the effectiveness of oral anticoagulants, estrogens, and oral contraceptives, necessitating increased dosages of these agents for therapeutic effect.

ADMINISTRATION AND DOSAGE: Psychic or physical dependence may result with prolonged use of meprobamate. The effect of therapy longer than four months has not been studied. Discontinue gradually after prolonged use to prevent symptoms of withdrawal. Onset of withdrawal symptoms is usually within 12 to 48 hours after cessation of therapy. Prescriptions should be given for the smallest amount possible to reduce the possibility of overdose. This agent is not recommended for use in children less than 6 years. Onset of the drug occurs one hour after oral administration. Administer with food to decrease symptoms of gastric distress.

IMPLEMENTATION CONSIDERATIONS:
—Obtain a complete health history, including the presence of hypersensitivity (especially to meprobamate, carisoprodol, mebutamate, tybamate, carbromal, or aspirin), possibility of pregnancy or lactation, history of intermittent porphyria or underlying systemic disease, concurrent use of medications (both prescription and over-the-counter drugs) and previous history of drug or alcohol habituation.

—Elderly and debilitated patients may require a decreased initial dosage with careful monitoring of individual response before dosages are altered.

—Abrupt termination of these agents can cause withdrawal symptoms of vomiting, ataxia, tremors, muscle twitching, confusion, hallucinations, and convulsive seizures (rare). The danger of seizures is greater in patients with a history of convulsive disorders or central nervous system dysfunction. Following lengthy high-dose treatment, drug should be tapered over a one-to-two-week period.

—Take lying, sitting and standing blood pressures.

—Obtain baseline laboratory studies and physical examination.

—Observe patient for signs and symptoms of depression or suicidal tendencies.

—Explore alternatives for coping with stress and change with the patient; for example, increased regular physical exercise, muscle relaxation exercises and hobbies may be suggested.

WHAT THE PATIENT NEEDS TO KNOW:

—Take this drug exactly as ordered. Do not stop taking medication suddenly. If you miss a regular dose of the medicine, take another dose if it is within one to two hours of the regular dosage time. If it is later than two hours, skip the dose and take the next dose at the regular time. Do not double the dosage.

—It is essential that you keep regular appointments with your medical care provider so that your progress can be checked and side effects of the drug can be monitored.

—This drug may cause dizziness, lightheadedness, drowsiness, and unsteadiness. It may decrease your ability to think or react clearly and quickly. You should not drive, operate dangerous machinery, or perform hazardous activities until you know how your body responds to the drug. These symptoms will often stop after you have taken the medicine for several weeks. Additionally, change positions from sitting and standing slowly to minimize these symptoms and prevent falls.

—Inform your health care provider if you are taking any other prescription or non-prescription drugs. Many different medications can change the way this drug will affect you. Therefore your provider may want to increase or decrease the dosage.

—You should not drink beer, wine, or liquor while you are taking this medicine.

—Use of caffeinated beverages (coffee, tea, cola drinks) can decrease the effect of the medicine.

—This medication is not intended for pregnant women. If you are pregnant, breast-feeding, or if you should become pregnant while taking this medicine, you should inform your health care provider immediately.

—Notify your health practitioner promptly if you notice any of the following side effects: mental confusion, sore throat with fever, unusual bruising or bleeding, unexplained excitement, either a very fast or slow heartbeat, wheezing, trouble with breathing, skin rash, or decreased amount of urine.

—This drug may be habit-forming and should be taken for the shortest possible time.

EVALUATION:

ADVERSE REACTIONS: *Cardiovascular:* arrhythmias, hypotensive crisis, palpitations, syncope, transient electrocardiogram changes. *CNS:* ataxia, dizziness, drowsiness, fast electroencephalographic activity, headache, impairment of visual accommodation, insomnia, paradoxical reactions of rage or euphoria, panic reaction, paresthesias, seizures in epileptics, slurrred speech, vertigo, weakness. *Gastrointestinal:* anorexia, diarrhea, dry mouth, glossitis, nausea, vomiting. *Hematopoietic:* agranulocytosis, aplastic anemia, leukopenia, and (rarely) thrombocytopenic purpura. *Hypersensitivity:* Reactions usually occur between the first and fourth doses. Milder reactions are characterized by pruritic, urticarial, or erythematous maculopapular rash that is generalized or found in groin. Other reactions have included leukopenia, acute non-thrombocytopenic purpura, petechiae, ecchymoses, eosinophilia, peripheral edema, adenopathy, fever, fixed drug eruption with cross-sensitivity between meprobamate-mebutamate and meprobamate-carbromal. More severe, rare reactions include hyperpyrexia, chills, angioneurotic edema, bronchospasm, oliguria, anuria, anaphylaxis, erythema multiforme, exfoliative dermatitis, stomatitis, proctitis, Stevens-Johnson syndrome, and bullous dermatitis. *Other:* exacerbation of acute intermittent porphyria, grand mal attack, respiratory depression, and circulatory collapse.

OVERDOSAGE: *Signs and symptoms:* There is a wide range of reactions to overdosage. Death has been reported with as little as 12 gm and survival with as much as 40 gm. Blood levels of 0.5 to 3 mg/100 ml indicate therapeutic range. Drowsiness, lethargy, stupor, ataxia, coma, shock, vasomotor and respiratory collapse and death may develop. *Treatment:* Referral for gastric lavage and supportive therapy as needed. Osmotic diuresis with mannitol, peritoneal dialysis and hemodialysis have been effective. Avoid dehydration.

PARAMETERS TO MONITOR: The effectiveness of prolonged use (more than four months) has not been studied. Therefore, careful consideration must be given to continuing therapy beyond that time. Some important factors to consider in determining the necessity for return visits include: alterations in laboratory tests, the possibility of developing dependence on the drugs, and the occurrence of withdrawal symptoms after prolonged use in high dosages. Baseline laboratory studies should consist of complete blood count, differential, platelet count, serum blood urea nitrogen (BUN), creatinine, aspartate aminotransferase (SGOT), alanine aminotransferase (SGPT), alkaline phosphatase, bilirubin, cholesterol, total protein, prothrombin time and urinalysis. In those patients with impaired renal or hepatic function, or in those receiving higher dosages than recommended, a repeat of these tests is advisable after three months and periodically thereafter.

Patient response to these agents will vary greatly. The timing of return visits will be determined by the therapeutic response of the patient as measured by changes in signs and symptoms of anxiety and depression, and performance of mental status and neurologic exams. Monitor pulse and blood pressure. Use of alcohol and other medications concurrently with meprobamate should be closely questioned. Interviews with the patient should be conducted in a manner that will allow therapeutic listening and counseling to aid the patient in long-term relief of anxiety, and development of coping mechanisms once medication is withdrawn.

CHLORMEZANONE

PRODUCTS (TRADE NAME):
Chlormezanone (Available in 200 mg tablets). **Trancopol Caplets** (Available in 100 and 200 mg tablets).
DRUG SPECIFICS:
Central nervous system depressant effects are similar to those of meprobamate. Onset is 15 to 30 minutes after oral dosage; half-life is 24 hours. Additional adverse reactions of xerostomia, jaundice, and inability to void have been reported. Begin with smallest possible dose and increase gradually. Not recommended in children younger than age 6 years.
ADMINISTRATION AND DOSAGE SPECIFICS:
Adults: 100 to 200 mg po three or four times each day.
Children 5 to 12 years: 50 to 100 mg po three or four times each day.

MEPROBAMATE

PRODUCTS (TRADE NAME):
Equanil (Available in 200 and 400 mg tablets, and 400 mg capsules). **Equanil Wyseals** (Available in 400 mg coated tablets with tartrazine). **Mepriam** (Available in 400 mg tablets). **Meprobamate** (Available in 200 and 400 mg tablets). **Meprospan** (Available in 200 and 400 mg sustained-release capsules). **Miltown** (Available in 200, 400 and 600 mg tablets). **Neuramate** (Available in 200 and 400 mg tablets). **Neurate-400** (Available in 400 mg tablets.) **Sedabamate, SK-Bamate, Tranmep** (Available in 400 mg tablets). **SK-Bamate** (Available in 200 and 400 mg tablets).
DRUG SPECIFICS:
Onset of action is within one hour after oral dosage. Half-life ranges from 6 to 16 hours. Not recommended for use in children younger than age 6 years.
ADMINISTRATION AND DOSAGE SPECIFICS:
Adults: 1200 to 1600 mg po three or four times per day. Not to exceed 2400 mg/day.
Children 6 to 12 years: 100 to 200 mg po two or three times each day.

TYBAMATE

PRODUCTS (TRADE NAME):
   Tybatran (Available in 250 and 350 mg capsules containing tartrazine).
DRUG SPECIFICS:
   Chemically and pharmacologically similar to meprobamate but is shorter acting. Peak blood levels reached in one to two hours with a half-life of three hours. Not recommended in children under age 6.
ADMINISTRATION AND DOSAGE SPECIFICS:
   Adults: 250 or 500 mg three or four times each day or 350 mg three times each day or 700 mg at bedtime. Do not exceed 3000 mg each day.
   Children 6 to 12 years: 20 to 35 mg/kg/day in three or four divided doses.

Carol Ann Vittek

ANTIANXIETY AGENTS:
DOXEPIN HYDROCHLORIDE

ACTION OF THE DRUG: Doxepin HCl is a tricyclic antidepressant that is believed to act on the central nervous system to produce increased concentrations of catecholamines at the synapses. These drugs have some anticonvulsant, anticholinergic, and sedative effects. They can also act as mild peripheral vasodilators.

ASSESSMENT:

INDICATIONS: Doxepin is utilized in the treatment of anxiety and/or depression caused by neuroses, organic disease or alcoholism.
   SUBJECTIVE: The provider may elicit a history of feelings of apprehension, uncertainty, fear, an unpleasant state of tension, a sense of impending doom, insomnia, irritability, hypersensitivity to stress, difficulty with concentration or nightmares. There may be complaints of easy fatigability, headaches, malaise, weakness, restlessness, or nervousness.
   Anxiety could also be manifested as gastrointestinal disturbances such as anorexia, indigestion, flatulence, frequent bowel movements, diarrhea, or nervous stomach. Episodes of chest pain, palpitations, tachycardia, shortness of breath, tightness in the chest, and increased respiratory rate can be symptomatic of anxiety. Additionally, urinary frequency, urgency, decreased sex drive, and menstrual irregularities may be present.
   OBJECTIVE: Alterations in the mental status exam may be seen such as inability to concentrate, slow speech or rapid speech. Other signs could include weight loss or weight gain, tremors, nail biting, restlessness, agitation, hyperven-

tilation, diaphoresis, hand wringing, tachycardia, premature atrial or ventricular contractions, or brisk deep tendon reflexes.

PLAN:

CONTRAINDICATIONS: Do not give in the presence of hypersensitivity to any tricyclic antidepressant; in patients with glaucoma or urinary retention; and in the immediate recovery phase after myocardial infarction. Generally these drugs should not be used concurrently with monoamine oxidase (MAO) inhibitors.

WARNINGS: In patients with convulsive disorders, seizures frequently may increase. New onset of seizures has also been reported. Cardiac arrhythmias, tachycardia, and increased conduction time have been reported. Cautious use of these agents is recommended in patients with a history of angina pectoris, myocardial infarction, hyperthyroidism, or other cardiac disorders. Excessive accumulation of the drug may occur in patients with hepatic or renal dysfunction. In clients with a history of psychosis, symptoms may be worsened. Use in pregnancy and lactation is not advised since this drug crosses the placental barrier and is present in breast milk. Doxepin should not be used with alcohol. Organic disease that may be manifested as anxiety must be ruled out. Alterations in serum glucose (increase or decrease), leukocyte count, differential white blood cell counts, and liver function tests have occurred.

PRECAUTIONS: Patients must be questioned and observed for suicidal tendencies. Drowsiness may impair mental alertness and response time. Warn patients against performing hazardous activities. An electrocardiogram should be performed before starting higher than normal doses with subsequent periodic repeat exams as dosage is adjusted. Stop the drug for as long an interval as possible prior to elective surgery. Administer in conjunction with counseling or psychotherapy for maximum benefit.

IMPLEMENTATION:

DRUG INTERACTIONS: Concurrent use with monoamine oxidase (MAO) inhibitors is contraindicated since hyperpyretic episodes, convulsions, hypertensive crises, and death have resulted. Additive anticholinergic side effects can occur when administered with antihistamines, narcotics, analgesics, benzodiazepines, phenothiazines, glutethimide, and other anticholinergics. Concomitant administration with acetazolamide, ammonium chloride, ascorbic acid, and sodium bicarbonate can increase the effect by enhancing renal tubular reabsorption of the drug. Given in doses greater than 150 mg daily, the antihypertensive effects of guanethidine or clonidine may be blocked. Use with sympathomimetics can cause hyperpyrexia, severe hypertension, or cardiac arrhythmias. Increased effect of either agent can occur when doxepin is administered simultaneously with alcohol, methylphenidate, phenothiazines, barbiturates, benzodiazepines, quinidine, and procainamide. Sinus tachycardia or cardiac arrhythmias may result when concurrently administered with thyroid preparations. Given with ethylchlorvynol, transient delirium may result. Potentiation of adverse reactions and a decrease in antidepressant effects can occur when administered with estrogens or oral contraceptives. Tricyclic antidepressants are antagonized by beta-adrenergic blockers. They may also diminish the hypotensive effect of reserpine. Reserpine can cause a stimulating response in the depressed patient.

PRODUCTS (TRADE NAME):

Adapin (Available in 10, 25, 50, 75 and 100 mg capsules which contain tartrazine.) **Sinequan** (Available in 10, 25, 50, 75, 100 and 150 mg capsules; and oral concentration with 10 mg/ml in 120 ml with dropper.)

ADMINISTRATION AND DOSAGE SPECIFICS:

Dosages should be individualized by titration. The desired antidepressant effect may not be realized for two to six weeks after initiation of therapy. Initiate therapy in the elderly (over age 60) and adolescents at lower dosages. A single daily dose at bedtime may be sufficient for maintenance; however, this may not be tolerated well in the elderly. Divided doses are recommended in elderly, adolescents, and patients with cardiac disease. Administer oral preparations with meals to reduce gastric irritation. Since withdrawal symptoms have been reported, medication should be tapered over a month or longer. Larger quantities of the drug should not be prescribed, especially in potentially suicidal patients. The elderly are particularly prone to orthostatic hypotension.

The antianxiety effect is rapid. No reports of dependency or withdrawal symptoms noted. Medication is not recommended for children less than age 12. Some capsules contain FD&C Yellow #5 which contains tartrazine, which may provoke allergy in some patients, especially those sensitive to aspirin.

Mix oral concentrate immediately before use with 120 ml of water, milk, or fruit juice. Do not mix with carbonated beverages or grape juice. Do not store diluted concentrate.

Mild symptoms: 10 to 25 mg po three times each day.

Moderate symptoms: 25 mg three times each day. Optimum dosage 75-150 mg each day. May be given as single bedtime dose of up to 150 mg.

Severe symptoms: 50 mg po three times each day. Maximum daily dosage 300 mg.

IMPLEMENTATION CONSIDERATIONS:

—Obtain a complete health history including the presence of hypersensitivity (especially to tricyclic antidepressants or aspirin), underlying systemic disease (such as glaucoma, urinary retention, prostatic hypertrophy, recent myocardial infarction, seizures), possibility of pregnancy or lactation, and concurrent use of other medications (especially MAO inhibitors.)

—When prolonged therapy has been in effect drug should be tapered to prevent withdrawal symptoms.

—Observe the patient for signs and symptoms of depression or suicidal tendencies.

—Xerostomia is a common side effect caused by persistently dry mucous membranes. Encourage frequent oral hygiene measures and use of sugarless gum, saliva substitutes, and an increase of fluid intake.

—Monitor symptoms of hypoglycemia and hyperglycemia in the diabetic patient.

—Explore support systems that are available to the patient to aid in resolving anxiety or depression. Assist patient in developing coping strategies to deal with stress and change such as a regular plan of physical exercise, muscle relaxation techniques, and hobbies.

WHAT THE PATIENT NEEDS TO KNOW:

—Take this drug exactly as ordered by health care provider. If you forget to take one dose of medicine, take it as soon as you remember, then return to your regular medication schedule. But if you miss a bedtime dose that is once a day, do not take it in the morning. Check with your health care provider.

—This drug can cause dizziness, lightheadedness, drowsiness and unsteadiness. It may decrease your ability to think or react clearly and quickly. You should not drive, operate dangerous machinery, or perform hazardous activities, until you know how your body responds to the drug. These symptoms will often stop after you have taken the medicine for several weeks. Additionally, change positions from lying or sitting slowly to minimize these symptoms and prevent falls.

—Inform your health care provider if you are taking any other prescription or non-prescription drugs. Many different medications can change the way this drug will affect you. Therefore your provider may want to increase or decrease the dosage.

—You should not drink beer, wine, or liquor while you are taking this medication.

—If you are pregnant, breast feeding, or if you should become pregnant while taking this medicine, you should inform your health care provider immediately.

—Keep this medication out of the reach of children and all others for whom it is not prescribed.

—This drug may make you feel unsteady, dizzy, or lightheaded when you change positions. To lessen these symptoms and prevent falls, change position slowly when moving from lying to sitting to standing. Also hold onto something to steady yourself. Keep your legs elevated when sitting. The use of firm support socks, pantyhose, or elastic stockings may also help prevent these symptoms.

—This drug can make your mouth feel very dry. Use sugarless gum, and brush and floss your teeth frequently. Rinse your mouth and drink at least two quarts of fluid each day if you have not been told to restrict fluids by your health provider.

—If you develop a fever, sore throat, and aching all over your body, or your skin or eyes look yellow, call your health care provider immediately.

EVALUATION:

ADVERSE REACTIONS: *Anticholinergic:* blurred vision, constipation, delayed micturition, dilation of the urinary tract, disturbance of accommodation, dry mouth, paralytic ileus, sublingual adenitis, urinary retention. *Cardiac:* arrhythmias, electrocardiogram changes (prolonged QT interval, T-wave and ST segment changes), heart block, hypertension, hypotension, myocardial infarction, palpitations, precipitation of congestive heart failure, stroke, syncope, tachycardia. *CNS:* agitation, anxiety, ataxia, changes in electroencephalographic patterns, confusion, decreased memory, delusion, disorientation, dizziness, drowsiness, exacerbation of psychosis, extrapyramidal symptoms, fatigue, feelings of unreality, hallucinations, headaches, incoordination, insomnia, nervousness, nightmares, numbness, panic, paresthesias, peripheral neuropathy, seizures, tinnitus, tremors, weakness. *Endocrine:* altered libido, breast enlargement, impotence, increased or decreased blood glucose levels, testicular swelling. *Gastrointestinal:* abdominal cramps, anorexia, black tongue, constipation, diarrhea, epigastric distress, jaundice, nausea, peculiar taste, stomatitis, vomiting. *Hematopoietic:* agranulocytosis, bone marrow depression, eosinophilia, leukopenia, purpura, thrombocytopenia. *Hypersensitivity:* cross-sensitivity with other tricyclics, drug fever, edema, petechiae, photosensitization, pruritus, skin rash, urticaria. *Other:* alopecia, diaphoresis, flushing, parotid swelling, unexplained sore throat and fever, weight loss or gain.

OVERDOSAGE: *Signs and symptoms:* Mild: Drowsiness, stupor, blurred vision, and excessive dryness of mouth may be an indication that mild overdosage is present. Severe: Respiratory depression, hypotension, coma, convulsions, cardiac arrhythmias and tachycardia may develop. Other signs and symptoms: urinary retention (bladder atony), decreased gastrointestinal motility (paralytic ileus), hyperthermia or hypothermia, hypertension, dilated pupils, hyperactive reflexes. *Treatment:* Refer for gastric lavage. Administer activated charcoal, give continuous lavage for 24 hours with saline. Provide general supportive measures. Electrocardiographic monitoring should be carried out until patients' sensorium has returned to normal and ECG is normal. Treat arrhythmias as needed. Central nervous system symptoms may be reversed with administration of 1 mg to 3 mg of physostigmine salicylate; repeat dosage as needed.

PARAMETERS TO MONITOR: Baseline laboratory determinations should include electrocardiogram (ECG), complete blood count, differential blood count, platelet count, serum glucose, blood urea nitrogen (BUN), creatinine, aspartate aminotransferase (SGOT), alanine aminotransferase (SGPT), bilirubin, total protein, albumin, prothrombin time, and urinalysis. Since dosages are individualized, repeat tests will be determined by each patient's therapeutic response and clinical picture. Orthostatic blood pressures should be determined. Cardiac rate and rhythm should also be evaluated. Weight, presence of edema, condition of skin (noting rashes or bruises particularly), and oral mucosa, mental status, and neurologic exams should be monitored with repeat visits. Explore the use of alcohol and other medications with the patient. Conduct interviews to allow for therapeutic listening and counseling to aid the patient in long-term relief of anxiety and development of coping mechanisms once medication is withdrawn. Also monitor for symptoms of dependency and suicidal tendencies.

Carol Ann Vittek

ANTIANXIETY AGENTS—HYDROXYZINE

ACTION OF THE DRUG: An anxiolytic agent that probably acts by suppressing activity of the hypothalamus and the brain stem and reticular formation. Also has antispasmodic, antihistaminic, antiemetic, anticholinergic, antisecretory, and skeletal muscle relaxant effects.

ASSESSMENT:

INDICATIONS: Can be used to alleviate tension and anxiety associated with temporary stressful situations, organic disease states, and alcoholism. Other indications include treatment of pruritus associated with allergic conditions, control of nausea and vomiting, prevention of motion sickness, and to decrease the amount of narcotic required for preoperative or postoperative sedation.

SUBJECTIVE: The provider may elicit a history of feelings of apprehension, uncertainty, fear, an unpleasant state of tension, a sense of impending doom, insomnia, irritability, hypersensitivity to stress, difficulty with concentration, or nightmares. There may be complaints of easy fatigability, headaches, malaise, weakness, restlessness, or nervousness.

Anxiety may also be manifested as gastrointestinal disturbances such as anorexia, indigestion, flatulence, frequent bowel movements, diarrhea, or nervous stomach. Episodes of chest pain, palpitations, tachycardia, shortness of breath, tightness in the chest, and increased respiratory rate can be symptomatic of anxiety. Additionally, urinary frequency, urgency, decreased sex drive, and menstrual irregularities may be present.

OBJECTIVE: Alterations in the mental status exam such as inability to concentrate, slow speech or rapid speech may be noted. Other signs could include weight loss or weight gain, tremors, nail biting, restlessness, agitation, hyperventilation, diaphoresis, hand wringing, tachycardia, premature atrial or ventricular contractions, or brisk deep tendon reflexes.

PLAN:

CONTRAINDICATIONS: Do not give in the presence of hypersensitivity to hydroxyzine, or during early pregnancy. The injectable form is for intramuscular use only. Not for use as the only agent in the treatment of psychosis or depression.

WARNINGS: Safety for use in lactating mothers is not established; therefore, use is not advised.

PRECAUTIONS: Drowsiness may impair mental alertness and response time. Elderly patients (over age 60) may be more sensitive to the normal adult dose. Careful intramuscular injection into a large muscle mass is required to prevent tissue damage. Administer in conjunction with counseling or psychotherapy for maximum benefits.

IMPLEMENTATION:

DRUG INTERACTIONS: Concurrent administration with any of the following agents may add to the effect of either agent: alcohol, general anesthetics, central nervous system depressants, tricyclic antidepressants, barbiturates, antihistamines, anticonvulsants, narcotics, prescription pain medications, sedatives, hypnotics, or tranquilizers. The anticholinergic activity of hydroxyzine can antagonize anticholinesterase drugs such as physostigmine, neostigmine, and edrophonium chloride. This product may produce interference with 17-hydroxycorticosteroid determinations.

ADMINISTRATION AND DOSAGE: Individualize dosages based on patient response. Elderly (over age 60) patients should be given lower than usual initial dosages. Central nervous system depressant drug dosages may require up to a 50 percent reduction when administered concomitantly with hydroxyzine. When given with phenytoin, increased dosages of the anticonvulsant may be necessitated. Prolonged use (over four months) as an antianxiety agent has not been studied. In adults, IM injection should be given in upper-outer quadrant of buttock or in the mid-lateral thigh. Gangrene has been reported when administered in a smaller muscle.

IMPLEMENTATION CONSIDERATIONS:
—Obtain a complete health history including the presence of hypersensitivity, underlying systemic disease, possibility of pregnancy, concurrent use of medications, and history of alcohol or drug abuse.

—Elderly patients may be more susceptible to side effects of drowsiness.

—IM injection must be given cautiously in a large muscle in order to prevent gangrene.

—Observe patient for signs and symptoms of depression or suicidal tendencies.

—Xerostomia may occur. Encourage frequent oral hygiene measures and the use of sugarless gum, saliva substitutes, and increase of fluid intake to prevent drying of oral mucosa.

—Assist patient in developing coping strategies to deal with stress and change such as regular planned physical exercise, muscle relaxation techniques and hobbies.

WHAT THE PATIENT NEEDS TO KNOW:
—Take this medication exactly as ordered. If you miss a regular dose of the medicine, take another dose if it is within one or two hours of the regular dosage time. If it is later than two hours, skip the dose, and take the next dose at the regular time. Do not double the dosage.

—This drug can cause dizziness, lightheadedness, drowsiness, and unsteadiness. It may decrease your ability to think or react clearly and quickly. You should not drive, operate dangerous machinery, or perform hazardous activities, until you know how your body responds to this drug. These symptoms will often stop after you have taken the medicine for several weeks. Additionally, change positions from lying and sitting to standing slowly in order to minimize these symptoms and prevent falls.

—It is essential that you keep regular appointments with your health care provider so that your progress can be checked and side effects of the drug can be monitored.

—You should not drink beer, wine, or liquor while you are taking this medicine.

—Use of caffeinated beverages (coffee, tea, cola drinks) can decrease the effect of the medicine.

—If you are pregnant, breast-feeding, or if you should become pregnant while taking this medicine, you should inform your health care provider immediately.

—This drug can make your mouth very dry. Use sugarless gum or ice chips and brush and floss your teeth frequently. Rinse your mouth and increase your fluid intake if your health care provider has not limited your fluids.

—Check with your health care practitioner if any unusual symptoms develop.

—Keep this medication out of the reach of children and all others for whom it is not prescribed.

EVALUATION:

ADVERSE REACTIONS: No serious side effects have been reported and confirmed when the recommended dosages are followed. *Cardiovascular:* postural hypotension. *CNS:* convulsions, drowsiness, headache, tremors. *Gastrointestinal:* dry mouth. *Hematopoietic:* agranulocytosis. *Hypersensitivity:* erythematous macular eruptions, erythema multiforme, pruritus, skin rash, urticaria. *Other:* intra-arterial, intravenous, or subcutaneous injection: pain and induration at the injection site, endarteritis, thrombosis, digital gangrene.

OVERDOSAGE: *Signs and symptoms:* Oversedation, hypotension, and central nervous system depression may be seen. *Treatment:* Referral for emesis induction or gastric lavage. General supportive measures should be provided. Use of epinephrine is contraindicated in therapy. Caffeine and sodium benzoate injection, U.S.P. may counteract central nervous system depression.

PARAMETERS TO MONITOR: Obtain baseline physical examination. Measure blood pressure in lying, sitting and standing positions. Observe for therapeutic response. On return visits, question the patient concerning use of alcohol, prescription or non-prescription drugs. Frequency of return visits will be determined by individual patient response as measured by relief of anxiety. Monitor the patient for suicidal tendencies. Conduct patient interviews to allow for therapeutic listening, and counsel the patient to aid in long-term relief of anxiety and development of coping mechanisms once medication is withdrawn.

HYDROXYZINE HYDROCHLORIDE

PRODUCTS (TRADE NAME):
Atarax (Available in 10, 25, 50, and 100 mg tablets; and 10 mg/5 ml syrup.) **Anxanil** (Available in 25 mg tablets). **Atozine** (Available in 10, 25, and 50 mg tablets). **Durrax** (Available in 10 and 25 mg tablets). **Hydroxyzine HCl** (Available in 10, 25, 50 and 100 mg tablets; 10 mg/5 ml syrup; and 25 mg/ml and 50 mg/ml

injection. **Vistail Injection** (As Hydroxyzine HCl preparations of 25 mg/ml and 50 mg/ml).

DRUG SPECIFICS:

Injectable preparations are for IM use only, and SQ, intra-arterial, or IV use may produce tissue necrosis and hemolysis. Give injections in deep large muscles only. Onset of action occurs 15 to 30 minutes after oral administration. Duration of action is four to six hours.

ADMINISTRATION AND DOSAGE SPECIFICS:

Anxiety:
Adults: 50 to 100 mg po four times each day.
Children over 6 years: 50 to 100 mg po each day in divided doses.
Children under 6 years: 50 mg each day in divided doses.
Pruritis:
Adults and children: 25 mg po three or four times each day.
Emesis:
Adults: 25 to 100 mg IM.
Children: 0.5 mg/lb IM.
For other specific dosages for IM uses see manufacturers' latest publications.

HYDROXYZINE PAMOATE

PRODUCTS (TRADE NAME):

Hydroxyzine Pamoate (Available in 25, 50, and 100 mg capsules.) **Hy-Pam** (Available in 25 and 50 mg capsules.) **Vamate** (Available in 25, 50, and 100 mg.) **Vistaril** (Available in 25, 50 and 100 mg capsules; 25 mg/5 ml oral suspension.

DRUG SPECIFICS:

Onset occurs 15 to 30 minutes after oral administration. Duration of action is four to six hours. Give IM injection in deep, large muscle only.

ADMINISTRATION AND DOSAGE SPECIFICS:

Anxiety:
Adults: 50 to 100 mg po four times each day.
Children over 6 years: 50 to 100 mg each day in divided doses.
Children under 6 years: 50 mg each day in divided doses.
Pruritus:
Adults or children: 25 mg three or four times each day.
Emesis:
Adults: 25 to 100 mg IM.
Children: 0.5 mg/lb IM.
For specific dosages for other IM use see manufacturers' latest publications.

Carol Ann Vittek

PSYCHOTHERAPEUTIC DRUGS—
ANTIDEPRESSANT AGENTS

MONOAMINE OXIDASE (MAO) INHIBITORS

ACTION OF THE DRUG: Monoamine oxidase (MAO) is an enzyme found in the mitochondria of cells located in nerve endings and other body tissues such as the kidney, liver and intestines. This enzyme normally acts as a catalyst by inactivating dopamine, norepinephrine, epinephrine and serotonin (biogenic amines) and therefore, regulating the intracellular levels of these neurotransmitters. MAO inhibitors block the inactivation of the biogenic amines resulting in an increased concentration of dopamine, epinephrine, norepinephrine and serotonin at neuronal synapses. The antidepressant effects of MAO inhibitors are thought to be directly related to this increased concentration of biogenic amines.

ASSESSMENT:

INDICATIONS: MAO inhibitors are used for relief of the symptoms of severe reactive or endogenous depression that have not responded to tricyclic antidepressant therapy, electroshock therapy, or other modes of psychotherapy. They may also be used for patients with manic-depressive disorders in the depressive phase when other modes of psychotherapy have been unsuccessful. Some drug forms are used as antihypertensives. (See cardiovascular section.)

SUBJECTIVE: Provider may elicit a history of insomnia, early morning awakening, anorexia, constipation, loss of motivation and fatigue.

OBJECTIVE: Patient may verbalize feelings of hopelessness and pessimism. May verbally degrade self. Responds slowly to questions and has slowed motor movements, decreased variability in facial expression and stooped posture.

PLAN:

CONTRAINDICATIONS: Do not use in the presence of hypersensitivity to a MAO-inhibitor, congestive heart failure, cerebrovascular disease, hyperthyroidism, pheochromocytoma, severe hepatic or renal impairment. Should not be used with patients who are elderly, debilitated, or under the age of 16 years.

WARNINGS: Because of drug interactions it was originally felt that MAO inhibitors could never be used concomitantly with tricyclic antidepressants. Some experimental studies show that, in certain patients and under the direction of a specialist, these drugs may be carefully combined. Risk-benefit ratio must be carefully considered before use in pregnant patients or nursing mothers since safe use of MAO inhibitors with these two population groups has not been established. Use with caution in patients with impaired hepatic or renal function, alcoholism, cardiovascular disease, hypertension, severe and/or frequent headaches, seizure disorder, Parkinson's disease, paranoid schizophrenia, and in patients who have had a sympathectomy (who may be more sensitive to the hypotensive effects of MAO inhibitors.)

PRECAUTIONS: All patients taking MAO inhibitors must be monitored for symptoms of postural hypotension. If this occurs, reduce the dose of the drug or discontinue use. Patients who are agitated or have schizophrenia may become more hyperactive. Manic-depressive patients may convert to the manic phase of their illness. This may be treated by discontinuing the drug for a brief period of time and then resuming the drug at a lower dose. Precaution must be used when prescribing MAO inhibitors to patients who are possibly suicidal. The smallest amount reasonable should be written on the prescription. Discontinue MAO inhibitors at least 2 weeks before elective surgery. If emergency surgery is indicated, doses of narcotics and anesthetics need to be reduced. All patients treated on an outpatient basis need to be closely monitored. The effects of MAO inhibitors continue for approximately 2 weeks after discontinuing the drug; therefore all drugs and foods that interact with MAO inhibitors need to be avoided during this 2-week period.

IMPLEMENTATION:

DRUG INTERACTIONS: MAO inhibitors potentiate the CNS depressant effect of alcohol, anesthetics, sedatives, hypnotics, and narcotics (particularly meperidine and may cause severe hypertension and hyperpyrexia.) Use with anticonvulsants may cause a change in the seizure pattern of the patient and dosage of anticonvulsant medication may have to be adjusted accordingly. The hypotensive effects of diuretics and antihypertensives may be enhanced when used with MAO inhibitors. (An exception is that a severe hypertensive reaction may occur with methyldopa, guanethidine or reserpine administration.) Hypertensive reactions or crisis may also be provoked with concurrent use of levodopa and at least one month should separate administration of these two drugs. Use with indirect-acting amines such as ephedrine, pseudoephedrine and amphetamines may cause sudden severe hypertension and hyperpyrexia. The hypoglycemic effects of insulin or oral hypoglycemics may be enhanced by MAO inhibitors, and dosages may need to be adjusted accordingly. Concurrent use of MAO inhibitors and tricyclic antidepressants has resulted in hyperpyrexia, severe convulsions, hypertensive crisis and death. It is imperative that a minimum of 7 days be allowed between discontinuation of a tricyclic and initiation of a MAO inhibitor (or 14 days between discontinuance of an MAO inhibitor and initiation of a tricyclic antidepressant). In moderate doses, these drugs have been used together by specialists in experimental control of refractory problems.

FOOD INTERACTIONS: Sudden and severe hypertension can result when MAO inhibitors are used with the following foods and beverages high in tyramine and other high pressor amines: alcoholic beverages such as beer and wines (particularly sherry, hearty red wines and Chianti), yeast extracts, meat tenderizers, soy sauce, beef or chicken liver, other meats; fish, sausage, pickled herring, bean pods, figs, raisins, bananas, avocados, sour cream, yogurt and cheese. Concurrent use of MAO inhibitors and large amounts of caffeine-containing products (coffee, tea, cola, chocolate, fava beans) can cause hypertension and cardiac arrhythmias.

ADMINISTRATION AND DOSAGE: MAO inhibitors are administered orally only and are well absorbed by this route. The desired antidepressant effect of the MAO inhibitors will usually occur between one to four weeks of drug therapy and there is no benefit in continuing the drug if results are not obtained during this period. When improvement is noted during the initial period of drug therapy, the dose should then be reduced gradually over a period of several weeks until an effective maintenance dose is reached. MAO inhibitors are usually not administered in the evening because of their psychomotor stimulating effect, which may produce insomnia. Maintenance dose of MAO inhibitors can be administered either in single or divided doses.

IMPLEMENTATION CONSIDERATIONS:

—Obtain a complete health history, including the presence of hypersensitivity, cardiovascular disease (especially hypertension or congestive heart failure), cerebrovascular disease, chronic headaches, Parkinson's disease, alcoholism, manic-depression, schizophrenia, hyperthyroidism, pheochromocytoma, impaired renal or hepatic function, previous sympathectomy, concurrent use of medications (especially tricyclic antidepressants), or possibility of pregnancy.

—MAO inhibitors are not recommended for children under 16 years of age, or elderly or debilitated patients.

—Because this drug has many contraindications, warnings, food and drug interactions, be certain to read these sections before prescribing drug.

—Watch for suicidal ideation in patient. Refer patient to specialists if necessary.

WHAT THE PATIENT NEEDS TO KNOW:

—Take this medication exactly as ordered by your health care provider. It may take up to four weeks before you begin to feel better. Therefore, it is important to take the drug in the exact amount and frequency ordered even though you notice no changes.

—This drug may cause very dangerous reactions if taken with certain foods or beverages. Do not eat foods such as cheese, yogurt, sour cream, raisins, bananas, avocados, bean pods, chicken livers or pickled herring. Also avoid meat tenderizers and soy sauce. Only very small amounts of coffee, tea, cola drinks and chocolate are permitted.

—This drug can increase the effects of alcohol and other drugs such as narcotics, sleeping pills, and amphetamines. Alcohol (including beer and wine) should be avoided. You should check with your health care practitioner before taking any other prescribed or over-the-counter medications.

—The effect of this drug continues for 2 weeks after you stop taking it. Therefore, if the drug is discontinued, you must not eat or drink the above specified foods or beverages during the 2-week time.

—Lightheadedness, dizziness, or feeling of faintness may occur, especially when getting up from a lying or sitting position. In order to reduce this feeling, move slowly when changing positions.

—This drug may cause drowsiness or make you feel less alert than usual. If you experience these feelings, avoid driving or other activities requiring alertness.

—If you plan to have surgery (including dental surgery) this drug should be discontinued 2 weeks before surgery. It is important to tell your provider if you plan surgery so that the drug may be discontinued in the proper manner.

—Notify your practitioner immediately or go to hospital emergency room if you develop fever, severe headache, nausea, vomiting, chest pain or rapid heartbeat.

—This is a dangerous drug. Keep it out of the reach of children and all others for whom it is not prescribed.

—Wear a Medic-Alert bracelet and carry a medical identification card specifying that you are taking this medication.

EVALUATION:

ADVERSE REACTIONS: *Cardiovascular:* orthostatic hypotension, tachycardia and other arrhythmias. *CNS:* ataxia, delirium, drowsiness, hallucinations, headache, hyperactivity, hypomania, insomnia, seizures, tremors, vertigo. *Gastrointestinal:* anorexia, constipation, diarrhea, hepatocellular hepatitis, nausea, vomiting. *Hematopoietic:* hypochromic anemia, leukopenia. *Hypersensitivity:* fever, photosensitivity, skin rash. *Musculoskeletal:* muscle twitching during sleep. *Urinary:* dysuria, incontinence. *Other:* blurred vision, dry mouth, edema, impotence, weight gain.

OVERDOSAGE: *Signs and symptoms:* Mental confusion, restlessness, hypotension, respiratory depression, tachycardia, seizures, shock which may persist for 1-2 weeks may develop. *Treatment:* Give supportive treatment. Maintain airway, give plasma infusions as indicated in severe hypotension.

PARAMETERS TO MONITOR: Obtain diet history, physical examination and liver function tests and blood cell count prior to initiating therapy. Repeat these at regular intervals during therapy. It is most important to obtain positional blood pressure readings and a baseline weight before starting treatment with MAO inhibitors. At each visit evaluate for therapeutic effects and orthostatic blood pressure changes. Monitor mental status (including affect, feelings, thought patterns), signs of fluid retention, peripheral edema and weight gain, insomnia, hyperactivity and tachycardia. If patient is a diabetic, assess for symptoms of hypoglycemia and obtain blood sugar levels at regular intervals. Reinforce dietary restrictions each visit. Observe closely for suicidal thoughts and for signs and symptoms of liver dysfunction.

ISOCARBOXAZID

PRODUCTS (TRADE NAME):
   Marplan (Available in 10 mg tablets.)
DRUG SPECIFICS: This product has a slow onset of action, and therapeutic effects may take several weeks to develop. Patient needs to be monitored very closely since

adverse effects can occur within hours. It is most effective in the treatment of neurotic or atypical depression.

ADMINISTRATION AND DOSAGE SPECIFICS:
   Initial: 30 mg po a day in single or divided doses.
   Maintenance: 10 to 20 mg po a day. Do not exceed 30 mg a day.

PHENELZINE SULFATE

PRODUCTS (TRADE NAME):
   Nardil (Available in 15 mg tablets.)
DRUG SPECIFICS:
   This product has a slow onset of action. The initial dose can be increased rapidly up to 60 mg a day according to patient tolerance. This dose, or a higher dose of 75 mg a day maximum, may be necessary for the first month of therapy to achieve relief of depressive symptoms in some patients. It is effective in moderate to severe neurotic or atypical depression, especially when anxiety is also a problem.

ADMINISTRATION AND DOSAGE SPECIFICS:
   Initial: 15 mg po three times a day up to 60 to 75 mg maximum.
   Maintenance: Reduce slowly to 15 mg po a day or every other day.

TRANYLCYPROMINE SULFATE

PRODUCTS (TRADE NAME):
   Parnate (Available in 10 mg tablets.)
DRUG SPECIFICS:
   This has a more rapid onset of action compared to other MAO inhibitors. Improvement in symptoms is usually seen in 1-3 weeks after therapy is begun. There is a higher incidence of hypertensive reactions with this drug than other MAO inhibitors. It is most effective in treatment of endogenous depression. If patient is concurrently receiving electroshock therapy, administer a maximum of 10 mg one to two times a day.

ADMINISTRATION AND DOSAGE SPECIFICS:
   Initial: 20 mg to 30 mg po per day in divided doses. (Usually give 10 to 20 mg in the morning and 10 mg in the afternoon.)
   Maintenance: 10 to 20 mg po per day.

Marsha Goodwin

ANTIDEPRESSANT AGENTS—
MISCELLANEOUS

TRAZODONE HYDROCHLORIDE

ACTION OF THE DRUG: Trazodone HCl is a non tricyclic/tetracyclic and non-MAO inhibitor antidepressant drug which inhibits the uptake of serotonin, a biogenic amine, at the neuronal synaptosomes in the brain and enhances the behavioral changes caused by 5-hydroxytryptophan, a serotonin precursor. The action of this drug is more selective than other types of antidepressants; i.e. there is less effect on the cardiac conduction system than with tricyclic/tetracyclic antidepressants and virtually no CNS stimulation which occurs frequently with MAO inhibitors.

ASSESSMENT:

INDICATIONS: Used for the relief of the symptoms of depression, with or without anxiety.
SUBJECTIVE: Patient may complain of a history of insomnia, early morning awakening, anorexia, constipation, loss of motivation and fatigue.
OBJECTIVE: Patient may verbalize feelings of hopelessness and pessimism. May degrade self verbally. Responds slowly to questions, exhibits slowed motor movements, decreased facial expression and stooped posture.

PLAN:

CONTRAINDICATIONS: Do not use in the presence of hypersensitivity. Drug is not recommended for use in a patient in the initial phase of recovery from a myocardial infarction. Safety in children under the age of 18 years has not been established.
WARNINGS: Risk-benefit ratio must be carefully considered before use in children less than 18 years, pregnant patients, or nursing mothers since use of this antidepressant has not been established for these population groups. Use with caution in patients with impaired hepatic and renal function or recovery phase of myocardial infarction. Other cardiovascular diseases may increase chances of arrhythmia development with use of trazodone.
PRECAUTIONS: Care must be used in prescribing this drug to patients who are possibly suicidal. The smallest amount reasonable should be written on the prescription. The drug should be discontinued 2 weeks before elective surgery whenever possible, since little is known about its interaction with anesthesia. It should not be used concurrently with electroshock therapy. Trazodone may produce drowsiness, dizziness and blurred vision. Do not use in tasks requiring alertness. Priapism has been reported. Patients with inappropriate or prolonged erection of the penis should stop taking this drug.

IMPLEMENTATION:

DRUG INTERACTIONS: Concurrent use of this antidepressant and antihypertensives can cause hypotension. The hypotensive effects of clonidine may be inhibited by trazodone. The effect of concomitant use of MAO inhibitors and this product is not known and dosage of both drugs should be kept at a low level, increasing as tolerated. Increased serum levels of digoxin or phenytoin have been reported with trazodone use. This drug may potentiate the effects of alcohol, barbiturates, and other CNS depressants. Discontinue drug as long as possible before general anesthesia as interactions are unknown. Elevation of liver enzymes may also be found.

PRODUCTS (TRADE NAME):

Desyrel (Available in 50 and 100 mg tablets).

ADMINISTRATION AND DOSAGE: This drug is administered orally and is well absorbed from the gastrointestinal tract. The absorption time is one hour on an empty stomach and two hours with food. The desired antidepressant effect usually occurs within 1 to 2 weeks after initiating therapy. If drowsiness occurs, the larger dose of the drug can be administered at bedtime.

Initial: 150 mg po per day in divided doses, increasing by 50 mg a day every 3-4 days to a maximum of 400 mg a day.

Maintenance: Individualize to the lowest dose both tolerated and effective.

IMPLEMENTATION CONSIDERATIONS:

—Obtain a complete health history including the presence of hypersensitivity, underlying systemic disease (especially hepatic, cardiovascular or renal), concurrent electroshock therapy or drug administration, and possibility of pregnancy.

—Occasional low WBC and neutrophil counts have been reported. Although not yet found to be clinically significant, discontinue drug if this occurs.

—This is a new drug; be on the alert for adverse reactions which are not known at the present time.

WHAT THE PATIENT NEEDS TO KNOW:

—Take this medication exactly as ordered by your health care provider. It is important that drug be continued as ordered even if you feel no better as it may take up to 2 weeks before you notice any changes.

—This drug can increase the effects of alcohol and sleeping pills. Avoid alcohol and check with your health practitioner before taking any other prescribed or over-the-counter medication.

—This drug may cause drowsiness or make you feel less alert than usual. If you experience these feelings, avoid driving or other activities that require alertness. If drowsiness persists, contact your practitioner.

—Lightheadedness or dizziness may occur when getting up from a lying or sitting position. In order to reduce this feeling, move slowly when you change positions.

—Keep this medication out of the reach of children and all others for whom it is not prescribed.

EVALUATION:

ADVERSE REACTIONS: This is a new drug. The following reactions are based on a study of 237 inpatients and 315 outpatients, half of whom were administered this antidepressant and the other half a placebo.

Autonomic: blurred vision, dry mouth. *Cardiovascular:* chest pain, orthostatic hypotension, sinus bradycardia (after long-term use). *CNS:* delusions, dizziness, drowsiness, hallucinations, hypomania, impaired speech, lightheadedness, muscle twitches, tinnitus. *Gastrointestinal:* bad taste in mouth, constipation, diarrhea, flatulence, hypersalivation, increased appetite, nausea, vomiting. *Hematopoietic:* anemia, leukopenia, neutropenia. *Hypersensitivity:* skin rash. *Urinary:* delayed urine flow, increased frequency. *Other:* early menses, hematuria, impotence, increased or decreased libido, missed periods, priapism, retrograde ejaculation, urinary frequency, weight gain or loss.

OVERDOSAGE: May cause an increase in frequency or severity of any adverse reaction. No deaths have occurred from intentional or accidental overdosage of this drug. *Treatment:* Gastric lavage and supportive therapy.

PARAMETERS TO MONITOR: Obtain baseline physical examination and liver function tests, complete blood count and electrocardiogram prior to initiating therapy and periodically during therapy. Discontinue drug if WBC or neutrophil count decreases. Take blood pressure in lying, sitting and standing positions. On each visit evaluate for therapeutic effects, and adverse reactions such as orthostatic hypotension. Monitor mental status (including affect, feelings, thought patterns). Assess for suicidal thoughts, prolonged penile erection, and signs and symptoms of liver dysfunction.

Marsha Goodwin

ANTIDEPRESSANT AGENTS—TRICYCLIC

ACTION OF THE DRUG: The antidepressant effect of the tricyclics in man is not completely understood. It is thought that the tricyclic antidepressants inhibit the uptake of norepinephrine and/or serotonin (biogenic amines) by the presynaptic neuronal membrane in the central nervous system, thereby increasing the concentration of these biogenic amines at the synapse.

ASSESSMENT:

INDICATIONS: Used primarily for relief of the symptoms of endogenous depression. May also be useful for exogenous depression which is not self-limiting or interfering with usual activities of daily living. Less frequently used for manic-depressive disorders as adjunctive therapy.

SUBJECTIVE: Provider may elicit a history of insomnia, early morning awakening, anorexia, constipation, loss of motivation, and fatigue.

OBJECTIVE: Patient may verbalize feelings of hopelessness and pessimism. Degrades self verbally. Responds slowly to questions and may have slowed motor movements, decreased facial expression and stooped posture.

PLAN:

CONTRAINDICATIONS: Do not give in the presence of prior hypersensitivity to a tricyclic antidepressant, myocardial infarction (during the acute recovery period), narrow-angle glaucoma, severe hepatic or renal failure. (Note exception under MAO inhibitors.) Should never be used concomitantly with MAO inhibitors.

WARNINGS: Risk-benefit ratio must be carefully considered before use in pregnant patients or nursing mothers, since safe use of tricyclic antidepressants with these two population groups has not been established. Cross-sensitivity occurs among the tricyclic antidepressants. Use with caution in patients with impaired hepatic or renal function; history of seizures, urinary retention, increased intra-ocular pressure; cardiovascular disease, asthma, hyperthyroidism, alcoholism, or manic-depression.

PRECAUTIONS: Manic-depressive patients may convert to the manic phase of their illness; patients with paranoid ideation and those with schizophrenia may develop exaggerated symptoms of their respective disorders. This may be avoided or treated by reduction in the dose of the tricyclic antidepressant or concomitant use of a major tranquilizer. If a tricyclic antidepressant is taken concurrently with any anticholinergic-type drug, the patient could develop paralytic ileus. Discontinue tricyclic antidepressants, if possible, several days before elective surgery. Precaution must be used when prescribing antidepressants to patients who are possibly suicidal. The smallest amount reasonable should be written on the prescription. Hazards of electroshock therapy may be increased if treatment is given to a patient on tricyclic antidepressants.

IMPLEMENTATION:

DRUG INTERACTIONS: Tricyclic antidepressants potentiate the CNS depressant effect of alcohol and other CNS depressants, particularly ethchlorvynol. (Reduction in the dose of either the tricyclic antidepressant or ethchlorvynol or both may be necessary if used concomitantly.) The effects of anticonvulsants may be decreased when used concomitantly with tricyclic antidepressants. (Dosage of the anticonvulsant may have to be increased to control seizures.) The antihypertensive effects, especially guanethidine and clonidine, may be blocked when used with most tricyclic antidepressants with the exception of doxepin (in doses less than 150 mg per day.) There may be a reduction in the antidepressant effect of tricyclics and an increase in their side effects when used concurrently with estrogen, including oral contraceptives containing estrogen. An increased incidence of cardiac arrhythmias has been found with concurrent use of thyroid medication and tricyclic antidepressants. Severe hypertension or hyperpyrexia may result when tricyclic antidepressants are used with MAO inhibitors or sympathomimetics.

ADMINISTRATION AND DOSAGE: Since the plasma concentrations of the tricyclic antidepressants have a wide variability and do not necessarily correlate well with the dose or therapeutic effects, the initial and maintenance dosages of these drugs are individualized according to the patient's age, physical health status plus the desired and/or untoward responses of the drug. The desired antidepressant effect of the drug will usually occur within one to four weeks after initiating therapy.

The initial dose may cause sedation, especially when using a tricyclic known to have moderate to strong sedative effects. Therefore, tricyclic antidepressant therapy may be initiated by a single bedtime dose, especially for depressed patients with a sleep disturbance. The drug dosage can then be titrated with the objective of gaining maximal therapeutic response with the lowest dosage and minimal side effects. A maintenance dose, administered in divided doses or as a single bedtime dose, may often be continued for 6 months to 1 year.

If a tricyclic antidepressant is given in large doses or over a prolonged period of time, discontinuation of the drug should be accomplished by gradual reduction over a period of four to eight weeks in order to avoid withdrawal symptoms of general listlessness, headache, and nausea.

Adolescent and geriatric patients tend to be more sensitive to the effects of tricyclics. They should, therefore, be started with lower doses, titrated slower, and give maintenace therapy in divided doses if possible. These suggestions might also be indicated for patients with cardiovascular disease.

In choosing a specific tricyclic antidepressant, consideration should be given to the degree of sedation and anticholinergic effects associated with the drug and the relation of these effects to the individual patient situation. Table 4-11 lists the tricyclic antidepressants according to degree of sedative and anticholinergic effects and gives the half-life for each drug. All of the tricyclic antidepressants are administered orally; amitriptyline and imipramine can also be given parenterally.

IMPLEMENTATION CONSIDERATIONS:

—Obtain a complete health history, including the presence of hypersensitivity, cardiovascular disease, asthma, hyperthyroidism, increased intraocular pressure,

TABLE 4-11. TRICYCLIC ANTIDEPRESSANTS GROUPED BY DEGREE OF SEDATION AND ANTICHOLINERGIC EFFECTS

Category	Drug	Half-life (hrs)
Strong Sedative-Anticholinergic	Amitriptyline	32-40
	Doxepin	8-25
Strong Sedative-Moderate Anticholinergic	Trimipramine	
Moderate Sedative-Anticholinergic	Amoxapine	8-30
	Nortriptyline	18-90
	Imipramine	6-20
Moderate Sedative-Mild Anticholinergic	Maprotiline*	20-80
Mild Sedative-Anticholinergic	Desipramine	12-55
No Significant Sedative-Moderate Anticholinergic	Protriptyline	55-100

*Chemically classified as a tetracyclic.

alcoholism, manic-depression, electroshock therapy, seizure disorder, impaired renal or liver function, urinary retention, or if there is possibility of pregnancy. Assess for prostatic hypertrophy in male patients over 50 years of age. Evaluate other medications taken concurrently, including over-the-counter preparations.

—Assess thoroughly for the presence of suicidal thoughts.

—Patients under 18 and over 60 are often unusually sensitive to the usual recommended dosages. It is imperative to begin these patients on a small dose and observe individual patient response before increasing the dosage.

—Since concurrent use of MAO inhibitors and tricyclic antidepressants have resulted in hyperpyrexia, severe convulsions, hypertensive crisis and death, it is important that a minimum of 7 days be allowed between discontinuance of a tricyclic and initiation of an MAO inhibitor or 14 days between discontinuance of an MAO inhibitor and initiation of a tricyclic antidepressant.

—Read thoroughly the general information under administration and dosage before prescribing this drug.

WHAT THE PATIENT NEEDS TO KNOW:

—Take this medication exactly as ordered. It may be taken with food in order to avoid gastric distress. It may take up to eight weeks before you begin to feel better. Therefore, it is important to take the drug in the exact amount and frequency specified even though you notice no changes initially.

—This drug should never be stopped suddenly because there could be an increase in your symptoms, as well as nausea, headache and feelings of listlessness. Do not stop the drug without talking to your health provider.

—This drug may cause drowsiness or make you feel less alert than usual. If you experience these feelings, avoid driving or other activities requiring alertness. This feeling should pass after taking the medication for a short time. Tell your health practitioner if drowsiness or decreased alertness persists longer than 2 weeks and interferes with your usual activities.

—Dryness of the mouth may occur when you start taking the drug. Chewing sugarless gum, sucking on hard candy, or rinsing your mouth frequently may help relieve the dryness.

—This drug will increase the effects of alcohol, sleeping pills and some medications for the relief of colds and hay fever. Avoid beer, wine or liquor and check with your health provider before taking any other medications.

—This is a very powerful drug and must be kept out of the reach of children and others for whom it is not prescribed. Do not leave it on dressers or low bedside tables.

—Lightheadedness, dizziness, or feeling of faintness occurs in some people taking this drug, especially older people. In order to reduce this feeling, move slowly, especially when changing from a lying or sitting position to standing upright.

—If you have surgery or dental work done requiring an anesthetic, this drug is usually discontinued several days before the surgery. It is important to work with your health care provider in developing a plan to gradually discontinue the medicine in the proper manner.

—Notify your health practitioner if you develop any new or troublesome symptoms. Especially report promptly the appearance of urinary retention, constipation, blurring vision, or excessive sleepiness.

—If you are taking this medication for a prolonged period of time it is wise to wear a Medic-Alert bracelet and carry a medical-identification card explaining that you are taking this drug.

EVALUATION:

ADVERSE REACTIONS: *Cardiovascular:* arrhythmias, heart block, palpitations, and orthostatic hypotension, especially in the elderly. *CNS:* confusion, delirium, headache, prolonged drowsiness, and seizures (rare.) *Gastrointestinal:* cholestatic jaundice (rare), constipation, increased appetite for sweets, nausea, paralytic ileus, vomiting, weight gain. *Hematopoietic:* agranulocytosis, eosinophilia, leukopenia, thrombocytopenia. *Hypersensitivity:* fever, photosensitivity, pruritus, skin rash. *Musculoskeletal:* muscle twitching, tremors. *Urinary:* hesitancy, retention. *Other:* altered liver function tests, blurred vision, delayed sexual orgasm, hyperglycemia, hypomania (manic-depressive patients), insomnia (in children), nervousness.

OVERDOSAGE: *Signs and symptoms:* Initially there is stimulation of the CNS exhibited by irritability, agitation, hallucinations, delirium, twitching, hypertonia, hyperreflexia, nystagmus, hyperpyrexia, hypertension and seizures (more frequently seen in children.) This initial CNS stimulation is followed by CNS depression exhibited by drowsiness, areflexia, hypothermia, hypotension, cardiac arrhythmias, respiratory depression, coma or cardiorespiratory arrest. *Treatment:* Refer for gastric lavage, and supportive therapy. Physostigmine salicylate may be used to counteract severe anticholinergic effects. Diazepam may be used to control seizures if they occur. Close monitoring of the patient's cardiac and respiratory status is indicated. A quiet environment should also be maintained during the initial phase.

PARAMETERS TO MONITOR: Obtain a complete physical examination and baseline laboratory studies prior to initiation of therapy. This should include liver and kidney function tests, complete blood count and electrocardiogram. A lying, sitting and standing blood pressure and pulse should also be monitored. During extended therapy, complete blood counts and liver function tests should be done every 2 months for the first 6 months, then at least every 6 months thereafter. For any patient over 35 or with a family history of glaucoma, obtain an intraocular pressure reading prior to and periodically during therapy. On each visit monitor the following things: mental status (including affect, feelings, thought patterns, sleep patterns), weight, pulse rate and rhythm, degree of anticholinergic side effects (dry mouth, blurred vision, constipation, urinary hesitancy or retention.) Evaluate for orthostatic hypotension particularly in the elderly. Observe closely for suicidal thoughts and for signs and symptoms of liver dysfunction and hyperglycemia.

AMITRIPTYLINE HCL

PRODUCTS (TRADE NAME):
Amitid (Available in 10, 25, 50, 75, and 100 mg tablets.) **Amitril** (Available in 10, 25, 50, 75, 100 and 150 mg tablets.) **Amitriptyline HCl, Elavil HCl** (Available in 10, 25, 50, 75, 100 and 150 mg tablets; and 10 mg/ml injection.) **Endep, SK-Amitriptyline** (Available in 10, 25, 50, 75, 100 and 150 mg tablets.)

DRUG SPECIFICS:
This product has a strong sedative effect, especially early in therapy. If administered at bedtime, drowsiness during the daytime may be minimized. It is most effective in the treatment of endogenous depression accompanied by anxiety.

ADMINISTRATION AND DOSAGE SPECIFICS:
Initial: 25 mg po two to four times daily.
Maintenance: 50 to 100 mg/day at bedtime or in divided doses. May also give 20 to 30 mg IM four times a day.

AMOXAPINE

PRODUCTS (TRADE NAME):
Asendin (Available in 50, 100 and 150 mg tablets.)

DRUG SPECIFICS:
The antidepressant effect is usually seen within two weeks after initiating therapy. Onset of action more rapid than with amitriptyline or imipramine. It is effective in the treatment of a wide variety of depressions including reactive, endogenous and psychotic depressions.

ADMINISTRATION AND DOSAGE SPECIFICS:
Initial: 50 mg po three times a day; increase to 100 mg po three times a day on third day.
Maintenance: 30 mg/day or less at bedtime.

DESIPRAMINE HCL

PRODUCTS (TRADE NAME):
Norpramin (Available in 25, 50, 75, 100, and 150 mg tablets.) **Pertofrane** (Available in 25 and 50 mg capsules.)

DRUG SPECIFICS:
Has mild sedative effect. Urinary retention rarely occurs. Orthostatic hypotension is common during the first few weeks of therapy. Instruct patient to change

positions slowly to prevent dizziness and falls. Is effective in the treatment of a variety of depressions, particularly endogenous type. Not recommended for use in children.

ADMINISTRATION AND DOSAGE SPECIFICS:

Initial: 25-50 mg po three times day. Give only 25 to 50 mg/day in adolescents and elderly.

Maintenance: Up to 200 mg/day.

DOXEPIN HCL

PRODUCTS (TRADE NAME):

Adapin (Available in 10, 25, 50, 75 and 100 mg capsules.) **Sinequan** (Available in 10, 25, 50, 75, 100 and 150 mg capsules, and 10 mg/ml oral concentrate.)

DRUG SPECIFICS:

Has a marked sedative effect, particularly during the initial phase of therapy. (See Antianxiety agents for more information.) In doses up to 150 mg/day this drug has not blocked the effects of guanethidine or other similar antihypertensive drugs. It is effective in treating psychotic and psychoneurotic depression with associated anxiety and somatic symptoms. Antianxiety effects usually occur within 1-2 weeks; antidepressant effects within several weeks. This drug is well tolerated in the elderly. It is not recommended for children under 12 years of age. The oral concentrate should be diluted in milk, fruit juice, or water prior to administration.

ADMINISTRATION AND DOSAGE SPECIFICS:

Initial: 25 mg po three times a day.

Maintenance: 50 to 150 mg/day at bedtime or in divided doses.

IMIPRAMINE HCL

PRODUCTS (TRADE NAME):

Antipress (Available in 25 mg tablets.) **Imavate** (Available in 25 and 50 mg tablets.) **Imipramine HCl, Janimine** (Available in 10, 25 and 50 mg tablets.) **Presamine** (Available in 25 and 50 mg tablets.) **SK-Pramine** (Available in 10, 25 and 50 mg tablets.) **Tofranil** (Available in 10, 25 and 50 mg tablets and 25 mg/2 ml injection.)

DRUG SPECIFICS:

This is most effective in treatment of endogenous depressions. It is the only tricyclic that is also used for treatment of enuresis in children.

ADMINISTRATION AND DOSAGE SPECIFICS:

Depression:

Initial: 25 mg po three to four times a day; or 25-50 mg IM three to four times a day. Reduce to 30 to 40 mg a day in divided doses for adolescents and elderly patients.

Maintenance: 50 to 150 mg/day po at bedtime.

Enuresis in children 6 years or older: 25 to 50 mg one hour before bedtime or 25 mg in midafternoon and 25 mg one hour before bedtime.

MAPROTILINE HCL

PRODUCTS (TRADE NAME):
Ludiomil (Available in 25 and 50 mg tablets.)
DRUG SPECIFICS:
This is a tricyclic antidepressant that is effective in the treatment of neurotic depression and manic-depressive disorders, depressed type. Antidepressive effects may occur within 1 week of initiating therapy. There is a lower incidence of cardiovascular adverse reactions and anticholinergic side effects with this drug compared to other tricyclic antidepressants. It is contraindicated in patients with known or suspected seizure disorder. It is not recommended in adolescents under 18 years of age. Dosage should be reduced if used with elderly patients.
ADMINISTRATION AND DOSAGE SPECIFICS:
Initial: 75 mg/day po in single or divided doses.
Maintenance: 150 to 225 mg/day po.

NORTRIPTYLINE HCL

PRODUCTS (TRADE NAME):
Aventyl HCl (Available in 10 and 25 mg capsules; 10 mg/5 ml liquid.) **Pamelor** (Available in 10, 25 and 75 mg capsules; 10 mg/5 ml solution.)
DRUG SPECIFICS:
This product is effective primarily in the treatment of patients with endogenous depression. It is not recommended in children under 12 years of age.
ADMINISTRATION AND DOSAGE SPECIFICS:
Initial: 25 mg po three to four times a day. Reduce to 30 or 50 mg a day in divided doses for adolescent or elderly patients and increase only as needed and tolerated.
Maintenance: Up to 100 mg/day po.

PROTRIPTYLINE HCL

PRODUCTS (TRADE NAME):
   Vivactil (Available in 5 and 10 mg tablets.)
DRUG SPECIFICS: This drug is effective primarily in the treatment of endogenous depression, particularly when the patient is withdrawn or listless. This drug has no sedative effect and stimulates the CNS more than other tricyclics. The last dose should not be taken later than mid afternoon and any increases in dosage should be made with the morning dose. There is an increased incidence of cardiovascular and anticholinergic side effects with this drug compared to other tricyclics; therefore close monitoring should be carried out in patients with a history of cardiovascular disease and patients who are elderly. It is not recommended in children under 12 years of age.
ADMINISTRATION AND DOSAGE SPECIFICS:
   Initial: 5 to 10 mg po three to four times daily. Reduce dose in adolescents and elderly to 5 mg three times a day.
   Maintenance: Not to exceed 60 mg/day.

TRIMIPRAMINE MALEATE

PRODUCTS (TRADE NAME):
   Surmontil (Available in 25 and 50 mg capsules.)
DRUG SPECIFICS:
   This product has a strong sedative effect. It is most effective in treatment of endogenous depression accompanied by anxiety. It has been shown to have effectiveness equal to amitriptyline in mild to moderately depressed patients, but less effective in more severely depressed patients. Not recommended in children under 12 years of age.
ADMINISTRATION AND DOSAGE SPECIFICS:
   Initial: 25 mg po three times a day. Reduce dosage to 25 mg twice a day in adolescent and elderly patients.
   Maintenance: 50 to 150 mg/day at bedtime. In adolescents and the elderly increase dose to maximum of 100 mg/day only as necessary and tolerated.

Marsha Goodwin

PSYCHOTHERAPEUTIC DRUGS—
ANTIMANIC AGENT

LITHIUM

ACTION OF THE DRUG: The exact mechanism of lithium is not known. The mood stabilizing effect of the drug may be attributed to its ability to alter sodium transport at the nerve endings, inhibit cyclic AMP formation in nerve cells, and enhance the uptake of serotonin and norepinephrine by nerve cells, thus increasing the inactivation of these neurotransmitters.

ASSESSMENT:

INDICATIONS: Lithium is specifically used for patients with manic-depressive psychosis in an acute manic phase. Also may be used to prevent recurrent episodes of mania in the manic-depressive patient. It has been used experimentally for the prophylaxis of cluster headaches.

SUBJECTIVE: Patient may present with history of excessive talkativeness, restlessness, hyperactivity, aggressiveness and perhaps delusions of grandeur.

OBJECTIVE: Practitioner may note agitation, euphoric mood, and continuous verbalization which may contain appropriate or inappropriate content. Patient may verbalize grandiose ideations. Hyperactive motor activity may also be demonstrated.

PLAN:

CONTRAINDICATIONS: This drug should not be used in patients with known hypersensitivity, severe cardiovascular disease, renal insufficiency, dehydration, sodium depletion, or severe debilitation. It should not be administered to patients concurrently receiving diuretics.

WARNINGS: Risk-benefit ratio must be very carefully considered before using in pregnant patients and nursing mothers. If a patient receiving lithium becomes pregnant, effort should be taken to discontinue the drug, especially during the first trimester, since birth defects may occur. Maintenance of adequate hydration and electrolyte balance is imperative during lithium therapy.

PRECAUTIONS: Serum lithium at the therapeutic level is relatively close to the toxic level. It is important to monitor serum lithium levels on a regular basis in order to avoid drug toxicity. Lithium is tolerated better by patients in an acute manic stage than in controlled stages when manifestations of mania have subsided. The dose of lithium may have to be adjusted according to the patient's manifestation of symptoms. Lithium should be used with caution in patients with seizure disorders, Parkinson's disease, cardiovascular disease, hypotension, diabetes mellitus, hypothyroidism, urinary retention, renal insufficiency, and severe infection.

IMPLEMENTATION:

DRUG INTERACTIONS: Concurrent use of lithium and diuretics can lead to lithium toxicity. Neurotoxicity may occur if lithium is taken concurrently with haloperidol and other antipsychotic agents. The therapeutic effects of lithium may be inhibited if administered concurrently with caffeine, theophylline, aminophylline, or sodium bicarbonate. The effects of lithium may be potentiated to the degree of toxicity if taken with methyldopa, tetracycline, or indomethacin. The pressor effects of norepinephrine may be inhibited if taken with lithium. The effects of skeletal muscle relaxants may be enhanced and prolonged by concurrent use of these drugs. Hypothyroidism may result from long-term use of iodide preparations and lithium.

PRODUCTS (TRADE NAME):
Cibalith-S (Available in 300 mg/5 ml syrup.) **Eskalith** (Available in 300 mg capsules or tablets.) **Lithane** (Available in 300 mg tablets.) **Lithobid** (Available in 300 mg slow-release tablets). **Lithium Carbonate** (Available in 300 mg capsules or tablets.) **Lithium Citrate** (Available in 300 mg/5 ml syrup.)

ADMINISTRATION AND DOSAGE: Lithium administered orally is rapidly absorbed in the gastrointestinal tract. The desired effect of lithium may take one to several weeks to occur. The drug is not protein bound to any significant degree; therefore, it is widely distributed in the body. Lithium is excreted by the kidneys, with a half-life of approximately 24 hours in a physically healthly adult. The half-life of lithium in the elderly may be increased to 36 hours; therefore, lower doses are indicated for this group. Excretion of lithium is inhibited in the presence of low serum sodium levels. The therapeutic serum level of lithium is 1 to 1.5 mEq/l. Lithium is not recommended for children under 12 years of age.

Acute manic: 600 mg po three times a day.

Prophylaxis: 300 mg po three to four times a day.

Prophylaxis of cluster headaches: 600 to 900 mg/day.

IMPLEMENTATION CONSIDERATIONS:

—Obtain a complete health history, including the presence of hypersensitivity, cardiovascular disease, renal insufficiency, dehydration, sodium depletion, hypotension, hypothyroidism, diabetes mellitus, Parkinson's disease, seizure disorder, urinary retention, possibility of pregnancy, and other medications being used concurrently (especially diuretics).

—Elderly patients are often more sensitive to lithium toxicity. It is important to begin these patients on lower doses and monitor therapeutic and adverse effects closely while increasing dosage.

—Patients who develop diarrhea, or become ill and do not eat, are at increased risk of toxicity and their condition should be followed closely.

WHAT THE PATIENT NEEDS TO KNOW:

—Take this medication exactly as ordered. It may take several weeks before you feel better. Therefore, it is important to take the drug in the exact amount and frequency ordered even though you may notice no difference. If the drug causes stomach upset, this may be reduced by taking it with milk or food.

—Lithium can become toxic and, therefore, harmful in the body if you get too much. If you become dehydrated from vomiting, diarrhea, or not eating, you are at greater risk for problems. Avoid activities which cause excessive sweating (strenuous exercise, sun bathing, hot tub baths), and things which produce excessive urination (drinking large amounts of caffeine in coffee, tea or cola drinks). Contact your health practitioner if you develop any illnesses or do not feel well.

—Some patients experience side effects to this product. They are usually mild and disappear with time. Notify your practitioner if you note any new or troublesome symptoms such as vomiting, nausea, shakiness, trembling, jerky movements of arms or legs, or generalized weakness.

—You will need to have frequent blood tests to measure the level of drug in your blood. This is important in keeping the drug at the proper level and reducing side effects. You will need these blood tests every few days when you first begin treatment, and then every one to two months.

—Keep this medication out of the reach of children and others for whom it is not prescribed.

—Wear a Medic-Alert bracelet and carry a medical identification card specifying that you are taking this medication.

EVALUATION:

ADVERSE REACTIONS: *Cardiovascular:* arrhythmias, ECG changes (flattening of T-waves, prominent U waves), hypotension. *CNS:* ataxia, confusion, coma, dizziness, drowsiness, extrapyramidal symptoms, motor retardation, restlessness, seizures, slurred speech, tinnitus. *Dermatologic:* cutaneous ulcerations, pruritus, rash. *Gastrointestinal:* abdominal pain, anorexia, diarrhea, vomiting. *Urinary:* incontinence or retention, polyuria. *Other:* albuminuria, blurred vision, hyperglycemia, hypothyroidism, leukocytosis, scotoma, weight gain.

OVERDOSAGE: *Signs and symptoms:* diarrhea, vomiting, muscle weakness, drowsiness and ataxia may develop. *Treatment:* Stop drug and refer for gastric lavage. Restore fluid and electrolyte balance and evaluate kidney function. Evaluate source of problem.

PARAMETERS TO MONITOR: Baseline physical examination and laboratory studies should be obtained prior to beginning therapy. Electrolytes, kidney function tests, ECG, glucose tolerance test should also be obtained and repeated periodically, especially if symptoms of diabetes mellitus occur. Thyroid studies may also be indicated if hypothyroidism is suspected. Serum lithium levels should be monitored closely, with the blood being drawn 12 hours after the last dose. Monitoring should be carried out every few days during the initial therapy and then a minimum of every 2 months after the patient is stabilized. The therapeutic serum lithium level is 1 to 1.5 mEq/l in most laboratories. On each visit observe for therapeutic effects. Monitor mental and emotional status. Observe for signs of dehydration and sodium depletion. Monitor weight, blood pressure (in lying, sitting and standing positions), and pulse rate and rhythm.

Marsha Goodwin

PSYCHOTHERAPEUTIC DRUGS— ANTIPSYCHOTIC AGENTS

BUTYROPHENONE—HALOPERIDOL

ACTION OF THE DRUG: The complete mechanism by which butyrophenones act is not well established. It is known that the drugs act potently and selectively as a blockade of dopamine at receptor sites in the brain, thereby enhancing the turnover of this particular neurotransmitter. Secondarily, butyrophenones act as a mild-to-moderate blockade of alpha-adrenergic receptors located in the sympathetic nervous system.

ASSESSMENT:

INDICATIONS: Used primarily for reducing or relieving symptoms of psychoses including schizophrenia and manic-depressive disorders in the manic phase. Also useful in the control of tics and verbal utterances associated with Gilles de la Tourette's disease in children and adults. Other uses of butyrophenones include control of extreme combativeness in mentally disturbed children.

SUBJECTIVE: Patient may present with a history of emotional upset, agitation, paranoid ideations, hallucinations, delusions, inability to think clearly, euphoric mood, and inability to cope with reality. There may also be a history of involuntary vocal utterances and muscle spasms.

OBJECTIVE: Patient has difficulty attending and responding to immediate environment. Inappropriate verbal responses to questions, non-verbal behavior and possibly inappropriate dress and general appearance may develop. Agitated and euphoric mood, or uncontrollable verbal utterances and tics may be present.

PLAN:

CONTRAINDICATIONS: This drug should not be used in patients with prior hypersensitivity, Parkinson's disease or severe mental depression. Severe hepatic or renal failure, jaundice, angina pectoris, blood dyscrasias, bone marrow depression, thyrotoxicosis, or drug-induced central nervous system depression are also contraindications.

WARNINGS: Risk-benefit ratio must be carefully considered before use in pregnant patients and nursing mothers. Use with caution in patients with impaired hepatic or renal function, chronic alcoholism, seizure disorder, hyperthyroidism, respiratory insufficiency, urinary retention, and a potential for glaucoma.

PRECAUTIONS: Allergic reaction to the tartrazine in Yellow #5 contained in the drug has occurred, especially in patients with a hypersensitivity to aspirin. Studies have shown that prolactin levels are increased by short-term use of this product, and persist during long-term therapy. Since approximatly one third of breast cancers are prolactin dependent, use of haloperidol in patients with a history of breast cancer must be carefully considered. Patients in the manic phase of manic-depression who are taking haloperidol may convert to the depressive phase quite rapidly and be potentially suicidal. Therefore, manic-depressive patients need to be monitored closely.

IMPLEMENTATION:

DRUG INTERACTIONS: Butyrophenones taken concurrently with CNS depressants, including alcohol, barbiturates, narcotics, and anesthetics, may potentiate the depressant effect. Butyrophenones taken concurrently with an antimuscarinic such as atropine may decrease the effect of butyrophenone, particularly in the schizophrenic patient, and also may cause increased intraocular pressure. Severe hypotension may occur when butyrophenones are taken concurrently with anti-hypertensive drugs or epinephrine. There may possibly be toxic neurologic effects and brain damage when lithium is taken concurrently with this product, although this interaction is not well established. The effect of amphetamines may be inhibited when taken concurrently, and the seizure threshold in an epileptic patient may be lowered.

PRODUCTS (TRADE NAME):

Haldol (Available in 0.5, 1, 2, 5 and 10 mg tablets; 2 mg/ml concentrate; and 5 mg/ml injection.)

ADMINISTRATION AND DOSAGE: Haloperidol is approximately 97% protein bound; and its metabolism and excretion may be slow. This drug may be administered orally or intramuscularly. The dosage has not been established in children under 12 years of age and therefore very low doses should be administered. Elderly or debilitated patients should also be given low doses and titrated slowly. The desired antipsychotic effect of haloperidol usually occurs within 3 weeks after initiating therapy. Once this desired effect is attained, the dose should be gradually reduced. The extrapyramidal side effects which are common with haloperidol especially early in therapy and with elderly females, tend to be dose-related. Adjustment of the dose may eliminate this side effect. If haloperidol is given over an extended period of time, discontinuance of the drug should be done gradually over several weeks to avoid symptoms of nausea, vomiting, trembling and dyskinesia.

Adults and children over 12 years: 0.5 mg to 5 mg po two to three times a day, up to 100 mg/day. May also give 2 to 5 mg IM every four to eight hours.

Children 3 to 12 years: 0.5 mg/day initially with increments of 0.5 mg at 5 to 7 day intervals as needed. Total dose may be divided and given 2 to 3 times a day.

IMPLEMENTATION CONSIDERATIONS:

—Obtain a complete health history, including the presence of hypersensitivity (especially to aspirin), cardiovascular disease (particularly angina), hepatic or renal failure, blood dyscrasias, bone marrow depression, hyperthyroidism, Parkinson's disease, mental depression, respiratory insufficiency, alcoholism, glaucoma, urinary retention, seizures, breast cancer, use of concurrent medications, or the possibility of pregnancy.

—Elderly or debilitated patients are often sensitive to the effects of usual recommended doses and are more prone to extrapyramidal side effects. It is important to begin these patients on a small dose and monitor for desired and adverse effects.

—Watch for suicidal tendencies.

WHAT THE PATIENT NEEDS TO KNOW:

—Take this medication exactly as ordered. It may take up to three weeks before you begin to feel better. Therefore, it is important to take the drug in the exact amount and frequency ordered even though you feel no different.

—This drug can increase the effects of alcohol and other drugs such as sleeping pills, prescribed pain medication, and some medicines for relief of colds and hay fever. Alcohol should be avoided and you should check with your health practitioner before taking any other drugs.

—This drug may cause drowsiness or make you feel less alert than usual, especially when you first start taking the drug. If you experience these feelings, avoid driving or other activities requiring alertness. Talk with your health provider if drowsiness or decreased alertness persist.

—Lightheadedness, dizziness, or feelings of faintness have occurred in some people taking this drug. In order to reduce the possibility of falling, move slowly when you change from a lying or sitting position.

—Some people taking this drug become more sensitive to the sun. To avoid sunburn, use a sunscreen lotion if out in the sun, or limit your exposure to the sun and sunlamps.

—If you are taking this drug in liquid form, avoid contact of the medicine with your skin or clothes since it can cause irritation.

—If the drug you are taking comes in a bottle with a medicine dropper, make sure you measure out the prescribed dose marked on the dropper. You can take the medicine alone or mixed with food, water or juice. If the drug causes gastric discomfort, taking it with food may help reduce this problem.

—This drug should not be discontinued suddenly because you could experience nausea, vomiting, trembling, and other symptoms. Therefore, always contact your health care provider before discontinuing this drug.

—Notify your health practitioner promptly if you notice urinary retention, arm or leg stiffness, shaking of hands, jerking of head or neck, skin rash, yellow tinge to skin and eyes, or small uncontrollable movements of the tongue.

—Keep this drug out of the reach of children and all others for whom it is not prescribed.

EVALUATION:

ADVERSE REACTIONS: *Cardiovascular:* orthostatic hypotension. *CNS:* drowsiness. *Extrapyramidal effects:* jerky, tic-like movements of head, face, or neck;

shaking hands, shuffling walk, stiffness of limbs, tardive dyskinesia. *Hematopoietic:* agranulocytosis. *Hepatic:* obstructive jaundice. *Hypersensitivity:* contact dermatitis. *Urinary:* retention. *Other:* blurred vision, breast engorgement, constipation, decreased libido, dry mouth, impotence, menstrual irregularity, nausea, vomiting.

OVERDOSAGE: *Signs and symptoms:* Severe extrapyramidal symptoms, hypotension, sedation, respiratory depression and coma may develop. *Treatment:* Refer for gastric lavage, or production of emesis with agents such as Ipecac. Maintain patent airway; help maintain blood pressure with plasma expanders and/or vasopressor agents. Anticholinergic antiparkinsonian drugs may be used to control extrapyramidal symptoms. Epinephrine should never be used as it may potentiate hypotension.

PARAMETERS TO MONITOR: Obtain baseline complete blood count, liver function tests and physical examination prior to initiating therapy, and repeat at periodic intervals during extended therapy. For a patient over 35 or with a family history of glaucoma, obtain an intraocular pressure reading before therapy is started. Regular breast examination should be done on female patients and the patient should be taught breast self-exam to be done monthly. On each visit check mental and emotional status, including thought patterns, delusions, hallucinations, inappropriate behavior. Observe for signs of jaundice. Evaluate for orthostatic hypotension by taking lying, sitting and standing blood pressures. Observe closely for extrapyramidal symptoms and signs of depression or suicidal ideation.

Marsha Goodwin

DIBENZOXAZEPINE—LOXAPINE

ACTION OF THE DRUG: The complete mechanism by which dibenzoxazepines act is not well established. The drugs are thought to inhibit subcortical areas of the brain, thus producing a tranquilizing effect and a decrease in aggressive behavior. These drugs are pharmacologically similar to the phenothiazines.

ASSESSMENT:

INDICATIONS: Used primarily for reducing or relieving symptoms associated with psychosis, particularly schizophrenia.

SUBJECTIVE: Practitioner may elicit a history of emotional unrest, agitation, paranoid ideations, visual, auditory and/or tactile hallucinations, delusions, inability to think clearly, severe mood swings, and inability to cope with reality.

OBJECTIVE: Patient may or may not verbalize paranoid thoughts. Often has difficulty attending and responding to immediate environment. Inappropriate verbal responses to questions, non-verbal behavior, and possibly inappropriate dress and general appearance may develop.

PLAN:

CONTRAINDICATIONS: This drug should not be used in the presence of hypersensitivity, in drug-induced central nervous system depression, or in coma from any etiology.

WARNINGS: Risk-benefit ratio must be carefully considered before use in pregnant patients and nursing mothers since sufficient data regarding safety in these populations are unavailable. Use with caution in patients with impaired hepatic or renal functions, symptomatic prostatic hypertrophy, Parkinson's disease, cardiovascular disease, and a potential for glaucoma.

PRECAUTIONS: Significant sedation may occur during initial therapy with dibenzoxazepine. Studies have shown that prolactin levels are increased by short-term use of dibenzoxazepine and persist during long-term use. Since approximately one-third of breast cancers are prolactin dependent, use of dibenzoxazepine in patients with a history of breast cancer must be carefully considered.

IMPLEMENTATION:

DRUG INTERACTIONS: Dibenzoxazepines are a relatively new category of antipsychotic agent, but are pharmacologically similar to phenothiazines. Therefore, these drugs may have the potential to interact with the same drugs as phenothiazines. (See phenothiazines).

PRODUCTS (TRADE NAME):
Loxitane (Available in 5, 10, 25, and 50 mg tablets; 25 mg/ml concentrate; and 50 mg/ml injection).

ADMINISTRATION AND DOSAGE: The half-life of this dibenzoxazepine is 3 to 4 hours and the effects may last as long as 12 hours. Elderly and debilitated patients should be started on low doses which are increased slowly. The dosage has not been established for children under 16 years of age and should not be given to this group. The absorption rate of this dibenzoxazepine administered orally may be delayed if taken concurrently with antacids or antidiarrheal agents. The oral concentrate should be diluted with fruit juice just prior to administration.

Initial: 10 mg po two to three times a day; or 12.5 to 50 mg IM every four to six hours.

Maintenance: May give 60 to 100 mg/day, up to a maximum of 250 mg/day.

IMPLEMENTATION CONSIDERATIONS:

—Obtain a complete health history including the presence of hypersensitivity, coronary artery disease, cerebral arteriosclerosis, prostatic hypertrophy, Parkinson's disease, impaired hepatic or renal function, alcoholism, glaucoma, urinary retention, breast cancer, seizures, possibility of pregnancy, or the concurrent use of other medications.

—Complete examination of the patient's eyes, including inspection of external structures and the lens, is warranted prior to beginning therapy.

—Elderly, emaciated or debilitated patients are often unusually sensitive to the normal dosages and should be started on reduced amounts. They are more prone to extrapyramidal and hypotensive side effects if medication is not increased slowly.

WHAT THE PATIENT NEEDS TO KNOW:

—Take this medication exactly as ordered. It may take several days before you notice a change in symptoms.

—This drug can increase the effects of alcohol, sleeping pills, and some pain medication. Therefore, alcohol should be avoided, and you should check with your health practitioner before taking any other medications.

—This drug may cause drowsiness or make you feel less alert than usual, particularly when you first begin taking the drug. If you experience this, do not drive or perform tasks requiring alertness. This usually passes after a short time. Tell your health practitioner if drowsiness or decreased alertness persist.

—Lightheadedness, dizziness, or feeling of faintness may occur in some people taking this drug. In order to reduce any of these feelings, move slowly when you change from the lying or sitting positions.

—Some people taking this drug also become unusually sensitive to the sun. To avoid sunburn, use a sunscreen lotion when you are in the sun, and limit your exposure when possible.

—If you are taking this drug in liquid form, avoid contact of the medicine with your skin or clothes, as it is quite irritating.

—Do not take any antacids or antidiarrheal medicine within one hour of the drug, as it will decrease the amount of medicine which your body absorbs.

—Dryness of the mouth may occur when you start taking this drug. Chewing gum, sucking on hard candy or rinsing your mouth frequently with water can help relieve this dryness.

—This drug may make you perspire less than usual. You need to be careful not to become overheated when you exercise vigorously or are in hot and humid weather.

—The drug should not be discontinued abruptly because you could experience nausea, vomiting, trembling and other symptoms. Always contact your health practitioner if there is some reason why you cannot take the medicine.

—Notify your health practitioner immediately if you notice urinary retention, change in vision, sore throat with fever, muscle spasms, trembling or shaking (particularly of hands), skin rash, or small uncontrollable movements of your tongue.

—Keep this medication out of the reach of children and all others for whom it is not prescribed.

—Wear a Medic-Alert bracelet and carry a medical identification card specifying that you are taking this drug.

EVALUATION:

ADVERSE REACTIONS: *Cardiovascular:* orthostatic hypotension, tachycardia. *CNS:* drowsiness, hyperactivity, seizures. *Extrapyramidal symptoms:* akathisia, dystonia, hyperreflexia, pseudoparkinsonism, tardive dyskinesia. *Hypersensitivity:*

skin rash. *Ophthalmologic:* blurred vision, opaque depositions on cornea and lens. *Urinary:* retention. *Other:* constipation, dry mouth, headache, photosensitivity.

OVERDOSAGE: *Signs and symptoms:* CNS depression, bradycardia, hypotension, increased extrapyramidal symptoms, and coma may develop. *Treatment:* Referral for gastric lavage, symptomatic and supportive treatment. Never use epinephrine to treat hypotension and cardiovascular depression as it may potentiate hypotension.

PARAMETERS TO MONITOR: Obtain baseline physical examination and complete blood count, liver function tests and ophthalmologic examination prior to beginning therapy. Tests should be repeated periodically throughout extended therapy. Periodic ECG tracings should also be done if changes in rate or rhythm are detected. If patient is over 35 or has a family history of glaucoma, obtain an intraocular pressure reading prior to therapy. The cornea and lens should also be inspected for abnormal deposition during therapy. At each visit, mental and emotional status should be evaluated, including thought patterns, delusions, hallucinations, and inappropriate behavior. Observe for therapeutic effects. Assess sitting, standing and lying blood pressures to evaluate presence of orthostatic hypotension, particularly in the elderly or debilitated patient. Observe closely for extrapyramidal symptoms, especially fine, involuntary movements of the tongue.

Marsha Goodwin

INDOLONE—MOLINDONE HCL

ACTION OF THE DRUG: The complete mechanism by which indolones act is not well established. The primary site of action is the ascending reticular activating system where stimuli are thought to be blocked. A tranquilizing effect is produced without relaxation of muscles or interference with coordination of body movements.

ASSESSMENT:

INDICATIONS: Used primarily for reducing or relieving symptoms associated with psychosis, particularly schizophrenia.

SUBJECTIVE: Practitioner may elicit a history of emotional unrest, agitation, paranoid ideations, visual, auditory and/or tactile hallucinations, delusions, inability to think clearly, severe mood swings, and inability to cope with reality.

OBJECTIVE: Patients may or may not verbalize paranoid thoughts. They often have difficulty attending and responding to immediate environment. Inappropriate verbal responses to questions, non-verbal behavior and possibly inappropriate dress and general appearance may be present.

PLAN:

CONTRAINDICATIONS: This drug should not be used in patients with a known history of drug hypersensitivity, drug-induced central nervous system depression, or coma from any etiology.

WARNINGS: Risk-benefit ratio must be carefully considered before use in pregnant patients and nursing mothers since there is insufficient data regarding safety in these groups. Use with caution in patients with impaired hepatic or renal function.

PRECAUTIONS: Significant drowsiness may occur during initial therapy with indolones. Studies have shown that prolactin levels are increased by short-term use of indolones and persist during long-term use. Since approximately one third of breast cancers are prolactin dependent, use of indolones in patients with a history of breast cancer must be carefully considered.

IMPLEMENTATION:

DRUG INTERACTIONS: Inhibition or potentiation of drugs given concurrently with indolones has not been documented at this time. Animal studies have been done testing for interactions between indolones and CNS depressants and levodopa. There have been no toxic effects reported as yet. The tablet form of indolone contains calcium sulfate and may interfere with the absorption of tetracycline and phenytoin.

PRODUCTS (TRADE NAME):
Moban (Available in 5, 10, 25, 50 and 100 mg tablets); and 20 mg/ml concentrate).

ADMINISTRATION AND DOSAGE: Indolones are well absorbed from the gastrointestinal tract and the effects of one dose may last for one to one and a half days. Elderly and debilitated patients should be started on low doses and increased slowly. The dosage has not been established for children under 12 years of age and therefore should not be given to this group.

Initial: 50 to 75 mg/day po.

Maintenance: 5 to 25 mg po three to four times a day, up to a maximum of 400 mg/day.

IMPLEMENTATION CONSIDERATIONS:

—Obtain a complete health history, including the presence of hypersensitivity, underlying disease (especially hepatic or renal failure, breast cancer, or CNS depression), concurrent use of other medications, and possibility of pregnancy.

—Elderly or debilitated patients may be overly sensitive to the effects of normal doses. It is important to begin these patients on small doses and monitor for desired and adverse effects.

—Watch for suicidal ideation.

WHAT THE PATIENT NEEDS TO KNOW:

—Take this drug exactly as ordered. If you miss a dose, take it as soon as possible unless it is close to the next scheduled dose. Do not double doses.

—If medication causes gastric upset, this may be minimized by taking it with food or milk.

—Do not stop taking this drug suddenly. Contact your health provider if you have any difficulty taking the medication, or notice the development of any new or troublesome symptoms.

—This drug may cause you to feel very drowsy or sleepy when you first start taking it. If you experience this, avoid driving or performing tasks requiring alertness until this passes. Notify your practitioner if drowsiness persists.

—Keep this medication out of the reach of children and all others for whom it is not prescribed.

EVALUATION:

ADVERSE REACTIONS: *Cardiovascular:* non-specific ECG changes (particularly T-wave changes), orthostatic hypotension. *CNS:* depression, drowsiness, euphoria, hyperactivity. *Extrapyramidal effects:* akathisia, dystonia, tardive dyskinesia, Parkinson's syndrome. *Hematopoietic:* leukocytosis, leukopenia. *Hypersensitivity:* skin rash. *Urinary:* retention. *Other:* blurred vision, dry mouth, increased libido, heavy menses, resumption of menses in amenorrheic patients.

OVERDOSAGE: *Signs and symptoms:* Exaggeration of adverse effects may develop, particularly sedation. *Treatment:* Refer for gastric lavage, supportive and symptomatic treatment.

PARAMETERS TO MONITOR: Baseline physical examination with lying, standing and sitting blood pressures should be obtained. Complete blood count and liver function tests should also be obtained prior to initiating therapy, and should be repeated at periodic intervals. Regular breast examination should be performed in female patients and the patient should be taught breast self-examination. Each month mental and emotional status should be evaluated. Observe for therapeutic effect. Sedation, symptoms of extrapyramidal and anticholinergic effects, and orthostatic hypotension should be assessed.

Marsha Goodwin

PSYCHOTHERAPEUTIC DRUGS—
COMBINATIONS

CHLORDIAZEPOXIDE AND AMITRIPTYLINE

PRODUCTS (TRADE NAME):
   Limbitrol 5/12.5 or 10/25 (Available in tablets with chlordiazepoxide 5 mg and amitriptyline HCl 12.5 mg or chlordiazepoxide 10 mg and amitriptyline HCl 25 mg.)

DRUG SPECIFICS:
   Limbitrol is used in the treatment of patients with moderate to severe depression associated with moderate to severe anxiety. Contraindications to the use of

this drug include hypersensitivity to benzodiazepines or tricyclic antidepressants, concomitant MAO inhibitor therapy, myocardial infarction (during acute recovery phase), children under the age of 12, pregnant or breast-feeding women. Use caution in giving to patients with a history of urinary retention, angle-closure glaucoma, or cardiovascular disease. Drug may cause arrhythmias, tachycardia, and prolongation of conduction time. Physical and psychological dependence may occur.

The elderly or debilitated patients, those with renal or hepatic disorders, hyperthyroidism, history of seizures, potentially suicidal patients, those taking thyroid medications, anticholinergics or sympathomimetics are all at special risk in using this medication.

Mental impairment and reflex-slowing are possible. Patient should be cautioned against performing jobs which require complete mental alertness.

Concurrent use with alcohol or other central nervous system depressants will increase the CNS depressant effect. Use with anticholinergics may cause acute glaucoma, urinary retention, severe constipation and paralytic ileus. Use with epinephrine may increase the pressor response and provoke arrhythmias. When used with guanethidine, the antihypertensive effect will be decreased. Use with MAO inhibitors may produce hyperpyrexia, excitability, convulsions, coma and death. Oral anticoagulant doses may be altered, requiring either increased or decreased doses. This agent may produce transient delirium when used with ethchlorvynol. Hyperpyrexia and severe hypertension may be provoked when used with sympathomimetic agents. Use with thyroid preparations may increase antidepressant effect, with the risk of developing arrhythmias also possible.

ADMINISTRATION AND DOSAGE SPECIFICS:

Recommended starting dose of 10/25: 3 or 4 tablets daily in divided doses with a maximum of 6 tablets daily. Some patients may respond to only 2 tablets daily.

Initial dosage of 5/12.5: 3-4 tablets daily in divided doses, may be used for those who do not tolerate higher doses. Use smallest amount of drug possible to maintain remission.

Mary Ann Bolter

PENTYLENETETRAZOL COMBINATIONS

PRODUCTS (TRADE NAME):
See Table 4-12.
DRUG SPECIFICS:

These drugs are used to enhance physical and mental activity in elderly patients. Pentylenetetrazol is a CNS stimulant. Some forms of this drug are also used for peripheral vestibular disorders, idiopathic vertigo and as a respiratory stimulant.

There are few side effects with recommended oral dosage. Insomnia, anorexia,

ADMINISTRATION AND DOSAGE SPECIFICS:

TABLE 4-12. COMPONENTS AND DOSAGE FOR PENTYLENETETRAZOL COMBINATIONS

Product	Components	Dosage
Cenalene (available as 100 mg tablets and 100 mg/ 5 ml elixir)	Pentylenetetrazol, 100 mg; thiamine, 1.67 mg; niacinamide, 7.5 mg; vitamin B$_{12}$ 2.5 mcg;	2 tsp or two tablets three times daily for 1 month; then 1 tsp or one tablet three times daily
Cerebro-Nicin	Pentylenetetrazol, 100 mg;	1 capsule three times daily
Alcohol (elixir) 15% (available in 100 mg capsules)	nicotinic acid 100 mg; niacinamide, 5 mg; vitamin C, 100 mg; thiamine, 25 mg; riboflavin, 2 mg; pyridoxine, 3 mg; L-glutamic acid 50 mg	1 capsule 3 times daily
D-Vaso, Tega-Vert Verticon (available in 50 mg tablets)	Pentylenetetrazol 150 mg; niacin, 50 mg; dimen- hydrinate, 25 mg	One to two tablets three times daily
Menic (available in 100 mg tablets)	Pentylenetetrazol, 100 mg; nicotinic acid, 50 mg	two tablets after each meal

nausea, vomiting and headache may occur. Overdosage produces toxic symptoms similar to those induced by CNS stimulants.

Any stimulant may interact with antihypertensive agents and other drugs commonly administered to elderly patients.

Pentylenetetrazol is contraindicated in patients with a history of severely impaired liver function, seizures or focal brain lesions. Guidelines have not been established for use in children, pregnancy and nursing mothers. Use high doses cautiously if patient has cardiac disease.

Mary Ann Bolter

PSYCHOTHERAPEUTIC DRUGS— MINIMAL BRAIN DYSFUNCTION AGENTS

DEANOL ACETAMIDOBENZOATE

ACTION OF THE DRUG: These products affect the central nervous system and cross the blood-brain barrier. Although it is not known for certain, they are probably converted to acetylcholine intracellularly.

ASSESSMENT:

INDICATIONS: *Children:* treatment of minimal brain damage, learning and behavior problems, hyperkinetic behavior and learning problems with a combination of reading and speech difficulties, impaired motor coordination, impulsive and compulsive behavior. *Adults:* chronic fatigue, neurasthenia, and mild neurotic depression.

SUBJECTIVE: Children may present with history of poor attention span, inability to concentrate, uncontrollable behavior, and difficulty in school both with behavior and learning.

OBJECTIVE: No objective findings may be observed. Some children demonstrate reading and speech difficulties which may be quantified.

PLAN:

CONTRAINDICATIONS: Should not be used in grand mal epilepsy or mixed epilepsy with grand mal components.

IMPLEMENTATION:

PRODUCTS (TRADE NAME):
Deaner (Available as 25, 100, 250 mg scored tablets.)
ADMINISTRATION AND DOSAGE:
Initial oral dose is 500 mg daily in AM. If improvement is noted after 3 weeks, maintenance dosage is from 250 to 500 mg, adjusted to the needs of the individual patient. Should not be administered to children under 6 years of age.
IMPLEMENTATION CONSIDERATIONS:
—Take a complete history of hypersensitivity, concurrent drug use, seizures, behavioral history, and nursing assessment of any other health problems.
—Spend time counseling family and client about purpose of the drug, as well as possible side effects.

WHAT THE PATIENT NEEDS TO KNOW:
—You will need to take this drug for several weeks before you begin to feel a difference.
—Most side effects to this drug are slight and will disappear with continued treatment, or reduction in dosage. All new symptoms should be reported to your health care provider before any changes in dosage are made.
—Do not take this drug later than 6 p.m.
—Taking the drug as prescribed and regular visits to your health care provider are important while you are taking this medication.

EVALUATION:

ADVERSE REACTIONS: There are frequently mild side effects which disappear with continued treatment or reduced dosage. *Cardiovascular:* postural hypotension (rarely). *CNS:* dull occipital headache early in therapy, insomnia, mild over-stimulation. *Gastrointestinal:* constipation. *Integumentary:* pruritus, transient rash. *Musculoskeletal:* Tenseness in neck: masseter and quadriceps muscles.

OVERDOSAGE: There may be persistence of adverse symptoms (listed above), which can be lessened by decreasing the dose.

PARAMETERS TO MONITOR: Identify through history major behavioral problems and monitor these same symptoms each visit to look for therapeutic effect. Contact with child's school may help evaluate effect of drug also.

Linda Ross

METHYLPHENIDATE HCL

ACTION OF THE DRUG: Methylphenidate HCL produces mild central nervous system stimulant with greater effects on mental than motor activities. Mode of action is on the cerebral cortex and subcortical structures, including the thalamus.

ASSESSMENT:

INDICATIONS: Adjunct in the treatment of hyperactivity associated with minimal brain dysfunction, narcolepsy, and children with perceptual problems.

SUBJECTIVE: "Hyperactivity" of a child, shortened attention span, aggressiveness, fatigue. May also be used to counteract overdosage from depressant drugs.

OBJECTIVE: Signs of hyperactivity, along with observation of depression and emotional lability.

PLAN

CONTRAINDICATIONS: This drug should not be used in patients who are breast-feeding, who have glaucoma, hypersensitivity to the drug, marked anxiety, tension and agitation, during pregnancy or someone planning to become pregnant.

WARNINGS: Do not use in children less than 6 years of age. Also not to be used for severe depression because it may exacerbate symptoms. Can cause allergic-type reaction, including bronchial asthma in susceptible individuals, particularly those who are allergic to aspirin because of the FD&C Yellow #5 (tartrazene) in the 5 and 10 mg tablet.

PRECAUTIONS: Patients with some degree of agitation may react adversely. With the behavioral syndrome of hyperactivity, a thorough neurological and laboratory workup should be completed before starting medication. This drug can lower the convulsive threshold in patients with a seizure disorder. Abrupt withdrawal can cause severe depression. Patients who abuse methylphenidate have injected the drug, causing infected abscesses at the site, or produced an embolus when mixed with a binder. Avoid hazardous activities (driving, piloting, operating heavy machinery) if drowsiness or dizziness occurs. Patients over sixty years of age may be more sensitive to stimulants; therefore, proceed with smaller doses.

IMPLEMENTATION:

DRUG INTERACTIONS: Decreases the effect of guanethidine by displacement from its site of action. May potentiate the effects of pressor agents and MAO inhibitors. May inhibit the metabolism of coumarin anticoagulants, anticonvulsants, phenylbutazone and tricyclic depressants.

PRODUCTS (TRADE NAME):

Methylphenidate HCl, Ritalin HCl (Available in 5, 15 and 20 mg tablets.)

ADMINISTRATION AND DOSAGE: Initial dose acts within 30-60 minutes of administration. Wears off within 4-5 hours. Store medicine in tight, light-resistant container in a dry place.

This drug is a controlled substance. Drug recommended for school days for help in learning environment, or other occasions when necessary. Tolerance may develop and require dose adjustment. Drug treatment should not and need not be indefinite and usually may be discontinued after puberty.

Adults: Dosage 10 mg tablet orally 2 or 3 times a day with maximum of 40 to 60 mg/day in certain patients.

Children 6 years and older: Initial oral dosage 0.25 mg/kg daily in equal portions before breakfast and lunch. Dosage can be doubled on a weekly basis, if no untoward effects are noted. Maximum dosage 2 mg/kg daily or 60 mg daily. Should be discontinued periodically to assess the child's condition.

IMPLEMENTATION CONSIDERATIONS:

—Obtain complete health history, including history of hypersensitivity, seizures, hypertension or any other health problem and possibility of pregnancy. Obtain history of any concomitant drug therapy.

—As baseline physical be certain to include height, weight and blood pressure.

—Obtain baseline laboratory studies, including complete blood count, differential and platelet count.

—Obtain periodic teacher and school report to see if there is change in behavior after medication is instituted. Communicate to teacher, with the parent's permission, the name of the drug, amount and expected effects.

—Counsel parents that under normal circumstances and with proper regulation, the drug is not habit-forming.

—Communicate to parents that drug does not sedate child.

—If a patient over sixty is taking the drug, they may be more sensitive to the drug. This requires smaller initial doses.

—Drug should be discontinued periodically to monitor therapeutic action, and to see if drug may be stopped permanently.

WHAT THE PATIENT NEEDS TO KNOW:
—Take this medication only as directed.
—For the best action take this medicine 30-40 minutes before meal time.

—Take the last dose of medicine before 6 pm to avoid problems falling asleep.

—If you are an hour late in taking your medicine, take the missed dose. Do not wait and take a double dose at the next time.

—Regular follow-up to your health provider is very important.

—Avoid certain foods and liquids during the time you are on this drug. Particularly avoid foods rich in tyramine such as: aged cheese of any kind, avocado, chocolate, canned fish, raisins and soy sauce. Also avoid beverages prepared from meat or yeast extracts, chocolate drinks, beer, Chianti, and vermouth.

—Do not discontinue drug abruptly, as this can cause severe depression or erratic behavior.

EVALUATION:

ADVERSE REACTIONS: *Cardiovascular:* angina, arrhythmias, blood pressure increase, tachycardia. *CNS:* blurred vision, chorea, convulsions, dyskinesia, headache, insomnia, nervousness. *Gastrointestinal:* abdominal pain, anorexia, nausea, weight loss. *Hematopoietic:* anemia, leukopenia, thrombocytopenic purpura. *Integumentary:* angioneurotic edema, atopic or nonspecific dermatitis, hives, hypersensitivity, photodermatitis, scalp hair loss, skin rashes, urticaria. *Musculoskeletal:* joint pains. *Other:* mood or mental changes. *Children:* abdominal pain, insomnia, loss of steady growth pattern, (however compensated by growth rebound when the drug is discontinued).

OVERDOSAGE: *Signs and symptoms:* agitation, coma, confusion, convulsions, dryness of mucous membranes, hallucinations, headache, mydriasis, rapid and irregular pulse, sweating, vomiting. *Treatment:* Referral for gastric lavage. Use supportive measures, protection against self-injury.

PARAMETERS TO MONITOR: Obtain blood pressure, pulse, height and weight, complete blood count at initial visit and every six months thereafter. Check with parent/teacher for effects of drug on behavior. Observe for signs and symptoms of therapeutic effects: less irritability, better attention span.

Linda Ross

PEMOLINE

ACTION OF THE DRUG: This product is a central nervous system stimulant which increases the concentration of choline, acetylcholine and dopamine in the brain. The exact site and mechanism of action in man is unknown.

ASSESSMENT:

INDICATIONS: Therapy for minimal brain dysfunction or attention span deficit in conjunction with a total therapeutic program. Has been used experimentally for treatment of narcolepsy and excessive daytime drowsiness.

SUBJECTIVE: Distractability, emotional lability, impulsiveness in children and adults, short attention span and overstimulation may be found in elderly patients.

OBJECTIVE: No objective signs may be found.

PLAN:

CONTRAINDICATIONS: Do not use with known hypersensitivity to drug, or in children under 6 years of age.

WARNINGS: Should not be administered to children with impaired renal function. Some suppression of predicted growth has been noted in long-term usage.

PRECAUTIONS: Use with caution in patients with emotional instability, hepatic function impairment, psychoses and renal function impairment. Excessive use of drug may cause a psychological dependence if used by an unstable person. The risk of unknown complications must be weighed against the benefit in patients who are pregnant or breast-feeding.

IMPLEMENTATION:

DRUG INTERACTIONS: Not studied fully in humans; however, patient should be monitored carefully when taking pemoline with other drugs which have central nervous system activity.

PRODUCTS (TRADE NAME):
Cylert (Available as 18.75, 37.5 and 75 mg tablet and 37.5 mg chewable tablet.)

ADMINISTRATION AND DOSAGE:
This drug is a controlled substance. It needs to be taken for 3-4 weeks for effect to be realized. The serum half-life is approximately 12 hours. When discontinuing drug, do so slowly, as there is the possibility of withdrawal symptoms. Chronic excessive use may result in psychic or physical dependence. Store medication between 15 and 30 degrees centigrade in a well-closed container.

Children 6 years and older: Initial dose 37.5 mg orally in the morning. Dosage can be increased weekly by 18.75 mg until desired clinical response is achieved. Usual effective dose is 56.25 mg 75 mg daily.

IMPLEMENTATION CONSIDERATIONS:
—Obtain a complete health history, including presence of hypersensitivity, history of any renal or liver disease, and the possibility of pregnancy.

—Obtain baseline laboratory studies: urinalysis, liver function studies, complete blood count.

—Obtain baseline height and weight in patients.

—Obtain a complete history of the behavior of the patient, and particularly note any indication of drug dependence or substance abuse.

—Note any other health problems which may be related.

WHAT THE PATIENT NEEDS TO KNOW:
—It is important to follow instructions in taking this medication. Do not take more than is prescribed at any one time.
—Do not discontinue medicine without checking with your health care provider.
—If morning dose is missed, take it as soon as possible. Do not take medicine just prior to your regular bedtime.
—Contact your health provider if there are any signs of yellowing of skin or eyes, seizures, hallucinations, uncontrolled movements, unusual nervousness, restlessness, rapid heartbeat, or any symptom that is new for you.
—You may lose some weight after beginning this drug. This is only a short-term effect, and your weight should return to normal within six months.
—If you are only taking one dose of medication each day, take it in the morning.

EVALUATION:

ADVERSE REACTIONS: *Cardiovascular:* shock, fatigue, increase in blood pressure, tachycardia. *CNS:* convulsions, dizziness, hallucinations, insomnia, irritability, uncontrolled movements of the eyes or other parts of the body. *Endocrine:* growth suppression. *Gastrointestinal:* anorexia, weight loss during first weeks, nausea, abdominal pain. *Hematopoietic:* jaundiced skin or eyes.

PARAMETERS TO MONITOR: Obtain height and weight each visit. Parent and child should keep a record at home on a twice-weekly basis. Baseline liver enzymes and urinalysis should be collected initially, repeated every six months. Assess behavior (improvement or not) in the school situation after beginning drug. Review dosage and time of administration with the parent and child.

Linda Ross

ANTIPSYCHOTIC AGENTS—PHENOTHIAZINES AND RELATED DRUGS

ACTION OF THE DRUG: A major action of phenothiazines is (1) to block dopamine at the postsynaptic receptor sites in the brain, thus enhancing the turnover of the neurotransmitter. They also decrease the uptake of other neurotransmitters, norepinephrine and serotonin, by the neurons. Intraneurally, the drugs decrease the level of cyclic AMP particularly in areas of the brain that control emotion and behavior. These changes are thought to produce the antipsychotic effects of the phenothiazines. (2) Phenothiazines also reduce sensory stimulation of the reticular activating system in the brain stem, thereby producing a sedative effect. (3) Antiemesis results from phenothiazine's inhibitory action in the chemoreceptor trigger zone.

ASSESSMENT:

INDICATIONS: Used primarily for reducing or relieving the symptoms of acute and chronic psychoses including schizophrenia, schizoaffective disorders, and involutional psychosis. May be useful in the treatment of several idiopathic or organic disorders in which the patient exhibits severe agitation or psychotic symptoms. Other uses of phenothiazines include the following: relief of nausea and vomiting, relief of intractable hiccoughs, reduction in agitation associated with alcohol withdrawal, and reduction in aggressiveness of mentally disturbed children.

SUBJECTIVE: Provider may elicit history of emotional unrest, agitation, paranoid ideation, visual, auditory and/or tactile hallucinations, delusions, inability to think clearly, severe mood swings, inability to cope with reality.

OBJECTIVE: Patients may or may not verbalize paranoid thoughts. Often have difficulty attending and responding to immediate environment. Inappropriate verbal responses to questions, non-verbal behavior, and possibly inappropriate dress and general appearance.

PLAN:

CONTRAINDICATIONS: Do not give in the presence of prior hypersensitivity to a phenothiazine, severe hepatic or renal failure, jaundice, chronic alcoholism, subcortical brain damage, cerebral arteriosclerosis, severe coronary artery disease, blood dyscrasias, bone marrow depression, and comatose states. Phenothiazines should not be used in children or adolescents who are vomiting and have other signs and symptoms suggestive of Reye's syndrome.

WARNINGS: Risk-benefit ratio must be carefully considered before use in pregnant patients since jaundice and extrapyramidal signs have occurred in the neonates of mothers using phenothiazines. The drug may also be excreted in the milk of nursing mothers, and risk to the child is not known. Cross-sensitivity occurs among the phenothiazines. Use with caution in patients with impaired hepatic or renal function, peptic ulcer disease, symptomatic prostatic hypertrophy, Parkinson's disease, cardiovascular disease, and those with a potential for glaucoma.

PRECAUTIONS: Patients with severe asthma, emphysema or acute respiratory infections (especially children) may develop hypoventilation secondary to the CNS depressant effects of phenothiazines. Phenothiazines may also depress the cough reflex and lead to aspiration in a patient who is vomiting. Studies have shown that prolactin levels are increased by short-term use of phenothiazines and elevations persist during long-term use. Since approximately one third of breast cancers are prolactin dependent, use of phenothiazines in patients with a history of breast cancer must be carefully considered.

IMPLEMENTATION:

DRUG INTERACTIONS: Phenothiazines taken concurrently with CNS depressants (alcohol, barbiturates, narcotics, and anesthetics) may potentiate and prolong the effects of either the CNS depressant or the phenothiazine. If patient is scheduled for elective surgery, anesthesiologist should be warned that patient has been receiving this drug. Reduction by 1/4 to 1/2 the dose of either the phenothiazine or the CNS depressant or both may be necessary. Other drugs whose effects may be potentiated when used concurrently with phenothiazines include antimuscarinics (particularly atropine), MAO inhibitors, and tricyclic antidepressants. Antacids and antidiarrheal drugs reduce the absorption rate. The effects of some drugs such as amphetamines, levodopa, guanethidine and other similar antihypertensives may be diminished when used concurrently. The seizure threshold in an epileptic patient may be lowered by phenothiazines. Phenothiazines may also interact with endogenous and exogenous substances and therefore alter certain diagnostic test results. For example, a patient taking phenothiazines may have a false-positive urine bilirubin, a false-positive or false-negative urine pregnancy test, or an abnormal metyrapone test since ACTH secretion can be reduced by phenothiazines.

ADMINISTRATION AND DOSAGE: Phenothiazines in general are highly protein bound; and their metabolism by the liver and excretion through the kidneys may be slow. The drug can be taken either orally or parenterally. The oral form of the phenothiazines is fairly well absorbed but the absorption rate will be delayed if taken concurrently with antacids or antidiarrheal agents. Stomach upset from the oral form of phenothiazines can be reduced or avoided by taking the drug with mild food or an 8 ounce glass of water. The desired antipsychotic effects of phenothiazines may take several weeks after therapy is initiated. The initial dose should be the lowest recommended amount, according to individual tolerance and severity of psychosis, until the psychotic symptoms are controlled. Titration of dose in the elderly or debilitated should be done gradually and with close monitoring of the patient. The dosage of phenothiazines that controls the patient's symptoms should be maintained for 2-3 weeks and then gradually reduced until the lowest effective maintenance dose is attained. If a phenothiazine is given in large doses or over a prolonged period of time, discontinuation of the drug should be accomplished by gradual reduction over several weeks in order to avoid symptoms of dyskinesia, nausea, vomiting, dizziness and trembling.

In choosing a specific phenothiazine in the treatment of psychosis, consideration should be given to the degree of sedative, extrapyramidal and hypotensive side effects associated with the drug, its potency (generally compared with chlorpromazine), and the relation of these side effects and potency level to the individual patient situation. Table 4-12 lists the phenothiazines according to their chemical structure (aliphatics, piperazines and piperidines), degree of sedation, extrapyramidal and hypotensive effects, and potency compared with chlorpromazine for each drug.

IMPLEMENTATION CONSIDERATIONS:
—Obtain a complete health history, including the presence of hypersensitivity to phenothiazines, history of coronary artery disease, cardiovascular disease, cerebral arteriosclerosis, asthma, emphysema, respiratory infections, bone marrow depression, blood dyscrasias, prostatic hypertrophy, Parkinson's disease, Reye's syndrome, impaired hepatic or renal function, alcoholism, peptic ulcer disease, glaucoma, urinary retention, breast cancer, seizures, concurrent use of other medications, or the possibility of pregnancy.

TABLE 4-12. POTENCY AND SIDE EFFECTS OF MAJOR PHENOTHIAZINES

Chemical Class	Sedation	Extrapyramidal Symptoms	Hypotension	Potency Compared With Chlorpromazine
A. Aliphatic				
Chlorpromazine	***	**	**	1
Promazine	**	**	**	0.5
Triflupromazine	***	**	**	4
B. Piperazine				
Acetophenazine	**	***	*	5
Carphenazine	**	***	*	4
Fluphenazine	*	***	*	50
Perphenazine	*	***	*	12
Prochlorperazine	**	***	*	10
Trifluoperazine	*	***	*	25
C. Piperidine				
Mesoridazine	***	*	**	2
Piperacetazine	**	*	*	10
Thioridazine	***	*	**	1

*Occurs infrequently
**Occurs occasionally
***Occurs frequently

—Patient should have a complete eye evaluation by a specialist, including the inspection of internal structures and the lens to establish baseline data.

—Elderly, debilitated or emaciated patients are often sensitive to the effects of usual recommended doses and are more prone to extrapyramidal and hypotensive side effects. It is important to begin these patients on a small dose and monitor for desired and adverse effects before increasing the dosage.

WHAT THE PATIENT NEEDS TO KNOW:

—Take this medication exactly as ordered. It may take several weeks before you begin to feel better. Therefore, it is important to continue taking the drug in the exact amount and frequency specified even though you may notice no changes.

—This drug can increase the effects of alcohol, sleeping pills and many other prescribed medications. Alcohol should be avoided and you should check with your health practitioner before taking any prescribed or over-the-counter drugs.

—This drug may cause drowsiness or make you feel less alert than usual, particularly when you first start taking the medicine. If you experience these feelings, avoid driving or other activities that require alertness. Talk with your health practitioner if drowsiness or decreased alertness persists.

—Lightheadedness, dizziness, or feelings of faintness occur in some people taking this drug. In order to reduce any of these feelings, move slowly when you get up from a lying or sitting position.

—Some people taking this drug become more sensitive to the sun. To avoid sunburn, use a sunscreen lotion if out in the sun, and limit your exposure to the sun or sunlamps.

—If you are taking this drug in liquid form, avoid contact of the medicine with your skin or clothes since it can cause irritation.

—If the medicine causes any gastric distress it may be reduced by taking drug with food, milk, or an 8 ounce glass of water. Do not take any antacids or antidiarrheal medicine within one hour of the drug.

—If the drug you are taking comes in a bottle with a medicine dropper, make sure you measure out the prescribed dose marked on the dropper and then dilute it in a glass of water or juice.

—Dryness of the mouth may occur when you start taking this drug. Chewing gum, sucking on hard candy, or rinsing your mouth frequently may help relieve this dryness.

—This drug may make you perspire less than usual. Therefore, you need to be careful not to become overheated when you exercise vigorously or in hot and humid weather.

—Notify your health provider promptly if urinary retention, change in vision, sore throat with fever, muscle spasms, trembling or shaking (particularly of hands), skin rash, yellow tinge to skin and eyes, small uncontrollable movements of the tongue, or other new or troublesome symptoms develop.

—Keep this medication out of the reach of children and all others for whom it is not prescribed.

—Wear a Medic-Alert bracelet and carry a medical identification card specifying that you are taking this medication.

EVALUATION:

ADVERSE REACTIONS: *Cardiovascular:* ECG changes (prolonged PR and QT intervals, T-wave blunting), orthostatic hypotension, tachycardia. *CNS:* cerebral edema, confusion, drowsiness, hyperactivity, insomnia, seizures. *Endocrine:* abnormal lactation, amenorrhea, breast engorgement, decreased libido, glycosuria, gynecomastia, hyperglycemia, increased appetite. *Extrapyramidal effects:* akathisia, dystonia, hyperreflexia, pseudoparkinsonism, tardive dyskinesia. *Hematopoietic:* agranulocytosis, leukopenia, pancytopenia, purpura, thrombocytopenia. *Hepatic:* obstructive jaundice. *Hypersensitivity:* anaphylactic reaction (rare), contact dermatitis, photosensitivity, urticaria. *Other:* altered urine pregnancy tests, urine bilirubin tests, thyroid and adrenal function tests, constipation, decreased perspiration, dry mouth, dyspnea, enuresis, nasal congestion, opaque deposits on cornea and lens, urinary retention.

OVERDOSAGE: *Signs and symptoms:* Exaggerated central nervous system depression, coma, severe hypotension, and extrapyramidal symptoms, seizures, or cardiac arrhythmias may appear. *Treatment:* Referral for gastric lavage, maintenance of patent airway and monitoring. Provide symptomatic relief. Benadryl or anticholinergic antiparkinsonism drugs may control extrapyramidal symptoms. Amphetamines or caffeine benzoate as a stimulant may be given, and a vasopressor used for hypotension. Never induce vomiting since aspiration may occur.

PARAMETERS TO MONITOR: Baseline complete blood counts, liver function tests (including urine for bilirubin) and ophthalmologic examination should be obtained prior to beginning therapy, and repeated at periodic intervals during extended therapy. In addition, periodic ECG tracing should be done if changes in pulse rate or rhythm are detected. For any patient over 35 or with a family history of glaucoma, obtain an intraocular pressure reading prior to therapy. The cornea and lens should be inspected for abnormal deposition during therapy and referral made to specialists if indicated. On each visit mental and emotional status should be evaluated including, thought patterns, delusions, hallucinations, or inappropriate behavior. Evaluate lying, sitting and standing blood pressures in order to identify orthostatic hypotension which may be especially pronounced in the elderly or debilitated patient. Observe closely for jaundice, and for fine, involuntary movements of the tongue or other extrapyramidal symptoms.

ALIPHATIC PHENOTHIAZINE: CHLORPROMAZINE HCL

PRODUCTS (TRADE NAME):
Chlorpromazine HCl (Available in 10, 25, 50, 100, 200 mg tablets and 100 mg/ml concentrate and 25 mg/ml injection.) **Promapar** (Available in 10, 25, 50, 100, 200 mg tablets.) **Thorazine** (Available in 10, 25, 50, 100, 200 mg tablets; 10 mg/5 ml syrup; 30 mg/ml and 100 mg/ml concentrate; 25 mg and 100 mg suppository; 25 mg/ml injection; and 30, 75, 150, 200 and 300 mg timed-release Spansules.) **Thor-Prom** (Available in 10, 25, 50, 100 and 200 mg tablets.)
DRUG SPECIFICS:
This is one of the first known phenothiazine products. It remains today a popular and inexpensive drug. It is used in psychotic disorders, control of the manic phase of manic-depressive reactions, preoperatively for restlessness, and in the treatment of intermittent porphyria, and tetanus. It is especially useful in treating behavioral problems of children who are combative, or for hyperactive children with excessive motor activity. It is also used in the management of nausea and vomiting in the same doses.
ADMINISTRATION AND DOSAGE SPECIFICS:
Adults: 30-300 mg/day po in divided doses; or 25 to 50 mg IM three times a day. Do not exceed 1000 mg/day.

Children over 6 months: 0.55 mg/kg po two to four times a day; or 0.55 mg/kg IM every 6-8 hours. May also give 1 mg/kg rectally three to four times a day.

ALIPHATIC PHENOTHIAZINE: PROMAZINE HCL

PRODUCTS (TRADE NAME):
Promazine (Available in 25 mg/ml and 50 mg/ml injection.) **Prozine** (Available in 50 mg/ml injection.) **Sparine** (Available in 10, 25, 50 and 100 mg tablets; 10 mg/ 5 ml syrup; 30 mg/ml concentrate; and 25 and 50 mg/ml injection.)
DRUG SPECIFICS:
Used primarily in the management of psychotic disorders. Oral medication is usually preferred, unless patient is hospitalized and postural hypotension can be monitored. Dosage must be titrated according to individual response. IM dose of 50 to 150 mg is usually sufficient to calm a severely agitated patient.
ADMINISTRATION AND DOSAGE SPECIFICS:
Adults: Give 10-200 mg po every 4 to 6 hours, up to a maximum of 100O mg/ day. May also give 10-200 mg IM every 4-6 hours.
Children over 12 years: Give 10-25 mg po every 4-6 hours.

ALPHETIC PHENOTHIAZENE: TRIFLUPROMAZINE HCL

PRODUCTS (TRADE NAME):
Vesprin (Available in 50 mg/5 ml suspension; and 10 and 20 mg/ml injection.)
DRUG SPECIFICS:
Used in the management of psychotic disorders and also for the treatment and prophylaxis of nausea and vomiting. May color the urine pink or reddish brown. Prolonged exposure to sunlight may produce photosensitivity.
ADMINISTRATION AND DOSAGE SPECIFICS:
Adults: 100 to 150 mg/day po; or 60 to 150 mg/day IM.
Children over 2 years: 2 mg/kg po, up to 150 mg/day; or 0.2 to 0.25 mg/kg IM, up to 10 mg/day.
Prophylaxis or treatment of nausea or vomiting: 5 to 15 mg IM every 4 hours; dose not to exceed 60 mg/day, or may take 20 mg po, with dose not to exceed 30 mg/day. Doses should be lower for elderly or debilitated.

PIPERAZINE PHENOTHIAZINE: ACETOPHENAZINE MALEATE

PRODUCTS (TRADE NAME):
    Tindal (Available in 20 mg tablet.)
DRUG SPECIFICS:
    Used in the management of psychotic disorders.
ADMINISTRATION AND DOSAGE SPECIFICS:
    Adults: 20 mg po three times a day.
    Children: 0.8 to 1.6 mg/kg/day po.

PIPERAZINE PHENOTHIAZINE: CARPHENAZINE MALEATE

PRODUCTS (TRADE NAME):
    Proketazine (Available in 25 mg tablets.)
DRUG SPECIFICS:
    Used in controlling symptoms of psychotic disorders. Usually an inexpensive preparation.
ADMINISTRATION AND DOSAGE SPECIFICS:
    Adults: 12.5 to 25 mg po two to three times/day, gradually increasing dosage as necessary at weekly intervals until maximum response is obtained. Then gradually decrease dosage until the lowest effective maintenance dose is obtained. Acutely upset patients may respond to 100 mg/day. Do not exceed 400 mg/day. Elderly and debilitated may need smaller doses.
    Children over 12 years: 12.5 to 50 mg po two to three times daily.

PIPERAZINE PHENOTHIAZENE: FLUPHENAZINE HCL

PRODUCTS (TRADE NAME):
    Permitil (Available in 0.25, 2.5, 5, and 10 mg tablets; 1 mg timed-release chronotabs; and 5 mg/ml concentrate.) **Prolixin** (Available in 1, 2.5, 5, and 10 mg tablets; 2.5 mg/5 ml elixir; and 2.5 mg/ 5 ml injection.)
DRUG SPECIFICS:
    Used in the control of psychotic symptoms. Prolixin contains tartrazine, a product which may produce an asthma-like allergic response in sensitive individuals.

Dosage must be titrated according to individual response to the medication. Use the smallest possible dosage. Geriatric and debilitated patients need smaller than normal dosages.

ADMINISTRATION AND DOSAGE SPECIFICS:

Adults: Give 0.5 to 10 mg po in divided doses administered at 8-hour intervals initially. Normal maintenance dose is 3 mg po daily, but occasionally higher doses are required. Do not exceed 20 mg/day po. If given IM, 1.25 mg is usual initial dose, with 2.5 to 10 mg IM divided and given in 6-to-8-hour intervals as needed. Do not exceed 10 mg/day IM.

Children: 0.25 to 0.75 mg po one to four times a day; IM dose same as for adults.

Geriatrics: 1 to 2.5 mg/day initially, with increases made according to individual responsiveness.

PIPERAZINE PHENOTHIAZINE: PERPHENAZINE

PRODUCTS (TRADE NAME):

Trilafon (Available in 2, 4, 8 and 16 mg tablets, 8 mg repeat-action tablets; 16 mg/5 ml concentrate; 5 mg/ml injection.)

DRUG SPECIFICS:

Used in the management of psychotic symptoms, and in the control of severe nausea and vomiting in adults. Drug causes excessive drowsiness, and reacts adversely with alcohol. Avoid prolonged exposure to sunlamps or sunlight, which may prompt photosensitivity. Urine may be discolored pink or reddish-brown. IV use of medication should be reserved for severe cases and given slowly by physician.

ADMINISTRATION AND DOSAGE SPECIFICS:

Adults and children over 12: 2-16 mg po two to four times daily; or 5 to 10 mg IM every 6 hours, up to 15 mg/day.

Control of nausea and vomiting: 8 to 16 mg daily po in divided doses. Reduce dosage as soon as possible. May give 5 mg IM in severe cases.

PIPERAZINE PHENOTHIAZINE: PROCHLORPERAZINE

PRODUCTS (TRADE NAME):

Compazine (Available in 5, 10 and 25 mg tablets; 10, 15, 30 and 75 mg sustained-release Spansules; 5 mg/5 ml syrup; 10 mg/ml concentrate; 2.5, 5 and 25 mg suppositories; and 5 mg/ml injection.) **Prochlorperazine** (Available in 5, 10 and 25 mg tablets; 5 mg/ml injection.)

DRUG SPECIFICS:

Used in the treatment of moderate to severe anxiety and tension, and for the management of psychotic disorders. Also used in the treatment of nausea and vomiting. May cause drowsiness. May discolor urine to pink or reddish-brown color. Avoid prolonged exposure to sunlamps or sunlight to avoid development of photosensitization. Dosage is same for nausea and psychiatric use.

ADMINISTRATION AND DOSAGE SPECIFICS:

Adults: 5 to 10 mg po three to four times a day, up to 150 mg/day; or 10 to 20 mg IM every four to six hours, up to 200 mg/day. May also give 25 mg rectally two times a day.

Children over 2 years old or 9 kg body weight: 0.1 mg/kg po four times a day, not to exceed 10 mg/day on first day or 20 mg/day on subsequent days; or 0.132 mg/kg/day IM; or 2.5 mg rectally one to three times a day, not to exceed 10 mg/day on first day or 20 mg/day on subsequent days.

PIPERAZINE PHENOTHIAZINE: TRIFLUOPERAZINE

PRODUCTS (TRADE NAME):

Stelazine (Available in 1, 2, 5, and 10 mg tablets; 10 mg/ml concentrate; and 2 mg/ml injection.) **Suprazine** (Available in 1, 2, 5 and 10 mg tablets.) **Trifluoperazine** (Available in 1, 2, 5, and 10 mg tablets, and 10 mg/ml concentrate.)

DRUG SPECIFICS:

Used for the management of psychotic disorders. Also used in the relief of anxiety, tension and agitation and listed by the FDA as "possibly effective" in these conditions. Give individual dose, increasing as needed until symptoms are relieved. Then titrate dosage to lowest possible dose based on individual response. Oral concentrate must be diluted, usually with milk, tomato or fruit juice, carbonated beverages, coffee, tea or water. It may also be mixed with puddings, soups, and other semi-solid foods. Give elderly patients small doses in order to avoid neuromuscular reactions and hypotension.

ADMINISTRATION AND DOSAGE SPECIFICS:

Adults: 1 to 5 mg po twice a day, up to 40 mg/day; or may give 1 to 2 mg IM every four to six hours, up to 10 mg/day.

Children over 6 years: 1 mg po one to two times a day; or may give 1 mg IM one to two times a day.

PIPERIDINE PHENOTHIAZINE: MESORIDAZINE

PRODUCTS (TRADE NAME):

Serentil (Available in 10, 25, 50 and 100 mg tablets; 25 mg/ml concentrate; and 25 mg/ml injection.)

DRUG SPECIFICS:

Used in the treatment of severe emotional withdrawal, anxiety, tension, hallucinatory behavior, and blunted affect in schizophrenic patients. Reduces hyperactivity and uncooperativeness in some patients with chronic brain syndrome and mental deficiencies. Also used to reduce symptoms present in alcoholism and psychoneurotic manifestations.

ADMINISTRATION AND DOSAGE SPECIFICS:

Adults and children over 12 years: 10 to 50 mg po two to three times a day, up to 400 mg/day; or 25 mg IM repeated in one half to one hour if necessary, up to 200 mg/day.

Alcoholism: 25 mg po twice daily initially. Maintenance dose is 50 to 200 mg/day.

Behavioral problems in chronic brain syndrome and mental deficiencies: 25 mg po three times daily initially. Maintenance is 75 to 300 mg/day.

Schizophrenia: 50 mg po three times daily. Maintenance dose is 100 to 400 mg/day.

PIPERIDINE PHENOTHIAZINE: PIPERACETAZINE

PRODUCTS (TRADE NAME):

Quide (Available in 10 and 25 mg tablets.)

DRUG SPECIFICS:

Used in the management of psychiatric disorders. Generally, it is a moderately priced drug. If side effects occur, reduce dosage or discontinue drug.

ADMINISTRATION AND DOSAGE SPECIFICS:

Adults and children over 12 years: 10 mg po two to four times a day, up to 160 mg/day within a 3 to 5 day period. Maintenance may be 160 mg/day in divided doses.

PIPERIDINE PHENOTHIAZINE: THIORIDAZINE HYDROCHLORIDE

PRODUCTS (TRADE NAME):

Mellaril, Millazine (Available in 10, 15, 25, 50, 100, 150 and 200 mg tablets; 30 and 100 mg/ml concentrate.) **Mellaril-S** (Available in 25 and 100 mg/5 ml suspensions.)

DRUG SPECIFICS:

Used for the treatment of psychotic disorders, and as adjunct to short-term therapy in moderate to marked depression and anxiety. Especially useful in geriatric patients with anxiety, agitation, tension, sleep disturbances, and mood depression or fear. May be used in hyperactive children or children with marked behavioral problems. Higher dosages should be reserved for hospitalized patients. After control is achieved, reduce dosage as soon as possible.

ADMINISTRATION AND DOSAGE SPECIFICS:

Adults: 25 to 100 mg po three times a day initially, then 10 to 200 mg po two to four times a day as maintenance. Do not exceed 800 mg/day.

Children over 2 years: 0.25 mg to 3 mg/kg po or 10 to 25 mg po two to three times a day.

Marsha Goodwin

ANTIPSYCHOTIC AGENTS— THIOXANTHENE DERIVATIVES

The thioxanthene derivatives are similar to phenothiazines, chemically and pharmacologically, and can be used interchangeably. (See Phenothiazines-general.) The thioxanthene derivative chlorprothixene is comparable to the aliphatic phenothiazines and thiothixene is comparable to the piperazine phenothiazines. (There is no drug in the thioxanthene group that is comparable to the piperidine phenothiazines.)

The only possible advantage to using a thioxanthene derivative instead of a comparable phenothiazine is with a psychotic patient who is withdrawn or exhibiting retarded behavior. Clinical evidence has shown that patients with certain types of apathetic psychosis have benefited from thioxanthene therapy.

CHLORPROTHIXENE

PRODUCTS (TRADE NAME):

Taractan (Available in 10, 25, 50 and 100 mg tablets; 20 mg/ml concentrate; and 12.5 mg/ml injection).

DRUG SPECIFICS:

The most prominent adverse effects of this drug are sedation, orthostatic hypotension, dry mouth, blurred vision, and urinary retention. Therefore, it is most important to monitor the patient's blood pressure in lying, sitting and standing positions and instruct the patient to change positions slowly, avoid driving and other activities requiring alertness. Health provider should be contacted if urinary retention occurs.

ADMINISTRATION AND DOSAGE SPECIFICS:

Adults: 25 to 50 mg po three to four times a day, up to 600 mg/day; or 25 to 50 mg IM three to four times a day.

Children over 12 years: 10 mg to 25 mg po three to four times a day.

Children 6 to 12 years: 25 to 50 mg IM three to four times a day.

THIOTHIXENE

PRODUCTS (TRADE NAME):

Navane (Available in 1, 2, 5, 10 and 20 mg capsules; 5 mg/ml concentrate; and 2 and 5 mg/ml injection).

DRUG SPECIFICS:

The most prominent adverse effects of this drug are drowsiness and extrapyramidal symptoms. Therefore it is important to monitor the patient for early signs of tardive dyskinesia and jerky movements, particularly of the hands. Patient should not drive or perform activities requiring alertness if drowsiness occurs. Contact health practitioner if fine, involuntary movement of the tongue occurs.

ADMINISTRATION AND DOSAGE SPECIFICS:

Adults and children over 12 years: 2 to 5 mg po two or three times a day initially. Maintenance dose is 20 to 60 mg a day in divided doses. 4 mg IM two to four times a day may also be given.

Marsha Goodwin

SEDATIVE HYPNOTICS— BARBITURATES

ACTION OF THE DRUG: (1) Barbiturates are central nervous system depressants. They act primarily on the brainstem reticular formation, reducing nerve impulses to the cerebral cortex. (2) Barbiturates also depress the respiratory system, the activity of nerves, muscle (smooth, skeletal and cardiac), and (3) they can also raise the seizure threshold. (4) They are hepatic microsomal enzyme inducers.

PLAN:

INDICATIONS: Barbiturates are used for short-term treatment of anxiety, agitation and insomnia due to transient psychosocial stresses, and at times when rest is mandatory, such as before surgery. High doses of the short-acting barbiturates can produce surgical anesthesia. Long-acting barbiturates are used to treat some forms of hyperbilirubinemia, and as anticonvulsants to control and prevent grand mal seizures. They are sometimes used to treat convulsions due to status epilepticus, tetanus, fever or drugs.

SUBJECTIVE: There may be non-specific complaints of anxiety or stress affecting any organ system, difficulty concentrating, fatigue, insomnia (difficulty falling or staying asleep), or a history of a specific causative factor; discomfort of minor physical conditions or intense emotional stress as with grief, mourning or anticipation. There may also be a history of seizure disorder.

OBJECTIVE: There may be signs of restlessness, tremor, fatigue, tearfulness, tachycardia, tachypnea, or there may be no objective signs. In patients with seizure disorders, abnormal EEG may be documented.

PLAN:

CONTRAINDICATIONS: Do not use in acute intermittent porphyria, suspected sleep apnea, previously addicted individuals, hypersensitivity, or marked impairment of hepatic function. Pulmonary insufficiency is a relative contraindication.

WARNINGS: A use period of greater than one week may result in further disturbances in the sleep cycle with rebound insomnia. Dependence can develop with indiscriminate use, and abrupt withdrawal is dangerous. Hypothermia may occur. If administered to a patient in pain, barbiturates may worsen it. Safety in pregnancy has not been established. Administration to steroid-dependent asthmatics may worsen asthma. Cross-tolerance exists between the barbiturates and there is a synergistic effect if they are taken with alcohol. Barbiturates induce hepatic microsomal enzymes, and therefore affect the activity of many hepatically metabolized drugs. They must be used with caution in patients with impaired cardiac, respiratory, hepatic or renal function.

PRECAUTIONS: Lower than recommended doses should be used for geriatric or debilitated patients. Careful monitoring is necessary when a patient on anticoagulants stops taking barbiturates, as serious bleeding may occur. Always discontinue the drug slowly in people who have been on long-term therapy.

IMPLEMENTATION:

DRUG INTERACTIONS: Because barbiturates cause hepatic microsomal enzyme induction, they increase the metabolism, and thus reduce the activity of anticoagulants, corticosteroids and digitalis preparations. They can decrease the oral absorption of griseofulvin. Monoamine oxidase inhibitors (isocarboxazid, phenelzine, tranylcypromine) may potentiate the depressant effects of the barbiturates. There may be significant additive effects if barbiturates are used concomitantly with alcohol, antihistamines, benzodiazepines, methotrimeprazine, narcotics and tranquilizers. Drugs that enhance the sedative-hypnotic action of the barbiturates are griseofulvin, muscle relaxants, narcotics, Rauwolfia alkaloids and tranquilizers.

ADMINISTRATION AND DOSAGE: All barbiturates exhibit the same sedative-hypnotic efficacy but they differ in onset time, duration and potency. The onset and duration are determined by the lipid solubility of the particular drug. In determining dosage, it is best to begin with the lowest possible effective dose and adjust upward according to individual patient response. The amount prescribed should be no greater than that needed for current treatment and less than a potentially lethal dose.

Table 4-14 compares the usual adult dose for sedation, hypnosis, the time for onset of action, and the duration of action for the different barbiturates.

IMPLEMENTATION CONSIDERATIONS:

—Obtain a thorough health history: medications which may produce drug interactions, other barbiturates (sometimes present in bronchodilators or antispasmodics), response to barbiturates taken in the past, hypersensitivity, pregnancy.

—Determine if there is any cardiac, respiratory, hepatic or renal disease.

—Elderly or debilitated patients may be more sensitive to barbiturates and should be started on lower doses. These groups are more prone to the side effects of hangover, confusion and delirium.

—The amount of sleep needed varies among individuals. Variations in sleep patterns are not a problem unless they impair a person's health or functioning.

—The normal aging process is associated with a reduction in stage 3 and stage 4 sleep and more frequent awakenings.

—Many of the symptoms typical of insomnia and anxiety are also characteristic of hyperthyroidism which should be ruled out.

—Sleep disturbances and somatic symptoms are also present in patients with depression which is better treated with other agents.

—Tolerance is usually proportional to the total amount of drug received.

—Barbiturates are controlled substances. Attempts should be made to avoid giving them to patients with a history of abuse or addiction.

—Barbiturates should not be administered to patients in pain.

—When parenterally administering barbiturates, use great caution to avoid intra-arterial injection or extravasation, as serious ischemia or gangrene could result.

—The therapeutic efficacy of an anticonvulsant dosage regimen takes several weeks before it can be assessed.

WHAT THE PATIENT NEEDS TO KNOW:

—Unless used to treat seizure disorders barbiturates are only for short-term use. There is sometimes a problem with tolerance, dependence and addiction with this medication.

—Medication should be taken exactly as prescribed. Do not keep it on the bedside table where it would be possible to accidently retake it. Flush medication down toilet when it is no longer needed. Do not share your medication with anyone.

TABLE 4-14. COMPARATIVE ACTION OF BARBITURATES

Generic Drug	Time for Onset of Action	Duration	Sedative Dose	Hypnotic Dose
Long-Acting:				
Phenobarbital	One hour	10-16 hours	30-120 mg po divided into 2-3 doses daily	50-320 mg po
Phenobarbital Sodium			30-120 mg divided into 2-3 rectal or parenteral doses	100-320 mg rectally or parenterally
Mephobarbital			32-200 mg po divided into 3-4 doses	100-200 mg po
Intermediate-Acting:				
Amobarbital	One hour	4-6 hours	50-300 mg po divided into 2-3 doses	65-200 mg po
Amobarbital Sodium	30-60 min.	8-10 hours	50-300 mg po or parenterally daily in divided doses	65-200 mg po or parenterally
Aprobarbital	20 min.	4-6 hours	120-160 mg po daily in divided doses	40-160 mg po
Butabarbital Sodium	30 min.	6-8 hours	40-120 mg po daily in divided doses	50-100 mg po
Talbutal	20 min.	4-6 hours	30-180 mg po daily in divided doses	120 mg po
Short-Acting				
Secobarbital	15-30 min.	3-6 hours	30-90 mg po in 2-3 divided doses daily	100 mg po
Secobarbital Sodium			90-200 mg po in divided doses 120-200 mg rectally	100 mg po; 120-200 mg rectally; 50-250 mg parenterally
Pentobarbital			90-120 mg po in divided doses	100 mg po
Pentobarbital Sodium			90-120 mg in divided doses po, or rectally	100 mg po, rectal; parenteral dose 150-200 mg IM
Hexobarbital	5-10 min.	3-4 hours	250-750 mg po in 2 divided doses	250-500 mg po

—Keep medication out of reach of children and all others for whom drug is not prescribed.

—Barbiturates frequently cause drowsiness and you must be cautious when driving, using hazardous machinery, or performing tasks which require alertness.

—Some barbiturates also produce daytime sedation which may interfere with home and child care responsibilities requiring alertness.

—Notify your health care practitioner immediately if you experience any rash, fever, unusual bleeding, bruising, sore throat, jaundice or abdominal pain. Some people experience side effects while taking this drug, so notify your provider of any new or uncomfortable symptoms.

—You may have excessive dreaming when drug is stopped. This should lessen each night.

—Tablets and capsules should be kept in a dry, tightly closed container.

—Elixirs should be kept in a tightly closed brown glass bottle.

—If you are taking blood thinners, stopping your barbiturate suddenly can cause problems with your blood clotting.

—If you are using this drug primarily to relax and go to sleep, investigate other alternative methods of relaxation to help reduce the need for medication.

EVALUATION:

ADVERSE REACTIONS: *CNS:* exacerbation of symptoms of certain organic brain disorders in elderly patients, dizziness, drowsiness, hangover, headache, lethargy, paradoxical restlessnness or excitement, unsteadiness. *Dermatologic:* photosensitivity, rash. *Gastrointestinal:* diarrhea, nausea, hepatitis with jaundice, vomiting. *Hematopoietic:* anemia, decreased platelets, unusual bleeding or bruising. *Hypersensitivity:* angioneurotic edema, asthma, Stevens-Johnson syndrome, urticaria. *Musculoskeletal:* joint and muscle pains, most often in the neck, shoulders and arms. *Other:* hypothermia, tolerance, withdrawal symptoms upon discontinuance.

OVERDOSAGE: *Signs and symptoms:* With acute overdose the patient may evidence exaggerated CNS depression, decreased respiration, constricted pupils, tachycardia, areflexia, shock or coma. Death may occur secondary to cardiorespiratory failure. *Treatment:* In conscious patients, vomiting should be induced with syrup of Ipecac. If unconscious, refer for gastric lavage and use of activated charcoal once airway is secured. Supportive therapy is indicated. Signs of chronic intoxication: ataxia, euphoria, withdrawal (increased frequency and intensity of dreaming, grand mal seizures twelve hours to twelve days after drug is stopped, anxiety, fear, panic, tremor, anorexia, vomiting, sweating, hyperreflexia, delirium and craving drug.) *Treatment:* hospitalization is necessary. Slow withdrawal, phenobarbital or phenytoin is sometimes used.

PARAMETERS TO MONITOR: Evaluate therapeutic effects and whether the degree of sedation is compatible with the patient's life style. Monitor how patient takes medications: amount, times, etc. Look for patterns of abuse. Observe for signs of intoxication, paradoxical reactions, tolerance, dependence, withdrawal and toxicity (jaundice, rash, sore throat, etc..) Complete blood counts and liver function tests should be done as a baseline, and repeated for patients on long-term barbiturate therapy. Also observe for porphyria, which is characterized by abdominal pain. When using these drugs for their anticonvulsant properties serum levels should be monitored.

AMOBARBITAL AND AMOBARBITAL SODIUM

PRODUCTS (TRADE NAME):
   Amobarbital Sodium (Available in 65 and 200 mg capsules and 15 and 30 mg powder for injection.) **Amytal** (Available in 15, 30, 50 and 100 mg tablets; 44 mg/5 ml elixir.) **Amytal Sodium** (Available in 65 mg and 200 mg capsules, 125, 250, and 500 mg powder for injection.)
DRUG SPECIFICS:
   This barbiturate has an intermediate duration of action about four to six hours. Onset of action occurs about one hour after oral hypnotic dose. Amobarbital sodium lasts slightly longer. For IV injection, do not exceed 1 ml/minute. For IM administration, inject slowly and deeply into a large muscle mass, not more than 5 ml at one site. Maximum IM dose is 0.5 gm. This drug is a Schedule II controlled substance. The elixir is 34% alcohol. It should be kept in an amber-colored glass bottle.
ADMINISTRATION AND DOSAGE SPECIFICS:
   Sedative:
   Adults: 50-300 mg daily po in two to three divided doses. 30-50 mg 2-3 times a day IM or IV.
   Children: 6 mg/kg po in three divided doses daily.
   Hypnotic:
   Adults: 65-200 mg po; 65-500 mg IV; 65–100 mg IM.
   Children six to twelve years old: 3-5 mg/kg po and IM, 65-500 mg IV.
   Anticonvulsant:
   Adults: 65-500 mg IV.
   Children older than 6 years: 65-500 mg per dose.
   Children 6 years and younger: 3-5 mg/kg IM or IV.

APROBARBITAL

PRODUCTS (TRADE NAME):
   Alurate (Available in 40 mg/5 ml elixir.)
DRUG SPECIFICS:
   Aprobarbital is an intermediate-acting Schedule III barbiturate. It is used for

sedation or treatment of mild or pronounced insomnia. Onset of action is approximately twenty minutes and it lasts four to six hours.

ADMINISTRATION AND DOSAGE SPECIFICS:

Sedative:
Adults: 40 mg po three times a day.
Hypnotic:
Adults: 40-160 mg po before bed.

BUTABARBITAL SODIUM

PRODUCTS (TRADE NAME):
Buticaps (Available in 15 mg and 30 mg capsules.) **Butabarbital Sodium, Butisol Sodium** (Available in 15 mg, 30 mg, 50 mg, 100 mg tablets; 30 mg/5 ml elixir.) **Sarisol No. 2** (Available in 30 mg tablets.)

DRUG SPECIFICS:
Butabarbital sodium is an intermediate-acting Schedule III barbiturate. It is used for sedation, mild anxiety and for insomnia when daytime sedation is also desirable. It is effective for no more than fourteen days. Its onset of action is thirty minutes and the duration is six to eight hours.

ADMINISTRATION AND DOSAGE SPECIFICS:

Sedative:
Adults: 45-120 mg po divided in three to four doses.
Children: 6 mg/kg po divided in three daily doses.
Hypnotic:
Adults: 50-100 mg po before bed.

MEPHOBARBITAL

PRODUCTS (TRADE NAME):
Mebaral (Available in 32, 50, 100 and 200 mg tablets.)

DRUG SPECIFICS:
Mephobarbital is a long-acting barbiturate which is converted to phenobarbital by hepatic microsomal enzymes. It is used as an anticonvulsant as well as a sedative. It is a weak hypnotic.

ADMINISTRATION AND DOSAGE SPECIFICS:

Sedative:
Adults: 32-100 mg po three times per day.
Children: 16-32 mg po three to four times per day.
Anticonvulsant:
Adults: 400 to 600 mg po daily.

Children over five: 32-64 mg three to four times po daily.
*Children under five:*16-32 mg three to four times po daily.

METHARBITAL

PRODUCTS (TRADE NAME):
Gemonil (Available in 100 mg scored tablets.)
DRUG SPECIFICS:
Metharbital is a long-acting barbiturate used to control grand mal, petit mal, myoclonic and mixed types of seizures. It is important to individualize dosage for optimal control. May be used alone or in conjunction with other antiepileptics.
ADMINISTRATION AND DOSAGE SPECIFICS:
Anticonvulsant: Adult: 100 mg po one to three times daily.
Children: 50 mg po one to three times daily. (Up to 5-15 mg/kg/day.)

PENTOBARBITAL AND PENTOBARBITAL SODIUM

PRODUCTS (TRADE NAME):
Nembutal (Available as 18.2 mg/5 ml elixir, equivalent to 20 mg pentobarbital sodium.) **Nembutal Sodium** (Available in 30, 50, 100 mg capsules; in 30, 60, 120, and 200 mg suppositories; 50 mg/ml injection.) **Pentobarbital Sodium** (Available in 50, 100 mg capsules; 50 mg/ml injection.)
DRUG SPECIFICS:
Pentobarbital is an effective, short-acting drug which is given orally. Pentobarbital sodium comes in po, parenteral or rectal forms. In order to avoid irritation when administering IM, no more than 250 mg (5 ml) should be injected at any one site. Inject into large muscle mass (upper quadrant of gluteus maximus.) This is a Schedule II controlled substance.
ADMINISTRATION AND DOSAGE SPECIFICS:
Sedative:
Adults: 30 mg po or rectally three or four times daily; 150 to 200 mg IM two to four times a day.
Children: 60 mg/kg po daily in three divided doses; 6 mg/kg daily in three divided doses, rectally. 2-4 mg/kg IM (up to 100 mg per dose.)
Hypnotic:
Adults: 100 mg po; 120-200 mg rectally, 150-200 mg IM; 100 mg initially IV, with small incremental doses to a total of 500 mg given slowly until the desired effect is obtained.

Anticonvulsant:
Adults: 100 mg IV initially; after one minute additional 1 small dose may be administered per minute up to a total of 500 mg.
Children: 3-5 mg/kg IM or IV.

PHENOBARBITAL AND PHENOBARBITAL SODIUM

PRODUCTS (TRADE NAME):

Barbita (Available in 16 mg tablet.) **Luminal Ovoids** (Available in 16, 32 mg tablets.) **Luminal Sodium** (Available in 130 mg/ml in 1 ml ampules.) **PBR/12 Capsules** (Available as 65 mg timed-release capsule.) **Phenobarbital** (Available as 8,16, 32, 65, 100 mg tablets; 15 mg/5 ml liquid, and 20 mg/5 ml Elixir.) **Phenobarbital Sodium** (Available in 30, 60, 130 mg/ml Tubex; and powder for injection.) **Sedadrops** (Available as 16 mg/ml drops.) **SK-Phenobarbital** (Available as 15, 30 mg tablets.) **Solfoton** (Available as 16 mg tablet or capsule.)

DRUG SPECIFICS:

IM and IV routes are usually used only when oral administration is impossible or impractical. Administer IM injection slowly and deeply into large muscle mass. Patient must be observed carefully during IV injection. Rate must not exceed 60-100 mg/minute.

ADMINISTRATION AND DOSAGE SPECIFICS:

Sedative:
Adults: 30-120 mg in 2-3 divided doses po, rectally, IM or IV.
Children: 6 mg/kg parenterally in three divided doses.*Hypnotic: Adult:* 100-320 mg parenterally, 100 mg rectally or 100-200 mg po.
Anticonvulsant:
Adults: 50-100 mg po two to three times daily, 200-300 mg rectally, 30-20 mg IM or IV.
Children: 3-5 mg/kg po, rectally, IM or IV.

PRIMIDONE

PRODUCTS (TRADE NAME):

Myidone (Available in 250 mg tablets.) **Mysoline** (Available in 50 mg and 250 mg tablets and in 250 mg/5 ml oral suspension.) **Primidone** (Available in 250 mg tablets.) **Primoline** (Available in 250 mg tablets.)

DRUG SPECIFICS:

Phenobarbital is a metabolite of primidone. These drugs may be used alone or in conjunction with other anticonvulsants to control grand mal, psychomotor and focal seizures. Dosage should be individualized and increased gradually.

ADMINISTRATION AND DOSAGE SPECIFICS:

Anticonvulsant:

Adults and children over 8 years: 250 mg once a day initially, increased by an additional 250 mg at one-week intervals until seizures are controlled, or total daily dose reaches 2 grams. Maintenance dose is 250-500 mg three times a day.

Children under 8 years: 125 mg once a day initially, increased by 125 mg at one-week intervals until control is obtained or daily dose reaches 1 gram.

SECOBARBITAL AND SECOBARBITAL SODIUM

PRODUCTS (TRADE NAME):

Seconal (Available in 22 mg/5 ml elixir.) **Seconal Sodium and Secobarbital Sodium** (Available in 50 and 100 mg capsules; 100 mg tablets; 30, 60, 120 and 200 mg suppositories; and 50 mg/ml for injection.)

DRUG SPECIFICS:

Secobarbital is a short-acting barbiturate that is administered orally, rectally or by deep IM injection. It may also be administered IV for control of convulsions in emergency situations, but IV rate should not exceed 50 mg/15 seconds and should be discontinued as soon as desired effect is obtained. Onset of action is fifteen to thirty minutes and duration is approximately three to six hours. This is a Schedule II controlled substance.

ADMINISTRATION AND DOSAGE SPECIFICS:

Sedation:

Adults: 30-50 mg po three to four times a day; may use up to 100 mg po at bedtime; 120-200 mg suppository; 50 mg/15 sec for IV use and discontinue when desired state of sedation is reached.

Children: 1.1-2.2 mg/kg IM; or 6 mg/kg/day po or rectally divided in 3 equal doses.

Hypnosis:

Adults: 100 mg po; 120-200 mg rectally; 100-200 mg IM. 50-250 mg IV.

Children: 3-5mg/kg IM (100 mg maximum.)

Anticonvulsant:

Adults: 5.5 mg/kg IM or IV repeated every 3-4 hours as needed.

Children: 3-5 mg/kg.

TALBUTAL

PRODUCTS (TRADE NAME):

Lotusate Caplets (Available in 120 mg tablets.)

DRUG SPECIFICS:

Talbutal is an intermediate-acting, Schedule III barbiturate. Onset of action is twenty minutes and duration of action is four to six hours.

ADMINISTRATION AND DOSAGE SPECIFICS:

Sedatives:
Adults: 30-60 mg po two to three times daily.
Hypnotic:
Adults: 120 mg po before bed.

Candis Morrison

SEDATIVE-HYPNOTICS— BENZODIAZEPINES

ACTION OF THE DRUG: The main action of these drugs is central nervous system depression, and although the exact mechanism is not known, they are thought to act on the hypothalamus and limbic system of the brain, decreasing the pressor response and increasing the arousal threshold.

ASSESSMENT:

INDICATIONS: These benzodiazepine compounds are used as hypnotic agents for treatment of insomnia characterized by difficulty falling, or staying asleep and/or early morning awakenings. The therapeutic objective is to prevent insomnia and restore normal sleep patterns. Used in patients with acute or chronic medical problems requiring restful sleep.

SUBJECTIVE: There may be complaints of restlessness, difficulty concentrating, anxiety, fatigue, insomnia (difficulty falling or staying asleep, or early morning awakening.) There may be a specific causative factor such as intense emotional reactions (grief, temporary stress or sleep schedule changes).

OBJECTIVE: There may be no objective signs, or such non-specific signs as restlessness, tremor, tearfulness, tachycardia or tachypnea.

PLAN:

CONTRAINDICATIONS: Do not use in cases of known hypersensitivity to a benzodiazepine, pregnancy, or children less than fifteen years of age.

WARNINGS: Some of the benzodiazepines are transformed by the liver into long-acting forms which may remain in the body for twenty-four hours or more and produce increasing sedation. Liver function may be impaired with prolonged use. Additive effects may occur if alcohol is consumed the day following administration. Ability to perform tasks requiring alertness may be impaired. There is an increased risk of congenital malformations and neonatal depression if used during pregnancy. Combined effects are possible if used with other CNS depressants. Elderly or debilitated patients are more sensitive to the drug. Dependence and withdrawal symptoms may occur if used for extended periods.

PRECAUTIONS: Use with caution in patients with impaired renal or hepatic function and in those with chronic obstructive pulmonary disease, and in those who may be addiction-prone. Avoid rapid withdrawal following prolonged administration.

IMPLEMENTATION:

DRUG INTERACTIONS: Alcohol, other sedatives and hypotics, antidepressants, anticonvulsants and narcotics may produce additive sedative effects if used concomitantly. Benzodiazepines may alter the effects of anticonvulsants. May alter laboratory tests in the following manner: increased SGOT, SGPT, alkaline phosphatase, total and indirect bilirubins.

ADMINISTRATION AND DOSAGE: Individualize dose for maximum benefit. Onset of action is approximately thirty to sixty minutes. Effects last seven to eight hours. Drug should be administered fifteen to thirty minutes before bedtime. Elderly or debilitated persons should receive no more than 15 mg.

IMPLEMENTATION CONSIDERATIONS:

—Take a thorough health history: other drugs which may produce drug interactions or additive sedative effects, pregnancy, or hypersensitivity.

—Assess the patient's renal, hepatic and pulmonary status.

—Alcohol can increase the sedation produced by these drugs and depress vital brain functions.

—Flurazepam is increasingly effective on the second or third night of consecutive use. For one to two nights after drug is discontinued, both time before patient falls asleep and total wake time may still be decreased.

—Use with caution in women in whom there is any chance of pregnancy.

—Avoid rapid withdrawal of drug following long-term therapy.

—These are Schedule IV controlled substances.

WHAT THE PATIENT NEEDS TO KNOW:

—Take medication only as prescribed.

—Continuous use of this drug is to be avoided.

—Keep medication away from children and individuals for whom drug is not prescribed.

—A hangover feeling may sometimes be experienced the day after taking the medication. Any driving or activities requiring alertness should be avoided until all drowsiness has disappeared.

—It is dangerous to drink alcohol within twenty-four hours after taking this drug. Do not take the medication if you are planning to drink.

—Smoking may decrease the length of time the drug helps you sleep.

—Avoid drinking caffeine for at least four hours before taking the medication as it decreases the ability of the drug to produce sleep.

EVALUATION:

ADVERSE REACTIONS: *Cardiovascular:* chest pains, hypotension, palpitations, shortness of breath. *CNS:* apprehension, ataxia, difficulty focusing or blurred vision, confusion, drowsiness, euphoria, falling, flushing, hallucinations, headaches, irritability, lethargy, lightheadedness, paradoxical reactions (excitement, stimulation, hyperactivity), restlessness, severe sedation, slurred speech, staggering, sweating, talkativeness, unsteadiness. *Gastrointestinal:* anorexia, bitter taste, dry mouth, diarrhea, heartburn, increased salivation, nausea, pain, vomiting. *Hematopoietic:* granulocytopenia, leukopenia. *Hypersensitivity:* pruritus, rash. *Musculoskeletal:* joint pains, weakness. *Other:* burning eyes, tolerance.

OVERDOSAGE: *Signs and symptoms:* Marked drowsiness, weakness, somnolence, impairment of stance and gait, confusion and coma may occur. *Treatment:* Immediately remove gastric contents through induction of vomiting or refer for gastric lavage. Institute supportive measures, including maintenance of airway and adequate ventilation. Monitor respiration, pulse and blood pressure.

PARAMETERS TO MONITOR: Observe therapeutic effect. Periodic complete blood counts are recommended. For any long-term use, SGOT, SGPT, alkaline phosphatase, BUN, creatinine and bilirubin tests are advisable, keeping in mind that the drug alters these laboratory values. Monitor how patient is taking medication and observe for any signs of overdosage or withdrawal.

FLURAZEPAM HCL

PRODUCTS (TRADE NAME):
   Dalmane (Available in 15 and 30 mg capsules).
DRUG SPECIFICS:
   Flurazepam has a longer use period (effective for twenty-eight consecutive nights) and less REM rebound than some other hypnotics. It does markedly suppress stage 4 and increase stage 2 sleep.
ADMINISTRATION AND DOSAGE SPECIFICS:
   Hypnotic: Give 15 or 30 mg po; in elderly or debilitated patients, 15 mg.

LORAZEPAM

PRODUCTS (TRADE NAME):
   Ativan (Available in 0.5, 1 and 2 mg tablets, and 2 and 4 mg/ml injection.)
DRUG SPECIFICS:
   This is an antianxiety agent used usually for mild or transient situational stress. Parenterally it is used as preanesthetic medication. It may be used concomitantly

with other narcotic analgesics, anesthetics, muscle relaxants, and atropine sulfate. Wean patient off medication slowly after long-term use.

ADMINISTRATION AND DOSAGE SPECIFICS:

Mild anxiety or insomnia: 2 to 4 mg po at bedtime.

Elderly or debilitated patients: 1 to 2 mg/day in divided doses.

Preanesthesia medications: O.05 mg/kg (maximum dose 4 mg) IM at least 2 hours before operative procedure.

Sedation: 2 mg total or O.02 mg/lb IV for adult patients under 50 years.

TEMAZEPAM

PRODUCTS (TRADE NAME):

Restoril (Available in 15 and 30 mg capsules).

DRUG SPECIFICS:

Induces sleep in twenty to forty minutes. Individualize dosage for maximum benefit.

ADMINISTRATION AND DOSAGE SPECIFICS:

Hypnotic:

Adults: 30 mg po before bedtime. In elderly or debilitated patients, 15 mg may be sufficient.

TRIAZOLAM

PRODUCTS (TRADE NAME):

Halcion (Available in 0.25 and 0.5 mg tablets.)

DRUG SPECIFICS:

Used primarily for short-term treatment of insomnia or early morning awakenings. Contraindicated in pregnancy so patient must be warned of potential risk to fetus if contemplating pregnancy. Do not prescribe more than a one month supply of medication. Elderly or debilitated patients should be given reduced doses to reduce chance of oversedation. Watch for suicidal tendencies, as symptoms of depression may be intensified by hypnotic drugs. This drug may cause dependency, and withdrawal symptoms may be observed after long-term use. Do not stop drug abruptly. Monitor patients on long-term therapy through periodic blood counts, blood chemistry analysis and urinalysis. Some nonspecific EEG changes may be detected. Additive effects maybe seen when administered with alcohol, antihistaminics, anticonvulsants, other CNS depressant or psychotropic drugs. Nausea, vomiting, drowsiness, headache, dizziness, nervousness and lightheadedness along with ataxia and coordination disorders may be noted. Mood alteration, visual disturbances and tachycardia have also been seen less commonly. Initiate therapy at lowest dosage levels and individualize therapy depending upon patient response.

ADMINISTRATION AND DOSAGE SPECIFICS:

Adults: 0.25 to 0.5 mg at bedtime is usual dose.
Geriatric or debilitated patients: 0.125 to 0.25 mg.

Candis Morrison

SEDATIVE-HYPNOTICS— CARBAMATES

ETHINAMATE

ACTION OF THE DRUG: Carbamates are non-barbiturate central nervous system depressants. Though the exact site and mechanism of action are yet unknown, it is thought to be similar to the barbiturates which act on the reticular activating system to reduce impulses to the cerebral cortex.

ASSESSMENT:

INDICATIONS: Ethinamate is useful for short periods (not proven effective for more than seven days) as a short-acting hypnotic. It is used when deep hypnosis is not needed.

SUBJECTIVE: There may be non-specific complaints of anxiety or stress, and any organ system may be affected. Complaints of difficulty concentrating, fatigue and insomnia are common. There may be a history of a specific causative factor; discomfort of minor physical conditions; or intense emotional stress as with grief or mourning.

OBJECTIVE: There may be no objective signs or non-specific signs such as restlessness, tremor, tearfulness, tachycardia and tachypnea.

PLAN:

CONTRAINDICATIONS: Do not use in the presence of hypersensitivity to the carbamates.

WARNINGS: Habituation and tolerance may occur. Withdrawal reactions in addicted persons may be associated with convulsions. There may be additive effects when drug is used with alcohol or other CNS depressants. Drug may impair mental alertness and ability to perform hazardous tasks. Safety in pregnancy has not been proven. Drug is not recommended for children under fifteen years of age.

PRECAUTIONS: Use with caution in addiction-prone persons or those whose reliance in following medication instructions cannot be guaranteed. Avoid use in depressed or potentially suicidal individuals. Limit repeat prescriptions. The lowest possible effective dose is recommended for elderly or debilitated patients. Use with caution in patients with hepatic impairment.

IMPLEMENTATION:

DRUG INTERACTIONS: There may be additive depressant effects if drug is taken concomitantly with alcohol, other sedatives, hypnotics, or any central nervous system depressants.

PRODUCTS (TRADE NAME):
Valmid Pulvules (Available in 500 mg capsules.)

ADMINISTRATION AND DOSAGE: Use of the lowest possible effective dose for the shortest period possible is the objective. The hypnotic dose induces sleep within fifteen to twenty minutes and lasts three to five hours.

Hypnosis: Usual adult dose is 500 mg -1 gm po twenty minutes before bedtime.

IMPLEMENTATION CONSIDERATIONS:

—Take a thorough health history: other medications which could interact with carbamate; pregnancy; presence of hypersensitivity.

—Carefully evaluate the patient's complaint of insomnia. This drug has a shorter duration of action than most other hypnotics; therefore, it would not be as helpful in patients complaining of early morning awakening.

—Due to the shorter duration of action, there is less chance of over-sedation and hangover than with other agents.

WHAT THE PATIENT NEEDS TO KNOW:
—This drug is usually only for short-term use.
—Take medication only as directed by health provider.
—Avoid alcohol or other sedatives while you are taking this medicine.
—Keep medication away from children or others for whom the medication is not prescribed.
—Do not drive or perform any tasks requiring alertness until all drowsiness has disappeared.
—This drug can be habit-forming if it is not taken as recommended.

EVALUATION:

ADVERSE REACTIONS: *CNS:* ataxia, confusion, dizziness, residual sedation. *Gastrointestinal:* epigastric burning. *Hematopoietic:* thrombocytopenia purpura. *Hypersensitivity:* fever, rash. *Other:* dependency, tolerance and withdrawal symptoms if there is long-term administration of high doses.

OVERDOSAGE: *Signs and symptoms:* The patient may show exaggerated CNS depression, depressed respiration and perhaps shock or coma. *Treatment:* In the conscious patient the drug should be removed from the stomach via induction of vomiting. If unconscious, refer for gastric lavage after an airway is secured. Dialysis can be effective. Give supportive care.

PARAMETERS TO MONITOR: Evaluate therapeutic effects of drug. Monitor how patient is using medication and the extent of sedation produced. After long-term use, monitor for signs of withdrawal: tremulousness, hyperactive reflexes, severe insomnia, agitation, syncope, confusion, disorientation, hallucination or seizures.

Candis Morrison

SEDATIVE HYPNOTICS— CHLORAL DERIVATIVES

ACTION OF THE DRUG: Chloral derivatives are central nervous system depressants, probably acting on the reticular activating system. They produce drowsiness and sleep within one hour.

ASSESSMENT:

INDICATIONS: Used as a sedative for periods of less than two weeks. Used as a hypnotic for short periods. Useful in the treatment of insomnia characterized by difficulty falling asleep and frequent nocturnal awakenings. Chloral derivatives are also used locally as antipruritics. Triclofos sodium is used as a pre-medication for obtaining sleep records in electroencephalograms. Chloral hydrate has been used for its analgesic and antispasmodic properties particularly postoperatively.

SUBJECTIVE: Restlessness, difficulty concentrating, anxiety, fatigue, insomnia (difficulty falling, or staying asleep, or early morning awakenings). May be associated with one or a combination of stresses including chronic diseases, planned surgery, aging, sleep schedule changes or a period of intense emotional involvement.

OBJECTIVE: There may be no objective signs, or such non-specific signs as restlessness, tremor, tearfulness, tachycardia or tachypnea.

PLAN:

CONTRAINDICATIONS: Do not use with marked impairment of renal or hepatic function, severe cardiac disease, allergy or sensitivity to chloral derivatives, women in labor or the neonate. Do not use the liquid forms in ulcer disease, gastritis or esophagitis.

WARNINGS: Chloral derivatives can impair mental alertness, coordination, judgment and reaction time. They can potentiate the effects of other CNS depressants, and when used with alcohol can cause sudden loss of consciousness. They cross the blood-brain and placental barriers, and small amounts are excreted in milk of nursing mothers. Long-term use is not recommended as they may be habit forming. Exercise caution in administering to patients known to be addiction prone. Both psychological and physiological dependence may develop with prolonged use.

Continued use of large doses causes peripheral vasodilation, hypotension, respiratory and myocardial depression, and possible renal damage.

PRECAUTIONS: Elderly and debilitated patients may be more sensitive to the effects of chloral derivatives; therefore, lower than recommended doses should be used until the response is determined. Lower doses should also be given to patients with hepatic or renal disease. Use with caution in patients with cardiac arrhythmias. Carefully monitor prothrombin times in patients taking oral anticoagulants concomitantly with chloral derivatives. Adjustment of the anticoagulant dose may be necessary. Caution should be exercised with use in patients known or thought to be addiction prone. Because of the habit-forming potential, avoid large doses and continuous use. Avoid or carefully monitor these drugs in pregnant and nursing mothers.

IMPLEMENTATION:

DRUG INTERACTIONS: The sedative effects of the chloral derivatives are enhanced by other sedatives, barbiturates, hypnotics, antianxiety drugs, antihistamines, narcotics, pain medications and phenothiazines. Alcohol consumed at or near the time a chloral derivative is taken may cause loss of consciousness, tachycardia, palpitations, facial flushing and dysphoria as a consequence of vasodilation. Chloral derivatives potentiate the action of oral anticoagulants and can cause hypoprothrombinemia. If intravenous furosemide (Lasix) is administered to a patient who has taken a chloral derivative within twenty-four hours, it produces diaphoresis, uneasiness and blood pressure changes.

Chloral derivatives are responsible for certain laboratory test interactions. They may increase serum SGPT, SGOT, bilirubin, urinary porphyrins and proteins and increase retention of BSP. They may cause false-positive increases in urinary catecholamines, corticosteroids, urea nitrogen, and uric acid; and may cause false-negatives in urine glucose. They may also cause a false positive Benedict's test for glycosuria. Mono amine oxidase inhibitor drugs may increase the effects of chloral derivatives and cause oversedation.

ADMINISTRATION AND DOSAGE: The period of effectiveness of the chloral derivatives is less than two weeks. Relief of symptoms with the lowest possible dose for the shortest period of time is the therapeutic objective. The onset and duration of action differ slightly between the three products in this category. Chloral Hydrate's effects begin in thirty to sixty minutes and last four to eight hours. Chloral Betaine's effects begin in thirty to sixty minutes but last six to eight hours. Triclofos produces effects in twenty to forty minutes and they last six to eight hours.

IMPLEMENTATION CONSIDERATIONS:

—Take a thorough health history: alcohol consumption patterns, drug history to determine that patient is not using any drugs which interact, and determine the possibility of pregnancy.

—Determine the status of the patient's renal, hepatic, cardiac and respiratory systems.

—Before prescribing, be certain that the patient is not scheduled to have any of the laboratory tests that chloral derivatives may distort.

—Chloral derivatives produce a false-positive Benedict's reagent test for glycosuria. In evaluating urine glucose levels this will need to be taken into account.

—These drugs are Schedule IV controlled substances.

—This group of sedative-hypnotic drugs has no, or minimal, effects on REM sleep.

—Many patients take higher dosages of hypnotics than they admit. Watch for nystagmus, incoordination, tremulousness and slurring of speech as signs of overdosage.

—Tolerance develops quickly to the hypnotic effect. Usage of these products should therefore be short-term.

WHAT THE PATIENT NEEDS TO KNOW:

—Take medications exactly as ordered.

—Never use this medicine at the same time as alcohol. Avoid drinking alcohol at least six full hours after taking a dose of medicine.

—This medication can cause drowsiness. Avoid performing hazardous work, or tasks requiring alertness until all drowsiness has disappeared.

—Take capsules with a full glass of liquid to decrease irritation to stomach.

—Syrup and elixirs should be taken in one-half glass of water, juice or milk.

—The effects of these drugs may be increased by other sedatives, hypnotics, antihistamines, narcotics and pain relievers. Inform your health provider of any drugs you plan to take while you are using this medication, as adjustments of dosage may be necessary.

—Keep drug in a tightly-closed container. Keep suppositories in refrigerator.

—Keep this medication away from children and all others for whom it was not prescribed.

EVALUATION:

ADVERSE REACTIONS: *CNS:* ataxia, confusion, delirium, disorientation, dizziness, excitement, hallucinations, hangover, headaches, incoherence, nightmares, paradoxical excitement, paranoid behavior, sleepwalking, vertigo. *Gastrointestinal:* abdominal pain, bad taste in mouth, diarrhea, flatulence, gastric irritation, heartburn, indigestion, nausea, vomiting. *Hematopoietic:* leukopenia, relative eosinophilia. *Hypersensitivity:* erythema, hives, skin rashes, urticaria. *Other:* ketonuria, malaise, psychological and physical dependence with long-term use, tolerance.

OVERDOSAGE: *Signs and symptoms:* The principal symptoms are gastric irritation and circulatory collapse. Coma, miosis, hypotension, respiratory depression, cardiac arrhythmias, hypothermia, pinpoint pupils, vomiting, areflexia or muscle flaccidity may be seen. Toxic oral dose is approximately 10 gm for adults. *Treatment:* Treatment is based on functional decomposition. In conscious patients, remove drug by induction of vomiting. Refer for gastric lavage if unconscious. Institute supportive measures as indicated. Maintain respiration, monitor cardiac functioning and maintain blood pressure with intravenous fluids.

PARAMETERS TO MONITOR: During prolonged use, complete blood counts are recommended, as well as urinalysis, blood urea nitrogen and creatinine to monitor renal function. Observe for signs and symptoms of tolerance, dependence, toxicity, gastric irritation, excessive central nervous system depression.

CHLORAL HYDRATE

PRODUCTS (TRADE NAME):
Aquachloral (Available in 325 and 650 mg suppositories.) **Chloral Hydrate** (Available in 250 and 500 mg capsules, 250 and 500 mg/5 ml syrup; 500 mg/5 ml elixir; 500 mg syppository.) **Noctec** (Available in 250 and 500 mg capsules, 500 mg/5 ml elixir.) **Oradrate, SK-Chloral Hydrate** (Available in 500 mg capsule.)

DRUG SPECIFICS:
Effects begin in thirty to sixty minutes and last for four to eight hours. Product has a disagreeable taste and causes gastric irritation. This may be minimized if capsules are taken after meals and elixir is taken in a glass of water, juice or soda.

ADMINISTRATION AND DOSAGE SPECIFICS:
Sedative:
Adults: 250 mg po three times a day after meals or rectally by suppositories 325-650 mg three times a day .
Children: 8.3 mg/kg po or rectally three times a day.
Hypnotic:
Adults: 500 mg to 1 gm po administered fifteen to thirty minutes before bedtime or rectally by suppositories 975 mg to 1.95 gm.
Children: 50 mg/kg. Maximum dose of 1 gm po or rectally.

TRICLOFOS SODIUM

PRODUCTS (TRADE NAME):
Triclos (Available in 750 mg coated tablets and 1.5 gm/15 ml liquid.)

DRUG SPECIFICS:
Triclofos has less of the disagreeable properties of chloral hydrate but is more expensive. Effective in twenty to forty minutes and lasts six to eight hours.

ADMINISTRATION AND DOSAGE SPECIFICS:
Hypnotic:
Adults: 1500 mg tablet or 15 ml liquid po fifteen to thirty minutes before bedtime.

Children less than 12 years: 0.1 ml/lb po. (Usually for sleep induction for electroencephalogram) 0.1 ml/lb po.

Candis Morrison

SEDATIVE HYPNOTICS—PARALDEHYDE

ACTION OF THE DRUG: Paraldehyde produces sedative and hypnotic effects similar to those of the barbiturates, by depressing the ascending reticular activating system. Sleep is induced in ten to fifteen minutes and lasts six to eight hours.

ASSESSMENT:

INDICATIONS: Paraldehyde is used in the treatment of delirium tremens, and other alcohol withdrawal symptoms. Occasionally used in the emergency treatment of convulsive disorders such as those arising from tetanus, status epilepticus, eclampsia, and toxicity of convulsive drugs. Paraldehyde has also been used to treat excitement in certain psychiatric disorders. It is preferred over barbiturates in elderly patients who have liver disease or who cannot tolerate the barbiturates.

SUBJECTIVE: Complaints may include: excitement, difficulty concentrating, anxiety, fatigue, worry, insomnia (difficulty falling asleep, staying asleep or early morning awakenings). Symptoms may be idiopathic, but are often associated with one or a combination of stresses including: drugs, alcohol, aging, sleep schedule changes, chronic diseases, or a period of intense emotional involvement.

OBJECTIVE: There may be non-specific signs such as restlessness, tremor, fatigue, tearfulness, tachycardia or tachypnea. Often no objective signs are evidenced.

PLAN:

CONTRAINDICATIONS: Lung congestion, gastrointestinal inflammation, or ulcer disease.

WARNINGS Chronic use can produce toxic hepatitis, metabolic acidosis, and nephrosis. In its oral form, the drug can be quite irritating to the throat and gastric mucosa. If administered parenterally, paraldehyde can cause necrosis and nerve injury (with intramuscular injection), or cyanosis, hypotension and cough (with undiluted intravenous injection). The drug has a low therapeutic index and decomposes on exposure to light and air. It reacts with plastic. The sedative effect can be intensified and prolonged in patients with severe liver damage. Paraldehyde may be psychologically and physically addicting.

PRECAUTIONS: Avoid long-term use. Use bed rails for inpatients and keep the patient on his side to prevent aspiration. Avoid use in pregnant women as the drug crosses the placental barrier and can depress neonatal respiration. The nurse must ensure that new, undecomposed medication is administered, following suggested procedures listed in following sections.

IMPLEMENTATION:

DRUG INTERACTIONS: Depressant effects may be increased if paraldehyde is taken concomitantly with other sedative or hypnotic agents.

PRODUCTS (TRADE NAME):

Paraldehyde, Paral (Available in 30 ml containers of liquid for oral or rectal use; 1 gm/ml for parenteral use. Never give undiluted drug IV.)

ADMINISTRATION AND DOSAGE: Can be given orally, rectally, intramuscularly or intravenously. The maximum dose by injection should not exceed 0.2 ml/kg. When given I.V., use a 5% solution DSW or NS.

Sedation:
Adults: 5-15 ml po or rectally; 5 ml IM.
Children: 0.15 ml/kg po, rectally or IM.
Hypnosis:
Adults: 10-30 ml po or rectally; 10 ml IM.
Children: 0.3 ml/kg po.

IMPLEMENTATION CONSIDERATIONS:

—The oral liquid may be diluted in milk or fruit juice to decrease the gastric irritation. This also serves to disguise the bad taste. Compliance should therefore be enhanced.

—Paraldehyde reacts with some plastics. When given intramuscularly, it should be in a glass syringe and injected deep into the gluteus maximus muscle to prevent formation of sterile abscesses and to enhance absorption.

—Paraldehyde decomposes on exposure to light. Use only new, freshly opened containers of paraldehyde. Do not use solution if it is not clear and colorless, or if it smells of acetic acid.

—Obtain a thorough health history: pregnancy, respiratory or hepatic disease, increased bronchial secretions.

—Paraldehyde is a Schedule IV controlled substance.

—Paraldehyde is not an analgesic, and in the presence of pain it may produce excitement or delirium.

—Paraldehyde may exacerbate gastritis, ulcer disease or esophagitis.

—Paraldehyde is an addicting drug.

—Paraldehyde must be diluted with an equal or double amount of vegetable oil for rectal administration.

—Exhaled breath will have the same penetrating odor as the drug. This occurs because 10-20% of the drug is excreted through the lungs.

WHAT THE PATIENT NEEDS TO KNOW:

—Taking this medicine with milk or juice may help hide the rather unpleasant taste. It will also lessen irritation to the mouth, throat and stomach.

—When you breathe out, you will be able to smell the medicine.

—Keep this drug in a tightly closed, dark brown glass bottle.

—This medicine should be kept out of the reach of children and others for whom it is not prescribed.

—Take this drug exactly as ordered. Suddenly stopping it when you have been taking it for a long time causes bad effects, such as shaking and hallucinations.

—This drug produces excessive drowsiness. You must not drive, operate dangerous machinery, do hazardous work or work requiring alertness while you are taking this medication.

—If you note any new or uncomfortable symptoms while you are taking this drug, report them to your health provider.

EVALUATION:

ADVERSE REACTIONS: *Cardiovascular:* dilation of the right heart, hypotension. *CNS:* ataxia, confusion, dizziness, headache, paradoxical excitement, residual sedation on awakening. *Gastrointestinal:* burning sensation, disagreeable taste, gastric irritation. *Respiratory:* increased bronchial secretions, pulmonary hemorrhage and edema. *Other:* acidosis, psychic and physical dependence.

OVERDOSAGE: *Signs and symptoms:* Overdosage is usually at a level that prolongs sleep without causing much respiratory depression. At higher doses hypotension, coma, respiratory depression, cardiac arrhythmias, hypothermia, miosis, vomiting, areflexia and muscle flaccidity may be seen. Rapid, labored respiratory excursions, acidosis, bleeding, azotemia, oliguria, albuminuria, leukocytosis, fatty changes in the liver, and toxic hepatitis and nephrosis, as well as pulmonary hemorrhages and edema have been reported. *Treatment:* Referral for gastric lavage, external heat, and central nervous system stimulants if necessary. Maintain adequate hydration and ventilation.

PARAMETERS TO MONITOR: Monitor respiratory function through both subjective symptoms (shortness of breath) and objective assessment (percussion and auscultation of chest, cough), as paraldehyde may increase bronchial secretions. Evaluation for signs and symptoms of gastrointestinal bleeding, for signs of oversedation or paradoxical excitement.

Candis Morrison

SEDATIVE HYPNOTICS— PIPERIDINE DERIVATIVES

ACTION OF THE DRUG: Piperidine derivatives produce hypnosis, probably through action on the reticular activating system of the brain, although the exact mechanism of action is not known. They also exhibit pronounced anticholinergic activity.

ASSESSMENT:

INDICATIONS: Used as hypnotics for periods of three to seven days. Not indicated for long-term administration.

SUBJECTIVE: Complaints of insomnia characterized by difficulty falling asleep or staying asleep, or early morning awakenings. These complaints may be idiopathic or may be associated with any stress in life. The patient may complain of feeling tired but still be unable to sleep.

OBJECTIVE: There may be no objective signs, or such non-specific signs as restlessness, tremor, or tearfulness.

PLAN:

CONTRAINDICATIONS: Do not use in the presence of known hypersensitivity or in patients with porphyria or glaucoma (especially if taking tricyclics as well).

WARNINGS: Additive effects are possible when these drugs are taken with other CNS depressants. Anticholinergic effects are possible. There is less safety margin than with barbiturates. Overdoses are extremely dangerous due to sequestration of the drug in body fat and subsequent irregular release. These drugs cross the placental barrier and appear in breast milk, and are not proven safe for use in children. Both physical and psychological dependence may occur. Sudden withdrawal is dangerous. Increased seizures may occur if used with patients on phenytoin. Decreased stage IV and REM sleep occurs.

PRECAUTIONS: These drugs may impair mental alertness, or cause oversedation. They should not be taken in larger than recommended amounts or for long periods. After periods of chronic administration, withdrawal must be undertaken slowly. Avoid use in addiction-prone individuals, or those in whom suicidal tendencies are suspected. For elderly or debilitated patients, the initial daily dose should be reduced.

IMPLEMENTATION:

DRUG INTERACTIONS: Concurrent use of other CNS depressants (including alcohol) can produce additive effects. Additive anticholinergic effects may occur with concomitant use of phenothiazines, belladonna alkaloids or tricyclic antidepressants. Since hepatic microsomal enzymes are induced, these drugs can increase metabolism of coumarin anticoagulants, decrease the effects of cortisone and related steroids and decrease the antifungal effects of griseofulvin. The control of seizure activity with phenytoin may be disrupted.

ADMINISTRATION AND DOSAGE: Glutethimide's effects occur in approximately thirty minutes and last four to eight hours. Methyprylon induces sleep within one hour which lasts five to eight hours. Start patient on lowest possible dose and increase as needed. Dosage should be individualized for best results.

IMPLEMENTATION CONSIDERATIONS:

—Obtain a complete health history: addiction potential of patient, reliability of patient, other conditions which may contraindicate drug because of its anticholinergic effect, other medications which may cause drug interactions, pregnancy, breast-feeding.

—Elderly or debilitated patients are more sensitive to CNS depressants and should be started on smaller doses.

—Prescribe only for short intervals and for total amount less than lethal dose. Usually a one-week supply is sufficient.

WHAT THE PATIENT NEEDS TO KNOW:

—These drugs may make your mouth feel dry, and/or cause constipation.

—Some people experience mild side effects while using this medication. If you notice any new or uncomfortable symptoms, notify your health care provider.

—Stop taking the drug and notify your health care provider if you have any skin rash.

—Keep drug in a dry, tightly closed container and out of reach of children or others for whom it is not prescribed.

—Drug loses its effectiveness after the period of recommended usage.

—When you stop taking this medication, there may be a marked increase in dreaming, nightmares or insomnia.

EVALUATION:

ADVERSE REACTIONS: *Cardiovascular:* hypotension. *CNS:* blurring of vision, hangover, paradoxical excitement. *Gastrointestinal:* anorexia, constipation, nausea, vomiting. *Hematopoietic:* aplastic anemia, leukopenia, megaloblastic anemia, porphyria, thrombocytopenic purpura. *Hypersensitivity:* exfoliative dermatitis, generalized skin rash, gingivitis, glossitis, purpuric urticaria. *Musculoskeletal:* osteomalacia with long-term use. *Other:* dryness of mouth, fatigue, fever, sore throat, stomatitis, urine retention, weakness.

OVERDOSAGE: *Signs and symptoms:* Sequestration in fat makes overdosage very serious and difficult to treat. Symptoms include: dryness of mouth, widely dilated and fixed pupils, adynamic ileus, bladder atony, CNS depression often progressing to profound and prolonged coma, hypothermia followed by fever, depressed response to painful stimuli, inadequate ventilation, cyanosis, sudden apnea, severe hypotension, tonic muscle spasm, twitching and convulsions. *Treatment:* Diagnosis and referral for early and vigorous cardiopulmonary support is necessary, including maintenance of patent airway with assisted ventilation later if necessary. Monitor vital signs, level of consciousness and cardiac activity. Maintain blood pressure with plasma volume expanders and pressor drugs as needed. Monitor blood levels. Vomiting should be induced if the patient is fully conscious. If the patient is unconscious, refer for gastric lavage (should be performed after there is assurance of an adequate airway with a cuffed endotracheal tube or tracheostomy). Drug extraction procedures must be continued for at least two hours after the patient regains consciousness. Since the drug is so highly lipid soluble and erratically released into the blood,

blood level rebound can cause coma to persist or recur. Lipid dialysis has been effective.

PARAMETERS TO MONITOR: Assess for therapeutic effect: relaxation and sedation. Also evaluate how patient is taking medication, signs of chronic overdosage (impaired memory and ability to concentrate, ataxia, tremors, hyporeflexia, slurred speech), signs of withdrawal (nausea, abdominal pain, tremors, convulsions, delirium, fever, chills, paresthesias of extremities, dysphagia, hallucinations, seizures, tachycardia). Maintain complete blood counts while patient is on medication.

GLUTETHIMIDE

PRODUCTS (TRADE NAME):
Doriden (Available in 200 and 500 mg tablet.) **Gluthethimide** (Available in 250 mg and 500 mg tablets and 500 mg capsules.)

DRUG SPECIFICS:
Effects begin in thirty minutes and last four to eight hours. Should be stored in light-resistant containers.

ADMINISTRATION AND DOSAGE SPECIFICS:
Sedative: 125 mg to 250 mg four times a day.
Hypnotic: 250 mg at bedtime for adults.

METHYPRYLON

PRODUCTS (TRADE NAME):
Noludar (Available in 50 mg and 200 mg tablets and 300 mg capsules.)

DRUG SPECIFICS:
Induces sleep within one hour, and lasts five to eight hours. Total daily intake should not exceed 400 mg. Greater amounts of drug do not significantly increase the hypnotic effects.

ADMINISTRATION AND DOSAGE SPECIFICS:
Hypnosis:
Adults: 200-400 mg po before bedtime.
Children: Start at 50 mg and increase to 200 mg if required. Do not use in children under three months of age.

Candis Morrison

SEDATIVE HYPNOTICS— QUINAZOLINES

METHAQUALONE

ACTION OF THE DRUG: The main effect of the quinazolines is central nervous system depression, thought to occur through action on the reticular activating system. The exact mechanism of action is not known. These drugs are also hepatic microsomal enzyme inducers.

ASSESSMENT:

INDICATIONS: Quinazolines are used as hypnotics in cases of insomnia, and in medical situations requiring restful sleep or sedation. They are probably safe for use in patients with hereditary porphyria.

SUBJECTIVE: There may be complaints of restlessness, difficulty concentrating, anxiety, fatigue, insomnia (difficulty falling asleep or staying asleep, or early morning awakening). There may be a specific causative factor such as intense emotional reactions (grief, temporary stress or sleep schedule changes).

OBJECTIVE: There may be no objective signs, or such non-specific signs as restlessness, tremor, tearfulness, tachycardia or tachypnea.

PLAN:

CONTRAINDICATIONS: Do not use in cases of known hypersensitivity, women who are or may become pregnant, and children less than twelve years of age.

WARNINGS: These drugs have high misuse potential and are easily habit forming. Alcohol and other CNS depressants can increase the sedative and depressant actions of quinazolines on brain function. These drugs can impair mental alertness, judgment, coordination and reaction time. After prolonged use, gradual withdrawal is necessary.

PRECAUTIONS: Use decreased dosages in those with impaired renal or hepatic function. Dosage for elderly or debilitated patients, or highly agitated persons, should be highly individualized. Avoid long and continuous use. Monitor coagulation studies carefully if patient is taking an anticoagulant.

IMPLEMENTATION:

DRUG INTERACTIONS: Additive effects may occur if these drugs are taken concomitantly with other sedatives, hypnotics, antihistamines, pain medications or narcotics. Quinazolines are hepatic microsomal enzyme inducers so they may interfere with and necessitate dosage adjustment for oral anticoagulants, steroids and griseofulvin. Quinazolines may cause alterations in laboratory tests in the following manner: decrease in iodine uptake and interference with Fring's test for urinary alkaloids.

PRODUCTS (TRADE NAME):

Mequin (Available in 300 mg tablets.) **Parest** (Available in 200 and 400 mg capsules, equivalent to 175 mg and 350 mg base.) **Quaalude** (Available in 150, 300 mg tablets.)

ADMINISTRATION AND DOSAGE: Qnset of sleep occurs in approximately thirty minutes and lasts five to eight hours. Half-life is ten to forty-two hours. The drugs may lose their effectiveness by the second week of continued administration. Begin with lowest possible effective dose.

Sedative:

Adults: 75 mg po three or four times a day.

Hypnotic: 150-400 mg po at bedtime.

IMPLEMENTATION CONSIDERATIONS:

—Obtain a thorough health history: hypersensitivity, drugs which may cause interactions; pregnancy; or breast-feeding.

—Prescribe only small amounts and reevaluate patient frequently.

—Use decreased dosage in those with impaired renal or hepatic function, and in older or debilitated patients.

—Evaluate client's reliability in following dosage instructions. Keep in mind the potential for drug abuse or use for suicide. These drugs are commonly abused. Prescribe only small amounts to reliable patients.

—Quinazolines depress REM sleep. This may cause increased dreaming after withdrawal, which should decrease on subsequent nights.

—These drugs are Schedule II controlled substance drugs. They are only available by a written, unrefillable prescription.

WHAT THE PATIENT NEEDS TO KNOW:

—Take this drug only as ordered. Do not increase dosage.

—Keep all medication out of the reach of children and those for whom it is not prescribed.

—The drug may cause drowsiness in ten to twenty minutes. Take only at bedtime. Avoid driving, operating dangerous machinery, or activities requiring alertness or physical coordination until all drowsiness has disappeared.

—Some people taking this drug experience side effects. If you have any new or uncomfortable symptoms, notify your practitioner. Notify health provider immediately if you notice overwhelming fatigue, weakness, fever, sore throat, unusual bleeding or bruising.

—Alcohol should be completely avoided for at least six hours before and after taking this drug.

EVALUATION:

ADVERSE REACTIONS: *CNS:* anxiety, dizziness, drowsiness, fatigue, hangover, headache, lightheadedness, paresthesia, peripheral neuropathy, restlessness, unsteady stance and gait. *Gastrointestinal:* dryness of mouth, diarrhea, nausea, pain, vomiting. *Hematopoietic:* aplastic anemia. Hypersensitivity: urticaria. *Musculoskeletal:* weakness. *Other:* bromhidrosis, dependency, diaphoresis, exanthema, tolerance.

OVERDOSAGE: *Signs and symptoms:* Marked drowsiness, confusion, dilated pupils, delirium, coma, restlessness, hypertonia, convulsions, shock and respiratory arrest may occur. Spontaneous vomiting with increased secretions may cause aspiration pneumonia or respiratory obstruction. Swelling, fluid retention and abnormal bleeding may occur. *Treatment:* Refer patient for initiation of prompt evacuation of gastric contents by lavage after airway has been ensured. Supportive therapy includes maintenance of adequate ventilation, support of blood pressure. Hemodialysis may be indicated. Analeptics are contraindicated.

PARAMETERS TO MONITOR: Monitor for therapeutic effect. Monitor how patient is taking drug, and for signs of abuse. Complete blood counts are recommended. Monitor for signs of toxicity (increased muscle tone, hyperreflexia, myoclonia). Also observe for signs of withdrawal: nausea, vomiting, anorexia, abdominal cramps, diaphoresis, nervousness, tremulousness, headache, anxiety, weakness, confusion, insomnia, nightmares, hallucinations, seizures.

Candis Morrison

SEDATIVE HYPNOTICS— TERTIARY ACETYLENIC ALCOHOLS

ETHCHLORVYNOL

ACTION OF THE DRUG: (1) The main action is to depress the central nervous system, probably at the level of the reticular activating system (although the exact mechanism is unknown). (2) There are also muscle relaxing and anticonvulsant properties.

ASSESSMENT:

INDICATIONS: Used primarily to produce sedation or induce sleep for short periods.

SUBJECTIVE: There may be complaints of restlessness, difficulty concentrating, anxiety, fatigue, insomnia (difficulty falling asleep or staying asleep, or early morning awakenings). There may be a specific causative factor such as intense emotional involvement, sleep schedule changes, or other temporary stresses.

OBJECTIVE: There may be no objective signs, or such non-specific signs as restlessness, tremor, tearfulness, tachycardia or tachypnea.

PLAN:

CONTRAINDICATIONS: Do not use in the presence of porphyria, known hypersensitivity to this product or aspirin, pain or for use in children under twelve years of age.

WARNINGS: Long-term use of larger than usual doses may result in physical and psychological dependence. Elderly or debilitated patients are more susceptible to hangover, dizziness, confusion, impaired memory, ataxia, loss of bladder control, and constipation. Ethchlorvynol may impair alertness and coordination necessary for the performance of potentially hazardous activities. Withdrawal, including convulsions, may occur if discontinued abruptly after long-term administration. Extensive tissue localization occurs, particularly in adipose tissue. Safety in pediatric age groups has not been established.

PRECAUTIONS: Use with caution in mentally depressed patients or those with suicidal tendencies. Use with caution in patients receiving tricyclic antidepressants, and those taking anticoagulants (dosage adjustment may be necessary). Prescribe only small amounts of drug at a time. If re-treatment is necessary, it should be instituted after a drug-free period of one or more weeks and after reevaluation of patient. Should not be used for insomnia in the presence of pain. Avoid this drug in the first or second trimester of pregnancy. Use sparingly in the third trimester. Safety in lactation is not established. Elderly or debilitated patients should receive the lowest effective dose.

IMPLEMENTATION:

DRUG INTERACTIONS: Alcohol, barbiturates, and other central nervous system depressants and MAO inhibitors can increase the depressant effects of the tertiary acetylenic alcohols. Ethchlorvynol taken concurrently with amitriptyline has caused transient delirium. It may depress anticipated response to dicumarol.

PRODUCTS (TRADE NAME):

Placidyl (Available in 100, 200, 500 and 750 mg capsules.)

ADMINISTRATION AND DOSAGE: Sleep is induced within fifteen minutes to one hour and lasts five hours. Peak effect occurs in approximately two hours. This drug should not be used for longer than a week. Begin with the lowest possible effective dose. This drug is not recomended for use in children.

Hypnotic:

Adults: 500 mg-1 gm po at bedtime. A single additional dose of 100-200 mg may be given if patient awakens during the night.

IMPLEMENTATION CONSIDERATIONS:

—Obtain a thorough health history: presence of medications which may cause drug interactions; pregnancy; hypersensitivity to drug.

—Patients who have hypersensitivity to aspirin frequently have allergic reactions, including asthma, when given this drug.

—If patient has had paradoxical restlessness or unpredictable behavior when taking barbiturates, alcohol, or other sedative-hypnotic drugs, it is likely that this drug will have similar effects.

—Assess status of hepatic and renal function.

—Before using this drug, evaluate reliability of patient, possibility for drug abuse, suicidal tendencies. Overdoses of this drug are especially dangerous.

—Use this drug for periods not exceeding one week.

—Withdrawal signs and symptoms can appear as long as nine days after drug is discontinued.

—This is a Schedule IV controlled substances.

WHAT THE PATIENT NEEDS TO KNOW:

—This medication is usually given for short term use. Take only as ordered.

—This drug is potentially habit-forming.

—Keep drug in dry, tightly closed container, out of the reach of children and others for whom it is not prescribed.

—If you have been taking this drug for longer than one week do not stop taking it suddenly. Gradually tapering off drug under guidance of your health provider is essential.

—Do not take alcohol or other sedatives while you are taking this drug. Two drugs together can produce too much depression.

—Avoid operating motor vehicles or dangerous machinery, or performing any tasks requiring alertness until all drowsiness has disappeared.

EVALUATION:

ADVERSE REACTIONS: *Cardiovascular:* hypotension. *CNS:* blurred vision, dizziness, excitement, facial numbness, hangover, prolonged sleep, toxic amblyopia. *Gastrointestinal:* aftertaste, cholestatic jaundice, constipation, indigestion, nausea, vomiting. *Hematopoietic:* thrombocytopenia. *Hypersensitivity:* rash, urticaria. *Musculoskeletal:* extreme muscular weakness. *Other:* loss of bladder control, psychological and physical dependence.

OVERDOSAGE: *Signs and symptoms:* Prolonged deep coma may occur, as well as severe respiratory depression, hypothermia, hypotension and relative bradycardia. *Treatment:* management is especially difficult due to the erratic absorption from the GI tract. Referral for immediate gastric evacuation is necessary, either through induction of vomiting in the conscious patient, or in the unconscious patient through gastric lavage preceded by tracheal intubation with a cuffed tube. Give supportive care. Dialysis may be necessary. Forced diuresis may help.

PARAMETERS TO MONITOR: Observe for therapeutic effects. Liver function and vision tests are recommended. Observe for signs of intoxication: slurred speech, hyperreflexia, diplopia, incoordination, tremors, ataxia, confusion, muscle weakness, toxic amblyopia, scotoma, nystagmus, peripheral neuropathy. Also observe for signs and symptoms of withdrawal which may occur up to nine days later: convulsions, delirium, schizoid reactions, perceptual disturbances, memory loss, ataxia, insomnia, slurred speech, anxiety, tremors, anorexia, nausea, vomiting, dizziness, sweating, muscle twitching, weight loss.

Candis Morrison

GASTROINTESTINAL DRUGS

ANTACIDS

ACTION OF THE DRUG: Antacids are over-the-counter drugs which neutralize hydrochloric acid and increase gastric pH, thus inhibiting pepsin. Antacids work in a variety of ways. Some antacids bring about hydrogen ion absorption, or buffering of the acid. Antacids may produce tightening of the gastric mucosa, and cardiac sphincter tone may be increased. Formation of gas which may be burped up is another mechanism by which antacids work.

ASSESSMENT:

INDICATIONS: Antacids are used adjunctively in the treatment of peptic ulcer disease, gastritis, gastric ulcer, peptic esophagitis, hiatal hernia, gastric hyperacidity, and esophageal reflux.

SUBJECTIVE: The patient may complain of sour stomach, burning pain in the region of the esophagus or stomach, a gnawing, aching feeling after meals, fullness, dyspepsia, acid eructations, nausea, vomiting, anorexia, diarrhea, loss of weight and/or thirst.

OBJECTIVE: Patients may be without objective signs. If a peptic ulcer is present, localized pain or tenderness in the epigastrium, vomiting, diarrhea, radiation of pain to the back, and abdominal distention may be present. An ulcer may be confirmed by gastrointestinal series, gastric analysis showing increased level of hydrochloric acid, or blood evident in stools tested for occult blood.

PLAN:

CONTRAINDICATIONS: Use extreme caution in administering antacids to patients with kidney failure. Any magnesium-containing antacids should be avoided with these patients. Those with a hypersensitivity to one of the components of the drugs, such as aluminum or magnesium, should avoid that particular drug. Milk of magnesia is contraindicated in patients complaining of abdominal pain, nausea, or vomiting.

WARNINGS: Fluid and electrolyte depletion may ensue as a result of diarrhea caused by some products. Rebound reflux, or hypersecretion caused by the elevation of gastric pH, should be of concern especially when caused by sodium bicarbonate administration. Hypermagnesemia (characterized by hypotension, nausea, vomiting, decreased reflexes, respiratory depression, and coma) has been reported when magnesium salts are a component in the antacid therapy. Cardiotoxicity in severe hypermagnesemia may also occur. Renal stones in those with renal dysfunction of varying degrees may also occur. (For additional warnings see specific product information.)

PRECAUTIONS: Antacids that alkalinize the urine present a potential danger for patients with decreased renal function. Patients on restricted fluid intake, and those debilitated or with decreased bowel motility (such as the elderly) may experience bowel obstruction when a constipating antacid is prescribed for an excessive period of time. Antacid forms containing aspirin should be avoided after heavy alcohol intake as hematemesis or melena may occur. Prolonged therapy with either a cathartic or constipating antacid may cause severe complications, including fluid and electrolyte imbalance or impaction. This may be avoided when different antacids are alternated. Parkinsonian patients may find after years of control that they suffer a relapse of symptoms when beginning antacid therapy (or the same patients may adjust quickly to the therapy and suffer a relapse when antacid therapy is withdrawn.)

IMPLEMENTATION:

DRUG INTERACTIONS: Antacids inhibit the absorption of tetracycline. Enteric coatings of various medications dissolve more quickly in the presence of antacids, leaving the upper gastrointestinal tract more susceptible to irritation. Weakly acidic drugs are less likely to be absorbed, whereas weakly basic drugs may be absorbed faster. Some antacids have been known to either bind with or alter the absorption rate of digoxin, digitoxin, iron, chlorpromazine, indomethacin, isoniazid, dicumeral, naproxen, amphetamines, chlordiazepoxide, diazepam, phenytoin, pseudoephedrine, and possibly propranolol. Antacids should not be used by those taking quinidine, amphetamines, or levodopa. Watch for toxic effects of aspirin resulting in an increase in their absorption rate when the coated form is taken with antacids such as aluminum-magnesium hydroxide gel. Dicumerol is absorbed 50% faster when taken concomitantly with antacids. Antacids which are quickly absorbed, such as sodium bicarbonate, magnesium hydroxide, calcium carbonate, and magnesium-aluminum hydroxide gel, may affect the pH of urine, resulting in a change in the rate of excretion. (Acid drugs will be excreted readily; basic drugs will be slowly excreted.)

ADMINISTRATION AND DOSAGE: Antacids are available in several different forms. Liquids or solutions are the preferred choice whenever possible since they more quickly neutralize acid. Suspensions, gels, chewable, effervescent and swallow tablets and powders are available through various manufacturers. When the patient feels unable to accept antacid therapy in another form, consider tablets last. The gastric emptying time of the peptic ulcer patient may vary. It is wise to individualize the antacid schedule to best accommodate this factor.

The neutralizing abilities of antacids vary. Table 5-1 lists common antacids and their neutralization capabilities.

IMPLEMENTATION CONSIDERATIONS:

—Obtain a complete health history including the presence of underlying disease (especially renal failure), and the presence of hypersensitivity to any chemical components of the antacid.

—Determine if any medications that might cause drug interactions are currently being taken by the patient. Even small amounts of certain drugs may be increased or delayed in their absorption when given with antacids.

—Baseline serum phosphate levels (and in some specific cases other electrolytes) should be acquired prior to long-term administration of any of the aluminum-containing antacids.

—Increase fluid intake and monitor carefully patients on constipative antacids such as those containing calcium or aluminum. Consider alternating them with

TABLE 5-1. MILLIEQUIVALENTS OF ACID NEUTRALIZED BY ANTAC-IDS

Antacid	Dosage	mEq Acid Neutralized
Aludrox	2 tablets	23 mEq acid
	2 teaspoonfuls (10 ml)	28 mEq acid
Amphojel	2 teaspoonfuls (10 ml)	13 mEq acid
	2 tablets (0.3 gm)	18 mEq acid
	1 tablet (0.6 gm)	18 mEq acid
Basaljel	2 teaspoonfuls	28 mEq acid
Extra Strength	1 teaspoonful (5 ml)	22 mEq acid
Basaljel	2 capsules or	26 mEq acid
	swallow tablets	28 mEq acid
Gelusil	2 teaspoonfuls	24 mEq acid
	2 tablets	22 mEq acid
Gelusil M	2 teaspoonfuls	30 mEq acids
	2 tablets	25 mEq acid
Gelusil II	2 teaspoonfuls	48 mEq acid
	2 tablets	42 mEq acid
Maalox	2 teaspoonfuls suspension	27 mEq acid
	No. 1 tablets, 2 tablets	17 mEq acid
	No. 2 tablet, 1 tablet	18 mEq acid
Maalox Plus	2 teaspoonfuls	27 mEq acid
	2 tablets	17 mEq acid
Maalox TC	1 teaspoonful	28.3 mEq acid
Riopan	1 teaspoonful suspension	3.5 mEq acid
	chew or swallow tablet	13.5 mEq acid
Riopan Plus	1 teaspoonful	13.5 mEq acid
(with	1 chewable tablet	13.5 mEq acid
simethicone)		
Titralac	1 teaspoonful	19 mEq acid
	2 tablets	15 mEq acid
Tums	1 tablet	19 mEq acid

antacids with cathartic-like actions such as those in the magnesium group. See these patients frequently and regularly.

—Antacids with a laxative effect should be taken at bedtime to allow adequate rest before the bowel is stimulated.

—If patient is concurrently on anticoagulant therapy, consider use of warfarin instead of dicumeral. Dicumeral undergoes increased absorption with concomitant antacid therapy.

—Assess flavor preferences of patients. Many patients will discontinue antacid therapy due to flavor dislikes. Studies have shown that many patients prefer Mylanta II primarily because of increased palatability. Products come in many flavors, and various drugs may be tried if compliance becomes a problem.

—For patients on restricted sodium intake (pregnant women, patients with congestive heart failure or other cardiac conditions, hypertension, edema, or renal failure) carefully assess the sodium content of various antacids. Table 5-2 presents a list of the sodium content of some common antacids.

WHAT THE PATIENT NEEDS TO KNOW:

—Take medications exactly as ordered. Generally take antacids one hour after meals. If you are being treated for peptic ulcer, gastric emptying time (usually between 1 and 3 hours) will dictate when you should take your antacid. Do not switch to another antacid or take new drugs without consulting your health provider. Other antacids may contain products which you should not use.

—Antacids may cause diarrhea or constipation. Report any significant difficulty to health care provider. Maintain a good fluid intake and increase the amount of fluids in your diet if constipation becomes a problem.

—Chew the chewable tablets thoroughly before swallowing. Follow with a full glass of water.

—Be sure to shake liquid preparations well before taking in order to ensure accurate dosage.

—If you are taking other medications at the same time, check with your health provider about whether the antacids will affect the medication. Spacing of other medication at different times may eliminate drug interactions. For example, isoniazid should be taken one hour before antacids.

—Store liquid forms in a cool place but do not freeze. Refrigeration makes them taste better.

—Time often decreases the reaction time of antacids. Do not use old medication.

—If your health provider tells you to take an aluminum-containing antacid, be sure your diet contains adequate amounts of dietary phosphorus (up to 1.5 gm/day.) Phosphorus is found in the protein of meat, almonds, beans, barley, bran, cheese, cocoa, chocolate, eggs, lentils, liver, milk, oatmeal, peanuts, peas, walnuts, whole wheat, rye, asparagus, beef, carrots, cabbage, celery, cauliflower, chards, chicken, clams, corn, cream, cucumbers, eggplant, fish, figs, prunes, pineapples, pumpkins, raisins, and string beans.

EVALUATION:

ADVERSE REACTIONS: Some adverse reactions will occur only with a particular category of antacids; others are common to most. For specifics, refer to the particular product information.

CNS: malaise. *Gastrointestinal:* anorexia, bowel obstruction, constipation, diarrhea, frequent burping, thirst. *Musculoskeletal:* muscle weakness, osteomalacia, osteoporosis (hypophosphatemia.) *Renal:* oliguria, renal stones.

TABLE 5-2. SODIUM CONTENT OF COMMON ANTACIDS

Drug	Milligrams of Sodium
Aluminum Carbonate Gel, Basic	
Basaljel	0.48 mg/ml (0.1 mEq/5 ml) suspension
	2.8 mg/capsule (0.12 mEq/cap)
	2.1 mg/tablet (O.09 mEq/tablet)
Extra Strength Basaljel	3.4 mg/ml (1.0 mEq/5 ml) suspension
Aluminum Hydroxide Gel	
Aluminum Hydroxide Gel	1.7 mg/ml
Amphojel	1.4 or 2.8 mg/tablet; not more than 0.3 mEq/5ml liquid (1.4 mg/ml)
Aluminum Phosphate Gel	
Phosphaljel	2.5 mg/ml
Calcium Carbonate	
Dicarbosil	2.7 mg/tablet
Tums	2.7 mg/tablet
Dihydroxyaluminum Aminoacetate	
Robalate	less than 1 mg/tablet
Dihydroxyaluminum Sodium Carbonate	
Rolaids	53 mg/tablet
Magaldrate	
Riopan	not more than 0.3 mg/tablet
	not more than 0.3 mg/5 ml suspension
Riopan Plus (with simethicone)	0.65 mg/tablet (or less); 0.13 g/ml (or less) suspension
Antacid Combination Products	
Aludrox	1.6 mg/tablet; 0.22 mg/ml suspension
A.M.T.	3.5 mg/tablet; 1.4 mg/ml suspension
BiSoDol	O.036 mg/tablet; 157 mg/5 gm powder
Creamalin	41 mg/tablet
Gelusil	0.8 mg/tablet; 0.7 mg/5 ml suspension
Gelusil II	2.1 mg/tablet; 1.3 mg/5 ml suspension

TABLE 5-2. *(Continued)*

Drug	Milligrams of Sodium
Gelusil M	1.3 mg/tablet; 1.2 mg/5 ml suspension
Maalox	1.35 mg/5 ml suspension
Maalox #1	0.84 mg/tablet
Maalox #2	1.84 mg/ml
Maalox Plus	1.4 mg/tablet; 0.5 mg/ml suspension
Mylanta	0.68 mg/5 ml liquid; 0.77 mg/tablet
Mylanta II	1.14 mg/5 ml liquid; 1.3 mg/tablet
Silain-Gel	0.96 mg/ml suspension; 7.68 mg/tablet
Trisogel	3.2 mg/ml capsule or suspension

OVERDOSAGE: In cases of extreme hypermagnesemia, cardiotoxicity with bradyarrhythmia, asystole, and hypotension may be seen. Coma, decreased reflexes, and respiratory depression may be found. Specific products may cause particular problems. Refer to specific product information.

PARAMETERS TO MONITOR: Obtain a complete history and baseline physical examination prior to starting antacid therapy. Baseline serum phosphate levels (and in some specific cases other electrolytes) should be drawn prior to the initiation of any of the aluminum-containing antacids.

Each visit, monitor patient's blood pressure. Evaluate for therapeutic effect. Assess for signs of electrolyte imbalance and ascertain whether diarrhea or constipation has been a problem. Assess for use of additional medications and compliance with antacid regimen. Does patient complain of the taste? Lack of effectiveness? Examine patient with special attention to tenderness in the abdominal region. Evaluation of urine and stool for occult blood, upper gastrointestinal series, and gastric analysis may be indicated if ulcer or renal problems are suspected.

Bimonthly serum phosphate levels are advised if long-term aluminum-containing antacids are prescribed, in order to guard against hypophosphatemia. Aluminum phosphate administration may reverse this effect. Obtain periodic serum electrolyte studies. Hemoglobin and hematocrit levels should be measured each visit until the patient seems stable, then every 3-6 months. Kidney function tests may be indicated if oliguria is found.

Reevaluate patients being treated for indigestion in two weeks. It is unlikely that indigestion will continue with antacid therapy for longer than this.

ALUMINUM CARBONATE GEL, BASIC

PRODUCTS (TRADE NAME):

Basaljel (Available in capsules or swallow tablets equivalent to 608 mg dried aluminum hydroxide gel or 500 mg aluminum hydroxide; or suspension equivalent to 400 mg aluminum hydroxide per 5 ml.) **Extra Strength Basaljel** (Available as 1000 mg aluminum hydroxide per 5 ml, capsules or tablets.)

DRUG SPECIFICS:

This antacid is used for the treatment of hyperacidity associated with peptic ulcer, gastritis, esophagitis, gastric hyperacidity, and hiatal hernia. Warnings and contraindications are similar to aluminum hydroxide gel.

ADMINISTRATION AND DOSAGE SPECIFICS:

Give 1-2 tablets or capsules, or 2 teaspoonfuls of suspension in water or fruit juice every 2 hours. May use up to 12 times/day.

For extra strength preparation, use 1 teaspoonful every 2 hour up to 12 times/day, or use 2 capsules or tablets up to 12 times/day.

ALUMINUM HYDROXIDE GEL

PRODUCTS (TRADE NAME):

Alternagel (Available in 600 mg/5 ml suspension). **Alu-Cap** (Available in 475 mg capsules.) **Aluminum Hydroxide** (Available in 487.5 mg tablets and 600 mg/5ml suspension.) **Aluminum Hydroxide Gel** (Available in suspension equivalent to 4% aluminium oxide.) **Alu-Tab** (Available in 600 mg tablet.) **Amphojel** (Available in 300 and 600 mg tablets, 320 mg plain or peppermint suspension.) **Dialume** (Available in 500 mg capsules.)

DRUG SPECIFICS:

Aluminium hydroxide gel is an antacid that helps delay the emptying of the stomach. It seems to have a greater effect on the binding of bile salts than other antacids. Although its neutralizing capabilities are greater than the other aluminum antacids, they are less than those of magnesium hydroxide, calcium carbonate, or sodium bicarbonate. It is more reactive in the gel form than in powder or tablet form. Aluminum hydroxide gel is the drug of choice in peptic ulcer disease.

Baseline serum phosphate levels should be obtained with bimonthly follow-up levels. Aluminum phosphate antacid may reverse any evidence of hypophosphatemia. Assess whether patient is experiencing significant constipation. Each visit, monitor bowel motility and adequacy of fluid intake.

WARNINGS:

Patients such as the elderly with decreased bowel motility may develop bowel obstruction associated with the constipative effects of this drug. Hypophosphatemia, as a result of the binding with dietary phosphates, may occur with long-term therapy.

DRUG INTERACTIONS:
Interferes with the absorption of barbiturates and anticholinergics. May bind with other drugs rendering them ineffective. Urine pH may be altered affecting the excretion rate. (Acidic drugs will be excreted easily, basic drugs will be excreted slowly.)

ADMINISTRATION AND DOSAGE SPECIFICS:
Oral: 5-10 ml every 2-4 hours, followed by a sip of water if desired.
Tablets: Two tablets (300 mg or 600 mg) 5-6 times daily. Chew thoroughly and follow with water.
For peptic ulcer: Take medication 1-3 hours after meals and at bedtime, according to individual gastric emptying time.

ALUMINUM PHOSPHATE GEL

PRODUCTS (TRADE NAME):
Phosphaljel (Available in 233 mg suspension.)

DRUG SPECIFICS:
Aluminum phosphate gel has half the neutralizing power of aluminum hydroxide gel but has a similar antacid, astringent, and demulcent power. This antacid is preferred for patients with diarrhea or those needing dietary phosphorus. It helps combat hypophosphatemia associated with the administration of other long-term aluminum-containing antacids.

ADMINISTRATION AND DOSAGE SPECIFICS:
Initially: 15-45 ml po with water four or more times/day.
Maintenance: 45 ml po after meals and at bedtime, or 30 mg six times/day.

CALCIUM CARBONATE

PRODUCTS (TRADE NAME):
Alka-2 (Available in 500 mg chewable tablets.) **Amitone** (Available in 350 mg chewable tablet.) **Calcium Carbonate** (Available in 650 mg tablets.) **Chooz** (Available in 500 mg chewable tablets.) **Dicarbosil, Equilet** (Available in 500 mg chewable tablet.) **Mallamint** (Available in 420 mg chewable tablet.) **Trialka** (Available in 350 mg tablets.) **Tums** (Available in 500 mg chewable tablets.)

DRUG SPECIFICS:
This is one of the most effective antacids available. It produces a rapid, prolonged and powerful neutralizing effect greater than aluminum hydroxide. It is primarily suited for short-term therapy and is given in small doses. Tums comes

in cherry, lemon, orange, wintergreen, and peppermint flavors. Dicarbosil comes in peppermint flavor, and Amitone is available in mint.

The constipating effects may be minimized by alternating it with doses of a magnesium-containing antacid such as magnesium carbonate.

Monitor blood calcium levels initially and in 2 weeks. Discourage long-term self-medication with this drug. Milk should not be taken with this antacid in order to prevent milk-alkali syndrome. This is characterized by nausea, vomiting, headache, mental confusion, anorexia, hypercalcemia, renal insufficiency, and metabolic alkalosis. Test urinary pH both initially and in subsequent visits.

WARNINGS:

Neurological symptoms, renal calculi, or a decrease in renal function associated with hypercalcemia may occur.

DRUG INTERACTIONS:

Calcium carbonate holds a great binding potential with other drugs.

ADMINISTRATION AND DOSAGE SPECIFICS:

Orally: 2-4 gm (30-40 gr) every hour. Tums should be taken 1 or 2 tablets at a time, chewed or dissolved slowly in the mouth between the cheek and gum.

DIHYDROXYALUMINUM AMINOACETATE

PRODUCTS (TRADE NAME):

Robalate (Available in 500 mg chewable tablets.)

DRUG SPECIFICS:

Acts more quickly and neutralizes more acid than aluminum hydroxide but is less effective than the liquid form of aluminum hydroxide. It is useful in the treatment of peptic ulcer, hyperacidity, gastritis, enteritis, pyrosis, and diarrhea.

ADMINISTRATION AND DOSAGE SPECIFICS:

Give 0.5 to 1 Gm po after meals and at bedtime. Use 1-2 Gm po every 2-4 hours for severe discomfort.

DIHYDROXYALUMINUM SODIUM CARBONATE

PRODUCTS (TRADE NAME):

Rolaids (Available in 334 mg chewable tablets.)

DRUG SPECIFICS:

Used interchangeably with dihydroxyaluminum aminoacetate.

ADMINISTRATION AND DOSAGE SPECIFICS:

1-2 tablets, chewed, as necessary.

MAGALDRATE

PRODUCTS (TRADE NAME):
Riopan (Available in 480 mg swallow tablets, chewable tablets, or suspension.)
DRUG SPECIFICS:
This antacid is a chemical combination of magnesium and aluminum hydroxide gel. It may either be more or less effective than magnesium hydroxide depending upon the buffering action desired. With a pH greater than 4.5 it will be less effective. However, with a pH less than 3.5 magaldrate will be found to be more potent. It does not cause alkalosis or acid rebound. Magaldrate is used for the relief of upset stomach and hyperacidity. It does have a mild constipative effect.
ADMINISTRATION AND DOSAGE SPECIFICS:
Orally: 1-2 tablets or 1-2 teaspoonfuls between meals and at bedtime. Swallow tablets should be swallowed with enough water to do so quickly. For severe symptoms, increase to hourly dosage. Do not take more than 20 teaspoonfuls or 20 tablets in 24 hours nor take maximum dosage for more than 2 weeks.

MAGNESIUM CARBONATE

PRODUCTS (TRADE NAME):
Magnesium Carbonate (Available in powder.)
DRUG SPECIFICS:
This is an antacid with a high neutralizing ability. Carbon dioxide forms in the stomach during the process of neutralization. It may be taken with aluminum hydroxide to counteract the cathartic effect. Take the same precautions as with other magnesium-containing antacids.
ADMINISTRATION AND DOSAGE SPECIFICS:
Orally: 0.5 to 2 gm po between meals with 1/2 glass of water. Chew tablets before swallowing.

MAGNESIUM HYDROXIDE (MAGNESIA)

PRODUCTS (TRADE NAME):
Milk of Magnesia (Available in 325 mg, 650 mg tablets, or liquid containing approximately 7.5% magnesium hydroxide.)
DRUG SPECIFICS:
Magnesium hydroxide is an antacid effective in the treatment of hyperacidity. It is helpful because of its cathartic effect in the counteraction of constipation as-

sociated with aluminum hydroxide. Alternate doses of the two are generally given. Osmotic diarrhea may occur when given alone. This drug should not be given to patients with abdominal pain, nausea, or vomiting. Available in regular and mint flavors.

ADMINISTRATION AND DOSAGE SPECIFICS:
Antacid:
Adult: Give 1-3 teaspoonfuls with water up to four times/day.
Children 1-12 years of age: Give 1/4 to 1/2 adult dosage up to four times/day.

MAGNESIUM OXIDE

PRODUCTS (TRADE NAME):
Mag-Ox 400 (Available in 400 mg tablets.) **Maox** (Available in 420 mg tablets.) **Magnesium Oxide** (Available in 140 mg capsules , 400 and 420 mg tablets, and as a powder.) **Par Mag, Uro-Mag** (Available in 140 mg capsules.)

DRUG SPECIFICS:
Magnesium oxide is a very effective non-systemic antacid. It acts more slowly than sodium bicarbonate, but has a more prolonged action and increased neutralizing ability. As with other magnesium antacids, osmotic diarrhea may develop but may be alleviated if alternated with aluminum or calcium salts. Hypermagnesemia may develop in patients with any renal insufficiency, and, thus, this product should be avoided in this patient group.

ADMINISTRATION AND DOSAGE SPECIFICS:
Oral: 250 mg po as required.
Sippy Powders: 1.3 Gms as required, to be alternated with one another to reduce the laxative effect of magnesium:
  Sippy Powder No. 1: Sodium Bicarbonate and Calcium Carbonate Powder
  Sippy Powder No. 2: Sodium Bicarbonate and Magnesium Oxide powder.

MAGNESIUM TRISILICATE

PRODUCTS (TRADE NAME):
Magnesium Trisilicate (Available in 488 mg tablet, or powder.)

DRUG SPECIFICS:
Magnesium trisilicate acts by adsorbing and protecting the stomach. It is slow to neutralize and is not absorbed well. The alkalinizing effect is minimal. It has a mild cathartic effect. Often magnesium trisilicate is combined with aluminum hydroxide. The real value of this antacid lies in the fact that even after excessive use the gastrointestinal pH remains at 7.

ADMINISTRATION AND DOSAGE SPECIFICS:
Orally: 1-4 gms four times per day. Tablets should be chewed thoroughly before swallowing. Follow with 60 ml water.

In combination with aluminum hyroxide: Give 5-30 ml in 1/2 glass water every 2-4 hours.

SODIUM BICARBONATE

PRODUCTS (TRADE NAME):
Bell/ans (Available in 520 mg tablets.) **Soda Mint** (Available in 325 and 487.5 mg tablets.) **Sodium Bicarbonate** (Available in 325 mg, 650 mg tablets and a powder.)

DRUG SPECIFICS:
Sodium bicarbonate is a systemic alkalinizing antacid with a short duration of action. It gives temporary relief of pain due to peptic ulcer and the discomfort of indigestion.

ADVERSE REACTIONS:
Routine use could cause an increase in acid secretions or acid rebound, or gastric distention could occur. In addition, repeated use may bring about systemic alkalosis and the formation of phosphate calculi in the kidney.

WARNINGS:
Avoid routine use for gastric distress. Avoid taking milk and calcium products with this medication as milk-alkali syndrome may be provoked. This is characterized by nausea, vomiting, mental confusion, and anorexia.

ADMINISTRATION AND DOSAGE SPECIFICS:
Give 0.3 to 2 gm po as necessary. Usually 1-4 times daily.

ANTACIDS—COMBINATIONS

ALUMINUM HYDROXIDE GEL AND MAGNESIUM HYDROXIDE

PRODUCTS (TRADE NAME):
Aludrox (Available as 233 mg aluminum hydroxide and 83 mg magnesium hydroxide tablet.) **Creamalin** (Available as 248 mg aluminum hydroxide and 75 mg magnesium hydroxide tablets.) **Maalox #1 and #2** (Available as 200/200 mg or 400/400 mg aluminum hydroxide and magnesium hydroxide suspension and tablets.) **Maalox TC** (Available in 600 mg aluminum hydroxide and 300 mg magnesium hydroxide suspension and tablets.)

DRUG SPECIFICS:

Aluminum hydroxide gel and magnesium hydroxide combine to produce a non-constipating, non-cathartic antacid for the relief of the hyperacidity of peptic ulcer, gastritis, peptic esophagitis, gastric hyperacidity, and hiatal hernia. There are a wide variety of combination productions on the market and only a few of the most commonly prescribed medications are included here. Maalox TC is a concentrated form of Maalox. It is capable of neutralizing a large amount of acid.

ADMINISTRATION AND DOSAGE SPECIFICS:

Aludrox and Creamalin: Two tablets or two teaspoonfuls every four hours as necessary. Suspension form may be followed by a sip of water.

Maalox: 2-4 teaspoonfuls suspension four times per day 20 minutes to one hour after meals and at bedtime.

No. 1 tablets: 2-4 tablets well chewed 20 minutes to 1 hour after meals and at bedtime.

No. 2 tablets: 1-2 tablets well chewed 20 minutes to 1 hour after meals and at bedtime. May follow with water.

Maalox TC: 1-2 teaspoonfuls as necessary between meals and at bedtime. This dosage may be increased for active peptic ulcers, but not more than 8 teaspoonfuls in 24 hours, nor the maximum dosage for more than 2 weeks, should be given. Available in peppermint flavor.

ALUMINUM HYDROXIDE GEL, MAGNESIUM HYROXIDE, SIMETHICONE

PRODUCTS (TRADE NAME):

Gelusil (Available in 200 mg aluminum hydroxide and 200 mg magnesium hydroxide and 25 mg simethicone tablets or liquid.) **Gelusil M** (Available in 300 mg aluminum hydroxide and 200 mg magnesium hydroxide with 25 mg simethicone in tablets.) **Gelusil II** (Available in 40 mg aluminum hydroxide and 400 mg magnesium hydroxide with 30 mg simethicone in tablets or liquid.) **Maalox Plus** (Available in 200 mg aluminum hydroxide and 200 mg magnesium hydroxide with 25 mg simethicone tablet.) **Mylanta** (Available in 200 mg aluminum hydroxide, 200 mg magnesium hydroxide and 20 mg simethicone liquid and tablets.) **Mylanta II** (Available in 400 mg aluminum hydroxide and 400 mg magnesium hydroxide, and 30 mg simethicone tablets or liquid.)

DRUG SPECIFICS:

These combination products utilize simethicone to reduce gas formation. There are a great many of these combination products and a variety of flavors. The medications presented here represent only a few of the more commonly prescribed drugs. Products with the higher concentration neutralize the most acid.

ADMINISTRATION AND DOSAGE SPECIFICS:

Suspension: 1-2 teaspoonfuls four times per day between meals and at bedtime.

Tablets: 1-2 tablets (well chewed) four times per day between meals and at bedtime.

Do not exceed 24 teaspoonfuls or tablets in a 24-hour period or use the maximum dosage for longer than 2 weeks.

CALCIUM CARBONATE AND GLYCINE

PRODUCTS (TRADE NAME):
Titralac (Available in tablets as precipitated calcium carbonate.)

DRUG SPECIFICS:
Calcium carbonate and glycine combine to form an insoluble antacid-protective for the relief of hyperacidity of heartburn, sour stomach, and acid indigestion and the relief of symptoms of peptic ulcer, gastritis, peptic esophagitis, gastric hyperacidity, and hiatal hernia. Constipation may be alleviated by alternating with doses of magnesium oxide.

CONTRAINDICATIONS:
Do not give to any patient whose ulcer is close to perforation due to the release of carbon dioxide.

WARNINGS:
Large doses or long-term therapy may cause a chalky formation in the bowel.

ADMINISTRATION AND DOSAGE SPECIFICS:
One teaspoonful or two tablets every hour after meals, chewed, swallowed or allowed to dissolve slowly in the mouth. Do not exceed 19 tablets or 8 teaspoonfuls in 24 hours.

CALCIUM CARBONATE AND MAGNESIUM HYDROXIDE

PRODUCTS (TRADE NAME):
Bisodol (Available with 194 mg calcium carbonate and 178 magnesium hydroxide tablets.)

DRUG SPECIFICS:
Calcium carbonate and magnesium hydroxide combine to form this antacid. Its neutralizing effect is powerful and prolonged. Constipation or diarrhea may occur, but the likelihood is less than if either of the antacids were taken alone.

ADMINISTRATION AND DOSAGE SPECIFICS:
One to two tablets every 2 hours. Chew tablets thoroughly and follow with a glass of water.

Bonnie K. Winterton

ANTICHOLINERGICS/ANTISPASMODICS

ACTION OF THE DRUG: These parasympatholytic drugs (natural and synthetic) act with antacids in prolonging the therapeutic benefits of both categories of drugs. Anticholinergics act to reduce spasms and intestinal motility, acid production and gastric motility and, consequently, reduce the associated pain. Gastric emptying time is slowed and neutralization is increased. Pancreatic secretions of fluid, electrolytes and enzymes are also suppressed. However, the adverse reactions resulting from the high dosages necessary to achieve antisecretory effects makes their utility questionable.

ASSESSMENT:

INDICATIONS: Used primarily in the treatment of peptic ulcer, pylorospasm, biliary colic, hypermotility, hyperacidity, irritable colon, and acute pancreatitis.

SUBJECTIVE: Patient may complain of chronic or periodic gnawing, burning, cramping, or aching pain in the abdomen. Heartburn, nausea, and vomiting may all occur 45-60 minutes after eating and become progressively worse throughout the day. Discomfort is least before breakfast and with food, or after vomiting. It is frequently worse during the night and may wake patient with the discomfort. Patient may complain of emotional or psychological stress, infections, physical trauma, or accident.

OBJECTIVE: Pain may be produced by palpation of the abdomen. Pain is located in the midline near the esophagus with point tenderness in the peptic or duodenal area (either on deep or superficial examination), possibly radiating to the back. Muscle guarding in the abdomen may be noted upon examination. Vomiting highly acidic gastric juice with little or no food may be documented. Blood in stools, bleeding, hypochromic anemia, and acid findings on gastric analysis may all be present. Upper gastrointestinal series x-rays may show ulcer crater or other evidence of irritation through radiologic examination, or duodenoscopy showing duodenal ulcer or duodenitis. In cases where no ulcer is documented on x-ray, a therapeutic trial of medication may be helpful in confirming suspicion of ulcer.

PLAN:

CONTRAINDICATIONS: Patients with glaucoma, prostatic disease, pyloric obstruction, gastric ulcer, cardiospasm, esophageal reflux, gastrointestinal hemorrhage, bladder neck obstruction, or serious myocardial disease should not receive anticholinergic therapy. Do not give products that also contain phenobarbital to patients with acute intermittent porphyria or sensitivity to phenobarbital (including reactions such as restlessness or excitement).

WARNINGS: These drugs easily cross the placental barrier and reach the blood of the fetus. Small amounts have also been found in mother's milk. Their use in pregnant women and breast-feeding women should be used only after serious medical consideration.

Fixed combinations of antacids and anticholinergics are dangerous and prohibited by the FDA.

If gastric retention occurs, evaluate patient for pyloric obstruction secondary to use of the drug. Diarrhea may be an early sign of intestinal obstruction. Heat prostration may occur in high environmental temperatures with use of these medications. Do not operate machinery or perform hazardous tasks since blurred vision and drowsiness are common with these preparations.

In preparations containing phenobarbital, it must be remembered that medication may be habit-forming. Do not administer to patients prone to addiction. Begin with small initial doses and use with caution in patients with hepatic dysfunction.

PRECAUTIONS: Long-term anticholinergic therapy may mask or alter the symptoms of gastrointestinal disease, so it may be difficult to determine recurrences. Special precautions are needed in administering the drug to patients with coronary heart disease, hypertension, congestive heart failure, autonomic neuropathy, hiatal hernia with reflux esophagitis, and cardiac arrhythmias. These drugs may increase heart rate, so caution should be used in any patient with tachycardia.

IMPLEMENTATION:

DRUG INTERACTIONS: Phenobarbital-containing anticholinergics may decrease the effects of anticoagulants, requiring higher doses of the anticoagulant. Anticoagulant dosage may need to be decreased when the phenobarbital product is discontinued.

ADMINISTRATION AND DOSAGE: Anticholinergics may be given orally or parenterally (when oral dosages cannot be retained or when immediate relief is needed.) It is generally better to begin the oral dosage as soon as feasible.

IMPLEMENTATION CONSIDERATIONS:

—Obtain a complete health history including the presence of hypersensitivity, underlying diseases, concurrent use of medications, and previous gastrointestinal history.

—Synthetic forms of these drugs are more expensive than the natural forms (belladonna, atropine, scopolamine.)

—Evaluate the patient as a candidate for this medication by weighing adverse reactions, contraindications, and warnings against potential benefits to be achieved.

—Central nervous system side effects are not to be expected with synthetic anticholinergic therapy. This is one of the advantages of the synthetic products.

—If complications arise and a repeat gastrointestinal series is warranted, discontinue anticholinergic therapy 72 hours prior to the radiographic exam.

—Diarrhea may be an early sign of intestinal obstruction. Evaluate seriously any complaint of diarrhea by patients on this medication.

WHAT THE PATIENT NEEDS TO KNOW:

—Take this medication exactly as ordered by your health provider.

—Keep this medication out of the reach of children and all others for whom it has not been prescribed.

—Unless otherwise directed, do not chew tablet forms of this drug.

—Many people experience mild side effects to this medication. Be certain to alert your health provider to any new or troublesome problems so that they may be evaluated. Especially report any severe diarrhea.

—High environmental temperatures may make you feel unusually hot and fatigued. Use care to avoid becoming overheated while on this drug.

EVALUATION:

ADVERSE REACTIONS: Adverse reactions are common in anticholinergic therapy due to the necessity of increasing the dosage to achieve consistent effect on the target organ. *Cardiovascular:* circulatory failure, rapid weak pulse. *CNS:* amnesia, blurring of vision (mild), coma, confusion, delirium, difficulty swallowing, difficulty talking, dilatation of pupils, drowsiness, euphoria, excitation, photophobia, relaxation, restlessness, sleep, staggering, stupor, talkativeness. *Dermatologic:* rash primarily over the face, neck, and upper trunk (especially in children), flushing of skin. *Gastrointestinal:* constipation, dry mouth (mild), great thirst. *Renal:* urinary urgency, difficulty emptying bladder. *Respiratory:* respiratory failure. *Other:* increased body temperature (to 107 degrees F. or more in infants and children), relief of fear.

Anticholinergics with phenobarbital: *CNS:* convulsions, delirium, excitement. *Musculoskeletal:* musculoskeletal pain. *Other:* various dermatologic and allergic responses.

OVERDOSAGE: Skeletal muscle paralysis will occur in overdosages. Poisoning is rarely fatal, however. Fatal dosages are considered to be 100 mg for adults and 10 mg for children. Many who have taken far more have survived.

With phenobarbital products: Early overdosage will produce sleepiness, mental confusion, unsteadiness. This progresses to prolonged coma, slow shallow respirations, flaccid muscles, absent deep reflexes. Death is often from pulmonary complications.

PARAMETERS TO MONITOR: Before initiating therapy, obtain complete baseline physical examination. Check stools for occult blood. Obtain complete blood count including hematocrit and hemoglobin. Gastric analysis showing acid should be obtained and HCl hypersecretion documented if possible. Upper gastrointestinal series should be performed to document ulcer. Ulcer may not be visualized, but other factors which may suggest an ulcer would be pylorospasm, hypermotility, hypersecretions or retained acid secretion, an irritability of the duodenal bulb (displacing the barium from this area), or point tenderness over the area of the duodenal bulb. Duodenoscopy may either show an ulcer or irritation of the duodenum. A trial with antacids or anticholinergics may be carried out with patients not documented to have an ulcer, but in which the index of suspicion is high.

ANTICHOLINERGICS—COMBINATION DRUGS

PRODUCTS (TRADE NAME):
Donnatal (Available in capsules, tablets or elixir, containing O.0194 mg atro-

pine, O.0065 mg hyoscine hydrobromide, 0.1037 hyoscyamine hydrobromide, and 15 or 16 mg phenobarbital.) **Donnatal No. 2** (Available in tablets containing O.0194 mg atropine, O.0065 hyoscine hydrobromide, 0.1037 hyoscyamine hydrobromide, and 32.4 mg phenobarbital.) **Donnatal Extentabs** (Available in O.0582 mg atropine sulfate, O.0195 mg hyoscine hydrobromide, 0.3111 mg hycosyamine sulfate, and 48.6 mg phenobarbital as a sustained-release tablet.) **Robinul-PH** (Available in tablets with 1 mg glycopyrrolate and 16.2 mg phenobarbital.) **Robinul-PH Forte** (Available in tablets with 2 mg glycopyrrolate and 16.2 mg phenobarbital.)

DRUG SPECIFICS:

These medications are only a few of the many combination products combining anticholinergic and sedative drugs. Because of the phenobarbital these products may be habit-forming.

ADMINISTRATION AND DOSAGE SPECIFICS:

Donnatal tablets or capsules: Give 3-8 capsules or tablets in equally divided doses, three to four times daily.

Elixir: Give 15-40 ml/day in equally divided doses.

Extentabs: Give 2 tablets every 12 hours.

Robinul tablets: Give 3 tablets/day in divided dosages.

Bonnie K. Winterton

ANTISPASMODICS

DICYCLOMINE HCL

PRODUCTS (TRADE NAME):

Antispas (Available in 10 mg/ml injection.) **Bentyl** (Available in 10 mg capsules, 20 mg tablets, 10 mg/5 ml syrup, and 10 mg/ml injection.) **Dicen** (Available in 10 mg/ml injection.) **Dibent** (Available in 20 mg tablets, 10 mg/ml injection.) **Dicyclomine Hydrochloride** (Available in 10 and 20 mg capsules, 20 mg tablets, 10 mg/5 ml syrup, and 10 mg/ml injection.) **Di-Spaz** (Available in 10 mg capsules, 10 mg/ml injection.) **Neoquess, Nospaz, Or-Tyl, Spasmoject** (Available in 10 mg/ml injection.)

DRUG SPECIFICS:

This synthetic antispasmodic controls spasms of the gastrointestinal tract. It is "probably effective" in the treatment of functional bowel and irritable bowel syndrome. The syrup is used primarily for treating infant colic.

ADMINISTRATION AND DOSAGE:

Adults: 10 to 20 mg po three or four times daily; or 20 mg IM every 4 to 6 hours.

Children: 10 mg po three or four times daily.

Infants: 5 mg syrup diluted with an equal volume of water, three or four times daily.

METHIXENE HCL

PRODUCTS (TRADE NAME):
   Trest (Available in 1 mg tablets.)
DRUG SPECIFICS:
   This is a synthetic antispasmodic used as adjunctive treatment in biliary dyskinesis, gastric ulcer, gastritis, gastroenteritis, duodenal ulcer, duodenitis, epigastric distress, functional bowel distress, irritable bowel, pylorospasm, and spastic colon.
ADMINISTRATION AND DOSAGE SPECIFICS:
   One or two tablets po three times daily.

OXYPHENCYCLIMINE HCL

PRODUCTS (TRADE NAME):
   Daricon (Available in 10 mg tablets)
DRUG SPECIFICS:
   Synthetic antispasmodic used in the adjunctive treatment of peptic ulcer disease.
ADMINISTRATION AND DOSAGE SPECIFICS:
   Adults and children over 12 years: 10 mg in the morning and at bedtime. Dosage may be increased to three times a day, or reduced to 5 mg twice a day as necessary.

THIPHENAMIL HCL

PRODUCTS (TRADE NAME):
   Trocinate (Available in 100 and 400 mg tablets.)
DRUG SPECIFICS:
   Synthetic antispasmodic used in the relief of pain and discomfort caused by smooth muscle spasm, associated with acute enterocolitis, spastic colitis, irritable colon, and functional gastric disorders. It is "probably effective" in the treatment of irritable bowel syndrome and neurogenic bowel problems.

ADMINISTRATION AND DOSAGE SPECIFICS:
Adults: 400 mg po, repeated in four hours as needed.

ANTICHOLINERGICS/ANTISPASMODICS— BELLADONNA ALKALOIDS

ATROPINE SULFATE

PRODUCTS (TRADE NAME):
   Atropine Sulfate (Available in 0.4 mg tablets, and 0.3, 0.4 and 0.6 mg soluble tablets, and in 0.2, 0.3, 0.4, 0.5, 0.6, 1.0, and 1.2 mg/ml in 1, 5 or 10 ml disposable syringes for injection.)

DRUG SPECIFICS:
   Among the most effective of the anticholinergic drugs. The side effects, unlike some anticholinergics, are minimal. Atropine produces a slight antispasmodic effect on the gallbladder and bile ducts and a relaxing effect on the ureter after it has been in spasm. (Parenteral use is reserved primarily for emergency cardiac or gastric problems.) Give same dosage po or SQ.

ADMINISTRATION AND DOSAGE SPECIFICS:
   Adults: 0.4 to 0.6 mg
   Children 7 to 16 lbs: 0.1 mg
   Children 17 to 24 lbs: 0.15 mg
   Children 24 to 40 lbs: 0.2 mg
   Children 40 to 65 lbs: 0.3 mg
   Children 65 to 90 lbs: 0.4 mg
   Children over 90 lbs: 0.4 to 0.6 mg.

BELLADONNA

PRODUCTS (TRADE NAME):
   Belladonna Extract (Available in 15 mg tablets.) **Belladonna Tincture** (Available in 30 mg alkaloid of belladonna liquid.)

DRUG SPECIFICS:
   A very effective anticholinergic with less side effects than many. Has the same therapeutic action as atropine.

ADMINISTRATION AND DOSAGE SPECIFICS:
   Belladonna Extract: 15 mg po 3 or 4 times daily.

Belladonna Tincture:
Adults: 0.6 to 1.0 ml 3 to 4 times daily.
Children: 0.03 ml/kg three times daily.

LEVOROTATORY ALKALOIDS OF BELLADONNA

PRODUCTS (TRADE NAME):
Bellafoline (Available in 0.25 mg tablets and 0.5 mg/ml injection.)
DRUG SPECIFICS:
This versatile product is used in a variety of smooth muscle spastic conditions and when excessive secretion is present. It is used in controlling spasm associated with colitis, intestinal and biliary colics, pylorospasm, peptic ulcer, and for dysmenorrhea, renal colic, enuresis and nocturia. It is used for vagal inhibition, motion sickness, parkinsonism, and to control bronchial asthma and hypersecretion in the respiratory tract.
ADMINISTRATION AND DOSAGE SPECIFICS:
Adults: 0.25 to 0.5 mg po 3 times daily or 0.5 to 1 ml SQ once or twice daily.
Children over 6 years of age: 0.125 to 0.25 mg po three times daily.

L-HYOSCYAMINE SULFATE

PRODUCTS (TRADE NAME):
Anaspaz (Available in 0.125 mg tablet.) **Cystospaz** (Available in 0.15 mg tablet.) **Cystospaz-M** (Available in 0.375 mg timed-released capsules.) **Levsin** (Available in 0.125 mg tablets, 0.125 mg per 5 ml elixir; 0.125 mg/ml drops, or 0.5 mg/ml injection.) **Levsinex Timecaps** (Available in 0.375 mg timed-release capsules.)
DRUG SPECIFICS:
This drug functions in reducing hypermotility and hyperacidity. It is used as an adjunct in the treatment of peptic ulcer, in controlling excess secretions and spasms associated with spastic colitis, cystitis, pylorospasm, mild diarrhea, diverticulitis, irritable bowel syndrome, colic in infants, and bowel problems of a neurogenic nature.
CONTRAINDICATIONS:
In addition to those mentioned in the general section of anticholinergic—antispasmodics, this drug should not be taken by patients with any gastrointestinal obstruction or atony, paralytic ileus, hemorrhage, severe or complicating ulcerative colitis, toxic megacolon and myasthenia gravis.
OVERDOSAGE:
With this drug, some normally adverse reactions to anticholinergics would be

indicative of overdosage. Watch for headaches, nausea, vomiting, blurred vision, dilated pupils, hot/dry skin, dizziness, dry mouth, and difficulty swallowing.

ADMINISTRATION AND DOSAGE SPECIFICS:

Adults: 0.125 to 0.25 mg every 3 to 4 hours po or SQ. Use 1-2 cc drops every four hours as needed. Use 0.375 mg in sustained-release tablets every 12 hours. In severe cases use 2 timecaps every 12 hours or 1 timecap every 8 hours. Parenterally give 0.25 to 0.5 mg SQ, IM, or IV 3–4 times daily, as needed.

Children up to 5 pounds: Use 3 drops every four hours as needed.

Children up to 7.5 pounds: Use 4 drops every four hours as needed.

Children up to 10 pounds: Use 5 drops or 0.5 to .75 ml elixir every four hours as needed.

Children up to 15 pounds: Use 6 drops every four hours as needed.

Children up to 20 pounds: Use 7 drops or 1.2 to 2.0 ml elixir every four hours as needed.

Children up to 30 pounds: Use 3.5 ml elixir every four hours as needed.

Children up to 50 pounds: Use 3/4 to 1 teaspoonful every four hours as needed.

SCOPOLAMINE HYDROBROMIDE (HYOSCINE HYDROBROMIDE)

PRODUCTS (TRADE NAME):

Scopolamine Hydrobromide (Available in 0.4 and 0.6 mg soluble tablets, 0.3, 0.4, and 1.0 mg/ml injection.)

DRUG SPECIFICS:

Similar to atropine in peripheral action, but parenteral dosages cause central nervous system depression resulting in drowsiness, euphoria, relief of fear, sleep, relaxation and amnesia. This drug is sometimes used to relieve motion sickness. Use cautiously in patients with Parkinsonism or spasticity.

ADMINISTRATION AND DOSAGE SPECIFICS:

Adults: 0.3 to 0.6 mg SQ or IM, 0.4 to 0.8 mg po.

Children: 0.006 mg/kg po or SQ.

ANTICHOLINERGICS/ANTISPASMODICS— QUATERNARY DERIVATIVES

ANISOTROPINE METHYLBROMIDE

PRODUCTS (TRADE NAME):

Anisotropine Methylbromide, Valpin 50 (Available in 50 mg tablets.)

DRUG SPECIFICS:

This anticholinergic acts to decrease gastric secretions and hypermotility. As with other anticholinergics, there is no real evidence that it is effective in treating gastric or peptic ulcer. Benefits should be weighed against side effects produced.

ADMINISTRATION AND DOSAGE SPECIFICS:

Adults: Give 50 mg (1 tablet) po three times daily.

CLIDINIUM BROMIDE

PRODUCTS (TRADE NAME):

Quarzan (Available in 2.5 and 5 mg capsules.)

DRUG SPECIFICS:

The anticholinergic effect of this drug is similar to that of atropine and propantheline bromide. In cases of suspected overdosage watch for restlessness, excitement, psychotic behavior, flushing, tachycardia, a decrease in blood pressure, circulatory failure, respiratory failure, paralysis, and coma.

ADMINISTRATION AND DOSAGE SPECIFICS:

Adults: Give 2.5 to 5 mg po three to four times daily before meals and at bedtime.
Debilitated or geriatric patients: Give 2.5 mg po three times/day before meals.

GLYCOPYRROLATE

PRODUCTS (TRADE NAME):

Glycopyrrolate (Available in 1 and 2 mg tablets.) **Robinul** (Available in 1 mg tablets and 0.2 mg/ml injection.) **Robinul Forte** (Available in 2 mg tablets.)

DRUG SPECIFICS:

Used orally as adjunctive treatment in peptic ulcer disease. (Parenteral use primarily for anesthesia.)

ADMINISTRATION AND DOSAGE SPECIFICS:

Peptic ulcer disease: 1 to 2 tablets two or three times daily.

HEXOCYCLIUM METHYLSULFATE

PRODUCTS (TRADE NAME):

Tral Filmtabs (Available in 25 mg tablets.) **Tral Gradumets** (Available in 50 mg timed release tablets.)

DRUG SPECIFICS:

Used adjunctively as treatment for peptic ulcer disease. In cases of suspected overdosage, watch for an atropine-like flush in the blush areas and an increase in mouth dryness. Extra-large doses may bring about respiratory paralysis and circulatory collapse.

ADMINISTRATION AND DOSAGE SPECIFICS:

Adults: 25 mg before meals and at bedtime. For timed-release capsule, take 50 mg before lunch and at bedtime. Do not chew.

ISOPROPAMIDE IODIDE

PRODUCTS (TRADE NAME):

Darbid (Available in 5 mg tablets.)

DRUG SPECIFICS:

This is a synthetic anticholinergic which suppresses gastric secretions and relieves hypermotility for 10 to 12 hours. It is used as adjunctive therapy in peptic ulcer treatment and "probably effective" in irritable bowel syndrome.

ADMINISTRATION AND DOSAGE SPECIFICS:

Adults: 5 to 10 mg every 12 hours. May use more frequently if symptoms are severe.

MEPENZOLATE BROMIDE

PRODUCTS (TRADE NAME):

Cantil (Available in 25 mg tablets.)

DRUG SPECIFICS:

This drug decreases gastric acid and pepsin secretion while slowing contractions of the colon. It is a synthetic anticholinergic drug used as an adjunct in the treatment of peptic ulcer disease but has not been shown to aid in the healing, prevention of recurrences, or complications of the disease.

ADMINISTRATION AND DOSAGE SPECIFICS:

Adults: 25 to 50 mg po with meals and at bedtime.

METHANTHELINE BROMIDE

PRODUCTS (TRADE NAME):

Banthine (Available in 50 mg tablets.)

DRUG SPECIFICS:
This drug is similar in action to atropine. The gastrointestinal action is to inhibit motility of the stomach and small intestine, delay stomach emptying time, and lessen secretions. Medication acts within 30-45 minutes and lasts 4-6 hours. Administer the smallest effective dosage possible.

WARNINGS:
Do not administer with antacids with adsorbent action (i.e. aluminum hydroxide.) Patients can be allergic to the bromide component.

ADVERSE EFFECTS:
Some dilatation of the pupils, dry mouth, inability to read fine print, constipation requiring laxatives, urinary retention (especially in those with prostatic hypertrophy), general malaise and weakness may occur. High dosages may result in impotency, respiratory paralysis, or other anticholinergic adverse reactions.

ADMINISTRATION AND DOSAGE SPECIFICS:
Adults: 50 mg initially, then 100 mg every 6 hours.
Children: 6 mg/kg body weight daily in four divided doses.

METHSCOPOLAMINE BROMIDE

PRODUCTS (TRADE NAME):
Pamine (Available in 2.5 mg tablets.)

DRUG SPECIFICS:
This drug is a synthetic substitute for atropine as an antispasmodic. It is used in the treatment of gastric and duodenal ulcers to relieve hypersecretion and hypertonicity. Patients with peptic ulcer and gastritis are helped as it reduces hypermotility and hyperacidity. It has been used to relieve excess salivary secretions and sweating. The action is more prolonged than atropine. It acts in 8 hours, yet is less potent.

ADVERSE REACTIONS:
In addition to others mentioned in the general section, constipation is also common with this drug. Less frequently, palpitations, nausea, or headache may be found. Patients can be allergic to the bromide component.

ADMINISTRATION AND DOSAGE SPECIFICS:
Adults: Give 2.5 mg 1/2 hour before eating and 2.5 to 5 mg at bedtime.

OXYPHENONIUM BROMIDE

PRODUCTS (TRADE NAME):
Antrenyl Bromide (Available in 5 mg tablets.)

DRUG SPECIFICS:
This drug has a greater effect on hypersecretions than methantheline but less

ability to control hypermotility than atropine. It is used as adjunctive therapy in the treatment of peptic ulcer disease. Patients can be allergic to the bromide component.

ADMINISTRATION AND DOSAGE SPECIFICS:

10 mg four times daily for several days, reducing the dosage according to effectiveness.

PROPANTHELINE BROMIDE

PRODUCTS (TRADE NAME):

Norpanth (Available in 15 mg tablet.) **Pro-Banthine** (Available in 7.5 and 15 mg tablets.) **ProBanthine Bromide, SK-Probantheline Bromide** (Available in 15 mg tablets.)

DRUG SPECIFICS:

An analog to methantheline bromide, this drug is more effective than methantheline in the reduction of volume and acidity of the stomach's secretions and in the less severe adverse reactions. It is often preferred over methantheline bromide because of these reasons. It is used adjunctively in the treatment of peptic ulcer disease. Parenteral forms are used in severe peptic ulcer problems and in preparing patients for diagnostic gastrointestinal radiography. Patients can be allergic to the bromide component.

ADMINISTRATION AND DOSAGE SPECIFICS:

Adults:

Orally: 15 mg with meals and 30 mg at bedtime, adjusted according to therapeutic response.

IM or IV: 30 mg every 6 hours depending on need. Maintenance is usually 15 mg.

TRIDIHEXETHYL CHLORIDE

PRODUCTS (TRADE NAME):

Panthilon (Available in 25 mg tablet.)

DRUG SPECIFICS:

This synthetic anticholinergic is effective in relaxing pain by reducing spasms of the gastrointestinal tract. Used adjunctively in the treatment of peptic ulcer and, "probably effective" in the treatment of irritable bowel syndrome.

ADMINISTRATION AND DOSAGE SPECIFICS:

Oral: 25 to 50 mg 3 or 4 times daily, or 75 mg sequels every 12 hours.

IM, IV or SQ: 10 to 20 mg every 6 hours. Switch to oral preparation as soon as possible.

Bonnie K. Winterton

ANTIDIARRHEALS

ACTION OF THE DRUG: Antidiarrheals reduce fluid content of the stool and decrease peristalsis and motility of the intestinal tract. They increase smooth muscle tone and diminish digestive secretions. The bismuth salts absorb toxins and provide a protective coating for the intestinal mucosa.

ASSESSMENT:

INDICATIONS: Used in nonspecific diarrhea, or diarrhea caused by antibiotics.

SUBJECTIVE: Frequent loose, watery stools, often with mild, cramping abdominal pain prior to bowel movements, are seen.

OBJECTIVE: Hyperactive bowel sounds may be found on auscultation; slight generalized abdominal tenderness with no rebound or localized tenderness on palpation.

PLAN:

CONTRAINDICATIONS: Do not use in the presence of pseudomembranous enterocolitis, glaucoma, advanced hepatic or renal disease, hypersensitivity to specific drugs, or infectious diarrhea caused by toxic organisms such as Salmonella and Shigella.

WARNINGS: Use with caution in patients with prostatic hypertrophy, or incipient glaucoma. The opiates, loperamide, and diphenoxylate may cause psychic or physical dependence if used in high dosages or for long periods. The non-specific antidiarrheal agents are used to provide symptomatic relief until the etiology of the diarrhea can be determined and specific therapy instituted. These agents should not be used in diarrhea caused by poison until the toxin has been removed from the gastrointestinal tract.

PRECAUTIONS: Safe use has not been established during pregnancy and benefit must be weighed against hazard in use. The opiates and diphenoxylate are excreted in breast milk and should not be used in nursing mothers.

IMPLEMENTATION:

DRUG INTERACTIONS: Diphenoxylate may potentiate the action of barbiturates and other central nervous system depressants.

ADMINISTRATION AND DOSAGE: All the antidiarrheal agents are administered orally. Individual dosages are listed with specific product information.

IMPLEMENTATION CONSIDERATIONS:

—Obtain a complete health history including evaluation for the underlying cause of diarrhea, presence of other systemic diseases, or other medications taken concurrently.

—Prolonged diarrhea can result in dehydration and electrolyte imbalance.

—Encourage fluid intake to help replace fluid lost in the stool.

—Observe patients being treated with Lomotil or other narcotics for signs of central nervous system depression.

—Dietary modifications are usually a part of management. Diet is restricted to clear liquids for 24 hours and then gradually foods are added as tolerated.

WHAT THE PATIENT NEEDS TO KNOW:

—The antidiarrheal agents are used for relief of symptoms and to prevent dehydration until the underlying cause can be found and treated.

—Diet should be restricted to clear liquids (tea, jello, broth, carbonated beverages) for 24 hours. Then begin adding bland foods. Continue addition of more solid foods if diarrhea does not reappear.

—Diarrhea that persists after 48 hours should not be self-treated. You should return to your health care provider for further evaluation and diagnosis.

—Some of these medications contain habit-forming drugs; therefore they should be used only at the dosage recommended, and for the length of time prescribed.

—Keep this medication out of the reach of children and others for whom drug is not prescribed.

EVALUATION:

ADVERSE REACTIONS: *Cardiovascular:* tachycardia. *CNS:* dizziness, drowsiness, fatigue, headache, sedation. *Dermatologic:* pruritis, urticaria. *EENT:* mydriasis. *Gastrointestinal:* abdominal distention, constipation, dry mouth, nausea, vomiting. *Genitourinary:* urinary retention. *Other:* physical dependence with long-term use.

OVERDOSAGE: *Signs and symptoms:* Dryness of skin, flushing, hyperthermia, tachycardia, pinpoint pupils, respiratory depression may be seen. *Treatment:* Administration of a narcotic antagonist will counteract these effects. Provide supportive therapy as indicated.

PARAMETERS TO MONITOR: Antidiarrheals should not be used long term. Monitor for therapeutic effect in controlling diarrhea, and for development of adverse effects.

BISMUTH SUBSALICYLATE

PRODUCTS (TRADE NAME):
Pepto-Bismol (Available in 300 mg tablets and 527 mg/30 ml liquid.)
DRUG SPECIFICS:
This non-prescription product contains large amounts of salicylate and should be used with caution by those already taking aspirin products. Obtain history of

any sensitivity to aspirin before prescribing. It may cause temporary darkening of the stool and tongue.

ADMINISTRATION AND DOSAGE SPECIFICS:

Adults: Give 30 ml or 2 tablets orally every 1/2 to 1 hour until symptoms are relieved or a maximum of 8 doses is taken.

Children over 10 years: Give 20 ml as above.

Children 6 to 10 years: Give 10 ml as above.

Children 3 to 6 years: Give 5 ml as above.

DIPHENOXYLATE HYDROCHLORIDE AND ATROPINE SULFATE

PRODUCTS (TRADE NAME):

Diphenoxylate HCl, Elmotil, Enoxa, Lofene (Available in 2.5 mg tablets.) **Lomotil** (Available in 2.5 mg tablets, 2.5 mg/5 ml liquid.) **Lonox, Lo-Trol, LowQuel, Nor-Mil, SK-Diphenoxylate** (Available in 2.5 mg tablets.)

DRUG SPECIFICS:

These are controlled substances, Schedule V. Addition of atropine sulfate helps to prevent abuse.

ADMINISTRATION AND DOSAGE SPECIFICS:

Adults: Give 2 tablets or 2 teaspoons 4 times a day until diarrhea is controlled.

Children 2 to 12 years: Give 0.3 mg to 0.4 mg/kg in divided doses using liquid form. Not to be used in those under 2 years.

DONNAGEL

PRODUCTS (TRADE NAME):

Donnagel (Available in kaolin 90 gr, pectin 2 gr, hyoscyamine sulfate 0.1037 mg, atropine sulfate O.0194 mg, hyoscine hydrobromide O.0065 mg, sodium benzoate 60 mg and alcohol 3.81% in 30 ml.) **Donnagel-PG** (Available in the same basic formula plus powdered opium 24 mg.)

DRUG SPECIFICS:

Because of the presence of the belladonna alkaloids, caution must be used in patients with glaucoma or bladder neck obstruction.

ADMINISTRATION AND DOSAGE SPECIFICS:

Donnagel:

Adults: 2 tablespoonfuls at once and 1 or 2 tablespoonfuls after each stool.

Children 30 lbs and over: 2 teaspoonfuls every 3 hours.

Children 20 lb: 1 teaspoonful every 3 hours.

Children 10 lbs: 1/2 teaspoonful every 3 hours.

Donnagel-PG:
Adults: 2 tablespoonfuls every 3 hours.
Children: Same as for plain Donnagel.

KAOLIN AND PECTIN MIXTURES

PRODUCTS (TRADE NAME):
  Kaolin with Pectin, Kaopectate, K-Pek, Pektamalt (Available in 3 oz, 8 oz and 12 oz bottles.)
DRUG SPECIFICS:
  These are non-prescription products widely used in self-treatment of diarrhea. Clinical effectiveness has not been established. Although stools may become formed, water loss is not decreased.
ADMINISTRATION AND DOSAGE SPECIFICS:
  Adults: 60 to 120 ml po after each bowel movement.
  Children over 12 years: 60 ml po after each bowel movement.
  Children 6 to 12 years: 30 to 60 ml as above.
  Children 3 to 6 years: 15 to 30 ml as above.

LACTOBACILLUS

PRODUCTS (TRADE NAME):
  Bacid (Available in capsules.) **Lactinex** (Available in tablets and granules.)
DRUG SPECIFICS:
  These non-prescription products are specifically used in the treatment of diarrhea caused by antibiotics although effectiveness has not been proven. They act to reestablish normal intestinal flora. They may be used prophylactically in those with a history of antibiotic-induced diarrhea.
ADMINISTRATION AND DOSAGE SPECIFICS:
  Adults: Give 2 capsules Bacid or 4 tablets, or use 1 packet of granules of Lactinex, two to four times a day, preferably with milk.

LOPERAMIDE HYDROCHLORIDE

PRODUCTS (TRADE NAME):
  Imodium (Available in 2 mg capsules.)
DRUG SPECIFICS:
  This is a controlled substance, Schedule V. It is more potent, and has a longer duration of action with less central nervous system depression than diphenoxylate.

ADMINISTRATION AND DOSAGE SPECIFICS:
Adults: Initially give 4 mg po, then 2 mg after each unformed stool; maximum of 16 mg po daily.

OPIUM TINCTURE

PRODUCTS (TRADE NAME):
Brown Mixture (Available in 12% paregoric/30 ml liquid.) **Opium Tincture** (Available in 10 mg/ml.) **Paregoric Tincture** (Available in 2 mg/5 ml liquid.)
DRUG SPECIFICS:
This is a controlled substance, Schedule III. It is given orally mixed with water. A white, milky fluid forms when they are mixed together.
ADMINISTRATION AND DOSAGE SPECIFICS:
Tincture of Opium:
Adult: Give 0.6 ml po four times a day.
Camphorated Opium Tincture:
Adults: 5 to 10 ml po four times a day until diarrhea subsides.
Children: 0.25 to 0.5 ml/kg po four times a day until diarrhea subsides.

Patricia Newton

ANTIFLATULENTS

SIMETHICONE

ACTION OF THE DRUG: An antiflatulent acts to break up gastrointestinal gas bubbles through a defoaming action so that they may be more easily expelled by belching or as flatus. Mucus surrounding the gas bubbles is dispersed, and the gas bubbles coalesce, freeing the gas. In this manner, gastric pain is reduced.

ASSESSMENT:

INDICATIONS: These products are used in the treatment of any problems producing bloating, flatulence, or postoperative gas pains. They may also be used for chronic air-swallowing, functional dyspepsia, peptic ulcer, spastic or irritable colon, and diverticulitis.
SUBJECTIVE: Patient may complain of being bloated, distended, feeling "full," gaseous, or frequent belching. Gas pains may also be noted, especially after surgery.

OBJECTIVE: Abdomen feels extra firm or hard to palpation, and pain may shift with the pressure of palpation. Abdominal distention may be detected by observation and percussion. Tympanic percussion notes are heard, as well as hyperactive bowel sounds.

PLAN:

CONTRAINDICATIONS: Use with caution if there has been previous difficulty with this product.

IMPLEMENTATION:

PRODUCTS (TRADE NAME):
Mylicon (Available in 40 mg chewable tablets or 40 mg/0.6 ml drops). **Mylicon-80** (Available in 80 mg chewable tablets). **Silain** (Available in 50 mg tablets).

ADMINISTRATION AND DOSAGE: Available in both drops and tablet form. Chew tablets thoroughly before swallowing. Shake drops well before using. Give 40 to 80 mg tablets after each meal and at bedtime, or use 40 mg (0.6 ml) drops 4 times daily after meals and at bedtime.

IMPLEMENTATION CONSIDERATIONS:
—Obtain a complete history including underlying diseases, previous gastrointestinal surgery, hypersensitivity, concurrent use of drugs, and previous response to therapy.
—Determine if there is a dietary origin to the flatulence and whether changing diet may decrease symptoms.
—Medication is often used in combination with antacid therapy.
—This medication is intended for short-term use only. More rigorous evaluation should be undertaken if symptoms do not disappear with medication.

WHAT THE PATIENT NEEDS TO KNOW:
—Take medication exactly as ordered. This medication will relieve abdominal pain by reducing gas. You will notice an increase in belching or passing of flatus and this assures you that the medicine is working.
—Chew tablets thoroughly before swallowing, or shake drops well before pouring dose.
—This medication is intended for short-term use. If your problem does not resolve within a short time, return to see your health provider.

EVALUATION:

PARAMETERS TO MONITOR: Monitor for therapeutic effect. Pain should disappear with systematic use.

Bonnie K. Winterton

DIGESTIVE ENZYMES

ACTION OF THE DRUG: Digestive enzymes promote digestion by acting as replacement therapy when enzymes are lacking, not secreted, or not absorbed properly. They are obtained from the pancreas of a hog. Healthy patients may find a decrease in intestinal gas following use of the product.

ASSESSMENT:

INDICATIONS: Digestive enzymes are often indicated for individuals with poor digestion, for predigestive purposes, and as replacement therapy. They may be used to relieve the symptoms associated with cystic fibrosis, cancer of the pancreas, or chronic inflammation of the pancreas causing malabsorption syndromes. Patients having had gastrointestinal bypass surgery may also benefit. Obstruction of the pancreatic or common bile duct by neoplasm may prompt need for this drug.

SUBJECTIVE: Patients may complain of sudden intense pain in the gastric region, hiccoughs, belching of gas, vomiting, constipation, pain radiating to the back, weakness, diarrhea, collapse, indigestion, good or ravenous appetite without weight gain, chronic cough, and respiratory infections.

OBJECTIVE: Meconium ileus, large volume mushy stools with an offensive odor, or undigested fat in stools may suggest cystic fibrosis in infants. Tenderness, rigidity over umbilical area, slow pulse, jaundice, and emaciation may all be found in adults with gastrointestinal problems.

PLAN:

CONTRAINDICATIONS: Those individuals hypersensitive to pork protein should avoid this therapy.

WARNINGS: Treat primary disorder in addition to providing this supplemental therapy.

PRECAUTIONS: Avoid inhaling the powder form or allowing it to come into contact with the skin as irritation may be produced. Do not use in pregnancy unless the potential benefits outweigh the unknown risks to fetus. It is also to be used with caution in breast-feeding women.

IMPLEMENTATION:

DRUG INTERACTIONS: Antacids containing calcium carbonate or magnesium hydroxide may cancel out the therapeutic effect of this medication. Serum iron levels due to iron supplements may be decreased by these preparations.

ADMINISTRATION AND DOSAGE: Digestive enzymes are administered with meals or snacks. They are available in tablet or capsule form which is swallowed, not chewed. It also comes in powder, or the capsules may be opened and sprinkled on food for those who have difficulty swallowing tablets. Medication granules are not to be taken without food as this will destroy the enzymes.

Therapeutic dosage may be determined after several weeks of therapy and adjusted accordingly. Different flavors are provided by the product manufacturers.

IMPLEMENTATION CONSIDERATIONS:

—Obtain a complete health history to identify the underlying cause of problem, concurrent use of medication, hypersensitivities, and previous therapy.

—Determine that the patient maintains a well-balanced diet of fats, proteins and carbohydrates. Medication should be incorporated into regular meal schedule.

—Determine the average quantity of dietary fat eaten daily. This may affect dosage levels.

—Provide for patient experimentation with various flavors.

—If sensitivity should occur, discontinue the drug.

WHAT THE PATIENT NEEDS TO KNOW:

—Take this medication exactly as ordered. Swallow capsules or tablets at mealtime, or open capsules of powder and sprinkle on food if you have difficulty swallowing pill.

—Always take granules with meals or snacks. Your body will destroy the granules and not receive any benefit from them if you don't provide food with them.

—When opening the powder and pouring it, be careful not to inhale it, or touch it with your hands. Direct exposure to the powder produces a strong irritation.

—Eat a well-balanced diet, with adequate amounts of fat, starch, and protein. You should develop and maintain a normal eating routine. This will help prevent indigestion.

—Experiment with various flavors of medication until you find the ones you like best.

—Report any discomfort or troublesome symptoms to your practitioner.

EVALUATION:

ADVERSE REACTIONS: If proper dietary balance of fat, protein, and starch is not maintained, temporary indigestion may develop. Nausea, abdominal cramps, and diarrhea have been reported in patients taking high doses. Inhalation of powder may provoke asthma.

OVERDOSAGE: Constipation or anorexia are indications of overdosage. Hyperuricosuria and hyperuricemia may be found with extremely high doses of the drug.

PARAMETERS TO MONITOR: Monitor for therapeutic effect and absence of adverse reactions. Questioning the patient about the appearance of stools may help in evaluating degree of malabsorption present. Examination of stools may also be valuable.

PANCREATIN

PRODUCTS (TRADE NAME):

Pancreatin (Available in 325 mg pancreatin tablet with 8,125 units amylase, 650 units lipase and 8,125 units protease; or 1000 mg pancreatin enteric-coated tablet with 25,000 units amylase, 2,000 units lipase, and 25,000 units protease). **Viokase** (Available in 325 mg pancreatin tablet with 48,000 units amylase, 6500 units lipase and 32,000 units protease; or a powder with 112,500 units amylase, 15,000 units lipase, and 75,000 units protease).

DRUG SPECIFICS:

This product tends to be cheaper than pancrelipase, although not as effective.

ADMINISTRATION AND DOSAGE SPECIFICS:

Give 325 mg to 1 gm with meals.

PANCRELIPASE

PRODUCTS (TRADE NAME):

Cotazym (Available in capsules containing 8,000 units lipase, 30,000 units protease, 30,000 units amylase, and other enzymes with 25 mg calcium carbonate; powder packets containing 16,000 units lipase, 60,000 units protease, 60,000 amylase, and other enzymes with 50 mg calcium carbonate per packet; and powder packets containing 40,000 units lipase, 150,000 units protease, 150,000 units amylase, and other enzymes with 50 mg calcium carbonate per packet). **Cotazym S** (Available in 5,000 units lipase, 20,000 units protease, and 20,000 amylase per packet.) **Ilozyme** (Available in 400 mg pancrelipase tablets, with 9,600 units lipase, 40,000 units protease, and 40,000 units amylase). **Ku-Zyme HP** (Available in capsules with 8,000 units lipase, 30,000 units protease and 30,000 units amylase). **Pancrease** (Available in capsules with 4,000 units lipase, 25,000 units protease, and 20,000 units amylase).

DRUG SPECIFICS:

Pancrelipase is a prescription drug combination of the pancreatic enzymes used in replacement therapy. It works more effectively than pancreatin. It provides a catalyst effect in the hydrolyzation of fats, proteins; and starch.

ADMINISTRATION AND DOSAGE:

The amount of dietary fat is the key to dosage. For every 17 Gm of fat, 300 mg of pancrelipase should be taken.

Use 1-3 capsules or tablets (or 1-2 packets) just before each meal or snack.

Bonnie K. Winterton

EMETICS

Emetics are drugs used in emergency situations to remove poisons from the stomach before they can be absorbed. They have largely replaced gastric lavage as the treatment of choice in management of poisoning or drug overdosage. Except in situations for which they are contraindicated, they are superior to lavage for rapid elimination of poisons before extensive absorption of gastric contents can occur. There are only two emetics commonly used in current clinical practice: apomorphine and syrup of ipecac. Apomorphine is given by injection and acts directly on the central nervous system. The nurse practitioner is more likely to use and to recommend the use of syrup of ipecac, an oral preparation, and it is the only drug discussed in this section.

SYRUP OF IPECAC

ACTION OF THE DRUG: Acts primarily as a gastric irritant to produce vomiting. Then, after absorption it stimulates the chemoreceptor trigger zone in the brain to induce vomiting.

ASSESSMENT:

INDICATIONS: This product is used when patients have ingested toxic substances, to empty the stomach before the toxins can be absorbed. (See Contraindications).

SUBJECTIVE: Patient has ingested a toxic substance that should be removed by vomiting.

OBJECTIVE: Patient is conscious, with no evidence of shock or convulsions.

PLAN:

CONTRAINDICATIONS: Never induce vomiting after ingestion of corrosive or caustic substances such as lye; regurgitation will only expose the esophagus to additional injury.

WARNINGS: Emetics should never be used in unconscious patients, in those who are convulsing, severely inebriated, in shock, or who have loss of the gag reflex. There is a difference of opinion as to use of the emetic if the ingested substance is a petroleum distillate (kerosene, gasoline, etc.). Previously considered a contraindication because of the possibility of aspiration of the vomitus and oils with resulting lipid pneumonia, many investigators now believe that the benefits outweigh the risks. The clinician must therefore weigh the benefits and risks and make a decision based on each individual situation.

PRECAUTIONS: Emetics may not be effective in those cases in which the ingested substance is an antiemetic.

Always clearly indicate ipecac *syrup* not the single word "ipecac," to avoid confusion with the fluid extract which is 14 times more concentrated.

IMPLEMENTATION:

DRUG INTERACTIONS: Should not be given with activated charcoal or with milk as they will adsorb the ipecac, neutralizing the emetic effect.

PRODUCT (TRADE NAMES):

Syrup of Ipecac (Available in 15, 30, 120, pt and gallon size; contains 7 grams ipecac per 100 ml.) Do not confuse with fluidextract ipecac which is 14 times more concentrated.

ADMINISTRATION AND DOSAGE: Syrup of ipecac is administered orally.

Children over one year of age: 1 tablespoonful (15 ml) followed by 2-3 glasses of water (200-300 ml).

Under one year of age: 2 teaspoonfuls followed by 1-2 glasses of water. Dose may be repeated once after 20 minutes if vomiting does not occur.

IMPLEMENTATION CONSIDERATIONS:

—Obtain a complete history from patient or anyone who can give details about what was ingested, when, and what has happened during that time.

—Consult with local poison control center if uncertain as how to proceed.

—If 2 doses do not produce vomiting within 30 minutes; referral and gastric lavage is necessary.

—After the emergency treatment, patient counseling is needed. If the ingestion was a deliberate drug overdosage, emotional support and adequate therapy for the underlying cause must be instituted. If an accidental overdosage of medication was taken, more teaching as to drug awareness and the need for careful regulation of dosage is in order. If this is an accidental ingestion of poison by a child there will be need for teaching basic safety rules and, frequently, a need for emotional support to reduce adult guilt and self-recrimination.

—Most parents should be encouraged to keep syrup of ipecac at home in their emergency medicine supply and be taught how and when to use it. This will avoid valuable delays in time as ipecac may be administered before starting for emergency room or health provider.

WHAT THE PATIENT NEEDS TO KNOW:

—It is wise to keep one-ounce bottles of syrup of ipecac readily available in your home in case of a poisoning emergency.

—Keep this medication out of the reach of children or others who might take it inadvertently.

—In case of an accidental episode of poisoning, first call the local poison control center, your health care provider, or hospital emergency room before using the syrup of ipecac.

—This product produces vomiting. If emptying of stomach has not occurred within 20 minutes, a second dose may be taken. Follow each dose with at least two glasses of water.

—Patient should be brought to emergency room or office immediately so that they may be adequately evaluated.

EVALUATION:

ADVERSE REACTIONS: Drug is not absorbed and has no systemic effect, unless vomiting does not occur within thirty minutes. If the drug is absorbed or excessive dose is ingested, it may cause cardiac arrhythmias, atrial fibrillation, or other cardio-toxic effect. For this reason, gastric lavage is necessary if vomiting does not occur within thirty minutes.

OVERDOSAGE: See above.

PARAMETERS TO MONITOR: The only parameter to monitor in connection with the syrup of ipecac is the occurrence of vomiting. Other parameters to monitor depend upon the ingested substance and its effect on the body. Practitioner should also assess whether this situation is likely to happen again, and take necessary counseling or teaching steps to reduce this possibility.

Patricia Newton

HISTAMINE H$_2$ RECEPTOR ANTAGONISTS

ACTION OF THE DRUG: These products are unique in their promotion of healing of gastric and duodenal ulcers. They act synergistically with antacids to produce a more alkaline gastrointestinal media. They block histamine, inhibit the secretion of gastric acid, and are rapidly absorbed, reaching peak of effectiveness in 45 to 90 minutes.

ASSESSMENT:

INDICATIONS: Histamine receptor antagonists promote healing of duodenal ulcers when used over 6 to 8 weeks. Relapse following discontinuation of medication is common. It is used in the prophylaxis and treatment of peptic esophagitis, benign gastric ulcers, duodenal ulcers, stress ulcers, and Zollinger-Ellison syndrome. It is being used experimentally in the treatment of patients with osteoarthritis who have an intolerance to aspirin and for patients with renal failure, and in prophylaxis of aspiration pneumonitis, acute upper GI bleeding, in the treatment of primary hyperparathyroidism, reflux esophagitis, hirsutism, herpes virus infection and tinea capitis.

SUBJECTIVE: Patient may complain of typical pain of peptic ulcer: gnawing, burning, aching pain (like hunger pangs) that comes and goes, which occur 45-60 minutes after meals, and is relieved by eating, vomiting, or antacids. Patient may also have complaints of diarrhea, chronic peptic ulcer disease uncontrolled by medication, hemorrhage, nausea, vomiting, weight loss, constipation, and fatigue.

OBJECTIVE: On examination, pain is often located in the midline near the esophagus with point tenderness in the peptic or duodenal area (on deep or superficial palpation), possibly radiating to the back. Muscle guarding may be noted upon examination. Vomiting highly acidic gastric juice with little or no food may also be documented. Blood in stools, bleeding, hypochromic anemia, and acid findings on gastric analysis may be found. X-ray may reveal an ulcer crater or show other evidence of gastrointestinal problems through radiologic exam or duodenoscopy.

PLAN:

WARNINGS: Leukopenia, elevated serum creatinine levels, and decreases in IgA and IgM have been reported following use of this drug.

PRECAUTIONS: Weigh potential benefits against unknown hazards when using in pregnant women, women of childbearing years, breast-feeding women and children under 16 years. A weak antiandrogenic effect without impairment of sexual abilities has been found with use of this drug. Gynecomastia has been noted in treatments lasting more than one month. Sperm count is decreased while cimetidine is administered. Ranitidine should be used cautiously in patients with renal or hepatic dysfunction. Weak cases of cardiac arrhythmias and hypotension are found when administered rapidly IV. Gastric malignancies may be masked by this therapy.

IMPLEMENTATION:

DRUG INTERACTIONS: Antacids may increase the absorption of cimetidine. Patients on warfarin may experience an increase in the anticoagulant effect when cimetidine is used concurrently. Cimetidine may increase the effects of phenytoin, beta-adrenergic blocking agents, lidocaine, benzodiazepine derivatives, and theophylline. Decreased white blood cell counts, including agranulocytosis have been reported in cimetidine-treated patients who also received other drugs and treatment known to produce neutropenia, especially antimetabolites and alkylating agents. Apnea, confusion and muscle twitching may be produced when cimetidine is administered with morphine. Carbamazepine toxicity may be precipitated with concurrent use of cimetidine. Serum digoxin levels may be reduced when digoxin and cimetidine are administered together. Cigarette smoking may neutralize the action of cimetidine. Ranitidine is less likely than cimetidine to interact with warfarin-type anticoagulants, theophylline or diazepam, although it does produce false-positive urine protein tests when Multistix is used.

ADMINISTRATION AND DOSAGE: May be administered IV or po. Administer orally with meals and at bedtime. IV infusions or injections should be diluted and injected over 1-2 minutes or given by infusion, and are most likely given to patients with hypersecretion of gastric acid or intractable pain from ulcers.

IMPLEMENTATION CONSIDERATIONS:

—Obtain a complete health history including the presence of underlying disease, hypersensitivities, past history of present illness, concurrent use of medications and any adverse reactions from previous treatment.

—This medication should be given for 2-6 weeks until endoscopy reveals healing.

—Remember that this drug may mask underlying malignancy.

WHAT THE PATIENT NEEDS TO KNOW:

—Take this medication exactly as ordered by your health Do not stop it without being advised to do so.

—During the treatment for your problem you will need to ma visits to your health provider for examination and laboratory tests important in assessing the healing process.

—Report any new or troublesome complaints to your practitioner s they may be adequately evaluated.

—Peptic and duodenal ulcers tend to recur. It will be important to try determine what causes your problem and to try to correct it. This medication is only part of your therapy. Controlling stress, avoiding sporadic eating and stressful living habits, and eliminating other diseases and infections are important.

—Keep this medication out of the reach of children and all others for whom it is not prescribed.

—Antacid therapy is helpful when taken with this medication. Be sure to keep antacids at home or office for use with the first appearance of gastric distress.

EVALUATION:

ADVERSE REACTIONS: Side effects are unusual, but patient may experience mild and self-limiting problems. *CNS:* dizziness, headaches, somnolence. *Gastrointestinal:* hemorrhage, mild and transient diarrhea. *Hematopoietic:* agranulocytosis, aplastic anemia, decreased white blood count, rash, thrombocytopenia. *Other:* galactorrhea, impotence, increase in plasma creatinine and serum transaminase, mild gynecomastia, muscle pain. Fever, interstitial nephritis, hepatitis, and pancreatitis are rare and clear up when the drug is discontinued.

OVERDOSAGE: Patients taking up to 10 gms of cimetidine have shown no symptoms of toxicity. Respiratory failure and tachycardia have been found in experimental studies on animals.

PARAMETERS TO MONITOR: Obtain a baseline history and laboratory studies. Evaluate patient for therapeutic effect by monitoring decrease in symptoms. Check prothrombin time every week if the patient is on anticoagulant therapy, especially with warfarin. Watch for an increase in the anticoagulant effect. Monitor plasma creatinine and serum transaminase levels for any increase. Unless complications exist, it is unnecessary to repeat any of the diagnostic work. When extended treatment seems necessary, blood work should be obtained periodically to check for adverse effects. On return visits, examine for rash and for the appearance of gynecomastia in males. Patients who continue to have gastric discomfort and do not have ulcer healing should be referred for further evaluation and management.

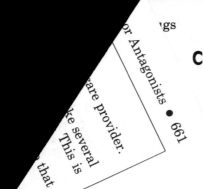

CIMETIDINE

...d 300 mg tablets, 300 mg/5 ml liquid, and 300

...tment of ulcers. Has more drug interactions

...GE SPECIFICS:

...00 mg po four times a day with meals and at bedtime,
...IV. Should be taken with antacids. In patients with hy-
...ic acid, give up to 2400 mg/day. For patients with renal failure,
...very 8-12 hours.

RANITIDINE

PRODUCTS (TRADE NAME):
   Zantac (Available in 150 mg tablets.)
DRUG SPECIFICS:
   New product which is similar in action to cimetidine but has fewer drug in-
teractions. Headache is a frequent side effect in these patients. SGPT values may
be increased with this product. Drug may be taken with food or antacids. Gastric
healing may occur within 2 weeks and gastroscopy at that time may show that
therapy can be terminated.
ADMINISTRATION AND DOSAGE SPECIFICS:
   Duodenal ulcer: 150 mg twice daily po. Do not give more than 150 mg/24 hours
if creatinine clearance is below 50 ml/min.
   Zollinger-Ellison syndrome: Give 150 mg po twice daily to decrease hyperse-
cretory conditions. May increase dosage as necessary up to 6 gm/day.

Bonnie K. Winterton

LAXATIVES—BULK-FORMING

ACTION OF THE DRUG: Laxatives are drugs that change fecal consistency, speed
passage of feces through the colon, and aid in elimination of stool from the rectum.
They are classified in five major categories, based on mechanism of action. Bulk-
forming laxatives is one of these categories. The bulk-forming agents absorb water
and expand, increasing both bulk and moisture content of the stool. The increased

bulk stimulates peristalsis and the absorbed water softens the stool. These agents are not absorbed systemically.

ASSESSMENT:

INDICATIONS: These drugs are used in simple constipation, and in atonic constipation from overuse of other cathartics. Bulk-forming laxatives are also particularly useful in postpartum, elderly, and debilitated patients. They have been used in treatment of diverticulosis and irritable bowel syndrome.

SUBJECTIVE: Patient may complain of increased hardness of stool or difficulty passing stool. Decreased frequency of stools, mild abdominal discomfort and distention, and occasionally mild anorexia may be present.

OBJECTIVE: Normal bowel sounds should be present, with no abdominal tenderness to palpation. Digital rectal examination may show hard stool in rectum. Abdominal examination may reveal a palpable colon; fecal material which is very firm, but which may be molded. (No other intra-abdominal mass may be so molded.)

PLAN:

CONTRAINDICATIONS: Do not use with abdominal pain, nausea, vomiting, other signs of appendicitis, or acute surgical abdomen. Other contraindications include fecal impaction, intestinal ulcerations, stenosis or obstruction, disabling adhesions, or dysphagia.

WARNINGS: Many of these products contain significant amounts of dextrose, galactose, and sucrose and should be avoided in patients with diabetes mellitus. Allergic reactions (urticaria, rhinitis, and asthma) may occur due to the plant gums present in these agents. This should be considered in patients with a history of allergic reactions, especially to plants.

PRECAUTIONS: These agents may become dry, thick, and hardened in the throat or within the intestine if they are swallowed without sufficient water. They can cause esophageal or intestinal obstruction or impaction if this occurs. The drugs should never be chewed or swallowed without one or more full glasses of water.

IMPLEMENTATION:

DRUG INTERACTIONS: Antibiotics, anticoagulants, digitalis preparations, and salicylates may have reduced effectiveness if used concurrently with bulk-forming agents because of binding and hindrance of absorption. A two-hour interval between dosages of these medications is recommended.

ADMINISTRATION AND DOSAGE: All of the bulk-forming laxatives are administered orally, with one or more glasses of liquid. Individual dosages are listed with specific product information.

IMPLEMENTATION CONSIDERATIONS:

—Obtain a complete health history including presence of diabetes, swallowing difficulty, asthma or seasonal allergies, allergy to specific plant gums.

—Constipation that persists should always be evaluated for serious organic causes. Changes in bowel habits, especially waking up at night to defecate, should always be investigated.

—Results from laxatives are obtained in 12 to 72 hours.

—Before giving medication for constipation, make certain patient is well hydrated.

—Begin education regarding usefulness of exercise, diet, and liquids in diet to reduce constipation.

WHAT THE PATIENT NEEDS TO KNOW:

—These agents require large amounts of fluid to work properly. They should never be chewed or swallowed without water. Take at least one full glass of liquid with each dose.

—These drugs should be taken exactly as specified by your health provider and are indicated for short-term use only. Overuse of laxatives robs the bowel of its ability to perform effectively on its own.

—Some agents are high in sodium or glucose. Check content if diet is restricted.

—Laxative should be used only as additional therapy to good, regular bowel habits, daily exercise, and the use of high bulk foods and fruits in diet to help maintain regularity.

—The bulk-forming laxatives should not be taken within two hours of any other medictions.

—Allergic reactions may occur. If rash, itching, nasal congestion, or wheezing occur, stop medication immediately and contact your health care provider.

—The laxative effect may occur within 12 hours or may take up to 3 days to appear.

EVALUATION:

ADVERSE REACTIONS: *Gastrointestinal:* abdominal cramps, diarrhea, esophageal, gastric, small intestine or colonic strictures and obstructions when taken without sufficient liquid, nausea, vomiting. *Hypersensitivity:* asthma, dermatitis, rhinitis, urticaria.

PARAMETERS TO MONITOR: Bulk-forming laxatives should be used only for very short periods and therefore should not require any patient monitoring. If for any reason they are used on a long-term basis, question patient about bowel habits, diet, and exercise and monitor for adverse reactions.

METHYLCELLULOSE

PRODUCTS (TRADE NAME):

Cologel (Available in 450 mg/5 ml liquid.) **Maltsuprex** (Available in 750 mg tablets, powder or liquid.)

DRUG SPECIFICS:

This product is indigestible, nonabsorbable, and does not interfere with intestinal absorption of nutrients. It produces a laxative effect in 12 to 72 hours. All doses should be taken with one full glass or more of liquid.

ADMINISTRATION AND DOSAGE SPECIFICS:

Adults: Give 5 to 20 ml liquid po three times a day with a full glass of water. Or 1 to 3 capsules or tablets may be taken po four times daily with meals and at bedtime.

Children: Take 5 to 10 ml liquid po once or twice daily.

PSYLLIUM SEED

PRODUCTS (TRADE NAME):

Effersyllium Instant Mix, Hydrocil Instant, Hydrocil Plain, Konsyl, L.A. Formula, Metamucil, Metamucil Instant Mix, Modane Bulk, Mucillium (Available in powder.) **Mucilose** (Available in 420 gm granules and flakes.) **Regacillium, Reguloid, Saraka, Siblin, Syllact, V-Lax** (Available in powder.)

DRUG SPECIFICS:

This product is made of whole or powdered seeds of a species of *Plantago,* and are indigestible, nonabsorbed, and do not interfere with absorption of nutrients. These laxatives are least likely to cause laxative abuse. Metamucil now comes in a sugar-free form for diabetics.

ADMINISTRATION AND DOSAGE SPECIFICS:

Adults: Take 1 to 2 teaspoonfuls po in full glass of water once, twice, or three times daily; follow by second glass of water.

Children over 6 years: Take 1 teaspoon in 1/2 glass of water at bedtime.

Patricia Newton

LAXATIVES—FECAL SOFTENERS (WETTING AGENTS)

ACTION OF THE DRUG: Laxatives are drugs that change fecal consistency, speed passage of feces through the colon, and aid in elimination of stool from the rectum. They are classified into five categories based on the mechanism of action. One of these categories includes fecal softeners or wetting agents. These act to soften stool by lowering surface tension, allowing the fecal mass to be penetrated by intestinal fluids. They also inhibit fluid and electrolyte reabsorption by the intestine.

ASSESSMENT:

INDICATIONS: Fecal softeners are helpful in relieving constipation produced by a delay in rectal emptying. They are also useful when it is important to reduce straining at stool, as in patients with hernia, cardiovascular disease, postpartum, or after rectal surgery.

SUBJECTIVE: Patients may complain of increased hardness of stool or difficulty passing stool. Decreased frequency of stools, abdominal discomfort, and distention may also be present.

OBJECTIVE: Normal bowel sounds are usually present, with no tenderness on palpation of the abdomen. Digital examination may reveal hard stool in the rectum.

PLAN:

CONTRAINDICATIONS: Do not use in patients with abdominal pain, nausea, vomiting, or other signs of appendicitis or surgical abdomen. Fecal impaction and intestinal obstruction are also contraindications.

WARNINGS: Never use concurrently with mineral oil or other laxatives, particularly phenolphthalein or danthron. The systemic absorption of the other agents will be enhanced, causing a greater risk of toxic effects.

IMPLEMENTATION:

DRUG INTERACTIONS: Fecal softeners enhance absorption of mineral oil and other laxatives.

PRODUCTS (TRADE NAME):

Docusate Calcium: **Docusate Calcium, Pro-Cal-Sof, Surfak** (Available in 240 mg capsules.) **Surfak** (Available in 50 mg capsules.)

Docusate Potassium: **Dialose** (Available in 100 mg capsules.) **Kasof** (Available in 240 mg capsules.)

Docusate Sodium: **Afko-Lube** (Available in 100 and 250 mg capsules, and 20 mg/5 ml syrup.) **Bu-Lax, Colace** (Available in 50, 100 and 250 mg capsules, 10 mg/ml drops, syrup of 20 mg/5 ml). **Comfolax, Diosuccin, Dio-Sul** (Available in 100 mg capsules.) **Disonate** (Available in 60, 100, and 240 mg capsules and 10 mg/ml drops.) **Docusate Sodium** (Available in 50, 100 and 250 mg capsules, 100 mg tablets, and 20 mg/5 ml and 50 mg/15 ml syrup.) **Doxinate** (Available in 60 mg and 240 mg capsules, 50 mg/ml solution.) **Laxinate 100** (Available in 100 mg capsules.) **Modane Soft** (Available in 120 mg capsules.) **Molatoc, Regutol, Stulex** (Available in 100 mg tablets.)

ADMINISTRATION AND DOSAGE:

Docusate calcium preparations:

Adults: 240 mg daily po.

Children: One to three 50 mg capsules daily.

Docusate potassium preparations:

Adults: 240 mg daily po.

Colace:

Adults: 50 to 200 mg daily po.
Children 6 to 12 years: 40 to 120 mg po daily.
Children 3 to 6 years: 20 to 60 mg po daily.
Comfolax:
Adults: 1 to 2 capsules daily by mouth.
Children 6 to 12 years: 40 to 120 mg po daily.

IMPLEMENTATION CONSIDERATIONS:

—Obtain a complete health history including presence of allergies or adverse reactions to laxative preparations, presence of systemic diseases, or edema, congestive heart failure, use of a sodium-restricted diet, and other drugs taken concurrently. Evaluate the patient potential for abuse.

—Constipation that persists should always be evaluated for serious organic causes. Any change in bowel habits should be investigated.

—When using fecal softeners to prevent constipation, be sure patient has adequate fluid intake, bulk in the diet, and daily exercise. Educate patient to danger of overuse of laxatives.

—Sodium salt products should be avoided in patients with edema, congestive heart failure, and sodium-restricted diets. The potassium salt should be avoided in patients with renal impairment.

WHAT THE PATIENT NEEDS TO KNOW:

—These drugs should be taken exactly as specified by your health care provider and are indicated for short-term use only. Overuse of laxatives robs the bowel of its ability to perform effectively on its own.

—Fecal softeners should be used only as additional therapy to good, regular bowel habits, daily exercise, and the use of high bulk in the diet to help maintain regularity. They do not treat pre-existing constipation, but prevent constipation from developing.

—Many of these agents contain sodium. Check content if your diet is restricted in sodium, or if you have swelling of ankles or hands.

—Take milk or fruit juice to mask the bitter taste.

—These preparations act within 24 to 48 hours.

—Your health provider can give you a list of food high in bulk which you can eat to assist you in maintaining bowel regularity.

EVALUATION:

ADVERSE REACTIONS: *Gastrointestinal:* diarrhea, mild abdominal cramping. *Other:* laxative dependence in long-term use.

PARAMETERS TO MONITOR: Discuss dietary habits with patients and need for laxatives and fecal softeners on regular basis. Monitor bowel habits with the goal of achieving regularity without drugs. Watch for laxative abuse.

Patricia Newton

LAXATIVES—HYPEROSMOLAR AND SALINE

ACTION OF THE DRUG: Laxatives are drugs that change fecal consistency, speed passage of feces through the colon, and aid in elimination of stool from the rectum. They are classified into five categories, based on mechanism of action. Hyperosmolar or saline laxatives make up one of these categories. Hyperosmolar laxatives, lactulose, and glycerin, produce an osmotic effect in the colon, distending the bowel from fluid accumulation, promoting peristalsis and bowel movement. The saline laxatives also produce an osmotic effect, drawing water into the intestinal lumen of the small intestine as well as the colon.

ASSESSMENT:

INDICATIONS: Saline laxatives are used to cleanse the bowel in preparation for endoscopic examination, x-ray studies, or surgery. They are used to hasten evacuation of worms after administration of anthelmintics, and after the ingestion of poisons to hasten elimination of toxic material. Lactulose and glycerin are used most frequently in the treatment of simple constipation.

SUBJECTIVE: Patient may complain of increased hardness of stool or difficulty passing stool. Decreased frequency of stools is not often important if stool is soft and easily passed, but is often considered important by the patient. Mild abdominal discomfort, distention, and occasionally mild anorexia may also be noted.

OBJECTIVE: Normal bowel sounds should be present in simple constipation. There is no abdominal tenderness to palpation. Digital rectal examination may find hard stool in the rectum. Abdominal examination may reveal palpable colon and fecal material which is very firm but moldable. (This helps in making the diagnosis as no other intra-abdominal mass may be molded.)

PLAN:

CONTRAINDICATIONS: Do not use in the presence of hypersensitivity to any of the drug components, abdominal pain, nausea, vomiting, or other signs of appendicitis or acute surgical abdomen. Fecal impaction, intestinal obstruction, and rectal fissures also present contraindications.

WARNINGS: Use with caution in patients with renal impairment, particularly the preparations containing magnesium and potassium salts. Sodium salts should not be used in cardiac patients with edema or signs of congestive heart failure. Sodium salts should be avoided by patients on low-sodium diets. The sodium salts may promote sodium retention with resultant edema in pregnancy. Lactulose should be used cautiously in diabetic patients or in those who need a low galactose diet.

PRECAUTIONS: Congestive heart failure has been precipitated in patients who use saline cathartics without careful supervision. Severe hyperkalemia and hypermagnesemia have been produced in patients with renal impairment who abuse these laxatives. Since they are available without prescription, patient education as to these serious side effects is especially important.

IMPLEMENTATION:

DRUG INTERACTIONS: Hyperosmolar saline laxatives should not be taken within one to three hours of tetracyclines as they may form nonabsorbable complexes.

ADMINISTRATION AND DOSAGE: Lactulose and the saline laxatives are administered orally, with individual dosages listed with specific product information. Glycerin is administered by rectal suppository or as an enema.

IMPLEMENTATION CONSIDERATIONS:

—Obtain a complete health history including history of hypersensitivities, underlying medical problems such as renal impairment, cardiac disease, congestive heart failure, previous adverse reaction to these preparations, or possibility of pregnancy.

—Constipation is a common complaint with many possible causes. To treat correctly, the etiology, age, physical condition, and preferences of the patient must be considered.

—Patients should be taught about the use of diet in correcting constipation: the use of bulk-forming foods, fruits, vegetables, and whole grain cereals. Encourage increased physical activity within patient capabilities. Proper bowel habits should be discussed and encouraged. Increased fluid intake is very important.

—Constipation that persists for several weeks should always be evaluated for more serious organic cause, especially changes in bowel habits, including getting up at night to defecate.

—Plan medication administration to allow the drug's effects to occur at a time that will not interfere with patient's rest or digestion.

WHAT THE PATIENT NEEDS TO KNOW:

—These drugs should be taken exactly as specified by your health care provider and are indicated for short-term use only. Overuse of laxatives robs the bowel of its ability to perform effectively on its own. Do not use in children under 6 years of age.

—Laxatives should be used only as additional therapy to good, regular bowel habits, daily exercise, and the use of high bulk in diet to help maintain regularity.

—The saline laxatives produce results within 2 to 8 hours and should not be taken at bedtime.

—Lactulose may require 24 to 48 hours to produce a normal bowel movement.

—The fastest effect is obtained when drug is taken on an empty stomach with a full glass of water.

—Flavor may be improved by taking medication with fruit juice or a citrusflavored carbonated beverage.

—Saline laxatives should not be taken daily, nor used in children under six years of age. If you have underlying heart or renal disease you must be especially careful in your use of these preparations.

EVALUATION:

ADVERSE REACTIONS: *Gastrointestinal:* abdominal cramping, nausea. *Metabolic:* fluid and electrolyte disturbance if used daily, or in renal impairment. *Other:* laxative dependence with excessive or long-term use.

OVERDOSAGE: *Signs and symptoms:* Hypermagnesemia occurs almost exclusively in patients with chronic renal insufficiency, and is aggravated by increased intake of magnesium. Paresthesias, vasodilatation, mild hypotension, muscle weakness, and decreased tendon reflexes may be found. In patients with cardiac disease or congestive heart failure, the increased sodium intake in the sodium-containing saline cathartics can precipitate or worsen congestive heart failure. *Treatment:* Symptomatic treatment of effects.

PARAMETERS TO MONITOR: Saline cathartics should not be taken over extended periods, seldom used more than once in any short period, and therefore would not usually require monitoring. Elderly, debilitated patients taking lactulose over long periods should have serum electrolytes monitored periodically and evaluated for adverse reactions.

LACTULOSE

PRODUCTS (TRADE NAME):
Chronulac (Available in 8 oz or 1 qt bottles of syrup.)
DRUG SPECIFICS:
Lactulose may require 24 to 48 hours to produce a normal bowel movement. It is used in the treatment of simple, chronic constipation. It is very poorly absorbed from the gastrointestinal tract and has no systemic effect. It is available without prescription.
ADMINISTRATION AND DOSAGE SPECIFICS:
Adults: Give 15 to 30 ml po daily. May be increased to 60 ml po daily if necessary.

MAGNESIUM SALTS

PRODUCTS (TRADE NAME):
Citroma, Citro-Nesia, Concentrated Milk of Magnesia, Milk of Magnesia, Magnesium Citrate, Magnesium Sulfate (Available in 4, 12, and 26 oz bottles or powder.)
DRUG SPECIFICS:
Laxative action begins within 2-6 hours. Magnesium sulfate is the most potent of the products within this group. Use with caution in patients with decreased renal function.

ADMINISTRATION AND DOSAGE SPECIFICS:
Concentrated milk of magnesia: Give 10 to 20 ml po.
Milk of magnesia: Give 30 to 60 ml po, usually at bedtime.
Magnesium citrate: Give 5 to 10 oz po at bedtime.
Magnesium sulfate: Give 15 mg (4 teaspoonfuls) in a glass of water.

SODIUM SALTS

PRODUCTS (TRADE NAME):
Fleet Enema (Available in 4 1/2 oz ready to use bottles.) **Phospho-Soda** (Available in 3 and 8 fluid oz bottles.) **Sodium Phosphate, Sodium Phosphate and Biphosphate** (Available in powder.)
DRUG SPECIFICS:
Up to 10% of the sodium in these products may be absorbed. This medication is available without prescription. Overuse may lead to hyperphosphotenvia.
ADMINISTRATION AND DOSAGE SPECIFICS:
For oral medication: Give 20 ml po mixed with 1/2 glass of water; follow with another full glass of water. Take this preferably on arising in the morning.
For enema: Use 4 ounces rectally for adults; 2 1/2 ounces for children over 2 years.

Patricia Newman

LAXATIVES—LUBRICANT

ACTION OF THE DRUG: Laxatives are drugs that change fecal consistency, speed passage of feces through the colon, and aid in elimination of stool from the rectum. They are classified into five categories based on the mechanism. One of these categories is lubricant laxatives. Lubricant laxatives create a barrier between the feces and the colon wall that prevents colonic reabsorption of fecal fluid, thus softening the stool. The lubricant effect also eases the passage of feces through the intestine.

ASSESSMENT:

INDICATIONS: Lubricant laxatives are used to soften stool in conditions where straining at stool should be avoided, as in myocardial infarction, aneurysm, stroke, hernia, or following abdominal or rectal surgery. They are also used to prevent discomfort and tearing or laceration of hemorrhoids or fissures.
SUBJECTIVE: Patient may complain of increased hardness of stool, or difficulty in passing stool. Rectal pain on attempting to pass hard, dry stool, and mild abdominal discomfort and distention may be present also.

OBJECTIVE: Normal bowel sounds should be present in simple constipation, with abdomen non-tender to palpation. Digital examination may reveal a hard stool in rectum. Inspection of rectal area may show fissures or hemorrhoids that cause pain with straining.

PLAN:

CONTRAINDICATIONS: Do not use in the presence of abdominal pain, nausea, vomiting, other signs of appendicitis or acute abdominal problems. Fecal impaction or intestinal obstruction also are contraindications for use.

WARNINGS: Use with caution in young children, or in elderly, or debilitated patients due to the possibility of lipid pneumonia resulting from aspiration of the oil. Droplets accumulate in the pharynx and are easily drawn into the lung. Chronic administration of mineral oil during pregnancy can reduce the vitamin K available to the fetus.

PRECAUTIONS: Chronic administration (more than two weeks) may decrease absorption of nutrients and fat-soluble vitamins (A, D, E, and K). Large doses may cause leakage of oil from the rectum, soiling of clothing, and pruritus.

IMPLEMENTATION:

DRUG INTERACTIONS: Lubricant laxatives may reduce the effectiveness of anticoagulants, contraceptives, digitalis, and fat-soluble vitamins if taken concurrently. They should not be taken with the fecal softeners because these agents enhance the systemic absorption of mineral oil, giving an increased laxative effect and toxicity to the liver.

PRODUCTS (TRADE NAME):

Agoral Plain (Available in liquid, jelly, emulsion or suspension in 8 and 16 oz bottles.) **Fleets Mineral Oil Enema** (Available in 4 oz bottle, ready to use). **Kondremul Plain, Mineral Oil, Neo-Cultol, Nujol, Petrogalar Plain, Zymenol** (Available in 8 and 16 oz bottles).

ADMINISTRATION AND DOSAGE: Mineral oil is used orally and also given rectally as an enema for retention and softening. It should be given at least two hours after meals.

Adults: Use 15 to 30 ml po orally at bedtime.

Children over 6 years: Use 5 to 15 ml po.

Rectally: Use 4 ounces administered as enema.

IMPLEMENTATION CONSIDERATIONS:

—Obtain a health history including history of allergy or adverse reaction to these preparations, concurrent use of other drugs which may cause drug interactions, presence of other systemic diseases, and possibility of pregnancy. Evaluate the patients potential for laxative abuse.

—For proper management, nurse must consider the reason for the medication, the age, physical condition, and preferences of the patient.

—Constipation that persists should always be evaluated for serious organic causes. Changes in bowel habits, including awakening at night to defecate, should be investigated.

—When treating constipation, be sure patient has adequate fluid intake, bulk in the diet, and daily exercise. Educate patient to dangers of overuse of laxatives.

—Time laxative administration so that it is not given within two hours of meals or medicine.

WHAT THE PATIENT NEEDS TO KNOW:

—These drugs should be taken exactly as specified by your health provider and are indicated for short-term use only. Overuse of laxatives robs the bowel of its ability to perform effectively on its own.

—Laxatives should be used only as additional therapy to good, regular bowel habits, daily exercise, and high bulk in the diet to help maintain regularity.

—Mineral oil should not be taken within two hours of taking food or other medication.

—Large doses may cause a leakage of oil from the rectum. The use of pads to protect clothing may be necessary if tight sphincter control is not present.

—Fruit juices or carbonated drinks may help disguise oily taste.

EVALUATION:

ADVERSE REACTIONS: *Gastrointestinal:* abdominal cramps, decreased absorption of nutrients and fat-soluble vitamins, diarrhea, nausea, slowed healing after rectal surgery and increased risk of infection due to seepage of oil from rectum, vomiting. *Other:* Laxative dependence with long-term or excessive use.

OVERDOSAGE: Lipid pneumonia caused by aspiration and deficiency syndromes reflecting decreased absorption of the fat-soluble vitamins may occur with long-term or excessive use. *Treatment:* symptomatic treatment of symptoms.

PARAMETERS TO MONITOR: These laxatives should be used only for very short periods and therefore would not require any patient monitoring. If for any reason they are used on a long-term basis, patients should be monitored for adverse reactions.

Patricia Newton

LAXATIVES—STIMULANT OR IRRITANT

ACTION OF THE DRUG: Laxatives are drugs that change fecal consistency, speed passage of feces through the colon, and aid in elimination of stool from the rectum. They are classified into five categories based on the mechanism of action. The first of these categories, stimulant or irritant laxatives, increase peristalsis by several mechanisms, depending upon the agent. Primary stimulation of colonic intramural nerve plexuses (senna preparations), stimulation of sensory nerves in the intestinal mucosa (bisacodyl), direct stimulation of smooth muscle and inhibition of water and electrolyte reabsorption from the intestinal lumen (castor oil).

ASSESSMENT:

INDICATIONS: Stimulant or irritant laxatives are useful for the treatment of constipation resulting from prolonged bedrest, poor dietary habits, or induced by other drugs. They are also used to cleanse the bowel in preparation for endoscopic examination, x-ray studies, or surgery.

SUBJECTIVE: Patient may complain of increased hardness of stool or difficulty passing stool. Decreased frequency of stools is not often important if stool is soft and easily passed, but is often considered important by the patient. Mild abdominal discomfort, distention, and occasionally mild anorexia may also be noted.

OBJECTIVE: Normal bowel sounds should be present in simple constipation. There is no abdominal tenderness to palpation. Digital rectal examination may find hard stool in the rectum. Abdominal examination may reveal palpable colon, fecal material which is very firm but moldable. (This helps in making the diagnosis as no other intra-abdominal mass may be molded.)

PLAN:

CONTRAINDICATIONS: Do not give laxatives with complaint of abdominal pain, nausea, vomiting, or if other signs of appendicitis or acute surgical abdomen are present. Fecal impaction and intestinal obstruction are also contraindications. Stimulant laxatives, especially castor oil, may cause uterine contractions in pregnancy.

WARNINGS: Stimulant laxatives containing anthraquinones (cascara, senna, danthron) are excreted in breast milk at levels that may cause laxative effect in the infant.

PRECAUTIONS: Overdosage or overusage may cause excessive fluid loss and electrolyte imbalance, particularly hypokalemia. Overuse can lead to atonic constipation and create laxative dependence. Patients need to be instructed in proper bowel habits, the need for fiber- and bulk-containing diet, and exercise programs. This group of laxatives are those most often abused, and all are available without prescription.

IMPLEMENTATION:

DRUG INTERACTIONS: Antacids or milk should not be taken with bisacodyl tablets as they cause a too-rapid dissolving of the enteric coating, resulting in gastric irritation. Some laxatives cause rapid transit through the bowel and so concurrent use of many medications which require time to dissolve may be adversely affected.

ADMINISTRATION AND DOSAGE: All of this group of laxatives are orally administered. Bisacodyl is also available as a suppository for rectal administration. Dosages vary and are listed with specific product information.

IMPLEMENTATION CONSIDERATIONS:

—Obtain a health history including history of allergy or adverse reaction to laxative preparations, presence of other systemic diseases, and possibility of pregnancy or breast feeding. Evaluate the patient's potential for abuse.

—Constipation that persists should always be evaluated for serious organic causes. Changes in bowel habits should always be investigated.

—When treating constipation, be sure patient has adequate fluid intake, bulk in the diet, and daily exercise. Educate patient to dangers of overuse of laxatives.

—The laxative effect of the phenolphthaleins may last up to 4 days.

—Constipation is a common complaint; for correct management the nurse must consider the etiology, age, and physical condition of the patient.

—This class of laxatives includes many of the chewing gum and chocolate types and is most often abused.

WHAT THE PATIENT NEEDS TO KNOW:

—These drugs should be taken exactly as specified by your health provider and are indicated for short-term use only. Overuse of laxatives robs the bowel of its ability to perform effectively on its own.

—Laxatives should be used only as additional therapy to good, regular bowel habits, daily exercise, and high bulk in diet to help maintain regularity.

—The stimulant laxatives act within 6 to 10 hours, except castor oil which acts within 1 to 3 hours.

—The laxative effect of phenolphthaleins may last up to 4 days.

—Many of the stimulant laxatives discolor alkaline urine red-pink and acid urine yellow-brown. They may cause a reddish color to feces.

—Bisacodyl enteric-coated tablets must be swallowed whole, never chewed or crushed, and never taken with milk or antacids.

EVALUATION:

ADVERSE REACTIONS: *CNS:* muscle weakness (following excessive use of laxatives). *Dermatologic:* dermatitis, pruritus. *Gastrointestinal:* abdominal cramps, diarrhea, discoloration of rectal mucosa with long-term use, nausea, vomiting. *Metabolic:* alkalosis, electrolyte imbalance (with excessive use), hypokalemia. *Other:* dependence on laxatives for bowel movement with excessive or long-term use.

OVERDOSAGE: Long-term, excessive use of stimulant laxatives may result in irritable bowel syndrome or a severe, prolonged diarrhea. These conditions may lead to hyponatremia, hypokalemia, dehydration, and protein-losing enteropathies. Cathartic colon, a syndrome resembling ulcerative colitis both radiologically and pathologically, may develop after chronic misuse. *Treatment:* Symptomatic treatment of imbalances and reeducation of the patient to prevent further laxative abuse.

PARAMETERS TO MONITOR: All of the stimulant laxatives should be used only for very short periods and therefore would not require any patient monitoring. If for any reason they are used on a long-term basis, serum electrolytes should be monitored periodically.

BISACODYL

PRODUCTS (TRADE NAME):
Biscolax (Available in 10 mg suppository.) **Cenalax, Deticol, Dulcolax** (Available in 5 mg tablets, and in 10 mg suppository). **Fleet Bisacodyl** (Available in 5 mg enteric-coated tablet, 10 mg suppository, and 1 1/2 oz Fleet enema). **Nuvac, Theralax** (Available in 10 mg suppository.)

DRUG SPECIFICS:
Enteric-coated tablets must be swallowed whole. Do not chew or crush. Do not take within one hour of antacids or milk. Drink at least one full glass of water with each dose. Suppository should be inserted at time bowel movement is desired; acts within 15 to 60 minutes. Enema is administered rectally at time evacuation is desired.

ADMINISTRATION AND DOSAGE SPECIFICS:
Adults: Give 10 to 15 mg po in evening or before breakfast. Up to 30 mg po may be safely used in preparation for special procedures.
Children: Give 5 to 10 mg po.
Children under 2 years: Give 2.5 mg suppository rectally.

CASCARA SAGRADA

PRODUCTS (TRADE NAME):
Cascara Sagrada (Available as aromatic fluidextract, plain fluidextract, which is 4 times more concentrated than the aromatic fluid extract, and as 325 mg tablets.)

DRUG SPECIFICS:
The fluidextract contains 18% alcohol. Under various brand names, some tablets are sugar-coated, others are uncoated. They may discolor alkaline urine red-pink, and acidic urine yellow-brown.

ADMINISTRATION AND DOSAGE SPECIFICS:
Adults: Aromatic: Give 5 ml daily with full glass of water. Plain: Give 1 ml po daily with glass of water. Tablet: Give one 325 mg tablet at bedtime.

CASTOR OIL

PRODUCTS (TRADE NAME):
Alphamul, Castor Oil, Emulsoil, Neoloid, Purge (Available in 30, 60, 120, 180, 240 ml liquid or emulsion.)

DRUG SPECIFICS

Give with juice or carbonated beverage to mask oily taste. Ice held in mouth also helps prevent tasting the drug. For best results give on empty stomach. Produces results within 3 hours. For emulsion preparation, shake well.

ADMINISTRATION AND DOSAGE SPECIFICS:

Adults: Give 15 to 60 ml po.

Children over 2 years: Give 5 to 15 ml po.

DANTHRON

PRODUCTS (TRADE NAME):

Danthron, Dorbane (Available in 75 mg tablets). **Modane Mild** (Available in 37.5 mg tablets). **Modane** (Available in 75 mg tablets or 37.5 mg/5 ml liquid).

DRUG SPECIFICS:

This preparation may discolor alkaline urine red-pink and acidic urine yellow-brown. It may discolor rectal mucosa in long-term use. Danthron is excreted in breast milk and should be avoided in nursing mothers.

ADMINISTRATION AND DOSAGE SPECIFICS:

Adults: Give 37.5 to 150 mg po with evening meal.

Children: Give 37.5 to 75 mg po with evening meal.

PHENOLPHTHALEIN

PRODUCTS (TRADE NAME):

Alophen Pills (Available in 60 mg tablet.) **Correctol** (Available in 65 mg/15 ml liquid.) **Espotabs** (Available in 97.5 mg tablet.) **Evac-U-Gen** (Available in 97.2 mg chewable tablet.) **Evac-U-Lax** (Available in 80 mg wafer.) **ExLax** (Available in 90 mg chew or swallow tablet.) **Feen-A-Mint** (Available in 97.2 mg mint or chewable tablet.) **Phenolax** (Available in 64.8 mg wafer.) **Prulet** (Available in 60 mg chewable tablet.)

DRUG SPECIFICS:

The laxative effect may last 3 to 4 days. It causes a reddish discoloration in alkaline feces and may discolor alkaline urine red-pink and acidic urine yellow-brown. It may cause a characteristic skin rash, and drug should be discontinued and patient advised to avoid exposure to sun until rash has disappeared. Most tablets are chewable.

ADMINISTRATION AND DOSAGE SPECIFICS:

Adults: Give 90 to 180 mg tablet, chewed well, night or morning.

Children: Give 45 to 90 mg tablet, chewed well, night or morning.

SENNA

PRODUCTS (TRADE NAME):

Black Draught (Available in 600 mg tablets and granules with 1/2 tsp equal to 1.65 gm). **Casafru** (Available in 120 and 240 ml syrup.) **Senexon** (Available in 100 mg tablet.) **Senokot** (Available in 187 mg tablets, 325 mg/5 ml granules, 218 mg/5 ml syrup, and 652 mg suppositories). **Senolax** (Available in 217 mg tablet.) **X-Prep** (Available in single dose powders or 2.5 oz liquid.)

DRUG SPECIFICS:

May cause yellow or yellow-green cast to feces, red-pink discoloration of alkaline urine; yellow-brown color in acid urine. After taking prescribed dose of X-Prep, diet should be confined to clear liquids. Drug is excreted in breast milk and should be avoided in nursing mothers.

ADMINISTRATION AND DOSAGE SPECIFICS:

Adults:

Black Draught: Give 1 to 3 tablets at bedtime; or 1/4 to 1/2 teaspoon granules with water.

Glysennid: Give 1 to 2 tablets at bedtime.

Senokot: Give 2 tablets, 1 teaspoon granules, or 10-15 ml syrup po at bedtime. Insert one suppository rectally at bedtime.

X-Prep: Take dissolved in juice between 2 and 4 of day prior to x-ray or surgical procedure.

Children: For all senna preparations, children use one-half of the usual adult dosage.

Patricia Newton

LAXATIVES—COMBINATION DRUGS

PRODUCTS (TRADE NAME):

(See Table 5-3.)

DRUG SPECIFICS:

The need for mixtures of laxatives has not been documented. With knowledge of the action of various laxatives, it is apparent that combinations are unnecessary and may produce harmful or undesirable effects. They also tend to be more expensive than drugs sold singly. A partial listing of available mixtures is provided for information and because they are still widely used by both patients and some practitioners, but it is not recommended that combinations be used.

Patricia Newton

TABLE 5-3. LAXATIVE COMBINATION DRUGS

Trade Name:	Available In:	Chemical Combinations:
Dialose	100 mg capsules	Docusate potassium, methylcellulose
DialosePlus	100 mg capsules	Docusate potassium, methylcellulose, casanthanol
Dorbantyl	50 mg capsules	Danthron, docusate sodium
Doxidan	60 mg capsules	Danthron, docusate calcium
Haley's MO	emulsion	Milk of magnesia, mineral oil
Hydrocil	powder	Psyllium, kara gum, dextrose
Peri-Colace	100 mg capsule	Casanthranol, docusate sodium
Senokot S	50 mg tablet	Senna, docusate sodium

MISCELLANEOUS GASTROINTESTINAL DRUGS

CHENODIOL (CHENODEOXYCHOLIC ACID)

ACTION OF THE DRUG: This relatively new product acts on the liver to suppress cholesterol and cholic acid synthesis. Biliary cholesterol desaturation is enhanced, and dissolution of radiolucent cholesterol gallstones eventually occurs. There is no effect on calcified or radiopaque gallstones or radiolucent bile pigment stones.

ASSESSMENT:

INDICATIONS: This product is useful in selected patients with radiolucent stones in well-opacifying gallbladders who are poor surgical risks due to concomitant disease or advanced age. Success is likely to be higher with small and floatable stones.

SUBJECTIVE: Obtain a history of abdominal pain, nausea, vomiting, and increased gas and flateus following high fat intake. Patient may have had previous similar episodes. Women tend to be affected more than men.

OBJECTIVE: Although there may be a positive Murphy's inspiratory arrest sign, diagnosis may be confirmed by cholecystogram or ultrasonogram.

PLAN:

CONTRAINDICATIONS: Do not use this medication in the presence of known liver or other gallbladder disease. It the gallbladder fails to visualize after two consecutive single doses of dye, or if radiopaque or radiolucent bile pigment stones are seen, medication should not be used. Although human data have yet to be obtained, it appears that this product may be harmful to the fetus. Pregnant women should not take this medication.

WARNINGS: This product may produce hepatic toxicity, ranging from mildly toxic to fatal hepatic failure. The product should only be used in patients without previous hepatic problems and careful monitoring of patient liver function is mandatory. Safety for use in breast-feeding women and children has not been established. There is also the possibility that chenodiol therapy might contribute to the development of colon cancers in susceptible individuals.

IMPLEMENTATION:

DRUG INTERACTIONS: Biliary cholesterol secretion and incidence of gallstones may be increased by estrogens, clofibrate and oral contraceptives. Therefore, these drugs may counteract the effectiveness of chenodiol. Bile acid sequestering agents such as cholestyramine and colestipol may reduce the absorption of chenodiol. Aluminum-based antacids may adsorb bile acids and reduce the absorption of chenodiol also.

PRODUCTS (TRADE NAME):
Chenix (Available in 250 mg tablets.)

ADMINISTRATION AND DOSAGE: Recommended dosage range is 13 to 16 mg/kg/day in 2 divided doses taken morning and evening. Increase dose by 250 mg/day each week until the recommended or tolerated dose is obtained. Dosages less than 10 mg/kg is usually ineffective and may, in fact, contribute to increased risk of cholecystectomy.

Adults 100-130 lbs: Give 3 tablets/day or 17 to 13 mg/kg.
Adults 131-165 lbs: Give 4 tablets/day or 17 to 13 mg/kg.
Adults 166-200 lbs: Give 5 tablets/day or 16 to 14 mg/kg.
Adults 201-235 lbs: Give 6 tablets/day or 16 to 14 mg/kg.
Adults 236-275 lbs: Give 7 tablets/day or 16 to 14 mg/kg.

IMPLEMENTATION CONSIDERATIONS:
—Take a complete health history, especially asking about any incidence of hepatic, biliary, or gallbladder dysfunction or problems. Document that patient is a poor surgical candidate, has advanced age, or is otherwise unable to undergo surgery. Rule out pregancy.
—If patient develops diarrhea, reduction of dosage will usually eliminate sym-

toms. Usually patient is able to resume higher dosages without recurrence of diarrhea.

—Stone recurrence can be expected within 5 years in 50% of all cases using chenodiol. Low cholesterol, low carbohydrate diets with increased dietary bran may help reduce biliary cholesterol. Weight reduction may help to postpone stone recurrence.

—Evaluation of patient compliance is important in considering this product as part of the therapeutic regimen. Patient must be reliable in keeping appointments, reporting problems, and undergoing periodic health evaluations.

WHAT THE PATIENT NEEDS TO KNOW:

—Take this medication exactly as prescribed by your health care practitioner.

—Keep this product out of the reach of children or others for whom it is not prescribed.

—It will be important while you are taking this product to return for tests and examinations periodically. This will help your health care practitioner learn how helpful this drug is in controlling your gallstones.

—This product is designed to help dissolve your gallstones. Once they have disappeared, there is still the possibility that new ones may form in future years. It is important to continue seeing your health provider even though you may no longer be taking this medication.

—Report any gallbladder symptoms (abdominal pain, nausea, vomiting), diarrhea, or any new or troublesome symptoms to your health care practitioner immediately.

—Your health care practitioner may give you a special diet to follow to (1) help you lose weight, (2) keep your cholesterol low, and (3) keep your bowels regular.

EVALUATION:

ADVERSE REACTIONS: *Gastrointestinal:* Dose-related diarrhea, may be seen, plus anorexia, constipation, cramps, dyspepsia, epigastric distress, flatulence, heartburn, nausea, nonspecific abdominal pain, and vomiting. Dose-related serum elevations may also be seen, especially SGPT. Serum total cholesterol and low density lipoprotein cholesterol levels may increase during therapy. *Hematopoietic:* nonspecific decreases in white cell count.

OVERDOSAGE: None reported.

PARAMETERS TO MONITOR: Obtain a complete history and physical examination prior to starting therapy. This should include good cholecystograms or ultrasonograms documenting extent and nature of stone formation. After one to three months of medication, repeat cholecystograms or ultrasonograms should document stone dissolution. These tests should be repeated every 6 to 9 months while patient is taking medication. (Use beyond 24 months has not been reported.) If stone dissolution is documented, therapy may be terminated with periodic radiologic evaluations to search for recurrence. If partial dissolution is not seen after 9 to 12 months of therapy, the chances of successful therapy are slim; medication should be terminated if no results are seen by 18 months. Serum aminotransferase levels should be monitored monthly for the first three months, and then every 3 months during therapy. Elevations of serum aminotransferase 1 1/2 to 3 times the upper limit of normal for a three month period of time should prompt the health care provider to discontinue the product. Cholesterol levels should also be monitored every 6 months, and medication discontinued if elevations develop.

Marilyn W. Edmunds

MISCELLANEOUS GASTROINTESTINAL DRUGS— ANTIALCOHOLIC

DISULFIRAM

ACTION OF THE DRUG: Disulfiram produces a severe sensitivity to alcohol which results in an extremely unpleasant reaction when even small amounts of alcohol are ingested. This drug promotes an excessive accumulation of acetaldehyde by inhibiting the normal liver enzyme activity after the conversion of alcohol to acetaldehyde. Increased levels of acetaldehyde produce the disulfiram reaction. The reaction is present until the metabolism of alcohol is completed. The intensity of the reaction is variable, but is usually proportional to the amounts of disulfiram and alcohol ingested.

ASSESSMENT:

INDICATIONS: Disulfiram is specific for the management of alcoholism. It is used as a deterrent to alcoholic intake which enables development of a state of enforced sobriety. This drug is an adjunct to psychiatric therapy or alcoholic counseling and used in patients who are motivated and fully cooperative.

SUBJECTIVE: Patient or others may complain of any of the following: loss of control over alcoholic consumption and/or increasing tolerance to the effects of alcohol. Use of alcohol may be used to relieve stress or tension. May also note continued intake of alcohol despite medical and social contraindications and disruptions in life style. Surreptitious drinking may be reported by the patient, family members, co-workers, or friends.

OBJECTIVE: Evidence of physiologic dependence manifested by a withdrawal syndrome when intake of alcohol is stopped or decreased. Presence of alcohol-associated illnesses: coagulation disorders, cerebellar degeneration, chronic gastritis, chronic pancreatitis, and certain types of liver disease, etc. One must first rule out other non-alcohol abuse conditions for the presenting illness. Further evidence may be obtained from increased blood alcohol levels, abnormal liver function tests, coagulation defects, or electroencephalographic abnormalities consistent with chronic alcohol abuse.

PLAN:

CONTRAINDICATIONS: Do not use if patient has used alcohol in any form in the last 12 hours. This includes use of cough mixtures, tonics, vinegars, sauces, after shave lotions, back rubbing solutions, creams, or other products containing alcohol. Do not use if there has been recent ingestion of paraldehyde or metronidazole, in the presence of severe myocardial disease or coronary occlusion, psychoses, or hypersensitivity to disulfiram. Do not use in pediatric patients. As safe use of disulfiram has not been established during pregnancy, it should be used only when the probable benefits outweigh the possible risks.

WARNINGS: Disulfiram should never be administered to a patient when he is in a state of alcoholic intoxication or without his full knowledge. The disulfiram-alcohol reaction occurs when any form of alcohol is combined with disulfiram. Even small amounts of alcohol can produce this reaction. See Implementation Considerations.

Patients with rubber contact dermatitis should be evaluated for hypersensitivity to thiuram derivatives prior to disulfiram therapy.

PRECAUTIONS: Cautious use of disulfiram should be followed in patients taking phenytoin and its congeners as the combination of these drugs can lead to a phenytoin intoxication. Disulfiram should be used with extreme caution in patients with any of the following conditions: diabetes mellitus, epilepsy, cerebral damage, hypothyroidism, chronic and acute nephritis, hepatic cirrhosis or insufficiency, conditions requiring multiple drug usage, coronary artery disease, and hypertension. In these patients there is the possibility of an accidental disulfiram-alcohol reaction.

Dependence on narcotics or sedatives may accompany or follow alcoholism. The possibility of initiating a new abuse must be considered. Disulfiram and barbiturates have been administered concurrently without untoward effects.

IMPLEMENTATION:

DRUG INTERACTIONS: Use with even small amounts of alcohol produces severe disulfiram-alcohol reactions. Concurrent use of disulfiram increases the effects of anticoagulants, phenytoins and barbiturates and may increase the side effects of isoniazid. Patients taking isoniazid should have disulfiram medication discontinued if changes in behavior or unsteady gait appear. Concurrent use with metronidazole and marijuana produces an additive effect, and may produce psychotic episodes. Exaggerated clinical effects of diazepam and chlordiazepoxide are produced with concurrent use of this drug. When benzodiazepine treatment is indicated, use alprazolam, lorazepam or oxazepam since they are not metabolized to active metabolites. Use with paraldehyde may produce disulfiram-alcohol reactions. Disulfiram may increase serum cholesterol and decrease VMA levels.

PRODUCTS (TRADE NAME):

Antabuse, Disulfiram (Available in 250 and 500 mg tablets.)

ADMINISTRATION AND DOSAGE: Disulfiram should not be administered until the patient has abstained from any form of alcohol for at least 12 hours.

The adult dosage is up to 500 mg daily for one to two weeks, followed by 125-

500 mg daily for maintenance. It may take up to 3 weeks for the drug to reach full effectiveness, and drug is still effective for up to 2 weeks after discontinuing therapy. The average maintenance dosage is 250 mg daily. Maintenance therapy is needed until the patient is fully recovered socially and a basis for permanent self-control has been established. This may take months or even years.

IMPLEMENTATION CONSIDERATIONS:

—Obtain a complete health history prior to treatment, including the presence of recent or current use of alcohol, metronidazole, or other drugs which may produce drug reactions, sensitivity to rubber, history of psychoses, severe myocardial disease, coronary occlusion, or hypersensitivity to disulfiram or other thiuram derivatives, or the possibility of pregnancy.

—The patient should give permission for disulfiram therapy. The patient and a responsible family member need to understand the consequences of this therapy.

—Disulfiram is an adjunct to supportive and psychiatric therapy and should be used only in patients that are cooperative and well motivated.

—Therapy cannot be initiated until the patient has abstained from any form of alcohol for at least 12 hours.

—Warn patient of disulfiram-alcohol reactions. This may occur for up to 2 weeks after a single dose of disulfiram. The longer a patient remains on this drug, the more sensitive he will become to alcohol.

—The disulfiram-alcohol reactions may be provoked by even small amounts of alcohol. Patient should be cautioned against hidden forms of alcohol: tonics, cough syrups, after shave lotions, vinegar, sauces, liniments, hair tonics, rubbing alcohol, certain high-alcohol flavoring extracts, or other alcohol-containing foods or products. A disulfiram-alcohol reaction may include the following symptoms: physiologic effects may include flushing and warming of the face, severe throbbing headache, shortness of breath, chest pain, nausea, vomiting, sweating, weakness, palpitations, hyperventilation, tachycardia, syncope, and confusion. Severe reactions could include arrhythmias, respiratory distress, cardiovascular collapse, myocardial infarction, acute congestive heart failure, convulsions, and death. The treatment of a severe disulfiram-alcohol reaction includes: treatment of shock, administration of oxygen, (carbogen (95% oxygen and 5% carbon dioxide), and ephedrine sulfate. Intravenous antihistamines have also been used. Monitoring of potassium levels is important especially in patients taking digitalis preparations, as hypokalemia has been reported.

—Disulfiram users should wear a bracelet or card identifying them as users of this drug and describing the symptoms most likely to occur in the disulfiram-alcohol reaction. Cards may be obtained from the pharmaceutical company to give to patients who are placed on this therapy.

—Side effects of disulfiram usually subside after two weeks of therapy.

—Crush tablets and mix with juice or other liquid and observe patient taking this if compliance is uncertain.

—Disulfiram is usually taken in the morning but may be taken in the evening if drowsiness is a problem.

—Disulfiram may increase serum cholesterol and decrease VMA levels.

—Cautious use of disulfiram should be followed in patients taking phenytoin and its congeners as the combination of these drugs can lead to phenytoin intoxication. Prior to initiating disulfiram therapy, a baseline phenytoin level should be obtained. Follow-up phenytoin levels are necessary after disulfiram therapy has been started to monitor for an increase or continuing rise in phenytoin levels. Adjustment of phenytoin therapy may be necessary.

—Patients taking isoniazid and disulfiram should be observed for the development of an unsteady gait or a marked change in mental status. Disulfiram should be discontinued if such symptoms appear.

—Disulfiram may prolong the prothrombin time so patients on oral anticoagulants may need the anticoagulant dosage adjusted upon beginning and ending disulfiram therapy.

—Dependence on narcotics or sedatives may accompany or follow alcoholism. The possibility of initiating a new abuse must be considered.

WHAT THE PATIENT NEEDS TO KNOW:
—Take this medication exactly as prescribed by health care practitioner. Tablets may be crushed and mixed with liquids if it is easier to take this way.

—Success with this therapy is dependent upon your cooperation and participation in additional psychiatric or alcoholic counseling.

—Avoid all forms of alcohol during therapy and for two weeks after therapy is discontinued. This means you will have to read the labels on things which you normally eat. Note particularly things like vanilla extract, hair tonics, rubbing alcohol, cough syrups, after shave lotions, vinegar, sauces, or other foods or products which contain alcohol.

—Some people experience mild side effects while taking this medication. Most of these disappear within 2 weeks after beginning therapy. Be certain to tell your health practitioner of any new or troublesome symptoms.

—Inform your physician if you plan to have any surgery requiring a general anesthetic while taking this drug.

—It is important to wear a Medic-Alert bracelet or carry a card identifying yourself as a disulfiram user.

—While you are taking this medication do not take any other medications, including medications you may buy over the counter, without the knowledge of your health practitioner.

—If you note any symptoms of an alcohol-disulfiram reaction, notify your health provider immediately. Symptoms to note are: flushing and warmth of face, severe throbbing headache, shortness of breath, chest pain, nausea, vomiting, sweating, weakness, palpitations, hyperventilation, tachycardia, syncope, and confusion. In some cases these symptoms may progress to even more severe problems and must not be ignored.

—Medication is usually taken in the morning, but may be taken in the evening if drowsiness is a problem.

EVALUATION:

ADVERSE REACTIONS: *CNS:* drowsiness, fatigue, headache, optic neuritis (with impaired vision, decreased color perception and blindness), peripheral neuritis, polyneuritis, psychotic reactions, restlessness, transient mild drowsiness. *Dermatologic:* acneiform eruptions, allergic dermatitis. *Gastrointestinal:* dry mouth, elevation of liver enzymes, hepatotoxicity, metallic or garlic-like aftertaste. *Genitourinary:* impotence. *Other:* acetonemia, arthropathy, disulfiram-alcohol reaction.

OVERDOSAGE: *Signs and symptoms:* behavioral disturbances, fatigue, impaired memory, headache, nausea, vomiting, diarrhea, confusion, impaired stance and gait, muscle weakness, temporary paralysis. *Treatment:* symptomatic.

PARAMETERS TO MONITOR: Patient should be actively involved in support and counseling to reduce psychological dependence on drug. Patient should be monitored for compliance with dosage regimen, and for development of adverse effects. Liver function tests should be done prior to therapy and 10-14 days after initiation of therapy. They should be repeated on a regular basis through therapy to detect any hepatic dysfunction due to the disulfiram. Baseline complete blood count and sequential multiple analysis (SMA-12) are necessary and should be repeated every 6 months. Assessment should be made for any problems related to interactions of other drugs the patient is taking (anticoagulants, isoniazid, phenytoin, etc.).

Mary Ann Bolter

6

HEMATOLOGIC AND NUTRITIONAL PREPARATIONS

ANTICOAGULANTS

COUMARIN AND INDANDIONE DERIVATIVES

ACTION OF THE DRUG: Coumarin and indandione derivatives inhibit synthesis of blood coagulation factors II, VII, IX, and X in the liver through interfering with vitamin K. These drugs have no thrombolytic effect; however, they may limit extension of existing thrombi.

ASSESSMENT:

INDICATIONS: Nurse practitioners do not generally initiate anticoagulant therapy; however they frequently have the responsibility of monitoring the patient receiving this therapy and making changes in maintenance doses. Heparin is the anticoagulant of choice when an immediate effect is needed. For long-term therapy, a coumarin or indandione derivative is used. Coumarin derivatives such as dicumarol and warfarin are used in the prophylaxis and treatment of venous thrombosis and its extension, treatment of atrial fibrillation with embolization, prophylaxis and treatment of pulmonary embolism and as adjunctive therapy in the treatment of coronary occlusion. The FDA has classified this drug as "possibly" effective as adjunctive therapy for treatment of transient cerebral ischemic attacks. Indandione derivatives (phenindione) are used in the treatment of pulmonary emboli and as prophylaxis and treatment of deep vein thrombosis, myocardial infarction, rheumatic heart disease with valve damage, and atrial arrhythmias.

SUBJECTIVE: Patient may present with a history of deep vein thrombosis, myocardial infarction, rheumatic heart disease with valve damage, atrial arrhythmias, or transient cerebral ischemic attacks.

OBJECTIVE: Clinical evidence of venous thrombosis, atrial fibrillation with embolization, coronary occlusion, transient cerebral ischemic attacks, acute and chronic consumption coagulopathies, and peripheral arterial embolism may be present. Also, some form of heparin may have been used during prior operative procedures which now warrant long-term therapy.

PLAN:

CONTRAINDICATIONS: Do not use coumarin derivatives in children, pregnant women, people with blood dyscrasias or hemorrhagic tendencies; recent or impending surgery of central nervous system or eye, or traumatic surgery resulting in large, open surfaces; bleeding tendencies associated with active ulceration or overt bleeding (gastrointestinal, genitourinary or respiratory-tract bleeding or ulceration, cerebrovascular hemorrhage, aneurysm, pericarditis, pericardial effusions, subacute bacterial endocarditis); or obstetrical complications such as threatened abortion, eclampsia, or preeclampsia. Drug should not be used if there are inadequate laboratory facilities or if patient is uncooperative in taking medications or keeping appointments for laboratory and health assessment. Also it should not be used if patient is an alcoholic, is senile, or has malignant hypertension, major regional or lumbar block anesthesia, or a psychosis which cannot be closely supervised. Coumarin derivatives should not be used in a patient undergoing diagnostic or therapeutic procedures with potential for uncontrolled bleeding.

WARNINGS: If heparin is being given simultaneously with a coumarin or indandione derivative, do not draw blood for prothrombin time within 5 hours of IV heparin administration, or 24 hours if heparin is given subcutaneously. Prothrombinopenic states may develop in infant of nursing mother. Increased risks are associated with patients having severe to moderate hepatic or renal insufficiency; infectious diseases or disturbances of intestinal flora (sprue, antibiotic therapy), trauma which could result in internal bleeding; surgery or trauma resulting in large, exposed raw surfaces, indwelling catheters; severe to moderate hypertension; severe allergic and anaphylactic disorders; severe diabetes, vasculitis, and polycythemia vera. Concurrent use of streptokinase or urokinase with anticoagulants may be hazardous. Anticoagulant therapy should not be stopped abruptly. Congestive heart failure patients may be more sensitive to these drugs.

PRECAUTIONS: Periodic determination of prothrombin time or other suitable coagulation tests are absolutely essential. Numerous factors, including travel, changes in diet, environment, physical state, and medication, may influence the patient's response to anticoagulants. Use cautiously during menses. Use with extreme caution in psychiatric, debilitated, or cachectic patients.

IMPLEMENTATION:

DRUG INTERACTIONS: The following drugs will increase prothombin time response: allopurinol, aminosalicylic acid, anabolic steroids, antibiotics, androgens, bromelains, chloral hydrate, chloramphenicol, chymotrypsin, cimetidine, clofibrate, dextran, dextrothyroxine, diazoxide, disulfiram, drugs affecting blood elements, glucagon, heparin sodium, methyldopa, methylphenidate, methylthiouracil, metronidazole, nalidixic acid, narcotics (with prolonged use), nortriptyline, oxolinic acid, oxyphenbutazone, phenylbutazone, propylthiouracil, quinidine, quinine, salicylates, thyroid drugs, triclofos sodium, and vitamin E.

The following drugs will decrease prothrombin time response: adrenocorticosteroids, antacids, antihistamines, antipyrine, barbiturates, carbamazepine, chlordiazepoxide, cholestyramine, contraceptives (oral), ethchlorvynol, estrogens, glutethimide, griseofulvin, haloperidol, meprobamate, primidone, rifampin, thiazide diuretics, and vitamin K.

Anticoagulant effects may be increased with acute alcohol intoxication and decreased with chronic alcohol abuse. Oral hypoglycemics may increase the effect of either the hypoglycemic or anticoagulant. Phenytoin used concurrently with dicumarol may increase or decrease the effects of both drugs. Concurrent use is not recommended. Concurrent use of streptokinase or urokinase with anticoagulants may be hazardous and is not recommended.

The following drugs will increase the risk of bleeding: alkylating agents, antimetabolites, corticosteroids, dipyridamole, ethacrynic acid, indomethacin, oxyphenbutazone, phenylbutazone, quinidine, salicylates, streptokinase, sulfinpyrazone, and urokinase.

ADMINISTRATION AND DOSAGE: Dosage is determined according to the patient's prothrombin time values. The preferred method is to report the ratio of prolonged therapeutic prothrombin time to the normal control value. The therapeutic range is usually 1 1/2 to 2 1/2 times the control value.

Dicumarol is given only by the oral route. Warfarin may be given by the oral or parenteral route. Phenindione, an indandione derivative, is given only by the oral route.

If anticoagulant therapy is initiated with heparin and continued with a coumarin or indandione derivative, it is recommended that both drugs be given concurrently until prothrombin time determinations indicate an adequate response to the coumarin or indandione derivative.

IMPLEMENTATION CONSIDERATIONS:

—Obtain a complete health history, including the presence of hypersensitivity, underlying systemic disease, current nature of the problem, and concurrent use of medications. Rule out conditions which would contraindicate use of some anticoagulants: alcoholism, blood dyscrasias, bleeding tendencies of gastrointestinal, genitourinary, or respiratory tracts, or malignant hypertension. (Refer to section on Contraindications for more information.)

—Understand the rationale for current therapy, and work with a competent physician in supervising patient therapy.

—If a female patient is taking a coumarin or indandione derivative, verify that she is neither pregnant nor a nursing mother.

—Obtain baseline complete blood count, prothrombin and/or partial thromboplastin time, liver and kidney function tests, complete urinalysis, and stool specimens.

—Patients with congestive heart failure may be more sensitive to coumarin and indandione derivatives.

—Watch for signs of overdosage of anticoagulants and internal bleeding as therapy progresses.

—Stress to patient and family the importance of complying with therapy and keeping follow-up appointments.

—Do not abruptly discontinue anticoagulant therapy.

WHAT THE PATIENT NEEDS TO KNOW:

—Take medication only as directed. If you miss a dose, take it as soon as possible. Do not take it if it is almost time for the next dose. Do not double doses. Keep record of all missed doses.

—You will need regular prothrombin time or coagulation tests and regular visits to health care provider in order to ensure that blood clotting stays within special and narrow limits. Dosage may need to be altered from time to time based upon results of laboratory tests.

—Do not take other medication without checking with your health provider. This means even aspirin or any over-the-counter medicines.

—Wear a Medic-Alert bracelet or necklace, and carry a medical information card with you explaining that you are taking an anticoagulant.

—Inform all doctors, dentists, or podiatrists whom you go to for care that you are taking an anticoagulant.

—Use caution in brushing teeth, trimming nails, and shaving. Use an electric razor when possible.

—Should you cut yourself, use pressure to stop bleeding. If bleeding persists after 10 minutes, call your health care provider.

—Do not engage in contact sports or other activities that could lead to injuries.

—Eat a normal, balanced diet. Do not eat excessive amounts of food which are high in vitamin K (tomatoes, onions, dark leafy greens, bananas, or fish.)

—Avoid drinking alcohol.

—Know the possible side effects of anticoagulants: active bleeding or signs of bleeding such as tarry stools, blood in the urine, bleeding gums, nosebleeds, dizziness, coughing up blood, abdominal or joint pains, unexplained bruising, or unusually heavy or unexpected menstrual periods in women.

—After anticoagulant therapy has been stopped, use caution until your body recovers its blood-clotting abilities.

EVALUATION:

ADVERSE REACTIONS:
Coumarin Derivatives:

Dicumarol: *Dermatologic:* alopecia, rashes, urticaria. *Gastrointestinal:* abdominal bloating, anorexia, cramping, diarrhea, flatus, mouth ulcers, nausea, vomiting. *Genitourinary:* hematuria. *Hematopoietic:* agranulocytosis, hemorrhage (with excessive dosage), leukopenia. *Other:* fever.

Warfarin: *Dermatologic:* alopecia, necrosis (purple toes syndrome), rash, urticaria. *Gastrointestinal:* cramping, diarrhea, intestinal obstruction, nausea, paralytic ileus, vomiting. *Genitourinary:* excessive uterine bleeding. *Hematopoietic:* hemorrhage with excessive dosage, leukopenia. *Other:* fever.

Indandione Derivatives:

Phenindione: *Cardiovascular:* myocarditis, tachycardia. *CNS:* headache. *EENT:* blurred vision, conjunctivitis, paralysis of ocular accommodation. *Dermatologic:* rash, severe exfoliative dermatitis. *Gastrointestinal:* diarrhea, jaundice, sore mouth and throat. *Genitourinary:* albuminuria, nephropathy with renal tubular necrosis. *Other:* fever.

OVERDOSAGE: *Signs and symptoms:* Early signs of overdosage or internal bleeding are: bleeding from gums while brushing teeth, excessive bleeding or oozing from cuts, unexplained bruising or nosebleeds, unusually heavy or unexpected menses in women. Signs suggesting internal bleeding are abdominal pain or swelling, back pain, bloody or tarry stools, bloody or cloudy urine, constipation (resulting from paralytic ileus or intestinal obstruction), coughing up blood, dizziness, severe or continuous headaches, vomiting blood or "coffee ground" substance. *Treatment:* For mild symptoms, omit one or more doses of the anticoagulant; administer 2.5 to 10 mg vitamin K, orally, if necessary. For persistent minor bleeding or frank bleeding, refer for treatment which usually includes giving 5 to 25 mg vitamin K slowly IV. If bleeding is severe or unresponsive to vitamin K, transfuse whole fresh, blood, fresh or fresh-frozen plasma.

PARAMETERS TO MONITOR: Obtain baseline complete blood count, prothrombin and/or partial thromboplastin time, liver and kidney function tests, complete urinalysis, and stools for occult blood prior to beginning therapy. Dosage of anticoagulant will be determined by prothombin time values.

When an oral anticoagulant is administered with heparin, coagulation tests and prothrombin activity should be determined at the onset of therapy. Heparin is given for an immediate effect. When the results of the prothrombin tests are known, give the first dose of the oral anticoagulant. Thereafter, obtain coagulation and prothrombin tests at regular intervals. When the oral anticoagulant shows proper effect and the prothrombin activity is in the therapeutic range, heparin therapy may be stopped and the oral anticoagulant therapy continued.

Initially, prothrombin tests are done daily until the results stabilize in the therapeutic range (1 1/2 to 2 1/2 times the normal control value.) After stabilization, the tests may be done at 1-4 week intervals, depending upon patient status.

With coumarin derivatives, stool tests for occult blood and urinalysis for hematuria are indicated at regular intervals. If an indandione derivative is prescribed, the following tests are indicated at regular intervals: complete blood count, liver and kidney function tests, stool tests for occult blood, and urinalysis for hematuria and proteinuria. Patients should be examined and questioned regularly regarding signs and symptoms of anticoagulant overdosage.

ANISINDIONE

PRODUCTS (TRADE NAME):
Miradon (Available in 50 mg tablets.)
DRUG SPECIFICS:
This is a relatively new product, similar in action to dicumarol. It is generally in the medium price range.
ADMINISTRATION AND DOSAGE SPECIFICS:
Give 300 mg first day, 200 mg the second day, 100 mg the third day, and 25 to 250 mg daily thereafter, as indicated by prothrombin time levels.

DICUMAROL (BISHYDROXYCOUMARIN)

PRODUCTS (TRADE NAME):
Dicumarol (Available in 25, 50 mg capsules and 25, 50, and 100 mg tablets.)

DRUG SPECIFICS:
Dicumarol is poorly and erratically absorbed from the gastrointestinal tract. The therapeutic effect on the prothrombin time is achieved in 1-5 days. After discontinuation of therapy, prothrombin activity returns to normal within 2 to 10 days.

ADMINISTRATION AND DOSAGE SPECIFICS:
Adults: 200 to 300 mg the first day, and then 25 to 200 mg daily, as indicated by prothrombin time levels. Keep prothrombin activity 25% or more of normal.

Children: Dosage has not been established.

PHENINDIONE

PRODUCTS (TRADE NAME):
Hedulin (Available in 20 and 50 mg tablets.)

DRUG SPECIFICS:
Phenindione may cause alkaline urine to change to orange color. Acidification of the urine eliminates this color change. The therapeutic effect on the prothrombin time is achieved in 18 to 48 hours. After discontinuation of this drug, the prothrombin activity returns to normal within 1 to 5 days. This class of drugs is usually reserved for those sensitive to the coumarin class of anticoagulants as it has more adverse side effects.

ADMINISTRATION AND DOSAGE SPECIFICS:
Adults: 300 mg as initial dose, then 200 mg the next day and 100 mg the third day. Then give 50-100 mg po daily as indicated by prothrombin time levels.

Children: Dosage has not been established.

PHENPROCOUMON

PRODUCTS (TRADE NAME):
Liquamar (Available in 3 mg tablets.)

DRUG SPECIFICS:
A popular and relatively inexpensive product.

ADMINISTRATION AND DOSAGE SPECIFICS:
Give 24 mg po initially, and 0.75 to 6 mg daily, depending upon prothrombin time levels.

WARFARIN POTASSIUM AND WARFARIN SODIUM

PRODUCTS (TRADE NAME):
Athrombin-K (Available in 5 mg warfarin potassium tablets.) **Coufarin** (Available in 2, 2.5, 5, 7.5, and 10 mg tablets.) **Coumadin Sodium** (Available in

2, 2.5, 5, 7.5 and 10 mg warfarin sodium tablets and 50 mg single injection units.)
Panwarfin (Available in 2, 2.5, 5, 7.5, and 10 mg warfarin sodium tablets.)
DRUG SPECIFICS:

These are the preferred anticoagulants when the patient is receiving antacids or phenytoin. The therapeutic effect on the prothrombin time is achieved in 36 to 72 hours (including oral, IM or IV routes.) After discontinuation of therapy, prothrombin activity returns to normal in 2 to 5 days.

ADMINISTRATION AND DOSAGE SPECIFICS:

Warfarin potassium: 10 to 15 mg po daily for 2-4 days, then 2 to 10 mg daily as indicated by prothrombin time levels.

Warfarin sodium: 10 to 15 mg IM or IV daily for 2-4 days, then 2 to 10 mg daily as indicated by prothrombin levels; or 10 to 15 mg po daily for 2-4 days, and then 2 to 10 mg po daily for maintenance as indicated by prothrombin levels.

Mary Ann Bolter

ANTICOAGULANTS—
HEPARIN SODIUM

ACTION OF THE DRUG: Heparin acts at multiple sites in the normal coagulation system to inhibit reactions that lead to the clotting of blood and the formation of fibrin clots. It potentiates the inhibitory action of antithrombin III (heparin cofactor) on several other coagulation factors, primarily Factor Xa, to impede thrombin generation. Heparin will not lyse existing clots.

ASSESSMENT:

INDICATIONS: Nurse practitioners do not generally initiate anticoagulant therapy, however they frequently have the responsibility of monitoring the patient receiving this therapy and making changes in maintenance doses. Heparin is the anticoagulant of choice when an immediate effect is needed. For long-term therapy, a coumarin or indandione derivative is used. Heparin sodium is used in the prevention of clotting in arterial and heart surgery. It is also used in prophylaxis and treatment of venous thrombosis and its extension and for pulmonary embolism. It is used in the prevention of postoperative deep venous thrombosis and pulmonary embolism in patients undergoing major abdominothoracic surgery. It is the standard therapy in cases of atrial fibrillation with embolization. It is used in the diagnosis and treatment of acute and chronic consumption coagulopathies (disseminated intravascular coagulation), in the prevention of cerebral thrombosis in evolving stroke, as adjunctive therapy in coronary occlusion with acute myocardial infarction, and in the prophylaxis and treatment of peripheral arterial embolism. It may also be used as an anticoagulant in blood transfusions, extracorporeal circulation, dialysis procedures, and in preserving blood samples for laboratory purposes.

SUBJECTIVE: Patient may present with a history of deep vein thrombosis, myocardial infarction, rheumatic heart disease with valve damage, atrial arrhythmias, or transient cerebral ischemic attacks.

OBJECTIVE: Clinical evidence of venous thrombosis (positive Homan's sign, swollen, erythematous, painful areas on venous tracts of legs), pulmonary embolization, atrial fibrillation with embolization, coronary occlusion, transient cerebral ischemic attacks, acute and chronic consumption coagulopathies, and peripheral arterial embolism may be present.

PLAN:

CONTRAINDICATIONS: Do not give in the presence of hypersensitivity to heparin, uncontrollable active bleeding states, or if there is an inability to perform suitable blood coagulation tests at required intervals.

WARNINGS: Dosage of this drug should be regulated by frequent blood coagulation tests. Heparin should be used with caution in disease states in which there is increased danger of hemorrhage; subacute bacterial endocarditis; arterial sclerosis, increased capillary permeability, during and immediately after spinal tap, spinal anesthesia or major surgery, especially involving brain, eye or spinal cord; hemophilia, purpuras, thrombocytopenia, inaccessible ulcerative lesions and continuous tube drainage of the stomach and small intestine. Use cautiously in pregnancy, especially in the last trimester and post partum. During febrile states, heparin dosage may need to be increased. If heparin is being given concurrently with other anticoagulants, wait 5 hours after IV administration, or 24 hours after SQ administration, before drawing blood for prothrombin time.

PRECAUTIONS: Heparin sodium is derived from animal tissue and should be used with caution in any patient with a history of allergy. Use this drug cautiously in the presence of hepatic or renal disease, hypertension, during menses, or in patients with indwelling catheters. A higher incidence of bleeding may be seen in women over the age of 60. Use with caution when administering ACD-converted blood, especially if it is given in multiple transfusions.

IMPLEMENTATION:

DRUG INTERACTIONS: The following drugs will increase the anticoagulant effect: other anticoagulants (coumarin or indandione derivatives), methimazole and propylthiouracil.

The following drugs will decrease the anticoagulant effect: antihistamines, digitalis, nicotine, and tetracyclines.

The following drugs will increase the risk of bleeding and hemorrhage: ACD-converted blood, acetylsalicylic acid, coumarin-derivative anticoagulants, dextran, dipyridamole, hydroxychloroquine sulfate, nonsteroidal anti-inflammatory/analgesic medications, streptokinase, urokinase.

The following drugs will increase the risk of gastrointestinal bleeding and hemorrhage: acetylsalicylic acid, corticotropin, ethacrynic acid, glucocorticoids, meclofenamate, mefenamic acid, nonsteroidal anti-inflmmatory/analgesic medications.

PRODUCTS (TRADE NAME):

Heparin Sodium, Lipo-Hepin, Lipo-Hepin/BL, Liquaemin Sodium, Pan-heprin (Available in 1,000, 5,000, 10,000 USP units per ml derived from beef lung; 1,000, 2,000, 2,500, 5,000, 7,500, 10,000, 15,000, 20,000, 30,000, 40,000 USP units per ml derived from porcine intestinal mucosa).

ADMINISTRATION AND DOSAGE: Dosage is adjusted according to the patient's coagulation test. The standard tests for determining heparin's general effect on clotting are the Lee-White whole blood clotting time, the whole blood activated partial thromboplastin time (WBAPTT), and the activated partial thromboplastin time (APTT). The most frequently used test is the APTT. Dosage is considered adequate when the whole blood clotting time is approximately 2 1/2 to 3 times the control value.

The dosages listed are given in USP heparin units which are not identical to international units (IU). Heparin is not effective by oral administration and should be given by intermittent IV route, IV infusion, or deep SQ (intrafat) injection. Do not give heparin intramuscularly due to the frequent development of hematomas, irritation and pain at the injection site.

The sites of intrafat injections should be rotated to avoid formation of hematomas. Do not attempt to aspirate blood prior to injection and do not move needle while solution is being injected. Injection sites should not be massaged before or after injection. Patients receiving heparin are not good candidates for IIM injections of other medications since hematomas and bleeding into adjacent areas may occur.

Do not use medication if solution is discolored or contains a precipitate. Heparin is strongly acidic, and is chemically incompatible with many other medications in solution. Do not piggyback other drugs into an infusion line while heparin is infusing. Do not mix any drug with heparin in a syringe when bolus therapy is given.

If intermittent IV therapy is being given, blood for partial thromboplastin time determination should be drawn 1/2 hour before next scheduled heparin dose. Blood for partial thromboplastin time determination can be drawn anytime after 8 hours of initiation of continuous intravenous heparin therapy. However, do not draw the blood from the tubing of the heparin infusion line or from the vein of infusion. Always draw blood from the arm not being used for heparin infusion.

IV infusions should be checked frequently, even if pumps are in good working order, to assure that proper dosage is being administered.

If anticoagulant therapy is initiated with heparin and continued with a coumarin or indandione derivative, it is recommended that both drugs be given concurrently until the prothrombin time determinations indicate an adequate response to the coumarin or indandione derivative.

Adults: Deep SQ (intrafat): 10,000-20,000 USP units initially. Then either 8,000 to 10,000 USP units every 8 hours, or 15,000 to 20,000 USP units every 12 hours. Loading dose of 5,000 USP units may be given IV.

IV: 10,000 USP units initially, then 5,000 to 10,000 USP units every 4 to 6 hours. May administer either undiluted or diluted with 50 to 100 ml of isotonic sodium chloride injection.

IV infusion: Give 20,000 to 40,000 USP units in 1,000 ml of isotonic sodium chloride solution to be given over 24-hour period. Loading dose of 5,000 USP units may be given by IV injection.

Children: IV: 50 USP units/kg initially, then 50 to 100 USP units/kg every 4 hours.

IV infusion: 50 USP units/kg as a bolus initially. Then 100 USP units/kg added and absorbed every 4 hours.

IMPLEMENTATION CONSIDERATIONS:

—Obtain a complete health history, including the presence of hypersensitivity, underlying systemic disease, current nature of the problem, and concurrent use of medications. Rule out conditions which would contraindicate use of heparin. (Refer to section on Containdications for more information).

—Understand the rationale for current therapy and work with a competent physician in supervising patient therapy.

—Heparin does not cross the placental barrier nor is it excreted in breast milk.

—Obtain baseline complete blood count, prothrombin and/or partial thromboplastin time, liver and kidney function tests, complete urinalysis, and stools for occult blood.

—Watch for signs of overdosage of anticoagulants and internal bleeding as therapy progresses.

—Stress to patient and family the importance of complying with therapy and keeping follow-up appointments.

—Do not abruptly discontinue anticoagulant therapy.

WHAT THE PATIENT NEEDS TO KNOW:

—Take medication only as directed. You will be supervised closely while you receive this drug. Report any unusual or troublesome symptoms promptly to your health care provider.

—You will be having regular blood tests and evaluation of the effectiveness of this drug. If you are switched over to oral preparations, the frequency of these laboratory tests will decrease.

—Don't take other medication without checking with your health care provider. This includes aspirin or any other over-the-counter medicines.

—If you stay on this drug for any length of time, wear a Medic-Alert bracelet or necklace and carry a medical information card with you, explaining that you are taking an anticoagulant.

—Inform all doctors, dentists, or podiatrists whom you go to for care that you are taking an anticoagulant.

—Use caution in brushing teeth, trimming nails, and shaving. Use an electric razor when possible.

—Should you cut yourself, use pressure to stop the bleeding. If bleeding persists after 10 minutes, call your health care provider.

—Eat a normal, balanced diet.

—Avoid drinking alcohol.

—Be careful in physical activities to avoid injuring yourself.

—Know the possible side effects of anticoagulants: active bleeding or signs of bleeding such as tarry stools, blood in the urine, bleeding gums, nosebleeds, dizziness, coughing up blood, abdominal or joint pains, unexplained bruising, or unusually heavy or unexpected menstrual periods in women.

—After anticoagulant therapy has been stopped, use caution in physical activities until your body recovers its blood clotting abilities.

EVALUATION:

ADVERSE REACTIONS: *Cardiovascular:* chest pain, elevated blood pressure. *CNS:* headache. *Dermatologic:* hematoma, irritation and pain at injection site. *EENT:* conjunctivitis, lacrimation, rhinitis. *Genitourinary:* frequent or persistent erection. *Hematopoietic:* hemorrhage. thrombocytopenia. *Respiratory:* shortness of breath, wheezing. *Other:* chills, fever, hair loss, hypersensitivity reaction.

OVERDOSAGE: *Signs and symptoms:* Early signs of overdosage or internal bleeding are: bleeding from gums while brushing teeth, excessive bleeding or oozing from cuts, unexplained bruising or nosebleeds, unusually heavy or unexpected menses in women. Signs suggesting internal bleeding are abdominal pain or swelling, back pain, bloody or tarry stools, bloody or cloudy urine, constipation (resulting from paralytic ileus or intestinal obstruction,) coughing up blood, dizziness, severe or continuous headaches, vomiting blood or "coffee ground" substance. *Treatment:* If overdosage is mild, response usually occurs with withdrawal of heparin. For severe overdosage, administer 1.0 to 1.5 mg of 1% protamine sulfate by slow infusion for every 100 units of heparin to be neutralized. Limit is 50 mg given very slowly in a 10-minute period.

PARAMETERS TO MONITOR: The dosage of heparin is determined by coagulation tests, usually the partial thromboplastin time. The goal of the therapy is to keep the patient's values at 2 1/2 to 3 times the normal value. On the first day of treatment the coagulation test should be done prior to each dose of heparin, and continued on a daily basis. If heparin is given by continuous IV infusion, the coagulation time should be determined every 4 hours in the early stages of treatment.

When an oral anticoagulant is administered with heparin, coagulation tests and prothrombin activity should be determined at the onset of therapy. Heparin is given for an immediate effect. When the results of the prothrombin tests are known, give the first dose of the oral anticoagulant. Thereafter, obtain coagulation and prothrombin tests at regular intervals. When the oral anticoagulant shows proper effect and the prothrombin activity is in the therapeutic range, heparin therapy may be stopped and the oral anticoagulant therapy continued.

Patients receiving heparin should have hematocrit and platelet count determinations at regular intervals. Additionally, stool tests for occult blood and urinalysis for hematuria are required on a scheduled basis.

Any patient on anticoagulant therapy should be examined and questioned frequently for signs and symptoms of anticoagulant overdosage.

Mary Ann Bolter

FOLIC ACID (FOLACIN; PTEROYLGLUTAMIC ACID; FOLATE)

ACTION OF THE DRUG: Folic acid is required for normal erythropoiesis and nucleoprotein synthesis. It is metabolized in the liver where it is converted to its metabolically active form (tetrahydrofolic acid) by hepatic dihydrofolate reductase.

ASSESSMENT:

INDICATIONS: Use of folic acid is indicated for the following conditions: treatment of megaloblastic and macrocytic anemias due to folic acid deficiency, alcoholism, hepatic disease, hemolytic anemia, infancy (especially those infants on artificial formulas), lactation, oral contraceptive use and pregnancy. Folic acid supplements may be needed in low birth weight infants, infants being nursed by mothers deficient in folic acid or infants with infections or prolonged diarrhea.

SUBJECTIVE: Any of the following data may be obtained: history of malabsorption syndrome or gastric resection; history of alcoholism; history of being on a fad diet; deprived and elderly patients; women who have had several successive pregnancies; complaints of irritability, forgetfulness and insomnia; patients currently receiving hemodialysis, history of long-term use of analgesics, corticosteroids, anticonvulsants, antimalarials or oral contraceptives.

OBJECTIVE: The following may be present: low hemoglobin, low red blood cell count, leukopenia, thrombocytopenia. Red cell mean corpuscular volume is normal or increased; peripheral white cells are hypersegmented, bone marrow is hyperplastic and megaloblastic. Free gastric hydrochloric acid is present at normal levels. Serum iron values are high; serum vitamin B_{12} levels may be normal. Serum folate activity is low; red cell folic acid is low.

PLAN:

CONTRAINDICATIONS: Folic acid is contraindicated as the sole therapeutic agent for the treatment of pernicious anemia. Folic acid will correct the hematologic abnormalities, but the neurologic deficiencies will continue irreversibly. Folic acid should not be given in doses larger than 0.4 mg daily until pernicious anemia has been ruled out, except during pregnancy and lactation. The use of folic acid is contraindicated in normocytic, refractory, aplastic, or undiagnosed anemias.

WARNINGS: Do not exceed recommended dietary allowances (RDA) if self-medicating with vitamin supplements.

PRECAUTIONS: Consider risk-benefit ratio in pregnant women and nursing mothers. Problems have not been documented with normal daily requirements.

IMPLEMENTATION:

DRUG INTERACTIONS: Chloramphenicol, methotrexate, pyrimethamine, triamterene, and trimethoprim act as folate antagonists, and they may cause decreased folic acid activity. *p*-Aminosalicylic acid and sulfasalazine may cause symptoms of folic acid deficiency. Concurrent use with ethotoin, mephenytoin, and phenytoin may decrease the hydantoin effect, leading to increased seizure activity. Oral contraceptives may impair folate metabolism and lead to folic acid deficiency. The effect is usually mild and unlikely to cause anemia or megaloblastic changes.

ADMINISTRATION AND DOSAGE: The recommended dietary allowances (FDA) of folic acid include: *Adult males and females:* 400 mcg. *Pregnant females:* 800 mcg. *Lactating females:* 500 mcg. *Children 4-16 years:* 200 mcg.

These recommended dietary allowances are usually provided by an adequate diet.

IMPLEMENTATION CONSIDERATIONS:

—Obtain a complete health and dietary history including presence of hypersensitivity, underlying systemic disease, past gastrointestinal surgery, alcoholism, and concurrent use of other medications, especially those which may cause folate deficiency or decrease folic acid activity.

—Diagnose precise nature of anemia prior to initiation of therapy with folic acid.

—With drug therapy, improvement in hematologic parameters should be seen within 2-5 days.

—Proper nutrition is essential, and dietary measures are preferable to drug therapy. Patients should be counseled regarding foods high in folic acid to attempt to assist in solving deficiency problem. Dietary folic acid is present in foods but must undergo hydrolysis, reduction and methylation in the GI tract before it is absorbed. Conversion to the active form may be vitamin B12 dependent. Supplies are maintained by enterohepatic recirculation and food. Oral synthetic folic acid is a little different pharmacologically, and is completely absorbed following administration, even in the presence of malabsorption syndromes.

—Stress the importance of remaining under medical supervision while receiving therapy. Patients may need adjustment of maintenance doses. They often fail to return for follow-up visits when they begin feeling better.

—Folic acid for parenteral use must be protected from light.

—Do not mix other medications in the same syringe for injection.

—Most folic acid products are available over the counter. Only the highest dosage forms usually require prescriptions.

WHAT THE PATIENT NEEDS TO KNOW:

—Take this medication exactly as ordered. You will need to be under medical supervision while taking this drug and will need to return to confirm that medication is effective.

—Diet is important in restoring proper folic acid levels and in preventing further deficiencies in the future. Foods high in folate include fresh, leafy green vegetables, other vegetables and fruits, yeast, and organ meats.

—Store vitamins in a cool, dry place. Protect solution from light.

—If a dose is missed, take it as soon as you are aware of the missed dose. Regularity in taking medication is mandatory.

—Never treat yourself with folic acid if you believe you have anemia. This could cover up the presence of other serious blood problems.

EVALUATION:

ADVERSE REACTIONS: Folic acid is reportedly nontoxic. *Hypersensitivity:* allergic reaction may consist of bronchospasm, erythema, malaise, pruritus, and rash.

OVERDOSAGE: Has not been reported. Large doses of folic acid may cause yellow discoloration of urine.

PARAMETERS TO MONITOR: Obtain complete physical and laboratory baseline prior to starting treatment. Within 2-5 days after initiation of therapy, there should be an improvement in the hematologic picture. Reticulocyte activity should increase. A complete blood count should be obtained 1-2 weeks after therapy has started and should be repeated at intervals determined by the patient's response to therapy. Red cell folic acid levels should be obtained within a month after folic acid therapy has begun. Other hematologic studies may be ordered at the health care provider's discretion. It is also important to review the patient's dietary habits and medication compliance at periodic intervals.

FOLIC ACID—DERIVATIVES

FOLIC ACID

PRODUCTS (TRADE NAME):

Folic Acid (Available in 0.1, 0.4, 0.8 and 1 mg tablets, and 10 mg/ml injections).
Folvite (Available in 0.1, 0.4, 0.8 and 1 mg tablets and 5 mg/ml injection.)

DRUG SPECIFICS:

Parenteral administration is usually reserved for conditions in which oral administration is not possible, such as nausea, vomiting, preoperative and postoperative conditions, malabsorption syndromes, gastric resection.

ADMINISTRATION AND DOSAGE SPECIFICS:

Adults:

Aid in diagnosis of folate deficiency: 100 to 200 mcg (0.1 to 0.2 mg) per day po for 10 days, plus low dietary folic acid and vitamin B12. May also give the equivalent of 100 to 200 mcg (0.1 to 0.2 mg) folic acid IM daily for 10 days with low dietary folic acid and vitamin B12.

Dietary supplement: 100 mcg (0.1 mg) per day (up to 1 mg per day in pregnancy). May be increased to 500 mcg (0.5 mg) or 1 mg daily if underlying condition causes increased requirements. For example, in tropical sprue 3 to 15 mg daily may be needed.

Treatment of deficiency: Initially give 250 mcg (0.25 mg) to 1 mg daily po, IM, IV, or deep SQ until hematologic response occurs. For maintenance, give 400 mcg (0.4 mg) to 1 mg daily.

Pregnant and lactating women: 800 mcg (0.8 mg) daily.

Children:

Dietary supplement: Give 100 mcg (0.1 mg) daily. May be increased to 500 mcg (0.5 mg) to 1 mg if condition causes increased requirements.

Treatment of deficiency: Initially give 250 mcg (0.25 mg) to 1 mg daily po, IM, IV, or deep SQ until hematologic response occurs. For maintenance, give 400 mcg (0.4 mg) daily in children 4 years old and over, up to 300 mcg (0.3 mg) daily in children up to age 4, and 100 mcg (0.1 mg) daily to infants.

LEUCOVORIN CALCIUM
(FOLINIC ACID, CITROVORUM FACTOR)

PRODUCTS (TRADE NAME):

Leucovoriin Calcium (Available in 3 mg/ml injections and powder for reconstitution at 10 mg/ml.) **Wellcovorin** (Available in 5 mg/ml injection, 5 mg and 25 mg tablets.)

DRUG SPECIFICS:

This product is often used in patients receiving chemotherapy with folic acid antagonists. In overdosages of methotrexate, administer leucovorin within one hour if possible, as it is usually ineffective after a delay of four hours. Consult updated product information for latest leucovorin rescue schedules.

ADMINISTRATION AND DOSAGE SPECIFICS:

Megaloblastic anemia: Give up to 1 mg daily IM or PO. Greater doses do not lead to increased efficacy.

Overdosage of folic acid antagonists: See latest product information for rescue schedules.

Mary Ann Bolter

HEPARIN ANTAGONIST

PROTAMINE SULFATE

ACTION OF THE DRUG: This is a strongly basic, low-molecular-weight protein which acts as an anticoagulant. It forms a stable salt in the presence of heparin, which is strongly acidic. This results in the loss of anticoagulant activity of the drugs. When used with heparin, these results occur almost immediately and may persist for 2 hours or more. This product is one of several protamines, all of which are rich in arginine.

ASSESSMENT:

INDICATIONS: Used in the treatment of heparin overdosage. It may also be used following surgical procedures to neutralize the effects of heparin given during extracorporeal circulation.

SUBJECTIVE-OBJECTIVE: Patient may show active bleeding at gums, cuts, nose, or have unexplained bleeding. Internal bleeding may be suspected with the appearance of abdominal pain or swelling, back pain, bloody or cloudy urine, bloody or tarry stools, coughing up blood, dizziness, severe or continuous headaches, vomiting blood or "coffee ground" substance. Women may have unusually heavy or unexpected menses.

PLAN:

WARNINGS: Only a physician should administer this drug. It should be given slowly by intravenous injection over a 1 to 3 minute time period in doses not exceeding 50 mg of protamine sulfate activity (5 ml) during any 10-minute period. Severe hypotension and anaphylactoid-like reactions may be provoked by too rapid administration. Risk-benefit ratio must be considered in the use of this drug for pregnant women and nursing mothers. Use cautiously in patients with any allergy to fish. Protamine has an anticoagulant effect if given in excessive doses.

PRECAUTIONS: Because of the anticoagulant activity of protamine, overdoses of this drug when used as a heparin antagonist will promote additional anticoagulation. It is unwise to give more than 100 mg in a short period of time unless there is definite information as to a larger quantity being required.

Protamine sulfate may be inactivated by blood. Thus, there may be a "rebound" effect created when large doses are used to neutralize heparin. This requires increased doses of protamine. Hyperheparinemia or bleeding may be seen in some patients 30 minutes to 18 hours following open heart surgery, even when adequate amounts of protamine have been given. This phenomenon warrants special attention being paid to the patient in order to diagnose and treat the problem.

IMPLEMENTATION:

PRODUCTS (TRADE NAME):
Protamine Sulfate (Available in 50 and 250 mg powder for injections and 10 mg/ml ampules for injection).

ADMINISTRATION AND DOSAGE: The onset of action for protamine sulfate is 0.5 to 1 minute. The duration of action is 2 hours.

Adults and children: 1 mg of protamine sulfate for every 90 USP units of beef lung heparin or for every 115 USP units of porcine intestinal mucosa heparin to be neutralized. Administer IV at a slow rate over 1 to 3 minutes. (Limit is 50 mg given in 10 minutes). Additional doses may be given if need is indicated by coagulation studies.

IMPLEMENTATION CONSIDERATIONS:
—Follow the physicians orders carefully in calculation and administration of this medication.
—Closely monitor the patient for signs of further anticoagulant activity, especially for a "rebound" phenomenon, and especially in patients who are undergoing

dialysis or who have had cardiac surgery. Have equipment readily available to treat shock.

—This drug contains no preservatives, so unused portion of medication in ampule should be discarded.

WHAT THE PATIENT NEEDS TO KNOW:
—Family and patient should know that this is a routine drug used in the neutralization of heparin.

EVALUATION:

ADVERSE REACTIONS: bradycardia, dyspnea, lassitude, sudden fall in blood pressure, and transitory flushing, and a feeling of warmth.

OVERDOSAGE: May see anticoagulant effects with overdosage.

PARAMETERS TO MONITOR: Monitor vital signs and watch for signs of bleeding. Blood coagulation tests are needed frequently.

Mary Ann Bolter

IRON-CONTAINING PRODUCTS

ACTION OF THE DRUG: Iron is an essential mineral for the synthesis of myoglobin and hemoglobin. It stimulates the hematopoietic system and increases hemoglobin in the correction of iron-deficiency states.

ASSESSMENT:

INDICATIONS: Used in the treatment of symptomatic iron-deficiency anemia only after the cause of the anemia has been identified. Used to prevent hypochromic anemia during infancy, childhood, pregnancy, breast-feeding, in patients recovering from megaloblastic anemia, and in patients who have had subtotal gastrectomy or gastrojejunostomy.

SUBJECTIVE: Patient may have no complaint, or may present with vague complaints such as lack of energy, fatigue, lassitude, faintness, dyspnea, shortness of breath, palpitations, and headache. Symptoms may be pronounced in states of high iron demand or blood loss such as pregnancy, lactation, epistaxis, melena, or hematuria. There may be a history of taking medications which may predispose patients to bleeding, gastrointestinal disease, or previous surgery.

OBJECTIVE: Signs of anemia consist of pallor of skin and mucosa, loss of papillae and cheilosis of the tongue, koilonychia, systolic flow murmur, and tachycardia. Corroborative laboratory results may include decreased hemoglobin, microcytic hypochromic indices on peripheral smear, low serum iron, and increased total iron binding capacity. Evidence of blood loss may be demonstrated by positive result of stool examination for quaiac.

PLAN:

CONTRAINDICATIONS: Do not use in the presence of hypersensitivity to any ingredient in the drug preparation, hemochromatosis, hemosiderosis, chronic hemolytic anemia (in the absence of iron deficiency), pyridoxine-responsive anemia, cirrhosis, peptic ulcer disease, regional enteritis, or ulcerative colitis.

WARNINGS: Do not treat the anemia without locating and treating the cause. Prolonged use of iron salts may result in iron storage disease. It is unnecessary to chronically take iron in the absence of iron-deficiency anemia. Treatment of iron deficiency in patients receiving hemodialysis may mask melena and interact with antacids given for phosphate binding. Hemosiderosis may occur readily in patients receiving cumulative parenteral doses of iron greater than 2.5 gm.

PRECAUTIONS: Hematologic laboratory values may be normally decreased in the elderly, leading to overprescribing of iron for geriatric patients. Liquid preparations can discolor teeth and should be taken through a straw after dilution with liquid. Taking iron preparations after a meal can reduce their absorption by 40% to 50%. Allergic-type reactions may be caused by tartrazine in some iron preparations. Although incidence of allergic reactions is low, they are frequently seen in persons with aspirin allergy and can be severe.

IMPLEMENTATION:

DRUG INTERACTIONS: Large iron doses may cause false-positive tests for occult blood using the o-toluidine test (Hematest, Occultest, Labstix.) The benzidine test is not affected. Absorption of oral iron is inhibited by antacids (particularly magnesium trisilicate-containing antacids), cholestyramine, pancreatic extracts, milk, and eggs. Patients receiving chloramphenicol concurrently with iron may show a delayed response to iron therapy. Absorption of iron increases with concurrent administration of ascorbic acid in doses of 200 mg per 30 mg of iron. Iron interferes with absorption of oral tetracyclines. Vitamin E decreases response to iron therapy. Concurrent administration of allopurinol may increase hepatic iron concentrations. Patients receiving methyldopa are subject to autoimmune hemolysis and have a greater risk of developing hemochromatosis.

ADMINISTRATION AND DOSAGE: Replacement of iron in iron-deficiency anemia should be 90 mg to 300 mg of elemental iron daily in divided doses (6 mg/kg/day.) Remission of symptoms should be apparent within two weeks and laboratory studies normal within two months if diagnosis and treatment are adequate. Therapy for 4 to 6 months is advised to replenish iron stores after the anemia has been corrected. Absorption is enhanced if taken on an empty stomach with water or in an acid environment, although stomach irritation can be minimized by taking after meals. Different oral preparations and multihematinics vary in cost and percentage of elemental iron. Product selection must be based on these factors: how well it is absorbed, how well it is tolerated, and the individual needs of the patient. All simple oral iron preparations are available over the counter. Parenteral iron is indicated when a disorder is present that limits gastrointestinal absorption, when the patient cannot tolerate oral iron, and/or whenthe anemia is severe (patient has less than 7.5 gm/100 ml hemoglobin.)

IMPLEMENTATION CONSIDERATIONS:

—Obtain a complete health history, including hypersensitivities, presence of underlying disease, previous gastrointestinal disorders or conditions in which iron would be contraindicated, conditions which interfere with iron absorption (gastrectomy, atrophic gastritis, alcoholism), concurrent use of medications, dietary intake and previous treatment modalities. History should pursue the cause of anemia.

—Identify the state of iron-deficiency anemia by measuring hemoglobin, indices, serum iron, total iron binding capacity, and reticulocyte count.

—The cause of the anemia must be identified and treated. Obtain stool specimens to examine for occult blood after patient has been on a red-meat-free diet for at least 3 days. While dietary inadequacies may contribute to iron deficiency, especially in those over age 75, blood loss is the primary cause. Menorrhagia and multiple pregnancies in women may be additive in producing anemia.

—In patients who do not comply properly with dosage regimen, extending the time of therapy may be required.

—The Recommended Daily Allowances for elemental iron are:

Adult males: 10 mg. *Adult females:* 18 mg (with an additional 10 mg during pregnancy or lactation). *Children:* 10-15 mg.

A diet high in natural iron should be encouraged to meet these requirements. Fish and meat are the best sources of dietary iron.

WHAT THE PATIENT NEEDS TO KNOW:

—Take this medication exactly as ordered. It should not be discontinued without advice from your health care provider. Continue to take iron as long as prescribed even though you may feel better in two weeks.

—Take iron between meals with one to two glasses of liquid. If stomach upset occurs, notify your health care provider and begin taking iron after meals, but never within an hour of bedtime.

—Do not take with antacids, milk, or dairy products.

—Do not take within two hours of taking tetracycline.

—Liquid preparations may discolor teeth. Dilute well with water, use a straw, and rinse mouth well with water after taking.

—Iron can cause dark green or black stools. Report constipation, diarrhea, nausea, or abdominal pain to health practitioner.

—Store medication in a tightly closed container, in a dry, cool place, and out of heat or sun.

—Keep this medication out of the reach of children and all others for whom it is not prescribed.

—A diet high in elementary iron should be taken. The best sources of iron are meat and fish. Iron may also be found in dried fruits.

EVALUATION:

ADVERSE REACTIONS: *Gastrointestinal:* anorexia, constipation, cramping, diarrhea, epigastric or abdominal pain, gastrointestinal irritation. *Hematopoietic:* hemochromatosis, hemosiderosis (rare), iron overload. *Other:* allergic-type reactions to any component of the iron preparation.

OVERDOSAGE: *Signs and symptoms:* Accidental overdosage and poisoning occur most often in children. Symptoms may occur one half hour to several hours after ingestion. Symptoms are mostly gastrointestinal and include lethargy, nausea, vomiting, abdominal pain, diarrhea, melena, and dyspnea. Coma and metabolic acidosis may occur. Erosion of the gastric mucosa may permit sufficient amounts of iron to be absorbed and cause systemic damage. Weak, rapid pulse, low blood pressure and shock are commonly present. *Treatment:* Induce vomiting and then feed eggs, milk, and bicarbonate of soda until gastric lavage can be performed. Refer for emergency care. Institute supportive care for shock, acidosis, and respiratory failure.

PARAMETERS TO MONITOR: Obtain a complete baseline physical and laboratory examination. Periodic blood work (hemoglobin, indices, reticulocyte count) should be obtained to evaluate therapeutic response. Monitor for subjective signs of improvement, development of adverse effects, and evidence of recurrent blood loss two to three weeks after initiating therapy, then at three months, six months, and one year. Subjective improvement should be evident within two to three weeks if it is going to occur. By two weeks there should be evidence of reticulocytosis and an increase in the hemoglobin by 0.1 to 0.2 gm/100 ml/day. If this clinical response is not evident, evaluate patient compliance. If patient is taking medication as ordered, discontinue the drug and reevaluate the source of blood loss causing the anemia.

FERROUS FUMARATE

PRODUCTS (TRADE NAME):

Ferrous Fumarate (Available in 300 mg tablets with 99 mg iron, and 325 mg tablet with 107 mg iron.) **Feostat** (Available in 100 mg chewable tablets with 33 mg iron, 100 mg suspension with 33 mg iron/5 ml, and 45 mg drops with 15 mg iron /0.6 ml.) **Fumasorb** (Available in 200 mg tablets with 66 mg iron.) **Fumerin** (Available in 195 mg tablets with 64 mg iron.) **Hemocyte** (Available in 324 mg tablets with 106 mg iron.) **Ircon, Palmiron, Toleron** (Available in 200 mg tablets with 66 mg iron.)

DRUG SPECIFICS:

Fewer reported side effects with this product and better tolerated than sulfate or gluconate. Contains 33% elemental iron.

ADMINISTRATION AND DOSAGE SPECIFICS:

Adults: 600-800 mg/day po in divided doses.
Children under 5 years: 100-300 mg/day po in 3-4 divided doses.

FERROUS GLUCONATE

PRODUCTS (TRADE NAME):

    Fergon (Available in 320 mg tablets with 37 mg iron, 435 mg timed release capsules with 50 mg iron, and 300 mg elixir with 35 mg iron/5 ml.) **Ferralet** (Available in 320 mg tablets with 37 mg iron.) **Ferrous-G** (Available in 325 mg elixir with 38 gm iron/5 ml.) **Ferrous Gluconate** (Available in 325 mg tablets or capsules with 38 mg iron.)

DRUG SPECIFICS:

    This product is less corrosive than ferrous sulfate. It is indicated for those patients who can not tolerate sulfate because of gastric irritation. It contains 11.6% elemental iron.

ADMINISTRATION AND DOSAGE SPECIFICS:

    Adults: 320 to 640 mg po three times daily.
    Children 6 to 12 years: 100 to 300 mg po three times daily.
    Children under 6 years: 120 to 300 mg po daily.

FERROUS SULFATE

PRODUCTS (TRADE NAME):

    Fero-Gradumet (Available in 525 mg timed-release capsules with 105 mg iron.) **Ferrous Sulfate** (Available in 195 mg tablet and capsules with 39 mg elemental iron, 300 mg tablets and capsules with 60 mg elemental iron, and 325 mg tablets and capsules with 65 mg elemental iron, 150 mg timed release tablets and capsules with 30 mg elemental iron, 225 mg timed-release tablets and capsules with 45 mg elemental iron, and 250 mg timed-release tablets and capsules with 50 mg elemental iron; and 220 mg elixir with 44 mg iron/5 ml). **Ferusal** (Available in 325 mg tablets with 65 mg iron.) **Mol-Iron** (Available in 195 mg tablet with 39 mg iron, 390 mg timed release chronosules with 78 mg iron, and 195 mg liquid with 39 mg iron/4 ml.)

DRUG SPECIFICS:

    Ferrous sulfate is the standard preparation against which all other iron salts are compared. It is considered the optimal compound because it is the least expensive and contains 20% elemental iron. Timed-release capsules are more costly and less well absorbed but reportedly have fewer side effects. Timed-release preparations have been found to become lodged in the gastrointestinal tract and cause local necrosis. The timed-release product is designed to slowly release iron in order to minimize gastrointestinal side effects, but this may decrease total amount of iron absorbed.

ADMINISTRATION AND DOSAGE SPECIFICS:

    Adults: 300-1200 mg po daily in divided doses.
    Children 6-12 years: 600 mg po daily in divided doses.

Children under 6 years: 1-3 ml of pediatric preparation.
Prophylaxis in poorly developed children: 3-6 mg/kg/day.
Prophylaxis in pregnancy: 300-600 mg po daily.

FERROUS SULFATE EXSICCATED

PRODUCTS (TRADE NAME):
Fer-In-Sol (Available in 190 mg tablets with 60 mg iron and 90 mg syrup with 18 mg iron/5 ml or 75 mg drops with 15 mg iron/0.6 ml.) **Feosol** (Available in 200 mg tablets with 65 mg iron, 220 mg liquid with 44 mg iron/5 ml, and 167 mg timed release spansules with 50 mg iron.)

DRUG SPECIFICS:
This product contains more elemental iron per mg of compound than other products. It is more costly than plain ferrous sulfate. The liquid preparation of Feosol cannot be mixed with juice.

ADMINISTRATION AND DOSAGE SPECIFICS:
Iron deficiency states: 90 to 30 mg elemental iron daily.

IRON DEXTRAN

PRODUCTS (TRADE NAME):
Feostat, Ferotran, Hematran, Hydextran, I.D. 50, Imferon, Irodex, K-FERON, NorFeran, Proferdex (Available in 50 mg iron/ml as ferric hydroxide and dextran.)

DRUG SPECIFICS:
Indications are the same as for oral iron but used in cases where oral iron administration is impossible or unsatisfactory. Parenteral iron has caused fatal anaphylactic-type reactions and must be used with care. IV administration should be given slowly, preceded by a test dose. Not recommended for use in children or pregnant women.

ADVERSE REACTIONS: *Local:* pain, inflammation, staining, flushing. *Immediate systemic reactions:* anaphylaxis, hypotension, malaise, pruritus, urticaria, dyspnea, convulsions, headaches, and paresthesias. *Delayed systemic reactions* (4-48 hours post-injection and lasting 3-7 days): lymphadenopathy, myalgia, arthralgia, fever, headache.

ADMINISTRATION AND DOSAGE SPECIFICS:
Test dose: 0.5 ml IV or IM one hour prior to the therapeutic dose to rule out hypersensitivity.

Calculate the total dose required to return hemoglobin and iron stores to normal using the following formula:

$$0.3 \times \text{weight in lbs} \times \left[100 - \frac{\text{hemoglobin in gm/100 ml} \times 100}{14.8} \right] = \text{mg iron}$$

For patients weighing less than 30 lb, reduce to 80% total calculated by formula.

The Z-track method should be used for injection into the gluteus maximus muscle only. Inject deeply using a 2 or 3 inch needle of 19-20 gauge.

For adults, give calculated daily dose IM until total dose calculated by the formula has been reached. For IV, 2 ml or less may be given daily until total dose has been reached. Administer slowly (1 ml/min) and undiluted.

Patients over 110 lbs (50 kg): Daily dose should not exceed 250 mg iron.

Patients under 110 lbs (50 kg): Daily dose should not exceed 100 mg iron.

Children under 20 lbs: Daily dose should not exceed 50 mg iron.

Infants under 10 lbs: Daily dose should not exceed 25 mg iron.

IRON WITH VITAMIN C

PRODUCTS (TRADE NAME):

C-Ron (Available in 33 mg ferrous fumarate and 50 mg ascorbic acid Freckles tablets, in 66 mg ferrous fumarate and 100 mg ascorbic acid tablets, and in 66 mg ferrous fumarate and 600 mg ascorbic acid Forte tablets.) **Fumaral Spancaps** (Available in 108 mg ferrous fumarate and 200 mg ascorbic acid timed-release tablets.) **Iron with C** (Available in 50 mg ferrous fumarate and 25 mg ascorbic acid tablets with tartrazine.) **Mol-Iron with C** (Available in 39 mg ferrous sulfate and 75 mg ascorbic acid tablets with tartrazine.) **Vitron-C** (Available in 66 mg ferrous fumarate and 125 mg ascorbic acid chewable tablets.)

DRUG SPECIFICS:

Ascorbic acid, when given in a ratio of 200 mg to 30 mg of iron, increases iron absorption by 30%. Vitamin C may also reduce the gastrointestinal effects frequently seen when iron is given alone. Many of the vitamin C with iron compounds contain tartrazine, which may cause allergic-type reactions. Iron is available in combination with almost all vitamins. Only a few of the products available are listed here.

ADMINISTRATION AND DOSAGE SPECIFICS:

Give as indicated by therapeutic problem.

Carol C. Sylvester

VITAMIN K PREPARATIONS

ACTION OF THE DRUG: Vitamin K enhances hepatic formation of active prothrombin (Factor II), proconvertin (Factor VII), plasma thromboplastin component

(Factor IX), and Stuart factor (Factor X), which are essential for normal blood clotting. The exact mechanism is unknown. Menadione (K_3) and phytonadione (K_1) are synthetic lipid-soluble forms of vitamin K. Menadiol sodium diphosphate (K_4) is changed in the body to menadione (K_3).

ASSESSMENT:

INDICATIONS: Nurse practitioners should not initiate vitamin K therapy. However, they may frequently assume responsibility for monitoring the patient receiving this therapy. Vitamin K is indicated for the treatment or prevention of various coagulation disorders resulting in impaired formation of Factors II, VII, IX, and X. The American Academy of Pediatrics recommends routine phytonadione (K1) administration at birth to prevent hemorrhagic disease of the newborn. Vitamin K will not counteract the anticoagulant activity of heparin.

SUBJECTIVE: The following subjective data may be present: history of medical or surgical disorders of the small bowel that interfere with the absorption of fat; long-term therapy with antibiotics or nonabsorbable sulfonamides that interfere with the synthesis of vitamin K, prolonged total parenteral nutrition; biliary obstruction; drug therapy with oral anticoagulants or substantial use of aspirin.

OBJECTIVE: Abnormal prolongation of the prothrombin time and abnormal tests for coagulation Factors VII, IX, and X may be present. Hematuria or positive stool guaiac may also be seen. Patient may have numerous bruises which are especially significant on back of arm and posterior and anterior chest.

PLAN:

CONTRAINDICATIONS: Do not give in the presence of hypersensitivity to the drug, hereditary hypoprothrombinemia, hemorrhage secondary to heparin therapy, or hepatocellular disease (unless it is caused by biliary obstruction.) Do not use for treatment of oral anticoagulant overdosage, and do not administer to the mother during the last few weeks of pregnancy as a prophylactic measure for hemorrhagic disease of the newborn.

WARNINGS: Severe reactions, including fatalities, have occurred with the use of intravenous phytonadione even when precautions have been taken (dilution of drug, slow infusion.) These reactions have resembled anaphylaxis even though some patients were receiving the drug for the first time. The intravenous route should be restricted to those situations in which another route is not feasible or the risk involved is justified.

PRECAUTIONS: Risk-benefit ratio must be considered in pregnant women and nursing mothers. Use with caution in those patients with G-6-PD deficiency to avoid hemolysis. Use large doses cautiously in patients with severe hepatic disease.

IMPLEMENTATION:

DRUG INTERACTIONS: Concurrent use with oral anticoagulants may decrease the effects of the anticoagulant. Mineral oil and cholestyramine resin inhibit gastrointestinal absorption of oral vitamin K.

ADMINISTRATION AND DOSAGE: In determining the dosage of vitamin K to be given, the amount of vitamin K from dietary and other sources should be considered. If the drug is being used to counteract hypoprothrombinemia caused by anticoagulants, use the smallest effective dose since excessive dosage may result in temporary refractoriness to subsequent anticoagulant therapy.

If bleeding is severe, treat with fresh whole blood or plasma. There is a delay in the onset of vitamin K activity. If the drug is being given orally, be aware that absorption is impaired in malabsorption syndrome and in infants who are breast-fed or are on milk-substitute formulas. Also, if the gastrointestinal supply of bile is inadequate, concurrent administration of bile salts may be necessary.

The preferred route of administration of vitamin K is the parenteral route. Intravenous administration is not recommended due to the risk of anaphylaxis.

IMPLEMENTATION CONSIDERATIONS:

—Obtain a complete health history, including the presence of hypersensitivity, pregnancy, breast-feeding, underlying systemic disease (or problems such as hereditary hypoprothrombinemia or hepatocellular disease not caused by biliary obstruction), and concurrent use of medications.

—Obtain liver function tests and prothrombin time values prior to initiation of therapy.

—Coagulation defects may be present if the patient is not responsive to the therapy, this needs to be pursued further.

—In patients taking anticoagulant therapy, the patient's dosage of medication may need to be altered following the use of vitamin K.

—Prothrombin time determinations are needed regularly to determine dosage effectiveness.

—Parenteral forms of this product should be protected from light.

WHAT THE PATIENT NEEDS TO KNOW:

—Take this medication exactly as ordered. If you miss a dose, take it as soon as you remember. Do not take it if it is almost time for the next dose. Do not double doses. Inform your health care provider if you miss doses.

—You will need to make regular return visits to see your health care provider while taking this therapy.

—Inform all physicians and dentists you see for care that you are taking this medication.

—Do not take other medications, including over-the-counter drugs, without first discussing them with your health care provider.

—Some forms of this drug may cause an unusual taste sensation.

—Keep this medication out of the reach of children and all others for whom it is not prescribed.

EVALUATION:

ADVERSE REACTIONS: Specifically for menadione(K_3)/menadiol sodium diphosphate (K_4) *CNS:* headache, kernicterus. *Dermatologic:* rash, urticaria. *Gas-*

trointestinal: gastric upset. *Other:* redness, pain or swelling at injection site. Specifically for phytonadione (K_1): *Cardiovascular:* brief hypotension, rapid and weak pulse. *CNS:* dizziness. *Dermatologic:* flushing, sweating. *Gastrointestinal:* unusual taste sensations. *Other:* redness, pain or swelling at injection site. Anaphylaxis and anaphylactoid reactions.

PARAMETERS TO MONITOR: Prothrombin time determinations are needed before therapy is begun and at periodic intervals to monitor the patient's responsiveness to and need for changes in vitamin K therapy.

MENADIONE (K_3) AND
MENADIOL SODIUM DIPHOSPHATE (K_4)

PRODUCTS (TRADE NAME):

Kappadione (Available in 10 mg/ml ampules.) **Menadione** (Available in 5 mg tablets.) **Synkavite** (Supplied in 5 mg tablets, and in 5 mg/ml, 10 mg/ml, and 37.5 mg/2 ml injections.)

DRUG SPECIFICS:

The oral form of this drug is readily absorbed from the gastrointestinal tract. The diphosphate product is approximately one half as potent as menadione. When given intravenously, infusion rate should not exceed 1 mg/minute. The effects of the intravenous route are more rapid but last for shorter periods than if the drug is given SQ or IM.

In newborns, especially premature infants, these drugs have been associated with hemolytic anemia, hyperbilirubinemia, and kernicterus.

ADMINISTRATION AND DOSAGE SPECIFICS:

Treatment of Hypoprothrombinemia:

Adults: 5 to 15 mg IM or SQ once or twice daily, or 5-10 mg per day po.

Children: 5-10 mg IM or SQ once or twice daily.

PHYTONADIONE
(K_1, PHYLLOQUINONE, METHYLPHYTYL
NAPTHOQUINONE)

PRODUCTS (TRADE NAME):

AquaMEPHYON, Konakion (Available in 2 mg/ml and 10 mg/1 ml ampules.) **Mephyton** (Available in 5 mg tablets.)

DRUG SPECIFICS:

For therapy in newborns this drug is less risky than menadione (K_3)/menadiol sodium disphosphate (K_4) drugs. Parenteral administration gives onset of action in 1-2 hours, with normal prothrombin levels often obtained in 12-14 hours. Konakion may only be given intramuscularly. Give AquaMEPHYTON SQ or IM if possible. IV route has greater risks.

ADMINISTRATION AND DOSAGE SPECIFICS:

AquaMEPHYTON Therapy:

Anticoagulant-induced prothrombin deficiency: 2.5 to 10 mg or up to 25 mg initially. Frequency and dosage of subsequent therapy is determined by prothrombin time response.

Prophylaxis of hemorrhagic disease of newborn: 0.5 to 1 mg IM.

Treatment of hemorrhagic disease of newborn: 1.0 mg SQ or IM. If bleeding is excessive, whole blood or component therapy is indicated. AquaMEPHYTON should be given concurrently with dosage based on prothrombin time response.

Hypoprothrombinemia due to other causes: Give 2.5 to 25 mg. The amount and route of administration depend upon the severity of the condition and the response obtained.

Konakion Therapy:

Hypoprothrombinemia due to oral anticoagulants: 5 to 10 mg IM initially; up to 20 mg IM if needed in adults.

Hypoprothrombinemia due to antibacterial therapy: 5 to 20 mg IM in adults.

Hypoprothrombinemia due to factors limiting absorption or synthesis: 2 to 20 mg IM in adults.

Hypoprothrombinemia due to other drugs: 2 to 20 mg IM in adults.

Neonatal hemorrhage due to hypoprothrombinemia: Give 1 to 2 mg IIM immediately after birth for prophylaxis; and 1 to 2 mg IM daily to control hemorrhage.

Mary Ann Bolter

VITAMINS

Vitamins are chemical compounds which are found naturally in plant and animal tissues, but which are not synthesized in the human body. They are necessary for life and essential to normal metabolism. They can act as coenzymes or regulate the synthesis of compounds. Vitamins are classified into two types: fat-soluble (which are stored in the body), and water-soluble (which are excreted in the urine). Usually, vitamins may be obtained in sufficient amounts from a well-balanced nutritious diet, except when certain conditions prevent their ingestion (i.e., intravenous therapy when a patient is taking nothing by mouth) or prevent their metabolism (as in disorders which inhibit fat metabolism). Such conditions may require vitamin supplementation until a normal diet can be resumed or underlying problem be corrected.

A deficiency of one vitamin in a diet which is otherwise adequate is rare. Signs and symptoms in a particular patient may point to a deficiency of one vitamin, but usually a deficiency of multiple vitamins will be found. With the common proliferation of multiple vitamin preparations on the market today which are easily available to consumers, and the active advertising campaigns through the media, hypervitaminosis is more likely to occur than deficiencies and this is also associated with more than one vitamin.

While debates occur over natural versus synthetic vitamin preparations, vitamins are vitamins and the cheapest preparation is as therapeutic as a more expensive preparation. There are still many mysteries about the action of vitamins in the body, and needless overconsumption of vitamins should be avoided.

VITAMIN A

ACTION OF THE DRUG: Vitamin A is a fat-soluble vitamin which is chemically a long-chain alcohol which comes in several isometric forms: retinol, retinene, carotene, and retinoic acid. Its best understood action is aiding visual adaptation in changes from light to darkness. Lesser understood actions include aiding in the stabilization and maintenance of cell membrane structure, especially epithelial cell membranes, therefore helping the body to resist infection; affecting the synthesis of protein which affects growth of skeletal and soft tissue; and playing an essential role in reproduction. A quantity sufficient to meet a two years requirement is stored in the normal adult Kupffer cells of the liver.

ASSESSMENT:

INDICATIONS: Vitamin A is used for the treatment of vitamin A deficiency which may be provoked by sprue, colitis, reginal enteritis, biliary tract or pancreatic disease or portal gastrostomy. It is used specifically for the treatment of xerophthalmia, a type of eye disease characteristic of vitamin A deficient patients. It is also used in the treatment of nyctalopia, a type of night blindness. Certain cases of hyperkeratosis of the skin and lowered resistance to infection in general, which are seen in vitamin A deficiencies, are also improved by this agent.

SUBJECTIVE: Complaints of mild to moderate vitamin A deficiency include drying of ocular secretions, clouding of vision, and photophobia which may progress to an inability to see in subdued light and/or a decrease in visual acuity immediately following exposure to bright light.

OBJECTIVE: Practitioner should assess for dryness of the cornea which may progress to small epithelial erosions on the cornea. These may become infected, eventually leading to corneal destruction and blindness. Dry skin, scale formation, keratinization of the epithelial cells and connective tissue, decreased resistance to infection, and retardation of bone growth and tooth formation should all be considered during the examination.

PLAN:

CONTRAINDICATIONS: Do not give in the presence of hypersensitivity to vitamin A or any ingredient used in its preparation, hypervitaminosis A, or malabsorption syndrome. Do not give intravenously.

WARNINGS: Avoid overdosage. Keep out of the reach of children or pets.

PRECAUTIONS: The body is able to store extra vitamin A. Blood level assays are not a direct measure of liver storage, and liver storage should be adequate before discontinuing replacement therapy. If vitamin A is given in high doses over a long period, the treatment should be interrupted at times in over to avoid hypervitaminosis. Any patient receiving 25,000 USP IU or over should be closely supervised. Pregnant women should not receive more than 6,000 IU daily, or may risk fetal abnormalities. Patients undergoing hemodialysis chronically may develop vitamin A toxicity and elevated plasma calcium and alkaline phosphatase concentrations. Oral vitamin A therapy has not been shown effective in the treatment of acne.

IMPLEMENTATION:

DRUG INTERACTIONS: Females on oral contraceptives often show significant elevation in plasma vitamin A levels and should be closely monitored for hypervitaminosis. Mineral oil interferes with absorption of fat-soluble vitamins. Certain antihyperlipidemic agents may also affect absorption of this product.

ADMINISTRATION AND DOSAGE: One IU or USP unit vitamin A is equivalent to 0.6 mcg of beta-carotene or 0.3 mcg retinol. This medication may be given in oral, IV, or IM forms depending upon the rapidity of needed replacement. See individual drugs for dosage specifics.

Recommended daily intake includes:

Children 0 to 9 years: 300-450 mcg/day

Children 9 to 18 years: 575-750 mcg/day

Adults 18 to 75 years and older: 750 mcg/day

Pregnancy 2nd and 3rd trimester: 750 mcg/day

Lactation: 1200 mcg/day

IMPLEMENTATION CONSIDERATIONS:

—Obtain a complete health history, including the presence of hypersensitivity, possibility of pregnancy, underlying systemic disease, and past vitamin therapy. Attempt to identify problem which led to vitamin A deficiency.

—Vitamin A intake from all sources must be included in an evaluation of diet, in order to prevent hypervitaminosis A during therapy. For instance, dietary intake from natural as well as fortified food sources, dietary supplements, self-administered drugs, and over-the-counter and prescription drug sources should be evaluated. Absorption of vitamin A requires dietary fat, bile salts and pancreatic lipase.

—Care must be taken to keep these and any other medications out of the reach of children and others for whom they are not prescribed. Parents should be given the local poison control phone number in case of accidental ingestion.

—Vitamin A products should be stored in tight, light-resistant containers.

—Intramuscular injections of vitamin A must be given slowly and deeply in the upper outer quadrant of the gluteus or deep in the outer aspect of the thigh. Change the site of injection with each dose.

—Teaching about proper dietary intake, with an emphasis on those foods rich in vitamin A, may be essential in preventing recurrence of deficiency. The nurse must ascertain if cultural dietary habits, food fads or lack of finances or other resources contributed in any way to inadequate nutrition.

—Some research indicates that vitamin A deficiency states may be associated with a high incidence of cancer.

WHAT THE PATIENT NEEDS TO KNOW:

—Take this medication as ordered. Do not exceed the recommended dosage. It is possible to take too many vitamins.

—Do not take any mineral oil while taking this vitamin.

—Keep this drug out of the reach of children and all others for whom medication is not prescribed. Overdosage with this medication is possible, and the poison control center should be notified if overdosage is suspected.

—In order to reduce the likelihood of vitamin A deficiency in the future, include natural sources of vitamin A in your diet every day. Some foods rich in vitamin A include: animal products such as dairy products, eggs, organ meats (all contain preformed vitamin A); deep orange, yellow, and green fruits and vegetables (contain carotene.) In addition, some fortified sources of vitamin A include infant formula, skim milk, margarine, and some cereals.

—Store medicine in tightly capped, light-resistant containers.

—Report any of the following problems to your health care provider: lack of appetite, nausea, vomiting, feeling unusually tired, drying or cracking of skin or lips, irritability, headache or loss of hair.

EVALUATION:

ADVERSE REACTIONS: Anaphylactic shock and death have occurred following IV administration.

OVERDOSAGE: In acute toxicity, signs of increased intracranial pressure develop within 8 to 12 hours, and cutaneous desquamation may follow within a few days. Acute toxicity has been provoked by single doses of 25,000 IU/kg. Infants may show toxicity signs after 75,000 IU and adults when they have received over 2 million IU. Chronic toxicity may develop after prolonged administration of 4,000 IU/kg over 6 to 15 months. *Signs and symptoms:* fatigue, malaise, lethargy, abdominal discomfort, anorexia, and vomiting. Specific signs include slow growth of skeletal bones, hard, painful cortical thickening over the radius and tibia, migratory arthralgia, premature closure of the epiphysis, irritability, headache, bulging fontanelles from increased intracranial pressure in infants, papilledema, exophthalmos, fissure of the lips, drying and cracking of the skin, alopecia, scaling, massive desquamation, increased pigmentation, hypomenorrhea, hepatosplenomegaly, jaundice, leukopenia. Laboratory studies will reveal Vitamin A plasma levels in excess of 1,200 IU/100 ml. *Treatment:* Discontinue intake of vitamin A, and symptoms promptly disappear.

PARAMETERS TO MONITOR: Evaluate for therapeutic signs: relief of symptoms and reduction in serum plasma levels of vitamin A. Evaluate other sources of vitamin A which patient may be taking. Watch for signs of hypervitaminosis which may be slow in onset and duration: headache, blurry vision or diplopia, nausea and vomiting, bone pain, peeling skin, fissures and sores at the corners of the mouth, and hair loss. In infants, symptoms of hypervitaminosis include drowsiness, vomiting, bulging fontanelles secondary to increased intracranial pressure. Chronic deficiency leads to failure to gain weight, loss of hair, coarseness of hair, liver enlargement and swelling of the extremities. Prolonged or severe hypervitaminosis may induce skeletal changes, i.e., cortical thickening of hands and feet, clinically manifested by tenderness and weakness. Hypervitaminosis is not common except in patients who are likely to engage in food fads, strange diets, and excessive use of health foods and vitamins.

VITAMIN A—PREPARATIONS

PRODUCTS: (TRADE NAME):

Aquasol A (Available in 5,000 IU/0.1 ml drops, 25,000 IU and 50,000 IU capsules, and 50,000 IU/ml injection.) **Alphalin Gelseals** (Available in 50,000 IU capsules.) **Vitamin A** (Available in 10,000 IU tablets, 10,000, 25,000 and 50,000 IU capsules, and 50,000 IU/ml injection.)

DRUG SPECIFICS:

Patients should be cautioned about overdosage potential. They should contact health provider if nausea, vomiting, anorexia, malaise, drying or cracking of skin or lips, irritability, headache, or loss of hair occur.

ADMINISTRATION AND DOSAGE SPECIFICS:

Adults and Children:

Treatment of severe deficiency state and xerophthalmia: 500,000 IU/day for 3 days, followed by 50,000 IU/day for 2 weeks.

Treatment of severe deficiency state: 100,000 IU/day for 3 days, followed by 50,000 IU/day for 2 weeks.

Follow-up therapy: 10,000 to 20,000 IU/day for 2 months.

Parenteral Therapy:

Adults: 100,000 IU/day for 3 days, followed by 50,000 IU/day for 2 weeks.

Children 1 to 8 years old: 17,5000 to 35,000 IU/day for 10 days.

Infants: 7,500 to 15,000 IU/day for 10 days.

ISOTRETINOIN (13-cis-Retinoic Acid)

PRODUCTS (TRADE NAME):

Accutane (Available in 10 and 40 mg capsules.)

DRUG SPECIFICS:

This vitamin A metabolite is effective in the treatment of cystic acne through reduction in sebum secretion. Sebaceous gland size and differentiation is inhibited as well as the keratinization process. The exact mechanism of action is unknown. It has also been used for a variety of other cutaneous disorders of keratinization, and for mycosis fungoides.

This product must not be taken by women who are pregnant since severe fetal abnormalities may be produced. Women in childbearing years should be protected by adequate contraception methods during the course of therapy. At least one quarter of patients taking this medication develop elevated plasma triglyceride levels, one fifth of the patients show a reduction in high density lipoproteins and about one tenth of the patients demonstrate an increase in cholesterol level. These laboratory tests should be obtained regularly, with alcoholic consumption being discontinued at least 36 hours before blood is drawn. Patients may develop a variety of musculoskeletal complaints (such as arthralgia, bone, joint, muscle pain and stiffness) while on this product. A few patients have also reported corneal opacities developing as a result of this drug.

Frequently an exacerbation of acne occurs during the initial period of therapy, followed by a reduction in numbers of cysts. Rarely, an exaggerated healing response may develop, with exuberant granulation and crusting of lesions. Do not give this product concurrently with minocycline or tetracycline, as a few cases of pseudotumor cerebri or papilledema have been reported.

Most adverse effects appear to be dose related, with the more pronounced effects occurring at doses greater than 1.0 mg/kg/day. Adverse effects are usually reversible. Most common side effects are: cheilitis, eye irritation, conjunctivitis, skin fragility, with associated dry skin, pruritus, dry nose, dry mouth, and epistaxis. Nausea, vomiting, mild abdominal pain, and lethargy may also be noted. Elevated sedimentation rate may be seen in 40% of patients. Some side effects may be decreased when medication is taken with meals. Store medication in tight, light-resistant containers between 59 and 86 degrees Fahrenheit.

ADMINISTRATION AND DOSAGE SPECIFICS:

Cystic acne: 1 to 2 mg/kg/day divided into 2 doses for 2 weeks. Dosage may then be adjusted for individual weight and severity of disease. Higher end of dosage range may be required for patients greater than 70 kg and whose cysts are primarily on the back and chest. Treatment should be continued for 15 to 20 weeks. Discontinue product when there is 70% reduction in number of cysts. If retreatment is warranted, allow at least 2 months to elapse before starting patient again on medication.

Carol Wilson

VITAMIN B₁ (THIAMINE HCL)

ACTION OF THE DRUG: Thiamine is a water-soluble vitamin, that functions as a coenzyme involved closely with carbohydrate metabolism. Thiamine participates in 24 different reactions, including the citric acid cycle. It also has been thought to have a role in neurophysiology. Thiamine is excreted in the urine.

ASSESSMENT:

INDICATIONS: Used for the treatment of beriberi which, although rare in the United States, does sometimes occur. It is usually found in conjunction with alcoholism, gastric lesions, and hyperemesis of pregnancy.

SUBJECTIVE: Thiamine deficiency (beriberi) symptoms may be present in association with conditions such as alcoholism and gastric lesions and following hyperemesis of pregnancy. Symptoms include anorexia, vomiting, fatigability, aching muscles, ataxia of gait, and emotional disturbances such as moodiness or depression.

OBJECTIVE: Chronic manifestations include heart failure and various neurologic manifestations. Acute signs include edema; in infants, loss of voice, sudden episodes of cyanosis and cardiac arrest, pseudomeningitis. Occidental beriberi (secondary to alcoholism) can manifest itself as heart failure with normal or increased cardiac output which is not responsive to traditional therapy. Mild peripheral neuritis may also be found.

PLAN:

CONTRAINDICATIONS: Do not give in the presence of hypersensitivity to thiamine HCl.

WARNINGS: Sensitivity reactions, particularly following parenteral administration, can be of a severe allergic type, including anaphylaxis. Fatalities may occur. Sensitivity tests should be done before administration of therapeutic dose. IV doses should be administered very slowly.

PRECAUTIONS: Specific thiamine deficiencies are rare; suspect multiple deficiencies to be present.

IMPLEMENTATION:

DRUG INTERACTIONS: Neutral or alkaline solutions will produce poor stability of thiamine preparations.

PRODUCTS (TRADE NAME):
Betalin-S (Available in 10, 25, 50, and 100 mg tablets; 2.25 mg/5 ml elixir in 10% alcohol solution; 100 mg/ml injection.) **Bewon** (Available in 0.25 mg/5 ml elixir with 16% alcohol solution.) **Thiamine HCl** (Available in 5, 10, 25, 50, 100, 250 and 500 mg tablets; 1 mg/5 ml elixir; 100 mg/ml injection.)

ADMINISTRATION AND DOSAGE: Medication may be given po, IM or IV. Daily average dose is 0.5 mg/1000 kcal intake, or usually 1 to 1.4 mg/day. Increased intakes are recommended during periods of increased metabolism such as fever, hyperthyroidism, pregnancy, muscular activity, or breast-feeding.

IMPLEMENTATION CONSIDERATIONS:
—Obtain a complete health history, including a complete diet history in order to determine the cause of thiamine deficiency. Ask about use of vitamin supplements; fortified food sources, self-administered, over-the-counter, and prescription drugs; intake of alcohol; gastrointestinal pathology; or possibility of pregnancy.

—Thiamine is easily leached out of food and destroyed by heat over 100 degrees centigrade. It is destroyed in food fried in hot pans or cooked for a long time under pressure. There is some loss of thiamine during dehydration of vegetables. Product is also sensitive to ultraviolet light.

—Thiamine deficiency alone is rare; suspect multiple deficiencies.

—Teach the patient good nutritional habits, stressing those foods which are high in thiamine. This will be important if dietary habits are instrumental in the development of the deficiency. Ascertain if cultural dietary habits, food fads, or lack of finances or other resources have contributed in any way to inadequate nutrition.

—IV doses should be administered very slowly.

—There is decreased absorption in alcoholics, often related to a coexisting folic acid deficiency. Correction of the folic acid deficiency will help increase absorption of thiamine.

WHAT THE PATIENT NEEDS TO KNOW:

—Take this medication only as prescribed.

—Protect product from light by keeping it in a tightly sealed, light-resistant container.

—Keep this drug out of the reach of children and all others for whom it is not prescribed.

—Care must be taken in food preparation to prevent loss of thiamine. It is easily leached out of foods by soaking or boiling foods in water; it can be destroyed in temperatures over 100 degrees centigrade; it can be destroyed in food fried in hot pans or cooked a long time under pressure. Some thiamine can be lost when vegetables are dehydrated.

—Food sources rich in thiamine include pork, whole grains, enriched breads, and cereals and legumes. Satisfactory sources include green vegetables, fish, meats, fruit, and milk.

EVALUATION:

ADVERSE REACTIONS: *Dermatologic:* feelings of warmth, pruritus, urticaria. *Gastrointestinal:* hemorrhage of the GI tract, nausea. *Hypersensitivity:* angioneurotic edema, pulmonary edema, sweating, tightness of the throat, weakness. *Other:* collapse, cyanosis, and in some cases death.

OVERDOSAGE: Excess thiamine is excreted by the kidney and there is no known kidney threshold. No toxicity problem is known.

PARAMETERS TO MONITOR: In deficiency states, a rise in the serum pyruvic acid is considered a diagnostic sign. Patient should be monitored for resolution of symptoms and change in nutritional behavior following teaching. Patient should also be evaluated for the development of adverse effects.

Carol Wilson

VITAMIN B₂ (RIBOFLAVIN)

ACTION OF THE DRUG: Riboflavin is a water-soluble vitamin that functions as a precursor of two essential enzymes which deal with intermediary metabolism of proteins, fats, and carbohydrates. It also functions in the citric acid cycle, is related to the release of energy to the cells, and is active in tissue respiratory systems.

ASSESSMENT:

INDICATIONS: Used for the prophylaxis or treatment of riboflavin deficiency.

SUBJECTIVE: Early symptoms include soreness and burning of the tongue, lips, and mouth, discomfort in eating and swallowing, photophobia, lacrimation, burning and itching of the eyes, visual fatigue, and loss of visual acuity.

OBJECTIVE: Late manifestations include pallor, maceration at the angles of the mouth; dryness, redness, and denudation along the line of closure (cheilosis) of the lips; loss of filiform papillae on the tongue and enlargement of fungiform papillae, with possible extensive fissuring. A dermatitis of a scaly and oily character may develop, often beginning in the skin folds with scrotum or vulva potentially being involved. Vascularization of the cornea may also develop.

PLAN:

PRECAUTIONS: Riboflavin is unstable in the presence of alkali or ultraviolet light.

IMPLEMENTATION:

DRUG INTERACTIONS: Riboflavin is only slightly soluble in water. The solubility may be increased by the addition of urea. Riboflavin can be depleted by oral contraceptives, even in low doses. This depletion has been shown through studies to be greater when patients have been taking oral contraceptives over a period of at least 3 years.

PRODUCTS (TRADE NAME):

Riobin-50 (Available in 50 mg/ml injection). **Riboflavin** (Available in 5, 10, 25, 50 and 100 mg tablets).

ADMINISTRATION AND DOSAGE: Requirements are generally based on the level of caloric intake with 0.6 mg for every 1000 kcal. Recommended allowances include: 0.4 mg to 0.6 mg for infants; 0.18 to 1.2 mg for children; 1.4 to 1.6 mg for males (depending on age); and 1.1 mg to 1.3 mg for females. Increased dosages should be given during pregnancy and breast-feeding.

Usually dose is 50 mg IM for deficiency states, and 5-10 mg daily as dietary supplement for adults and children over 12 years of age.

IMPLEMENTATION CONSIDERATIONS:

—Obtain a complete health and dietary history from patient in order to determine the cause of the deficiency. Single vitamin deficiencies are rare; consider multiple deficiencies. Assess dietary intake from natural as well as fortified food sources, dietary supplements, and self-administered over-the-counter preparations or prescription drugs. Evaluate cultural dietary habits, adherence to food fads, or lack of financial or other resources which may have provoked development of deficiency. Assess whether female patient is currently taking or has recently taken oral contraceptives and for how long.

—Riboflavin is fairly heat stable but will leach out into cooking water.
—This vitamin is excreted by the kidneys and gives a yellow color to the urine.
—Riboflavin is unstable in the presence of alkali or in the presence of ultraviolet light.
—Teach the patient good nutritional habits and stress those foods which are high in riboflavin. This will be important if dietary habits were instrumental in the development of the deficiency.
—Patients who have been taking oral contraceptives for longer than 2 years might be placed on prophylactic therapy.

WHAT THE PATIENT NEEDS TO KNOW:
—Take this medication exactly as prescribed.
—Protect this product from light by keeping it in a tightly closed, light-resistant container.
—Keep this drug out of the reach of children and all others for whom it has not been prescribed.
—Care must be taken in food preparation to prevent loss of riboflavin. It is easily leached out of foods prepared in water.
—This medication turns the urine a yellow color.
—Food sources naturally rich in riboflavin include milk, eggs, liver, kidney, heart, green leafy vegetables, and enriched breads and cereals.

EVALUATION:

ADVERSE REACTIONS: None known.
PARAMETERS TO MONITOR: Watch for disappearance of deficiency symptoms. Assess patient's compliance with good nutritional patterns and medication supplements.

Carol Wilson

VITAMIN B₃ (NICOTINIC ACID, NIACIN OR NICOTINAMIDE—NIACINAMIDE)

ACTION OF THE DRUG: Vitamin B_3 is a water-soluble vitamin. Niacin is an essential component of two coenzymes (NAD and NADP) which transfer hydrogen in intracellular respiration. These coenzymes convert lactic acid to pyruvic acid and function in energy release and in amino acid metabolism. The body converts approximately 60 mg tryptophan to about 1 mg niacin. Nicotinic acid has two actions: peripheral vasodilation and serum cholesterol-reducing properties. (See section on Antihyperlipidemic drugs for additional information.)

ASSESSMENT:

INDICATIONS: Niacin is used for the prevention or treatment of deficiency states. Deficiency can be caused by limited dietary intake of niacin, excessive dietary intake of leucine (which increases the daily need for niacin), generalized anorexia related to disease or other problems, or malabsorptive syndrome. The deficiency disease is pellagra, which is rare but may be more prevalent where corn is the major staple. It is usually found in conjunction with other vitamin deficiencies. Niacin is also used as adjunctive therapy in treatment of conditions associated with hyperbetalipoproteinemia.

SUBJECTIVE: Deficiency symptoms are characterized by mucous membrane, cutaneous, gastrointestinal, and CNS manifestations. Gastrointestinal discomfort, anorexia, irritability, anxiety, and mental changes such as hallucinations, lassitude, apprehension, and depression may be especially prominent.

OBJECTIVE: Gastrointestinal symptoms include glossitis, stomatitis, swollen, beefy, red tongue, and diarrhea. (Inflammation of mucous membranes may result in glossitis and diarrhea.) Dermatitis of different body parts exposed to sun or trauma may develop as well as lesions on the skin from sun, fire or heat. Mental changes which are subjective early in deficiency may progress to disorientation, loss of memory, confusion, hysteria, and sometimes maniacal outbursts.

PLAN:

CONTRAINDICATIONS: Do not give in the presence of known hypersensitivity or idiosyncrasy to niacin, arterial bleeding, severe hypotension, hemorrhaging, hepatic dysfunction, or active, acute peptic ulcer.

WARNINGS: Not recommended for use in children. In pregnant or breastfeeding women, weigh the therapeutic benefits against the potential hazards to mother and child. There is no substantiated evidence that use of megadoses has any affect on schizophrenia.

PRECAUTIONS: Gallbladder disease, history of jaundice, liver disorders or peptic ulcer all require close medical supervision with this drug. Diabetics may require adjustment of diet and insulin dosage if decreased tolerance develops. Use with caution in patients with gout because of the occurrence of elevated uric acid levels. Because of the presence of the sensitizing agent, tartrazine, patients with allergies (especially to aspirin) may develop hypersensitivity reactions.

IMPLEMENTATION:

DRUG INTERACTIONS: Sympathetic blocking agents (antihypertensives) may increase vasodilatory effect leading to postural hypotension.

ADMINISTRATION AND DOSAGE: Recommended intakes are 8 mg/1000 kcal for infants and 6.6 mg/1000 kcal for children and adolescents. Not less than 8 mg/day should be given. Recommended dose for adults is 13 mg/day for women and 18 mg/day for men.

IMPLEMENTATION CONSIDERATIONS:

—Obtain a complete health history, including assessment of underlying gallbladder disease, jaundice or liver disease, peptic ulcer, diabetes or gout, arterial bleeding, history of hypersensitivity, and the possibility of pregnancy. Obtain a complete dietary history, including dietary supplements, natural and fortified food sources, self-administered over-the-counter or prescription drugs, especially antihypertensive medications. Assess cultural habits, food fad involvement, and financial or other resource limitations which may have led to this deficiency.

—Flushing is a frequent side effect of this medication. If the patient feels weak or dizzy, he or she should lie down until feeling better. The health care provider should then be notified. Usually, this reaction does not necessitate discontinuing the drug.

—Teach the patient principles of sound nutrition, including those foods which contain ample quantities of niacin.

WHAT THE PATIENT NEEDS TO KNOW:

—Take this medication exactly as ordered.

—Keep this medicine out of the reach of children and all others for whom it is not prescribed.

—Promptly inform your health care practitioner about any side effects you may experience.

—Foods rich in niacin are lean meats, peanuts, yeast, and cereal (especially bran and germ.) Other good sources include eggs, liver, red meat, whole grain, and enriched bread.

EVALUATION:

ADVERSE REACTIONS: *Dermatologic:* dry skin, keratosis nigricans, pruritus, skin rash. *Gastrointestinal:* abnormal liver function tests, activation of peptic ulcer, gastrointestinal disorders, jaundice. *Other:* allergies, decreased glucose tolerance, feelings of warmth, headache, hypotension, tingling of the skin, toxic amblyopia, transient flushing.

OVERDOSAGE: There may be some evidence that long-term, high-dosage nicotinic acid therapy may produce laboratory signs of diabetes and hepatic injury. Activation of peptic ulcer with use of unbuffered acid may also develop.

PARAMETERS TO MONITOR: Evaluate for therapeutic effects seen by disappearance of symptoms. Assess for development of adverse effects. Frequent liver function tests and blood glucose levels should be obtained, especially in the initial stages of therapy. Close supervision of diabetic diets and insulin doses should be maintained. Uric acid levels in patients predisposed to gout should also be followed.

NICOTINIC ACID (NIACIN)

PRODUCTS (TRADE NAME):
Diacin (Available in 200 mg timed release capsules.) **Niac** (Available in 300 mg timed release capsules.) **Nico-400,** (Available in 400 mg timed release capsules.) **Nicobid** (Available in 125, 250, and 500 mg timed release capsule.) **Nicolar** (Available in 500 mg tablets.) **Nico-Span** (Available in 400 mg timed release capsules.) **Nicotinex** (Available in 50 mg/5 ml elixir.) **Nicotinic Acid** (Available in 50, 100 and 500 mg tablets; 125, 250, and 400 mg timed release capsules, and 50 and 100 mg/ml injection.) **Span-Niacin-150** (Available in 150 mg timed release capsules.) **Tega-Span** (Available in 400 mg timed release capsules.)

DRUG SPECIFICS:
Used in the treatment of deficiency states and in the treatment of hyperlipidemia. Medication is usually given orally. Parenteral therapy may be given if patient is unable to take orally. May be given IM, SQ or IV, the IV route with slow drip preferred when parenteral medication is necessary.

ADMINISTRATION AND DOSAGE SPECIFICS:
Deficiency states: 50 to 100 mg daily.
Pellagra: Up to 500 mg/day.
Hyperlipidemia: 1 to 2 gm 3 times daily. Maximum dose is 6 gm/day.

NICOTINAMIDE (NIACINAMIDE)

PRODUCTS (TRADE NAME):
Nicotinamide (Available in 50, 100, 500 mg tablets and 500 mg capsules; and 100 mg/ml injection.)

DRUG SPECIFICS:
This product is used by the body as a vitamin source although it does not have the hypolipidemic or vasodilating effects of niacin. It is used in the prophylaxis and treatment of pellagra.

ADMINISTRATION AND DOSAGE SPECIFICS:
500 mg po daily, or may give 100 to 200 mg 1 to 5 times daily parenterally, depending upon the severity of the symptoms.

Carol Wilson

VITAMIN B$_5$ (CALCIUM PANTOTHENATE)

ACTION OF THE DRUG: Vitamin B$_5$, or pantothenic acid, is essential for the synthesis of coenzyme A, which has a role in the release of energy in fats, proteins and carbohydrates. It participates in the oxidation of several substances and is essential for the synthesis of porphyrin, fat, and cholesterol.

ASSESSMENT:

INDICATIONS: This vitamin has been used in the treatment of paralytic ileus following surgery, possibly acting to stimulate gastrointestinal motility. Other suggested benefits for humans have not been confirmed in controlled studies.

SUBJECTIVE: Volunteers who participated in deficiency studies experienced headache, fatigue, weakness, impaired motor coordination, muscle cramps, emotional lability, nausea, gastrointestinal distress or burning and cramps, tenderness in the heels, and insomnia.

OBJECTIVE: The most consistent objective finding is vomiting.

PLAN:

PRECAUTIONS: Vitamin is unstable in the presence of acids, bases, and heat.

IMPLEMENTATION:

PRODUCTS (TRADE NAMES):
Calcium Pantothenate (Available in 30, 100 and 218 mg tablets). **Durasil** (Available in 10 mg calcium pantothenate tablets with 200 mg aluminum hydroxide and 200 mg magnesium trisilicate). **Pantholin** (Available in 10 mg tablets).

ADMINISTRATION AND DOSAGE: Therapeutic dosage is not known. Dietary intake of the adult population is 5 to 20 mg/day. A daily intake of 5 to 10 mg is thought to be adequate, with the lower level suggested for children and the upper level suggested for pregnant and breast-feeding women. A dosage of 2 mg/day has been suggested for infants and 4 to 7 mg/day for adolescents.

Usual dose is 10 mg/day although 20 to 100 mg/day have been employed for therapeutic and experimental purposes.

IMPLEMENTATION CONSIDERATIONS:
—Obtain a complete health history, including the presence of underlying or systemic disease, hypersensitivities, and a complete diet survey including general nutritional status.

—This vitamin is abundant in many foods, and specific deficiency of this vitamin is difficult to produce. If patient has a documented deficiency of other vitamins, observe for symptoms that may be related to this vitamin also.

—Vitamin is unstable in the presence of acids, bases, and heat.

—Provide patient teaching regarding foods which are high in this vitamin.

—Evaluate patient behavior to determine if cultural factors, adherence to food fads, lack of education, and lack of financial or other resources might be responsible for dietary problems.

—Human milk contains 2.2 mg/liter, and cow's milk contains 3.4 mg/liter of calcium.

WHAT THE PATIENT NEEDS TO KNOW:
—Take this medication exactly as ordered.
—Keep this product out of the reach of children and all others for whom it is not prescribed.
—Care must be taken in food preparation to prevent the loss of pantothenic acid. When food is cooked above the boiling point, considerable loss of this vitamin occurs. Less loss occurs through moderate cooking or baking. Much of the original vitamin content is lost from frozen meat in the liquid which drips off during thawing.
—This vitamin is available naturally in all plant and animal tissues. Rich sources include yeast, liver, kidney, egg yolk, wheat bran and fresh vegetables. Human milk contains 2.2 mg/liter and cow's milk 3.4 mg/liter.

EVALUATION:

PARAMETERS TO MONITOR: Observe for development of good nutritional habits and general improvement in health. Patient should be able to explain what he or she should eat and to present a diet recall which includes daily essential nutrients.

Carol Wilson

VITAMIN B₆ (PYRIDOXINE HCL)

ACTION OF THE DRUG: Vitamin B_6 is a water-soluble vitamin that functions as a coenzyme in the metabolism of protein, carbohydrates and fat. In amino acid metabolism, it is involved in decarboxylation, conversion of tryptophan to niacin or serotonin, deamination, transamination, and transulfuration of amino acid. In carbohydrate metabolism, it breaks down glucose to glucose-l-phosphate.

ASSESSMENT:

INDICATIONS: Pyridoxine is used in the treatment of pyridoxine deficiency seen in inborn errors of metabolism such as vitamin B_6 dependency; vitamin B_6–responsive chronic anemia, vitamin B_6–responsive xanthurenic aciduria and crystathioninuria; and homocystinuria. Patients most likely to develop pyridoxine deficiency include the elderly, pregnant or breast-feeding women, and women of childbearing age. Women taking oral contraceptives, alcoholics, and those whose diets are of poor quality and quantity or whose diets are rich in refined foods are also at risk.
SUBJECTIVE: Symptoms of deficiency include weakness, nervousness, irritability, and difficulty in walking. There may also be personality changes in adults such as depression and a loss of sense of responsibility.

OBJECTIVE: Manifestations of deficiency include microcytic hypochromic anemia and kidney stones. There may also be pyridoxine-responsive anemia and diarrhea as well as seizures.

PLAN:

CONTRAINDICATIONS: Do not give in the presence of hypersensitivity to pyridoxine.

WARNINGS: Protect preparation from exposure to ultraviolet light. Use in breast-feeding women may inhibit lactation due to suppression of prolactin.

PRECAUTIONS: Alcohol ingestion and alcoholic liver disease can interfere with the normal processes of vitamin B_6 metabolism. Women taking oral contraceptives may need vitamin B_6 supplementation. Pyridoxine is resistant to normal heat but decomposes in alkalis and ultraviolet light. Pyridoxine needs in pregnancy may be increased, but this has not been conclusively proven.

IMPLEMENTATION:

DRUG INTERACTIONS: Oral contraceptives may induce pyridoxine deficiency. Concurrent use with levodopa will decrease the anti-parkinsonian effect of levodopa. Pyridoxine may prevent chloramphenicol-induced optic neuritis. Demonstrated antagonists to pyridoxine include deoxypyridoxine, isoniazid, hydralazine hydrochloride, and penicillamine. These antagonists promote enough interference with pyridoxine to provoke signs of deficiency.

PRODUCTS (TRADE NAMES):
Beesix (Available in 100 mg/ml injection.) **Hexa-Betalin** (Available in 10 and 50 mg tablets, and 100 mg/ml injection.) **Pyridoxine HCl** (Available in 5, 10, 25, 50, 100, 200, 250, and 500 mg tablets, and 100 mg/ml injection.) **TexSix T.R.** (Available in 100 mg timed release capsules.)

ADMINISTRATION AND DOSAGE: Recommended daily allowances range from 2 to 2.2 mg. Preparation may be given po, IM, or IV.

Dietary deficiency: Give 10-20 mg/day for 3 weeks, then 2-5 mg/day for several weeks.

Adjunctive therapy to isoniazid treatment: Give 100 mg/day for 3 weeks, then 50 mg daily. 10 mg/day may be sufficient for prophylactic therapy.

Vitamin B_6 dependency states: May give up to 600 mg/day initially, dropping to 50 mg/day for life.

IMPLEMENTATION CONSIDERATIONS:
—Obtain a complete health history, including the presence of hypersensitivities, underlying systemic disease, concurrent use of alcohol or medications, especially oral contraceptives or isoniazid, and possibility of pregnancy. Obtain a complete dietary history to evaluate nutritional pattern. Assess dietary intake from natural as well as fortified food sources, dietary supplements, and self-administered drugs, whether over the counter or prescription.

—Teach patients principles of good nutrition, including those foods which are the best sources of pyridoxine. Ascertain if cultural dietary habits, food fads, lack of education, finances, or other resources have contributed in any way to inadequate nutrition.

—Parenteral route may be used when patient is vomiting or otherwise unable to take medication orally.

WHAT THE PATIENT NEEDS TO KNOW:
—Vitamin should be taken exactly as ordered.
—Keep this preparation out of the reach of children and all others for whom it is not prescribed.
—Product should be kept in a tightly sealed, light-resistant container.
—Good food sources of pyridoxine include yeast, wheat, corn, egg yolk, liver, kidney and muscle meats. Limited amounts are available from milk and vegetables.
—Appropriate food preparation is important in preserving this vitamin. Freezing of vegetables results in a 20% loss of pyridoxine, and the milling of wheat results in a 90% loss.
—Check with your health care provider before drinking alcohol while taking this vitamin.

EVALUATION:

ADVERSE REACTIONS: Even with dosages exceeding 1000 mg/day, no adverse effects are usually found. Seizures may be aggravated in selected patients, with EEG pattern changes developing in others. Isolated incidents of lethargy, excessive energy, insomnia, or low serum folic acid levels have been found.

OVERDOSAGE: Adults taking doses exceeding 200 mg/day for a month may develop pyridoxine dependency.

PARAMETERS TO MONITOR: Assess for therapeutic effects, i.e., the disappearance of symptoms. Evaluate the general nutritional pattern of patient and whether behavior patterns are likely to prompt recurrence of pyridoxine deficiency in the future.

Carol Wilson

VITAMIN B$_{12}$ (CYANOCOBALAMIN; CYANOCOBALAMIN CRYSTALLINE)

ACTION OF THE DRUG: Vitamin B$_{12}$ is a water-soluble vitamin containing cobalt. It is produced by the bacterium *Streptomyces griseus*. It functions in many metabolic processes in protein, fat, and carbohydrate metabolism. The coenzymes of B$_{12}$ are also part of the erythrocyte-maturing factor of the liver and are required in the synthesis of DNA. Vitamin B$_{12}$ has a hematopoietic activity identical to the antianemia factor of the liver, and it is essential for growth, cell reproduction, and nucleoprotein and myelin synthesis. Vitamin B_{12} also interacts with folate in metabolic functions, and a deficiency in B_{12} renders folate useless in the body.

ASSESSMENT:

INDICATIONS: Vitamin B_{12} is used in the treatment of all B_{12} deficiency conditions including pernicious anemia (with or without neurologic manifestations); malabsorption syndromes; certain macrocytic or megaloblastic anemias; hemorrhage; blind-loop syndrome; infection due to fish tapeworm (*Diphyllobothrium latum*); nutritional macrocytic anemias of infancy, pregnancy and chronic liver disease complicated by deficiency of vitamin B_{12}; malignancy; thyrotoxicosis and renal disorders. Vitamin B_{12} is also used as the flushing dose in Schilling's test.

SUBJECTIVE: Symptoms of deficiency are rare, occurring mainly in those persons on strict vegetarian diets since vitamin B_{12} is found only in animal products. Symptoms include dyspepsia, sore tongue, breathlessness, and a characteristic stiff back, dubbed a "poker" or "vegan" back.

OBJECTIVE: Pathology may be demonstrated only through biopsy, showing nervous system lesions presenting as patchy, diffuse, and progressive demyelination producing an insidious neuropathy which moves peripherally to centrally. Children of women with long-standing deficiency may be born with congenital vitamin B_{12} deficiency showing megaloblastic anemia, neurologic anomalies, homocystinuria, and methylmalonic aciduria.

PLAN:

CONTRAINDICATIONS: Do not give in the presence of hypersensitivity to cobalt and/or vitamin B_{12}.

WARNINGS: Sudden and severe optic atrophy may develop in patients with early Leber's disease (hereditary optic nerve atrophy) or those predisposed to optic nerve atrophy. The presence of infection, uremia, concurrent iron or folic acid deficiencies, concomitant treatment with drugs having bone marrow suppressant properties (such as chloramphenicol), or misdiagnosis should be considered if an inadequate therapeutic response is found. Safety for use during pregnancy, breast-feeding, or with children has not been established.

PRECAUTIONS: Irreparable neurologic damage may occur if deficiency state continues longer than 3 months or when treatment for pernicious anemia includes only folic acid. If colchicine, *p*-aminosalicylic acid are used, or excessive alcohol intake occurs for more than two weeks, malabsorption of vitamin B_{12} may occur. In severe megaloblastic conditions, monitor serum potassium levels at the beginning of therapy due to the possibility of hypokalemia.

IMPLEMENTATION:

DRUG INTERACTIONS: Alcohol, colchicine, and *p*-aminosalicylic acid lower vitamin B_{12} absorption. Chloramphenicol and neomycin lower the response to vitamin B_{12} therapy. When the patient is treated with methotrexate, pyrimethamine, or most antibiotics, diagnostic microbiological blood assays of folic acid and vitamin B_{12} are nullified.

ADMINISTRATION AND DOSAGE: Drugs and dosages differ for treatment of nutritional deficiency and for treatment of pernicious anemia and cannot be used interchangeably. Consult specific product information for appropriate medication. Recommended daily allowance for cyanocobalamin for adults is 3 mcg.

IMPLEMENTATION CONSIDERATIONS:

—Obtain a complete health history, including the presence of underlying or systemic disease, diet intake from natural as well as fortified food sources, any dietary supplements, and self-administered over-the-counter or prescription drugs. Assess dietary patterns for any evidence of partial or complete vegetarianism, recent use of antibiotics, and pattern of alcoholic intake.

—Teach patient principles of sound nutrition, including those foods which are good sources of vitamin B_{12}. Ascertain if cultural dietary habits or lack of finances or other resources have contributed in any way to inadequate nutrition.

—It is uncommon to find patients with only a single vitamin deficiency. Investigate the possibility of multiple vitamin deficiency being present.

—Vitamin B_{12} is unstable in solution in the presence of alkali.

WHAT THE PATIENT NEEDS TO KNOW:

—Take this medication exactly as prescribed.

—Keep this medication out of the reach of children and others for whom it has not been prescribed.

—Inform your health care provider if you need to take any antibiotics while on this medication.

—Alcoholic intake will interfere with the absorption of this medicine and should be avoided during therapy.

—In order to avoid further deficiency problems, eat a diet high in vitamin B_{12}. The best food sources include organ meats, bivalves such as clams and oysters, nonfat dry milk, seafoods such as lobster, scallops, flounder, haddock, swordfish, and tuna, and fermented cheese such as Camembert and Limburger.

EVALUATION:

ADVERSE REACTIONS: *Hypersensitivity:* Allergy is rare. Patient may report itching, feeling of swelling of the entire body, transitory exanthema, polycythemia vera, peripheral vascular thrombosis, pulmonary edema, congestive heart failure, and anaphylactic shock (proceeding to death in a few cases.) A few patients may experience mild pain, localized skin irritation, or mild transient diarrhea following injection of cyanocobalamin.

OVERDOSAGE: This product is not toxic, even in large doses.

PARAMETERS TO MONITOR: In patients with suspected deficiency states, CBC with indices and electrolytes should be obtained prior to placing patient on vitamin B_{12} therapy. These studies should be repeated periodically throughout the treatment period. In patients with suspected pernicious anemia, confirmatory diagnostic studies should be conducted prior to initiation of therapy, and hemoglobin, hematocrit, RBC with indices, and reticulocyte count should be regularly obtained during therapy. B_{12} and folic acid levels should be obtained before beginning treatment and between the 5th and 7th day following initiation of therapy. Serum potassium levels should be monitored especially closely at the beginning of therapy, and supplementary doses of potassium may be indicated.

CYANOCOBALAMIN

PRODUCTS (TRADE NAMES):

Kaybovite (Available in 100 mcg soluble tablets.) **Redisol** (Available in 25 and 50 mcg tablets.) **Vitamin B_{12}** (Available in 25, 50, 100, and 250 mcg tablets and in 25, 50 and 100 mcg soluble tablets, and 25 mcg capsules.)

DRUG SPECIFICS:

With the exception of Redisol, these products are usually relatively inexpensive. They are used only for treatment of nutritional deficiency.

ADMINISTRATION AND DOSAGE SPECIFICS:

Nutritional deficiency: Give 25 to 250 mcg/day po.

CYANOCOBALAMIN, CRYSTALLINE

PRODUCTS (TRADE NAME):

Betalin 12 (Available in 100 and 1000 mcg/ml injections.) **Berubigen, Cabadon M, Crysti-12 1000, Crystimin 1000, Cyanoject, Cyomin, Dodex, Kaybovite-1000, Pernavit** (Available in 1000 mcg/ml injection.) **Redisol** (Available in 500 mcg tablets and in 100 and 1000 mcg/ml injections.) **Rubesol 1000** (Available in 1000 mcg/ml injection.) **Rubramin PC** (Available in 100 and 1000 mcg/ml injections.) **Ruvite** (Available in 1000 mcg/ml injection.) **Vitamin B_{12}** (Available in 500 and 1000 mcg tablets, and in 30, 100, 120, and 1000 mcg/ml injections.) **Vi-Twel** (Available in 1000 mcg/ml injection.)

DRUG SPECIFICS:

May give an interdermal test dose to check for sensitivity to cyanocobalamin prior to starting therapy. In pernicious anemia parenteral therapy for the duration of the patient's life is usually indicated. Oral absorption is inconsistent and should not be relied upon. In other vitamin B_{12} deficiency states, route of administration must be determined depending upon etiology of the problem.

ADMINISTRATION AND DOSAGE SPECIFICS:

Vitamin B_{12} deficiency: 1000 mcg/day po. If patients have normal gastrointestinal absorption give 15 mcg/day along with other multiple vitamins. In other cases, give 30 mcg IM or SQ daily for 5 to 10 days, and then 100 to 200 mcg monthly. Higher doses may be indicated in severe illness.

Schilling's test: Give 1000 mcg IM as a flushing dose.

HYDROXOCOBALAMIN, CRYSTALLINE

PRODUCTS (TRADE NAME):

alphaREDISOL, Alpha-Ruvite, Codroxomin, Crysti-12 Gel, Droxomin, Droxovite, Hydrobexan, Hydro-Cobex, Hydroxo-12, Hydroxocobalamin, LA-12, Neo-Betalin 12, Rubesol-H 1000 (Available in 1000 mcg/ml injection.)

DRUG SPECIFICS:

This relatively inexpensive preparation has the advantage of slower absorption at injection site, more concentrated uptake by the liver, and less urinary excretion than cyanocobalamin. Administer by IM route only. Concurrent administration with folic acid is usually indicated.

ADMINISTRATION AND DOSAGE SPECIFICS:

Deficiency: Give 30 mcg/day for 5 to 10 days, followed by 100 to 200 mcg every month.

Carol Wilson

VITAMIN C (ASCORBIC ACID, CALCIUM ASCORBATE, SODIUM ASCORBATE)

ACTION OF THE DRUG: Ascorbic acid has multiple functions, some of which are understood more than others. It functions in a number of enzyme systems and is involved in intracellular oxidation-reduction potentials. It aids in the conversion of folic acid and the degradation and metabolism of certain amino acids, and facilitates the absorption of iron and calcium and inhibits the absorption of copper in the gastrointestinal tract. Ascorbic acid works as an antioxidant in protecting vitamins A and E and polyunsaturated fatty acids. It is also necessary for the formation of the ground substance of bones, teeth, connective tissue and capillaries and for the synthesis of collagen. Ascorbic acid aids in wound healing and may be involved in blood clotting. It is known to facilitate the transfer of iron to ferritin. During certain types of stress the requirement for ascorbic acid is increased, but this action is not well understood. The role of ascorbic acid in preventing and treating colds, cancer, and atherosclerosis is controversial, being reported but unproven. As a water-soluble vitamin, it is present in extracellular fluids, muscle, connective tissue, and the aqueous humor of the eye. It is present in the highest concentration in glandular tissues such as the adrenal cortex, pituitary, pancreas, liver, and spleen.

ASSESSMENT:

INDICATIONS: Ascorbic acid is used for the treatment of debilitated patients, especially postoperatively in elderly patients with fractures and as supplementation for burn victims or patients undergoing severe stress. Infection, smoking, chronic illness, and febrile states may increase the need for vitamin C. It is used adjunctly with iron therapy, especially in patients with hemovascular disorders, and in patients on prolonged intravenous therapy. Premature infants require relatively large doses. It is also useful for the prophylaxis and treatment of scurvy, the deficiency syndrome.

SUBJECTIVE: Cases of deficiency produce the disease scurvy. With modern refrigeration and processing methods of citrus fruits, it is rarely seen in the United States but may be found when other vitamin deficiencies are present. Symptoms include tender, painful muscles, joints, and bones, muscle cramps, loss of appetite, fatigue, weakness, and sore gums.

OBJECTIVE: In deficiency states, impaired bone formation, disrupted metabolism of tyrosine and tryptophan, delayed formation of glycoproteins, and conversion of proline to collagen are seen. Wound healing is impaired, and hemorrhagic manifestations are demonstrated by subperiosteal bleeding and petechial hemorrhages. Vasomotor instability, ecchymosis, hemarthrosis, faulty bone and tooth development, loosened teeth, and gingivitis also may develop.

PLAN:

PRECAUTIONS: Ascorbic acid interferes with the effectiveness of disulfiram given to patients to encourage abstention from alcoholic beverages. Too rapid intravenous administration of ascorbic acid is to be avoided. Therapy of above-normal doses should be avoided with pregnant women because of the chance that the fetus may adapt to elevated dosages which then fall off at the time of delivery.

IMPLEMENTATION:

DRUG INTERACTIONS: Ascorbic acid may have varying effects on anticoagulants, either inhibiting the action of some or prolonging the intensity and duration of others. Aminosalicylic acid increases the chance of aminosalicylic acid crystalluria and increases the effect of salicylates through elevated renal tubular reabsorption. There is also an increased chance of crystallization of sulfonamides in urine when administered concurrently. Ascorbic acid decreases the effect of amphetamines and tricyclic antidepressants by decreasing renal tubular reabsorption. Calcium ascorbate may cause cardiac arrhythmias in patients receiving digitalis. Ascorbic acid is chemically incompatible with potassium penicillin G and should not be mixed in the same syringe. Smoking may lead to increased vitamin C requirements through decreasing ascorbic acid serum levels. Intermittent use of ascorbic acid in patients taking ethinyl estradiol may increase the risk of contraceptive failure. Large doses of Vitamin C may interfere with urine testing by causing false-negative results using Benedict's solution or copper reduction method or by causing false-negative urine glucose tests with the glucose oxidase method.

ADMINISTRATION AND DOSAGE: Vitamin C comes in three major forms: ascorbic acid (which may by given orally or parenterally), sodium ascorbate and calcium ascorbate (which come only in parenteral forms.) Recommended daily allowance is 60 mg for adults.

IMPLEMENTATION CONSIDERATIONS:

—Obtain a complete health history, including the presence of underlying pathology or systemic disease. Assess dietary intake from natural as well as fortified food sources, dietary supplements, and self-administered over-the counter or prescription drugs, especially aminosalicylic acid, amphetamines, or antidepressants.

—Teach patient the principles of sound nutrition, including those foods which are good sources of vitamin C. Ascertain if cultural dietary habits or lack of finances or other resources has contributed in any way to inadequate nutrition.

—Foods should be protected from air, light, and excessive heat or natural Vitamin C may be destroyed (e.g., boiling of vegetables for long periods or leaving juice uncovered in refrigerator leads to destruction of the vitamin.)

—Avoid too-rapid intravenous administration of vitamin C.

WHAT THE PATIENT NEEDS TO KNOW:

—Take this medication exactly as ordered by your health care provider.

—Keep this medication out of the reach of children and others for whom it has not been prescribed.

—Inform your health care provider if you need to take any other medications while you are receiving vitamin C therapy.

—Vitamin C is easily destroyed by air, heat, and light. Keep this medication tightly capped in its own container. Foods high in vitamin C should not be boiled for long periods of time or left uncovered in the refrigerator. Ask your nurse practitioner about methods of food preparation which are best.

—Good food sources of vitamin C include green, leafy vegetables, oranges, grapefruits, strawberries, cauliflower, cantaloupe, beef liver, asparagus, and potatoes.

EVALUATION:

ADVERSE REACTIONS: Patients may experience mild, transient soreness at injection sites whether medication is given intramuscularly or subcutaneously. They may also experience temporary episodes of faintness or dizziness when intravenous injections are given too rapidly. Excessive doses are usually rapidly excreted into the urine.

OVERDOSAGE: Doses in excess of 1 to 3 gm daily may result in acidosis, gastrointestinal complaints, glycosuria, oxaluria, and development of renal stones, especially in patients prone to oxaluria, hyperuricemia, and cystinuria. Patients who chronically overuse vitamins may develop a state of conditioned need.

PARAMETERS TO MONITOR: If patient is taking ascorbic acid for a deficiency state, monitor for disappearance of symptoms. Urine pH should be followed closely when ascorbic acid is used for urinary acidification. Monitor improvement in dietary habits or adequacy of nutrition.

ASCORBIC ACID

PRODUCTS (TRADE NAME):
Arco-Cee (Available in 750 mg timed release tablets.) **Ascorbicap** (Available in 500 mg timed release capsules.) **Ascorbic Acid** (Available in 25, 50, 100, 250, 500, and 1000 mg tablets; 100, 250, 500 and 1000 mg chewable tablets; 250, 500, and 1000 mg timed release tablets; 500 mg timed release capsules; 20 mg/ml syrup; and 100, 200, and 250 mg/ml injection.) **Cemill** (Available in 250 and 500 mg timed release tablets.) **Best-C, Cetane-Timed, Cevi-Bid, C-Long Granucaps, C-Span** (Available in 500 mg timed release capsules.) **Cevalin** (Available in 100, 250, and 500 mg tablets, and in 50, 100, and 500 mg/ml injection.) **CeVi-Sol** (Available in 35 mg/0.6 ml drops.) **Cecon** (Available in 100 mg/ml drops.) **Flavorcee** (Available in 100 and 250 mg chewable tablets.) **Vitacee** (Available in 25, 50, 100, 250, and 500 mg tablets.)

DRUG SPECIFICS:
Ascorbic acid is the most widely used vitamin C preparation, coming in both oral and parenteral forms. It is the only vitamin C preparation recommended for urine acidification. The cost varies widely according to manufacturer.

ADMINISTRATION AND DOSAGE SPECIFICS:
Prophylactically: Give 50 to 100 mg as indicated.
Therapeutically: Give 100 mg or more as needed.
Urine acidification: 4 to 12 gm/day. Give every 4 hours in divided doses.
Extensive injury therapy: Give 200 to 500 mg daily.
Parenterally: 100 to 250 mg once or twice daily up to maximum of 1 to 2 gm daily.

CALCIUM ASCORBATE

PRODUCTS (TRADE NAME):
Calscorbate (Available in 100 mg/ml injection.)

DRUG SPECIFICS:
This product is generally given IV since subcutaneous administration (and possibly even intramuscular injection) may cause necrosis, especially in infants. This product is fairly expensive.

ADMINISTRATION AND DOSAGE SPECIFICS:
Parenterally: Give slowly 100 to 250 mg once or twice daily up to a maximum of 1 to 2 gm/day.

SODIUM ASCORBATE

PRODUCTS (TRADE NAME):
    Cenolate (Available in 562.5 mg/ml injection, equivalent to 500 mg/ml ascorbic acid.) **Cevita, Sodium Ascorbate** (Available in 250 mg/ml injection.)

DRUG SPECIFICS:
    These parenterally preparations are relatively inexpensive. They should not be used, however, in patients who are on a sodium-restricted diet. This form of vitamin C is not effective in acidifying the urine.

ADMINISTRATION AND DOSAGE SPECIFICS:
    Parenterally: Give slowly 100 to 250 mg once or twice daily up to a maximum of 1 to 2 gm/day.

Carol Wilson

VITAMIN D (ERGOCALCIFEROL, CHOLECALCIFEROL)

ACTION OF THE DRUG: Vitamin D is a term applied to the group of fat soluble chemically similar sterols. The three main categories within this group include (1) ergocalciferol (vitamin D_2) which is very limited in nature in both distribution and concentration but which can be artificially manufactured by ultraviolet irradiation on ergot and yeasts, (2) cholecalciferol (vitamin D_3) which occurs naturally in fish liver oils, and can be formed in animals and man by ultraviolet irradiation on the skin; and (3) Other lesser compounds (D_4, D_5, D_6, D_7, which are formed by irradiation of sterols. The term "vitamin D" has therefore become a rather ambiguous term.

    The main action of this group of sterols is the movement of calcium and phosphorus ions into three main sites: small intestine (to promote absorption of calcium and phosphorus from the gut); kidney (to affect phosphate reabsorption in the proximal convoluted tubules and, to a lesser extent, to stimulate calcium and sodium reabsorption); and bone (to facilitate the mineralization of newly formed bone.) Other actions not yet proved definitively include involvement in muscle metabolism and suppression of size and hormone secretion of the parathyroid gland. (In hypoparathyroidism these agents increase serum calcium levels and decrease serum phosphorus levels.)

ASSESSMENT:

    INDICATIONS: These preparations are used for the treatment of childhood rickets and adult osteomalacia, hypoparathyroidism and familial hypophosphatemia.

    SUBJECTIVE: Evaluate for signs of deficiency. In childhood, rickets may be demonstrated by complaints of excessive sweating and gastrointestinal disturbances. These may be the first symptoms, preceding any objective findings. In adult cases of osteomalacia, patients may complain of skeletal pain and progressive muscular weakness.

OBJECTIVE: Evaluate children for signs of bone deformities, craniotabes and bossing of the skull, "rachitic rosary," bowlegs after the age of 2 years, and development of a potbelly appearance. In infants, late closure of the fontanelles, bending of the long bones, and enlargement of the epiphysis of the long bones and costochondral junctions may be seen. Fingers may show swelling of the shafts of the phalanges while the joints are normal in size. Greenstick fractures, waddling gait, and delayed eruption of teeth may also be seen in children. In adults with osteomalacia, pelvic deformities, spontaneous fractures secondary to thinning of the long bones, decreased serum inorganic phosphorus and plasma calcium, and increased alkaline phosphatase may be seen. Vitamin D levels are below 50 IU/100 ml.

PLAN:

CONTRAINDICATIONS: Do not give in the presence of abnormal sensitivity to the toxic effects of vitamin D, hypervitaminosis D, hypercalcemia, malabsorption syndrome, and decreased renal function.

WARNINGS: Some infants have developed idiopathic hypercalcemia (hypersensitivity to vitamin D.) Safe use of over 400 IU/day has not been established for use during pregnancy. Avoid overdosage. Keep out of the reach of children.

PRECAUTIONS: Use large doses with extreme caution in the elderly. Several fatalities have occurred due to prolonged use of excessive doses. The effects of the drug can persist as long as two months after therapy has been discontinued. In patients with hyperphosphatemia (frequently seen in renal osteodystrophy), normal serum phosphorus levels should be maintained through dietary phosphate restriction and/or the administration of aluminum gels as intestinal phosphate binders. This is necessary in order to prevent metastatic calcification. Use with caution in patients with history of renal stones.

IMPLEMENTATION:

DRUG INTERACTIONS: Mineral oil and some of the antihyperlipidemic agents may interfere with the absorption of fat-soluble vitamins. Thiazide diuretics and vitamin D together contribute to hypercalcemia. There is a possible connection between phenytoin and phenobarbital use leading to hypocalcemia, which in turn may contribute to rickets or osteomalacia.

ADMINISTRATION AND DOSAGE: Dosage must be individualized and given under close supervision because the margin between therapeutic and toxic level is narrow. Calcium intake should be sufficient to achieve a serum calcium level between 9 to 10 mg/100 ml. In rickets, up to 12,000 to 500,000 IU/day can be taken. In hypoparathyroidism initially give 50,000 to 200,000 IU/day with a maintenance dose of 50,000 to 400,000 IU/day.

IMPLEMENTATION CONSIDERATIONS:
—Obtain a complete health history, including the presence of hypersensitivity, other drugs taken concurrently, and the presence of underlying thyroid, parathyroid, cardiovascular, renal, malabsorption, carcinoma, or other systemic disease.

—Obtain a complete diet survey in order to discover the cause of vitamin D deficiency. Vitamin D intake from all sources must be included in the dietary evaluation. Dietary intake from natural as well as fortified food sources, dietary supplements, and self-administered drugs must all be assessed.

—Intramuscular administration of vitamin D preparations must be slow and deep into the gluteus muscle. Avoid injection into veins.

—There is a time lag of 12 to 24 hours between administration and initiation of action in the body.

—Teach the patient good nutritional habits and especially stress the foods which are high in vitamin D. This will be important if dietary habits were instrumental in the development of the deficiency. Ascertain if cultural dietary habits or lack of finances or other resources contributed in any way to inadequate nutrition.

WHAT THE PATIENT NEEDS TO KNOW:

—Take this drug precisely as ordered. Do not increase dosage or stop taking medication without being advised to do so.

—Avoid the use of mineral oil while taking this medication.

—Keep this drug out of the reach of children and all others for whom it is not prescribed. Even vitamins may be lethal when taken in overdosage. If overdosage is suspected, call your poison control center promptly.

—Most people obtain all the vitamin D they need from food within their diet. Natural sources of vitamin D are few, and the majority of vitamin D must be obtained from fortified sources. Fortified foods which are high in this vitamin are milk, evaporated milk, infant formula, powdered skim milk, and human milk. Also, cereals, margarine, and diet foods contain vitamin D supplements.

—Protect drug from light by keeping in light-resistant container.

EVALUATION:

OVERDOSAGE: Toxicity symptoms include: anorexia, nausea, weakness, weight loss, vague aches and stiffness, constipation, diarrhea, convulsions, anemia, mild acidosis, impairment of renal function preceded by polyuria, nocturia, polydipsia, hypercalciuria, and azotemia. These renal effects are usually reversible. Hypertension, mental retardation, nephrocalcinosis, generalized vascular calcification, irreversible renal insufficiency (which can be fatal), albuminuria, urinary casts, widespread calcification of the soft tissues (heart, lungs, blood vessels, renal tubules) and osteoporosis may all be seen in adults. Dwarfism may be present in infants and children secondary to decreased average rate of linear growth of bones and increased mineralization of bones. Most toxic effects persist for several months for adults at doses of 100,000 IU or more daily or for children at doses of 20,000 IU or more daily. Reactions gradually disappear if treatment is discontinued at the first sign of symptoms. Treatment of overdosage is low calcium diet, increase in oral fluids, acidification of the urine, and supportive therapy for symptoms. Deaths are secondary to renal or cardiovascular system failure.

PARAMETERS TO MONITOR: Obtain a complete history, physical, and laboratory evaluation as baseline. Observe patient for therapeutic effects. Alleviation of symptoms of deficiency should occur. Periodic serum calcium and urinary calcium tests should be done, as well as potassium and BUN tests every two weeks. Normal serum calcium and phosphate levels should be seen within 2 weeks. Bone x-rays should be obtained once a month until the condition is corrected and stabilized. Evidence of bone healing should be obvious on x-ray within 4 weeks after therapy is initiated. Evaluate dietary patterns after teaching patient about good nutrition. Monitor for appearance of toxicity signs and symptoms and observe to determine individual tolerances of dosage. Hypervitaminosis D, secondary to hypercalcemia, produces symptoms of weakness, lethargy, anorexia, nausea and vomiting, excessive thirst and urination, irritability, depression, constipation, diarrhea, weakness, vague aches, and stiffness. Signs to watch for include excessive weight loss, hyperphosphatemia or hypophosphatemia, decreased alkaline phosphatase, renal damage secondary to calcium deposits in the kidney, and calcium deposits in skin, heart, lung, pancreas, stomach, and other soft tissue. Calcification of tympanic membrane may result in deafness.

CALCIFEDIOL

PRODUCTS (TRADE NAME):
   Calderol (Available in 20 and 50 mcg capsules.)
DRUG SPECIFICS:
   A vitamin D_3 product used primarily in the management of patients on chronic renal dialysis who have metabolic bone disease or hypocalcemia. Obtain serum calcium levels weekly. If hypercalcemia is noted, discontinue until normocalcemia develops.
   ADMINISTRATION AND DOSAGE SPECIFICS:
   Give 300 to 350 mcg/week administered on a daily or every-other-day routine. Usually can give 20 to 50 mcg/day or 100 to 200 mcg every other day.

CALCITRIOL

PRODUCTS (TRADE NAME):
   Rocaltrol (Available in 0.25 and 0.5 mcg capsules.)
DRUG SPECIFICS:
   A Vitamin D_3 product used to reduce elevated parathyroid hormone levels. Used primarily in patients on chronic renal dialysis. Obtain serum calcium levels at least twice weekly during initial therapy. Discontinue drug at any sign of hypercalcemia.

ADMINISTRATION AND DOSAGE SPECIFICS:

Initially give 0.25 mcg/day. May be increased by 0.25 mcg/day at 2- to 4-week intervals until satisfactory response is obtained.

Some patients may respond to doses of 0.25 mcg every other day. Patients undergoing hemodialysis may require doses of 0.5 to 1 mcg/day.

DIHYDROTACHYSTEROL (DHT)

PRODUCTS (TRADE NAME):

Dihydrotachysterol (Available in 0.125, 0.2 and 0.4 mg tablets.) **Hytakerol** (Available in 0.125 mg capsules and 0.25 mg/ml solution.)

DRUG SPECIFICS:

Used in the treatment of hypoparathyroidism and all forms of tetany. May be supplemented with oral calcium.

ADMINISTRATION AND DOSAGE SPECIFICS:

Initial dosage: 0.75 to 2.5 mg daily for several days.

Maintenance dosage: 0.2 to 1 mg daily, titrated by serum calcium levels. Average dose is 0.6 mg.

ERGOCALCIFEROL (D₂)

PRODUCTS (TRADE NAME):

Calciferol (Available in 50,000 IU tablets and in 500,000 IU ml injection.) **Deltalin Gelseals** (Available in 50,000 IU capsules.) **Drisdol** (Available in 50,000 IU capsules and 8,000 IU ml liquid.) **Vitamin D** (Available in 25,000 and 50,000 IU capsules.)

DRUG SPECIFICS:

This product is used primarily in the treatment of familial hypophosphatemia and hypoparathyroidism. One mg of ergocalciferol provides 40,000 units of vitamin D activity. Recommended daily allowance is 200 IU for adults, or 400 IU for all age groups. The range between therapeutic and toxic doses is narrow, and adequate supervision of patient during therapy is mandatory. Patients with malabsorption problems, or GI, liver, or biliary disease may require IM administration.

ADMINISTRATION AND DOSAGE SPECIFICS:

Vitamin D resistant rickets: 50,000 to 500,000 IU daily.

Hypoparathyroidism: 50,000 to 400,000 IU of vitamin D daily plus 4 gm of calcium lactate, administered 6 times daily.

Carol Wilson

VITAMIN E

ACTION OF THE DRUG: Vitamin E is a fat-soluble vitamin consisting of naturally occurring tocopherols. Deficiencies of vitamin E have produced specific disease in animals, but this has not been proven in man. Vitamin E is considered an essential nutrient for man even though its specific functions are not yet understood. Vitamin E may function as an antioxidant, preventing damage to cellular membranes. It stabilizes red blood cell walls and protects them from hemolysis. It may also enhance vitamin A utilization and suppress platelet aggregation.

ASSESSMENT:

INDICATIONS: Many purported uses are controversial and unproven. The only established use is for the prevention or treatment of vitamin E deficiency. It has been used for the treatment of neonatal bronchopulmonary dysplasia, intermittent claudication, fibrocystic breast disease, and premenstrual syndrome (PMS types A, D, and C.) It may be used investigationally in premature infants (especially twins), or in severely protein-calorie-deficient infants or patients with prolonged fat malabsorption syndromes.

SUBJECTIVE: No complaints noted for deficiency states. If patients complain of premenstrual tension, symptoms of anxiety, depression, bloating, weight gain, weakness or dizziness may accompany behavior changes following ovulation until menses begins.

OBJECTIVE: The only symptoms which have been shown to occur regularly from deficiency of vitamin E in humans is a normochromic, normocytic anemia in the premature infant. Also, children who suffer from malabsorption syndrome have shown creatinuria, ceroid pigmentation of smooth muscle, and multifocal degeneration of striated muscle. Patients with fibrocystic disease may demonstrate multiple benign breast cysts by palpation or mammography. Patients with PMS-C may show low blood sugar levels premenstrually.

PLAN:

PRECAUTIONS: Appears to be the least toxic of the fat-soluble vitamins. No signs and symptoms of toxicity or hypervitaminosis have been identified as yet in humans.

IMPLEMENTATION:

PRODUCTS (TRADE NAMES):
Aquasol E (Available in 50 IU/ml drops and in 100 and 400 IU capsules). **E-Ferol Succinate** (Available in 200 and 400 IU capsules). **Eprolin Gelseals** (Available in 50 IU capsules). **Pheryl-E** (Available in 100 and 400 IU tablets). **Vitamin E** (Available in 50, 100, 200, 400, 600, 800, and 1000 IU capsules; 100, 200, 400, and 1000 IU tablets, 200 and 400 IU chewable tablets; and 200 IU/ml injection).

Preparations contain vitamin E in several forms of varying potency, and both with and without alcohol.

ADMINISTRATION AND DOSAGE: The recommended dietary allowance published by the National Academy of Science maintains that prescription of a fixed tocopherol level for man is unrealistic. A range of 10-20 IU of vitamin E should represent adequate levels for an adult diet. For premenstrual syndrome (PMS), 300 IU of an alcohol free product are taken po daily.

IMPLEMENTATION CONSIDERATIONS:

—Obtain a complete health history, including the presence of any hypersensitivities, underlying systemic disease, past vitamin therapy, and possibility of pregnancy. Since the question of vitamin E deficiency in man is controversial, ascertain what the patient knows or thinks about vitamin E and the possibility of a deficiency state.

—Food sources of vitamin E are primarily from plants. The highest amounts are found in vegetable oils such as soybean, corn, etc., with meat and dairy products providing less. An accurate assessment of tocopherol levels in food is difficult to obtain. The amount in the body depends upon the initial concentration of vitamin E and the processing, storage and preparation of the food.

—Since hypervitaminosis with vitamin E has not been identified, advice to patients regarding dietary intake is difficult and should simply be based on principles of overall sound nutrition at this point. The nurse should, however, evaluate intake of vitamin E from dietary supplements, self-administered drugs, and over-the-counter and prescription drug sources.

—Although vitamin E has not yet been proven effective in the treatment of fibrocystic disease, some clinicians are still prescribing 600 IU po per day for non-surgical therapy. The patient is also placed on a caffeine-free diet.

—Vitamin E (D-L-alpha-decopharol acetate) without alcohol has been used in the treatment of premenstrual syndrome associated with anxiety (PMS-A), depression (PMS-D), and low carbohydrates (PMS-C). It has not been found to be effective in the treatment of PMS-H associated with bloating, fluid retention and weight gain.

WHAT THE PATIENT NEEDS TO KNOW:

—Take this medication as ordered. Do not exceed the recommended dosage. Although hypervitaminosis has not yet been established with vitamin E, it is always wise not to exceed recommended dosage.

—Keep this drug out of the reach of children and all others for whom it is not prescribed. Although generally non-toxic, the poison control center should be notified if an unknown or excessive quantity of medication has been taken.

—Vitamin E products should be stored in tightly closed, light-resistant containers.

—Overall good nutrition requires a variety of foods. Vegetable oils are good sources of vitamin E, and meats and dairy products also provide some vitamin E.

—If taking vitamin E as therapy in fibrocystic breast disease, all caffeine must also be eliminated from the diet.

EVALUATION:

ADVERSE REACTIONS: None reported in humans.
PARAMETERS TO MONITOR: Monitor that patients are not obsessively using vitamins, especially as a replacement for eating a good diet.

Carol Wilson

MINERALS

CALCIUM

ACTION OF THE DRUG: Calcium is a major mineral in the body and is essential for muscular and neurological integrity, especially in the cardiac system. Calcium functions in the synthesis and remodeling of skeletal tissues (bones and teeth); activates several enzymes that influence cell membrane permeability; activates enzyme systems responsible for contractile properties of muscle; aids in blood clotting by stimulating the release of thromboplastin and the conversion of fibrinogen to fibrin; activates pancreatic lipase; influences the intestinal absorption of cobalamin; and in extracellular fluids is involved in the transmisson of acetylcholine. In intracellular fluid calcium is necessary for pancreatic secretion of insulin when stimulated by glucose. A recently identified function is the regulation of lymphocyte and phagocyte function through interaction with calmodulin.

Calcium is a mineral which exists in the body, with 99% found in bone and 1% in body fluids and striated muscle. It may be found in three forms in body fluids: 35% in combination with protein, 60% ionized and free, and 5% in combination with other substances (citrate bicarbonate and phosphate.) Calcium accounts for 1.5 to 2% of total body weight. Only 40% of dietary calcium is absorbed. Plasma levels tend to run higher in children than in adults.

ASSESSMENT:

INDICATIONS: Calcium is used as a supplement when dietary levels of calcium are inadequate. Calcium requirements may be increased in pregnant and breast-feeding women, adolescent, and postmenopausal women. Calcium is also used in the treatment of neonatal hypocalcemia and for the prevention and treatment of postmenopausal and senile osteoporosis. It may also be used as a supplement to parenterally administered calcium in cases of hypoparathyroidism, pseudohypoparathyroidism, rickets, and osteomalacia.

SUBJECTIVE: Patient may be without subjective complaints. A history of spontaneous fractures in the elderly should make the clinician suspicious.

OBJECTIVE: Often no signs are seen, although newborn tetany may be seen in some infants. In patients with low calcium levels, carpal spasm may be elicited by compressing the upper arm with a blood pressure cuff, causing ischemia to the distal nerves. The patient may report a tingling sensation and inadvertently flex his arm. (This is a positive Trousseau sign.)

PLAN:

CONTRAINDICATIONS: Do not give in the presence of renal calculi.
PRECAUTIONS: Excessive amounts of calcium may lead to hypercalcemia and hypercalciuria, especially in hyperthyroid patients. Serum and renal calcium levels should be monitored in order to detect development of renal stones.

IMPLEMENTATION:

DRUG INTERACTIONS: Vitamin D is essential for the absorption of calcium in the body. Calcium status is affected by the calcium/phosphorus ratio in the body and by the level of protein in the diet. Phytic acid (found in bran and whole grain cereals) and oxalic acid (found in spinach and rhubarb) may interfere with calcium absorption by combining with it to form insoluble salts in the intestine. Calcium compounds and calcium-rich substances such as milk interfere with the absorption of oral tetracyclines, and concomitant use should be avoided. Administration of corticosteroids may also decrease the absorption of calcium.

ADMINISTRATION AND DOSAGE: Calcium products come in combination with various other chemicals, with a concentration of between 6% and 40%. Preparations are both parenteral or oral. Parenteral calcium salts may be compared as summarized in Table 6-1.

Recommended daily allowances are 800 mg/day for adults, 1200 mg/day for adolescents, 800 mg/day for children, and 360-540 mg/day for infants from birth to one year.

TABLE 6-1. CALCIUM CONTENT OF VARIOUS CALCIUM SALTS

Salt	mEq Calcium/GM	% Calcium
Oral:		
Calcium carbonate	Variable	40%
Calcium glubionate	Variable	6%
Calcium gluconate	Variable	9%
Calcium lactate	Variable	13%
Dibasic calcium Phosphate	Variable	30%
Parenteral:		
Calcium chloride	13.6 mEq	27%
Calcium gluconate	4.5 mEq	9%
Calcium gluceptate	4.5 mEq	9%
Calcium levulinate	6.9 mEq	13%

IMPLEMENTATION CONSIDERATIONS:

—Obtain a complete health history, including the presence of underlying or systemic disease, dietary intake of calcium from natural as well as fortified food sources, dietary supplements, and self-administered over-the-counter and prescription drugs. Evaluate dietary patterns, including intake of protein, phosphorus, and vitamin D. Assess for history of renal calculi.

—Evaluate whether patient may have increased requirements for calcium: adolescence, breast-feeding, or pregnancy.

—Teach patient principles of sound nutrition, including those foods which are good sources of calcium. Ascertain if cultural dietary habits, food preferences, fad diets, or lack of finances or other resources have contributed in any way to inadequate nutrition.

WHAT THE PATIENT NEEDS TO KNOW:

—Take this medication exactly as ordered by your health care provider. Do not exceed recommended dosage.

—Keep this medication out of the reach of children and others for whom it is not prescribed.

—If you begin taking any other medications while using this product, notify your health care provider.

—Milk and dairy products are the richest sources of calcium. Egg yolks and most dark green, leafy vegetables are also good sources.

—Calcium supplements are constipating. Maintain a high dietary fiber content to minimize this effect.

EVALUATION:

ADVERSE REACTIONS: Watch for symptoms of hypercalcemia such as polyuria, constipation, abdominal pain, dryness of mouth, anorexia, nausea and vomiting.

PARAMETERS TO MONITOR: 24-hour urine calcium levels or Sulkowitch tests may document low calcium levels. Monitoring of plasma and urinary calcium levels should be done in order to monitor for therapeutic effect. Elevations in urinary calcium often precede elevated serum calcium levels.

CALCIUM CARBONATE

PRODUCTS (TRADE NAME):

Calcium Carbonate (Available in 650 mg tablets which are equivalent to 260 mg calcium or in 120 gm or 1 lb packets of powder.) **Os-Cal 500** (Available in 1.25 gm tablets which are equivalent to 500 mg calcium.)

DRUG SPECIFICS:

This oral preparation is usually inexpensive and well tolerated. Contains 40% concentration of calcium, the largest of any calcium product.

ADMINISTRATION AND DOSAGE SPECIFICS:
Give 1 to 1.5 gm po three times daily with meals.

CALCIUM CHLORIDE

PRODUCTS (TRADE NAME):
Calcium Chloride (Available in 10% solution for injection. Comes in 10 ml ampules, vials and syringes.)
DRUG SPECIFICS:
Calcium chloride is very irritating to veins and tissues, with severe necrosis and sloughing resulting from extravasation. For emergency cardiac resuscitation, inject into ventricular cavity and not into myocardium.
ADMINISTRATION AND DOSAGE SPECIFICS:
Cardiac resuscitation: Give 200 to 800 mg injected into ventricular cavity. Intravenous therapy may be continued with rate not to exceed 1 ml/min.

CALCIUM GLUBIONATE

PRODUCTS (TRADE NAME):
Neo-Calglucon (Available in 1.8 gm syrup, equivalent to 115 mg calcium per 5 ml.)
DRUG SPECIFICS:
Oral preparation contains 6% calcium. Administer before meals to increase absorption.
ADMINISTRATION AND DOSAGE SPECIFICS:
Adults (including pregnant and breast-feeding women) and children 4 years or older: 15 ml three times daily.
Children under four years of age: 10 ml three times daily.
Infants: 5 ml five times daily.

CALCIUM GLUCEPTATE

PRODUCTS (TRADE NAME):
Calcium Gluceptate (Available in 1.1 gm/5 ml injection.)
DRUG SPECIFICS:
This prescription preparation is used most frequently following exchange transfusions in newborns—(1.1 gm (5 ml) contains 90 mg (4.5 mEq) of calcium.

ADMINISTRATION AND DOSAGE SPECIFICS:

Hypocalcemia: Give 2 to 5 ml IM in the gluteal region (or in the lateral thigh of infants), or give 5 to 20 ml IV.

Exchange transfusions: Give 0.5 ml after every 100 ml of blood exchanged.

CALCIUM GLUCONATE

PRODUCTS (TRADE NAME):

Calcium Gluconate (Available in 500 mg (45 mg calcium), 650 mg (58.5 mg calcium), or 1 gm (90 mg calcium) tablets; in 120 gm or 1 lb powder packets; or in 10% solution for injection.) **Kalcinate** (Available in 10% solution (10 ml equals 4.5 mEq calcium) for injection.)

DRUG SPECIFICS:

Comes in both oral and parenteral forms. IV infusion is preferred over IM injection and is used frequently in emergency situations. Check equivalency of all oral products since they vary from preparation to preparation. In parenteral forms, 10 ml contains 90 mg (4.5 mEq) calcium. IV preparations are available by prescription only. IV calcium should be avoided in patients toxic to digoxin.

ADMINISTRATION AND DOSAGE SPECIFICS:

Orally: Give 1 to 2 gm several times daily.

Parenterally: 1 to 15 gm daily intravenously for adults; 500 mg/kg/day in divided doses for children.

CALCIUM LACTATE

PRODUCTS (TRADE NAME):

Calcium Lactate (Available in 325 mg tablets equivalent to 42.25 mg calcium, in 650 mg tablets equivalent to 84.5 mg calcium, and in 1 pound packets of powder.)

DRUG SPECIFICS:

Product contains 13% calcium and is given as an oral preparation. It is available without prescription.

ADMINISTRATION AND DOSAGE SPECIFICS:

Give 325 mg to 1.3 gm three times daily with meals.

DIBASIC CALCIUM PHOSPHATE

PRODUCTS (TRADE NAME):

Ca-Plus (Available in 280 mg calcium tablets.) **Dibasic Calcium Phosphate**

(Available in 500 mg (115 mg calcium) tablets, and 1 lb packages of powder.) **Elecal** (Available in tablets containing 250 mg calcium and 15 mg magnesium.) **Florical** (Available in capsules containing 145.6 mg calcium and 8.3 mg sodium fluoride.) **Glycate** (Available in tablets with 120 mg calcium carbonate and 150 mg aminoacetic acid.)

DRUG SPECIFICS:

Some of these preparations are combination products and are made from various ingredients such as oyster shell flour, soy protein, and torula yeast. Cost varies widely with manufacturer.

ADMINISTRATION AND DOSAGE SPECIFICS:

Usual dose is 500 mg to 1.5 gm two or three times daily.

Carol Wilson

MINERALS—FLUORIDE

ACTION OF THE DRUG: Fluoride is concentrated in bones and teeth and is present in soft tissues only in minute amounts. It is an essential trace element but has not been proven to be essential to life. Fluoride is incorporated into the surface enamel of teeth in higher concentrations than in deeper layers. This fortification of the enamel provides greater resistance to dissolution or demineralization by acids produced in dental plaque. It has therefore been found useful in reducing dental caries.

ASSESSMENT:

INDICATIONS: Fluoride is recommended for prevention of dental caries. It may be used topically or systemically. It is primarily administered in localities with unfluoridated water supplies or to individuals having a genetic tendency for dental caries. It also has been used experimentally in the treatment of osteoporosis, although this use has not been approved by the FDA.

SUBJECTIVE-OBJECTIVE: There are no signs or symptoms of deficiency. Incidence of substantial dental pain and decay may prompt the health practitioner to consider this product.

PLAN:

CONTRAINDICATIONS: Do not give in the presence of hypersensitivity to fluoride. Use of sodium fluoride should be avoided in patients on a sodium-restricted diet.

PRECAUTIONS: Excessive intake may lead to dental fluorosis with mottling of tooth enamel. Some products may contain tartrazine which may provoke allergic reactions in sensitive individuals.

IMPLEMENTATION:

DRUG INTERACTIONS: Systemic fluoride may produce calcium fluoride, a poorly absorbed product, when taken with dairy foods.

ADMINISTRATION AND DOSAGE: Product is available in gels, pastes, drops, tablets, capsules, and mouth rinses. The preparation and quantity chosen should be adjusted to the fluoride level of the local water supply. Contact the county water commissioner for this information. If local fluoride is less than 0.3 ppm, use the following schedule:

   0.25 mg/day for children 2 weeks to 2 years of age
   0.5 mg/day for children 2 to 3 years of age
   1.0 mg/day for children older than 3 years
If local fluoride is between 0.3 and 0.7 ppm, use the following schedule:
   0.25 mg/day for 2 to 3 years of age
   0.5 mg/day for children 3 to 16 years of age

IMPLEMENTATION CONSIDERATIONS:

—Obtain a complete health history including presence of underlying disease. Pay particular attention to allergies, dental history, dental development, and dental injuries.

—Assess whether older children and adults live in areas where water supplies are fluoridated.

—Assess whether older children and adults receive periodic topical fluoride treatment from dental practitioners.

—For infants, assess whether mother lives in an area where water supplies are fluoridated. Evaluate whether mother is breast-feeding or if formula is prepared with fluoridated water.

—Stress to patients that overdosage of this product can cause mottled teeth.

—Assess intake from any dietary supplements, formula, or self-administered over-the-counter or prescription drugs.

WHAT THE PATIENT NEEDS TO KNOW:

—Take this product as ordered. Tablets and drops may be dissolved in water used for making infant formula or added to food or juices. Tablets may also be swallowed, chewed, or allowed to dissolve slowly in the mouth. Products are best taken following meals.

For rinses and gels, brush teeth thoroughly and then apply to clean teeth. Do not swallow product. Do not rinse mouth, eat, or drink for 30 minutes after treatment.

—Use plastic containers for diluting drops or rinses. Avoid use of glass.

—Milk may decrease absorption of oral products, so avoid taking with milk or dairy products.

—This is a medication which should be kept out of the reach of children and others for whom it has not been prescribed.

—Overdosage of this medication will cause discoloration and mottling of the teeth.

—Inform your dentist at the next scheduled visit that you are taking this medication, and report to the dentist any signs of tooth discoloration.

EVALUATION:

ADVERSE REACTIONS: Atopic dermatitis, eczema, gastric distress, headache, urticaria, and weakness may be seen in hypersensitive individuals.

OVERDOSAGE: Excessive salivation, gastrointestinal disturbances, and nausea are seen in acute overdosage. Symptoms are usually severe enough to cause emesis, which resolves problems. Mottling of teeth is seen in chronic overdosage.

PARAMETERS TO MONITOR: Assess compliance in using product. Examine teeth for evidence of discoloration.

FLUORIDE (ORAL)

PRODUCTS (TRADE NAME):

Fluorineed (Available in 1 mg tablets.) **Fluoritab, Flura** (Available in 1 mg tablets and in 0.25 mg drops.) **Flura-Loz** (Available in 1 mg tablets.) **Karidium** (Available in 1 mg tablets and in 0.125 mg drops.) **Luride** (Available in 0.25 and 0.5 mg tablets and in 0.125 mg drops.) **Luride Lozi-Tabs, Pedi-Dent** (Available in 1 mg tablets.) **Phos-Flur** (Available in 0.2 mg/ml rinse/supplement). **Pediaflor** (Available in 0.5 mg/ml drops).

NURSING DRUG SPECIFICS:

Adjust dosage according to local water fluoride level.

ADMINISTRATION AND DOSAGE SPECIFICS:

General oral dosages: (Adjust for local fluoride levels. See general section on dosage and administration).

Children over 3 years: 1 mg daily.

Children 3 years old and under: 0.5 mg daily.

FLUORIDE (TOPICAL)

PRODUCTS (TRADE NAME):

Flura Drops (Available in 0.02% rinse.) **Fluoral** (Available in 2.3% paste.) **Fluorigard** (Available in 0.02% rinse.) **Fluorinse** (Available in 0.09% rinse.) **Gel-Kam, Gel-Tin** (Available in 0.1% gel.) **Karigel** (Available in 0.5% Gel). **Point-Two** (Available in 0.09% rinse). **Thera-Flur** (Available in 0.5% gel drops).

DRUG SPECIFICS:

These products may be used between professional dental fluoride treatments by patients who have excessive problems with tooth decay. Use after thoroughly brushing teeth and rinsing mouth with water. Hold preparation in mouth for at least one minute, then spit out. Do not swallow. Do not eat, drink, smoke, or rinse mouth for at least 15 to 30 minutes after treatment in order to obtain maximum benefit.

ADMINISTRATION AND DOSAGE SPECIFICS:
Adults and children over 12 years: Use 10 ml once daily.
Children 6 to 12 years: Use 5 to 10 ml once daily.

Carol Wilson

MINERALS—MAGNESIUM

ACTION OF THE DRUG: Magnesium is an electrolyte essential to several enzyme systems. It is important in maintaining osmotic pressure, ion balance, bone structure, and muscular contraction and nerve conduction. This electrolyte is stored within soft tissues, muscle, bone and cells of adults, although it may be difficult to mobilize when plasma levels fall.

ASSESSMENT:

INDICATIONS: Magnesium deficiencies are seen primarily when malabsorption syndromes are present. It is used primarily in general dietary supplementation. Magnesium is usually used with other vitamins when multiple deficiencies are suspected.

SUBJECTIVE-OBJECTIVE: Deficiency states have been associated with convulsions, retarded growth, digestive disturbances, spasticity of muscles and nerves, accelerated heart beat, arrhythmias, nervous conditions and vasodilation.

PLAN:

PRECAUTIONS: Excessive intake may produce a laxative effect.

IMPLEMENTATION:

PRODUCTS (TRADE NAME):
Almora, Magonate (Available in 500 mg tablets of magnesium gluconate.)
Mg-PLUS (Available in 133 mg magnesium-protein complex tablets.)

ADMINISTRATION AND DOSAGE: RDA for adult males is 350 mg; adult females, 330 mg. As a dietary supplement give 27 to 133 mg one to three times daily.

IMPLEMENTATION CONSIDERATIONS:
—Obtain a complete health history, including the presence of underlying or systemic disease.

—Assess dietary intake from natural as well as fortified food sources, any dietary supplements, and self-administered over-the-counter or prescription drugs.

—Teach patients principles of sound nutrition, including those foods which are good sources of magnesium. Ascertain if cultural dietary habits, food fads, lack of finances or other resources have contributed in any way to an unbalanced diet.

—Administer with caution to patients with renal dysfunction.

> **WHAT THE PATIENT NEEDS TO KNOW:**
> —Take this medication exactly as prescribed.
> —Keep this medication out of the reach of children and others for whom it has not been prescribed.
> —Magnesium is available in adequate quantities in meat, milk, fruits and vegetables to make special dietary planning unnecessary.

EVALUATION:

ADVERSE REACTIONS: None identified.
OVERDOSAGE: Magnesium may produce diarrhea if taken in excess.
PARAMETERS TO MONITOR: Check for adequacy of diet and compliance in taking medication.

Marilyn W. Edmunds

MINERALS—MANGANESE

ACTION OF THE DRUG: Manganese works in the activation of many enzymes, assists in normal skeletal and connective tissue development, helps in the initiation of protein synthesis, and plays a part in the synthesis of cholesterol and fatty acids. It is distributed throughout the body tissues and fluids with the highest concentrations found in bones, liver, kidney, pancreas, and pituitary. Its need in human nutrition has been documented, although no precise recommended daily allowances have been established.

ASSESSMENT:

INDICATIONS: It is used in dietary supplementation. It is usually used with other vitamins when multiple deficiencies are suspected.
SUBJECTIVE-OBJECTIVE: Deficiency states have been produced through controlled experimentation only. Subjects experience weight loss, changes in beard and hair growth (usually a slowing of growth), and occasional nausea and vomiting. Hypocholesterolemia has also been noted during laboratory evaluation. No symptoms of deficiency have been noted in infants and children.

PLAN:

CONTRAINDICATIONS-WARNINGS-PRECAUTIONS: The studies which have been done have produced no information in these areas.

IMPLEMENTATION:

PRODUCTS (TRADE NAME):
Mn-PLUS (Available in 5 mg tablets.)
ADMINISTRATION AND DOSAGE: No RDA has been determined. Suggested daily intake includes 0.5 to 0.7 mg po for infants, 2.5 to 5.0 mg po for adolescents, and 3 to 7 mg po for adults.
IMPLEMENTATION CONSIDERATIONS:
—Obtain a complete health history, including the presence of underlying or systemic disease.
—Assess dietary intake from natural as well as fortified food sources, any dietary supplements, and self-administered over-the-counter or prescription drugs.
—Teach patients principles of sound nutrition, including those foods which are good sources of manganese. Ascertain if cultural dietary habits, food fads, lack of finances or other resources have contributed in any way to an unbalanced diet.

WHAT THE PATIENT NEEDS TO KNOW:
—Take this medication exactly as prescribed.
—Keep this medication out of the reach of children and others for whom it has not been prescribed.
—Nuts and whole wheat cereals and grains are foods richest in manganese. Tea and cloves are exceptionally rich. Meat, fish, and dairy products have low amounts of manganese.

EVALUATION:

ADVERSE REACTIONS: None identified.
OVERDOSAGE: Manganese is one of the least toxic of the trace elements. There is no toxicity in infants or in children. The only poisoning occurs in miners who have long histories of chronic inhalation.
PARAMETERS TO MONITOR: Check for adequacy of diet and compliance in taking medication.

Carol Wilson

MINERALS—ZINC

ACTION OF THE DRUG: Zinc is an essential constituent of many enzymes and is essential for normal growth and tissue repair. Zinc functions in the mineralization of bone and in the detoxification and oxidation of methanol and ethylene glycol, and it plays a role in the synthesis of DNA and the synthesis of protein from amino acids. It is important in wound healing and functions in the mobilization of vitamin A from liver stores. Zinc is present in all cells and tissues of the body with the highest concentration in the testes, bone, and hair. It is also present in erythrocytes (75%-85% of total), leukocytes (3%), and in plasma (12%-22%). The turnover rate in these tissues varies according to the body tissue: the rate is constant in the hair, slow in bone, and rapid in the liver, spleen, pituitary, kidneys, and testes.

ASSESSMENT:

INDICATIONS: Zinc has been used for the prevention of zinc deficiency and in the treatment of delayed wound healing. It has been used experimentally in the treatment of rheumatoid arthritis and acne but is not FDA approved for these purposes.

SUBJECTIVE: Patients may complain of abnormalities of taste and smell, rough skin, and anorexia with profound disinterest in food.

OBJECTIVE: Patients may demonstrate sexual immaturity, delayed wound healing, and decreased absorption of dietary folate. In severe deficiency states, iron deficiency anemia, hepatosplenomegaly, dwarfism, and hypogonadism may also be seen.

PLAN:

WARNINGS: Exceeding the prescribed dosages may produce restlessness, nausea, and excessive vomiting leading to dehydration. Doses in excess of 2 grams will produce emesis.

IMPLEMENTATION:

DRUG INTERACTIONS: Calcium competes with zinc for absorption. Phylates form insoluble complexes with zinc and interfere with its absorption. Zinc impairs the absorption of tetracycline derivatives.

PRODUCTS (TRADE NAME):
Orazinc (Available in 110 mg capsules providing 25 mg zinc and 220 mg capsules providing 50 mg zinc.) **Verazinc** (Available in 220 mg capsules providing 50 mg zinc.) **Zinc** (Available in 66 mg tablets providing 15 mg zinc.) **Zinkaps-110, Zinkaps-220** (Available in 110 mg capsules providing 25 mg zinc and 220 mg capsules providing 50 mg zinc.) **Zinc Sulfate** (Available in 200 mg tablets providing 45 mg zinc, and 220 mg capsules providing 50 mg zinc). **Zinc-220** (Available in 220 mg capsules providing 80 mg zinc). **Zincate** (Available in 200 mg zinc sulfate providing 45 mg zinc.)

ADMINISTRATION AND DOSAGE: Minimum daily requirements include: infants to one year 3 to 5 mg/day; children one to ten years 10 mg/day; adolescents 11 to 18 years 15 mg/day; adults 15 mg/day; pregnant women 20 mg/day; lactating women 25 mg/day.

IMPLEMENTATION CONSIDERATIONS:
—Obtain a complete health history, including the presence of underlying or systemic disease.

—Assess dietary intake from natural as well as fortified food sources, any dietary supplements, self-administered over-the-counter drugs, or prescription drugs.

—Teach patient principles of sound nutrition, including those foods which are good sources of zinc. Ascertain if cultural dietary habits, food fads, lack of finances, or other resources have contributed in any way to inadequate nutrition.

—Ascertain whether patient is on any type of calcium supplement or is taking tetracycline drugs which may interfere with medication absorption.

—In patients who are susceptible to gastric upset, taking product with milk or food may be helpful in reducing nausea. Some studies suggest that certain foods decrease absorption of zinc.

—Products are over the counter except for 200 mg dosages which require prescriptions.

WHAT THE PATIENT NEEDS TO KNOW:

—Take medication as ordered. If gastric upset occurs, take with food or milk.

—Seafoods and meats are rich sources of natural zinc; cereals and legumes also have significant amounts of this mineral.

—Keep this medication out of the reach of children and others for whom it has not been prescribed.

EVALUATION:

ADVERSE REACTIONS: Gastric ulceration, nausea, and vomiting.

OVERDOSAGE: Acute zinc intoxication produces drowsiness, lethargy, lightheadedness, difficulty in writing, staggering gait, restlessness, and excessive vomiting leading to dehydration.

PARAMETERS TO MONITOR: Evaluate adequacy of dietary patterns, compliance with medication schedule, and presence of adverse effects.

Carol Wilson

MINERALS AND ELECTROLYTES

ORAL ELECTROLYTE SOLUTIONS

ACTION OF THE DRUG: Oral electrolyte mixtures are solutions of water and calories in the form of carbohydrates, with such minerals and electrolytes as sodium, potassium, chloride, calcium, and phosphorus. These are given in the event that oral food intake has been suspended, or for the prevention of dehydration and electrolyte loss, especially in diarrhea. Fluid deficits can result from inadequate intake, excessive loss, or both. Causes include vomiting, bowel obstruction (which causes a pooling of fluid and electrolytes), diarrhea, and fever (producing increased utilization of fluid and electrolytes). The body attempts to compensate for the reduced circulating volume by pulling in extracellular fluid first and then intracellular fluid. This contributes to imbalance of both fluid and electrolytes.

ASSESSMENT:

INDICATIONS: Oral electrolyte mixtures are used for the supply of both fluid and electrolytes to prevent dehydration when oral intake is temporarily halted, and to replace moderate losses of fluids and electrolytes. They are especially useful in managing dehydration from diarrhea in infants.

SUBJECTIVE: Symptoms of dehydration are usually present. Fatigue and a general feeling of malaise coupled with thirst are found. Patient may give a history compatible with progressive or acute dehydration.

OBJECTIVE: Signs of dehydration include weight loss, longitudinal wrinkles in the tongue, dry skin, lack of sweat, dry mucous membranes, decreased urinary output, lowered blood pressure, rapid pulse, increased respirations, and decreased venous pressure. In infants dehydration may also include sunken fontanelles and loss of skin turgor.

PLAN:

CONTRAINDICATIONS: These solutions are contraindicated when there is severe or continuing diarrhea or other major fluid loss which requires intravenous replacement and, in intractable vomiting, adynamic ileus, intestinal obstruction or bowel perforation, decreased renal function, or when the homeostatic mechanism of the body is impaired.

WARNINGS: Do not exceed the prescribed amount. If the patient is experiencing thirst after taking recommended dose, additional fluids in the form of water or other nonelectrolyte fluids should be given.

IMPLEMENTATION:

PRODUCTS (TRADE NAME):

Lytren Solution (Available in 32 oz ready-to-use containers which supply 30 mEq sodium, 25 mEq potassium, 4 mg calcium, 4 mg magnesium, 25 mEq chloride, 36 mg citrate, 4 mg sulfate, and 5 mg phosphate and providing 9 calories per fluid ounce.) **Pedialyte Solution** (Available in 32 oz ready-to-use containers which supply 30 mEq sodium, 20 mEq potassium, 4 mg calcium, 4 mg magnesium, 30 mg chloride, 28 mg citrate in a 5% dextrose solution and providing 6 calories per fluid ounce.)

ADMINISTRATION AND DOSAGE: Dosage should be based on water requirements calculated on the basis of total body surface area for infants and young children. As a general guide use 1500 ml/M² for maintenance during illness and 2400 ml/M² for maintenance and replacement of mild to moderate losses (as in diarrhea or vomiting.)

Replacement in Mild to Moderate Fluid Losses:
Children 5 to 10 years of age: 1-2 quarts/day.
Older children and adults: 2-3 quarts/day.

IMPLEMENTATION CONSIDERATIONS:

—Obtain a complete health history, including the presence of underlying or systemic disease.

—Obtain a complete history of the present illness including specifics on vomiting, diarrhea, fever, or other factors which might contribute to the total fluid imbalance.

—Obtain a complete dietary history, focusing upon the episode during the illness, so that an accurate assessment may be made of the nutritional and/or fluid status.

—Obtain details of history including self-treatment or self-medication during the illness.

—Obtain an accurate weight and compare to other recorded weights to assess weight loss status which may be attributable to present illness.

—Stress to the patient or parent which fluids or foods, if any, are to be given in what amount and in what combinations.

—Alert patient or parent to the signs and symptoms of dehydration and when to seek further medical attention.

WHAT THE PATIENT NEEDS TO KNOW:

—Take this medication only as prescribed. Do not exceed recommended doses.

—Keep this medication out of the reach of individuals for whom it has not been prescribed.

—Your health care provider will give you specific instructions regarding taking other food or liquids.

—Notify your health care provider if further signs of dehydration or illness appear or if the underlying problem does not resolve.

EVALUATION:

PARAMETERS TO MONITOR: Evaluate signs and symptoms of dehydration: assess urinary output and specific gravity, weight, skin turgor, vital signs, orthostatic blood pressure changes and status of fontanelles. Obtain serum electrolytes and monitor throughout therapy. As therapy progresses, watch for disappearance of signs and resolution of vomiting and diarrhea.

Carol Wilson

MINERALS AND ELECTROLYTES— POTASSIUM (ORAL)

ACTION OF THE DRUG: Potassium is the principal intracellular cation of most body tissues, participating in the maintenance of normal renal function, contraction of muscle, and the transmission of nerve impulses.

ASSESSMENT:

INDICATIONS: Prophylactic administration of potassium may be used in the therapy of nephrotic syndrome, hepatic cirrhosis accompanied by ascites, and in hyperaldosteronism patients who maintain normal renal function. Potassium products are used for the prevention or replacement of potassium loss which may occur as a result of long-term diuretic therapy, digitalis intoxication, low dietary intake of potassium, loss of potassium due to vomiting and diarrhea, diabetic acidosis, metabolic alkalosis, corticosteroid therapy, increased renal excretion of potassium due to acidosis, certain renal tubular disorders characterized by potassium wasting, adrenal cortical hyperactivity or certain cases of uremia, administration of potassium-free fluids which increase extracellular fluid volume, or diseases producing increased secretion of glucocorticoids or aldosterone.

SUBJECTIVE: Look for signs of potassium depletion: fatigue, weakness, and history of diuretic use or other source of potassium loss.

OBJECTIVE: Assess for gradual development of flaccid paralysis and/or impaired ability to concentrate urine. Serial electrocardiographic studies are helpful in documenting disturbances in cardiac rhythm, primarily ectopic beats and prominent U waves.

PLAN:

CONTRAINDICATIONS: Do not give in the presence of congestive heart failure or severe renal impairment with oliguria, anuria, or azotemia. Avoid use in patients who have edema with sodium retention, untreated Addison's disease, acute dehydration, heat cramps, or hyperkalemia from any cause.

WARNINGS: Serious and sometimes fatal stenotic and/or ulcerative lesions of the small bowel have been produced by highly localized concentrations of potassium chloride tablets as they dissolve.

PRECAUTIONS: In the individual with normal renal function it is difficult to produce potassium intoxication from oral administration since increased concentration of potassium produces increased renal excretion of the ion. However, many of the patients receiving potassium have minor defects in kidney function. Additionally, the amount of dietary potassium taken daily is unknown. It is always wise to treat conservatively and to watch for hyperkalemia since high serum concentrations of the potassium ion may produce cardiac arrhythmias, cardiac depression, and cardiac arrest. Additional risk is taken in using potassium in patients with atrioventricular conduction disturbances provoked by digitalis intoxication. All potassium products should be used cautiously in patients with decompensated cardiac disease, nephrotic disease, cirrhosis, systemic acidosis, or in patients receiving corticosteroids.

IMPLEMENTATION:

DRUG INTERACTIONS: Do not use in patients receiving potassium sparing agents such as aldosterone antagonists or triamterene.

ADMINISTRATION AND DOSAGE: The usual adult dietary intake of potassium ranges between 40 and 60 mEq per day. The loss of 200 mEq or more of potassium from the total body store is sufficient to produce hypokalemia.

Dosage must be titrated to the individual needs of each patient and closely monitored during therapy, especially in the initial stages of therapy. For patients on concurrent diuretic therapy, 20 mEq per day is usually adequate for the prevention of hypokalemia. In cases of potassium depletion, 40 to 100 mEq per day or more may be required for replacement. Potassium overdosage may result from any dosage and the patient must be closely observed for clinical effect.

Potassium comes in various salt combinations, with potassium chloride being the form most frequently prescribed. It may be ordered in either % KCl or in mEq, according to the following standard:

10 mEq potassium and chloride per 15 ml is equivalent to 5% KCl
20 mEq potassium and chloride per 15 ml is equivalent to 10% KCl
30 mEq potassium and chloride per 15 ml is equivalent to 15% KCl
40 mEq potassium and chloride per 15 ml is equivalent to 20% KCl

Potassium also comes as potassium gluconate, potassium citrate, potassium acetate, potassium bicarbonate, or in combinations, and with additions of vitamin C, ammonium chloride, citric acid, betaine HCl, and *l*-lysine monohydrochloride.

IMPLEMENTATION CONSIDERATIONS:

—Obtain a complete health history, including the presence of underlying or systemic disease, especially of cardiovascular, hepatic, or renal origin. Evaluate the concurrent use of other drugs and previous drug history.

—Because of the taste of this product, long-term compliance is often a problem. Adequate explanation to the patient about the need for this supplementation is mandatory.

—All medications must be diluted properly or taken with plenty of liquid to reduce risk of complications.

—Keep elixir and oral liquids in light-resistant, well-sealed containers.

—For patients with whom compliance is a problem, a single dose of potassium supplement might be added to individual jello cups and set with the jello. Each serving of jello then contains one dose of potassium.

WHAT THE PATIENT NEEDS TO KNOW:

—Take this medication exactly as prescribed: amount, dilution, and frequency are all carefully dictated by your own specific needs.

—The liquid form of this drug is quite salty. Taking it in a glass of tomato juice or other liquid which you might normally salt may be a helpful method of making it more palatable.

—Many health care providers advocate eating a potassium-rich diet as well as taking this type of supplement. If a potassium-rich diet is ordered, the foods which might be included are bananas, citrus fruits (especially tomatoes and oranges), apricots, and dried fruits such as raisins, prunes, and dates. Cantaloupe and watermelon in season are also good sources of potassium. Nuts, dried beans, beef, and fowl also contain ample quantities of potassium.

—This drug may have a mild laxative effect in some individuals.

—Inform your health care provider promptly if you are taking the tablet form of this drug and note any difficulty swallowing.

—Check with your health care provider if you are also using a salt substitute, as your dosage of potassium may need to be altered. Many salt substitutes contain potassium.

—Frequent blood determinations of potassium level will be done during the course of the therapy so that required alterations in dosage can be made.

—Keep all tablets in a dry, tightly closed container. Keep all elixirs and oral liquids in light-resistant, well-sealed containers.

—Keep this medication out of the reach of children and all others for whom it is not prescribed.

—Notify health care provider immediately of any new or troublesome symptoms which arise while taking this medication.

—In patients with hypochloremic alkalosis, commonly seen with diuretic use, only use the chloride salt of potassium as a supplement.

EVALUATION:

ADVERSE REACTIONS: Gastric irritation may develop, demonstrated by nausea, vomiting, diarrhea, and abdominal discomfort. GI bleeding may sometimes be provoked, and tarry stools should alert the patient to report to the health care practitioner.

OVERDOSAGE: Potassium intoxication may result from overdosage of potassium or from a change in the patient's underlying condition which makes an accumulation of potassium possible. Signs and symptoms of potassium intoxication include flaccid paralysis, paresthesias of the hands and feet, mental confusion, restlessness, listlessness, weakness, and heaviness of the legs. Hypotension and cardiac arrhythmias leading to heart block may also develop. Potentially fatal arrhythmias may develop if potassium cannot be excreted (or if it is administered too rapidly intravenously.) Detection of hyperkalemia mandates immediate treatment because lethal levels may be reached in a few hours in untreated patients. Patients should be referred to qualified physicians for management of this condition.

PARAMETERS TO MONITOR: A complete physical examination should be given and serum electrolytes should be obtained prior to beginning therapy. Baseline health status should be documented and future changes compared against it. Monitor therapeutic response through assessment of clinical status of patient and subjective complaints. Periodic measurements of serum potassium levels and serial electrocardiograms are also warranted, especially if overdosage or depletion of potassium stores is suspected. Hyperkalemia may be demonstrated on the electrocardiogram even prior to the development of clinical symptoms. Watch for disappearance of the P wave, changes in the ST segment, and the appearance of tall, peaked T waves (particularly in the right precordial leads.) Widening and slurring of the QRS complex with development of a biphasic curve may also develop, often rapidly progressing to cardiac arrest. Extended use of potassium supplements necessitates periodic red cell count and hemoglobin measurements to detect the development of anemia.

POTASSIUM CHLORIDE

PRODUCTS (TRADE NAME):

Liquids: **Cena-K, Kaochlor 10%, Kaochlor S-F** (Available in 20 mEq potassium and chloride per 15 ml, or 10% KCl.) **Kaon-CL 20%** (Available in 40 mEq potassium and chloride per 15 ml, or 20% KCl.) **Kay Ciel** (Available in 20 mEq potassium and chloride per 15 ml, or 10% KCl.) **Klor-10%** (Available in 20 mEq potassium and chloride per 15 ml, or 10% KCl.) **KLOR-CON** (Available in 40 mEq potassium and chloride per 15 ml, or 20% KCl.) **Potassium Chloride** (Available in 5%, 10%, and 20% solutions.) **Rum-K** (Available in 30 mEq potassium and chloride per 15 ml, or 15% KCl.) **SK-Potassium Chloride** (Available in 20 and 40 mEq potassium and chloride per 15 ml, or 10% and 20% KCl.)

Powders: **Kato** (Available in 20 mEq KCl per packet.) **Kay Ciel** (Available in 20 mEq KCl per packet.) **K-Lor** (Available in 15 mEq or 20 mEq KCl per packet.) **KLOR-CON** (Available in 20 mEq KCl per packet.) **K-Lyte/Cl** (Available in 25 mEq KCl per dose.) **Potassium Chloride** (Available in 20 mEq KCl per packet.)

Tablets: **Kaon-CL** (Available in 6.7 mEq (500 mg) or 10 mEq (750 mg) KCl wax matrix tablets.) **Klotrix, K-Tab** (Available in 10 mEq (750 mg) KCl wax matrix tablets.) **Potassium Chloride** (Available in 4 mEq (300 mg) or 13.4 mEq (1 gm) KCl enteric-coated tablets.) **Slow-K** (Available in 8 mEq (600 mg) KCl wax matrix tablets.)

DRUG SPECIFICS:

There is wide variation in prices, flavors, and sizes of these products. Make certain medication is diluted with water or juice or is taken with adequate quantities of liquid.

ADMINISTRATION AND DOSAGE SPECIFICS:

Titrate to individual requirements. Usual dose is 20 mEq/day for prophylaxis, and 40 to 100 mEq/day for treatment of potassium depletion.

POTASSIUM GLUCONATE, POTASSIUM CITRATE, POTASSIUM ACETATE, POTASSIUM BICARBONATE

PRODUCTS (TRADE NAME):

Effervescent tablets: **Kaochlor-Eff, KEFF** (Available in 20 mEq potassium and chloride, from potassium chloride, carbonate, and bicarbonate and betaine HCl.) **K-Lyte** (Available as 25 mEq potassium, as bicabonate and citrate.) **KLyte/CL** (Available in 25 mEq potassium and chloride, from potassium chloride and bicarbonate, *l*-lysine monohydrochloride and citric acid.) **K-Lyte/CL 50** (Available in 50 mEq potassium and chloride, from potassium chloride and bicarbonate, *l*-lysine monohydrochloride and citric acid.) **K-Lyte DS** (Available in 50 mEq potassium, as bicarbonate, citrate and citric acid.)

Liquids: **Bi-K** (Available in 20 mEq potassium gluconate and potassium citrate per 15 ml.) **Duo-K** (Available in 20 mEq potassium and 3.4 mEq chloride from potassium gluconate and potassium chloride, per 15 ml.) **Kaon, Kao-Nor, Kaylixir** (Available in 20 mEq potassium as potassium gluconate, per 15 ml.) **Kolyum** (Available in 20 mEq potassium and 3.4 mEq chloride, from potassium gluconate and potassium chloride, per 15 ml.) **Potassium Gluconate** (Available in 20 mEq potassium as potassium gluconate, per 15 ml.) **Trikates, Tri-K** (Available in 45 mEq potassium, from potassium acetate, potassium bicarbonate, and potassium citrate, per 15 ml.) **Twin-K** (Available 20 mEq potassium, as potassium gluconate and potassium citrate per 15 ml.) **Twin-K-Cl** (Available in 15 mEq potassium and 4 mEq chloride, as potassium gluconate, potassium citrate, and ammonium chloride, per 15 ml.)

Powders: **Klorvess Effervescent Granules** (Available in 20 mEq each potassium and chloride, from potassium chloride and bicarbonate and *l*-lysine monohydrochloride, per packet.) **Kolyum** (Available in 20 mEq potassium and 3.4 mEq chloride, from potassium gluconate and potassium chloride, per packet.)

Tablets: **Kaon** (Available in 5 mEq potassium as gluconate tablets.) **KaoNor** (Available in 2.5 mEq (595 mg) potassium gluconate tablets.) **OSTO-K** (Available in 1 mEq (39 mg) potassium, from chloride, citrate and gluconate, with 10 mg vitamin C in chewable tablets.) **Potassium Gluconate** (Available in 2 mEq (486 mg) potassium gluconate tablets.)

DRUG SPECIFICS:

These products, most of which require prescriptions, are utilized primarily in patients in whom chloride is restricted. Because some of these products do contain chloride, it is important to carefully choose the potassium salt desired. There is wide variability in the cost of these products, tending in general to be more expensive than potassium chloride products. Effervescent tablets must be dissolved completely in water before administration.

ADMINISTRATION AND DOSAGE SPECIFICS:

Titrate dosage to individual needs. Usual dose is 20 mEq per day for prophylaxis and 40 to 100 mEq per day for treatment of potassium depletion.

MINERALS AND ELECTROLYTES— SALT SUBSTITUTES

PRODUCTS (TRADE NAME):

Adolph's Salt Substitute (Available as 97.1% KCl with less than 10 mg sodium per 100 gm.) **Adolph's Seasoned Salt Substitute** (Available as 67.4% KCl with less than 20 mg Na per 100 gm.) **Morton Salt Substitute** (Available as 96% KCl with less than 10 mg Na per 100 gm in seasoned or unseasoned product.) **NoSalt** (Available as KCl with less than 10 mg Na per 100 mg.) **Neocurtasal** (Available as KCl with less than 0.5 mg Na in each 5 gm.) **Nu-Salt** (Available as KCl and with less than 10 mg sodium per 100 gm.)

DRUG SPECIFICS:

Salt substitutes are over-the-counter preparations that can be used in making both cooked and uncooked food more palatable for patients who are on low salt diets. Patients who may profit from this product are those with hypertension, congestive heart failure, and other processes which may cause edema (pregnancy, obesity, cirrhosis, corticosteroid therapy, and renal disease.)

These potassium chloride products come in salt shaker dispensers and are used in slightly less than normal amounts as a replacement for sodium chloride. They are not acceptable for patients who must also restrict potassium. They are contraindicated in patients with severe kidney disease or oliguria. Symptoms of hyponatremia (from overrestriction of sodium) or hyperkalemia (from excessive use) should be assessed. Long-term use may necessitate iodine supplements in some patients as these products do not contain iodine.

Marilyn W. Edmunds

MINERALS AND ELECTROLYTES— SYSTEMIC ALKALINIZERS

SODIUM BICARBONATE(ORAL)

ACTION OF THE DRUG: Sodium bicarbonate is used as a gastric, systemic, and urinary alkalinizer.

ASSESSMENT:

INDICATIONS: Often used by general public for the treatment and relief of the symptoms of occasional overeating and indigestion. (See sections on gastrointestinal and urinary tract products for other specific actions.) Extensive or prolonged use may produce electrolyte imbalance and systemic alkalosis.

SUBJECTIVE-OBJECTIVE: Symptoms of overeating and indigestion may be present: feelings of fullness, heartburn, burping, water brash, pyrosis.

PLAN:

CONTRAINDICATIONS: Do not use chronically or for prolonged treatment. Because sodium bicarbonate is completely soluble in gastric secretions, large doses or prolonged therapy may lead to sodium overload or systemic alkalosis.

WARNINGS: Use with caution in patients on low sodium diets, patients receiving diuretic therapy, and patients who have a tendency to retain fluids.

IMPLEMENTATION:

DRUG INTERACTIONS: Chronic administration with milk or calcium leads to an increase in calcium absorption and may precipitate a milk-alkali syndrome, possibly enhanced by a salt-losing neuropathy.

PRODUCTS (TRADE NAME):

Sodium Bicarbonate (Available in 325 mg, 487.5 mg, and 650 mg tablets and in 120, 240, and 300 gm powder).

ADMINISTRATION AND DOSAGE: Usual dose is from 325 mg to 2 gm given 2-4 times daily. Daily maximum intake should not exceed 16 gm.

IMPLEMENTATION CONSIDERATION:

—Obtain a complete health history, including the presence of underlying or systemic disease.

—Ascertain whether patient is currently on diuretic or other medications.

—Assess whether patient is currently on a low-sodium diet.

—Obtain a complete dietary history, including whether cultural habits, food fads, lack of money, or other resources may be responsible for causing gastric upset, overeating, or indigestion.

—Ascertain if patient is currently taking any calcium products (antacids, etc.) and the amount of milk and dairy products in the diet.

—Ascertain whether patient has been taking over-the-counter or prescription drugs which contain sodium bicarbonate, and for how long.

—Preparation contains 12 mEq of sodium per gram and may be dangerous to patients who cannot tolerate additional sodium.

—A milk-alkali syndrome may be provoked by chronic administration of this medication with milk or calcium. This syndrome is characterized by renal insufficiency, hypercalcemia, and metabolic acidosis. The syndrome improves when the antacid and calcium are discontinued. Symptoms include nausea, vomiting, headache, mental confusion, and anorexia.

WHAT THE PATIENT NEEDS TO KNOW:

—Take this medication exactly as prescribed. Overuse is to be strictly avoided.

—Keep this medication out of the reach of children and others for whom it has not been prescribed.

—Product should not be used while you are on a low-salt diet, receiving diuretic therapy, or taking any calcium products.

—Although there are few problems resulting from the use of this drug, report any unusual symptoms such as nausea, vomiting, headache, lack of appetite, and confusion to your health care provider promptly.

EVALUATION:

ADVERSE REACTIONS: Gastric distention and flatulence may occur with effervescent sodium bicarbonate. Acid rebound phenomenon may also be provoked.

Some commercial forms of sodium bicarbonate contain aspirin. Taking these products after heavy alcohol intake can lead to hematemesis and melena.

PARAMETERS TO MONITOR: Assess compliance with moderate dosing therapy. Discontinue at earliest possible time. Obtain serum electrolytes if alkalosis is suspected.

Carol Wilson

7

HORMONES

ADRENOCORTICAL STEROIDS

GLUCOCORTICOIDS

ACTION OF THE DRUG: (1) The major action of the glucocorticoids is the stimulation of protein synthesis of enzymes responsible for three systemic effects: anti-inflammatory, immunosuppressant, and metabolic. The latter action causes the catabolism of protein fats and carbohydrates into glucagon and ultimately raises the serum glucose level. (2) Naturally-occurring glucocorticoids (cortisone and hydrocortisone) also have moderate mineralocorticoid activity which causes reabsorption of sodium and excretion of potassium.

ASSESSMENT:

INDICATIONS:
Indications for systemic use:
In physiological doses: replacement of missing hormones in adrenal insufficiency (Addison's disease).

In pharmacological doses: (more commonly) suppression of inflammatory, allergic, or immunological responses, with antineoplastics for treatment of hematologic and malignant diseases. This class of drugs is not curative; it is to be used adjunctively with the primary method of treatment.

Examples of situations in which glucocorticoids might be used are as follows:

Acute emergencies: CNS emergencies: encephalitis, meningitis, fulminating bacterial infections, shock.

Acute hypersensitivity reactions: anaphylaxis, drug-infusion reactions, organ transplant, status asthmaticus.

Allergic state: atopic dermatitis, angioneurotic edema, bronchial asthma, contact dermatitis, exfoliative dermatitis, intractable hay fever, perennial aller gic rhinitis, serum sickness.

Collagen diseases: dermatomyositis, pemphigus, periarteritis nodosa, rheumatic fever (especially with carditis), rheumatoid arthritis, scleroderma, systemic lupus erythematosus.

Connective tissue disease: ankylosing spondylitis, bursitis, epicondylitis, post-traumatic osteo arthritis, psoritic arthritis, tenosynovitis.

Diagnostic testing of adrenocortical hyperfunction.

Edematous states: remission of proteinuria in nephrotic syndrome (without uremia).

Hematologic and neoplastic diseases: acquired hemolytic anemia, agranulocytosis, aplastic anemia, autoimmune hemolytic anemia, congenital hypoplastic anemia, erythroblastopenia, idiopathic and secondary thrombocytopenia, Hodgkin's disease, leukemia (especially lymphatic system types), lymphosarcoma, non-neoplastic blood dyscrasias, various solid tumors.

Ophthalmologic diseases: chorioretinitis, diffuse posterior uveitis and choroiditis, herpes zoster ophthalmicus, iritis and iridocyclitis, optic neuritis, retrolental fibroplasia, severe anterior segment inflammation, sympathetic ophthalmia.

Respiratory diseases: berylliosis, fulminating or disseminated pulmonary tuberculosis, Loffler's syndrome, symptomatic sarcoidosis.

Miscellaneous: acute Bell's palsy, chronic kidney disease, chronic ulcerative colitis, severe trichinosis, thromboembolic diseases.

Indications for local steroids:

Intra-articular, soft tissue, intrabursal: indicated as adjunctive treatment for short-term administration to support patients during acute, exacerbations of: acute gouty arthritis, acute and subacute bursitis, acute, nonspecific tenosynovitis, epicondylitis, osteoarthritis, post-traumatic osteoarthritis, rheumatoid arthritis.

Intralesional, subcutaneous dermatologic problems: alopecia areata, discoid lupus erythematosus, gangalia, granuloma annulare (unresponsive to topical treatment), keloids, lichen planus, lichen simplex chronicus, psoriatic plaques, status dermatitis.

Indications for topical use:

Acute and chronic dermatoses: anogenital pruritus; atopic, seborrheic, some types of chronic eczematous dermatitis; cutaneous manifestations of systemic collagen diseases (lupus dermatomyositis, pemphigus), infantile eczema, inter-triginous psoriasis, neurodermatitis.

Rectum: ulcerative colitis, proctitis, sigmoiditis, other inflammatory conditions of the distal intestine.

Otic diseases: steroid-responsive inflammatory conditions of external ear (otitis externa).

Ophthalmologic diseases: acute glaucoma, acne rosacea, allergic blepharitis, chemical or thermal burns, conjunctivitis, herpes zoster keratitis, iridocyclitis, penetration of foreign body, punctate keratitis, uveitis.

PLAN:

CONTRAINDICATIONS:

Systemic: Do not give in presence of systemic fungal infections, hypersensitivity.

Local: Do not give in septic joints without anti-infective treatment.

WARNINGS: Although glucocorticoids are exceptionally potent drugs, short-term administration of even extremely large doses is not likely to net long-term sequelae. However, moderate and long-term administration (longer than six days systemic treatment) places the patient at high risk to a large number of serious adverse effects and the risk/benefit ratio must be carefully considered. (See adverse effects.) The immediate and long-term effects of the drug are exceedingly variable and depend on the individual disease, route of administration, dose, frequency, duration, and time of administration.

Corticosteroid drugs cannot be withdrawn without gradual weaning. Sudden withdrawal leads to steroid withdrawal syndrome (anorexia, nausea and vomiting, lethargy, headache, fever, joint pain, desquamation, myalgia, weight loss and hypotension). Abrupt cessation may also result in rebound of the condition being treated.

When the drug is administered for longer than one to two weeks at pharmacological doses, pituitary release of ACTH is suppressed, producing secondary adrenocortical insufficiency. Patients undergoing physiological, emotional, or psychological stress may need support via additional amounts of steroids. This suppression may last up to two years following discontinuation of the drug.

Normal or large doses, especially of cortisone and hydrocortisone, can cause hypertension, sodium and water retention, and potassium loss. All corticosteroids promote calcium excretion.

Corticosteroids mask infection and increase the patient's susceptibility to them. Corticosteroids are particularly dangerous to use in patients with a history of tuberculosis. The disease can be reactivated; therefore, administer Isoniazide to these patients. In patients with active, fulminating, or disseminated tuberculosis, or any infection, use steroids only in conjunction with a total anti-infective regimen. Due to the altered antibody response, patients receiving corticosteroids should not be immunized against smallpox or other diseases.

Because of the multisystem ramifications of corticosteroid administration, careful consideration of the risk/benefit must be undertaken before prescribing systemic steroids to patients with the following problems: cardiac disease, congestive heart failure, diverticulitis, emotional instability, open angle glaucoma, diminished hepatic function, herpes simplex of the eye, hyperlipidemia, hypertension, hypothyroidism, myasthenia gravis, osteoporosis, peptic ulcer, gastritis, esophagitis, decreased renal function, tuberculosis, ulcerative colitis, convulsions, thrombophlebitis, psychosis, vaccinia, varicella, Cushing's syndrome, conditions causing thinning of cornea or sclera, and fresh intestinal anastomosis.

Although corticosteroids do cross the placental barrier, there is no research to document problems in humans. Fetal abnormalities have been noted in animal studies. Ratio of benefits to risks should be weighed. Mother and infant should be closely monitored for hypoadrenalism at the time of and following birth if steroid therapy has been administered.

There have been no documented problems in steroid use with nursing mothers. However, high-dose steroid consumption in the mother may result in growth suppression of the infant.

PRECAUTIONS:

Systemic dosage:

Existing active or latent psychological disorders may be aggravated or activated with prolonged dosage. Physiologic effects of corticosteroids may be exaggerated in patients with hypothyroidism and cirrhosis. Prolonged dosage may produce osteoporosis leading to vertebral collapse. The use of aspirin should be questioned and carefully monitored in patients receiving corticosteroids with hypoprothrombinemia. The lowest possible dose of corticosteroids which produces the desired effect should be used. Drug-induced secondary adrenal insufficiency can be minimized with alternate-day dosage regimens and then gradual reduction of drug. The growth of children receiving corticosteroids should be carefully monitored. The use of antacids with and between doses of large amounts of steroids has been recommended by some clinicians.

Local administration:

Intraarticular administration (particularly into large joints) may result in systemic absorption. Frequent intra-articular injection may be destructive to the joint. Aspiration of joint fluid is recommended prior to corticosteroid administration to rule out sepsis. Steroids should not be injected into an unstable joint. Patients should be urged not to overuse the joint following corticosteroid injection, despite the symptomatic relief.

Ophthalmological use:

Note that corneal fungal infections are particularly likely to develop coincidentally with extensive corticosteroid ophthalmological use. Therefore, fungal infection must be considered in any persistent corneal irritation in patients when the drug has been or is being used.

IMPLEMENTATION:

DRUG INTERACTIONS: Corticosteroids increase the effects of: barbiturates, sedatives, narcotics, and anticoagulants. They decrease the effects of insulin and oral hypoglycemics, coumarin anticoagulants, ioniazid, choline-like drugs (reduce effectiveness in treatment of glaucoma), aspirin (higher doses necessary which has led to salicylism after discontinuation of steroids), and broad spectrum antibiotics (may result in resistant strains). Drugs which increase the effects of steroids are: indomethacin, aspirin, troleandromycin, and oral contraceptives, especially estrogen (estrogen increases the antiinflammatory effect of hydrocortisone by slowing its breakdown in the liver). Drugs which decrease the effects of steroids include ephedrine, barbiturates, phenytoin, antihistamines, chloral hydrate, rifampin, glutethimide, phenylbutazone (increases effect and then reduces it), and propranolol.

Some drugs produce exaggerated side effects when given with steroids. These include: alcohol, aspirin and anti-inflammatory drugs (ulcerogenic), amphotericin B, thiazides and other potassium-wasting diuretics (excessive potassium loss), stimulants such as adrenalin, amphetamines and ephedrine, anticholinergics (increased intraocular pressure), and cardiac glycosides (enhances possibility of arrhythmias and digitalis toxicity).

Steroids also increase the laboratory serum levels of amylase, CO_2, glucose, and sodium. Corticosteroids may also increase thyroid ^{131}I uptake. Corticosteroids decrease the laboratory levels of serum calcium, potassium, platelets, T_3 and T_4.

ADMINISTRATION AND DOSAGE: Various corticosteroids may be administered by the following routes: oral, inhalation, intranasal, intravenous, intramuscular, subcutaneous, intrabursal, intradermal, intrasynovial, intralesional, soft tissue injection, topical, and per rectum.

Dosages vary radically; they are individualized by the diagnosis, severity, prognosis, probable duration of the disease, patient response, and tolerance. Individuals may respond better to one form than another in a somewhat unpredictable manner. The general rule, regardless of route of administration, is to initially prescribe as high a dose as necessary to obtain a favorable response, then decrease the amount gradually to the lowest level that will maintain the therapeutic effect and yet minimize complications.

Systemic administration:

Dosage regimens are of two types: (1) Physiological: for replacement of glucocorticoids in adrenal insufficiency 20 mg hydrocortisone/day. (2) Pharmacologic: For prednisone or prednisolone massive: 15-30 mg/kg/day; high: 1-3 mg/kg/day; moderate: 500 mcg/kg/day; maintenance: 5-15 mg/day.

All patients receiving systemic corticosteroids should be monitored often and the dose adjusted to reflect remissions, exacerbations, the individual response, or occurrence of stress (injury, infection, surgery, emotional crisis, etc.). Patients should be monitored for one or two years following high dosage or long-term treatment. While receiving steroids, patients should be given prescriptions which cannot be refilled in order to prevent unmonitored steroid consumption.

Pediatric administration is determined more by the disease, condition of the child, and response to the drug than by weight, although guidelines are often given. Inhibition of growth occurs in a large percentage of children taking pharmacological doses of steroids. Alternate day treatment with an oral intermediate-acting steroid (such as prednisone, prednisolone or methylprednisolone) may help decrease this untoward effect. A comparison of available systemic corticosteroids is presented in Table 7-1.

Generally, prednisone is considered the drug of choice for an anti-inflammatory immunosuppressant effect. Antacids are recommended with and/or between doses to minimize peptic ulcer complication. Systemic corticosteroids are administered orally except in emergency circumstances or when the patient is unable to take oral medication. Onset of action is 2-8 hours and the effects last for 24 hours. Oral corticosteroids are almost completely absorbed in the GI tract.

For long-term administration, the alternate-day regimen of an intermediateacting (12-36 hours) adrenocorticoid is recommended. Preferred drugs are prednisone or prednisolone. By giving one double dose every other day in the morning, the suppressive action of the HPA (hypothalamic-pituitary-adrenal) axis is minimized. Further, the dose should be given in the morning to stimulate the natural

TABLE 7-1. COMPARISON OF SYSTEMIC CORTICOSTEROIDS

Drug	Approx EQV Glucocorticoid Dose	Availability			Relative Potency*	Mineralocorticoid Effects Na+ and H_2O Retention
		Oral	IM	IV		
Short-Acting						
Cortisone	25	X	X		0.8	2+
Hydrocortisone	20	X	X	X	1	2+
Intermediate-Acting						
Prednisolone	5	X	X	X	3-4	1+
Prednisone	5	X			3-4	1+
Methylprednisolone	4	X	X	X	5	±
Triamcinolone	4	X	X		5	±
Long-Acting						
Betamethasone	0.6	X	X	X	20-30	±
Dexamethasone	0.75	X	X	X	20-30	±
Fluprednisolone	1.5-2	X				±
Paramethasone	2	X			6-10	±

*Anti-inflammatory and immunosuppressant effects

circadian rhythm of endogenous steroid blood levels. It is to be noted that some patients' symptoms cannot be controlled by the alternate-day regimen. In these cases, occasionally administering a larger-than-double dose on alternate days and/ or giving other supportive treatment on off days may help. When neither of these options is satisfactory, it is appropriate to attempt to administer the entire daily dose in the morning rather than in divided doses. Again, there are some patients (particularly those with rheumatoid arthritis or ulcerative colitis) who are not relieved by anything but high-divided doses. The latter regimen unfortunately places the patient at much higher risk for HPA axis suppression and the full gamut of side effects.

To shift a patient from individual divided doses to alternate-day treatment: (1) Document a stable hypothalamic-pituitary-adrenal axis. (2) Give twice the therapeutic daily dose (which has been found to be effective in relieving symptoms) as a single dose on alternate days in the morning. Gradually decrease to maintenance; or decrease the daily dose to maintenance prior to switching, then give twice the maintenance dose on alternate days. To establish the maintenance dose every morning as a single dose, gradually increase the dose on even days while decreasing the dose on odd days until twice the daily dose is being taken on even days.

It is vital that the drug be withdrawn gradually after administration for any period longer than one week. After long treatment, reduce dosage by 2.5 mg of prednisone (or its equivalent) at 7-day intervals until the physiologic dose is reached. The final daily doses must be given with breakfast to allow the body to revert to the early morning pattern for glucocorticoid release.

During tapering to maintenance or withdrawal, the patient must be watched carefully and taught signs of adrenal insufficiency (weakness, hypotension, anorexia). If this occurs, or the disease flares up, the steroid dose is increased until symptoms subside. Tapering then begins again on a more gradual regimen.

When the physiologic dose has been reached, substitute hydrocortisone 20 mg to be given in the morning. Maintain this dose for 2-3 weeks. After 2-3 weeks decrease the dose by 2.5 mg a week. That is, reduce to 17.5 mg/day for the next week, 15 mg/day the next week, etc., until 10 mg/day is reached. Test the patient for normal hypothalamic-pituitary-adrenal axis function. At this point, the drug may be discontinued. Note: After this regimen the patient may still need to be supported with additional steroids in periods of stress for up to one year.

After shorter steroid courses (1-2 weeks), reduce the dose on a daily basis by 50% decrements. Keep the same scheduled intervals.

Local injections:

Treatment by intra-articular, intrabursal, intralesional, subcutaneous or intradermal routes greatly reduces the incidence of systemic side effects of hypothalamic-pituitary-adrenal axis suppression, although with large doses, the possibilities must not be ignored. In many cases, a single injection yields sufficient anti-inflammatory effects to alleviate symptoms. The slowly absorbed forms (acetate, acetonide, diacetate, hexacetonide, tebutate) of appropriate corticosteroids generally result in relief for 1-2 weeks.

Appropriate joints for injection include the knee, ankle, wrist, elbow, shoulder, phalanges, and hip joints. Spinal and other joints without synovial spaces are not appropriate. Other considerations in administering intra-articular steroids are as follows: (1) Inject the cavity in its most superficial aspect, avoiding large vessels and nerves. (2) Always examine aspirate for sepsis. If infected, begin antibiotic therapy. Do not inject with steroids. (3) Do not inject non-stable joint. (4) Warn the patient not to overuse the joint. It will feel comfortable, but will still be inflamed. (5) It is sometimes appropriate to inject the joint or surrounding tissues with an anesthetic (not containing preservatives) prior to steroid injection. See individual drug directions. (6) Frequent intra-articular injection may result in damage to the joint tissue.

Only corticosteroid preparations which are specifically designated should be used for ophthalmological or otic administration. To apply eye ointment: pull lower lid away to form a pouch. Squeeze a thin one-centimeter strip into the pouch. Close the eye for one to two minutes. Warn patient that vision will be blurred for a short time. To apply otic drops: Carefully clean and dry the ear canal with a cotton-tipped applicator. Lie down with affected ear up and instill the solution directly into the canal, making certain not to contaminate dropper. Maintain the position for five minutes. Repeat on the other side if necessary. Alternately, use a cotton or gauze wick saturated with solution. Keep the wick moist by adding solution every four hours. Replace the wick every 12 to 24 hours.

IMPLEMENTATION CONSIDERATIONS:

—Obtain a complete health history, including history of infection (especially systemic fungal infections), positive tuberculin test or tuberculosis, hypersensitivity, underlying medical diseases, medications taken concurrently which may produce drug interactions, and possibility of pregnancy.

—Doses are quite variable and patients must be closely observed for response in order to make dosage adjustments.

—Generic forms of the drugs are considerably less expensive.

—All patients on corticosteroids should be monitored often and the dose adjusted to reflect remissions, exacerbations, the individual response, or occurrence of stress (injury, infection, surgery, emotional crisis, etc.). Patients should be monitored for one or two years following high doses or long-term treatment.

—While receiving steroids, patients should be given prescriptions which cannot be refilled in order to prevent unmonitored steroid consumption.

—Review information under Administration and Dosage regarding specific steps to follow in using corticosteroids for systemic, and local injection, and topical applications.

WHAT THE PATIENT NEEDS TO KNOW:

—You will need to come to your health care provider frequently to check progress during and after steroid therapy.

—There are no restrictions on driving vehicles, operating machinery, or sun exposure related to this drug.

—Nicotine raises the blood level of naturally produced cortisone; therefore heavy smoking may add to the expected action.

—Alcohol may enhance the tendency of the medication to cause ulcers. Drinking of alcohol should be discontinued or minimal during the course of therapy.

—This drug may decrease your resistance to infection and the ability to tolerate stress, injury, or surgery (including dental surgery). Inform your health care provider, dentist, or physician that you are on a steroid medication if you should encounter any of these situations.

—You may need additional steroids during times of injury, illness, emotional, or psychological stress for up to 2 years after prolonged treatment with steroids.

—You and your family should know the signs and symptoms of adrenal insufficiency: nausea and vomiting, aching of bones and muscles, headache, increased temperature, and diarrhea. Notify your health care provider immediately if you note any of these problems.

—This drug must not be stopped suddenly. Your body will slowly grow to depend on it and cannot survive well without it.

—Wear a Medic-Alert bracelet or carry other identifying information during and after treatment.

—Do not receive any immunizations without consulting your health care provider first.

—Take oral medication with food to minimize stomach upset.

—You may need to take a diet rich in potassium and low in sodium. Ask your health care provider to give you a list of foods to take and foods to avoid.

—Tablets should be kept in tightly corked brown bottles away from the heat.

—Inform your health care provider if you become pregnant, or begin to take medications from another health care provider, especially aspirin, diuretics, digitalis preparations, insulin, oral hypoglycemics, phenobarbital, rifampin, pheny-toin, and somatotropin.

—If you are taking buffered prednisone and tetracycline, you cannot take the two within 1/2 hour of each other.

—If a dose is missed:

a. If you are on an alternate-day schedule: Take the dose as soon as possible and go back to the regular schedule. If you remember in the evening, take the dose the next morning. Skip a day and start a new schedule.

b. If you are on a daily dose: Take the dose as soon as possible. If you do not remember until the next day, take the normal dose and return to normal schedule.

c. If you are on divided doses (taking medication more than once a day): Take the dose as soon as possible, then go back to the normal schedule. If you forget until the next dose, double that dose and go back to the regular schedule.

—Call your health care provider if you experience rapid weight gain, black or tarry stools, unusual bleeding or bruising, signs of low potassium or hypokalemia (anorexia, lethargy, confusion, nausea, or muscle weakness).

—Avoid eating licorice. It contains glycyrrhizic acid which can produce hypokalemia or low potassium.

—Make every attempt to avoid falls or bumps. Steroids can cause your bones to break more easily.

With ophthalmologic use, the patient needs to know:

a. Do not use the steroid preparation for different problems you may have in the future.

b. Call the health care provider immediately if you have trouble seeing properly: blurring of vision, or narrowing of vision.

—Do not give this medication to other members of your family.

EVALUATION:

ADVERSE REACTIONS: *Systemic Administration:* The side effects of systemic corticosteroids in pharmacologic doses are predictable exaggerations of functions of the corticosteroids normally produced by the adrenals, or the results of hypothalamicpituitary-adrenal axis suppression. Some adverse reactions are quite common, others are more unusual. Adverse reactions which might develop are listed in Table 7-2.

TABLE 7-2. POSSIBLE ADVERSE REACTIONS FROM CORTICOSTEROIDS

System	Major Problems	Subjective Signs	Treatment Options
Endocrine	Atrophy of adrenal cortex* (can occur after 10 days)	Signs of adrenal insufficiency: abdominal and back pain, dizziness, low fever, nausea, muscle pain.	Alternate-day dose; most of dose in AM
	Anterior pituitary suppression:*	Flushing, irregular menses, headache.	Reassurance that symptoms will subside when treatment ends
	Diabetes* (catabolism of fat, protein, glycogen, resulting in hyperglycemia)	Polyuria, polydipsia, polyphagia	Diabetic diet; antidiabetic agents.
	Fluid/electrolyte imbalance* (from overlapping mineralocorticoid effect)	Edema of feet and hands	Decrease sodium in diet, increase potassium intake or give supplement. Weigh frequently; check blood pressure.
	Hypokalemia	Muscle cramps, irregular heart rate	Dietary K+ supplement
	Redisposition of lipids:* androgenic effects from sex hormones.	Moon facies, buffalo hump, truncal obesity, striae, hirsutism, acne.	Anticipatory guidance, emotional support. Assure patient that

TABLE 7-2. POSSIBLE ADVERSE REACTIONS FROM CORTICOSTEROIDS

System	Major Problems	Subjective Signs	Treatment Options
			androgenic effects will abate as dosage is decreased.
Gastrointestinal	Gastritis,* peptic ulcer* (unrelated to local irritation of oral tablets), esophagitis, pancreatitis	Epigastric burning, back pain, food intolerance, indigestion, weight gain, increased appetite, distention, nausea, vomiting, diarrhea, constipation	Bland diet or small frequent meals; antacids (not aluminum hydroxide since this renders oral glucocorticoids unavailable); diet counseling
Immune	Absence of signs of infection:* uninhibited invasion and proliferation of virus, bacteria, fungus; inhibition of fibroplasia with delayed wound healing.	Wounds do not heal; high susceptibility to infection	Observe carefully for any signs or symptoms of infections; treat appropriately.
Musculoskeletal	Muscle wasting* (catabolism of protein)	Muscle weakness, atrophy of muscle	High-protein diet; evaluate muscle strength periodically
	Osteoporosis	Back pain, bone pain	Urge patient to keep active, help patient evaluate environment for hazards.
Neurologic	Mood changes, emotional lability EEG changes Pseudotumor cerebri	Euphoria, insomnia, nervousness, irritability, psychotic episodes, depression, sense of well-being, restlessness, inability to concentrate, vertigo, headache	Decrease dose if possible; reassure patient symptoms are drug related and time limited; reassure, support family; evaluate mental status each visit.
Ophthalmologic	Induces/aggravates glaucoma by decreasing aqueous outflow Cataracts Optic nerve damage Increased susceptibility	Headache, halos around lights, large pupils, diminished visual acuity, visual field defects, blurred vision,	Treat symptomatically (weigh benefit to risk).

TABLE 7-2. POSSIBLE ADVERSE REACTIONS FROM CORTICOSTEROIDS

System	Major Problems	Subjective Signs	Treatment Options
	to viral or fungal infection	droopy eyelids, eye pain.	
	Corneal perforation (when used in conditions that cause cornea to thin)	Persistent corneal irritation	Gradually discontinue steroids
Vascular (especially with cortisone)	Thrombosis, thromboembolism, thrombophlebitis, hypercholestrolemia, atherosclerosis	Leg pain	Weigh risk-benefit ratio; discontinue if indicated.
Others	Hypertension		Treat symptomatically if long term, but use potassium-sparing antihypertensives.
	Collagen tissue breakdown can activate latent tuberculosis by liberating organisms from deposits in pulmonary tissue.	Cough, weight loss	Some clinicians recommend prophylactic antitubercular therapy in anyone with history of tuberculosis or positive skin test.
	Hypersensitivity reactions		IV epinephrine

*Most common side effects.

Pediatric adverse reactions: Major adverse effects involve linear growth suppression and posterior, subcapsular, cataract formation following very-long-term therapy (longer than one year). Pseudotumor cerebri (benign intracranial hypertension) has been reported, usually following rapid decreases in dose or change in steroid.

Small physiologic doses or short-term emergency pharmacologic doses generally do not cause adverse effects.

OVERDOSAGE: *Systemic:* Moderate overdosage results in edema, flushing of face, nervousness, gastric irritation, and weakness. Severe overdosage produces severe headache, convulsions, heart failure (in susceptible individuals), psychological aberrations. *Treatment:* Decrease dose if possible and/or treat symptomatically. In life-threatening situations, extremely large doses have been administered with excellent results.

PARAMETERS TO MONITOR: Before beginning therapy, obtain baseline history and physical examination, documenting current patient status. A thorough examination for a patient to be placed on long-term therapy would specifically note weight, height, blood pressure, electrocardiogram, chest and spinal x-rays, hypothalamic-pituitary-adrenal axis function test, upper GI series (in patients with history of GI problems), serum electrolytes, and glucose. An ophthalmological consultation is also indicated for patients to be placed on long-term steroid therapy.

To monitor during treatment: On each visit monitor for therapeutic effect on underlying problem and for occurrence of adverse effects. Note sudden increases in weight, blood pressure, edema, muscle strength and wasting, intake and output. Monitor signs and symptoms of adrenal suppression: abdominal and back pain, dizziness, low fever, nausea and vomiting, prolonged loss of appetite and weight loss; signs and symptoms of Cushing's disease: moon face, buffalo hump, striae. Signs and symptoms of infections or other concurrent health problems, mental status. On each visit or alternate visit, obtain blood and urine tests for glucose, ketones, potassium and a stool for occult blood.

There should be regular evaluation by an ophthalmologist to rule out subcapsular cataracts, increased intraocular pressure, corneal abrasion, or infection. Hypothalamic-pituitary-adrenal axis function tests should be performed, particularly following withdrawal of high doses or long-term treatment. Prothrombin time should be monitored if patient is on anticoagulants. Growth and development should be monitored in children.

BECLOMETHASONE—INHALANT

PRODUCTS (TRADE NAME):

Beclovent, Vanceril (Available in 10 mg aerosol containers which deliver about 200 inhalations. Each inhalation yields 50 mcg.)

DRUG SPECIFICS:

Beclomethasone is a steroid inhalant that has extremely potent topical anti-inflammatory action with minimal systemic absorption. It should only be used for those patients (1) needing symptomatic control of asthma who are on systemic steroids in order to decrease or eliminate oral treatment; (2) who are unresponsive to other, more conservative treatment, (3) who cannot take systemic steroids; or (4) who have experienced side effects with steroids. This drug is not indicated in (1) nonasthmatic bronchitis, (2) those who are not steroid dependent; (3) patients controllable without steroids; and (4) for treatment of status asthmaticus. (This is not a bronchodilator and cannot be used for rapid relief of bronchospasm.)

It may take several months of treatment to achieve maximum results; however, pulmonary function tests should show improvement in 1-4 weeks. The client should be instructed to contact the health care provider immediately if asthma attacks develop which are not responsive to the combination of bronchodilator and beclomethasone. A patient using a bronchodilator should use it several minutes before the beclomethasone to increase bronchial penetration of the latter.

Cortisol levels should be followed regularly. After weaning completely from systemic steroids to beclomethasone, the cortisol level should be normal in the morning. Adrenal suppression can occur with therapy.

WARNINGS:

Patients have died while transfering to beclomethasone from systemic steroids (due to chronic adrenal insufficiency). The steroid dose must be very slowly withdrawn. The patient is also at risk during any episodes of stress because beclomathasone does not contain steroidal support for coping. Therefore, patient should resume taking oral steroids in large doses throughout and after the weaning process during illness, injury, or other stress.

At the time of steroid withdrawal and transfer to beclomethasone, some patients have complained of withdrawal symptoms such as joint pain, lassitude, and depression. Patients should be encouraged to continue with the inhaler provided objective signs of adrenal insufficiency (hypotension, weight loss) are not evident. If these signs appear, temporarily increase the steroid dose.

Oral fungus has been reported in 75% of patients and requires treatment with antifungals. This may be prevented by instructing the patient to drink a glass of water following inhalation therapy.

This product is not for children under six years, and may be teratogenic if given to pregnant women. The long-term effects have not been evaluated.

ADMINISTRATION AND DOSAGE SPECIFICS:

Directions for inhalant administration: Shake the cannister well and exhale as fully as possible. Place mouthpiece about one inch in front of lips (do not close lips on inhaler). Inhale and exhale deeply several times and then inhale deeply while pressing the cannister with first finger. Hold breath as long as possible and exhale slowly. Wait one minute between inhalations. Rinse inhaler with cool water once daily. Drug will continue to be released after 200 doses but container should be discarded as accuracy of delivered dose is decreased.

Adults: 2 inhalations (100 mcg) three to four times daily.

For severe asthma: Start with 600-800 mcg (12-16 inhalations) and adjust downward with response. Maximum is not more than 20 inhalations per day. (This will cause hypothalamic-pituitary-adrenal axis suppression.)

To wean from systemic steroids: Asthma must be currently stable. Use beclomethasone concurrently with the usual dose for 1-2 weeks. Then gradually decrease dose on alternate days, then decrease daily dose. Decrease by no more than 2.5 mg of prednisone (or equivalent) each 1-2 weeks.

Children 6-12 years: 1-2 inhalations three to four times daily or 2-4 inhalations twice daily. Maximum is not more than 10 inhalations/day.

BETAMETHASONE AND BETAMETHASONE SODIUM PHOSPHATE—SYSTEMIC

PRODUCTS (TRADE NAME):
    Celestone (Available in .6 mg/5 ml syrup, and .6 mg tablet.) **Celestone Phosphate** (Available as betamethasone sodium phosphate injection, 4 mg/ml.)

DRUG SPECIFICS:
    A synthetic fluorinated glucocorticoid similar to dexamethasone in its enhanced immunosuppressant anti-inflammatory activity with relatively little sodium and water retention. Betamethasone does promote weight gain and is more ulcerogenic than other steroids. Give antacids or small frequent meals to minimize this.
    Betamethasone sodium phosphate is an injection indicated in emergency situations or when oral therapy is not feasible. (Do not confuse with betamethasone phosphate and acetate combination (Soluspan) which should not be used intravenously.) Protect drug from freezing and light.

ADMINISTRATION AND DOSAGE SPECIFICS:
    Adults: Oral, IM or IV rose ranges from 600 mcg 7.2 mg daily in single or divided doses.
    Rheumatic fever: Initially give 6 to 8.4 mg/day.
    COPD, inflammatory eye disease, dermatosis, allergies: Initially give 2.4-3.6 mg/day; reduce to maintenance dosage 1.2 to 3.4 mg/day.
    Rheumatoid arthritis, bursitis (short-term): Initial oral dose: 1.2 to 2.4 mg/day; reduce to .6 to 1.2 mg per day as soon as feasible.
    Systemic lupus erythematosus: Initially give 3.6 to 4.8 mg/day (higher if needed to control symptoms); reduce to maintenance 1.2 to 3.6 mg/day.
    Pediatric: Dose determined by severity of the disease and the response rather than age or weight.

BETAMETHASONE SODIUM PHOSPHATE AND BETAMETHASONE ACETATE COMBINATION—SYSTEMIC

PRODUCTS (TRADE NAME):
    Celestone Soluspan Injection (Available with 3 mg betamethasone sodium phosphate and 3 mg betamethasone acetate mg/ml injection.)

DRUG SPECIFICS:
    This form of betamethasone, used for systemic action, is very slowly absorbed and is therefore not appropriate for emergency use. Do not mix with diluents or local anesthetics containing preservatives. Inject medication deep intramuscularly to prevent muscle atrophy. Do not administer intravenously.

ADMINISTRATION AND DOSAGE SPECIFICS:

Intramuscular: Dose depends on severity and disease, and ranges from 1.5 mg to 12 mg IM every one to two weeks up to .5 mg to 9 mg per day in severe systemic diseases. Maintenance is 6 mg/week.

For diagnostic test of adrenogenital syndrome: .6 to 1.2 mg/day IM.

BETAMETHASONE SODIUM PHOSPHATE, BETAMETHASONE PHOSPHATE AND ACETATE COMBINATION—LOCAL

PRODUCTS (TRADE NAME):

Celestone Phosphate (Available in 4 mg/ml injection.) **Celestone Soluspan** (Available in 6 mg/ml injection.)

DRUG SPECIFICS:

Celestone Phosphate, used locally, is absorbed fast and effects last up to seven days. Celestone Soluspan is absorbed slowly and effects last from one to two weeks. After intra-articular injection into large joints, monitor for possibility of systemic absorption. (See betamethasone and betamethasone phosphate and acetate combination for systemic administration.)

Do not administer subcutaneously although preparation may be given intradermally. Do not administer with anesthetics or diluents containing parabens or other preservatives because of danger of flocculation.

One or two percent lidocaine hydrochloride may be mixed in the syringe and injected into the joint or surrounding tissues before or with the steroid injection.

ADMINISTRATION AND DOSAGE SPECIFICS:

Intrasynovial or Intra-articular: Dose depends on joint size, location, and problem: Large joint (hip, knee): 1 to 2 ml; Small joint : .25 to 1 ml; Ganglia: .5 ml; Bursa: 1 ml; Acute gouty arthritis: .5 to 1 ml; Repeat dose as needed.

Intralesional: Dose depends on expected response of the problem. A single dose should not exceed 6 mg. Average dose: .20 ml/sq cm. Repeat at one week intervals.

Tendons: .25 to .5 ml into tendon sheath. Three to four local injections at intervals of one to two weeks is usually sufficient.

CORTISONE ACETATE—SYSTEMIC

PRODUCTS (TRADE NAME):

Cortisone Acetate (Available as 5, 10, 25 mg tablets, 25 and 50 mg/ml suspension.)**Cortone Acetate** (Available as 25 mg tablets, 25, 50 mg/ml suspension.)

DRUG SPECIFICS:

This is a natural steroid secreted by the adrenal cortex. It (or hydrocortisone) is the systemic drug of choice for replacement of adrenocortical insufficiency since it has both glucocorticoid and mineralocorticoid properties. However, such a patient may also need concurrent administration of a potent mineralocorticoid.

For patients requiring only the anti-inflammatory or immunosuppressive properties, a synthetic steroid is more appropriate to minimize sodium and water retention and other adverse effects.

Oral administration generally has a faster onset and is given in three or four divided doses per day. Intramuscular administration has a slower onset but lasts longer; it may be given once or twice a day. Do not use intravenously.

ADMINISTRATION AND DOSAGE SPECIFICS:

Addison's Disease:
Adults:
Chronic: 10-25 mg/day (with sodium chloride and desoxycorticosterone).
Acute: 100-300 mg/day until the crisis passes.
Children: .7 mg/kg body weight in four divided doses.
For other serious diseases if a synthetic steroid is not available or appropriate:
Adults: 100-300 mg/day in divided doses. Administer more if necessary; wean as soon as possible but not in more than 10 mg decrements.
Children: 2.5-10 mg/kg in divided doses.

DEXAMETHASONE—ORAL—SYSTEMIC

PRODUCTS (TRADE NAME):

Decadron (Available in .25, .5, .75, 1.5, and 4 mg tablets; or .5 mg/ml elixir.) **Dexamethasone** (Available in .25, .5, .75, 1.5, and 4 mg tablets, and .5 mg/5 ml elixir.) **Dexone** (Available in .5, .75, 1.5 and 4 mg tablets.) **Hexadrol** (Available in .5, .75, 1.5, and 4 mg tablets; and .5 mg/5 ml elixir.) **SK-Dexamethasone** (Available in 0.5, 0.75 and 1.5 mg tablets.)

DRUG SPECIFICS:

A very powerful (.75 mg = 5 mg prednisone or 20 mg hydrocortisone) synthetic corticosteroid which is particularly useful in decreasing cerebral edema. *Precaution:* dexamethasone has minimal sodium- and water-retaining properties. Consequently, usual parameters of overdosage (edema, weight gain, etc.,) are not present. Other signs of overdosage may be extremely subtle. This drug is ulcerogenic (like many other forms of glucocorticoids.) Consider antacids to prevent hemorrhage or ulcer.

ADMINISTRATION AND DOSAGE SPECIFICS:

Adults: 750 mcg -9 mg in two to four divided doses per day.
Children: .023 -.33 mg/kg body weight/day in four divided doses or as determined by severity of condition.

Diagnostic test for Cushing's disease:
1. Obtain baseline 24-hour urine for 17-hydroxycorticosteroid concentration.
2. Give 500 mcg dexamethasone orally evey six hours for 48 hours.
3. During the second 24 hours of dexamethasone administration another 24-hour urine is collected and analyzed. The 17-hour hydroxycorticosteroid level is depressed normally but is unchanged in Cushing's disease.

DEXAMETHASONE AND DEXAMETHASONE PHOSPHATE—OPHTHALMIC/OTIC

PRODUCTS (TRADE NAME):
Decadron Phosphate Ophthalmic (Available as .05% ointment and .1% solution.) **Decadron Phosphate Otic or Ophthalmic Solution** (Available in 1% dropper bottle.) **Maxidex Ophthalmic** (Available in .05% ointment.) **Maxidex Ophthalmic Suspension** (Available in .1% solution.)
DRUG SPECIFICS:
Anti-inflammatory topical preparation appropriate for ophthalmic or otic use in such conditions as uveitis, iridocyclitis, inflammatory conditions of the eyelids, conjunctiva, cornea, anterior segment of the globe, corneal injury from chemical or thermal burns, penetration of foreign bodies. Otic indications include inflammatory conditions of the canal. Dexamethasone has a greater anti-inflammatory effect than dexamethasone sodium phosphate.

At night, ointment may be used as an adjunct to solution or suspension used in the daytime to provide prolonged contact with eye. Relapses usually respond to re-treatment.
ADMINISTRATION AND DOSAGE SPECIFICS:
Adults and Children:
Ophthalmic ointment: Initially squeeze a one-centimeter thin strip in conjunctival sac 3 to 4 times a day. For maintenance, use one to two applications per day.
Ophthalmic solution: Instill one to two drops solution into conjunctival sacs 3 to 6 times a day. Then reduce to one to two drops 3 to 4 times a day. Taper dose after continued favorable response to twice and then once a day dosage.
Otic Instillation: Instill one to two drops into affected ear 3 to 4 times a day. See section on Administration and Dosage for technique to use.

DEXAMETHASONE SODIUM PHOSPHATE—INHALANT

PRODUCTS (TRADE NAME):
Decadron Phosphate Respihaler (Available in 100 mcg per metered spray.)
DRUG SPECIFICS:
Dexamethasone for inhalation is used in patients with refractory bronchial

asthma and bronchospasm who have not responded to conventional therapy. It should not be used for the relief of mild asthma which will respond to theophylline or sympathomimetics, or in status asthmaticus when more powerful measures are indicated. Dexamethasone is absorbed systemically more than beclomethasone and adverse effects may occur. If the patient is already on systemic steroids, the dose should be diminished or discontinued before oral inhalation is instituted. This must, of course, be carried out gradually. The drug is contraindicated in persons with hypersensitivity to dexamethasone, and systemic or respiratory fungal infection. See beclomethasone for direction on the use of an inhaler, mouth washing, and the use of the inhalant with bronchodilators.

ADMINISTRATION AND DOSAGE SPECIFICS:

Refractory Bronchial Asthma:

Adults: Initially give 300 mcg (3 inhalations) three or four times/day. Maximum dose is 12 inhalations/day. (More than this results in systemic absorption of 400-500 mcg of dexamethasone.) After satisfactory results, begin tapering. Many patients do well on 2 inhalations per day.

Children: 200 mcg (2 inhalations) three or four times/day. Maximum dose is 8 inhalations.

DEXAMETHASONE SODIUM PHOSPHATE—INJECTION

PRODUCTS (TRADE NAME):

Dalalone, Decadrol, Decadron Phosphate, Decajet (Available in 4 mg/ml injections.) **Decameth, Delladec, Demasone, Dexasone, Dexon, Dexone, Dezone** (Available in 4 mg/ml injections.) **Hexodrol Phosphate** (Available in 4 mg/ml and 10 mg/ml injections.)

DRUG SPECIFICS:

The intramuscular and particularly the intravenous administration of dexamethasone is absorbed very quickly and is thus indicated in emergency situations or when the client is unable to take oral medication. The intravenous dose should be the same as the oral dose. The dose depends on disease and condition. See Dexamethasone.

ADMINISTRATION AND DOSAGE SPECIFICS:

Adults: Generally give .75mg to 9mg/day IM or IV in single or divided doses. Give less for mild problems and more in severe problems. In life-threatening conditions, the dose can be massively increased (40 mg every 2-6 hours for up to three days.)

Acute self-limited allergic conditions or acute exacerbation of chronic allergy: Day one: 4 to 8 mg IM; Day two, three: 3 mg po in 2 divided doses; Day four: 1.5 mg po in 2 divided doses; Day five, six: 750 mcg po in the morning; Day seven: discontinue the drug; Day eight: evaluate the patient.

Children: .006 to .04 mg/kg per day or as condition or response warrants.

DEXAMETHASONE SODIUM PHOSPHATE—INTRANASAL

PRODUCTS (TRADE NAME):

Turbinaire Decadron Phosphate (Available with or without nasal attachment to provide .1 mg/metered spray.)

DRUG SPECIFICS:

This inhalant form of medication is useful in allergic or inflammatory nasal conditions and in treating nasal polyps, excluding those in the sinuses. In large or long-term usage beware of systemic side effects; otherwise, problems are unusual with the exception of nasal irritation or dryness. This drug is contraindicated in patients with sensitivity to fluorocarbons and should be used with caution in any type of upper respiratory infection. Remind patient to save nasal attachment for refills. Shake well before using.

ADMINISTRATION AND DOSAGE SPECIFICS:

For nasal polyps, inflammation of nose:

Adults: Spray one to two times into each nostril two or three times a day, up to twelve sprays.

Children 6 years and older: One to two metered sprays into each nostril twice a day, up to eight sprays.

Children under 5 years: No established dose.

DEXAMETHASONE SODIUM PHOSPHATE—LOCAL

PRODUCTS (TRADE NAME):

Decadron Phosphate, Deksone, Dexasone, Dezone (Available in 4 mg/ml injections.) **Hexadrol Phosphate** (Available in 4, 10, 20, 24 mg/ml injections.)

DRUG SPECIFICS:

A potent corticosteroid which produces rapid local anti-inflammatory relief. It is used for injection when affected joints or sites are limited to 1-2 problem areas. Note that frequent intra-articular dosage may result in joint tissue damage. Also note that systemic absorption may occur following large installation into bigger joints. See general statement on Corticosteroid Administration.

ADMINISTRATION AND DOSAGE SPECIFICS:

Intra-articular, soft tissue injection: 800 mcg to 16 mg injected into the synovial space. The dose varies with location and severity of inflammation. Suggested doses:

Knee: 2 to 4 mg; repeat if needed in 2-3 weeks.

Smaller joints: 800 mcg to 1 mg; repeat if necessary in 2-3 weeks.

Bursae: 2 to 3 mg; repeat in 3-5 days if necessary.

Ganglia: 1 to 2 mg; repeat in 3-5 days if necessary.

Soft tissue infiltration: 2 to 6 mg.

Tendon sheath: 400 mcg to 1 mg.

Acute, subacute bursitis, or nonspecific tenosynovitis: Use dexamethasone plus lidocaine mixed and/or diluted with up to 5 parts of sterile water for injection or 0.9% sodium chloride injection.

Intralesional: 0.8 to 1.6 mg per injection site, may be repeated in 1-3 weeks.
Intramuscular: 8 to 16 mg; may be repeated in 1-3 weeks.
Children: Dosage has not been established.

FLUOROMETHOLONE—OPHTHALMIC/TOPICAL

PRODUCTS (TRADE NAME):
   FML Liquifilm (Available in .1% suspension in 5 and 10 ml.)
DRUG SPECIFICS:
   This preparation is less likely to cause increased intraocular pressure with long-term use than any other ophthalmic anti-inflammatory except medrysone.
   Indicated in inflammatory, allergic conditions of the cornea, conjunctiva, sclera and anterior uvea. See general statement regarding ophthalmic use.
   To apply: Drop medication into conjunctival sac, gently close eye, keep closed for one to two minutes.
ADMINISTRATION AND DOSAGE SPECIFICS:
   Adults: Apply one to two drops every hours for first one to two days. Then taper to four times a day, three times a day, two times a day, then discontinue.

HYDROCORTISONE (CORTISOL)—SYSTEMIC

PRODUCTS (TRADE NAME):
   Cortef (Available in 5, 10, 20 mg tablets and 50 mg/ml injection.) **Cortef Oral Suspension** (Available in 10 mg/5 ml hydrocortisone cypionate.) **Hydrocortisone, Hydrocortone** (Available in 10, 20 mg tablets and 25 mg/ml injection.)
DRUG SPECIFICS:
   A natural glucocorticoid (cortisol is converted to hydrocortisone in order to become active) which is most useful in treatment of adrenocortical insufficiency (along with a mineralocorticoid if indicated.) Can be used for its inflammatory properties but causes sodium and water retention. Do not administer intravenously. May give one-third or one-half the oral dosage IM every 12 hours. In certain life-threatening emergencies, excessive dosages may be justified and multiples of the oral dosage may be administered.
   The oral suspension with hydrocortisone cypionate is more slowly absorbed from the GI tract. Dosage is the same.
ADMINISTRATION AND DOSAGE SPECIFICS:
   Initial dose depends upon severity of the disease.

Adults: 20 to 240 mg/day in single dose or up to four divided doses.
Children: 560 mcg to 8 mg/kg/day in single dose or up to four divided doses.

HYDROCORTISONE ACETATE—LOCAL INJECTION

PRODUCTS (TRADE NAME):
Biosone, Cortef Acetate (Available in 50 mg/ml injections.) **Cortril Acetate** (Available in 25 mg/ml injections.) **Hydrocortisone Acetate** (Available in 25 mg/ml.) **Hydrocortone Acetate** (Available in 25, 50 mg/ml injections.)
DRUG SPECIFICS:
This form is much less soluble than hydrocortisone and is therefore useful as a local anti-inflammatory agent because of its prolonged effect. Systemic absorption is completed in 24-48 hours and relief is afforded for one to four weeks. Do not administer IV.

A local anesthetic such as procaine hydrochloride may be infiltrated into the soft tissues surrounding the joint or directly into the joint prior to steroid administration.
ADMINISTRATION AND DOSAGE SPECIFICS:
Adults: Dose depends on joint size and severity of the symptoms. Suggested doses include:
Large joint (hip, knee): 15 to 75 mg; repeat in 1-4 weeks as necessary.
Small joint (fingers): 5 to 25 mg; repeat in 1-4 weeks as necessary.
Bursae: 25-50 mg; repeat in 3 to 5 days if needed.
Ganglia: 10 to 25 mg; repeat in 3 to 5 days if needed.
Soft tissue infiltrate: 25 to 75 mg.
Tendon sheath: 5 to 12.5 mg.

HYDROCORTISONE ACETATE—OPHTHALMIC/OTIC

PRODUCTS (TRADE NAME):
Hydrocortisone Acetate (Available in ophthalmic/otic .5%, 1.5% ointments; 2.5% suspension.)
DRUG SPECIFICS:
A regimen of suspension in the day and ointment before sleep can provide maximum contact to affected tissues. See Administration section regarding ophthalmic/otic topical preparations.
ADMINISTRATION AND DOSAGE SPECIFICS:
Ophthalmic—Adults and Children:
Ointment: Apply thin strip, one centimeter in length, two to four times a day.

Suspension: Instill one drop every hour in the daytime and every two hours at night; then apply one drop three to four times a day.

The duration of treatment for either route depends on the severity of the problem. Course lasts from a few days to several weeks.

Otic—Adults and Children:

Ointment: Apply with a cotton-tipped applicator to the cleansed canal two or three times a day; then reduce to twice a day; then once a day.

Suspension: Clean and dry canal. Instill drops into the canal via dropper initially three to four times a day, then gradually reduce dose. Can be used via a gauze wick. Keep wet with medication. Remove wick every twelve to twenty-four hours and replace.

HYDROCORTISONE SODIUM SUCCINATE—SYSTEMIC

PRODUCTS (TRADE NAME):

A-hydroCort, Hycorace, Solu-Cortef (Available in 100, 250, 500 and 1000 mg vials.)

DRUG SPECIFICS:

See Hydrocortisone. This is the parenteral form of the drug. Note: Do not confuse with Solu-Medrol (methylprednisolone.)

The advantage of this form is that it is extremely soluble and high doses can be given in a small amount of diluent. Plasma levels peak within one hour; it is excreted within twelve hours (short-acting.) Thus, it is the preferred emergency form of the drug. After the patient is stabilized, it is recommended that the drug be switched to a longer acting preparation or an oral form.

ADMINISTRATION AND DOSAGE SPECIFICS:

Adults: 10 to 500 mg infused over two to ten hours intravenously, or 15 to 240 mg IM every twelve hours depending on the disease. In shock, give 500 mg to 2 gm every two to six hours IV.

Children: Give .16 mg to 1 mg/kg one to two times a day as indicated or depending on condition.

METHYLPREDNISOLONE ACETATE—LOCAL

PRODUCTS (TRADE NAME):

Depo-Medrol (Available in 20, 40, and 80 mg/ml injection.) **Depo-Pred 40, D-Med-40, Duralone-40, Duralone-80, Dura Meth, Med-Depo** (Available in 40 mg/ml injection.) **Methylprednisolone Acetate** (Available in 20, 40, 80 mg/ml.) **MPrednisol-80, Pre-Dep, Rep-Pred-80** (Available in 80 mg/ml injection.)

DRUG SPECIFICS:

This is a potent synthetic steroid useful for anti-inflammatory action in fairly severe conditions. It is not for intravenous use. Do not dilute or mix with other drugs.

Methylprednisolone acetate is very slowly absorbed and is thus inappropriate when immediate, short-term action is needed. Intra-articularly, the therapeutic effect continues for one to three weeks. Do not dilute or mix with other drugs.

Note: Dermal atrophy may occur with large doses. Use multiple small injections into lesions.

ADMINISTRATION AND DOSAGE SPECIFICS:

Intra-articular use:

Adults: 10-80 mg. (Large joint: 10 to 80 mg; Medium joint: 10 to 40 mg; Small joint: 4 to 10 mg.)

Children: No local injection recommended.

Bursae, ganglia, soft tissue instillation: 4 to 30 mg.

Intralesional use: 20 to 60 mg.

Repeat above dosages in one to five weeks if necessary.

PREDNISOLONE—SYSTEMIC

PRODUCTS (TRADE NAME):

Delta-Cortef, Cortalone (Available in 5 mg tablets.) **Fernisolone P** (Available in 5 mg tablets.) **Panisolone** (Available in 1, 5 mg tablets.) **Prednisolone** (Available in 1 and 5 mg tablets.) **Predoxine-5, Sterane** (Available in 5 mg tablets.)

DRUG SPECIFICS:

An intermediate-acting, synthetic corticosteroid primarily used for its anti-inflammatory or immunosuppressant properties. It is very similar to prednisone. It has minimal mineralocorticoid activity and, hence, relatively few side effects except for GI distress. Administer antacids or antiulcer regimen concurrently. Use prednisolone cautiously with diabetics.

Prednisolone is suitable for alternate-day dose regimen. Note that it is five times more potent than cortisone.

ADMINISTRATION AND DOSAGE SPECIFICS:

Adults: 5 to 60 mg/day in single or in 2 to 4 divided doses.

Children: .4 mg to 2 mg/kg/day in single or divided doses or in the amount warranted by severity of the disease.

PREDNISOLONE ACETATE—LOCAL

PRODUCTS (TRADE NAME):

Fernisolone (Available in 25 mg/ml injection.) **Key-Pred** (Available in 25 and

50 mg/ml injections.) **Meticortelone Acetate** (Available in 25 mg/ml injection.) **Pred-Cor, Savacort** (Available in 50 mg, 100 mg/ml injections.)

DRUG SPECIFICS:

See Administration section for information on local injections and Prednisolone section for specific comments.

ADMINISTRATION AND DOSAGE SPECIFICS:

Intra-articular, Intralesional, Soft tissue, Intrabursal, Intrasynovial:

Adults: 5 to 100 mg. Large joints: 25 mg; Smaller joints: 6 mg; Bursae: 6-12 mg; Ganglia, tendon sheaths: 6 mg or as indicated by response or severity. May be repeated every several days to every four weeks.

Children: Dosage not established.

PREDNISOLONE ACETATE—SYSTEMIC

PRODUCTS (TRADE NAME):

Articulose-50 (Available in 50 mg/ml injection.) Fernisolone (Available in 25 mg/ml injection.) **Key-Pred** (Available in 25, 50, and 100 mg/ml injections.) **Meticortelone Acetate** (Available in 25 mg/ml injection.) **Predcore** (Available in 25 and 50 mg/ml injections.) **Prednisolone Acetate** (Available in 25, 50 and 100 mg/ml injections.) **Savacort** (Available in 50 and 100 mg/ml injections.) **Sterane** (Available in 25 mg/ml injection.)

DRUG SPECIFICS:

This is the intramuscular form of prednisolone. It has limited use because it has a fairly slow onset and must be administered at least twice a day. It is not used as often as other more potent synthetics. Patients are usually shifted to a longer-acting or oral form as soon as possible.

ADMINISTRATION AND DOSAGE SPECIFICS:

Adults: Initially give 4 to 60 mg/day IM at twelve hour intervals, then 10-400 mg per day in 2 doses.

Children: 0.040 to 0.250 mg/kg IM one to two times daily or as determined by severity.

PREDNISOLONE SODIUM PHOSPHATE—LOCAL

PRODUCTS (TRADE NAME):

Hydeltrasol, Key-Pred-SP (Available in 20 mg/ml injection.)

DRUG SPECIFICS:

This is a slowly absorbed prednisolone salt, useful in local inflammatory problems. Normal duration of action is three days to three weeks. See drug monograph and comments regarding prednisolone.

ADMINISTRATION AND DOSAGE SPECIFICS:
Adults: Generally give 2 to 30 mg repeated in 3 days to 3 weeks if needed. Large joints (knee, hip): 10 to 20 mg; Small joints: 4 to 5 mg; Bursae: 10 to 15 mg; Ganglia: 5 to 15 mg; Soft tissue: 10 to 30 mg; Tendon sheath: 2 to 5 mg.
Children: Dosage not established.

PREDNISOLONE SODIUM PHOSPHATE—OPHTHALMIC/OTIC

PRODUCTS (TRADE NAME):
Hydeltrasol (Available in 0.25% otic or ophthalmic ointment, or 0.5% solution.) **Inflamase Ophthalmic** (Available as 0.125 or 1% solution.) **Metreton Ophthalmic** (Available as .5% solution.)
DRUG SPECIFICS:
The ophthalmologic ointment is convenient with use of an eye pad or in those conditions which need prolonged contact with ocular tissue. See drug monograph and also section on prednisolone—systemic.
ADMINISTRATION AND DOSAGE SPECIFICS:
Adults and children:
Otic ointment: Apply a thin coat with cotton-tipped applicator two to three times a day. After favorable response, gradually decrease the number of daily applications.
Ophthalmic ointment: Squeeze a one centimeter strip into pouch of conjunctiva and close eye for one minute. Use three to four times a day. After favorable response, reduce gradually.
Otic solution: May be instilled directly into the cleansed canal two to three times a day or via cotton wick packed into the canal. Keep the wick moist and replace it every 12 to 24 hours.
Ophthalmic solution: Instill one to two drops in each eye. In severe conditions, use once per hour in the day and once every two hours at night until favorable response is obtained; then reduce to four times a day; then twice a day; then once a day as maintenance; then discontinue.

PREDNISOLONE SODIUM PHOSPHATE—SYSTEMIC

PRODUCTS (TRADE NAME):
Hydeltrasol, Key-Pred-SP, Prednisolone Phosphate, PSP-IV, Sol-Predalone (Available in 20 mg/ml.)
DRUG SPECIFICS:
This form can be used intravenously or intramuscularly. See Administration section and section on prednisolone for remarks.

The onset is rapid and peaks within one hour. The absorption in intramuscular administration is particularly fast. As noted in the discussion of prednisolone acetate, the parenteral forms are not used as often in emergency situations as other synthetics which are more potent or longer lasting. Since steroids are only administered parenterally in emergencies, or when the client is comatose or unable to take oral medications, the usefulness is limited.

ADMINISTRATION AND DOSAGE SPECIFICS:

Adults: Initially give 4 to 60 mg, then 10 to 400 mg/day by infusion or in two IM doses. In emergency situations the dose can be up to 400 mg/day.

Children: 0.04 to 0.25 mg/kg IV or IM one to two times a day or as condition warrants.

PREDNISOLONE TEBUTATE—LOCAL

PRODUCTS (TRADE NAME):

Hydeltra-T.B.A., Metalone T.B.A., Nor-Pred T.B.A., Predcor-TBA (Available in 20 mg/ml injection.)

DRUG SPECIFICS:

One of the slowest acting prednisolone salts, thus making it a good drug for most of the diseases responsive to local administration. See section on Prednisolone and instructions for local administration in drug monograph.

Do not administer intravenously. Shake well before drawing into the syringe. The onset is slow, 1-2 days. The duration of therapeutic effects is 1-3 weeks.

A local injection of anesthetic may be infiltrated into the soft tissue around the articular space and/or into the synovial space itself before steroid administration.

ADMINISTRATION AND DOSAGE SPECIFICS:

Adults: 4 to 40 mg, generally repeated at 2 to 3 week intervals if necessary. (Severe cases can be injected weekly, but consider possibility of damage to joint tissues.) Specific recommendations: Knee or hip: 20 to 40 mg; Smaller joints: 8 to 10 mg; Bursae: 20 to 30 mg; Ganglia: 10 to 20 mg; Soft tissues: 4 to 10 mg in tendon sheath inflammation; 10 to 20 mg nasal polyps; 20 to 60 mg soft tissue injury.

PREDNISONE—SYSTEMIC

PRODUCTS (TRADE NAME):

Cortran (Available in 5 mg tablets.) **Deltasone** (Available in 2.5, 5, 10, 20, 50 mg tablets.) **Fernisone** (Available in 5 mg tablets.) **Meticorten** (Available in 1, 5 mg tablets.) **Orasone** (Available in 1, 5, 10, 20, 50 mg tablets.) **Panasol, Prednicen-M** (Available in 5 mg tablets.) **Prednisone** (Available in 1, 2.5, 5, 10, 20, and 50 mg tablets.)

DRUG SPECIFICS:

Prednisone is an oral synthetic corticosteroid which is fairly high in glucocorticoid and low in mineralocorticoid activity. It is the most commonly prescribed steroid for anti-inflammatory and immunosuppressant effects. The mineralocorticoid activity is one-half that of cortisone or hydrocortisone; therefore, it may cause mild to moderate fluid retention. It is suitable for alternate-day treatment. See drug monograph. Prednisone peaks in 1-2 hours and lasts 1 1/4 to 1 1/2 days. The dose is highly individualized.

ADMINISTRATION AND DOSAGE SPECIFICS:

Adults: In acute, severe conditions give 5 to 250 mg/day in single or divided doses until favorable response is obtained. Gradually reduce the dosage by 5 to 10 mg/week to establish maintenance dose (5 to 10 mg) every day or every other day.

Children: 0.14 mg to 2 mg/kg in single or divided doses or as determined by severity.

TRIAMCINOLONE—SYSTEMIC

PRODUCTS (TRADE NAME):

Aristcort (Available in 1, 2, 4, 8, 16 mg tablets and 2 mg/5ml syrup.) **Kenacort** (Available in 2, 4, 8 mg tablets and 4 mg/5 ml syrup. **SK-Triamcinolone** (Available in 2, 4, 8 mg tablets.) **Spencort** (Available in 4 mg tablets.) **Triamcinolone** (Available in 4 mg tablets.)

DRUG SPECIFICS:

A synthetic, intermediate-acting steroid slightly more potent than prednisone, but with less mineralocorticoid activity. Use caution when using in patients with decreased renal function. Mild diuresis with sodium loss occurs during the first few days of treatment. Patients with decreased glomerular filtration rates may become edematous. May produce myopathy, weakness, and anorexia. High protein intake should be encouraged. Also depression, syncope, and anaphylactoid reactions may occur.

Dosage is highly individualized. Onset of action is several hours; duration is one or more weeks.

ADMINISTRATION AND DOSAGE SPECIFICS:

Adults: Initially give 4 to 48 mg day in single dose or up to four divided doses.

Children: Give 0.416 mg to 1.76 mg/kg in single or divided doses, or as needed. Dosage generally based on severity and response.

TRIAMCINOLONE ACETONIDE—LOCAL

PRODUCTS (TRADE NAME):

Acetospan, Cenocort A-40 (Available in 40 mg/ml syspension for injection.)

Kenalog-10, Kenalog-40 (Available in 10 and 40 mg/ml injections.) **Tramcort-40, Triamcinolone Acetate, Triamonide 40, Tri-Kort, Trilog** (Available in 40 mg/ml suspension for injection.)

DRUG SPECIFICS:

This is a slowly-absorbed, long-acting salt of triamcinolone. The effects persist for several weeks. Local administration of triamcinolone has been reported to cause transient flushing, dizziness, local depigmentation, and (rarely) local irritation. There also have been reports of exacerbation of symptoms. Instillation into a septic joint causes great increase in swelling, pain, and restriction of joint movement. Intradermal instillation has caused vesicular ulceration and scarring. Avoid superficial injection and use strict aseptic technique.

Procaine hydrochloride may be infiltrated into the soft tissue or joint space prior to steroid administration. See drug monograph.

ADMINISTRATION AND DOSAGE SPECIFICS:

Adults and children over 6 years: Intrabursal use: 2.5 to 40 mg; Large joints: 15 to 40 mg; Small joints: 2.5 mg to 10 mg. Intradermal, intralesional use: 1 mg/injection site, repeat at weekly or less intervals. Use TB syringe. Multiple sites may be injected if they are farther than one centimeter apart, not to exceed 30 mg at one time. Soft tissue, tendon sheath: use 2.5 to 10 mg.

TRIAMCINOLONE ACETONIDE—TOPICAL

PRODUCTS (TRADE NAME):

Aristocort, Aristocort A, Kenalog, Triamcinalone Acetonide (Available in 0.025%, 0.5% ointment or cream; 0.025%, 0.1% lotion; 0.1% gel or foam; 0.2 mg/per 3 second spray.)

DRUG SPECIFICS:

This is a fluorinated steroid which is considered high potency in its highest strength. It is not to be used on the face as it has caused a paradoxical skin reaction in long-term use; nor is it to be used ophthalmologically. Use particular caution in administering this preparation to clients with decreased renal function. See Triamcinalone—systemic and General Statement relating to topical preparations.

ADMINISTRATION AND DOSAGE SPECIFICS:

Adults: Apply to the affected area 2 to 4 times a day.

Children: Use weaker strenths and apply 1 to 2 times a day.

TRIAMCINOLONE DIACETATE—LOCAL

PRODUCTS (TRADE NAME):

Amcort, Aristocort Forte Parenteral, Articulose L.A. (Available in 40 mg/

ml injection.) **Aristocort Intralesional** (Available in 25 mg/ml injection.) **Cenocort Forte, Cino 40, Spencort Fortified, Tracilon, Triacin-40, Triacort, Triamcinolone, Triam-Forte, Triamolone 40, Trilone, Tristoject** (Available in 40 mg/ml injection.)

DRUG SPECIFICS:

Patients have complained of increased pain in the joint following intra-articular administration. This setback is generally followed by prompt relief. Note: 5 mg of triamcinolone diacetate is equivalent to 4 mg of triamcinolone. See Triamcinolone Acetonide and general drug monograph.

ADMINISTRATION AND DOSAGE SPECIFICS:

Adults and Children over 6 years:

Intra-articular, intrasynovial: 5 to 40 mg depending on severity and location. General recommendations: Knee: 25 mg; Fingers: 2 to 5 mg. Duration of relief is usually from one to eight weeks. Severely inflamed joints may require more frequent treatment.

Intralesional, sublesional: (Use 25 mg/ml strength, or dilute it further to 12.5 mg or 2.5 mg/ml.) Use 5 to 48 mg. The average limit is 25 mg/lesion or 12.5 mg/injection site. Weekly limit is 75 mg/week. Usually 2 to 3 intralesional injections at 1-2 week intervals will be effective. The remissions last from several weeks to eleven months.

TRIAMCINOLONE HEXACETONIDE—LOCAL

PRODUCT (TRADE NAME):

Aristospan Intra-articular (Available in 20 mg/ml suspension for injection.) **Aristospan Intralesional** (Available in 5 mg/ml suspension for injection and may be diluted further as needed.)

DRUG SPECIFICS:

This form of triamcinolone salt is similar to acetonide and diacetate; however, intra-articularly, it is restricted to rheumatoid arthritis and osteoarthritis. It is the slowest acting of the salts. Otherwise, the information and directions given for Triamcinolone acetonide apply.

ADMINISTRATION AND DOSAGE SPECIFICS:

Adult:

Intra-articular use: Large joints: 10 to 20 mg; Small joints: 2 to 6 mg. May be repeated in 3 to 4 weeks. More often is not recommended.

Intralesional use: Up to 0.5 mg/square inch of affected area. Additional injection may be administered depending on condition or response of the patient.

Children: No recommended dosage.

GLUCOCORTICOID/ANTIBACTERIAL COMBINATIONS

HYDROCORTISONE PLUS IODOCHLORHYDROXYQUIN—TOPICAL

PRODUCTS (TRADE NAME):

Domeform HC, Vioform-Hydrocortisone (Available in 3% iodo with .5% hydrocortisone or 3% iodo with 1% hydrocortisone cream, lotion and ointment.)

DRUG SPECIFICS:

See General Statement regarding topical glucocorticoids. See Hydrocortisone plus Antibiotics for additional information.

This combination is possibly useful in eczema, cutaneous or mucocutaneous *Candida* infections, and other inflammatory skin conditions. Note: Patients sensitive to iodine preparations may show reactions to this drug. Use with caution in herpex simplex, TB, viral infections and all others listed in General Statement. Warn the patient that this preparation may stain fabric, nails, hair and skin. If ointment is used occlusively, the medication may cause increased steroid absorption.

ADMINISTRATION AND DOSAGE SPECIFICS:

Adults and Children:

Cream: Use for moist, weepy lesions. The dosage with the least hydrocortisone is the best for extensive use. Apply 2-4 times per day.

Lotion: For intertriginous use. Shake well. Apply as for cream.

Ointment: For dry, scaling lesions. Apply as for cream.

OTHER GLUCOCORTICOID/ANTIBIOTICS—TOPICAL

PRODUCTS (TRADE NAME):

Cordran N (Available with neomycin and flurandrenolide .05%.) **Neo Decadron** (Available with neomycin and dexamethasone in cream and ointment). **Neo Synalar** (Available with neomycin 0.5%, fluocinalone acetonide .025% in cream and ointment.)

DRUG SPECIFICS:

See General Statement for topical corticosteroids. See Hydrocortisone plus Antibiotics for additional information.

ADMINISTRATION AND DOSAGE SPECIFICS:

Cream: Rub in scanty amount 2 to 3 times a day.

Ointment: Apply a thin film 2 to 3 times a day.

GLUCOCORTICOID/ANTIBIOTIC COMBINATIONS

HYDROCORTISONE PLUS ANTIBIOTICS—OPHTHALMIC/ OTIC

PRODUCTS (TRADE NAME):

Ak-Neo-Cort Suspension, Cor-Oticin Suspension, Ophthel Suspension (Available in 1.5 % suspension with neomycin 0.5%, hydrocortisone 1.5% as drops.) **Cortisporin Otic or Ophthalmic Solution or Ointment** (Available with neomycin 0.5%, polymyxin B 10,000 units, and hydrocortisone 1% as drops or ointment.) **Neo-Cortef** (Available in 1.5% hydrocortisone, 0.5% neomycin drops and 0.5% or 1.5% hydrocortisone acetate and 0.5% neomycin drops.) **NeoDecadron** (Available in 0.1% dexamethasone phosphate and 0.5% neomycin in drops or 0.05% dexamethasone phosphate and 0.5% neomycin as ointment.) **Neo-Delta-Cortef** (Available in 0.25 or 0.5% hydrocortisone acetate, 0.5% neomycin, in drops or ointment.) **NeoMedrol** (Available in 0.1% methylprednisolone and 0.5% neomycin in ointment.)

DRUG SPECIFICS:

Steroid/antibiotic combinations are used when a bacteriocidal agent and an anti-inflammatory agent are needed. Such preparations are convenient, however, many authorities recommend prescribing the two separately in order to select exactly the appropriate antibiotic and steroid strength and potency which are indicated. Such preparations are contraindicated with bullous myringitis, herpes simplex, herpes zoster oticus, TB, fungal infections, vaccinia, varicella, and other viruses in chronic otitis media or perforation. Do not use preparations more than 10 days.

Note: Neomycin is a "not uncommon" skin sensitizer. Watch for hypersensitivity reaction: itching, redness, and swelling. The Food and Drug Administration considers such combination products as "possibly effective: pending more conclusive evidence of usefulness". Cortisporin is not effective against *Pseudomonas*.

ADMINISTRATION AND DOSAGE SPECIFICS:

Otic:

Adults: Apply 4 drops to the canal every six to eight hours.

Children: Apply 3 drops to canal every six hours.

Ophthalmic: Apply to eye 3 to 4 times per day.

HYDROCORTISONE PLUS ANTIBIOTICS—TOPICAL

PRODUCTS (TRADE NAME):

Cortisporin Ointment (Available with neomycin, polymixin B, hydrocortisone.) **Neo Cortef** (Available with neomycin sulfate, hydrocortisone.) **Neo Cort Dome** (Available as neomycin plus hydrocortisone as a rectal preparation.)

DRUG SPECIFICS:
Combinations of antibiotics and steroids are considered by the Food and Drug Administration to be "possibly effective" in treating bacterial inflammatory skin conditions. See General Statement regarding cautions for all topical steroids. This medication may be used occlusively. See notes on occlusive dressings in the General Statement.

ADMINISTRATION AND DOSAGE SPECIFICS:
Adults and children: Apply to affected area 2 to 3 times a day. Withdraw gradually if medication has been used chronically.

TRIAMCINOLONE PLUS ANTIFUNGALS—TOPICAL

PRODUCTS (TRADE NAME):
Mycolog (Contains nystatin, neomycin, gramcidin, ethylenediamine, and triamcinalone in a cream and ointment.)

DRUG SPECIFICS:
The Food and Drug Administration considers this preparation as "possibly effective" against an infection sensitive to the antifungal when an anti-inflammatory agent is also indicated. Use with caution in any fungal infection except candidiasis. See General Statement regarding topical glucocorticoids. See Hydrocortisone plus Antibiotics for additional information. Ethylenediamine is associated with high incidence of contact dermatitis. Patients developing this reaction may also become sensitive to aminophylline.

Caution: Ototoxicity and nephrotoxicity have been reported if this preparation has been overused or applied to a large area of denuded skin. It may be used occlusively.

ADMINISTRATION AND DOSAGE SPECIFICS:
Adults and children: Apply to affected areas 2 to 3 times a day.

GLUCOCORTICOID COMBINATIONS

HYDROCORTISONE EMOLLIENTS—TOPICAL/ANORECTAL

PRODUCTS (TRADE NAME):
Anusol-HC (Available with hydrocortisone 5 mg/gm, bismuth, benzyl benzoate, Peruvian balsam and zinc oxide in a cream 5 mg/gm; and in 10 mg suppositories.)

DRUG SPECIFICS:
This is a glucocorticoid emollient for treatment of pain, itching or discomfort from hemorrhoids, pruritus ani, proctitis and other miscellaneous problems. This is not an antibacterial preparation, thus is not to be used solely in rectal infections.

See General Statement. Stains on clothing may be removed with household detergent.

ADMINISTRATION AND DOSAGE SPECIFICS:

Adults:

Cream: Apply to the exterior anorectal area and gently rub in. Apply internally with special applicator. Apply 3 to 4 times a day for 3 to 6 days or until the infection subsides.

Suppository: Insert one suppository per rectum in the morning and one before bedtime.

Molly Craig Billingsley

ANTIDIABETIC DRUGS

INSULIN

ACTION OF THE DRUG: (1) The main action of insulin is to stimulate carbohydrate metabolism by promoting cellular uptake of glucose and other monosaccharides. (2) Insulin also reduces the rate of glycogenolysis, increases glycogen synthesis, and decreases glyconeogenesis by the liver. (3) Insulin promotes lipogenesis and inhibits lipolysis by adipose cells. Insulin is commonly extracted from either beef or pork pancreas, however, human insulin is now available, derived from a recombinant DNA technology using strains of E. coli.

ASSESSMENT:

INDICATIONS: Used in the management of insulin-dependent, diabetes mellitus (IDDM) and in diabetes mellitus that cannot be controlled by diet alone. Useful in treatment of non-insulin-dependent diabetes mellitus (NIDDM) which fail to respond to oral hypoglycemic therapy. Used as a substitute for oral hypoglycemic therapy for patients with NIDDM diabetes complicated by ketosis, major surgery, infection, or trauma. Utilized in the management of gestational diabetics.

SUBJECTIVE: History (in someone not previously diagnosed as diabetic, or a poorly controlled or out-of-control diabetic) of polyuria, polydipsia, polyphagia, weight loss, blurred vision, fatigue. In severe cases of hyperglycemia, symptoms of systemic acidosis such as nausea and vomiting may be present.

In patients taking insulin, look for history of hypoglycemia: sudden onset of nervousness, hunger, weakness, cold clammy sweat, lethargy. Symptoms relieved by intake of fast-acting sugar.

OBJECTIVE: Signs of ketoacidosis: elevated fasting blood sugar (greater than 150 mg%), glycosuria, ketonuria, Kussmaul's respiration, tachycardia, acetone breath. Signs of hyperglycemia: elevated fasting blood sugar, glycosuria, increased urinary output, increased thirst, or coma.

Signs of hypoglycemia: serum glucose less than 60 m̲ ̲ ̲
and acetone, pallor, diaphoresis, change in level of cons̲ ̲ ̲
rations.

• Hormones
cutaneously 15̲ ̲ ̲
intravenous̲ ̲ ̲
Ins̲ ̲ ̲
dos̲
804

PLAN:

CONTRAINDICATIONS: Hypersensitivity to insulin. ̲ ̲
sulin is a combination of beef and pork insulin. Pure pork insulir̲ ̲
"purified" insulin, single component, is substituted because i̲ ̲
immunogenic.

WARNINGS: Use with caution in patients with impaired ̲ ̲ ̲ ̲ ̲ ̲ic function, decreased renal function, hypothyroidism and patients with nausea or vomiting. Insulin requirements decrease with these conditions and hypoglycemia may be induced. Insulin requirements are often increased during second and third trimesters of pregnancy. Stress, infection, fever, trauma, surgery, hyperthyroidism, and ketoacidosis all increase insulin requirements.

PRECAUTIONS: Hypoglycemia may develop especially with insulin overdosage, increased work or exercise, omission or delay of a meal, or in illness associated with vomiting, diarrhea, or delayed digestion. Decline of insulin requirements may induce hypoglycemia. Meals must be correlated with the activity of the insulin (i.e., onset, peak, and duration).

Insulin allergy (transient local itching, swelling and erythema at the injection site) frequently develops during initiation of therapy. Incidence has decreased with the advent of "single peak" insulin. Lipodystrophy, atrophy or hypertrophy of subcutaneous fat tissue may occur at frequently used injection sites.

Insulin resistance (requirements for more than 200 units of insulin per day) is rare and may be attributed to infection, inflammatory diseases, obesity and stress. To avoid hypoglycemia closely monitor the patient with insulin resistance who is being treated with a concentrated insulin injection. Long-acting insulins are not adequate in the treatment and management of acidosis and emergencies.

IMPLEMENTATION:

DRUG INTERACTIONS: Insulin requirements may be increased by insulin antagonists such as oral contraceptives, corticosteroids, epinephrine, and thyroid preparations utilized for replacement therapy. Thiazide diuretics may cause elevation in glucose levels. Monoamine oxidase inhibitors, phenylbutazone, tetracycline, alcohol, and anabolic steroids may potentiate the hypoglycemic effects of insulin. Serum potassium levels may be affected by insulin (it promotes movement of potassium into cells and lowers serum potassium levels); therefore, careful monitoring of potassium levels should take place when insulin is administered with cardiotonic glycosides. Concurrent use of insulin and propranolol requires close observation since propranolol can mask the signs and symptoms of hypoglycemia due to its antiadrenergic effects.

ADMINISTRATION AND DOSAGE: Insulin is a protein and therefore inactivated by gastrointestinal enzymes. Thus, insulin is generally administered sub-

30 minutes before meals. Only regular insulin can be administered ly, as is done during ketoacidosis or diabetic coma emergencies. lin therapy is individualized according to patient response. Titration of ge to gain maximal therapeutic response with the lowest dosage is an objective. Controversy exists concerning the degree of glycemic control. Generally, a minimal goal of therapy is to avoid extremes of ketoacidosis and hypoglycemia.

The different insulin preparations and their onset, peak and duration of action are given in Table 7-3.

TABLE 7-3. INSULIN PREPARATIONS

Action	Preparation	Action In Hours Onset	Peak	Duration

Rapid or short	Insulin Injection
	  Insulin (regular)
	  Actrapid
	  Regular Iletin I
	  Beef Regular Iletin
	  Humulin-R
	  Pork Regular Iletin II
	  Purified Pork Insulin
	  Velosulin
	  Regular Iletin U-500
	    (concentrated)
		½-1	2-4	6-8

	Prompt Insulin, Zinc Suspension
	  Semilente Iletin
	  Semilente Insulin
	  Semitard
		½-1½	5-8	12-14

Intermediate	Isophane Insulin Suspension
	  Humulin N
	  Insulatard NPH
	  Isophane Insulin (NPH)
	  NPH Iletin I
	  Beef NPH Iletin II
	  Pork NPH Iletin II
	  Protaphane NPH
		1-2	8-12	24-28

	Insulin Zinc Suspension
	  Lentard
	  Lente Insulin
	  Lente Iletin I
	  Lente Iletin II
	  Monotard
	  Purified Beef Insulin Zinc
		1-3	9-12	24-28

TABLE 7-3. INSULIN PREPARATIONS

Action	Preparation	Action In Hours Onset	Peak	Duration
Long	Protamine Zinc Insulin Suspension	4-8	14-24	36
	Protamine Zinc Insulin			
	Protamine Zinc and Iletin I			
	Beef Protamine, Zinc and Iletin II			
	Pork Protamine, Zinc and Iletin II			
	Extended Insulin Zinc Suspension	4-8	10-30	36+
	Ultralente Insulin			
	Ultralente Iletin I			
	Ultratard			

The insulin vial in use may be stored outside the refrigerator for one month provided it is not exposed to extreme temperature. An extra supply of insulin should be stored in the refrigerator. Expiration dates need to be checked regularly. Injection of cold insulin may be irritating to the tissues.

For insulin suspensions, gently roll the vial and invert from end-to-end before withdrawal in order to return particles to suspension. Vigorous shaking may result in air bubbles and cause difficult withdrawal.

IMPLEMENTATION CONSIDERATIONS:

—The management of diabetes mellitus is dependent on client education. Control and maintenance require that the patient be knowledgeable about his or her diet, the need for weight control, the nature of the disease, urine testing, signs and symptoms of hypoglycemia and hyperglycemia, and the appropriate actions to take as well as the importance of hygiene, exercise, and procedures on sick days.

—Monitor the patient for signs of pregnancy, infection, and kidney, liver, or thyroid disease since they will alter the requirement for insulin.

—Teach about rotation of injection sites to prevent lipodystrophy.

—Ascertain what other drugs the patient is taking that may interact with insulin.

—Patients over 60 are often sensitive to hypoglycemia. Observe for confusion and abnormal behavior since repeated episodes of hypoglycemia may cause brain damage.

—Teach the patient proper injection technique, including rotation site and storage of insulin. Errors in administration are common among patients. Routine follow-up and assessment of technique is important. Having clients periodically give the health care provider a demonstration of the technique they are using may be helpful.

—Inform the patient that local allergic reactions such as swelling, redness, stinging, or warmth at the injection site usually disappear after a few weeks of therapy.

—If hypoglycemia occurs, the patient should be taught to administer a carbohydrate (monosaccharide) immediately. The family should also be involved in patient teaching about therapy for hypoglycemia. If the patient is unconscious, honey or Karo syrup may be applied under the tongue or to the buccal mucosa. Provide additional carbohydrate such as bread, crackers, or milk for the next two hours. Provide a sandwich if a snack or meal would not be regularly taken within an hour. Glucagon may be administered by a family member or provider.

—Osmotic changes in the lens due to alterations in blood glucose can cause blurred vision. All changes in the lens may not resolve with therapy. Advise the patient to delay eye examination until glycemic control is achieved, generally 6-8 weeks following the initiation of insulin therapy.

—The Somogyi effect (rebound elevation of glucose levels triggered by hypoglycemia) can lead to overtreatment of the client with insulin when less insulin is actually indicated. Analyze the pattern of glycosuria and serum glucose levels. A series of negative urine test results followed by an elevated glucose level could indicate that a hypoglycemic reaction has occurred and the body has responded with release of epinephrine and glucagon.

WHAT THE PATIENT NEEDS TO KNOW:

—Adherence to a diet (regularity of meals, snacks, and caloric requirements) and maintenance of ideal body weight promotes glycemic control and prevents hypoglycemia.

—Knowledge of the signs and symptoms of hypoglycemia (too little sugar) and hyperglycemia (too much sugar), their causes, prevention, and treatment are vital. Notify health care provider if any of the following occur:

	Hyperglycemia	**Hypoglycemia**
Onset	Gradual (days)	Sudden (minutes to hours)
Causes	Insufficient insulin, stress, illness, infection, excessive food intake, decreased exercise without decreased food intake	Excess insulin, increased exercise without increased food intake, decreased food intake
Signs and Symptoms	Polyuria (urinating more); polydipsia (thirsty); polyphagia (hungry); drowsiness, weakness, dry mouth, dry skin, nausea, vomiting, abdominal pain, increased	Weakness, lethargy, dizziness, nervousness, hunger, shaky feeling

Antidiabetic Drugs • 807

	respiratory depth and rate, sweet smelling breath, coma	
Treatment	Administer regular insulin; drink lots of water See health care provider.	Eat simple sugar: soda, candy, juice. See health care provider.

—Insulin can cause increase (hypertrophy) or decrease (atrophy) in size of fatty tissue when injected into the same site frequently. A plan for rotation of insulin injection sites should be developed, followed, and recorded.

—Utilization of the proper syringe and correct type, strength, and dosage of insulin is necessary to avoid dosage errors.

—Alcohol consumption may cause hypoglycemic reactions. Discuss with your health care provider use of alcoholic beverages. Alcoholic beverages may be included in meal plans provided the caloric value is considered.

—Control of blood sugar levels can be monitored by daily urine testing. Knowledge of the proper technique, which has been demonstrated by your health care provider, recording, and interpretation of results will assist you and your health care provider with data to manage the disease successfully.

—Daily home blood glucose monitoring may be indicated. Request information from your health care provider.

—Insulin requirements increase when you are under stress or become ill, especially with an infection. Faithfully test your urine when ill and do not stop taking your insulin. Take a liquid diet if you have an upset stomach, nausea or vomiting. Notify your health care provider for adjustment of insulin dosage.

—Be prepared for emergency situations by (1) carrying an identification card; (2) wearing a Medic-Alert bracelet or necklace; and (3) carrying a readily available source of sugar at all times.

—When traveling, carry an extra supply of insulin, syringe, and needles with you in case you become separated from your luggage. Adjustment to time zone changes needs to be made to avoid hypoglycemia.

—Care should be taken to be alert for hypoglycemia when driving, operating machinery, or engaging in activities requiring alertness.

EVALUATION:

ADVERSE REACTIONS: *Dermatologic:* lipodystrophy, local itching, swelling, erythema at injection site. *Endocrine:* symptoms of insulin allergy, resistance, hypoglycemia. hyperglycemia.

OVERDOSAGE: *Signs and symptoms:* Hypoglycemia (blood sugar level below 60 mg/100 ml) or an excessively rapid fall in blood glucose levels. The main signs and symptoms are due to alteration in central nervous system function and may include lethargy, confusion, behavior change, sensorimotor disturbances, and coma.

Excess epinephrine release causes nervousness, tremors, sweating, palpitations, and tachycardia.

PARAMETERS TO MONITOR: The therapeutic objective of insulin therapy is to decrease blood glucose to levels which will decrease symptoms of hyperglycemia and prevent hypoglycemia. Urine testing for glucose is commonly used to measure adequacy of control. Double-voided specimens should be tested before each meal and at bedtime during periods of insulin dosage change, acute illness, or surgery. Once control has been achieved, urine sugar can be monitored before breakfast and before the evening meal, especially to determine peak effect of intermediate-acting insulin. Diabetics on short-acting insulin need to test urine before lunch and at bedtime depending on when the insulin was taken. Urine ketones should be measured during acute illness or periods of increased glycosuria and in ketosis-prone diabetics. Review of these records provides information regarding control between office visits.

Monitor fasting blood sugars when insulin therpy is being initiated until diabetes is stable. Blood glucose should be evaluated each time insulin dose is changed. Blood glucose levels may be monitored to determine the peak effect of insulin, e.g., 6-8 hours after NPH administration.

Two-hour postprandial blood glucose tests measure glucose after some degree of stress. A standard glucose level needs to be consumed with the meal in order for accurate evaluation of Beta cell function.

Establish a flowchart of symptoms which seem to be most consistent with each patient experiencing hypo or hyperglycemic reactions, as well as many common problems seen with diabetes. Monitor these individual symptoms each visit and record on the flowchart. Weight gain or loss should always be evaluated since alterations in weight may increase or decrease insulin requirements respectively.

INSULIN INJECTION

PRODUCTS (TRADE NAME:)

Actrapid (Available in 100 units/ml from purified pork). **Beef Regular Iletin II** (Available in 100 units/ml from purified beef.) **Humulin R** (Available in 100 units/ml from human insulin of recombinant DNA origin.) **Insulin** (Available in 40 units/ml and 100 units/ml from pork.) **Pork Regular Iletin II, Purified Pork Insulin** (Available in 100 units/ml from purified pork.) **Regular (Concentrated) Iletin II** (Available in 500 units/ml from purified pork.) **Regular Iletin Ipb** (Available in 40 units/ml and 100 units/ml from beef and pork.) **Velosulin** (Available in 100 units/ml from purified pork.)

DRUG SPECIFICS:

Rapid-acting insulin is indicated for use during acidosis and other acute situations (infection, surgery) when the patient's food intake is variable. Often used in combination with longer-acting insulins to achieve greater control. Regular insulin may be administered IV. Pork preparations may be utilized for insulin allergy or for patients with insulin resistance. Humulin may be used for patients with insulin allergy.

Concentrated Regular Iletin U-500 should not be administered IV.

ADMINISTRATION AND DOSAGE SPECIFICS:

May be administered with NPH and crystalline PZI insulin in any proportion. Regular insulin may also be utilized in divided dose therapy. The dose is determined by the amount of glucose and acetone in the urine. "Double-voided urines" are used to determine sliding scale or "rainbow coverage," and a predetermined number of units of insulin is administered for each degree of glycosuria. An example of a sliding scale may be the following:

Urine Glucose Level	Amount of Insulin
0 to 1+	No insulin
2+	5 units regular insulin
3+	10 units regular insulin
4+	20 units regular insulin

If ketones are present, add 5 units to the dose.

Urine testing alone may be inadequate for informed therapeutic decision making. Direct information about the blood glucose itself may be obtained routinely using available technology for home blood glucose monitoring. Indications for home blood glucose monitoring are the following: abnormal renal threshold, pregnancy, brittle diabetes, existing complications, and impending complications.

INSULIN ZINC SUSPENSION

PRODUCTS (TRADE NAME):

Lentard (Available in 100 units/ml from purified pork and beef in 10 ml vials.) **Lente Insulin** (Available in 40 or 100 units/ml from beef in 10 ml vials). **Lente Iletin Insulin I** (Available in beef and pork in 40 or 100 units/ml in 10 ml vials). **Lente Iletin II** (Available 100 units/ml from purified beef or from purified pork in 10 ml vials.) **Monotard** (Available in 100 units/ml from purified pork in 10 ml vials.) **Purified Beef Insulin Zinc** (Available in 100 units/ml from purified beef in 10 ml vials.)

DRUG SPECIFICS:

Intermediate-acting insulin. Not suitable for emergency use.

ADMINISTRATION AND DOSAGE SPECIFICS:

May be mixed with Semilente or Ultralente in any ratio.

Initial therapy: 10 to 15 units subcutaneously before breakfast daily, with increase in dosage of 3 to 5 units until control is achieved.

INSULIN ZINC SUSPENSION, EXTENDED

PRODUCTS (TRADE NAME):
  Ultralente Iletin I (Available in 40 or 100 units/ml from beef and pork in 10 ml vials.) **Ultralente Insulin** (Available in 100 units/ml from beef in 10 ml vials.) **Ultratard** (Available in 100 units/ml from purified beef in 10 ml vials.)
DRUG SPECIFICS:
  Long-acting insulin with larger particles of zinc insulin. Not useful in management of emergency situations or diabetic coma. Duration of action increases hazard of hypoglycemia. Do not administer IV.
ADMINISTRATION AND DOSAGE SPECIFICS:
  This product may be mixed with Semilente or Lente insulin in any ratio.

INSULIN ZINC SUSPENSION, PROMPT

PRODUCTS (TRADE NAME):
  Semilente Iletin I (Available as beef or pork in 40 or 100 units/ml in 10 ml vials.) **Semilente Insulin** (Available as beef in 100 units/ml in 10 ml vials). **Semitard** (Available as purified pork in 100 units/ml in 10 ml vials).
DRUG SPECIFICS:
  Rapid-acting insulin. May be used in combination with longer-acting insulins. Not suitable for IV injection or emergency use. May be mixed with Lente or Ultralente in any proportion.
ADMINISTRATION AND DOSAGE SPECIFICS:
  Titrate according to individual blood and urine sugar level.

ISOPHANE INSULIN SUSPENSION (NPH)

PRODUCTS (TRADE NAME):
  Beef NPH Iletin II (Available in 100 units/ml from purified beef in 10 ml vials.) **Humulin N** (Available in 100 units/ml from human insulin of recombinant DNA origin). **Insulatard NPH** (Available in 100 units/ml from purified pork in 10 ml vials.) **Isophane Insulin NPH** (Available in 40 or 100 units/ml from purified beef or 100 units/ml from purified pork in 10 ml vials.) **NPH Iletin I** (Available in 40 units/ml or 100 units/ml from beef and pork in 10 ml vials). **Pork NPH Iletin II** (Available in 100 units/ml from purified pork in 10 ml vials.) **Protaphane NPH** (Available in 100 units/ml from purified pork in 10 ml vials.)
DRUG SPECIFICS:
  Intermediate-acting insulins. Most commonly used insulin for daily maintenance and control of diabetes mellitus. Pork preparations are less immunogenic.

ADMINISTRATION AND DOSAGE SPECIFICS:

Initial therapy: 10 to 15 units subcutaneously before breakfast daily, with increase in dosage of 3 to 5 units until control is achieved. A short-acting insulin (regular) may be added in any ratio to improve control. A combination of regular insulin and NPH is frequently utilized to manage late-morning glycosuria. A split dosage of NPH in the morning and early evening may be instituted to control early morning glycosuria. Late evening snack is necessary to prevent hypoglycemia during sleep.

ISOPHANE INSULIN SUSPENSION AND INSULIN INJECTION

PRODUCTS (TRADE NAME):

Mixtard (Available in 100 units/ml of purified pork injection.)

DRUG SPECIFICS:

This is a combination drug with 70% isophane insulin and 30% insulin. Onset of action is 30 minutes to 1 hour with a prolonged duration of up to 24 hours. Combination drugs are not generally recommended because drug flexibility is then lost. However, some patients may be stabilized upon this combination if they have difficulty mixing other insulin preparations because of poor eyesight, etc.

ADMINISTRATION AND DOSAGE SPECIFICS:

Titrate according to individual blood and urine sugar level. Give once in the morning before eating.

PROTAMINE ZINC INSULIN (PZI) SUSPENSION

PRODUCTS (TRADE NAME):

Beef Protamine Zinc and Iletin II (Available in 40 and 100 units/ml from beef and pork in 10 ml vials.) **Pork Protamine, Zinc and Iletin II** (Available in 100 units/ml from purified pork in 10 ml vials.) **Protamine Zinc and Iletin II** (Available in 100 units/ml from purified pork in 10 ml vials.) **Protamine Zinc Insulin** (Available in 100 units/ml from beef in 10 ml vials.)

DRUG SPECIFICS:

Long-acting insulin. Not suitable for emergency use. Used less often due to duration of action and increased hazard of hypoglycemia.

ADMINISTRATION AND DOSAGE SPECIFICS:

May mix with regular insulin. Ratios of less than 1:1 have the same time/activity as PZI alone. As the proportion of regular insulin to PZI insulin nears 2:1, the time activity curve approaches that of NPH.

Sheila Fitzgerald

SULFONYLUREAS

ACTION OF THE DRUG: (1) The primary action of the sulfonylureas is to stimulate insulin release by the beta cells of the pancreas. As a result, functional islet-cell tissue is necessary in patients receiving these drugs. (2) The sulfonylureas have also been found to increase the peripheral utilization of insulin as well as suppress gluconeogenesis and glycogenolysis.

ASSESSMENT:

INDICATIONS: Used in the management of non-insulin dependent adult onset diabetics who generally are over 40 years of age; whose insulin requirement is less than 20 units per day; whose diabetes mellitus cannot be adequately controlled by diet and weight loss; and in whom the use of insulin is unacceptable.

SUBJECTIVE: History of polyuria, polydipsia, polyphagia, weight loss, blurred vision, and fatigue. History of hypoglycemia: nervousness, hunger, weakness, cold clammy sweat, lethargy; symptoms relieved by intake of fast-acting sugar.

OBJECTIVE: Signs of hyperglycemia: elevated fasting blood sugar, glycosuria. Signs of hypoglycemia: serum glucose less than 60 mg%, negative urine glucose, pallor, diaphoresis, change in level of consciousness, shallow respirations.

PLAN:

CONTRAINDICATIONS: Hypersensitivity to sulfa drugs. Should not be used in insulin-dependent, ketosis-prone diabetics, juvenile-onset diabetes, or labile (brittle) diabetes.

Discontinue oral hypoglycemics and initiate insulin therapy in diabetics who have surgery, severe trauma, infection, fever, ketosis, acidosis or coma.

Oral hypoglycemics are not a substitute for diet therapy and weight control. Elimination of the sulfonylureas occurs via renal excretion; therefore, it is contraindicated in serious renal insufficiency. Use with caution in patients with impaired hepatic, thyroid, and endocrine function. The safe use of sulfonylureas during pregnancy has not been established. May cause hypoglycemia in breast-feeding infants.

PRECAUTIONS: Elderly or debilitated patients may be more sensitive to therapy; therefore, start with a lower initial dose and monitor urine and blood sugars carefully. There is a disulfiram-like interaction in some patients between alcohol and the oral hypoglycemics; they should not be prescribed for alcoholics. An excess of ADH and resultant water retention and hyponatremia may occur with the sulfonylureas and should be used with caution in patients who retain water.

IMPLEMENTATION:

DRUG INTERACTIONS: Alcohol consumption may result in a disulfiram-like reaction. In addition, alcohol decreases gluconeogenesis and the release of glucose from the liver. Hypoglycemic effects of the sulfonylureas are potentiated by oral anticoagulants, propranolol, phenylbutazone, chloramphenicol, and probenecid by decreasing liver metabolism. Sulfonamide-type antibacterial agents and salicylates displace the sulfonylureas from protein-binding sites, which leads to high blood levels of the active drug. Barbiturates, sedatives and hypnotics may have a prolonged effect when taken concurrently with the sulfonylureas due to a decreased rate of elimination from the body. Thiazide diuretics oppose the secretion of insulin from the beta cells and decrease the effectiveness of sulfonylureas.

ADMINISTRATION AND DOSAGE: Sulfonylurea therapy is most useful in the treatment of symptomatic, non-insulin-dependent, non-ketosis-prone diabetics in whom some beta cell function is preserved. Therapy is individualized according to patient response. Titration of dosage to gain maximal therapeutic response with the lowest dosage is the objective.

The sulfonylureas are administered orally. Duration of hypoglycemic effect is the main difference between the different sulfonylureas. The duration of action, serum half-life, dose range and approximate doses/day is given in Table 7-4.

IMPLEMENTATION CONSIDERATIONS:

—The management of diabetes mellitus is dependent on client education. Control and maintenance require that the patient be knowledgeable about his or her diet, the need for weight control, the nature of the disease, urine testing, signs and symptoms of hypoglycemia and hyperglycemia, and the appropriate action to take as well as the importance of hygiene, exercise, and sick-day procedures.

—Take a thorough health history. Ascertain what other drugs the patient is taking that may interact with the sulfonylureas, and ascertain if the patient has any allergy to sulfa drugs, or if the patient is pregnant, has renal insufficiency, impaired liver function, or history of ketoacidosis.

—Infection, trauma, surgery, pregnancy, or any physical or emotional stress increases the requirement for insulin. During these periods, discontinuation of the oral agents and administration of insulin injections may be required.

—Hypoglycemia may occur with increased dosage, omission of meals, and increased exercise.

—If hypoglycemia occurs, administer a carbohydrate (monosaccharide) immediately. If the patient is unconscious, honey or corn syrup may be applied under the tongue or to the buccal mucosa. Glucagon may be administered by a family member if available. Provide additional carbohydrate for the next two hours in the form of bread, crackers, or milk. Give a sandwich if a snack or meal is not scheduled to be taken within an hour.

—The University Group Diabetic Program (UGDP) has raised questions con-

TABLE 7-4. COMPARISON OF SULFONYLUREAS

Drug	Duration of Action (hr)	Serum Half-life (hr)	Dose Range (gm)	Doses/ Day
Tolbutamide (Orinase)	6-12	4-5	0.25-3.0	2-3
Acetohexamide (Dymelor)	12-24	6-8	0.25-1.5	1-2
Tolazamide (Tolinase)	10-15	6-8	0.1-1.0	1-2
Chlorpropamide (Diabinese)	60	35	0.1-0.5	1

cerning the safety and efficacy of the oral hypoglycemic agents. In particular, the study implicated tolbutamide as having significant toxicity. To date, these findings have been questioned and remain a source of debate.

—No transition period is necessary when transferring patients from one oral hypoglycemic to another.

—Rashes may develop with initiation of therapy. These are usually transient. If they persist, the oral agent should be discontinued.

—Cholestatic jaundice has been reported in a small number of patients on oral hypoglycemic therapy. Discontinuation of the drug reverses liver damage that may occur.

WHAT THE PATIENT NEEDS TO KNOW:

—Adherence to a diet (regularity of meals, snacks, and caloric requirements) as well as maintenance of ideal body weight promotes sugar control and prevents low blood sugar (hypoglycemia.)

—Knowledge of the signs and symptoms of low blood sugar (hypoglycemia) and high blood sugar (hyperglycemia) their causes, prevention, and treatment are vital. Notify your health care provider if any of the following occur:

	Hyperglycemia	Hypoglycemia
Onset	Gradual (days)	Sudden (minutes to hours)
Causes	Insufficient insulin, stress, illness, infection, excessive food intake, decreased exercise without decreased food intake	Excess insulin, increased exercise without increased food intake, decreased food intake
Signs and Symptoms	Polyuria (excessive urination); polydipsia (excessive thirst); polyphagia (excessive hunger); drowsiness, weakness, dry mouth, dry skin, nausea and vomiting, abdominal pain, increased respiratory rate and depth, fruity smelling breath, coma	Weakness, lethargy, dizziness, nervousness, hunger, shaky feeling.
Treatment	Administration of regular insulin; drink lots of water.	Ingestion of simple sugar: soda, candy or juice. Family member or health care provider can give 0.5 to 1 mg glucagon SQ or IM if available.

—Notify your health care provider if you become pregnant, develop an infection or require surgery.

—Report jaundice, dark urine, light-colored stools, fever, sore throat, fatigue, or any unusual bleeding or bruising.

—Monitor blood sugar control by urine testing, especially during periods of illness, infection, trauma, or physical or emotional stress. Record results and bring this record with you when you visit your health provider.

—Avoid alcohol. Hypoglycemia, severe nausea and vomiting, dizziness, headache, sweating, and flushing may develop.

—Be prepared for emergency situations by (1) carrying an identification card, (2) wearing a Medic-Alert bracelet or necklace, and (3) carrying a readily available source of sugar at all times.

—Allergic skin reactions may develop with initiation of oral hypoglycemic therapy. Red raised rashes are generally transient and will disappear with continued drug therapy.

EVALUATION:

ADVERSE REACTIONS: *Dermatologic:* allergic reactions manifested by urticaria, rash, pruritus, and erythema are generally transient and develop with initiation of therapy. Photosensitivity is rare. *Gastrointestinal:* heartburn, nausea, vomiting, abdominal pain, diarrhea due to increased gastric acid secretion. *Hematopoietic:* bone marrow toxicity with leukopenia, thrombocytopenia, and hemolytic anemia (rare.) *Other:* hepatic toxicity, cholestatic jaundice (manifested by jaundice, dark urine, light-colored stools.)

OVERDOSAGE: Hypoglycemia is caused by an abnormally low blood sugar level (less than 60 mg per 100 ml) or an excessively rapid fall in blood glucose levels. The main causes are overdosage of insulin and omission of meals. *Signs and symptoms:* lethargy, confusion, behavior changes, sensorimotor changes and coma, nervousness, tremors, sweating, palpitations, and tachycardia. Prolonged hypoglycemia may occur in patients on chlorpropamide due to its long duration of action.

PARAMETERS TO MONITOR: Monitor weight gain or loss at each visit. Review urine testing records. Urine testing for glucose is commonly used to measure adequacy of control. Double-voided specimens should be tested before each meal and at bedtime during initiation of therapy, periods of stress, illness, or injury. Once control has been achieved, urine sugars can be monitored daily before breakfast. Evaluate urine for ketonuria during periods of illness, stress, and surgery. Evaluate liver function tests of any patient suspected of liver toxicity. Develop a flow chart to observe for signs and symptoms of therapeutic effect: reduction in blood sugar, elimination of polyuria, polyphagia, polydipsia, fatigue. Also record signs and symptoms commonly associated with chronic diabetes: neuropathies, presence of cataracts, acceleration of atherosclerotic changes. Observe closely for symptoms of gradually developing renal insufficiency. Evaluate CBC and electrocardiogram annually.

ACETOHEXAMIDE

PRODUCTS (TRADE NAME):
Dymelor (Available in 250 or 500 mg tablets.)

DRUG SPECIFICS:
Duration of action 12-24 hours.
ADMINISTRATION AND DOSAGE SPECIFICS:
Dosage may range between 0.25 and 1.5 gm/day. Daily dosage may be utilized for patients who require less than 1 gm/day. Those who require more than 1.5 gm/day benefit from twice-a-day dosages.

For patients on 20 units or less of insulin, insulin may be discontinued and the oral agent initiated. When patients require 20-40 units of insulin/day, initiate the oral agent and reduce insulin by 50%. Reduce insulin gradually and monitor urine sugar as a guide to response.

No transition period is necessary when transferring patients from one oral hypoglycemic to another.

CHLORPROPAMIDE

PRODUCTS (TRADE NAME):
Chlorpropamide (Available in 250 mg tablets.) **Diabinese** (Available in 100 mg or 250 mg tablets.)
DRUG SPECIFICS:
Duration of action is up to 60 hours. Drug is extensively bound to plasma protein and a maximum blood level is not achieved until about 4 days after the initiation of therapy. Overdosage and adverse reactions such as cholestatic jaundice are much more likely with this drug because of the long duration of action. This drug is usually used once the patient has demonstrated good control on a shorter-acting oral hypoglycemic agent.
ADMINISTRATION AND DOSAGE SPECIFICS:
Initial therapy is generally 250 mg as a single dose. Maintenance dosage ranges between 100 and 250 mg daily. Severe diabetes may require 500 mg/day.

For patients on 20 units or less of insulin, insulin may be discontinued and the chlorpropamide initiated. When patients require 20 to 40 units of insulin per day, initiate the oral agent and reduce insulin by 50%. Reduce insulin gradually and monitor urine sugar as a guide to response.

No transition period is necessary when transferring patients from one oral hypoglycemic to another.

TOLAZAMIDE

PRODUCTS (TRADE NAME):
Tolinase (Available in 100, 250 and 500 mg tablets.)

DRUG SPECIFICS:
Duration of action is 10-15 hours.

ADMINISTRATION AND DOSAGE SPECIFICS:
Initial dose is generally 100 mg/day if fasting blood sugar is less than 100 ml/ 200 mg %, or 250 mg/day if fasting blood sugar is greater than 200 mg/100 ml. Titrate dose to obtain desired blood level response. If more than 500 mg/day is required, divided doses should be administered.

For patients on 20 units or less of insulin, insulin may be discontinued and the oral agent initiated. When patients require 20-40 units of insulin/day, initiate the oral agent and reduce insulin by 50%. Reduce insulin gradually and monitor urine sugar as a guide to response.

No transition period is necessary when transferring patients from one oral hypoglycemic to another.

TOLBUTAMIDE

PRODUCTS (TRADE NAME):
Orinase (Available in 250 and 500 mg tablets.) **SK-Tolbutamide, Tolbutamide** (Available in 500 mg tablets.)

DRUG SPECIFICS:
This is the drug about which there is the greatest unresolved debate concerning associated toxicity. Action lasts 6-12 hours. Dosage is titrated based on blood glucose levels.

ADMINISTRATION AND DOSAGE SPECIFICS:
Average initial dose is 1-2 gm/day. This is increased or decreased based on desired blood glucose levels. Maintenance dose is generally 0.25-3.0 gm in divided doses.

For patients on 20 units or less of insulin, insulin may be discontinued and the oral agent initiated. When patients require 20-40 units of insulin/day, initiate the oral agent and reduce insulin by 50%. Reduce insulin gradually and monitor urine sugar as a guide to response.

No transition period is necessary when transferring patients from one oral hypoglycemic to another.

Sheila Fitzgerald

GLUCOSE-ELEVATING AGENTS

GLUCAGON

ACTION OF THE DRUG: Glucagon is a hormone produced by the alpha cells of the pancreas. It stimulates glycogenolysis, gluconeogenesis and lipolysis in the liver, thus providing sources of glucose to assist in overcoming hypoglycemia. Glucagon is only effective in combating hypoglycemia when the liver has a reserve of glycogen; it is not useful in starvation states, adrenal insufficiency, or chronic hypoglycemia.

ASSESSMENT:

INDICATIONS: Used in the management of severe hypoglycemic reactions in diabetics or to terminate insulin-induced shock in psychiatric patients. Failure to respond (regain consciousness) 5-20 minutes after parenteral injection may be an indication for IV administration of glucose.

SUBJECTIVE: Sudden onset of weakness, lethargy, dizziness, and nervousness particularly in known diabetics.

OBJECTIVE: Signs of hypoglycemia: serum glucose less than 60 mg%, loss of consciousness, shallow respirations, diaphoresis.

PLAN:

CONTRAINDICATIONS: Hypersensitivity may develop since glucagon is a protein.

PRECAUTIONS: Liver glycogen must be available in the treatment of hypoglycemic shock. IV glucose or glucose by gavage should be considered in the hypoglycemic patient. Glucagon given with solutions containing sodium or calcium chloride will precipitate. Use in dextrose solutions is acceptable.

IMPLEMENTATION:

DRUG INTERACTIONS: The hyperglycemic effect of glucagon antagonizes the hypoglycemic effect of oral sulfonylureas. Glucagon creates an additive hyperglycemic effect when administered to patients on corticosteroids, epinephrine, estrogen or phenytoin.

PRODUCTS (TRADE NAME):
Glucagon (Available in 1 unit (1 mg) vial as a dry powder with 1 ml diluent, or 10 mg (10 unit) vials with 10 ml diluent.)

ADMINISTRATION AND DOSAGE SPECIFICS:
Family members are taught to administer 0.5 to 1 mg subcutaneously or intramuscularly. IV glucagon may be administered by the health care provider. A response is usually produced in 5-20 minutes. Repeat dosage may be administered 1-2 times if response is delayed. If refrigerated, the 10 mg vial may be used up to 3 months after mixture.

IMPLEMENTATION CONSIDERATIONS:
—Supplemental carbohydrate should be administered to the patient once a response occurs and consciousness is restored. This will restore liver glycogen and prevent secondary hypoglycemia. Food or drink (milk, cheese, meat, crackers, other protein) may be given when the patient is responsive.

—Since prolonged hypoglycemia creates cerebral complications, the use of parenteral glucose must be considered by the health care provider.

—Check expiration date prior to administration.

WHAT THE PATIENT NEEDS TO KNOW:
—The patient, family, and friends need to know how to recognize the signs and symptoms of hypoglycemia and what actions to take.
—If loss of consciousness occurs, a responsible family member or friend needs to know how to administer and monitor the effects of glucagon.
—The health care provider must be informed of hypoglycemic reactions so that doses of insulin can be adjusted.
—After the patient has revived, supplemental sugar should be given.
—If a second injection is required due to lack of patient response, medical assistance should be sought.
—Careful attention to regularity of meals and snacks, administration of the correct dose of insulin, and urine testing will help promote the control of diabetes and reduce the incidence of hypoglycemia.
—Have a fast-acting sugar available at all times to take if you feel hypoglycemic.

EVALUATION:

ADVERSE REACTIONS: *Gastrointestinal:* nausea and vomiting may occur, but this is rare.
PARAMETERS TO MONITOR: Signs and symptoms of hypoglycemia: acute onset of weakness, lethargy, dizziness, nervousness, hunger, blurred vision, diaphoresis, headache, disorientation, unconsciousness, or convulsions.
Indices of effect: response to injection within 5-20 minutes, increase in blood sugar level.

Sheila Fitzgerald

PITUITARY DRUGS
ANTERIOR PITUITARY HORMONES

CORTICOTROPIN

ACTION OF THE DRUG: Corticotropin is an anterior pituitary hormone (or synthetic derivative) that stimulates the adrenal cortex (in the absence of adrenal pathology) to produce and secrete its entire gamut of hormones. These include glucocorticoids and mineralocorticoids. The physiologic effects are similar to those of cortisone.

ASSESSMENT:

INDICATIONS: Corticotropin is a drug largely given by medical specialists.

It is unlikely that non-physicians would be prescribing this drug. However, nurse practitioners often have the responsibility of evaluating patient response for those patients receiving this drug. Corticotropin is most useful in the diagnosis of idiopathic thrombocytopenic purpura and adrenal insufficiency. It has been used to speed resolution of acute episodes of multiple sclerosis; however, it does not affect the natural progression or outcome of the disease. It has also been used in the treatment of acute myasthenia gravis, but only under controlled situations. It can be used as replacement therapy in hypopituitarism; however, usually the individual hormones are replaced directly. Generally, it is only used therapeutically when more conventional treatment fails.

It is of limited use in some of the same diseases treated with glucocorticoids, provided the adrenal cortex is functioning. However, the glucocorticoids are nearly always preferred because cortisone and its derivatives are more available, more easily regulated, tapered, and predicted and are available in longer acting, more convenient forms. Corticotropin must be given by injection.

If high doses of corticosteroids are needed, they must be given directly, since the adrenal cortex can secrete only 10-20 mg of cortisol per hour regardless of the amount of corticotropic stimulation.

It is also important to note that corticotropin is not appropriate in emergency situations. Following corticotropic stimulation, the blood cortisol levels increase slowly over several hours to maximum level several days after treatment has begun.

SUBJECTIVE-OBJECTIVE: Patient comes with a history of idiopathic thrombocytopenia purpura, adrenal insufficiency, multiple sclerosis, myasthenia gravis oro hypopituitarism. Patient should be under medical care by a specialist. Objective findings on physical examination and laboratory tests should confirm preexisting disease.

PLAN:

CONTRAINDICATIONS: See drug monograph on adrenocortical steroids. Do not use in patients with scleroderma, osteoporosis, Cushing's syndrome, recent surgery, congestive heart failure, sensitivity to porcine proteins, primary adrenocortical insufficiency, ocular herpes simplex, hypertension, and ulcer diseases.

WARNINGS: Short-term doses are unlikely to cause harmful side effects. In patients receiving prolonged corticotropin treatment, additional support with rapidly-acting corticosteroids is necessary during periods of stress. Do not administer therapeutically until adrenal cortical functioning has been verified. Prolonged use may cause hypothalamic-pituitary-adrenal axis suppression. Patients may develop cushinoid features yet respond to stress like those with Addison's disease. The drug must be withdrawn gradually.

Safe use in pregnant women or in women of childbearing age has not been documented. Infants of women who took the drug during pregnancy should be monitored for adrenal insufficiency. Long-term administration in children has been found to retard bone growth similar to glucocorticoids.

Hypersensitivity reactions have been reported even in patients who have not been previously treated. Symptoms include skin reactions, nausea and vomiting, shock, circulatory failure, and death. Immediate emergency support is required.

PRECAUTIONS: Patients with hypothyroidism and cirrhosis show enhanced effects of corticotropin. Use with caution in patients with diabetes, hypotension, psychosis, diverticulitis, ulcerative colitis, those patients at risk for perforation, abscess or pyogenic infections, thromboembolic disorders, and myasthenia gravis (except in intensive care settings). Use only in life-threatening emergencies in patients with viral or bacterial infections (without antibiotics) or in uncontrolled hypertension. Patients with a history of or with active tuberculosis or positive tuberculin test should be very closely observed. The drug manufacturer recommends preventive antituberculin therapy; however, many clinicians do not think this is necessary.

IMPLEMENTATION:

DRUG INTERACTIONS: See section on interactions of glucocorticoids.

ADMINISTRATION AND DOSAGE: Generally, the lowest possible dose which will achieve the desired response should be used. See section on corticosteroids. Chronic doses of more than 40 units per day may result in uncontrollable side effects.

The amount necessary to produce the desired effects is dependent on the diagnosis, severity, prognosis, and probable duration of the problem. Prior to beginning therapy, adrenal responsiveness to the drug via the proposed route must be verified.

The drug can only be administered parenterally, via intramuscular or subcutaneous route, when given for therapeutic purposes. (Oral ACTH is destroyed by gastric juices and topical administration is totally ineffective). Intravenous injection or infusion is only used for diagnostic testing of idiopathic thrombocytopenia.

The response to therapeutic administration is extremely variable because of idiosyncrasies in the adrenal cortex. Note that maximal stimulation occurs only after several days of treatment. The patient must be monitored for signs of remission or exacerbation which dictate dose adjustment. The patient must be supported with corticosteroids during periods of stress.

For therapeutic adjunctive treatment of inflammation: Administer 20 units IM or SQ four times a day.

For verification of adrenal responsiveness: Administer as much as 80 units IM or SQ in single or divided doses.

IMPLEMENTATION CONSIDERATIONS:

—See drug monograph on glucocorticoids. In addition, before starting therapy, skin test all clients with suspected porcine allergy.

WHAT THE PATIENT NEEDS TO KNOW:

—See drug monograph on glucocorticoids relative to systemic steroid consumption.

EVALUATION:

ADVERSE REACTIONS: See drug monograph on glucocorticoids. Also, in treatment of myasthenia gravis, corticotropin may cause severe muscle weakness, including the muscles of respiration, for 2-3 days after treatment. Consequently, ventilatory assistance must be immediately available. Strength recovers and condition improves within a week of cessation of treatment, and improvement lasts for 6 weeks to 3 months.

Note: Corticotropin causes adrenal cortical hyperplasia rather than atrophy like glucocorticoids. It also causes pituitary-hypothalamic insufficiency thus, patients must be supported with glucocorticoids during stress.

Hyperpigmentation and adverse androgenic effects (acne, hirsutism, amenorrhea) are likely to occur more often with ACTH than glucocorticoids.

OVERDOSAGE: See drug monograph on glucocorticoids.

PARAMETERS TO MONITOR: See drug monograph on glucocorticoids.

CORTICOTROPIN

PRODUCTS (TRADE NAME):

ACTH (Available in 40, 80 units/ml for injection.) **Acthar** (Available in 25 and 40 unit vials for injection.) **Corticotropin** (Available in 40 and 80 units/ml for injection.)

DRUG SPECIFICS:

See general drug monograph. Very rapid absorption and utilization necessitates administration every six hours to maintain desired production.

ADMINISTRATION AND DOSAGE SPECIFICS:

Therapeutic range: Use 20 to 100 units IM or SQ. Initially try 10 to 12.5 units 4 times a day. If there is no clinical effect in 72-96 hours, the dosage is increased by 5 units every few days to 25 units 4 times a day. In certain circumstances this can be increased to 200 units a day. Dose is lowered gradually as soon as possible.

Children: There is no official recommendation for infants and young children. They have been noted to require a larger dose per body weight than older children. 1.6 units/kg/day has been suggested by some clinicians.

Diagnostic Range: 10-25 units aqueous solution in 500 ml of 5% dextrose in water over a period of 8 hours. Make certain preparation is labeled that it can be given IV.

CORTICOTROPIN REPOSITORY

PRODUCTS (TRADE NAME):

ACTH-Gel, Corticotropin Gel, Cortopic Gel, Cortrophin Gel, Cotopic Gel,

HP Acthar Gel (Available in 40 or 80 units/ml for injection.)
DRUG SPECIFICS:

See general drug monograph. This form is slowly absorbed and can be administered in a single daily dose via the intramuscular route. The dose is individually adjusted.

ADMINISTRATION AND DOSAGE SPECIFICS:

Adults: 40 to 80 units IM every 24 to 72 hours.

Children: No official recommendation. Some clinicians suggest 0.8 units/kg/day in a single daily dose.

CORTICOTROPIN ZINC HYDROXIDE

PRODUCTS (TRADE NAME):

Cortrophin-Zinc (Available in 40 units corticotropin and 2 mg zinc per mil suspension).

DRUG SPECIFICS:

See general drug monograph.

ADMINISTRATION AND DOSAGE SPECIFICS:

Adults: 40 units IM or SQ every 12 to 24 hours.

COSYNTROPIN

PRODUCTS (TRADE NAME):

Cortrosyn (Available in 0.25 mg injection.)

DRUG SPECIFICS:

This relatively new product is a synthetic subunit of ACTH but exhibits all the pharmacologic properties of the natural ACTH. Cosyntropin 0.25 mg is equivalent in action to 25 units natural ACTH. This drug will also produce increased growth hormone, adipokinesis and melanotropic effects. It is used primarily as a preliminary diagnostic agent in patients presumed to have adrenocortical insufficiency before other more expensive tests are employed. Because it contains no protein, it is usually less likely to produce allergies in patients than natural ACTH. Rare hypersensitivity reactions do occur.

ADMINISTRATION AND DOSAGE SPECIFICS:

Adrenocortical insufficiency testing: Give 0.25 to 0.75 mg IM or IV. Children less than age 2 may respond to dose of 0.125 mg. This dose should provide a rapid screening test of adrenal function. Test may also be implementedj using 0.25 mg with dextrose or saline IV infustion. Give 40 mcg/hour over 6 hours to provide a greater stimulus to adrenal glands.

Molly Craig Billingsley

POSTERIOR PITUITARY HORMONES

ANTIDIURETIC HORMONES

ACTION OF THE DRUG: There are three basic actions of this class of drugs. Not all of the drugs exhibit all the actions; the relevant drugs are listed in parentheses.

(1) Smooth muscle contraction of the digestive tract and uterus (vasopressin and pituitary extract).

(2) Contraction of smooth muscle in vascular bed (vasopressor effect manifested in vasopressin, lypressin and pituitary extract).

(3) Promotion of water reabsorption and concentration of urine (vasopressin, pituitary extract, lypressin, desmopressin acetate).

ASSESSMENT:

INDICATIONS: The most common indication for this group of drugs is in treatment of diabetes insipidus caused by a posterior pituitary hormone deficiency. Although nurse practitioners would rarely be prescribing this medication, they may share in the responsibility of monitoring the progress of patients on this medication. Vasopressin is of secondary use in stimulating peristalsis in the prevention or treatment of intestinal paresis or postoperative abdominal distention, distention complicating pneumonia, or prior to GI x-rays to dispel gas shadows. Vasopressin tannate is also used to differentiate diabetes insipidus of neurohypophysial, nephrogenic, or psychogenic origins.

SUBJECTIVE-OBJECTIVE: Patient presents with previous history of excessive thirst and the passage of large amounts of urine with no excess of sugar. Patient should be under care of medical specialist and have laboratory documentation of preexisting problem.

PLAN:

CONTRAINDICATIONS: Do not give to patients with epilepsy, cardiorenal disease with hypertension, angina, coronary thrombosis, toxemia, advanced arteriosclerotic cardiovascular disease, first stage of labor, chronic nephritis with increased BUN, abnormal sensitivity to the drugs.

WARNINGS: Use with extreme caution in patients with vascular disease. Even very small doses have been known to precipitate chest pain. Note the possibility of water intoxication: drowsiness, listlessness, headache, convulsions, and coma. Discontinue the drug and restrict fluid intake until specific gravity is above 1.015 and polyuria occurs. The elderly and young children respond very sensitively. Monitor response and progress very carefully in these age groups.

This group of drugs is not appropriate for treatment of polyuria secondary to renal disease, nephrogenic diabetes insipidus, hypokalemia, hypercalcemia, or as a side effect of lithium or demeclocycline.

Safe use in pregnancy has not been established. These drugs must not be used intravenously.

PRECAUTIONS: Use with caution with patients with epilepsy, migraines, asthma, and any condition in which rapid addition of extracellular fluid to the blood volume is dangerous. See individual remarks on each drug.

IMPLEMENTATION:

DRUG INTERACTIONS: The following drugs alter the effect of vasopressin, vasopressin tannate, and lypressin: oral antidiabetic agents, chlorpropamide, urea, fludrocortisone increase the effects and cyclophosphamide, large doses of epinephrine, demeclocycline, heparin, and alcohol decrease the effect. The antidiuretic effect of desmopressin is decreased by lithium, large doses of epinephrine, demeclocycline, heparin, and alcohol. The antidiuretic effects of desmopressin may be increased by chlorpropamide, urea, and fludrocortisone.

ADMINISTRATION AND DOSAGE: See specific product information. Generally, in treatment of diabetes insipidus, vasopressin is useful in initial or emergency treatment but impractical for long-term treatment. Intranasally, it sometimes is appropriate for mild diabetes insipidus.

Vasopressin tannate is the most effective drug of longest duration. It is the drug of choice for children, adults with severe disease, and for overnight control. It is also appropriate for long-term treatment. Lypressin is preferred by many with mild diabetes insipidus because it is intranasal. It can be used if patient is allergic to vasopressin. Desmopressin acetate is a potent antidiuretic with longer duration of action and fewer adverse effects than vasopressin, the drug of choice for mild to moderate diabetes insipidus. It is also administered intranasally.

There are no oral forms of this group of drugs. They are administered intramuscularly or subcutaneously in severe forms of disease (vasopressin, pituitary injection, vasopressin tannate) or intranasally in mild to moderate forms of disease (desmopressin acetate, vasopressin, lypressin).

The dosages are individualized to the diurnal rhythm of water metabolism and adequate duration of sleep. Generally, the administration should coincide with onset of polyuria or excessive thirst and before sleep.

Note: 1-2 glasses of water at the time of administration reduces incidence of side effects.

IMPLEMENTATION CONSIDERATIONS:
—Obtain a complete health history, including the presence of epilepsy, cardiorenal disease, hypertension, angina, coronary thrombosis, toxemia, advanced arteriosclerotic vascular disease, chronic nephritis, a history of hypersensitivity to antidiuretic hormone, other drugs taken concurrently which may cause drug interactions, or the possibility of pregnancy.

—Obtain baseline blood pressure, urine for specific gravity, weight.

—Document usual pattern of water turnover and sleep duration.

—Monitor children and elderly very carefully for response to the drugs, especially desmopressin acetate.

—The side effects with low doses of these drugs are mild and infrequent. Effects become more troublesome as the dosage increases.

WHAT THE PATIENT NEEDS TO KNOW:

—This medication should be taken exactly as ordered by your health care provider.

—Your health care provider will teach you how to measure your fluid intake, the amount and specific gravity of your urine, and accurate record keeping which needs to be reviewed by your health care provider.

—Continued appointments to monitor your therapy while on this drug are important.

—Be aware of the possibility of developing water intoxication: drowsiness, listlessness, headache, convulsions, and coma. Drug should be discontinued and your health care provider notified at once if you note any of these symptoms.

—Also watch for signs of dehydration: failure to urinate, dry skin and mouth, complaints of thirst, furrowed tongue.

—If you experience any symptoms which are new or troublesome, notify your health care provider promptly.

EVALUATION:

ADVERSE REACTIONS: Side effects of small doses of vasopressin include: abdominal cramps. anaphylaxis, bronchial constriction, cardiac arrest, circumoral pallor. diarrhea, flateus. intestinal hyperactivity, nausea, "pounding" headaches. sweating. tremor. urticaria, uterine cramps, vertigo, vomiting.

Side effects of larger doses include allergic reaction, bradycardia, heart block, coronary insufficiency, hypertension, minor arrhythmias, myocardial infarction, vascular collapse.

Side effects of lypressin nasal spray are rare and mild. They include abdominal cramps, conjunctivitis, headache, heartburn, increased bowel movements, irritation and pruritus of mucosa, nasal conjestion, nasal drip, nasal ulcerations, rhinorrhea, secondary postnasal drip.

Side effects of desmopressin acetate are also rare. With high doses, patients have complained of flushing, transient headaches, nausea, nasal congestion, rhinitis, and vulvar pain. Hypertension has been reported with high doses; however, this and other side effects decrease when dosage is decreased.

OVERDOSAGE: *Signs and symptoms:* substernal tightness, coughing, transient dyspnea, pronounced but transient fluid retention, hypernatremia, blanching, abdominal cramps, and nausea. Recovery is spontaneous.

PARAMETERS TO MONITOR: Obtain complete baseline studies prior to instituting therapy. Then monitor for therapeutic and adverse effects. Monitor blood pressure twice a day for excessive increases or lack of response (decreasing blood pressure) while on vasopressin. Monitor increased continence, decreased urinary frequency. Follow intake and output. Check duration and amount of sleep per day. Be aware of early signs of water intoxication.

DESMOPRESSIN ACETATE

PRODUCTS (TRADE NAME):
    DDAVP (Available in 0.1 mg/ml nasal solution.)
DRUG SPECIFICS:
    This is a synthetic antidiuretic inhalant. It is the drug of choice for mild to moderate diabetes insipidus. It offers prolonged antidiuretic activity without vasopressor or oxytocic side effects. It is generally the most acceptable drug to patients because of its route of administration.
    Before instituting this drug, the patient should return to baseline levels. Give 2.5-10 mcg in the evening. Note the effect and increase nightly by 2.5 mcg until satisfactory sleep duration is attained. If the daily urine volume is greater than 2 liters after nocturia is controlled, add a morning dose of 10 mcg and adjust until 1.5-2 liters per day. Occasionally, a third dose is necessary in the afternoon. At times, excessive fluid retention may necessitate treatment with furosemide. Stress firmly the need for fluid intake restriction, especially in children and elderly patients.
    For intranasal administration: Deposit high in nasal cavity. The dosage is adjusted using intake and output and duration of sleep as parameters.
ADMINISTRATION AND DOSAGE SPECIFICS:
    For cranial diabetes insipidus, temporary polyuria, polydipsia secondary to trauma to or surgery of the pituitary:
    Adults: Give 0.1 to 0.4 ml/day in 1, 2, or 3 unequal doses. Most patients require about .2 ml/ day in unequal doses.
    Children 3 months to 12 years: Give 0.05 to 0.3 ml/day in single or divided doses. A third of the patients can be controlled in one dose.

LYPRESSIN

PRODUCTS (TRADE NAME):
    Diapid (Available in 0.185 mg/ml nasal spray.)
DRUG SPECIFICS:
    Lypressin is a synthetic derivative of antidiuretic hormone. It is the treatment preferred for mild diabetes insipidus and is especially useful in patients who have become unresponsive to other forms of treatment or who experience allergic or untoward effects from natural posterior pituitary extracts.
    The onset of action is about one hour, and the antidiuretic effects last from 3 to 8 hours. The effectiveness is decreased in rhinorrhea and upper respiratory infections. The dose may need to be increased at that time. The patient must be observed for dehydration. Check tongue, mucous membranes and ask about complaints of thirst.

ADMINISTRATION AND DOSAGE SPECIFICS:
Adults and children:
For neurohypophysial diabetes insipidus: Hold bottle upright with head vertical. Use 1 to 2 sprays in one or both nostrils 3-4 times a day or at onset of polyuria or thirst. (Note: More than 2 sprays per nostril results in unabsorbed wastage. Therefore, if an increase in dosage is necessary, increase the frequency of administration.) An additional dose may be given before sleep if necessary.

POSTERIOR PITUITARY INJECTION

PRODUCTS (TRADE NAME):
Pituitrin (S) (Available in 10 units/ml injection for surgical use).
DRUG SPECIFICS:
This is the natural extract of posterior pituitary glands and contains considerable vasopressor, oxytocic and antidiuretic activity. Because of its rapid pressor effects and short duration, it is considered a fairly hazardous drug, and most clinicians use a more refined preparation to achieve the desired response. Its clinical use is restricted to severe refractory diabetes insipidus and rarely other problems.

If it is utilized, observe the patient carefully for allergies and have oxygen and supportive medications ready. Take blood pressure frequently for one hour to monitor decreased cardiac output and coronary blood flow.
ADMINISTRATION AND DOSAGE SPECIFICS:
For refractory diabetes insipidus, postoperative ileus, to stimulate expulsion of gas for pyelography, homeostasis with esophageal varices, uterine stimulation, adjunctive treatment for shock, and after expulsion of the placenta: 5 to 20 units IM (preferred) or SQ. For postpartum hemorrhage give 10 units.

VASOPRESSIN (8-ARGININE VASOPRESSIN)

PRODUCTS (TRADE NAME):
Pitressin Synthetic (Available in 20 pressor units/ml for injection).
DRUG SPECIFICS:
This is a natural posterior pituitary hormone with antidiuretic properties much greater than its vasopressor oxytocic actions.

The intranasal route is not particularly efficient since vasopressin is not well absorbed via the nasal mucosa. However, some cases of mild diabetes insipidus have been adequately controlled in this way.
ADMINISTRATION AND DOSAGE SPECIFICS:
Initial or Emergency Treatment of Diabetes Insipidus:
Adults: 5 to 10 units (0.25-0.5 ml) IM or SQ, 2-4 times a day; maximum dose 60 units.

Children: 2.5 to 10 units (0.125-0.5 ml) IM or SQ, 2-4 times a day.

Intranasal therapy: Use intranasally via cotton pledgets or as a nasal spray. Dose is individually determined.

Prevention or Treatment of Abdominal Distention:

Adults: 5 units IM, then increase to 10 units every 3 to 4 hours if necessary.

Children: Administer proportionately less IM.

Before Abdominal X-rays, to Dispel Gas:

Adults: Administer enema; then at 2 hours and at 1/2 hour before the procedure, give 10 units IM or SQ.

VASOPRESSIN TANNATE

PRODUCTS (TRADE NAME):
Pitressin Tannate in Oil (Available in 5 pressor units/ml injection).

DRUG SPECIFICS:
A natural, water-insoluble derivative of vasopressin which has a longer duration of action and is of use in long-term treatment of diabetes insipidus in children and some adults. See General Statement.

Note: Shake well before withdrawing the dose. This form of drug particularly must be completely dissolved. It must be given IM. It is not absorbed by the nasal mucosa. Following administration, the effects of this drug are cumulative hence, the total response cannot be determined for several days.

ADMINISTRATION AND DOSAGE SPECIFICS:
Treatment of Neurohypophysial Diabetes Insipidus:

Adults: Give 1.5 to 5 units (0.3-1.0 ml) deep IM every 1 to 3 days. Adjust to maintain specific gravity of urine at greater than 1.005. The administration should be at the onset of polyuria and given before sleep if possible.

Children: Give 1.25 to 2.5 units (0.25-0.5 ml) every 3 to 5 days.

Molly Craig Billingsley

OXYTOCICS

ACTION OF THE DRUG: Included in this section are natural and synthetic posterior pituitary oxytocics and ergots. They have many similarities but also some differences. Refer to the specific drugs as well as the general monograph. These drugs act directly on the smooth musculature of (1) the uterus, especially at or near gestation, to produce firm regular contractions; (2) the vasculature system to produce vasoconstriction; and (3) the mammary gland cells in the postpartum phase, to stimulate the flow of milk.

ASSESSMENT:

INDICATIONS: Selected drugs from this group are used under the supervision of a physician when indicated in the stimulation or induction of labor at term (when there are medical problems threatening the life of the mother or fetus); in the management of delivery of the shoulder of the infant; in assisting expulsion of the placenta; in the control of postpartum bleeding or uterine atony; in the relief of breast engorgement related to static lactation; in the stimulation of uterine contraction following cesarean section or other uterine surgery; or in the promotion of incomplete abortion (adjunctively).

The ergots are used to prevent or control hemorrhage following the delivery of the placenta and in the postpartum period.

SUBJECTIVE: Patient may be past anticipated due date for baby, or give history of failure to empty breasts of milk-producing swollen, painful breasts. History of incomplete abortion, cesarean section or excessive bleeding postpartum also prompt consideration of this drug.

OBJECTIVE: Relaxed uterus, excessive bleeding. Breasts may be swollen with skin pulled taunt, and be tender to touch.

PLAN:

CONTRAINDICATIONS: Do not use when benefits versus risk for mother or infant favor caeserian section, or in fetal distress when delivery is not imminent. Avoid prolonged use in uterine inertia, in patients with cephalopelvic disproportion, fetal malpresentation, undilated or unripe cervix, history placing patient at risk to uterine rupture (uterine scar, grand multiparity), cardiovascular disease, factors predisposing to thromboplastin or amniotic fluid embolism, hypersensitivity, severe toxemia, cord presentation, or prolapse.

Ergot contraindications: Induction of labor, augmentation of spontaneous abortion, toxemia, hypersensitivity, cardiac disease, venoatrial shunts, mitral valve stenosis, obliterative vascular disease, renal or hepatic impairment, uterine sepsis.

WARNINGS: Injudicious use of either oxytocic or ergot preparations have been credited with fetal and maternal death or injury, subarachnoid hemorrhage, and uterine rupture.

Oxytocins: Use with constant supervision, extreme caution and a thorough knowledge of the drug. Do not use via more than one route. Do not use when labor is progressing on its own. Do not give undiluted or in excessive concentrations. Do not administer buccally to unconscious women.

Ergot Preparations: Do not use in first or second stages of labor or before the placenta is delivered. Previously hypertensive patients may be particularly sensitive to the drug, leading to CVA, arrhythmia, and headache.

PRECAUTIONS:

Oxytocins: The uterine contractions produced by oxytocics should be comparable to those of spontaneous normal labor. In multiparous women, use only after the cervix is completely dilated. Have drugs ready in case of hypertensive episodes. Note the antidiuretic effect (oxytocin has slight ADH properties) and monitor for water intoxication.

Ergots: Prolonged use should be avoided because of the danger of ergotism. If used in the early third stage of labor, the drug could cause captivation of the placenta. If patient is calcium deficient and does not respond, cautiously give intravenous calcium salts.

IMPLEMENTATION:

DRUG INTERACTIONS: The following drugs increase the effects of oxytocics: cyclophosphamide, vasoconstrictors, and local anesthetics. These two groups of drugs may be additive or synergistic with either group of oxytocics. Beware of intractable hypertension, rupture of cerebral vasculature.

ADMINISTRATION AND DOSAGE:

Oxytocins: These drugs are generally used for the induction or stimulation of labor because of their rapid onset of action at gestational term. When accompanied by amniotomy, oxytocin produces successful induction of labor in 80-90% of cases. It is still the drug of choice for induction in many areas of the country however, the prostaglandins are now preferred in some regions.

This product is usually given by intravenous infusion pump. The buccal tablets are available but are not as extensively used as they were at one time because the effects are more difficult to predict and control.

Ergot: Ergonovine is now the drug of choice for control of postpartum bleeding. It can be given sublingually, intramuscularly, or intravenously in emergency situations. Note: Some calcium-deficient women will not respond to ergonovine. Using care, restore calcium via intravenous injection if indicated.

Methylergonovine is the synthetic homolog and has been found to produce fewer vasoconstrictive or hypertensive side effects than ergonovine. It is noted that intravenous administration of either drug increases the danger of side effects.

IMPLEMENTATION CONSIDERATIONS:

When using oxytocins:

—Obtain a complete health history, including presence of cephalopelvic disproportion, abnormal fetal position, previous uterine surgery, fetal distress, placental abnormalities. Determine maturity of the fetus and whether the patient is also receiving cyclophosphamide or other vasoconstrictors. Ask about previous hypersensitivity.

—Hypersensitivity reactions are least likely to occur with intravenous infusion or diluted doses.

When using ergot preparations:

—Obtain a complete health history, including presence of liver disease, sepsis, obliterative vascular disease, renal disease, and cardiac disease. Ask about hypersensitivity to drug or concurrent administration of cyclophosphamide or other vasoconstrictors.

—Validate that the placenta has been delivered.

—Watch for the symptoms of ergotism: vomiting, diarrhea, unquenchable thirst, tingling, itching and coldness of the skin, a rapid and weak pulse, confusion, and unconsciousness.

—Ergotrate might stimulate cramping. If this becomes too uncomfortable, either decrease the dose or treat symptomatically.

—Most common side effects are nausea and vomiting. These can sometimes be alleviated with prior administration of a phenothiazine antiemetic.

—If overdosage occurs, producing a continuous contraction, discontinue the drug immediately. It may be necessary to give a general anesthestic to relax the uterus, particularly if the fetus is threatened.

WHAT THE PATIENT NEEDS TO KNOW:

—This drug is given to augment the body's natural action during and following labor.

—Patient will be watched continually throughout this treatment.

—Contractions should not be more intense than normal unaugmented contractions.

—Ergotrate might stimulate cramping. Should this become intense, notify your health care provider.

EVALUATION:

ADVERSE REACTIONS:

Oxytocin: Cardiovascular: cardiac arrhythmia, cardiovascular spasm, edema, fetal and neonatal bradycardia, precordial pain, premature ventricular contractions. *CNS:* anxiety. *Dermatologic:* redness of skin during administration. *Endocrine:* severe water intoxication due to long-term intravenous infusion. *Gastrointestinal:* nausea and vomiting. *Hypersensitivity:* anaphylaxis (usually rare and generally associated with parenteral administration (IM) of natural oxytocin or in concentrated intravenous injection.) *Reproductive:* pelvic hematoma, postpartum hemorrhage. *Respiratory:* cyanosis, dyspnea. *Other:* Fetal problems are unusual but consist of hypoxia, intracranial hemorrhage, premature ventricular contractions, and tachycardia.

Ergotrates: In the appropriate dosage and in the absence of contraindications, the ergots are fairly safe. Most common problems are nausea and vomiting. Other more unusual reactions would be allergic reactions, bradycardia, hypotension, rise in blood pressure (usually in conjunction with caudal or spinal anesthesia or in intravenous ergotrate administration), shock, drug-induced gangrene, or cerebral-spinal symptoms and spasms.

OVERDOSAGE:

Oxytocin: Excessive doses can produce uterine hypertonicity, spasm, tetanic contractions, and ruptures. Lesser overdoses in labor yield a sustained forceful contraction without rest. *Treatment:* Discontinue the drug immediately. May need to give general anesthesia to relax uterus.

Ergots: Overdosage during labor yields a similar picture: uterine tetany with compromise of uteroplacental circulation, rupture, cervical and perineal lacerations, and amniotic fluid embolism. Gradual onset of ergotism is manifested by nausea, vomiting, weak pulse, cramps, blood pressure increase or decrease, diarrhea, drowsiness, dizziness, headache, and confusion. Gastrointestinal and central nervous system effects may precede vascular problems in hands and feet. Also unquenchable thirst, tingling, dyspnea, itching, and coldness of skin. *Treatment:* Withdrawal of the drug and symptomatic assistance. Administer heparin to hold clotting at 3 times normal value. May administer vasodilators to regulate pulse and blood pressure.

PARAMETERS TO MONITOR:

Oxytocin during induction: Monitor for therapeutic effect and development of adverse reactions. Monitor blood pressure and pulse frequently, plus continuous fetal heart rate monitoring. Monitor dilation of cervix, progression of contractions: frequency, force, duration, resting uterine tone. Drastic increases in these parameters warrant discontinuing drug. The contractions should not be over 50 mm Hg. Note urinary output and edema. Guard against water intoxication. Closely watch the rate of intravenous solution and oxytocin.

Ergots Postpartum: Monitor for therapeutic effect and development of adverse reactions. Monitor height, consistency, and location of fundus. Check amount and color of lochia. Monitor vital signs for shock, hypertension. Note any sudden change in vital signs. Note frequent periods of uterine relaxation. Observe for excessive cramping, which suggests a need to decrease the dose.

ERGONOVINE MALEATE

PRODUCTS (TRADE NAME):

Ergonovine Maleate, Ergotrate Maleate (Available in 0.2 mg tablets, 0.2 mg/ml injection.)

DRUG SPECIFICS:

This is a natural alkaloid which is a derivative of ergot (a fungus). It stimulates the contraction of the uterine musculature. It is *not* used for induction of labor but is useful in the prevention or control of postpartum hemorrhage secondary to uterine atony or subinvolution. Note similarity in names between ergotamine and ergonovine; they are not the same although they may be listed the same in some books.

Severe cramping indicates that the drug is working; however it may necessitate dosage adjustment.

Protect the ampule from light, store in a cool place, and discard after 60 days.

ADMINISTRATION AND DOSAGE SPECIFICS:

Sublingually: Appropriate in nonemergency situations and for prophylaxis after leaving the labor and delivery suite: 200-400 mcg (0.2 to 0.4 mg) 2 to 4 times a day for 48 hours postpartum.

IM: Administered postpartally to facilitate uterine contraction and decrease bleeding; give 0.2 mg IM.

IV: Generally used only in emergency situations due to high incidence of side effects, especially hypertension.

METHYLERGONOVINE MALEATE

PRODUCTS (TRADE NAME):
Methergine(Available in 0.2 mg/ml ampule, 0.2 mg tablets.)

DRUG SPECIFICS:
This is a synthetic homolog of ergonovine which produces stronger and more prolonged contractions. It is used for the same situations as ergonovine. The choice of methylergonovine versus ergonovine is a personal preference of the clinician, although methylergonovine has fewer hypertensive or vasoconstrictive side effects. See General Statement.

Protect vials from heat and light and discard colored vials. Onset of action after IV administration is immediate; following intramuscular administration it is 2-5 minutes, and orally it is 5-10 minutes.

ADMINISTRATION AND DOSAGE SPECIFICS:
Prevention or Control of Postpartum Hemorrhage:

IV: Use only in emergencies because of possibility of inducing CVA or hypertension. Give 0.2 mg over a period of not less than 1 minute with continuous blood pressure monitoring. Some clinicians recommend dilution to a volume of 5 ml with .9% sodium chloride.

IM: Give 0.2 mg not more often than every 2 to 4 hours or not more than a total of 5 doses. Following IV or IM dose for subinvolution to facilitate involution of the uterus.

Dosage: 1 tablet po (0.2 mg) 3-4 times a day for 2-7 days.

OXYTOCIN

PRODUCTS (TRADE NAME):
Oxytocin, Pitocin, Syntocinon (Available in 10 units/ml for injection.) **Syntocinon Nasal** (Available in 40 units/ml in 2 and 5 ml squeeze bottles.)

DRUG SPECIFICS:
Pitocin is a natural posterior pituitary extract which is primarily used in induction or stimulation of labor at term and secondarily in the stimulation of milk flow. It is the drug of choice in many areas of the country for induction of labor. Syntocinon is a synthetic derivative without the cardiovascular or vasopressor effects. The nasal form is useful for initial milk let-down.

Never administer intravenously undiluted or in high concentrations.

ADMINISTRATION AND DOSAGE SPECIFICS:
For induction of labor: 10 units in 1 liter of 5% dextrose in water or isotonic saline as an intravenous infusion. Initially give 1-2 milliunits/minute. If no response within 15 minutes, gradually increase to a maximum of 20 milliunits per minute. The total induction dose ranges from 600 to 12,000 milliunits, with the average being 4,000 milliunits.

For postpartum bleeding: Give 3 to 10 units in one IM dose following delivery of the placenta. Or may give 10 to 40 units in 1000 ml isotonic saline intravenously at a rate to control the bleeding.

To stimulate milk flow: One spray nasally into one or both nostrils 2-3 minutes before nursing or pumping breasts. Hold squeeze bottle upright with patient sitting straight up.

OXYTOCIN CITRATE

PRODUCTS (TRADE NAME):
   Pitocin Citrate (Available in 200 unit buccal tablets).
DRUG SPECIFICS:
   This is a synthetic oxytocic identical to natural oxytocin. It is used to induce or stimulate labor at term. It is not widely used.
   Accidental swallowing is not harmful; the drug is inactivated by the trypsin in the GI tract.
   If patient complains of mouth dryness, instruct her to rinse her mouth with cold water. Remove and then replace the tablet. Alternate cheek pouches when dosage is continued. Onset of action is 30 minutes.
ADMINISTRATION AND DOSAGE SPECIFICS:
   For induction or stimulation of labor: Individualize dose according to response. Total dose for induction and completion of labor is 1500 to 2000 units, given in increments of one buccal tablet every 30 minutes. When the desired response is attained, maintain the same number of tablets in the buccal spaces until delivery. Maximum dose is 3000 units.

Molly Craig Billingsley

SEX HORMONES

ANDROGENS

ACTION OF THE DRUG: The main action of androgens is the development of secondary male sex characteristics. Androgens are anabolic. The balance of androgenic and anabolic activity varies with the specific synthetic compound. Androgens are also antineoplastic when used in certain breast cancers in women. Erythropoiesis is increased with the administration of androgens.

ASSESSMENT:

INDICATIONS: Androgens are used in hypogonadism, hypopituitarism, dwarfism, eunuchism, cryptorchidism, oligospermia, and general androgen deficiency in males. They are used to restore positive nitrogen balance in patients with chronic, debilitating illness or trauma; in treatment of anemia secondary to renal failure, and in other blood dyscrasias where increased erythropoiesis is needed; and palliatively for treatment of advanced breast cancer in postmenopausal women, and for endometriosis in younger women. They have been used additionally to suppress lactation. It is not likely that nurse practitioners would prescribe this medication; however, they may be responsible for helping monitor the therapeutic effects of patients receiving this medication.

SUBJECTIVE: Patient may complain of impotence, reduced libido, weight loss, male climacteric, castration, or there may be a history of traumatic castration or failure to develop secondary sex characteristics by 15-17 years of age.

OBJECTIVE: Prepubertal and pubertal males: hypogonadism, high-pitched voice, narrow shoulders, long arms, and other signs of lack of masculine characteristics, eunuchism, cryptorchidism, dwarfism, hypopituitarism, or oligospermia. Adult male: Practitioner may see atrophy of gonads, impotence during sleep studies, documented weight loss, muscle wasting, castration, or may detect osteoporosis, anemia (aplastic, red-cell aplasia, hemolytic, associated with renal failure or other chronic illness).

PLAN:

CONTRAINDICATIONS: Do not give in the presence of prostatic carcinoma, obstructing benign prostatic hypertrophy, or breast cancer in males. Do not give to patients with history of myocardial infarction, nephrosis or liver dysfunction or to patients with hypercalcemia. Do not use in pregnant, breast-feeding women, and premature or newborn infants.

WARNINGS: Androgens must be used cautiously in children and pubertal males because drug may cause premature epiphyseal closure resulting in short stature. Edema may be increased in patients with renal, hepatic, or cardiac dysfunction.

Some virilization can be expected in women who are given large doses for treatment of breast cancer. Some changes may remain after the drug is discontinued. If cholestatic jaundice develops or liver function decreases, the drug should be discontinued. Hypercalcemia may result when androgens are used in breast cancer or immobilized patients. Liver cancer has occurred in long-term therapy with 17-alkyl derivatives.

PRECAUTIONS: In young males who are being treated for hypogonadism or other androgen-deficiency conditions, skeletal growth should be monitored and dose adjusted to avoid premature epiphyseal closure. Renal and cardiac conditions may worsen because of edema. Serum cholesterol may be affected, either decreasing or increasing levels, and should be monitored serially in patients with a history of cardiac disease. Good liver function is necessary for metabolizing the drug.

Stomatitis may result from buccal administration. In older men with prostatism, urinary obstruction may result. Prolonged therapy may result in oligospermia. If priapism occurs, discontinue therapy. In women treated for breast cancer, signs of masculinization such as acne, facial hair, deepening of voice, increased libido, and clitoral hypertrophy may result. Diabetic patients may need to adjust antidiabetic drug doses. In long-term therapy, serum calcium, liver function, and cardiac function should be monitored.

IMPLEMENTATION:

DRUG INTERACTIONS: Anabolic steroids may increase the effects of anticoagulants, antidiabetics, oxyphenbutazone, and phenylbutazone. Corticosteroids given concurrently with androgens increase the possibility of edema. Barbiturates decrease therapeutic effects of androgens because of increased breakdown in the liver. Androgens may affect lab tests in the following manner: increased serum sodium, potassium, nitrogen, phosphorus, calcium, 17-ketosteroids, and hematocrit. Decreased liver function and thyroid-binding globulin are also seen. There are variable effects on serum cholesterol.

ADMINISTRATION AND DOSAGE: Androgens can be given by mouth, buccally, and sublingually, depending on the specific drug and reason for therapy. Dosages vary from 2 to 10 mg daily for replacement therapy. Higher divided doses are given for antineoplastic effect.

IMPLEMENTATION CONSIDERATIONS:

—Obtain a complete health history, including the presence of carcinoma, cardiac, renal, or liver dysfunction, other drugs taken concurrently, and possibility of pregnancy.

—When given for hypogonadism, careful descriptions of secondary sex characteristics and measurements should be recorded for a baseline in order to monitor therapeutic effects.

—Unless otherwise contraindicated, the patient should have a diet intake high in calories, proteins, minerals, and vitamins because of the anabolic effects of the androgens.

—Patients should be taught before starting drug therapy about different side effects to report and about possible physical and behavioral changes which may develop.

—The patient should be taught to use oral hygiene measures after sublingual or buccal administration. Patients must be instructed not to swallow the pill, and not to eat, drink, smoke, or chew until buccal tablets are absorbed.

—The drug should be discontinued if cholestatic jaundice or priapism occurs.

—Therapeutic response may be slow, requiring three or more months to affect symptoms.

—Androgens may change laboratory results on glucose tolerance, serum cholesterol, liver and thyroid function, hematocrit and 17-ketosteroid levels.

—Patients on anticoagulants may need the anticoagulant dosage lowered and should be monitored very closely.

WHAT THE PATIENT NEEDS TO KNOW:
—Take this medication as instructed by your health practitioner.
—Response to the drug may take several weeks or months.
—Eat a diet high in calories, protein, vitamins, and minerals unless otherwise instructed by your health care practitioner.
—Report any new or troublesome symptoms which may develop. For men: fluid retention, especially in feet and hands, enlargement of breasts, shortness of breath, excessive physical or sexual stimulation, prolonged or painful erection of penis, impotence, urinary retention, yellowing of skin or eyes. For women: yellowing of skin or eyes, fluid retention especially in feet and hands, shortness of breath, changes in vaginal bleeding, increased sex drive, masculinization of appearance. (Signs of masculinization in women usually, but not always, are reversed when the drug is discontinued.)
—If medicine is taken sublingually (under the tongue) or buccally (putting medicine in cheek), you should rinse mouth and brush teeth after taking medicine.
—Response to the drug may take several weeks or months to evaluate.
—It is important to return for clinic appointments and blood work when requested by the health care provider.

EVALUATION:

ADVERSE REACTIONS: *Cardiovascular:* edema due to sodium retention (usually only with large doses), increase in serum cholesterol. *Dermatologic:* acne, hirsutism, male pattern of baldness. *Gastrointestinal:* cholestatic hepatitis with jaundice, liver cancer (rare), buccal irritation, diarrhea, nausea, vomiting. *Genitourinary:* Female: clitoral enlargement, masculinization; Male: decrease in sperm count, excessive sexual stimulation, gynecomastia, impotence, priapism, urinary retention. Children: precocious puberty. *Musculoskeletal:* Children may develop short stature due to premature epiphyseal closure.

OVERDOSAGE: *Signs and symptoms:* Increased virilization develops. *Treatment:* none.

PARAMETERS TO MONITOR: Obtain complete history, physical and laboratory evaluation prior to institution of therapy. Blood pressure and weight should be checked. Physical examination should include thorough genitourinary, skin and behavioral evaluation. Order liver function tests, serum calcium, cholesterol, and CBC as baseline. Frequency of visits depends on the reason for therapy. Most patients probably should be seen monthly to monitor therapeutic effects and adverse reactions. Liver function and serum cholesterol should be monitored. Observe for jaundice or pruritus. Monitor for edema and weight gain, especially in patients with a history of cardiac, asthma, or renal disease. Patient can be instructed to weigh himself weekly and report significant changes. If patients take medication sublingually or buccally, mouth should be inspected carefully on each visit. Serum calcium should be checked following administration of large doses. Diabetic patients should be monitored for hypoglycemia. Antidiabetic medicines may need dosage adjustment.

ANDROGENS—ORAL

DANAZOL

PRODUCTS (TRADE NAME):
Danocrine (Available in 50, 100, and 200 mg capsules.)
DRUG SPECIFICS:
This is a synthetic androgen used to treat endometriosis, fibrocystic breast disease, and hereditary angioedema through suppression of pituitary gonadotrophins and therefore reduction in menstruation. Both uterine and ectopic endometrium atrophy when used for endometriosis. Contraindicated in abnormal, undiagnosed vaginal bleeding, pregnancy, breast-feeding women, patients with impaired hepatic, cardiac, or renal function. Rule out cancer before prescribing. Lower doses require a non-hormonal contraceptive method because ovulation may not be suppressed. Watch closely for virilization.
ADMINISTRATION AND DOSAGE SPECIFICS:
Endometriosis: Give 400 mg po twice a day for 3-6 months. May continue for 9 months. Use only for those who cannot tolerate other drugs or who fail to respond. Begin therapy during menstruation to rule out pregnancy. Use lowest effective dose.
Fibrocystic breast disease: Give 50 to 200 mg po twice a day for 4-6 months. Begin during menstruation. Use only when pain is severe.
Hereditary angioedema: Begin with 200 mg po two or three times a day. After symptoms are relieved, reduce dosage by 1/2 every 1-3 months. Adjust dosage to prevent episodes of edema.

FLUOXYMESTERONE

PRODUCTS (TRADE NAME):
Halotestin (Available in 2, 5, and 10 mg tablets.) **Ora-Testryl** (Available in 5 mg tablets.) **Android-f** (Available in 10 mg tablets.)
DRUG SPECIFICS:
Gastrointestinal disturbances are more frequent with this product than with other oral androgens.
ADMINISTRATION AND DOSAGE SPECIFICS:
Hypogonadism: Give 2 to 10 mg/day po.
Breast cancer: Give 15 to 30 mg/day po in divided doses.

METHYLTESTOSTERONE

PRODUCTS (TRADE NAME):
Android (Available in 10 and 25 mg tablets, 5 mg buccal tablets.) **Metandren** (Available in 10 and 25 mg tablets and 5 and 10 mg buccal tablets.) **Methyltestosterone, Oreton Methyl** (Available in 10 and 25 mg tablets and 10 mg buccal tablets.) **Testred** (Available in 10 mg capsules.) **Virilon** (Available in 10 mg timed release capsules and in generic preparations.)
DRUG SPECIFICS:
Teach patients that no drinking, eating, smoking, or chewing should be done until tablet is absorbed buccally. Patients should rinse mouth and brush teeth following absorption. Check mouth each visit for signs of local irritation.
ADMINISTRATION AND DOSAGE SPECIFICS:
Male eunuchism: Give 10 to 40 mg/day po; 5-20 mg buccal.
Androgen deficiency: Give 10 to 40 mg/day po; 5-20 mg buccal.
Undescended testicle after puberty: Give 30 mg/day po; 15 mg buccal.
Female breast cancer: Give 200 mg/day po; 100 mg buccal.

TESTOSTERONE PROPIONATE

PRODUCTS (TRADE NAME):
Oreton Propionate (Available in 10 mg buccal tablets.)
DRUG SPECIFICS:
Useful in adult hypogonadism. This product will not produce full sexual maturity in prepubertal androgen deficiencies. Teach patient that no drinking, eating, smoking, or chewing should be done until buccal tablet is absorbed. Patients should rinse mouth and brush teeth each time after buccal absorption. Check mouth each visit for signs of local buccal irritation.
ADMINISTRATION AND DOSAGE SPECIFICS:
Male eunuchism: Give 10 to 40 mg/day po; 5-20 mg buccal.
Androgen deficiency: Give 10 to 40 mg/day po; 5-20 mg buccal.
Undescended testicle after puberty: Give 30 mg/day po; 15 mg buccal.
Female breast cancer: Give 200 mg/day po; 100 mg buccal.

L. Colette Jones

ESTROGENS

ACTION OF THE DRUG: Exogenous estrogens cause: (1) development of both primary and secondary sex characteristics including growth and development of the uterine musculature and endothelium, vaginal epithelium, and fallopian tubes; development of breasts, including growth of ducts, nipples, and stroma; fat deposition and enlargement and darkening of the areolae; increased cervical mucus and decreased vaginal pH; increased uterine motility; growth of axillary and pubic hair; (2) uterine bleeding after withdrawal of the drug or with long-term therapy; (3) decreased long-bone growth in prepubertal and pubertal girls; (4) decreased calcium loss from bones. They suppress the release of gonadotropins (FSH and LH) from the pituitary through a poorly defined feedback mechanism. Estrogens are anabolic and cause retention of salt, water, and nitrogen, an increase in serum lipoproteins and triglycerides, and a decrease in cholesterol. They suppress ovulation when given in adequate doses. Excretion is through the kidneys.

ASSESSMENT:

INDICATIONS: Estrogens are used for therapy in menopause or other conditions in which the natural estrogens are decreased, such as hypopituitarism, ovarian failure, primary amenorrhea, sexual infantilism, oophorectomy, and kraurosis vulvae. They are used in infertility workups to test integrity of the endometrium and for palliative therapy in prostatic and breast cancer that is at least five years postmenopausal. Probably effective for treatment of postmenopausal osteoporosis when used with other measures.

SUBJECTIVE: For all ages obtain a detailed menstrual history and history of any thromboembolic events, migraine headaches, liver or kidney problems. For pubertal ages ask about primary amenorrhea and sexual infantilism. For women of childbearing age, ask about history of ovarian failure, need for contraception, and dysmenorrhea. For patients of perimenopausal age obtain history of hot flashes, menstrual irregularities, dyspareunia, vaginal discharge, vulvar pruritus, urinary frequency, breast diseases, history of oophorectomy, or hysterectomy.

OBJECTIVE: For all ages obtain blood pressure and Papanicolaou smear. Assess for body contour, hair distribution, breast development and presence of masses, renal and hepatic function, and perform a complete internal and external examination of genitalia. For pubertal patients examine for underdeveloped secondary sex characteristics. For women of childbearing age also complete abdominal exam, look for signs of endometriosis, and rule out structural problems in menstrual dysfunction. In menopausal women assess for atrophic vaginitis, fibroids, genital bleeding, decalcification of bones, redistribution of body contours, breast cancer, balding, or appearance of beard. In men for whom estrogen therapy is contemplated, advanced prostate or breast cancer is usually present.

PLAN:

CONTRAINDICATIONS: Do not use in the presence of pregnancy, breast-feeding, estrogen-dependent neoplasms (except in selected postmenopausal women with breast cancer). Estrogen is also contraindicated in patients with gallbladder disease, thromboembolic disease or thrombophlebitis, metastatic bone disease, undiagnosed abnormal vaginal bleeding, and porphyria. Relatively contraindicated in uterine fibroids, hypertension, cardiac disease, liver or renal dysfunction, depression, migraine headaches, and benign cystic breast disease.

WARNINGS: There is an increased dose-related risk of thromboembolic disease, especially in premenopausal women. For this reason, estrogens are no longer used for suppression of lactation. They should not be used during pregnancy, especially the first three months, because of the risk of congenital anomalies and of vaginal adenosis and/or vaginal or cervical cancer when female offspring reach childbearing age. There is an increased risk of gallbladder disease with long-term use. Postmenopausal estrogen therapy is associated with a 5 to 15 times increased risk of endometrial cancer, the risk being related to the length of treatment. Rare, benign hepatic adenomas that can rupture with injury have been associated with oral contraceptives. Administration of estrogen may result in hypercalcemia in patients with breast or bone cancer. Blood pressure may increase and glucose tolerance decrease following estrogen therapy.

PRECAUTIONS: Estrogen therapy affects many systems. When used before puberty, short stature and decreased growth can result. Use in adult women can increase the risk for thromboembolic disease, migraine headaches, hypertension, diabetes, certain benign and malignant tumors. Because estrogens are metabolized in the liver and excreted through the kidneys, renal or hepatic dysfunction can alter their actions. Fibroid tumors of the uterus (leiomyomas) may increase in size. Because fluid is retained, symptoms of hypertension, asthma, epilepsy, migraine, and heart or kidney dysfunction may be increased. Topical estrogens are readily absorbed and may have systemic effects.

IMPLEMENTATION:

DRUG INTERACTIONS: Rifampin and barbiturates may reduce estrogenic effect. Estrogens may reduce the effects of oral anticoagulants, tricyclic antidepressants, anticonvulsants, and antidiabetic agents. They may potentiate anti-inflammatory or glycosuric effects of hydrocortisone and the effect of meperidine. Many diagnostic test results are altered: BSP is increased; some thyroid function tests (PBI and T_4) are elevated while T_3 is decreased; serum glucose, cortisone levels, prothrombin and some clotting factors (VII, VIII, IX, X), sodium, calcium, pyridoxine, folate levels, cholesterol, and total serum lipids may be altered.

ADMINISTRATION AND DOSAGE: Estrogens can be given orally, intramuscularly, or topically. For control of menopausal symptoms, ovarian failure, or post-oophorectomy symptoms, they are usually given cyclically with one tablet daily for 3 weeks, followed by one week off the drug. Combining cyclic estrogen therapy with an overlapping cycle of progestins usually produces cyclic uterine bleeding and may decrease the excess risk of uterine cancer. Usually, the lowest effective dose is given for the shortest period of time. High doses or long-term therapy should be tapered gradually. Topical (vaginal) estrogens are readily absorbed and may result in systemic effects.

IMPLEMENTATION CONSIDERATIONS:
—Obtain a complete health history to rule out presence of pregnancy, breast-feeding or breast disease, uterine fibroids, abnormal vaginal bleeding, cancer,

thromboembolic events, migraine headaches, gallbladder, liver, or kidney disease. Take a good menstrual history and history of menopausal symptoms and signs.

—Perform a thorough physical examination, including genitalia, Papanicolaou smear, blood pressure, weight, and eye exam.

—Observe for edema. Patients on replacement therapy should be monitored regularly.

—Monitor for thrombophlebitis.

—Monitor men for feminizing characteristics and impotence.

WHAT THE PATIENT NEEDS TO KNOW:

—Estrogenic drugs, by law, must be dispensed with a patient package insert entitled "What You Should Know About Estrogens." When you receive your prescription be certain to look for this package insert and to read it thoroughly.

—Some patients experience side effects when taking this medication. If you experience any of the following symptoms, stop taking the medication and notify your health care provider immediately: chest pain, abdominal or leg pain or swelling, sudden severe headaches, visual changes, sudden loss of coordination, sudden shortness of breath, slurred speech.

—Discontinue drug immediately if you believe you are pregnant.

—Less dangerous symptoms that require care or consultation with your health provider are: changes in vaginal bleeding or discharge, skin rash, breast lumps, jaundice, increased blood pressure, abdominal pain, and mental depression.

—Nausea and breast tenderness may occur early in therapy but should be reduced after 1-3 weeks. Taking oral medicines with food may reduce nausea.

—Less common side effects are changes in libido (sex drive), photosensitivity, chloasma (facial skin changes often seen in pregnancy), and vomiting.

—Use of estrogens for replacement is associated with an increased risk of developing endometrial cancer. Any vaginal bleeding after menopause should be reported. (Cyclic uterine bleeding may occur with some types of therapy.)

—If surgery is anticipated, the surgeon should be notified so that doses may be changed or discontinued temporarily.

—Patients of all ages should be monitored regularly while on any estrogen preparation.

—Pills should be taken exactly as directed and kept out of the reach of children or anyone for whom they are not prescribed.

EVALUATION:

ADVERSE REACTIONS: *Cardiovascular:* edema, hypertension, thrombophlebitis or embolism. *CNS:* mental depression, increase in migraine headaches, stroke. *Dermatologic:* chloasma, skin rash. *Endocrine:* decreased glucose tolerance. *Eye:* change in corneal contour, intolerance to contact lenses. *Gastrointestinal:* abdominal cramping, cholestatic jaundice, diarrhea, liver adenoma (rare), nausea, vomiting. *Reproductive:* breast tenderness and enlargement, changes in vaginal bleeding, dysmenorrhea, endometrial cancer, exacerbation of estrogen-dependent malignancies, increase in size of uterine fibroids, vaginal candidiasis. *Other:* changes in weight, libido.

OVERDOSAGE: *Signs and symptoms:* An oral overdose may produce nausea. No serious side effects have been noted from accidental ingestion of oral contraceptives by children. Females may have withdrawal vaginal bleeding after an overdose.

PARAMETERS TO MONITOR: In the absence of side effects, patients on estrogen replacement should be seen every six months to one year for a complete health history and physical including breast, abdominal, pelvic examination with Papanicolaou smear, weight, blood pressure, and monitoring of renal and hepatic function. Those on oral contraceptives should be seen after 1-3 months of therapy, then at 6-12 month intervals to monitor for adverse reactions and proper administration. Patient education regarding side effects should be reinforced.

Counseling and active listening to women undergoing menopause may enhance well-being and allow a reduction of dose or discontinuation of the drug. Efforts should be made to assess and treat psychosocial problems related to menopause. Adequate calcium and Vitamin D intake and exercise enhances the prevention of postmenopausal bone decalcification.

Young women with primary amenorrhea may need referral for counseling. When used for palliative therapy in cancer, side effects and efficacy of treatment should be monitored frequently, depending on the stage of the illness. The nurse should monitor the patient's adjustment to a terminal illness and provide support.

CHLOROTRIANISENE

PRODUCTS (TRADE NAME):
TACE (Available in 12, 25 and 72 mg capsules.)
DRUG SPECIFICS:
This is a long-acting estrogen that is retained and released gradually from adipose tissue. For this reason it is not widely used.
ADMINISTRATION AND DOSAGE SPECIFICS:
Postpartum breast engorgement: Give 12 mg po 4 times a day for 7 days or 50 mg every 6 hours for 6 doses, beginning within 8 hours post partum. The 72 mg capsule can be given twice a day for 2 days.
Prostatic cancer: Give 12 to 25 mg po daily (palliative.)
Menopausal vasomotor symptoms, atrophic vaginitis or kraurosis vulvae: Give 12 to 25 mg po daily in 30 day cycles for 1 or 2 cycles.
Female hypogonadism: Give 12 to 25 mg po daily in 21-day cycles. May be combined with progestin therapy.

CONJUGATED ESTROGENS—ORAL

PRODUCTS (TRADE NAME):
   Conjugated Estrogen (Available in 0.3, 0.625, 1.25, and 2.5 mg tablets.) **Evestrone** (Available in 0.625 mg tablets.) **Premarin** (Available in 0.3, 0.625, 1.25 and 2.5 mg tablets.)

DRUG SPECIFICS:
   Contains 50-65% sodium estrone sulfate and 20-35% sodium equilin sulfate. These are naturally occurring and extracted from the urine of pregnant mares. It is required that oral estrogen products have a package insert which can be given to patients. They are available as generic drugs. Store in closed containers.

ADMINISTRATION AND DOSAGE SPECIFICS:
   Medication should be given for 3 weeks on a daily basis, with one week off the medication.
   Menopause (natural or surgical) vasomotor symptoms: Start on 1.25 mg po daily. Adjust to lowest dose that controls symptoms.
   Female hypogonadism: Use 2.5 to 7.5 mg po daily. Cycle 20 days on, 10 days off, until bleeding occurs.
   Atrophic vaginitis: Use 0.3 to 1.25 mg po daily. Adjust for therapeutic response.
   Osteoporosis: Cycle 1.25 mg po daily for 3 weeks, 1 week off. "Probably effective" if used with calcium and vitamin D.
   Breast cancer: Give 10 mg po 3 times a day for at least 3 months (palliative.)
   Prostatic cancer: Give 1.25 to 2.5 mg po 3 times a day (palliative.)

DIETHYLSTILBESTROL (DES)

PRODUCTS (TRADE NAME):
   Diethylstilbestrol (Available in 0.1, 0.25, 0.5, 1 and 5 mg regular or enteric coated tablets and 0.1 and 0.5 mg suppositories.)

DRUG SPECIFICS:
   This usually inexpensive product is used primarily in menopausal or postmenopausal women for the control of symptoms. It may also be used in inoperative breast or prostatic cancer which is progressing. Much attention has also been paid to the use of DES for postcoital contraception in emergency treatment. Perform a pregnancy test prior to use. It is not to be used for routine birth control and repeated courses should be avoided. Effectiveness as an emergency birth control product rests upon the time interval between coitus and when therapy is begun. See section on Estrogen-Vaginal Suppositories for more information.

ADMINISTRATION AND DOSAGE SPECIFICS:
   Female hypogonadism, female castration or primary ovarian failure: 0.2 to 0.5 mg daily given cyclically.
   Menopausal-related vasomotor symptoms, atrophic vaginitis, or kraurosis vulvae: 0.2 to 0.5 mg daily on cyclic short-term basis only.

Severe atrophic vaginitis: 0.2-2 mg/day given cyclically; may give for several years. May also use 1 mg/day of vaginal suppository form for 10 to 14 days concomitantly with the oral form. If only suppository form is utilized, dosage is up to 5 to 7 mg weekly.

Prostatic carcinoma (progressive and inoperable): Give 3 mg/day initially, decreasing to 1 mg/day as therapy progresses.

Breast cancer (progressive and inoperable): Give 15 mg/day in postmenopausal women and selected men.

Postcoital contraception: Give 25 mg twice daily for 5 consecutive days, beginning within 24 hours after coitus. Do not give later than 72 hours after coitus. Should not be used as a routine method of birth control.

ESTERIFIED ESTROGENS

PRODUCTS (TRADE NAME):

Estratab (Available in 0.3, 0.625, 1.25, and 2.5 mg tablets.) **Evex** (Available in 0.625 and 1.25 mg tablets.) **Menest** (Available in 0.3, 0.625, 1.25, and 2.5 mg tablets.)

DRUG SPECIFICS:

These products contain 75-85% sodium estrone sulfate and 6-15% sodium equilin sulfate. They are available as a generic drug. Store medication in a tightly closed container.

ADMINISTRATION AND DOSAGE SPECIFICS:

Vasomotor menopausal (natural or surgical) symptoms: Use 0.3 to 3.75 mg po/day. Adjust to lowest dose that controls symptoms for short-term therapy. Cycle with a progestin for replacement.

Female hypogonadism: Use 2.5 to 7.5 mg po daily. Cycle 20 days on medication, 10 days off, until bleeding occurs.

Atrophic vaginitis and kraurosis vulvae: Use 0.3 to 1.25 mg po daily. Cycling recommended.

Breast cancer: Use 10 mg three times a day for 2-3 months (palliative).

Prostatic cancer: Use 1.25 to 2.5 mg po three times a day (palliative).

ESTRADIOL

PRODUCTS (TRADE NAME):

Estrace (Available in 1 and 2 mg tablets.)

DRUG SPECIFICS:

See oral estrogens.

ADMINISTRATION AND DOSAGE SPECIFICS:

Vasomotor menopausal symptoms, atrophic vaginitis, kraurosis vulvae, or re-placement therapy in hypogonadism or female castration, ovarian failure: Give 1-2 mg po per day cycled 3 weeks on and 1 week off. Use lowest therapeutic dosage. Use short-term therapy only for relief of kraurosis vulvae, atrophic vaginitis, and vasomotor symptoms.

ESTROPIPATE OR PIPERAZINE ESTRONE SULFATE

PRODUCTS (TRADE NAME):

Ogen (Available in 0.625, 1.25, 2.5 and 5 mg tablets.)

DRUG SPECIFICS:

This drug is composed of crystalline estrone and piperazine for stability.

ADMINISTRATION AND DOSAGE SPECIFICS:

Atrophic vaginitis, kraurosis vulvae, or vasomotor menopausal symptoms: Cycle 3 weeks on, 1 week off with 0.625 to 5 mg per day. Use lowest dose to control symptoms.

Female hypogonadism, primary ovarian failure: Cycle with 0.625 to 5 mg per day. Several cycles may be necessary for therapeutic effect.

ETHINYL ESTRADIOL

PRODUCTS (TRADE NAME):

Estinyl (Available in 0.02, 0.05, and 0.5 mg tablets.) **Feminone** (Available in 0.05 mg tablet.)

DRUG SPECIFICS:

This is the most active synthetic estrogen known.

ADMINISTRATION AND DOSAGE SPECIFICS:

Vasomotor menopausal symptoms: Use 0.02 to 0.05 mg po per day cycled 3 weeks on, 1 week off. Use decreasing doses as menopause progresses. Use lowest effective dose.

Female hypogonadism: Use 0.05 mg 1-3 times per day for 2 weeks. Cycle with 2 weeks of progesterone for 2-3 cycles, then discontinue 2 months to observe ther-apeutic effect.

Female breast cancer: Use 1 mg three times a day (palliative.)

Prostatic cancer: Use 0.15 mg to 2 mg po per day (palliative.)

QUINESTROL

PRODUCTS (TRADE NAME):
Estrovis (Available in 100 mcg tablets.)
DRUG SPECIFICS:
See oral conjugated estrogens and general monograph about oral estrogens. This drug is lipid soluble and stored in body fat, resulting in slower release over several days.
ADMINISTRATION AND DOSAGE SPECIFICS:
Vasomotor menopausal symptoms, atrophic vaginitis, kraurosis vulvae, female hypogonadism or castration, primary ovarian failure: Give 1 tablet per day for 7 days, then 1 tablet weekly. Adjust dose to 2 tablets weekly if needed for therapeutic response.

VAGINAL CREAMS

PRODUCTS (TRADE NAME):
DV, Estraguard (Available in .01% cream.) **Ogen** (Available in 1.5 mg/gm cream.) **Ortho Dienestrol** (Available in .01% cream.) **Premarin** (Available in 0.625 mg/gm cream.)
DRUG SPECIFICS:
These preparations are used vaginally and on the vulvae to treat atrophic epithelial changes due to low estrogen levels. See Estrogen section for further information, warnings, and precautions. Can be absorbed systemically and produce side effects. Most effective when used at bedtime. Contain various synthetic estrogens.
ADMINISTRATION AND DOSAGE SPECIFICS:
Give 2 to 4 gm daily. Use applicator which is included, or rub on topically. Reduce to the lowest dosage for shortest time that will control symptoms.

VAGINAL SUPPOSITORIES

PRODUCTS (TRADE NAME):
Diethylstilbestrol (Available in 0.1 and 0.5 mg suppositories.) **DV** (Available as dienestrol 0.7 mg suppositories.)
DRUG SPECIFICS:
This medication is used vaginally to treat atrophic epithelial changes due to low estrogen levels. It is most effective when inserted before bedtime. See drug

monograph on Estrogens for warnings and precautions. Enough estrogen can be absorbed vaginally to give a systemic action.

ADMINISTRATION AND DOSAGE SPECIFICS:

Insert 1 or 2 tablets vaginally with applicator before retiring each night for 2 weeks. Use lowest dose for shortest time that will control symptoms, i.e., may reduce dose to one suppository nightly after 2 weeks.

L. Colette Jones

ORAL CONTRACEPTIVES

ACTION OF THE DRUG: Oral contraceptives are combination drugs that contain both an estrogen and a progestin. The principal action is to prevent ovulation through inhibition of the follicle-stimulating hormone (FSH) and the luteinizing hormone (LH). The progestin-only "mini-pill" inhibits ovulation by the same mechanism but is more variable in suppressing the gonadotropins. The progestins in both types of oral contraceptive pills have several other contraceptive effects: creating a thick cervical mucus hostile to sperm; decelerating ovum transport by decreasing motility of the fallopian tubes; and inhibiting implantation.

ASSESSMENT:

INDICATIONS: Oral contraceptives are used for the prevention of pregnancy when a highly effective method is needed and heterosexual activity is regular. Some of the products with higher mestrahol content are now used principally for the treatment of hypermenorrhea, endometriosis, and to produce withdrawal bleeding.

SUBJECTIVE: Determine the need for contraception. Take a thorough menstrual, contraceptive, and reproductive history. Check for history of endometriosis, gallbladder disease, abnormal vaginal bleeding, cancer, diabetes, high blood pressure, migraines, cholestatic jaundice, liver tumors, stroke or other thromboembolic events, uterine fibroids, depression, porphyria, smoking, and drug history. Make certain the patient is not breast-feeding or pregnant. Assess knowledge of contraceptive methods and sexual activity.

OBJECTIVE: Perform a gynecological and breast examination to rule out organic disease, structural problems, or pregnancy. Papanicolaou smear should be obtained. Inspect patient for body type, acne, and hair distribution. Use urine dipstick to screen for diabetes. Obtain blood pressure and weight.

PLAN:

CONTRAINDICATIONS: *Absolute contraindications:* history or presence of thromboembolic disorders, cerebrovascular accident, coronary artery disease, hepatic adenoma, malignancy of breast or reproductive system, known impairment of liver function, pregnancy.

In the following three paragraphs, * indicates contraindications to estrogen-containing pills which may not be contraindications to progestin-only pills or may be less of a contraindication to progestin-only pills than to combined pills. ** indicates some believe this to be an absolute contraindication.

Strong relative contraindications: severe headaches (particularly vascular or migraine),* hypertension (with resting diastolic BP of 90 or greater on three or more separate visits, or an accurate measurement of 110 or more on a single visit),* diabetes,* prediabetes or a strong family history of diabetes, gallbladder disease, including cholecystectomy,* previous cholestasis during pregnancy, congenital hyperbilirubinemia (Gilbert's disease), mononucleosis (acute phase), sickle cell disease (SS) or sickle C disease (SC),* undiagnosed, abnormal vaginal bleeding,** elective surgery (planned in next 4 weeks or major surgery requiring immobilization),* long leg casts or major injury to lower leg, patient over 40 years of age,* patient over 35 years of age with a history of heavy smoking,* impaired liver function within the past year.

Other relative contraindications: termination of term pregnancy within past 10-14 days,* weight gain of 10 pounds or more while on the "pill",* failure to have established regular menstrual cycles,* profile suggestive of anovulation and infertility problems (late onset of menses and very irregular, painless menses),* presence of or history of cardiac or renal disease,* conditions likely to make patient unreliable at following dosage instructions (mental retardation, major psychiatric problems, alcoholism, history of repeatedly taking pills incorrectly),* lactation (oral contraceptives may be initiated as weaning begins and may be an aid in decreasing the flow of milk)*.

May initiate the pill for women with these problems and observe carefully for worsening or improvement of the problem: depression,* hypertension (with resting diastolic BP at a single visit of 90-99),* presence of or history of chloasma or hair loss related to pregnancy,* asthma,* epilepsy,* uterine fibromyoma,* acne, varicose veins,* history of hepatitis (but liver function tests normal now and for at least one year).

WARNINGS: The use of oral contraceptives is associated with an increased risk of thromboembolic disorders, strokes, myocardial infarctions, visual disorders, hepatic tumors, gallbladder disease, hypertension, and fetal abnormalities. Smoking further increases the risk of thromboembolic events. This risk increases with age and more than 15 cigarettes per day. Women who take contraceptives should be advised not to smoke.

If possible, pills should be discontinued 4 weeks prior to surgery or during prolonged immobilization. Oral contraceptives should not be given during pregnancy or if pregnancy is planned within three months because of the increased risk of fetal malformation. Prediabetic or diabetic patients should be monitored closely for a decrease in glucose tolerance. Triglycerides and phospholipid may also increase. Migraines may begin or may be exacerbated by birth control pills. Hypertension may worsen, especially with increased age. Although breakthrough bleeding may be a side effect, non-functional causes should be investigated. Bleeding irregularities are more common with progestin-only pills.

There is some risk of infertility after discontinuation of oral contraceptives, especially in women who have had irregular or scanty periods prior to taking pills.

Oral contraceptives interfere with lactation and are found in breast milk. In general, defer initiation until the infant is weaned.

PRECAUTIONS: Pills may cause fluid retention, thus aggravating cardiac or renal problems, migraines, seizure disorders or asthma. Significant mental depression is a reason for discontinuing pills until other causes have been determined. Uterine fibroids may increase in size with combination pills. If jaundice develops, discontinue pills. Because hormones are metabolized in the liver, patients with prior history of liver disease should be monitored closely. Pyridoxine and folate levels may be depressed, especially in women who become pregnant after discontinuing oral contraceptives. Some pills contain tartrazine which may trigger allergic reactions, especially in persons who are also aspirin sensitive. Do not prescribe pills for pregnant mothers or nursing mothers. Advise using another form of contraception for three or more months after discontinuation to reduce the risk of fetal defects if pregnancy should occur right away.

IMPLEMENTATION:

DRUG INTERACTIONS: There may be an increase in breakthrough bleeding and a decrease in contraceptive effectiveness in patients on rifampin, nitrofurantoin, ampicillin, isoniazid, neomycin, penicillin V, chloramphenicol, phenytoin, phenylbutazone, primidone, barbiturates, tetracyclines, sulfonamides, and carbamazepine.

Oral contraceptives may decrease the effectiveness of oral anticoagulants, antihypertensives, anticonvulsants, tricyclic antidepressants, oral hypoglycemics, and vitamins. Given with troleandomycin, the effect may be additive in causing jaundice.

Oral contraceptives may change some lab results: BSP, thyroid, urinary pregnanediol, serum glucose, ceruloplasmin, cortisone, phospholipids, clotting factors, sodium, pyridoxine, folate, amino acids, alkaline phosphatase, and nitrogen.

ADMINISTRATION AND DOSAGE: To be effective, oral contraceptives must be taken at a regular time each day. This is particularly true with progestin-only pills. Taking medication with meals will reduce the nausea common in the first cycles.

Combination pills: All oral combination contraceptives are to be taken for 21 days. Usually therapy is initiated the 5th day after or the Sunday after menstruation starts. Another method of contraception should be used for the first 7-10 days of the first cycle. Pills are packaged in a one-month packet with the days named or numbered. Following the 21-day therapy, some preparations have 7 pills to be taken daily that contain an inert substance or iron. Others prescribe 7 days without pills before starting another 28-day cycle. During the "rest," vaginal bleeding should occur.

Combination pills vary in the type and relative amounts of estrogen and progestin. All contain a combination of one estrogen and one progestin. Two estrogens, ethinyl estradiol and mestranol, are used. Mestranol is half as strong as ethinyl estradiol. Several progestins are used in combination with them. Some progestins are estrogenic, anti-estrogenic, and/or androgenic in effect. A dose of 50 mcg or less of estrogen is used to initiate therapy. Less than this dose may cause breakthrough bleeding, but increasingly, doses of less than 50 mcg are being prescribed. New combinations are introduced frequently.

Progestin-only pills: Medication is taken daily on a continuous basis.

IMPLEMENTATION CONSIDERATIONS:

—Obtain a complete health history, including past menstrual, reproductive, and contraceptive history, underlying systemic disease, other medications taken concurrently which may cause drug interactions, and specific information on cardiovascular, hepatic, and renal function.

—Patients must be taught precisely how to take oral contraceptives and what to do if a pill is missed.

—Side effects vary in severity. They may be a result of the relative strengths of estrogen and progestin. Side effects may be eliminated by changing to a different combination of estrogen and progestin. Some spotting can be tolerated in younger women.

—Pregnancy should not be attempted until three or more months after discontinuation of these pills.

—Patients should be screened carefully for any contraindications.

—Patients who have trouble remembering to take other medications are not good candidates for oral contraceptives.

—Patients must be fully informed about action, side effects, and the risk of adverse reactions. Other methods of contraception should be explained so that an informed choice can be made. Side effects should be reviewed at each visit.

—Prescribe three months of pills first, then have patient return. If there are no contraindications, a year's supply can be given. Patients should always have an extra month's supply on hand.

—"Resting" for a period of time without pills is no longer recommended. It does not seem to decrease the chance of becoming permanently anovulatory.

—Smokers should be advised to quit while on the pill because of the increased risk of thromboembolic events. This risk increases with age.

—Pills should be discontinued at least 4 weeks before surgery and if on prolonged bedrest.

WHAT THE PATIENT NEEDS TO KNOW:

—Take pills exactly as prescribed. If a pill is missed, follow the directions given by the health care provider. This may include using a backup method for a period of time. Another method should also be used in the first three weeks of the first cycle and if vomiting for several days occurs due to illness.

—Certain side effects should be reported to your health care provider immediately: pain in chest, groin, or legs; sudden, severe headaches; sudden slurring of speech; sudden loss of coordination; sudden visual changes; sudden shortness of breath. Other symptoms may require attention but are not emergencies: changes in vaginal bleeding; hypertension; breast lumps; jaundice; vaginal discharge; stomach or side pains; mental depression. Other side effects may be present but not serious: nausea, loss of appetite, acne, stomach cramps, edema of ankles and feet, breast swelling and tenderness, tiredness, brown spots on skin, changes in libido, changes in weight, increased body hair, some hair loss on scalp, sensitivity to the sun. If these persist or trouble you, report them to your health care provider.

—It is important to return for scheduled check-ups.

—Stop the pill immediately if you think you are pregnant or miss two periods. Do not take while breast-feeding.

—Keep one extra month's supply of pills on hand so there is no chance of running out and breaking the cycles.

—You should not smoke while taking the pill.

—All other medications you are taking should be reported to your health care provider because of possible drug interactions.

—For women under 40, the risk of death from complications from the pill is less than the risk of death from complications of pregnancy. (Patients should not be so frightened of taking the pill that they fail to recognize that it is safer statistically to take the pill than to be pregnant.)

EVALUATION:

ADVERSE REACTIONS: *Cardiovascular:* heart attack, pulmonary embolism, stroke, other thromboembolic events including retinal thrombosis, hypertension, edema. *CNS:* headache, irritability, mental depression, nervous tension, onset or worsening of migraines. *Dermatologic:* acne, chloasma. *Gastrointestinal:* benign liver tumors, bloating, cholestatic jaundice, nausea, vomiting. *Reproductive:* amenorrhea and/or infertility on discontinuation, breast enlargement and tenderness, galactorrhea, increase in size of fibroids. *Other:* onset or worsening of diabetes, weight gain.

Most adverse reactions are caused by hormonal imbalance and can be summarized in Table 7-5.

TABLE 7-5. SIDE EFFECTS OF ESTROGENS DUE TO HORMONAL IMBALANCE

Estrogen Excess: nausea, dizziness; edema and abdominal or leg pain with cyclic weight gain, bloating; leukorrhea; increase in fibroid size; chloasma; uterine cramps; irritability; increased fat deposition; cervical exotropia; poor contact lens fit; telangiectasia; vascular-type headache; hypertension; lactation suppression; headaches while taking pill; cystic breast changes; breast tenderness; increased breast size; thrombophlebitis; cerebrovascular infarction; myocardial infarction; hepatic adenoma.

Progestin Excess: increased appetite and weight gain (noncyclic); tiredness, fatigue, and weakness; depression and decrease in libido; oily scalp, acne; loss of hair; cholestatic jaundice; decreased length of menstrual flow; hypertension; headaches during "resting" phase of cycle; candidal vaginitis; increase in breast size (alveolar tissue); breast tenderness; decreased carbohydrate tolerance; dilated leg veins; pelvic congestion syndrome.

Androgen Excess: increased appetite and weight gain; hirsutism; acne; oily skin, rash; increased libido; cholestatic jaundice; pruritus.

TABLE 7-5. *(Continued)*

Estrogen Deficiency: irritability, nervousness; hot flashes, vasomotor symptoms; uterine prolapse, pelvic relaxation symptoms; early and mid-cycle spotting; decreased amount of menstrual flow; no withdrawal bleeding; decreased libido; diminished breast size; dry vaginal mucosa, atrophic vaginitis and dyspareunia; headaches; depression.

Progestin Deficiency: late breakthrough bleeding and spotting; heavy menstrual flow and clots; delayed onset of menses; dysmenorrhea; weight loss.

OVERDOSAGE: *Signs and symptoms:* headache, nausea, vomiting, breast tenderness and enlargement, withdrawal bleeding. *Treatment:* none. Problems are self-limiting.

PARAMETERS TO MONITOR: A complete history and physical examination should precede the prescribing of oral contraceptives, and this should be repeated at least yearly. Particular attention should be given to breasts, abdomen, pelvic organs, Papanicolaou smear, blood pressure, and weight. Cardiovascular, pulmonary, renal, or hepatic function studies should be obtained if there are any questions as to patient's underlying health. In the absence of adverse reactions, the patient should be seen 3-6 months after initiation of therapy, and if no changes in therapy are indicated, patient can be seen yearly. Each visit should include an interim history of possible side effects or adverse reactions, a review of proper administration, and a reminder of signs and symptoms to report.

ESTROGEN–PROGESTIN CONTRACEPTIVES

PRODUCTS (TRADE NAME):

A sample of products including the combination of estrogen and progestin are presented in Table 7-6. This list is not intended to be all-inclusive as new preparations are released and products are withdrawn frequently. Consult latest sources for new drug information.

DRUG SPECIFICS:

See general drug monograph for oral contraceptives.

ADMINISTRATION AND DOSAGE SPECIFICS:

Take one pill each day for 21 days beginning with the regimen the health care provider suggests, either starting the Sunday after a period begins or starting 5 days after the onset of the period. If there are 7 inert pills, take them following the 21 day cycle. If not, start a new pack after 7 days.

If one pill is missed, the forgotten one should be taken and a back-up contraceptive method used. If 2 pills are missed, 2 should be taken for 2 consecutive days and another method used until the end of the cycle. If 3 are missed, a new pack should be started on the 8th day or the first Sunday after the last pill was taken.

TABLE 7-6. COMPOSITION OF COMBINATION ORAL CONTRACEPTIVES

Trade Name	Estrogen	Progestin
Brevicon 21-day	ethinyl estradiol 35 mcg	norethindrone 0.5 mg
Brevicon 28-day	ethinyl estradiol 35 mcg	
Demulen 1/35 21-day	ethinyl estradiol 35 mcg	
Demulen 1/35 28-day	ethinyl estradiol 35 mcg	
Demulen and	ethinyl estradiol 50 mcg	ethynodiol diacetate 1 mg
Demulen 2%		
Enovid 5 mg	mestranol 75 mcg	norethynodrel 5 mg
Enovid 10 mg*	mestranol 150 mcg	norethynodrel 10 mg
Enovid-E	mestranol 100 mcg	norethynodrel 2.5 mg
Enovid-E 21	mestranol 100 mcg	norethynodrel 2.5 mg
Loestrin 21 1/20	ethinyl estradiol 20 mcg	norethindrone acetate 1 mg
Loestrin Fe 1/20	ethinyl estradiol 20 mcg	norethindrone acetate 1 mg
Loestrin 21 1.5/30	ethinyl estradiol 30 mcg	norethindrone acetate 1.5 mg
Loestrin Fe 1.5/30	ethinyl estradiol 30 mcg	norethindrone acetate 1.5 mg
LoOvral	ethinyl estradiol 30 mcg	norgestrel 0.3 mg
LoOvral 1-2%	ethinyl estradiol 30 mcg	norgestrel 0.3 mg
Modicon	ethinyl estradiol 35 mcg	norethindrone 0.5 mg
Modicon 28	ethinyl estradiol 35 mcg	northindrone 0.5 mg
Nordette	ethinyl estradiol 30 mcg	levonorgestrel 0.15 mg
Nordette-28	ethinyl estradiol 30 mcg	levonorgestrel 0.15 mg
Norinyl 1+35 21	ethinyl estradiol 35 mcg	norethindrone 1 mg
Norinyl 1+35 28	ethinyl estradiol 35 mcg	norethindrone 1 mg
Norinyl 1+50 21	mestranol 50 mcg	norethindrone 1 mg
Norinyl 1+50 2%	mestranol 50 mcg	norethindrone 1 mg
Norinyl 1+80 21	mestranol 80 mcg	norethindrone 1 mg
Norinyl 1+80 28	mestranol 80 mcg	norethindrone 1 mg
Norinyl 2 mg*	mestranol 100 mcg	norethindrone 2 mg
Norlestrin 21 1/50	ethinyl estradiol 50 mcg	norethindrone acetate 1 mg
Norlestrin 28 1/50	ethinyl estradiol 50 mcg	norethindrone acetate 1 mg
Norlestrin Fe 1/50	ethinyl estradiol 50 mcg	norethindrone acetate 1 mg
Norlestrin 21 2.5/50	ethinyl estradiol 0.05 mcg	norethindrone acetate 2.5 mg
Norlestrin Fe 2.5/50	ethinyl estradiol 50 mcg	norethindrone acetate 2.5 mg
Ortho-Novum 1/35-21	ethinyl estradiol 35 mcg	norethindrone 1 mg
Ortho-Novum 1/35-28	ethinyl estradiol 35 mcg	norethindrone 1 mg
Ortho-Novum 10/11 21	10 tablets of ethinyl estradiol 35 mcg _and_	norethindrone 0.5 mg followed by 11 tablets of ethinyl estradiol 35 mcg and norethindrone 1 mg
Ortho-Novum 10/11 28	10 tablets of ethinyl estradiol 35 mcg _and_	norethindrone 0.5 mg followed by 11 tablets of ethinyl estradiol 35 mcg and norethindrone 1 mg

TABLE 7-6. *(Continued)*

Trade Name	Estrogen	Progestin
Ortho-Novum 1/50-21	mestranol 50 mcg	norethindrone 1 mg
Ortho-Novum 1/50-28	mestranol 50 mcg	norethindrone 1 mg
Ortho-Novum 1/80-21	mestranol 80 mcg	norethindrone 1 mg
Ortho-Novum 1/80-28	mestranol 80 mcg	norethindrone 1 mg
Ortho-Novum 2 mg 21*	mestranol 100 mcg	norethindrone 2 mg
Ovcon-35	ethinyl estradiol 35 mcg	norethindrone 0.4 mg
Ovcon-50	ethinyl estradiol 50 mcg	norethindrone 1 mg
Ovral	ethinyl estradiol 50 mcg	norgestrel 0.5 mg
Ovral 28	ethinyl estradiol 50 mcg	norgestrel 0.5 mg
Ovulen	mestranol 100 mcg	ethynodiol diacetate 1 mg
Ovulen-21	mestranol 100 mcg	ethynodiol diacetate 1 mg
Ovulen-28	mestranol 100 mcg	ethynodiol diacetate 1 mg

*Also recommended for treatment of endometriosis, hypermenorrhea, and to produce withdrawal bleeding

Another birth control method must be used for 7 to 14 days, depending on the dosage. Follow instructions listed on package inserts.

PROGESTIN-ONLY CONTRACEPTIVES (MINI-PILLS)

PRODUCTS (TRADE NAME):
   Micronor, Nor-Q.D. (Available with 0.35 mg norethindrone). **Ovrette** (Available with 0.075 mg norgestrel).
DRUG SPECIFICS:
   Because progestin-only mini-pills must be taken at the same time each day to be most effective, they should be prescribed only for patients who are judged reliable in medication compliance. They are slightly less effective than the combination oral contraceptives in preventing pregnancy but are more effective than any other method. Incidence of pregnancy is highest in the first six months of use. It would be ideal to use an additional method of contraception during the first month or two in patients who want to incur no risk of pregnancy. Breakthrough bleeding is more common than with combination pills therefore, undiagnosed genital bleeding is an important contraindication, especially in older women. The mini-pill is particularly appropriate for those who have unacceptable side effects from the estrogens in combined

pills. Ovrette contains tartrazine, a product which may produce asthma-like symptoms in sensitive individuals.

ADMINISTRATION AND DOSAGE SPECIFICS:

For contraception: Take one pill at the same time every day continually. Do not stop during menses. If a pill is missed, take one as soon as remembered and continue at the regular time. If two are missed, take two a day for 2 days. In both cases, use a second method of birth control until menses occurs. If there is no menses for 45 days, have a pregnancy test done.

L. Colette Jones

PROGESTINS

ACTION OF THE DRUG: (1) Progestins cause the endometrium to become secretory following growth stimulated by estrogens. (2) They maintain the endometrium and vaginal epithelium and decrease uterine motility during pregnancy. (3) Acting with estrogen, they cause the acini of the breasts to become secretory and more vascular. (4) Some progestins have estrogenic or androgenic effects. (5) With doses of 5 mg or more of progesterone daily, a body temperature increase of 1 degree F is produced. (6) Progestins suppress pituitary gonadotropins through a feedback mechanism. (7) They can suppress ovulation, control uterine bleeding due to hormonal imbalance, increase sodium excretion, and cause a negative nitrogen balance.

ASSESSMENT:

INDICATIONS: Progestins are used for contraception, control of excessive uterine bleeding due to hormonal imbalance, treatment of secondary amenorrhea, abnormal bleeding due to hormone imbalance, and to control pain in endometriosis. They may be used in the diagnosis and treatment of infertility. Their use is palliative for endometrial cancer. When used for contraception, progestin-only preparations are known as "mini-pills." Progestins may be used in conjunction with estrogens for hormone replacement in natural or surgical menopause. Combination therapy may reduce the increased risk of endometrial cancer when estrogens are given alone.

SUBJECTIVE: Obtain menstrual history and assess for possibility of pregnancy, need for contraception, history of menorrhagia, perimenopausal symptoms, mental depression, migraines, thromboembolic disease, stroke, diabetes, infertility, renal or liver disease.

OBJECTIVE: On pelvic examination there should be no evidence of organic pathology (fibroids, cancer), no signs of pregnancy, undiagnosed or excessive vaginal bleeding, low hematocrit, abnormal Papanicolaou smear, signs of fluid retention, breast lumps, or impaired liver function.

PLAN:

CONTRAINDICATIONS: Do not use in the presence of pregnancy, breast-feeding, thromboembolic disease or history, poor liver function, undiagnosed uterine bleeding, breast or genital cancer. Not to be used for diagnosis of pregnancy.

WARNINGS: Progestins should not be used in pregnancy or as a diagnostic test of pregnancy because of teratogenic effects. They may also cause delay in the spontaneous abortion of a defective fetus.

PRECAUTIONS: Because progestins are metabolized in the liver, they should not be used in patients with impaired liver function. Progestins are secreted in breast milk with unknown effects on the infant. They increase the risk of thromboembolic events. They should not be used or continued when there is any undiagnosed vaginal bleeding until malignancy is ruled out. Possible fluid retention may exacerbate asthma, cardiac or renal disease, epilepsy, or migraine headaches. A few patients may experience mental depression. Administration of progestins is sometimes accompanied by a decrease in glucose tolerance.

IMPLEMENTATION:

DRUG INTERACTIONS: Progestins alter several laboratory tests: pregnanediol is increased as are BUN, serum acid phosphatase, and plasma amino acids.

ADMINISTRATION AND DOSAGE: Naturally occurring progestins (progesterone) are poorly absorbed orally; hence, oral progestins are synthetic products. Tablets are given daily. Progestins are quickly metabolized in the liver, but daily doses are effective. When given with estrogen for hormone replacement, progestins are added on mid cycle and given from about the 16th to the 25th day.

IMPLEMENTATION CONSIDERATIONS:

—Obtain a complete health history including a thorough menstrual and reproductive history, presence of mental depression, migraines, thromboembolic disease, cancer of breast or genitals, diabetes, liver disease, adverse reaction to other drugs containing progesterones (i.e., birth control pills), and possibility of pregnancy.

—Obtain blood pressure, weight, complete gynecological examination to rule out organic diseases of uterus and breast.

—Since progestins are metabolized in the liver, any compromise of hepatic function may cause jaundice.

—Patients receiving preparations with estrogenic effects must be monitored for thromboembolic events.

WHAT THE PATIENT NEEDS TO KNOW:

—When used for a short period to treat dysfunctional bleeding, progestins should first stop the bleeding and then cause the endometrial lining to shed when the drug is withdrawn. Improvement of heavy bleeding should occur in 24-48 hours.

—Breakthrough or withdrawal bleeding can occur, especially in long-term use for contraception.

—Report abnormal or unexplained vaginal bleeding to your health care provider.

—You should not take progestins if there is a history of breast or genital cancer except as palliative treatment in advanced disease.

—Possible side effects include weight gain, changes in menstruation or spotting between periods, and photosensitivity.

—Health care provider should be notified promptly if any of the following occur: sudden leg or chest pain, sudden shortness of breath, bloody sputum, severe headaches, loss of consciousness, slurred speech, visual changes, tenderness or swelling of legs, jaundice, dark urine or light-colored stools, or feelings of depression.

—This medication should not be used in pregnancy. Discontinue the drug immediately if pregnancy is suspected. If the drug is taken in the first four months of pregnancy, there may be adverse effects upon the fetus.

—Minor side effects may include nausea, spotting, and breast tenderness. Nausea should decrease after the first few menstrual cycles.

—Diabetic patients should tell their health provider if they begin developing positive urine tests so that antidiabetic medication can be adjusted.

EVALUATION:

ADVERSE REACTIONS: *Cardiovascular:* fluid retention (may aggravate cardiac conditions), heart attack, thromboembolic events including pulmonary embolism. *CNS:* dizziness, headache, mental depression, stroke. *Dermatologic:* chloasma, rashes. *Endocrine:* decrease in glucose tolerance, weight gain or loss. *Gastrointestinal:* cholestatic jaundice, diarrhea, nausea, vomiting. *Reproductive:* amenorrhea, breast tenderness or enlargement, decreased libido, galactorrhea, increased vaginal discharge, spotting, withdrawal bleeding. *Other:* fetal abnormalities, hirsutism, masculinization of female fetus.

OVERDOSAGE: *Signs and symptoms:* change in menses, nausea, vomiting, withdrawal bleeding. *Treatment:* symptomatic.

PARAMETERS TO MONITOR: In the absence of adverse reactions, patients should be seen every 6-12 months. Timing and characteristics of any vaginal bleeding should be noted to determine if response is therapeutic or adverse. Question patient about renal or liver problems. Do complete breast and pelvic exam with Papanicolaou smear. Emphasis on possible thromboembolic complications depends on estrogenic effects of particular drug. Observe for edema, weight gain, increased blood pressure.

MEDROXYPROGESTERONE ACETATE

PRODUCTS (TRADE NAME):
Amen, Curretab (Available in 10 mg tablets.) **Provera** (Available in 2.5 and 10 mg tablets.)
DRUG SPECIFICS:
This product has a wide range of cost, depending upon the manufacturer. The duration of action of this product is long and somewhat variable.

ADMINISTRATION AND DOSAGE SPECIFICS:

Secondary amenorrhea, abnormal uterine bleeding due to hormonal imbalance (no organic pathology): Give 5-10 mg po daily for 5-10 days, beginning on 16th or 21st day of menstrual cycle. Maximum therapeutic effect will be seen with 10 mg/day for 10 days beginning on 16th day of cycle. Withdrawal bleeding should occur 3-7 days after last dose. When given in combination with estrogens to reproduce a normal cycle, estrogen is given from the 1st to the 25th day, and progestin added from the 16th to the 25th day.

NORETHINDRONE

PRODUCTS (TRADE NAME):

Norlutin (Available in 5 mg scored tablets).

DRUG SPECIFICS:

This medication represents the only ingredient in some "mini-pill" contraceptives (Micronor and Nor-Q.D.). See general drug monograph on oral contraceptives for dosages. Take with meals to reduce nausea. Store in closed container. It is mandatory to give patient a package insert when prescription is dispensed. This medication is mildly androgenic and could cause masculinization of a female fetus.

ADMINISTRATION AND DOSAGE SPECIFICS:

Amenorrhea or uterine bleeding due to hormonal imbalance: Give 5 to 20 mg per day on the 5th to 25th day of the menstrual cycle.

Endometriosis: Give 10 mg per day for 2 weeks, increasing 5 mg at 2-week intervals until a total dose of 30 mg is reached. Continue 6-9 months or until breakthrough bleeding occurs. Then it can be stopped temporarily. The object of therapy is to prevent menstruation.

NORETHINDRONE ACETATE

PRODUCTS (TRADE NAME):

Norlutate (Available in 5 mg scored tablets).

DRUG SPECIFICS:

This medication is twice as strong as norethindrone. It is mildly androgenic and could cause masculinization of a female fetus. Take with meals to reduce nausea. Store in a closed container. It is mandatory that package insert be given to patient when prescription is dispensed.

ADMINISTRATION AND DOSAGE SPECIFICS:

Amenorrhea or uterine bleeding due to hormonal imbalance: Give 2.5 to 10 mg per day on 5th to 25th day of the menstrual cycle.

Endometriosis: Give 5 mg for 2 weeks, increasing 2.5 mg at 2-week intervals until a dose of 15 mg per day is reached. Continue 6-9 months or until breakthrough bleeding occurs. Then it can be stopped temporarily. The object of therapy is to prevent menstruation.

L. Colette Jones

THYROID PREPARATIONS

ANTITHYROID PRODUCTS

ACTION OF THE DRUG: The main action of antithyroid products is to inhibit the synthesis of thyroid hormones. They are the main drugs used in the treatment of hyperthyroidism. These agents do not inactivate or inhibit the thyroid hormones, thyroxine T_4 or triiodothyronine T_3, which are already stored or circulating in the blood.

ASSESSMENT:

INDICATIONS: These products are used in the treatment of hyperthyroidism or to improve hyperthyroidism in preparation for surgery or radioactive iodine therapy. Treatment is designed to alter the physiological changes in hyperthyroidism, such as increased catabolism, calorigenesis, and enhanced sensitivity to catecholamines, due to excess secretion of thyroid hormones: While it may not be common for the nurse to prescribe this medication, it is frequently the responsibility of the nurse practitioner to monitor the progress of the patient taking this medication.

SUBJECTIVE: History of nervousness and/or tremor, palpitations, weight loss with increased appetite, heat intolerance and excessive sweating, emotional lability, and muscle weakness.

OBJECTIVE: Exophthalmos, lid lag, thyroid enlargement (a bruit may be heard in severe cases of hyperthyroidism, Grave's disease), tachycardia, increased blood pressure, tremor, brisk reflexes, warm, moist, smooth skin, proximal muscle weakness. Weight loss and the signs of congestive heart failure may be the predominant manifestations of hyperthyroidism in the elderly.

Laboratory findings may show: elevated free T_4 index, increased T_3, decreased TSH.

PLAN:

CONTRAINDICATIONS: Do not give in presence of hypersensitivity to antithyroid products.

WARNINGS: Careful consideration should be given to the decision to use antithyroid drugs in pregnant women, because the drugs cross the placental barrier and could induce goiter or cretinism in the developing fetus. These drugs are also excreted in breast milk and the postpartum patient should not breast-feed her infant.

PRECAUTIONS: Agranulocytosis may develop. Sore throats, fever, skin eruptions, headaches, or general malaise should be monitored and reported. A maculopapular skin rash may occur but usually does not require discontinuation of medication. Hepatocellular damage is a rare side effect.

IMPLEMENTATION:

DRUG INTERACTIONS: The effect of anticoagulants are potentiated by propylthiouracil. Caution should be taken in administering antithyroid drugs to patients who are receiving additional drugs known to cause agranulocytosis, e.g., hydantoins.

ADMINISTRATION AND DOSAGE: The therapeutic objective is to correct the hypermetabolic state with a minimum of side effects and with the smallest incidence of hypothyroidism. Clinical response to the antithyroid drugs usually takes 1-2 weeks since they do not affect release of thyroid hormone. Response is dependent on the inhibition of thyroid hormone synthesis, the amount of preformed hormone in the gland, and the peripheral rate of conversion of the thyroid hormones. Generally, therapy is maintained for 12-24 months and then reduced to see if a remission occurs. Titration of dosage to gain maximal therapeutic response with the lowest dosage is the objective.

IMPLEMENTATION CONSIDERATIONS:

—Obtain a complete health history: hypersensitivity to antithyroid drugs, other medications taken concurrently which could cause drug interactions, possibility of pregnancy, or breast-feeding.

—Encourage compliance to therapy to avoid hyperthyroidism. The antithyroid drugs have a high incidence of achieving remission if taken correctly for 1-2 years.

—Instruct patient to report to health care provider any signs or symptoms of illness, particularly sore throat, skin rash, enlargement of cervical lymph nodes, fever, headache, general malaise, unusual bleeding, or bruising. A reduction or withdrawal of medication may be necessary.

—Propranolol, a beta-adrenergic blocking agent, may be used to control cardiovascular symptoms in severe hyperthyroidism.

WHAT THE PATIENT NEEDS TO KNOW:

—Take this medication exactly as directed by your health care provider.

—Since clinical response usually takes from 1-2 weeks to achieve, do not increase dosage until each dosage level can be individually evaluated.

—Some patients experience side effects from this drug. Report fever, sore throat, malaise, unusual bleeding or bruising, headache, skin rash, and enlargement of cervical lymph nodes (in the neck) to your health care provider at once.

—Bed rest, adequate diet, and avoidance of occupational and domestic stress are also useful modalities of therapy.

EVALUATION:

ADVERSE REACTIONS: *CNS:* drowsiness, headaches, neuritis, paresthesia, vertigo. *Gastrointestinal:* epigastric distress, jaundice, nausea, vomiting. *Hematopoietic:* agranulocytosis (rare), leukopenia (10% of patients), thrombocytopenia. *Hypersensitivity:* skin rash, urticaria. *Musculoskeletal:* arthralgia, myalgia. *Other:* edema, loss of hair, lymphadenopathy.

OVERDOSAGE: *Signs and symptoms:* Hypothyroidism may occur as a result of prolonged therapy. Agranulocytosis is a rare but serious occurrence. In addition, hepatitis, neuropathies, CNS stimulation or depression, and exfoliative dermatitis may occur. *Treatment:* Antithyroid drugs must be discontinued when fever, agranulocytosis, pancytopenia, hepatitis, or exfoliative dermatitis occur. Antibiotics, blood transfusions, and corticosteroids may be used to treat bone marrow depression. Hepatitis may be treated with rest and adequate diet.

PARAMETERS TO MONITOR: Laboratory blood work should be done prior to initiating antithyroid therapy and periodically once the patient is on a maintenance dose. Before initiating therapy, a WBC with differential is done and then repeated with any sign of infection. Serum T_4 and T_3 levels are monitored initially and after two weeks of therapy until a euthyroid state is achieved, usually 3-5 months. Once the patient has been euthyroid for 6-12 months, a decision may be made to reduce dosage and ascertain whether a remission has occurred. If remission is achieved, therapy is discontinued. Consultation and referral to a physician is warranted during the initiation and decision to maintain or end therapy.

During each visit monitor for signs and symptoms of infection, as well as correction of the hypermetabolic state: decreased pulse, decreased blood pressure, weight gain, elimination of nervousness and tremor. Evaluate for hepatitis, agranulocytosis, and gastrointestinal irritation.

METHIMAZOLE

PRODUCTS (TRADE NAME):
Tapazole (Available in 5 and 10 mg tablets.)

DRUG SPECIFICS:
Methimazole does not inhibit peripheral conversion of thyroxine to T3. It is more potent than propylthiouracil (PTU), and doses are one-tenth those of PTU. It acts more rapidly but less consistently than PTU.

ADMINISTRATION AND DOSAGE SPECIFICS:
Mild hyperthyroidism: Initial dosage 15 mg.
Moderate hyperthyroidism: Initial dosage 30 to 40 mg.
Severe hyperthyroidism: Initial dosage 60 mg divided into 3 doses given every 8 hours.
Maintenance Dose: 5 to 15 mg po daily.

PROPYLTHIOURACIL (PTU)

PRODUCTS (TRADE NAME):
   Propylthiouracil (Available in 50 mg tablets.)
DRUG SPECIFICS:
   PTU interferes with synthesis of and blocks peripheral conversion of T_4 to T_3. It may cause hypoprothrombinemia and bleeding.
ADMINISTRATION AND DOSAGE SPECIFICS:
   Usual dosage: Ranges between 100 to 150 mg po three times daily at 8-hour intervals. Initial dose is 300 mg po daily at 8-hour intervals with adjustments in dosage made after two weeks depending on free T_4 levels and symptoms. Continue therapy 6-18 months before tapering.
   Severe hyperthyroidism: The initial dosage is often 400 mg po daily.

Sheila Fitzgerald

THYROID HORMONES

ACTION OF THE DRUG: The main action of thyroid hormones is to increase metabolic rate. The mechanism of action is not completely understood. Increases in oxygen consumption, body temperature, heart and respiratory rate, cardiac output, and carbohydrate, lipid and protein metabolism are due to the increased metabolic rate. In addition, thyroid hormones influence growth and development of the skeletal system, especially ossification in the epiphyses of long bones.

ASSESSMENT:

INDICATIONS: Thyroid hormones are used in replacement therapy in management of hypothyroidism, myxedema, cretinism, and/or non-toxic goiter due to deficiency of thyroid hormones, atrophy, congenital defects, the effects of surgery, antithyroid products, or radiation. They are also used in treatment of chronic thyroiditis and thyrotropin-dependent tumors. The non-physician health practitioner should work closely with a physician during diagnosis and initial management of the patient with hypothyroidism. The nurse practitioner may take primary responsibility in monitoring the patient for effects of drug therapy and educating the patient about his or her disease.
   SUBJECTIVE: History of fatigue, weakness, lethargy, moderate weight gain (around 10 pounds) with minimal appetite, cold intolerance, menorrhagia, dry skin, coarse hair, hoarseness, impaired memory, constipation. These symptoms are insidious and non-specific and are due to decreased cellular metabolic processes or accumulation of a mucopolysaccharide in the subcutaneous tissue.
   OBJECTIVE: Skin changes include signs of myxedema: non-pitting edema, doughy skin, puffy face, large tongue, decreased body hair, cool dry skin. The thyroid

gland may be normal in size, enlarged, or not palpable depending on cause of hypothyroidism. Neurologic signs include: slow mentation, muscle weakness, slowed relaxation phase of the deep tendon reflexes, dull facial expression, or carpal tunnel syndrome. Cardiac signs include: bradycardia, decreased blood pressure. X-ray may indicate pericardial effusion or dilatation.

Laboratory findings are: reduced free T_4 index, elevated serum TSH. In moderate to severe hypothyroidism serum cholesterol, triglycerides, CPK, LDH, and SGOT may be elevated. An anemia of chronic disease may also be present.

PLAN:

CONTRAINDICATIONS: Do not use in presence of uncorrected adrenal insufficiency and acute myocardial infarction uncomplicated by hypothyroidism.

WARNINGS: Thyroid preparations have been used for treatment of obesity; large doses may cause serious toxicity. Careful consideration should be given as to whether to use thyroid preparations in pregnant and nursing mothers, as these drugs cross the placental barrier and may be found in breast milk. Use with caution in patients over 50 who are at risk for coronary disease or in patients with underlying coronary artery disease; angina, sinus tachycardia, or arrhythmias may be produced. When treating patients for hypothyroidism who have cardiovascular disease, the initial dosage should be reduced. Development of angina, hypertension, tachycardia, cardiac arrhythmias, and cardiac decompensation will necessitate a decrease in dosage. Adrenal insufficiency is difficult to exclude in severe or prolonged hypothyroidism; therefore, supplemental corticosteroids may be necessary to prevent precipitation of acute adrenocortical insufficiency. In the hypothyroid state, water excretion is decreased; overhydration and hyponatremia may occur.

IMPLEMENTATION:

DRUG INTERACTIONS: Catecholamines and epinephrine enhance cardiovascular effects of thyroid hormones and may precipitate coronary insufficiency in patients with coronary artery disease. Thyroid preparations may increase requirements for antidiabetic agents. When decreasing dosage of thyroid hormones, monitor for hypoglycemic reactions. Potentiation of anticoagulant effects may be caused by thyroid replacement due to increased hypoprothrombinemia. Cholestyramine decreases absorption of thyroid hormones from the GI tract, causing a decreased effect. Severe hypertension and tachycardia may result with concurrent use of ketamine. Corticosteroid requirements are increased due to increased tissue demands for patients on thyroid preparations. Effects of tricyclic antidepressants are enhanced by thyroid hormones.

ADMINISTRATION AND DOSAGE: Patients with hypothyroidism are very sensitive to thyroid preparations; therefore, treatment should begin in small doses and be increased gradually. A reduction in dosage and gradual upward adjustment may be necessary when side effects occur; withdraw therapy for 2-6 days, then resume at lower dose.

Age, presence of cardiac disease, and severity of symptoms need to be considered when initiating therapy. Titration of dosage to gain maximal therapeutic responses with the lowest dosage is the objective. The usual maintenance dose in treatment of hypothyroidism is .5-2 gm as a single daily dose before breakfast.

T_4 (thyroxine) is the treatment of choice for hypothyroidism because of its purity and long duration of action. Because T_4 has a slow onset of action, therapeutic effects may not occur for 3-4 weeks. T_3 (triiodothyronine), which has a rapid onset, may be administered if rapid correction of hypothyroidism is necessary.

The equivalent strengths of the various thyroid products are shown below to assist in changing from one product to another.

Drug	Dosage
Liotrix (T_4 and T_3)	50-60 mcg T_4 and 12.5-15 mcg T_3
Liothyronine (T_3)	25 mcg
Levothyroxine (T_4)	100 mcg (0.1 mcg)
Thyroglobulin	65 mg
Thyroid USP	65 mg

IMPLEMENTATION CONSIDERATIONS:

—Obtain a complete health history: other drugs which may produce drug interactions, presence of diabetes mellitus, cardiovascular disease, adrenocortical insufficiency, pregnancy.

—Dosage may need to be altered, depending upon the presence of other underlying disease.

—Clients over 50 are often very sensitive to thyroid hormones. It is important to begin client on a small dose and observe for signs and symptoms of cardiovascular disease before increasing dosage.

—Instruct the patient to take the medication at the same time every day, preferably before breakfast. If taken late in the day, insomnia may result.

—Inform patient that response to therapy is not immediate and that most patients begin to feel better within 2 weeks, and therapeutic results are often achieved in 3 months.

—Teach patients the signs and symptoms of hypothyroidism and hyperthyroidism so that they can monitor underdosage or overdosage themselves. Refer to Table 7-7.

—If symptoms of overdosage occur, stop medication for several days and initiate therapy at a lower dose.

—Since thyroid hormones may increase demands for antidiabetic agents, instruct diabetics to test urine for sugar and acetone three times a day until the response to the medication is stabilized.

WHAT THE PATIENT NEEDS TO KNOW:

—Take medications exactly as directed by health care provider. Take the medication at the same time every day, preferably before breakfast. If it is taken too late in the day it may make it difficult to go to sleep.

—Response to this medicine is not immediate. Symptoms should improve within 2 weeks. Do not increase medication unless instructed by health care provider. Taking the medication and compliance with therapy is extremely important.

—Report any changes in urine sugar and acetone test results if being treated concurrently for diabetes mellitus.

—Report bleeding or excessive bruising if on anticoagulant therapy.

—Check with the health care provider when taking any other medications. This will decrease the chance of drug interactions.

—Report signs and symptoms of overdosage (hyperthyroidism) or underdosage (hypothyroidism) to your health care provider promptly. See Table 7-7.

TABLE 7-7. SIGNS AND SYMPTOMS OF HYPERTHYROIDISM AND HYPOTHYROIDISM

Hyperthyroidism	Hypothyroidism
weight loss	weight gain
decreased or absent menstruation	excessive menstrual bleeding
rapid or pounding heart rates	low heart rate
heat intolerance	cold intolerance
nervousness/irritability	tiredness/weakness
diarrhea	constipation
sweaty skin	dry puffy skin
inability to fall asleep	sleepiness
fever	
chest pain	

EVALUATION:

ADVERSE REACTIONS: *Cardiovascular:* angina pectoris, arrhythmias, hypertension, palpitations, tachycardia. *CNS:* hand tremors, headache, heat intolerance, insomnia, irritability, nervousness. *Dermatologic:* sweating. *Gastrointestinal:* diarrhea, vomiting, weight loss. *Genitourinary:* menstrual irregularities. *Hypersensitivity:* rash, hives (rare.) *Other:* glycosuria, hyperglycemia, increased prothrombin time, increased serum cholesterol levels.

OVERDOSAGE: *Signs and symptoms:* Hypertension, tachycardia, palpitations, dyspnea, headache, irritability, nervousness, insomnia, tremors, diarrhea, nausea and vomiting may all occur due to increased metabolic rate. Angina pectoris or congestive heart failure may occur or be aggravated. *Treatment:* Cessation or reduction of therapy may be indicated. A lower dosage may be reinstituted several days later. Propranolol may be used to control tachycardia or arrhythmias.

PARAMETERS TO MONITOR: Periodic blood work should be done prior to initiating thyroid hormone therapy and once the patient is on a maintenance dose. These tests include: Free T_4, TSH level, T_3-Resin uptake (RT3U.) Periodic evaluation of electrolytes, blood glucose levels, serum cholesterol, ECG, CPK, SGOT, and LDH should occur, especially if overdosage is suspected. Monitor TSH and Free T_4 until patient is stable and then every 6 months.

If secondary hypothyroidism is suspected, evaluate adrenal function with an ACTH stimulation test. Evaluate for disappearance of signs and symptoms of hypothyroidism as therapeutic effect is exerted. Each visit look for resolution of fatigue, weight loss, normalization of myxedematous skin changes. Evaluate for signs and symptoms of overdosage. (See Table 7-7.)

LEVOTHYROXINE SODIUM (T_4, L-THYROXINE)

PRODUCTS (TRADE NAME):
Levothroid (Available in 0.025, 0.05, 0.1, 0.125, 0.15, 0.175, 0.2, 0.3 mg tablets and 100 and 200 mcg/ml injection.) **Noroxine** (Available in 0.2 mg tablets and 100 mcg/ml injection.) **Synthroid** (Available in 0.025, 0.05, 0.1, 0.15, 0.2, 0.3 mg tablets, 100 and 20o mcg/ml injection.)

DRUG SPECIFICS:
This medication is a synthetic preparation of thyroid hormone. It is the drug of choice because the effect is predictable. Avoid taking with food as absorption is incomplete and variable. Initiate therapy slowly in older patients and those with long-standing hypothyroidism, myxedematous infiltration or cardiovascular disease.

ADMINISTRATION AND DOSAGE SPECIFICS:
Initial therapy: Give 0.05 to 0.1 mg po daily with increases in dosage of 0.05 to 0.1 mg at 2 week intervals until therapeutic effect is achieved.
Maintenance dosage: 0.1 to 0.2 mg/day po.

LIOTHYRONINE SODIUM (T_3)

PRODUCTS (TRADE NAME):
Cytomel (Available in 5, 25, and 50 mcg tablets.)

DRUG SPECIFICS:
Liothyronine sodium contains a synthetic form of thyroid hormone. The advantage of this drug is the rapid effect and short duration of action which allows fast dosage adjustment and quick reversibility of overdosage. Monitor for cardiac side effects because rapid action increases metabolic demand. Therapeutic effects are achieved in 24-72 hours and persist up to 72 hours after withdrawal of drug. When transferring from other thyroid hormones to liothyronine, discontinue other preparation and initiate a low daily dose of liothyronine.

ADMINISTRATION AND DOSAGE SPECIFICS:
Mild hypothyroidism: Initiate therapy at 25 mcg daily and increase by 12.5 to 25 mcg every 1-2 weeks until effects are achieved. Maintenance dose is usually 25 to 100 mcg/day.

Myxedema: Initiate therapy at 5 mcg daily and increase by 5 to 10 mcg every 1-2 weeks. Maintenance dose is usually 50 to 100 mcg/day.

LIOTRIX

PRODUCTS (TRADE NAME):
Euthroid, Thyrolar (Available in the following tablets):

Tablet Size	Availability		Thyroid Equivalency
	T_4 (mcg)	T_3 (mcg)	
Euthroid Tablets 1/2	30	7.5	30 mg
Euthroid Tablets 1	60	15	60 mg
Euthroid Tablets 2	120	30	120 mg
Euthroid Tablets 3	180	45	180 mg
Thyrolar Tablets 1/4	12.5	3.1	15 mg
Thyrolar Tablets 1/2	25	6.25	30 mg
Thyrolar Tablets 1	50	12.5	60 mg
Thyrolar Tablets 2	100	25	120 mg
Thyrolar Tablets 3	150	37.5	180 mg

DRUG SPECIFICS:
Liotrix is a combination of synthetic levothyroxine sodium (T_4) and liothyronine sodium (T_3) in a 4:1 ratio. Predictable therapeutic effect is an advantage as a choice of therapy. Transfer of patients from one drug to another requires caution due to the differences in amounts of components. Euthyroid contains tartrazine, a product which may produce asthma-like reactions in sensitive individuals.

ADMINISTRATION AND DOSAGE SPECIFICS:
Initiate therapy with one 1/2 (Euthroid or Thyrolar) tablet and increase by one 1/2 tablet at 1-2 week intervals.

THYROGLOBULIN

PRODUCTS (TRADE NAME):
Proloid (Available in 32, 65, 100, 130, and 200, mg tablets.)

DRUG SPECIFICS:
Thyroglobulin contains levothyroxine (T_4) and liothyronine (T_3). Because it is a natural product, its hormonal content is variable. In addition, because of its slow onset of action, it is not useful in the treatment of myxedema.

ADMINISTRATION AND DOSAGE SPECIFICS:
Start with 16-32 mg/day po and increase every 1-2 weeks until therapeutic effect is achieved. Maintenance is usually 32-200 mg/day.

THYROID, DESICCATED

PRODUCTS (TRADE NAME):
Armour Thyroid (Available in 16, 32, 65, 98, 130, 195, 260, and 325 mg tablets.) **Thyrar** (Available in 32, 65, 130 mg bovine tablets.) **Thyroid Strong** (Available in 32, 65, 130, 195 mg plain and sugar coated tablets.) **Thyroid USP** (Available in 16, 32, 65, 130, 195, and 325 mg regular or enteric coated tablets.) **Thyro-Teric** (Available in 65 mg tablets.) **S-P-T** (Available in 65, 130, 195 and 325 mg pork capsules.) **Westroid** (Available in 16, 32, 65, 130, 195, 260, and 325 mg tablets.)

DRUG SPECIFICS:
Desiccated thyroid contains T_4 and T_3 thyroid hormones in their natural state. Because these drugs are composed of desiccated animal thyroid glands, the hormonal content is variable and T_3 and T_4 levels fluctuate; therefore, avoid varying brands.

ADMINISTRATION AND DOSAGE SPECIFICS:
Myxedema or hypothyroidism with cardiovascular disease: Start with 16 mg/day, increase after 2 weeks to 30 mg/day; after 2 more weeks increase to 65 mg/day. Monitor after first and second months of therapy at 65 mg/day. If indicated, increase dose in increments of 30-60 mg. Maintenance is usually 65-195 mg/day.

Hypothyroidism without Myxedema: Initiate therapy at 65 mg/day with increases of 65 mg/month until therapeutic effects are achieved. Maintenance is usually 65-195 mg/day.

Sheila Fitzgerald

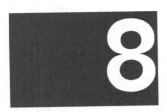

RESPIRATORY DRUGS

ANTIHISTAMINES

ACTION OF THE DRUG: (1) The main action of antihistamines is to competitively block the action of histamine by occupying the H_1 receptor sites of the effector structures (i.e., vascular and nonvascular smooth muscle, salivary, and respiratory mucosal glands.) The result is to antagonize the vasodilation, increase capillary permeability, and reduce the edema caused by histamine. (2) Antihistamines also inhibit the release of acetylcholine, exerting an anticholinergic (drying) effect, particularly in the bronchioles and gastrointestinal system. (3) The antihistamines also exert a sedative effect on the CNS.

ASSESSMENT:

INDICATIONS: These preparations are used in the primary treatment of allergic perennial or seasonal rhinitis. Also used in vasomotor rhinitis, though therapeutic effect is not predictable. They are used to relieve symptoms of allergic disorders, particularly urticaria, angioedema, serum sickness, reactions to blood or plasma, adjunctive therapy in anaphylactic reactions, and to relieve dermatographism. Used in combination cold remedies to decrease mucus secretion and at bedtime for sedation.

There are five main groups of antihistamines, with varying characteristics and actions. These groups, and specific drugs within each group are summarized in Table 8-1.

SUBJECTIVE: May elicit history of allergic reactions (systemic or topical), with allergic nasal congestion (usually seasonal in onset) runny nose, or cough related to colds or allergy.

OBJECTIVE: Signs of rhinitis: sneezing, nasal discharge, inflamed nasal mucosa. May also have edema, skin lesions, dermatographism, conjunctivitis, rhinitis, eczema, insect bites, or contact dermatitis. Presence of cough due to cold or allergy may also be present. Nasal mucosa may be swollen, boggy and pale, and there may be nasal obstruction or clear watery discharge. Sinus pressure may be elicited on palpation of frontal or maxillary sinuses.

PLAN:

CONTRAINDICATIONS: Do not give in presence of hypersensitivity to antihistamines, or to patients with symptoms of lower respiratory tract infection, or with monoamine oxidase inhibitor (MAO) therapy. Antihistamines are contraindicted in asthma, narrow angle glaucoma, prostatic hypertrophy, pyloroduodenal obstruction, stenosing peptic ulcer, bladder neck obstruction, and in elderly or debilitated persons. These drugs can be found in breast milk and may adversely affect infant as well as inhibit lactation. It should not be used in premature or newborn infants. Use in young children may cause hallucinations, convulsions, and even death. Doxylamine and pyridoxine may produce teratogenic effects in the fetus. Phenothiazine antihistamines are contraindicated in patients with CNS depression secondary to alcohol, barbiturates, analgesics or narcotics; comatose patients; acutely

TABLE 8-1. MAJOR ANTIHISTAMINE GROUPS

Major Group	Specific Drugs
Alkylamines	Brompheniramine
	Chlorpheniramine
	Dexchlorpheniramine
	Dimethindene
	Triprolidine
Ethanolamines	Bromodiphenhydramine
	Carbinoxamine
	Clemastine
	Diphenhydramine
	Doxylamine
Ethylenediamines	Pyrilamine
	Tripelennamine
Phenothiazines	Methdilazine
	Promethazine
	Trimeprazine
Miscellaneous	Azatadine
	Cyproheptadine
	Diphenylpyraline

ill or dehydrated children, and patients who have previously experienced pheno-thiazine-induced jaundice, bone marrow depression, allergic reactions, or other idio-syncratic reactions. Use with caution in children with a family history of sleep apnea, SIDS, or a child with symptoms of Reye's syndrome.

WARNINGS: Caution should be used in prescribing these drugs to patients with cardiovascular or renal disease, hypertension, urinary retention, diabetes, acute or chronic respiratory dysfunction, and hyperthyroidism. Use with asthma and lower respiratory tract infections may cause drying of the respiratory tract and increased thickening of secretions. The antihistamines should be used with extreme caution in persons with convulsive disorders and in persons who engage in activities requiring mental alertness. In children, antihistamines can cause paradoxical ex-citement instead of depression. Hypersensitivity reactions are more likely to develop following parenteral administration of drugs than oral administration. Elderly pa-tients are more likely to develop extra pyramidal side effects such as dizziness, syncope, confusion, akathisia, dyskinesia and parkinsonism.

PRECAUTIONS: Hypersensitivity reactions are not uncommon in persons who use topical antihistamine preparations. If any dermatologic reactions occur, the drug should be discontinued at once. The CNS depressant effects of these drugs may be potentiated if patients exceed the recommended doses. Also the sedative effects of these drugs make operating heavy machinery and driving particularly hazardous. Some products contain tartrazine which may produce an asthma-like reaction in sensitive individuals. Phenothiazines elevate prolactin levels and, there-fore, may be linked to development of prolactin-dependant breast cancer. These drugs, if given to patients with glucose-6-phosphate dehydrogenase (G-6-PD) deficiency may produce hemolysis at times of infection or stress.

IMPLEMENTATION:

DRUG INTERACTIONS: The sedative effect commonly associated with antihistamines is potentiated by concurrent use of other central nervous system depressants such as hypnotics, sedatives, tranquilizers, depressant analgesics, and alcohol. They also have an additive effect with anticholinergic drugs. Antihistamines can intensify the anticholinergic side effects of the MAO inhibitors as well as the tricyclic antidepressants. The effects of epinephrine may be enhanced by use of diphenhydramine, tripelennamine and d-chlorpheniramine. The antihistamines, when used concurrently with ototoxic drugs (e.g., large doses of aspirin or other salicylates, streptomycin), may mask ototoxic effects. By enzyme induction the antihistamines can decrease the effect of the corticosteroids, estradiol, progesterone, and testosterone. They may also antagonize the effects of anticholinesterase drugs.

ADMINISTRATION AND DOSAGE: The majority of the antihistamines are administered orally. Many are available over the counter although the highest dosage forms are available only by prescription. Most manufacturers have at least one preparation which can be obtained by prescription, thus people with Medicare-Medicaid benefits are able to obtain these with their cards. These drugs should only be taken when needed. Type and dosage of antihistamine should be chosen according to the desired effect and individual being treated. For example, ethanolamine derivatives have a high incidence of drowsiness and probably should not be prescribed for a machine operator. If tolerance to one type of antihistamine develops, switching to another type may restore responsiveness. Do not chew sustained release tablets or capsules. Gastrointestinal side effects can be minimized by administering oral doses with meals or milk. The oral route is usually well absorbed, precluding the need for the parenteral route. Parenteral administration is cautiously used because of the irritating nature of the drug. When IM preparations are used (i.e. diphenhydramine) they should be injected deeply into the muscle to prevent these irritating effects. IV administration of these agents should be done slowly, with the patient in the recumbent position. Long-term use of the topical nasal antihistamines increases the risk of sensitization, often causing a rebound effect.

IMPLEMENTATION CONSIDERATIONS:

—Obtain a compete health history, including presence of hypersensitivity, other drugs which may produce interactions, presence of asthma, glaucoma, peptic ulcer, prostatic hypertrophy, bladder neck obstruction, respiratory or cardiac disease, and possibility of pregnancy.

—All antihistamines produce a degree of drowsiness, and the patient must be cautioned to avoid situations in which alertness is required.

—These drugs may cause dizziness, thickening of secretions, and upset or painful stomach which may require health care provider attention if reactions continue.

—Many of the antihistamines can be purchased over the counter, while others require prescriptions. Make certain the patient has a prescription if it is needed.

—For parenteral use, give drugs IM rather than SQ because of their highly irritating properties.

—A wide variation exists in the occurrence of side effects among antihistamines. Even though a patient experiences many side effects from one agent, another antihistamine may produce few adverse reactions.

—Tolerance may develop after use of a histamine, and another should be tried for better control of symptoms if one product seems to grow less effective over time.

—Respiratory stimulants given during treatment for overdosage may only hasten the onset of convulsions.

—Before patient may be skin-tested for allergies, they should discontinue the use of antihistamines for 48 hours.

WHAT THE PATIENT NEEDS TO KNOW:

—This drug should be taken exactly as ordered. Do not attempt to change dosage or alter medication schedule.

—Some antihistamines are available over the counter, while others require a prescription.

—These drugs may cause drowsiness, and you should not drive or perform any actions requiring alertness until you are certain how this medication will affect you. Use caution at all times while taking this medication. Feelings of drowsiness usually disappear with continued use of the drug.

—These drugs may cause you to have a dry mouth, to have thick secretions, feel a little dizzy, or to note some stomach discomfort. Notify your health care provider if any of these symptoms become severe or bothersome.

—If this medication causes stomach upset, this can be decreased by taking medication with meals or milk.

—Do not take any other medications without the knowledge of your health care provider. It is especially important to avoid alcohol or sedative drugs while you are on this medication.

—Keep this medication out of the reach of children and others for whom it is not prescribed. Overdosages of this medication may be very serious.

—When using topical preparations, do not apply the medicine on open, raw sores or wounds.

EVALUATION:

ADVERSE REACTIONS: *Cardiovascular:* arrhythmias, extrasystoles, headache, hypertension, hypotension (especially in the elderly), palpitations, tachycardia. *CNS:* acute labyrinthitis, blurred vision, confusion, convulsions, disturbed coordination, dizziness, drowsiness, double vision, euphoria, excitation, fatigue, headache, hysteria, incoordination, insomnia, irritability, nervousness, neuritis, pallor, paradoxial excitation in children, paresthesia, personality changes, photosensitivity, restlessness, sedation, syncope, tinnitus, tremor, vertigo, weakness. *Gastrointestinal:* anorexia, constipation, diarrhea, dry mouth, epigastric distress, increased appetite, nausea, vomiting, weight gain. *Genitourinary:* decreased libido, difficult or painful urination, early menstruation, impotence, urinary retention or frequency. *Hematopoietic:* agranulocytosis, hemolytic anemia, leukopenia, pancytopenia, thrombocytopenia. *Hypersensitivity:* anaphylactic shock, photosensitization, rash, skin lesions, urticaria. *Respiratory:* chest tightness, nasal congestion or stuffiness, shortness of breath, thickening of bronchial secretions, wheezing. *Other:* chills, temporary reduction in male sperm count, unusual increase in sweating.

OVERDOSAGE: *Signs and symptoms:* Antihistamine overdosage is potentially fatal, particularly in children. The symptoms of overdosage are caused by concurrent CNS stimulation and depression. Stimulation is more likely in children. Hallucinations, incoordination, tonic-clonic convulsions and death may occur. Atropine-like symptoms (dry mouth, fixed dilated pupils, flushing) often develop. Central nervous system depression may be demonstrated by cerebral coma, respiratory depression, progressive coma, and cardiovascular collapse. Gastrointestinal symptoms may also occur. *Treatment:* If overdosage is due to a phenothiazine, give activated charcoal and gastric lavage. In overdosage from other preparations, induce vomiting by making patient gag after drinking a glass of milk or water or give syrup of ipecac if spontaneous vomiting has not occurred. Special precautions to prevent aspiration, especially in children, are needed. If vomiting is unsuccessful, referral for gastric lavage is indicated (best within 3 hours of ingestion, but may be done later if large amounts of milk or cream are given.) Use isotonic or one-half isotonic saline for lavage solution. Saline cathartics such as milk of magnesia draw water into the bowel and are helpful for their ability to cause rapid dilution of stomach contents. Maintain supportive and symptomatic treatment as indicated. Convulsions can be treated with short-acting barbiturates. Do not use stimulants.

PARAMETERS TO MONITOR: During the initial visit a complete history should be obtained in addition to vital signs. If long-term therapy is anticipated, the patient should be monitored at three-month intervals. Monitor for therapeutic effect: decrease in swelling, decreased in pruritus, rhinitis, decreased vascularity of eyes. Assess for presence of adverse reactions: wheezing, fever, sputum production (tenacious, thick dry sputum,) cough, dull percussion notes in chest, and absent or distant breath sounds. Monitor blood pressure, cardiac rate and rhythm, and character of respirations each visit. Watch for the appearance of lower respiratory tract symptoms and the development of drug tolerance. If patients are on long-term therapy, periodic complete blood counts should be obtained to detect development of blood dyscrasias.

ALKYLAMINES

BROMPHENIRAMINE MALEATE

PRODUCTS (TRADE NAME):
Bromamine (Available in 4 mg tablets.) **Bromphen, Brompheniramine Maleate** (Available in 4 mg tablets, 8 and 12 mg sustained release tablets, and 2 mg/5 ml elixir.) **Dimetane** (Available in 4 mg tablets; 2 mg/5 ml elixir.) **Dimetane**

Extentabs (Available in 8 and 12 mg sustained release tablets.) **Veltane** (Available in 4 mg tablets.)

DRUG SPECIFICS:

Drugs from the alkylamine group are useful and effective at low dosages and are practical for daytime use. They may cause both CNS stimulation (excitation) and depression (drowsiness.) The individual response is variable. Studies have shown that brompheniramine maleate may impair performance approximately 90 minutes after ingestion. Dimetane tablets and elixir are the only products available over the counter.

ADMINISTRATION AND DOSAGE SPECIFICS:

Adults: 4 to 8 mg three to four times daily po, or 8 to 12 mg of sustained release tablets po every 8-12 hours.

Children over 6 years: 4 mg po three to four times daily.

Children under 6 years: 0.5 mg/kg/day po.

CHLORPHENIRAMINE MALEATE

PRODUCTS (TRADE NAME):

Alermine (Available in 4 mg tablets.) **Aller-Chlor** (Available in 8 and 12 mg sustained release capsules.) **Allerid-O.D. 8 or 12** (Available in 8 and 12 mg sustained release capsules.) **Chlor-Niramine** (Available in 4 mg tablet.) **Chloramate Unicelles** (Available in 12 mg sustained release capsules.) **Chlorpheniramine Maleate** (Available in 4 mg tablets, 8 and 12 mg sustained release tablets and capsules and 2 mg/5 ml syrup.) **Chlo-Amine** (Available in 2 mg chewable tablets.) **Chlortab** (Available in 4 mg tablets and 8 or 12 mg sustained release tablets.) **Chlor-Trimeton** (Available in 4 mg tablets, 8 or 12 mg sustained release tablets and 2 mg/5 ml syrup.) **Hal-Chlor** (Available in 4 mg tablets.) **Histex** (Available in 12 mg sustained release capsules.) **Histrey** (Available in 4 mg tablets.) **Phenetron** (Available in 4 mg tablets, 8 and 12 mg sustained release tablets and 2 mg/5 ml syrup.) **Phenetron Lanacaps** (Available in 8 and 12 mg sustained release capsules.) **T.D. Alermine** (Available in 8 and 12 mg sustained release capsules.) **Teldrin** (Available in 8 and 12 mg sustained release capsules.) **Trymegen** (Available in 4 mg tablets.)

DRUG SPECIFICS:

Products from the alkylamines group are useful and effective at low dosages and are practical for daytime use. They may cause both CNS stimulation (excitation) and depression (drowsiness.) The individual response is variable. Sustained release forms are not for use in children under the age of 6. There is low incidence of side effects. Products may cause tingling, weakness, feeling of heaviness of hands. Chlor-Trimeton and Teldrin products are available over the counter except for the 12 mg Chlor-Trimeton Repetabs.

ADMINISTRATION AND DOSAGE SPECIFICS:

Adults: 2 to 4 mg three to four times daily po or 8 to 12 mg sustained release every 8-12 hours po during the day or at bedtime.

Children 6-12 years: 2 mg po three to four times daily or 8 mg of sustained release during the day or at bedtime.

Children 2-6 years: 1 mg po three to four times daily.

DEXCHLORPHENIRAMINE MALEATE

PRODUCTS (TRADE NAME):

Polaramine (Available in 2 mg tablets, 4 and 6 mg sustained release tablets, and 2 mg/5 ml syrup.)

DRUG SPECIFICS:

Products from the alkylamine group are useful and effective at low dosages and are practical for daytime use. They may cause both CNS stimulation (excitation) and depression (drowsiness.) However, drowsiness is usually mild. The individual response is variable. Repetabs should not be used for infants. This drug is available by prescription only.

ADMINISTRATION AND DOSAGE SPECIFICS:

Adults: 2 mg po three to four times daily, or 4-6 mg po sustained release tablets twice daily.

Children under 12: Give 1/2 adult dose.

Infants: Give 1/4 adult dose.

DIMETHINDENE MALEATE

PRODUCTS (TRADE NAME):

Triten Tab-In (Available in 2.5 mg sustained release tablets.)

DRUG SPECIFICS:

Products from the alkylamine group are useful and effective at low dosages and are practical for daytime use. They may cause both CNS stimulation (excitation) and depression (drowsiness.) The individual response is variable. Common side effects include drowsiness, gastrointestinal disturbances, dry mouth, and urinary frequency. Do not use in children under the age of 6. Available by prescription only.

ADMINISTRATION AND DOSAGE SPECIFICS:

Adults and children over 6 years: 2.5 mg po once or twice daily.

TRIPROLIDINE HYDROCHLORIDE

PRODUCTS (TRADE NAME):

Actidil (Available in 2.5 mg tablets and 1.25 mg/5 ml syrup.) **Triprolidine HCl** (Available in 1.25 mg/ml syrup.)

DRUG SPECIFICS:

Products from the alkylamine group are useful and effective at low dosages and are practical for daytime use. They may cause both CNS stimulation (excitation) and depression (drowsiness.) The individual response is variable. Triprolidine HCl has been shown to impair performance immediately after absorption. Compared to other products it has a low incidence of side effects. Onset is rapid. Available by prescription only.

ADMINISTRATION AND DOSAGE SPECIFICS:

Adults: 2.5 mg po three to four times daily.
Children 6-12 years: 1.25 mg po three to four times daily.
Children 4-6 years: 0.9 mg po three to four times daily.
Children 2-4 years: 0.6 mg po three to four times daily.
Children 4 months-2 years: 0.3 mg po three to four times daily.

ETHANOLAMINES

BROMODIPHENHYDRAMINE HYDROCHLORIDE

PRODUCTS (TRADE NAME):

Ambodryl Kapseals (Available in 25 mg capsules.)

DRUG SPECIFICS:

Ethanolamines have the highest incidence of drowsiness but gastrointestinal side effects are minimal. Available by prescription only.

ADMINISTRATION AND DOSAGE SPECIFICS:

Adults: 25 mg po every 4-6 hours; maximum of 150 mg in 24 hours.

CARBINOXAMINE MALEATE

PRODUCTS (TRADE NAME):

Clistin (Available in 4 mg tablets, 8 and 12 mg sustained release tablets.)

DRUG SPECIFICS:

Ethanolamines have the highest incidence of drowsiness but gastrointestinal side effects are minimal. Individualize dosage since some patients may respond to as little as 4 mg daily. Contains tartrazine which may produce asthma-like reactions in sensitive individuals. Available by prescription only.

ADMINISTRATION AND DOSAGE SPECIFICS:

Adults: 4 to 8 mg po three or four times daily, or 8 to 12 mg po sustained release tablets every 8-12 hours. Maximum 24 mg in 24 hours.
Children over 6 years: 4 to 6 mg po three or four times daily.

Children 3-6 years: 2 to 4 mg po three or four times daily.
Children 1-3 years: 2 mg po three or four times daily.

CLEMASTINE FUMARATE

PRODUCTS (TRADE NAME):
Tavist (Available in 2.68 mg tablets.) **Tavist-1**(Available in 1.34 mg tablets.)
DRUG SPECIFICS:
Ethanolamines have the highest incidence of drowsiness but gastrointestinal side effects are minimal. Do not use in children under the age of 12. Available by prescription only.
ADMINISTRATION AND DOSAGE SPECIFICS:
Adults and children over 12 years: 1.34 mg po twice daily. Higher dose available for dermatologic conditions.

DIPHENHYDRAMINE HYDROCHLORIDE

PRODUCTS (TRADE NAME):
Benadryl (Available in 25 and 50 mg capsules; 12.5 mg/5 ml elixir with 14% alcohol, lotion or ointment, and 10 mg or 50 mg/ml injection.) **Bendylate** (Available in 25 and 50 mg capsules, 10 or 50 mg/ml injection.) **Caladryl** (Available in 12.5 mg/5 ml elixir, and in 1% Benadryl cream or lotion.) **Diphenhydramine HCl** (Available in 25 and 50 mg capsules, 10 and 50 mg/ml injection.) **Fenylhist** (Available in 13.3 mg/5 ml syrup.) **Nordryl** (Available in 10 or 50 mg/ml injection.) **SK-Diphenhydramine** (Available in 25 and 50 mg capsules.) **Surfadil** (Available in 1% benadryl cream or lotion.) **Valdrene** (Available in 50 mg tablets.) **Zalydryl** (Available in lotion form equivalent to 2% Benadryl, 2% zinc oxide and 2% alcohol.)
DRUG SPECIFICS:
Ethanolamine products have the highest incidence of drowsiness but gastrointestinal side effects are minimal. Diphenhydramine is an antihistamine which blocks histamine receptors on peripheral effector cells. It has anticholinergic, antitussive, antiemetic and sedative properties. It is used often in allergic conjunctivitis, allergic reactions to blood or plasma, allergic rhinitis, uncomplicated angioedema, pruritus, and urticaria, insomnia, motion sickness, vasomotor rhinitis, anaphylactic reactions, adjunctively to epinephrine and antiparkinsonian therapy. The drug is not indicated for treatment of lower respiratory disease, in newborn or premature infants, and in pregnant or nursing mothers. It has a high incidence of CNS depressant effects associated with its use. Diphenhydramine HCl may cause tingling, weakness, and a feeling of heaviness in the hands. Drowsiness decreases with length of usage. Use of these agents in the elderly or debilitated is more likely to produce CNS

depressant effects. Most of these products are available by prescription only. Protect products from light.

ADMINISTRATION AND DOSAGE SPECIFICS:

Adults: 25 to 50 mg po three or four times daily.

Children over 20 pounds: 12.5 to 25 mg po three or four times daily or 5 mg/kg/day po.

DOXYLAMINE SUCCINATE

PRODUCTS (TRADE NAME):

Decapryn (Available in 12.5 and 25 mg tablets and 6.25 mg/5 ml syrup.)

DRUG SPECIFICS:

Ethanolamines have the highest incidence of drowsiness but gastrointestinal side effects are minimal. Doxylamine succinate produces a high level of sedation. Tablets are available by prescription only, but syrup can be purchased over the counter. Not for use in children under the age of 6 years.

ADMINISTRATION AND DOSAGE SPECIFICS:

Adults: 12.5 to 25 mg po every 4-6 hours; maximum of 150 mg in 24 hours.

Children 6 to 12 years: 6.25 to 12.5 mg po every 4-6 hours or 2 mg/kg/day.

PYRILAMINE MALEATE

PRODUCTS (TRADE NAME):

Pyrilamine Maleate (Available in 25 mg tablets.)

DRUG SPECIFICS:

This drug has a high incidence of gastrointestinal upset and produces moderate sedation. It can cause paradoxical excitation and hyperirritability. This antihistamine is available over the counter. It is not for use in children under the age of 6 years.

ADMINISTRATION AND DOSAGE SPECIFICS:

Adults: 25 to 100 mg po two to four times a day.

Children 6 to 12 years: 12.5 to 25 mg po two to four times a day.

TRIPELENNAMINE HCL

PRODUCTS (TRADE NAME):

PBZ (Available in 25 and 50 mg tablets, 50 mg long-acting tablets and 37.5

mg/5 ml elixir.) **PBZ-SR** (Available in 100 mg sustained release tablets.) **Tripelennamine Hydrochloride** (Available in 50 mg tablets.)

DRUG SPECIFICS:

There is a low incidence of side effects. The most common effects are drowsiness and dry mouth. The elixir is very palatable. Available by prescription only.

ADMINISTRATION AND DOSAGE SPECIFICS:

Adults: 25 to 50 mg po every 4-6 hours, maximum 600 mg po in 24 hours, or give 100 mg sustained release tablet in the morning and at night. (May rarely be required every 8 hours.)

Children over 5 years: 50 mg po morning and night; maximum 300 mg in 24 hours.

Children and infants: 5 mg/kg/day po.

PHENOTHIAZINES

METHDILAZINE HYDROCHLORIDE

PRODUCTS (TRADE NAME):

Tacaryl (Available in 4 mg chewable tablets, 8 mg tablets and 4 mg/5 ml syrup.)

DRUG SPECIFICS:

The phenothiazine group has a strong central nervous system depressant effect (drowsiness.) Phenothiazines may suppress the cough reflex or obscure signs of intestinal obstruction, brain tumor, or overdosage from toxic drugs. They are contraindicated in comatose patients and in states of CNS depression, phenothiazine hypersensitivity or allergy, jaundice, bone marrow depression, and acutely ill or dehydrated children since they may develop impairment in muscle contractility. (See section on phenothiazines.) Chew chewable tablets well. Available by prescription only.

ADMINISTRATION AND DOSAGE SPECIFICS:

Adults: 8 mg po two to four times daily.

Children over 3 years: 4 mg po two to four times daily.

PROMETHAZINE HYDROCHLORIDE

PRODUCTS (TRADE NAME):

Phenergan, Promethazine HCl (Available in 12.5, 25, and 50 mg tablets; 6.25 mg/5 ml syrup, 12.5 mg, 25 mg/5 ml and 50 mg suppositories, and 25 mg/ml and 50 mg/ml for IM injection.) **Remsed** (Available in 50 mg tablets.)

DRUG SPECIFICS:

The phenothiazine group has a strong central nervous system depressant effect (drowsiness.) They potentiate the action of barbiturates and narcotics. Dosage of barbiturates should be reduced by at least one half; and narcotic dosage reduced by one fourth to one half when given in combination with promethazine. Phenothiazines may suppress the cough reflex or obscure signs of intestinal obstruction, brain tumor, or overdosage from toxic drugs. They are contraindicated in comatose patients and in states of CNS depression, in phenothiazine hypersensitivity or allergy, jaundice, bone marrow depression, acutely ill or dehydrated children since they may develop impairment in muscle contractility. (See section on phenothiazines.) Promethazine HCl has a high incidence of side effects, including severe drowsiness. It is a very potent drug with a prolonged action. Use cautiously in ambulatory patients. Available by prescription only.

ADMINISTRATION AND DOSAGE SPECIFICS:

Allergy symptoms:
Adults: 25 mg po or IM at bedtime. May also give 12.5 mg po before meals and at bedtime if needed.
Children under 12 years: Give 6.25 or 12.5 mg po 3 times daily; may also give 12.5 mg IV or IM.
Sedation:
Adults: 25 to 50 mg po or IM at bedtime.
Children: 12.5 to 25 mg po, IM or rectally at bedtime.

TRIMEPRAZINE

PRODUCTS (TRADE NAME):

Temaril (Available in 2.5 mg tablets, 5 mg sustained release capsules and 2.5 mg/5 ml syrup.)

DRUG SPECIFICS:

Phenothiazines have a strong central nervous system depressant effect (drowsiness.) They may suppress the cough reflex or obscure signs of intestinal obstruction, brain tumor, or overdosage from toxic drugs. They are contraindicated in comatose patients and in states of CNS depression, phenothiazine hypersensitivity or allergy, jaundice, bone marrow depression, and acutely ill or dehydrated children since they may develop impairment in muscle contractility. (See section on phenothiazines.) With trimeprazine, drowsiness decreases with continued use. It may also cause dry mouth and dizziness. Use lowest effective dose. This medication is available by prescription only. Sustained release capsules are not for use in children 6 years and under.

ADMINISTRATION AND DOSAGE SPECIFICS:

Adults: 2.5 mg po four times a day.
Children 3-12 years: 2.5 mg po four times daily; maximum 10 mg in 24 hours.
Children 6 months-3 years: 1.25 mg po at bedtime or three times a day if necessary. Maximum of 5 mg po in 24 hours.

ANTIHISTAMINE—MISCELLANEOUS

AZATADINE MALEATE

PRODUCTS (TRADE NAME):
   Optimine (Available in 1 mg tablets.)
DRUG SPECIFICS:
   Not for use in children under 12 years of age. Dosage should be individualized. This drug has a prolonged action and is available by prescription only.
ADMINISTRATION AND DOSAGE SPECIFICS:
   Adults: 1 to 2 mg po twice daily.

CYPROHEPTADINE HYDROCHLORIDE

PRODUCTS (TRADE NAME):
   Cyproheptadine Hydrochloride, Periactin (Available in 4 mg tablets and 2 mg/5 ml syrup.)
DRUG SPECIFICS:
   May cause dryness of mouth and drowsiness. Contraindicated in angle closure glaucoma, urinary retention, intestinal obstruction, and in the elderly or debilitated. Available by prescription only.
ADMINISTRATION AND DOSAGE SPECIFICS:
   Adults: 4 to 20 mg po daily; maximum 0.5 mg/kg.
   Children 7-14 years: 4 mg po three times daily; maximum 16 mg in 24 hours.
   Children 2-6 years: 2 mg po three times daily; maximum 12 mg in 24 hours, or 0.25 mg/kg/day.

DIPHENYLPYRALINE HYDROCHLORIDE

PRODUCTS (TRADE NAME):
   Diafen (Available in 2 mg tablets.) **Hispril Spansules** (Available in 5 mg timed release capsules.)
DRUG SPECIFICS:
   This drug has a low incidence of side effects, the most common being drowsiness, headaches, dizziness, and dryness of mouth. This product is available by prescription only.
ADMINISTRATION AND DOSAGE SPECIFICS:
   Adults: 2 mg po every 4 hours, or 5 mg timed release capsule every 12 hours. Maximum 0.5 mg/kg daily.

Children over 6 years: 2 mg po every 6 hours, or 5 mg timed release capsule once daily. Maximum of 6 mg daily.

Children 2-6 years: 1 to 2 mg po every 8 hours. Maximum of 4 mg in 24 hours. Do not use timed release form in this age group.

Irene McCrea

ANTITUSSIVES—NARCOTIC AND NON-NARCOTIC

ACTION OF THE DRUG: The main action of narcotic antitussives is to suppress the cough reflex by acting directly on the cough center located in the medulla of the brain. Non-narcotic antitussives reduce the cough reflex at its source by anesthetizing stretch receptors in respiratory passages, lungs, and pleura, and decreasing their activity.

ASSESSMENT:

INDICATIONS: For symptomatic relief of overactive or nonproductive cough.

SUBJECTIVE: History of nonproductive cough or overactive cough which may keep the patient awake at night or cause muscular pain.

OBJECTIVE: Persistent, nonproductive cough without adventitious lung sounds.

PLAN:

CONTRAINDICATIONS: Do not use in patients with hypersensitivity to narcotic products or who have chronic pulmonary disease.

WARNINGS: Caution should be used in prescribing these products to pregnant women. Narcotics may produce drug dependence. See Central Nervous System drug monographs on narcotics.

PRECAUTIONS: May affect alertness, so caution needs to be exercised after taking medication.

IMPLEMENTATION:

DRUG INTERACTIONS: Narcotic antitussives have an additive effect with other CNS depressants so a reduced dosage should be used. Use caution in combining drugs. Potentiates the analgesic effect of aspirin and may be used with aspirin unless otherwise advised.

ADMINISTRATION AND DOSAGE: Only oral dosage forms are used as antitussives. They should be used for short periods of time due to the possibility of addiction. Some narcotic antitussives are schedule C-II drugs with strict controls.

IMPLEMENTATION CONSIDERATIONS:

—Obtain a complete health history: hypersensitivities to the drug, presence of chronic pulmonary disease, other drugs or alcohol which patient is taking that may cause drug interactions, or possibility of pregnancy.

—This drug should be used for only a short period of time due to the possibility of addiction.

WHAT THE PATIENT NEEDS TO KNOW:
—Narcotics can cause drowsiness, and caution needs to be used when performing any task requiring alertness.
—Overuse of this medication may cause severe constipation and addiction.
—This medication will increase the effect of aspirin and may be used with aspirin unless you are advised otherwise.
—This drug will increase the effects of alcohol and other drugs which slow the nervous system. Check with your health care provider before taking any other medications while you are taking this drug.
—Nausea may occur the first few minutes after you take this medication. This should go away if you lie down.
—The drug may occasionally cause lightheadedness, dizziness, or fainting when getting up from a lying or sitting position. Changing position slowly will help decrease this problem.
—Keep this medication out of the reach of children and others for whom it is not prescribed.
—Take drug with food or milk to avoid stomach upset.

EVALUATION:

ADVERSE REACTIONS: constipation, drowsiness, dry mouth, nausea, postural hypotension. (See section on narcotics in chapter on central nervous system drugs.)

OVERDOSAGE: Usually not a problem. Respiratory depression and oversedation may occur. (See section on narcotics in chapter on central nervous system drugs.)

PARAMETERS TO MONITOR: Watch for therapeutic effect: resolution of cough, decrease in frequency and duration of coughing spells, ability to sleep better at night. Also monitor adverse reactions. The drug should be used only for short periods of time and should not necessitate long-term monitoring.

NARCOTIC ANTITUSSIVES

CODEINE

PRODUCTS (TRADE NAME):
Codeine Sulfate (Available in 15, 30 and 60 mg tablets and soluble tablets.)
Codeine Phosphate (Available in 15, 30, and 60 mg soluble tablets.)

DRUG SPECIFICS:

The average antitussive dose ranges from 10-20 mg and is effective at this level. Protect codeine from light. This medication is available by prescription only.

ADMINISTRATION AND DOSAGE SPECIFICS:

Adults: 10 to 20 mg po every 4-6 hours; maximum 120 mg po in 24 hours.

Children 6-12 years: 5 to 10 mg po every 4-6 hours; maximum 60 mg in 24 hours.

Children 2-6 years: 2.5 to 5 mg po every 4-6 hours; maximum 30 mg in 24 hours.

HYDROCODONE BITARTRATE

PRODUCTS (TRADE NAME):

Dicodid (Available in 5 mg tablets.)

DRUG SPECIFICS:

Not for use in children under the age of 12.

ADMINISTRATION AND DOSAGE SPECIFICS:

Adults: 5 to 10 mg po 3-4 times daily.

Irene McCrea

NARCOTIC ANTITUSSIVES WITH EXPECTORANTS

DRUG SPECIFICS:

There is a lack of objective information to support the clinical effectiveness of expectorants (Table 8-2). Some products may be available without prescription, although not as over-the-counter preparations. They are under the legal control of the pharmacist and their availability varies from state to state. These products contain as much as 40% alcohol.

TABLE 8-2. NARCOTIC ANTITUSSIVES WITH EXPECTORANTS

Products (Trade Name):	Components	Dosage
Cheracol Syrup	Codeine phosphate 10 mg; guaifenesin 100 mg; alcohol 3.5%	5 ml every 3-4 hours
Cotussis (syrup)	Codeine phosphate 10 mg; terpin hydrate 20 mg; alcohol 20%	5-10 ml every 3 hours

TABLE 8-2. *(Continued)*

Products (Trade Name):	Components	Dosage
Dilaudid Cough Syrup*	Hydromorphone HCl 1 mg; guaifenesin 100 mg; alcohol 5%; tartrazine	5 ml every 3-4 hours
Hycotuss Expectorant (syrup)*	Hydrocodone bitartrate 5 mg; guaifenesin 100 mg; alcohol 10%	5 ml after meals and at bedtime
Nortussin with Codeine (liquid)	Codeine phosphate 10 mg; guaifenesin 100 mg; alcohol 3.5%	10 ml every 4 hours
Prunicodeine (liquid)	Codeine sulfate 10 mg; terpin hydrate 29 mg; alcohol 25%	5 ml every 3 hours
Terpin Hydrate with Codeine (elixir)	Codeine 10 mg; terpin hydrate 85 mg; alcohol 40%	5 ml three to four times daily
Tolu-Sed (syrup)	Codeine phosphate 10 mg; guaifenesin 100 mg; alcohol 10%	10 ml every 4 hours

*Available by prescription only.

Irene McCrae

NON-NARCOTIC ANTITUSSIVES

BENZONATATE

PRODUCTS (TRADE NAME):
Tessalon Perles (Available in 100 mg capsules.)
DRUG SPECIFICS:
Benzonatate acts to reduce the cough reflex at its source by anesthetizing stretch receptors in respiratory passages, lungs, and pleura and decreasing their activity. Caution should be used in prescribing this product for pregnant women or nursing mothers. Do not chew drug since local anesthesia of the mouth will develop. This product is available by prescription only. Adverse reactions include burning sensation of the eyes, constipation, dizziness, gastrointestinal upset, headaches, hypersensitivity, itching, nasal congestion, nausea, numbness in the chest, sedation, skin rash, or vague sensation of chilliness. *Overdosage:* CNS stimulation may cause restlessness, tremors, and clonic convulsions followed by CNS depression. *Treat-*

ment: Evacuate stomach contents and administer large amounts of activated charcoal. Care may be needed to prevent aspiration. CNS stimulants should not be used.

ADMINISTRATION AND DOSAGE SPECIFICS:

Adults and children over 10 years: 100 mg po three times daily as needed; maximum of 600 mg in 24 hours.

CHLORPHEDIANOL HYDROCHLORIDE

PRODUCTS (TRADE NAME):

Ulo (Available in syrup 25 mg/5 ml.)

DRUG SPECIFICS:

Potency is comparable to narcotic cough suppressants without tolerance, addiction, or respiratory depression. Onset is slower and duration of effect is longer. May cause some local anesthesia and anticholinergic effects. Not recommended for use in pregnancy or with infants. Often used in treatment of nonproductive cough. Use cautiously in patients on CNS stimulants or depressants and in debilitated patients. May cause excitation, hyperirritability, hallucinations, and nightmares which pass a few hours after drug is taken. Hypersensitivity and rash are rare. Large doses may cause dryness of the mouth, vertigo, visual disturbances, nausea, vomiting, and drowsiness. Drowsiness may be a problem in driving or in tasks requiring alertness. Available by prescription only.

ADMINISTRATION AND DOSAGE SPECIFICS:

Adults: 25 mg po three to four times daily as needed.

Children 6-12 years: 12.5 to 25 mg po three to four times daily as needed.

Children 2-6 years: 12.5 mg po three to four times daily as needed.

DEXTROMETHORPHAN HYDROBROMIDE

PRODUCTS (TRADE NAME):

Benylin DM Cough (Available in syrup 10 mg/5 ml.) **Chloraseptic Cough Control** (Available in 10 mg lozenges with phenol and sodium phenolate.) **Congespirin** (Available in 5 mg/5 ml syrup.) **Formula 44 Cough Control Discs** (Available in 5 mg lozenges with benzocaine, menthol, anethole, and peppermint.) **Hold 4 Hour** (Available in 7.5 mg lozenges with benzocaine.) **Pertussin 8 Hour Cough Formula** (Available in 15 mg/5 ml syrup.) **Romilar CF 8 hr Cough Formula** (Available in 15 mg/5 ml syrup and 2.5 mg/5 ml syrup for children.) **Sucrets Cough Control** (Available in 7.5 mg lozenges with benzocaine.)

DRUG SPECIFICS:

An effective antitussive that centrally depresses the cough center in the medulla and controls cough spasms. Dextromethorphan may cause gastrointestinal upset but has little or no analgesic effect, does not lead to tolerance, has no hypnotic effect, does not depress respirations, and is less likely to cause constipation than narcotic antitussives. Contraindicated in patients who are hypersensitive to the drug or who are taking MAO inhibitors. Not recommended for use in children under the age of 6 unless under supervision of health care provider. Major drug used in over the counter medications. Benzocaine additive can cause allergic reactions.

ADMINISTRATION AND DOSAGE SPECIFICS:

Adults: 10 to 20 mg po every 4 hours or 30 mg po every 6-8 hours; maximum of 120 mg daily.

Children 6-12 years: 5 to 10 mg po every 4 hours or 15 mg po every 6-8 hours; maximum of 60 mg daily.

Children 2-6 years: 2.5 to 5 mg po every 4 hours or 7.5 mg po every 6-8 hours; maximum of 30 mg daily.

DIPHENHYDRAMINE HYDROCHLORIDE

PRODUCTS (TRADE NAME):

Benylin Cough, Diphenadril, Diphenallin Cough, Diphen Cough, Diphenhydramine Hydrochloride Cough, Eldadryl Cough, Noradryl Cough, Robalyn, Tusstat (Available in 12.5 mg/5 ml syrup.) **Valdrene** (Available in 13.3 mg/5 ml syrup.)

DRUG SPECIFICS:

This drug is a potent antihistamine and a safe effective antitussive. (See drug monograph on Antihistamines.) Available by prescription only.

ADMINISTRATION AND DOSAGE SPECIFICS:

Adults: 25 mg po every 4 hours; maximum of 150 mg daily.

Children 6-12 years: 12.5 mg po every 4 hours; maximum of 75 mg daily.

Children 2-6 years: 6.25 mg po every 4 hours; maximum of 37.5 mg daily.

LEVOPROPOXYPHENE

PRODUCTS (TRADE NAME):

Novrad (Available in 100 mg capsules).

DRUG SPECIFICS:

A centrally acting cough suppressant for symptomatic treatment of cough. May cause CNS stimulation or depression and may cause drowsiness which affects the ability to drive or perform tasks requiring alertness. Can cause dizziness, drowsiness, epigastric distress, nausea, nervousness, and skin rash. Overdosage can lead to uncontrolled muscle tremor, agitation, and vomiting and can progress to sedation. Gastric lavage and supportive measures are indicated. Narcotic antagonists are not useful in overdosage. Available by prescription only.

ADMINISTRATION AND DOSAGE SPECIFICS:

Adults: 100 mg po every 4 hours; maximum of 600 mg daily.

Children: 0.5 mg/lb po every 4 hours; maximum daily dose of 75 mg in child of 25 pounds, 150 mg in child of 50 pounds, and 200 mg in child of 75-100 pounds.

NOSCAPINE

PRODUCTS (TRADE NAME):

Tusscapine (Available in 15 mg chewable tablets and 15 mg/5 ml syrup.)

DRUG SPECIFICS:

A nonnarcotic opium alkaloid related to papaverine with antitussive potency equal to codeine. It rarely causes allergy or side effects. Nausea and drowsiness may accompany high doses. Drowsiness may affect driving or tasks requiring alertness. Available over the counter.

ADMINISTRATION AND DOSAGE SPECIFICS:

Adults: 15 to 30 mg po every 4-6 hours or 5-10 ml three to four times daily; maximum of 120 mg in 24 hours.

Children 6-12 years: 15 mg po three to four times daily; maximum of 60 mg in 24 hours.

Children 2-6 years: 2.5 to 5 ml three to four times daily; maximum of 4 doses in 24 hours.

Irene McCrea

NON-NARCOTICS ANTITUSSIVES WITH EXPECTORANTS

DRUG SPECIFICS:

The products in Table 8-3 are available over the counter as liquids. Additional dosage forms are noted. One product, Silexin, is sugar- and alcohol-free.

TABLE 8-3. NON-NARCOTIC ANTITUSSIVES WITH EXPECTORANTS

Products	Components	Dosage
Anti-Tuss DM	Dextromethorphan hbr 15 mg; guaifenesin 100 mg; alcohol 1.4%.	10 ml every 6-8 hours

TABLE 8-3. *(Continued)*

Products	Components	Dosage
Cheracol D	Dextromethorphan hbr 10 mg; guaifenesin 100 mg; alcohol 4.75%.	10 ml every 4 hours
Dextro-Tuss GG (syrup)	Dextromethorphan hbr 15 mg; guaifenesin 100 mg; alcohol 1.4%.	10 ml every 6-8 hours
Glycotuss dM (tablets and syrup)	Dextromethorphan hbr 10 mg; guaifenesin 100 mg; alcohol 4.75%.	10 ml or 1-2 tablets every 4 hours
2/G-DM	Dextromethorphan hbr 15 mg; guaifenesin 100 mg; alcohol 5%.	10 ml every 6-8 hours
Novahistine Cough Formula	Dextromethorphan hbr 10 mg; guaifenesin 100 mg; alcohol 7.5%.	10 ml every 4 hours
Robitussin DM (syrup and lozenges)	Dextromethorphan hbr 7.5 mg; guaifenesin 50 mg.	1 lozenge every 3-4 hours or 10 ml every 6-8 hours
Romilar CF	Dextromethorphan hbr 15 mg; alcohol 20%.	10 ml every 6-8 hours
Silexin	Dextromethorphan hbr 5 mg; guaifenesin 50 mg.	10 ml every 3-8 hours
Tolu-Sed DM	Dextromethorphan hbr 10 mg; guaifenesin 100 mg; alcohol 10%.	10 ml every 4 hours
Vicks Cough Syrup	Dextromethorphan hbr 3.5 mg; guaifenesin 25 mg; sodium citrate 200 mg; alcohol 5%.	15 ml every 4 hours

Irene McCrae

ANTITUSSIVE COMBINATIONS

DRUG SPECIFICS:

This category contains narcotic or nonnarcotic antitussives in combination with anticholinergic, decongestant, analgesic or antihistamine agents. Prescription products are marked "Rx". Dosages in Table 8-4 are for adults. Some liquid preparations contain as much as 25% alcohol. See sections on Actions, Contraindications, etc. of individual agents for more information.

TABLE 8-4. ANTITUSSIVE COMBINATIONS

Products (Trade Name):	Components	Dosage
Colrex Compound (Rx)(capsules)	Codeine phosphate 16 mg; chlorpheniramine maleate 2 mg; phenylephrine HCl 10 mg; acetaminophen 325 mg.	1-2 capsules 3-4 times daily
Comtrex (tablets, capsules)	Dextromethorphan HBr 12.5 mg; chlorpheniramine maleate 1 mg; phenylpropanolamine HCl 12.5 mg; acetaminophen 325 mg.	2 capsules or tablets every 4 hours
Contac Severe Cold Formula (capsules)	Dextromethorphan HBr 15 mg; chlorpheniramine maleate 1 mg; pseudoephedrine HCl 30 mg; acetaminophen 500 mg.	2 tablets every 6 hours
CoTylenol Cold Formula (tablets, capsules and liquid)	Dextromethorphan HBr 15 mg; pseudoephedrine HCl 30 mg; acetaminophen 325 mg; plus alcohol 7.5% in liquid preparation.	2 tablets, capsules or 30 ml every 6 hours
Day Care (capsules and liquid)	Dextromethorphan HBr 10 mg; phenylpropanolamine HCl 12.5 mg; acetaminophen 325 mg; and alcohol 7.5% in liquid preparation.	2 capsules or 30 ml every 4 hours
Hycodan (Rx) (syrup and tablets)	Hydrocodone bitartrate 5 mg; homatropine methylbromide 1.5 mg.	5 ml or one tablet after meals and at bed time
Hycomine (Rx) (syrup)	Hydrocodone bitartrate 5 mg; phenylpropanolamine HCl 25 mg.	5 ml every 4 hours

TABLE 8-4. *(Continued)*

Products (Trade Name):	Components	Dosage
Novahistine Cough and Cold Formula (liquid)	Dextromethorphan HBr 10 mg; mg; chlorpheniramine maleate 2 mg; pseudoephedrine HCl 30 mg; alcohol 5%	10 ml every 4 hours
Novahistine DH (Rx) (liquid)	Codeine phosphate 10 mg; chlorpheniramine maleate 2 mg; phenylpropanolamine HCl 18.75 mg; alcohol 5%.	10 ml every 4 hours
NyQuil (liquid)	Dextromethorphan HBr 2.5 mg; ephedrine sulfate 1.33 mg; doxylamine succinate 1.33 mg; acetaminophen 100 mg; alcohol 25%.	30 ml at bedtime
Rhinex DM (syrup)	Dextromethorphan HBr 7.5 mg; chlorpheniramine maleate 1 mg; phenylephrine HCl 12.5 mg; guaifenesin 50 mg; ammonium Cl 100 mg; alcohol 5%.	2 tbsp. every 4 hours
Romilar III (syrup)	Dextromethorphan HBr 5 mg; phenylpropanolamine HCl 12.5 mg; alcohol 20%.	10 ml every 4 hours
Triaminic-DM (liquid)	Dextromethorphan HBr 10 mg; phenylpropanolamine HCl 12.5 mg.	10 ml every 4 hours
Tuss-Ade (Rx) (capsules)	Caramiphen edisylate 40 mg; phenylpropanolamine HCl 75 mg.	1 capsule every 12 hours

Irene McCrae

ASTHMA DRUGS—PROPHYLACTIC

CROMOLYN SODIUM (DISODIUM CROMOGLYCATE)

ACTION OF THE DRUG: (1) The main action of this drug is indirect antiasthmatic activity due to inhibition of degranulation of sensitized mast cells. (2) This drug inhibits the release of histamine and the slow-reacting substance of anaphylaxis (SRS-A) induced by inhaling specific antigens. (3) It may provide some hyposensitization after long-term use by preventing the release of phospholipase A. This enzyme assists in the release of chemical mediators from nonsensitized mast cells.

ASSESSMENT:

INDICATIONS: Cromolyn sodium should be used as an adjunct in the management of bronchial asthma in selected patients. This drug has no direct antihistaminic, anti-inflammatory, or bronchodilator activity. Thus, it is effective as a prophylactic agent only and should not be used in an acute attack of asthma. It is used investigationally in patients with food allergies to prevent GI and systemic reactions, in patients with allergic rhinitis, eczema and other dermatitis, chronic urticaria, and in post-exercise brochospasm.

SUBJECTIVE: History of allergies, asthma, bronchitis, emphysema; recurrent acute or chronic attacks of wheezing, cough with or without mucoid sputum, dyspnea, fatigue, intolerance for exercise, and, in severe cases, cyanosis. Acute upper or lower respiratory tract infections may precede onset of acute symptoms.

OBJECTIVE: Signs of bronchospasm or obstructive respiratory disease: prolonged expiration, wheezing, use of accessory respiratory muscles, profuse perspiration, coughing with or without sputum, hyperresonant percussion note, rales, inspiratory and expiratory rhonchi, distant breath sounds, decreased expiratory excursion, distended chest, bulging neck veins, overaerated lung fields, and flattened diaphragm on chest x-ray. Signs of decreased gas exchange: tachycardia, headache, restlessness, depression, apathy, and, in severe cases, unconsciousness.

PLAN:

CONTRAINDICATIONS: This drug should not be used with patients who have demonstrated a hypersensitivity to cromolyn sodium.

WARNINGS: Because of its method of excretion, the drug should be used with care in patients with renal or hepatic dysfunction. It should be discontinued immediately if the patient develops eosinophilic pneumonia. In test animals used in research, proliferative arterial lesions have been demonstrated with its usage. Safety in children and during pregnancy has not been established.

PRECAUTIONS: Occasionally, cough and bronchospasm may follow administration of cromolyn sodium. Thus, some patients may not be able to continue using it even with concurrent administration of bronchodilators. Caution should be used when decreasing the dosage or discontinuing its use because this procedure can cause asthmatic symptoms to recur.

IMPLEMENTATION:

DRUG INTERACTIONS: No drug interactions have currently been reported.

PRODUCTS (TRADE NAME):

Intal (Available in 20 mg capsules for inhalation. Spinhaler supplied separately.)

ADMINISTRATION AND DOSAGE: This drug is not absorbed and thus it is ineffective when taken orally. It is available in 20 mg capsules for inhalation using an oral inhaler called a Spinhaler. For adults and children 5 years and over use 20 mg inhaled at four equal intervals per day. Dosage can be decreased gradually to the minimum effective level, usually 20 mg three times daily. Improvement in symptoms can be expected within 4 weeks of using cromolyn sodium.

IMPLEMENTATION CONSIDERATIONS:

—Cromolyn sodium has been reported to be more effective in children than with in adults.

—Initiate administration of this drug when acute attack of asthma is over, airway is clear, and patient can inspire adequately.

—Instruct the patient concerning proper use and care of the inhaler. Have the patient return a demonstration of the procedure.

—Protect the capsules from light, moisture, and heat.

—Supervise the patient carefully when reducing the dosage or discontinuing the drug.

—Patients receiving corticosteroids and bronchodilators may continue them when cromolyn sodium is introduced. If improvement is seen in signs and symptoms, an attempt to reduce the dosage of the corticosteroids should be made. Institution of a regimen using alternate days of steroids is recommended.

—The amount of drug that is used by the lung is dependent on proper use of the inhaler, the degree of bronchospasm present, and the amount of secretion in the tracheobronchial tree. Only about 5 to 10 percent of the inhaled drug reaches the lung.

—Use caution when prescribing this drug for patients with hepatic or renal dysfunction and for women who are pregnant.

—Reevaluate drug regimen if no effect is achieved within four weeks.

WHAT THE PATIENT NEEDS TO KNOW:

—The capsules should not be swallowed.

—Capsules should be protected from light, heat, and moisture.

—Clear airway of as much mucus as possible before taking the drug.

—Avoid using this drug if you cannot take a deep breath and hold it or if you feel you are having an asthma attack.

—This drug must be administered *every* day at *regular* intervals.

—If a bronchodilator is being used at the same time, use it first, wait several minutes, then take this medication.

—Throat irritation, dryness of the mouth, and hoarseness may be prevented by rinsing and gargling after each dose.

—Proper use and cleaning of the Spinhaler must be understood to get effective results.

—Consult with health care provider on how to stop taking medication because suddenly stopping can make you have an acute attack of asthma.

—Notify health care provider if symptoms do not improve or you feel you are getting worse.

—Avoid breathing out moisture into inhaler. Since the drug is a powder, moisture may cause particle clumping and may interfere with correct dosage.

EVALUATION:

ADVERSE REACTIONS: *CNS:* dizziness, headache, peripheral neuritis, vertigo. *Dermatologic:* angioedema, photodermatitis, rash, urticaria. *Gastrointestinal:*

nausea. *Genitourinary:* dysuria, **nephrosis**, urinary frequency. *Respiratory:* bronchospasm, cough, hemoptysis, laryngeal edema, nasal congestion, wheezing. *Other:* anaphylaxis, anemia, joint swelling and pain, lacrimation, periarthritic vasculitis, pericarditis, polymiositis, swollen parotid gland.

OVERDOSAGE: *Signs and symptoms:* Because of its rapid elimination from the body, cromolyn sodium is practically nontoxic except for those who have a hypersensitivity to the drug. Overdosage is not common and produces symptoms that are an exaggeration of the adverse effects. No antidote is available. Patients should be treated supportively.

PARAMETERS TO MONITOR: It is recommended that pulmonary function tests be performed prior to initiation of cromolyn sodium therapy. The rationale for this recommendation is that the patient should have significant reversible airway obstruction. Since the drug should be given when a patient's condition is stable, a visit should be scheduled two weeks after initial administration and at least once more within the first four weeks for evaluation of the effectiveness of the preparation. Intervals thereafter depend on the condition of the patient. Parameters to monitor each visit: weight, vital signs, signs and symptoms of adverse reactions. Also observe for signs and symptoms of therapeutic effect: increased length of time between acute attacks; absence of prolonged expiration, wheezing, use of accessory muscles, coughing, hyperresonant percussion note, rales, rhonchi, distant breath sounds, and decreased expiratory excursion.

Mary F. Rapson

BRONCHODILATORS

SYMPATHOMIMETICS

ACTION OF THE DRUG: (1) The main action of sympathomimetic bronchodilators is to relax bronchial smooth muscle by stimulating beta-2-adrenergic receptors. (2) They also produce a systemic vasopressor response especially vasoconstriction in blood vessels of the bronchial mucosa which results in reduction of mucosal and submucosal edema. This action is due to stimulation of alpha receptors. (3) Sympathomimetic bronchodilator stimulation of beta-1 receptors also results in increased myocardial contractility and conduction. The sympathomimetic drugs vary in their selectivity for alpha and beta; some are relatively selective for the beta-2-receptors and some are nonselective. The degree of selectivity of each drug influences choice for therapy and the potential side effects for which each patient should be monitored.

ASSESSMENT:

INDICATIONS: Used for symptomatic treatment of bronchospasm occurring in acute and chronic asthma, bronchitis, and emphysema.

SUBJECTIVE: History of allergies, asthma, bronchitis, emphysema, recurrent acute or chronic attacks of wheezing, cough with or without mucoid sputum, dyspnea, fatigue, intolerance for exercise, and, in severe cases, cyanosis. Acute upper or lower respiratory tract infection may precede onset of acute symptoms.

OBJECTIVE: Signs of bronchospasm or obstructive respiratory disease: prolonged expiration, wheezing, use of accessory respiratory muscles, profuse perspiration, coughing with or without sputum, hyperresonant percussion note, rales, inspiratory and expiratory rhonchi, distant breath sounds, decreased expiratory excursion, distended chest, bulging neck veins, overaerated lung fields, and flattened diaphragm on chest x-ray. Signs of decreased gas exchange: tachycardia, headache, restlessness, depression, apathy, and, in severe cases, unconsciousness.

PLAN:

CONTRAINDICATIONS: To relieve bronchial spasm, beta-2 type receptors in bronchial smooth muscles must be stimulated. One of the drawbacks of adrenergic bronchodilators is that their effects are not limited to beta-2 type receptors. Some also stimulate beta-1 receptors, which increase heart rate and force of cardiac contraction, and alpha receptors, which control vasoconstriction. Thus, these drugs should be given with extreme care to individuals with coronary artery disease, cardiac arrhythmias, other organic heart disease, hypertension, hyperthyroidism, diabetes, glaucoma, or history of seizures.

WARNINGS: Use of sympathomimetics with inhalation anesthesia containing halogenated hydrocarbons such as halothane, methoxyflurane, and enflurane, or with a gas such as cyclopropane, may increase risk of arrhythmias. These drugs should not be used in patients receiving MAO inhibitor medicines. A sharp rise in blood pressure secondary to use of MAO inhibitors may result in cerebral or other types of hemorrhage. Adrenergic drugs may produce CNS stimulation and should be used with caution in patients having a history of seizures and psychoneurosis. They should be given with care to elderly patients, especially those with enlarged prostates. Safety is not established for use in pregnancy, so sympathomimetics should be used only when need outweighs the risk of administering them. Usage in breast-feeding mothers is not recommended.

PRECAUTIONS: Dosage must be carefully adjusted for patients having hyperthyroidism, hypertension, and coronary disease and for individuals sensitive to sympathomimetics to prevent tachycardia, palpitation, increased blood pressure, nausea, headache, or other central nervous system symptoms. Concurrent administration of more than one sympathomimetic is contraindicated, but alternation of two different drugs may be necessary. Tolerance may occur after too frequent administration of the drugs. In relation to use of inhalants, occasionally patients have developed severe paradoxical airway resistance with excessive use of these preparations. In these situations the drug should be discontinued immediately and other therapy instituted. Patients may experience less relief from aerosols after excessive use. Irritation of the bronchial tree and oropharynx may occur with use of powdered formulations. Following excessive administration of inhalation therapy, deaths have been reported. Cardiac arrest, arrhythmias, and concurrent use of corticosteroids were noted in these cases.

IMPLEMENTATION:

DRUG INTERACTIONS: Thyroid drugs, tricyclic antidepressants (MAO inhibitors), some antihistamines (diphenhydramine, tripelennamine, etc.), and amphetamines potentiate effects of sympathomimetic drugs. Concomitant use of one sympathomimetic drug with another may cause deleterious results. If given to patients on digitalis or diuretics, sympathomimetics may precipitate arrhythmias. General anesthetics mentioned under "WARNINGS" should not be given with the adrenergic drugs since they may also cause arrhythmias. Beta-adrenergic blocking agents such as propranolol may block bronchodilatory effects of these beta-receptor drugs. Sympathomimetics can antagonize the response of antihypertensives such as guanethidine, reserpine, and hydralazine.

ADMINISTRATION AND DOSAGE: The routes of administration of these bronchodilators vary according to the acuteness of the disease and the preparation used. They may be given parenterally, orally, or by oral inhalation (nebulizers, IPPB.) See individual drugs for specific information on administration and dosage.

IMPLEMENTATION CONSIDERATIONS:

—Obtain a thorough health history: determine if patient is pregnant, breast-feeding, or elderly; has a history of hyperthyroidism, heart disease, hypertension, diabetes, glaucoma, seizures or psychoneurotic disease; is taking other drugs which may interact with the bronchodilators; or has a history of allergy.

—Monitor the patient's pulse and blood pressure to determine the cardiac effects of the drug.

—Responses to therapy are variable among patients. Be prepared with alternative therapy if first approach is not effective.

—Patients should be monitored for increasing tolerance and concomitant diminished response to the drug.

—Careful instructions should be given to patients using inhalation method of administration. Demonstrations as well as written instructions are helpful.

—Monitor patient for paradoxical bronchospasm and discontinue the drug immediately if it develops.

—Adrenergic bronchodilators may cause transient increases in urinary epinephrine.

WHAT THE PATIENT NEEDS TO KNOW:

—Take the medication only as directed by your health care provider. Do not change dosage yourself.

—Excessive use of this drug may have severe side effects.

—Contact your health care provider if desired effect is not being achieved from the drug.

—Report the following symptoms to the health care provider: bronchial irritation, dizziness, chest pain, insomnia, or change in symptoms.

—Increased fluid intake, especially water, will reduce the thickness of mucus and help the medication work better.

—Do not take any other medications without checking first with your health care provider.

—To prevent difficulty falling asleep, take the last dose a few hours before bedtime.

—Your health care provider will demonstrate how to take this medication if you are taking it by an inhalation method.

—Protect drug from light and discard colored solutions.

EVALUATION:

ADVERSE REACTIONS: *Cardiovascular:* anginal pain, arrhythmias, cardiorespiratory arrest, hypotension, increased heart rate, increased myocardial contractility. *CNS:* anorexia, anxiety, dysuria, headache, insomnia, nausea, pallor, perspiration, polyuria, restlessness, tremors, vomiting, weakness, *Gastrointestinal:* decrease in muscle tone and motility in tract. *Genitourinary:* urinary hesitancy and retention. *Other:* increased glycogenesis and lipolysis, increased glucosinemia.

OVERDOSAGE: *Signs and symptoms:* Severe hypertension, palpitations, tachycardia, chest pain, delirium, convulsions, coma, nausea, vomiting, headache, bradycardia, insomnia, tremors, anxiety. *Treatment:* Toxic symptoms will generally be controlled or eliminated with discontinuation or reduction in dosage of the drug. A beta-blocker, i.e., propranolol, may be indicated if toxic effects are pronounced. An alpha-blocker may be used if it is necessary to block alpha-adrenergic actions.

PARAMETERS TO MONITOR: The acuteness of the respiratory attack dictates the parameters to monitor. In selected situations it may be useful to perform pulmonary function tests and blood gases. Baseline laboratory data is important to monitor effectiveness of the drug and its side effects. These tests should include chest x-ray, electrocardiogram, complete blood count, electrolytes, glucose and urinalysis. Frequency of ordering these tests and of return visits is dependent upon the frequency and acuteness of respiratory attacks. Parameters to monitor each visit: weight, pulse, heart rhythm, blood pressure, respiratory rate, signs and symptoms of adverse reactions. Also observe for signs and symptoms of therapeutic effect: increased duration between acute attacks; absence of prolonged expiration, wheezing, use of accessory muscles, coughing, hyperresonant percussion note, rales, rhonchi, distant breath sounds, and decreased expiratory excursion.

ALBUTEROL

PRODUCTS (TRADE NAME):
Proventil, Ventolin Inhaler (Available in 17 gm metered dose aerosol unit. Contains about 200 inhalations with 90 mcg/delivery, and 2 and 4 mg tablets.)
DRUG SPECIFICS:
This agent was recently introduced in the United States and is known internationally by the name salbutamol. Albuterol is relatively selective for beta-2 receptors and thus has fewer cardiac side effects than non-selective beta adrenergic drugs, and a longer duration of bronchodilation than isoproterenol. High doses, however, may produce prolonged cardiac.

ADMINISTRATION AND DOSAGE SPECIFICS:
Adults and children over 12 years: 1 to 2 inhalations every 4 to 6 hours.
Not recommended for children under twelve years of age.

EPHEDRINE SULFATE

PRODUCTS (TRADE NAME):
Ephedrine Sulfate (Available in 25 and 50 mg capsules, 25 and 50 mg/ml injections, and 11 mg/5 ml and 20 mg/5 ml syrup.)

DRUG SPECIFICS:
This drug is more stable and has a longer duration than epinephrine. It is used in the treatment of milder forms of chronic obstructive pulmonary disease.

ADMINISTRATION AND DOSAGE SPECIFICS:
Adults: 25 to 50 mg po every 3 to 4 hours or 25 to 50 mg SQ or IM every 3 to 4 hours.
Children 6 to 12 years: 6.25 to 12.5 mg po every 4 to 6 hours.
Children 2 to 6 years: 0.3 to 0.5 mg/kg po every 4 to 6 hours.

EPINEPHRINE

PRODUCTS (TRADE NAME):
Adrenalin Chloride (Available in 1:1000 solution in 1 ml ampules and 30 ml vials, in 1:100 solution for nebulizer in 7.5 ml.) **Asthma Haler, Bronitin, Bronkaid Mist Suspension** (Available in 0.3 mg aerosol). **Epinephrine Chloride** (Available in 1:1000 solution in 1 ml ampules, 30 ml vials and 2 ml syringe.) **Medihaler-Epi** (Available as aerosol: 0.3 mg epinephrine bitartrate in 15 ml vial with adapter.) **Primatene Mist Suspension** (Available as aerosol: 0.3 or 0.2 mg epinephrine per spray in 10 or 15 ml units with mouthpiece.) **Sus-Phrine** (Available in 1:200 suspension in 5 ml vials and 0.3 ml ampules.) **Vaponefrin** (Available in 2.25% epinephrine base solution for nebulizer in 7.5, 15, 30 ml and pocket nebulizer sizes.)

DRUG SPECIFICS:
This drug is reserved for acute attacks of bronchospasm. It has rapid onset of action (3-10 minutes) when administered parenterally or by inhalation. Epinephrine is absorbed well from mucous membranes. A high concentration of the drug is obtained from the pharynx and respiratory tract rather than systemically. It is destroyed by digestive enzymes and becomes ineffective if administered orally. Epinephrine can be prepared synthetically or obtained from animals and is available in suspension and in crystalline form. Solutions react to light, air, and heat and can change color with oxidation. No more inhalations should be used than are

necessary to create symptomatic relief. One to two minutes should be allowed between inhalations if successive dosage is needed. Do not give I.V.

ADMINISTRATION AND DOSAGE SPECIFICS:
For Adrenalin Chloride and Epinephrine Chloride:
Adults: 0.2 to 1.0 mg SQ or IM.
Children: 0.01 mg/kg or 0.3 mg/M² to a maximum of 0.5 mg.
For Sus-Phrine:
Adults: 0.1 to 0.3 ml SQ.
Children: 0.005 ml/kg SQ.
For Inhalation Products:
Number of inhalations varies according to condition of patient. Use for acute bronchospasm and use minimum number of sprays to provide relief.

ETHYLNOREPINEPHRINE HYDROCHLORIDE

PRODUCTS (TRADE NAME):
Bronkephrine (Available in 2 mg/ml in 1 ml ampules for injection.)
DRUG SPECIFICS:
This nonselective beta-adrenergic bronchodilator is similar to epinephrine but does not have significant pressor effects. It is used for severe asthma in those who do not respond to isoproterenol or epinephrine. It is appropriate for use in children and diabetics.

ADMINISTRATION AND DOSAGE SPECIFICS:
Adults: 0.5-1.0 ml SQ or IM.
Children: Determined by age and weight. 0.1-0.5 ml SQ or IM is average.

ISOPROTERNOL HYDROCHLORIDE

PRODUCTS (TRADE NAME):
Aerolone (Available in 1:400 solution for nebulization.) **Dispos-a-Med** (Available in 1:200 and 1:400 solution for nebulization.) **Isoproterenol HCl** (Available in 1:400 aerosol.) **Isuprel** (Available as 10 mg sublingual tablets; solutions for nebulizers in 1:100 and 1:200 dosages, and for Mistometer with 15 ml and 22.5 ml vials with nebulizer delivering a dose of 131 mcg, and 0.2 mg/ml injection.) **Medihaler-Iso** (Available in 15 ml and 22.5 ml aerosol delivering .08 mg per release. **Norisodrine Sulfate** (Available in 10 and 25 mg powder for inhalers and 0.25% solution delivering 120 mcg per release in 15 ml nebulizer.)
DRUG SPECIFICS
This drug is selective for beta receptors and has no appreciable effect on alpha-adrenergic receptors. It is a more active bronchodilator than epinephrine and shrinks

mucous membranes and reduces mucus secretion. It is helpful for the patient who is no longer benefiting from use of epinephrine. An effect of this drug is decreased blood pressure in contrast to increased blood pressure caused by other adrenergic agents. To minimize dryness of the mouth, it is useful to rinse mouth with water after inhalation therapy. Alert patients that their saliva and sputum may be pink after inhalation therapy due to the color of the drug.

ADMINISTRATION AND DOSAGE SPECIFICS:

Adults: 10 to 20 mg sublingually, not to exceed 60 mg per day.
Children: 5 to 10 mg sublingually, not to exceed 30 mg per day.
Inhalation: 1 to 5 treatments as needed daily.

METAPROTERENOL SULFATE

PRODUCTS (TRADE NAME):

Alupent, Metaprel (Available in 10, 20 mg tablets, 10 mg/5 ml syrup, 225 mg aerosol in propellant, and 5% solution for nebulization.)

DRUG SPECIFICS:

Metaproterenol sulfate, a synthetic drug, has more selectivity for beta-2-receptors of the bronchi and less effect on beta-1-receptors of the heart than isoproterenol. This drug has a more prolonged action and fewer side effects than other sympathomimetic bronchodilators. In addition, it is more effective when administered orally than isoproterenol because it is well absorbed from the gastrointestinal tract. Usually, it is not necessary to repeat treatment more often than every three to four hours in acute attacks of bronchospasm. In chronic bronchospasm, this dosage is sufficient. This product was formerly sold over-the-counter but prescription is now required.

ADMINISTRATION AND DOSAGE:

Adults: 20 mg po 3 or 4 times daily.
Children over 9 years or over 60 lbs: 20 mg po 3 or 4 times daily.
Children 6 to 9 years or less than 60 lbs: 10 mg po 3 or 4 times daily.

TERBUTALINE SULFATE

PRODUCTS (TRADE NAME):

Brethine (Available in 2.5 and 5 mg tablets and 1 mg/ml injection.) **Bricanyl** (Available in 2.5 and 5 mg tablets and 1 mg/ml injection.)

DRUG SPECIFICS:

This drug is relatively selective for the beta-2-receptors of the bronchial tree, peripheral vascular beds, and the uterus. Its actions are similar to isoproterenol and it is often effective when other drugs are not.

ADMINISTRATION AND DOSAGE SPECIFICS:

Adults: 5 mg po at 6 hour intervals, 3 times during the day. If side effects occur, drug can be reduced to 2.5 mg 3 times daily and still achieve therapeutic effect. If no response occurs after second dose, consider another medication. May also give 0.25 mg SQ. Dose may be repeated in 15 to 30 minutes if no significant effect is achieved from the first dose.

Children 12-15 years old: 2.5 mg po 3 times daily; or 2.5 mg SQ 3 times daily, not to exceed 7.5 mg SQ in 24 hours. Not recommended for children under twelve years of age.

Mary F. Rapson

BRONCHODILATORS

XANTHINE DERIVATIVES

ACTION OF THE DRUG: (1) The main action of xanthine derivative bronchodilators is to relax smooth muscle in the bronchi and blood vessels in the lungs. (2) They act directly on the kidneys to produce diuresis. (3) These drugs produce CNS effects. (4) Other actions include myocardial stimulation, increased respiration, lipolysis, glycogenolysis, and release of epinephrine from the adrenal medulla.

ASSESSMENT:

INDICATIONS: Used for symptomatic treatment of bronchospasm occurring in acute and chronic bronchial asthma, bronchitis, and emphysema.

SUBJECTIVE: History of allergies, asthma, bronchitis, emphysema, recurrent acute or chronic attacks of wheezing, cough with or without mucoid sputum, dyspnea, fatigue, intolerance for exercise, and, in severe cases, cyanosis. Acute upper or lower respiratory tract infections may precede onset of acute symptoms.

OBJECTIVE: Signs of bronchospasm or obstructive respiratory disease: prolonged expiration, wheezing, use of accessory respiratory muscles, profuse perspiration, coughing with or without sputum, hyperresonant percussion note, rales, inspiratory and expiratory rhonchi, distant breath sounds, decreased expiratory excursion, distended chest, bulging neck veins, overaerated lung fields, and flattened diaphragm on chest x-ray. Signs of decreased gas exchange: tachycardia, headache, restlessness, depression, apathy, and, in severe cases, unconsciousness.

PLAN:

CONTRAINDICATIONS: These drugs should not be given to persons demonstrating hypersensitivity to any xanthine. They should not be prescribed for patients with severe renal or liver impairment or those with heart disease in which cardiac stimulation would be dangerous.

WARNINGS: Caution should be used in administering these drugs to those with peptic ulcer, hypoxemia, severe hypertension, and glaucoma. Safety has not been established for use in pregnancy. Xanthine derivative bronchodilators should be administered cautiously in children and elderly patients because of CNS effects of the drugs. These preparations may worsen preexisting arrhythmias. Excessive doses may be associated with toxicity. Early signs of toxicity may be G.I. upset, anorexia, irritability and tremor, however, the patient may also present with cardiac arrhythmias or seizures.

PRECAUTIONS: The half-life of xanthine bronchodilators is shorter in smokers than nonsmokers, which may necessitate use of higher doses with smokers. Rectal irritation may appear when suppositories are given. Use of formulations containing alcohol are not necessary and may be harmful. When changing xanthine preparations, dosage adjustments must be made based on the theophylline base content of each drug.

IMPLEMENTATION:

DRUG INTERACTIONS: Xanthines may enhance the CNS stimulation caused by ephedrine, sympathomimetics and amphetamines. Erythromycin, lincomycin, and clindamycin may increase blood levels of theophylline. Beta-blocking agents such as propranolol, metoprolol, and nadolol may antagonize the effect of xanthines. The diuretic action of some types of diuretics is increased with these preparations. Xanthines may increase the risk of toxicity with use of digitalis glycoside. Concurrent use of xanthines with reserpine may produce tachycardia. Large doses of these agents may counteract the effectiveness of oral anticoagulants. Xanthines may increase excretion of lithium carbonate. The use of furosemide with theophylline increases the serum levels of theophylline and may cause toxicity. Cimeticline will significantly decrease theophylline clearance. Phenytoin leads to a decrease in theophylline levels.

ADMINISTRATION AND DOSAGE: These products are available in a number of dosage forms: capsules, coated tablets, sustained release tablets and capsules, aqueous solutions and suspensions, hydroalcoholic elixirs, suppositories, rectal solutions, and IV injections. Proper prescription requires consideration of many factors. The efficacy of the drug is directly related to the theophylline blood levels achieved from its administration. The desired therapeutic range is considered to be 10 mcg 20 mcg per milliliter of serum. Factors affecting blood levels are differing levels of theophylline in each product, variance in rates of absorption, metabolism and elimination of each drug, diet, smoking cigarettes and marijuana, and age of the patient receiving the medication. Avoid IM injections as they are very painful.

Prescription of the correct dosage can be aided by closer scrutiny of these factors. The theophylline-base content varies in xanthine products. The preparations are not therapeutically equal and may cause difficulty when patients are changed from one product to another. The critical factor is to monitor the theophylline blood levels to achieve a desired therapeutic effect. Appropriate dosage should produce a serum theophylline level between 10 and 20 mcg/ml. If serum theophylline level is between 5 and 10 mcg/ml, and patient is compliant increase dose by about 25%. Patient will have to be reevaluated very soon if level is between 5 and 7.5 mcg/ml, but may not need further evaluation for 6 to 12 months if level is between 7.5 and 10 mcg/ml. If serum theophylline level is between 20 and 25 mcg/ml, decrease dose by about 10% and recheck in 6 to 12 months. If level is between 25 and 30 mcg/ml, skip next dose and decrease subsequent dosage by 25%. If serum level is over 30 mcg/ml, skip next 2 doses and decrease dose by 50%, followed by repeated measurements of theophylline levels to make certain therapeutic range is maintained.

The rate of absorption of oral theophylline is dependent upon the dosage form used. Oral liquids have the fastest absorption time, followed by uncoated tablets. Enteric-coated or sustained release tablets and capsules produce inconsistent blood levels and should usually be reserved for use at night. Food does not influence absorption of theophylline. Rectal absorption is a slow method of absorption and is sometimes unpredictable with suppositories. Rectal absorption is very fast by solution, slower and more unpredictable by suppository.

The variance in rates of metabolism and excretion of theophylline is also problematic. Xanthines are metabolized in the liver and excreted by the kidney. The serum half-life of the drugs can range from 3 hours to 12 hours in adults and 4 hours to 9 hours in children. Heart failure, liver dysfunction and pulmonary edema can impede clearance, and smoking can increase clearance of theophylline from the body. The half-life of theophylline is shortened by a high-protein, low-carbohydrate diet and consumption of charcoal-broiled beef. Children under 9 years of age require larger doses/kg of theophylline than adults to maintain appropriate therapeutic blood levels of the drug. Thus, dosage must be prescribed on an individualized basis and carefully monitored. Frequently, an initial loading dose is indicated. Do not use sustained release products to load patient. Because of this need for individualized titration of the agents, use of fixed combination bronchodilator products, i.e., sympathomimetic, xanthine, and expectorant, are not recommended. Use of fixed combination products does not allow flexibility in changing dosages for individual drugs and may increase toxicity of some of the drugs. Concurrent use of selected sympathomimetic and xanthine dilators administered individually however may have a synergistic effect. See individual xanthine preparations for specifics concerning dosage and administration.

IMPLEMENTATION CONSIDERATIONS:

—Obtain a complete health history: presence of pregnancy, age (especially the very young or elderly), smoker or nonsmoker, hypersensitivity to xanthine, renal or liver dysfunction, heart disease, peptic ulcer, hypoxemia, severe hypertension, or glaucoma.

—Be alert for signs of toxicity, such as development of seizures, tachycardia or ventricular arrhythmias, vomiting, dizziness, and irritability.

—Prescribe drugs according to therapeutic blood levels of theophylline, consideration of the theophylline base in each preparation, and the clinical response of each patient.

—Observe patients for CNS stimulation, especially small children and the elderly.

—Consider the effect of cigarette smoking on the clinical response of each patient.

—To minimize GI symptoms, administer drug with food and water.

—Avoid use of alcoholic preparations.

WHAT THE PATIENT NEEDS TO KNOW:

—Report the following symptoms to the health care provider: seizures, rapid heart beat, irregular heart beat, vomiting, dizziness, and irritability.

—Avoid using large amounts of caffeine-containing beverages such as tea, coffee, cocoa, and cola drinks.

—Some other medications will interfere with the drug action if taken at the same time. Avoid taking any other drugs without first checking with your health care provider. This includes drugs which you may buy over the counter and which may also have an effect on the respiratory system (i.e., cough syrups, hay fever and allergy medicine.)

—Take medicine with a glass of water or with meals to avoid an upset stomach.

—Take medicine exactly as prescribed. This usually means taking medication every six hours except when you are taking sustained action drugs.

—If a dose is missed and noticed within an hour, take the prescribed dose. If remembered after an hour, skip the dose and stay on the original dosing schedule.

—Some suppositories must be refrigerated while others may not have this requirement. Check with the pharmacist when you have your prescription filled.

—If you are using rectal suppositories and burning or irritation of the rectal area occurs, notify your health care provider.

EVALUATION:

ADVERSE REACTIONS: *Cardiovascular:* decreased pulmonary vascular resistance, ECG changes, circulatory failure, extrasystoles, flushing, marked hypotension, palpitations, tachycardia. *CNS:* agitation, convulsions, headache, insomnia, irritability, muscle twitching, reflex hyperexcitability, restlessness. *Gastrointestinal:* diarrhea, epigastric or substernal pain, hematemesis, intestinal bleeding, irritation of peptic ulcer, nausea, vomiting. *Renal:* albuminuria, diuresis which may cause dehydration, increased excretion of red blood cells. *Respiratory:* tachypnea. *Other:* altered laboratory values, fever, hyperglycemia, inappropriate secretion of ADH syndrome, leukocytosis, rash.

OVERDOSAGE: *Signs and symptoms:* Anorexia, vomiting, nausea, agitation, vertigo, wakefulness, restlessness, irritability, headache, convulsions and ventricular arrhythmias are frequently the first signs of toxicity. Later symptoms include confusion, respiratory failure, shock, bizarre behavior, extreme thirst, delirium, and hyperthermia. Excessive overdosage may lead to seizures and death without warning symptoms. Children are at particular risk for this phenomenon.

PARAMETERS TO MONITOR: The acuteness of the respiratory attack dictates the parameters to monitor. The initial data base should include at least a chest x-ray, electrocardiogram, electrolytes (including glucose), complete blood count and urinalysis. During the initial visit, the health care provider should check vital signs, amount and characteristics of the sputum, level of fatigue and breath sounds. Pulmonary function tests and arterial blood gases may also be appropriate. At times, sputum should be sent for culture and sensitivity if an infection is suspected. If loading doses of the drug are given, the patient should be seen in one week, with each succeeding visit arranged according to response to the medication and relief of symptoms. *Parameters to monitor each visit:* weight, pulse, heart rhythm, heart sounds, blood pressure, respiratory rate, signs and symptoms of adverse reactions. Also observe for signs and symptoms of therapeutic effect: increased vital capacity; normal or near normal blood gases; lengthening of time between acute attacks; absence of prolonged expiration, wheezing, use of accessory muscles, coughing, hyperresonant percussion note, rales, rhonchi, distant breath sounds; and decreased expiratory excursion.

AMINOPHYLLINE (THEOPHYLLINE ETHYLENEDIAMINE)

PRODUCTS (TRADE NAME):

Aminodur Dura-tabs (Available in 300 mg timed release tablets, equivalent to 236 mg theophylline.) **Aminophylline** (Available in 105 mg/5 ml oral liquid, equivalent to 90 mg theophylline, and 100 and 200 mg tablets, equivalent to 79 and 158 mg theophylline, 250 and 500 mg suppositories, equivalent to 198, and 395 mg theophylline, and in 500 mg IM injection, equivalent to 395 mg theophylline per 2 ml.) **Amoline** (Available in 100 and 200 mg tablets, equivalent to 79 and 158 mg theophylline.) **Lixaminol** (Available in 250 mg elixir, equivalent to 215 mg theophylline/15 ml.) **Phyllocontin** (Available in 225 mg timed release capsules.) **Somophylline** (Available in 105 mg/5 ml oral liquid, equivalent to 90 mg theophylline/5 ml, and as 300 mg rectal solution, equivalent to 255 mg theophylline/5 ml.) **Truphylline** (Available in 250 and 500 mg suppositories, equivalent to 198 and 395 mg theophylline, and 500 mg suppositories, equivalent to 395 theophylline.)

DRUG SPECIFICS:

Aminophylline is a synthetic preparation. It plays a significant role in management of conditions with bronchial constriction and spasm. It is especially useful when differentiation cannot be made between bronchospasm and pulmonary edema. This agent is frequently prescribed by its generic name and contains 78% theophylline and 12% ethylenediamine. Oral aminophylhine offers no advantages over plain theophylline and exposes the patient to an additional agent which may itself cause allergic reactions. IM injection is painful and should be avoided.

ADMINISTRATION AND DOSAGE SPECIFICS:

Asthmatic Attacks:

Adults: 500 mg po stat; 200 to 315 mg po every 6-8 hours maintenance; For rectal suppositories usual dose is 500 mg once or twice a day not to exceed 1 gm/day, or 500 mg IM as necessary. With rectal solutions use 300 mg 1 to 3 times a day or 450 mg two times daily. Timed release tablets can be given in 300 mg to 600 mg every 8 to 12 hours.

Children: 7.5 mg/kg po stat; 5 to 6 mg/kg po every 6-8 hours maintenance; or give 7 mg/kg rectal suppository, or use rectal solutions in 5 mg/kg not to exceed every six hours. Timed release tablets are not recommended for children under twelve years of age.

DYPHYLLINE (DIHYDROXYPROPYL THEOPHYLLINE)

PRODUCTS (TRADE NAME):
Dilin (Available in 250 mg/ml in 2 ml ampules for injection.) **Dilor** (Available in 200 and 400 mg tablets, 160 mg/15 ml elixir with 18% alcohol, and 250 mg/ml injection.) **Droxine** (Available in 400 mg long-acting tablets and 100 mg/5 ml liquid.) **Dyflex** (Available in 200 and 400 mg tablets.) **Dyphylline** (Available in 200 mg and 400 mg tablets and 250 mg/ml injection.)**Lufyllin** (Available in 200 and 400 mg tablets, 100 mg/15 ml elixir with 20% alcohol, and 250 mg/ml for injection.) **Neothylline** (Available in 200 and 400 mg tablets, and 250 mg/ml for injection.)

DRUG SPECIFICS:
Dyphylline is incompletely absorbed. Therapeutic range has not been established. It has a short half-life, requiring frequent dosing.

ADMINISTRATION AND DOSAGE SPECIFICS:
Adults: Give up to 15 mg/kg po every 6 hours. Individualized dosage should be titrated depending upon the condition of the patient and the effect of the drug. For IM dosage, give 250 to 500 mg injected slowly.

Children 40 to 100 lbs: 80 to 240 mg for acute attacks; 27 to 80 mg for maintenance in 3-4 hours.

Children under 40 lbs: 40 to 80 mg for acute attacks; 13 to 17 mg in 3-4 hours for maintenance.

For IM dosage, give 2 to 3 mg/pound daily in divided doses.

OXTRIPHYLLINE (CHOLINE THEOPHYLLINATE)

PRODUCTS (TRADE NAME):
Choledyl (Available in 100 and 200 mg tablets, equivalent to 64 and 128 mg theophylline, 100 mg/5ml elixir, equivalent to 64 mg theophylline, in 20% alcohol, and 50 mg/5 ml pediatric syrup, equivalent to 32 mg theophylline.) **Choledyl SA** (Available in 400 and 600 mg sustained release tablets.) **Oxtriphylline** (Available in 100 mg/5 ml elixir, equivalent to 64 mg theophylline, with 20% alcohol.)

DRUG SPECIFICS:
Oxtriphylline has the same actions as aminophylline and may not be less irritating to the gastric mucosa, is completely absorbed from the gastrointestinal tract. The liquid formulation may taste better than theophylline liquid and may be better accepted by some patients.

ADMINISTRATION AND DOSAGE SPECIFICS:
Adults: 200 mg po four times daily.
Children 2 to 12 years: 100 mg/60 lb four times daily.
Sustained Action: 400 to 600 mg two times daily.

THEOPHYLLINE

PRODUCTS (TRADE NAME):
Aerolate (Available in 160 mg/15 ml liquid, alcohol free, and in 65, 130 and 260 mg timed release capsules.) **Bronkodyl** (Available in 100 and 200 mg capsules, 300 mg sustained release capsules, and 80 mg/15 ml elixir, with 20% alcohol.) **Elixophyllin** (Available in 100 and 200 mg capsules; 125 and 250 mg timed release capsules; and 80 mg/15 ml elixir, with 20% alcohol.) **Lanophyllin** (Available in 80 mg/15 ml elixir, with 20% alcohol.) **Quibron-T/SR Dividose** (Available in 300 mg tablet and 300 mg sustained release tablets.) **Slo-Phyllin** (Available in 100 and 200 mg tablets, 80 mg/ml syrup and 60, 125 and 250 mg sustained release capsles.) **Somophyllin T** (Available in 50, 100, 200 and 250 mg capsules.) **Somophyllin-CRT** (Available in 50, 100, and 250 mg sustained release capsules.) **Theo-clear** (Available in 100 and 200 mg tablets and 65, 130 and 260 mg timed release capsules, and 80 mg/15 ml syrup.) **Theo-dur** (Available in 100, 200 and 300 mg timed release capsules.) **Theolair** (Available in 125 and 250 mg tablets and in 80 mg/15 ml liquid, alcohol free.) **Theon** (Available in 150 mg/15 ml liquid with 10% alcohol.) **Theophyl** (Available in 100 mg chewable tablets and 125 and 250 mg timed release capsules.) **Theophyl-225** (Available in 225 mg tablets.) **Theostat** (Available in 100 and 200 mg tablets and 80 mg/15 ml syrup.) **Theophylline** (Available in 100 and 200 mg capsules, 100, 200 and 300 mg tablets, and 80 mg/15 ml elixir.)
DRUG SPECIFICS:
This drug plays a significant role in management of conditions with bronchial constriction and spasm. It is especially useful when differentiation cannot be made between bronchospasm and pulmonary edema.
ADMINISTRATION AND DOSAGE:
Dosage must be individualized using standard mg/kg formulas. Usual doses are:
Adults: 200 to 250 mg po every 6 hours.
Children: Administer 3 to 6 mg/kg every 6 hours.
For timed release capsules:
Aerolate: Give 65 to 260 mg po every 12 hours po.
Theo-dur:
Adults: give 300 mg po every 12 hours po.
Children 12 to 16: 200 mg po every 12 hours po.
Children 9 to 12: 150 mg po every 12 hours po.
Children under 9: 100 mg po every 12 hours po.

THEOPHYLLINE SODIUM GLYCINATE

PRODUCTS (TRADE NAME):
Synophylate (Available in 330 mg tablets, equivalent to 165 mg theophylline,

or as 330 mg/15 ml elixir, equivalent to 165 mg theophylline, in 20% alcohol.)
DRUG SPECIFICS:
This drug, with 49% theophylline, has the typical actions of theophylline with the advantage that it is less irritating to the gastric mucosa. Thus, larger doses of theophylline may be given than are possible with other theophylline preparations.
ADMINISTRATION AND DOSAGE SPECIFICS:
Adults: 330 to 660 mg po 2 to 3 times daily after meals.
Children 6 to 12 years: 220 to 330 mg po 2 to 3 times daily.
Children under 6 years: 27.5 to 55 mg/10 lbs po 2 to 3 times daily.

Mary F. Rapson

XANTHINE COMBINATION PRODUCTS

DRUG SPECIFICS:
A partial list of xanthine combination products which are most commonly used is given in Table 8-5. See specific drug monographs for details on drug actions. These products usually contain some form of theophylline in combination with ephedrine, guaifenesin and/or phenobarbital. They are considerably more expensive than plain theophylline. The theophylline component causes bronchodilation, vasodilation, myocardial stimulation, and mild diuresis. Ephedrine causes bronchodilation. Guaifenesin is an expectorant.

Combination products are associated with a higher incidence of toxicity, and have not been shown to be more effective. Warn the patient that side effects may include insomnia and nervousness. Ephedrine may decrease the effects of antihypertensive drugs. Serious disturbances of heart rhythm may develop if ephedrine is taken concurrently with digitalis preparations. Ephedrine in combination with ergot-related preparations, mono-amine oxidase (MAO) inhibitors, or tricyclic antidepressants may cause dangerous increases in blood pressure.

While taking these preparations, decrease intake of coffee, tea and caffeine products to lessen nervousness. Increase fluid intake. Theophylline is more effective on an empty stomach, but this could cause gastric irritation. Preparations may be taken with antacids. Smoking does not directly interfere with these drugs; however, it does aggravate bronchitis, asthma, and emphysema. Theophylline may decrease the effects of antigout medications and lithium.

Warn patients not to self-medicate with over-the-counter bronchodilators without medical approval. When serum theophylline levels exceed 20 mcg/ml, toxicity is probable. Obtain theophylline level if indicated. In calculating dosage, use ideal body weight for obese patients. "Rx" means prescription is required.

TABLE 8-5. XANTHINE COMBINATION PRODUCTS

Products (Trade Name)	Components	Dosage
Dyflex G (Rx) (tablets, liquid)	Dyphylline 200 mg; guaifenesin 200 mg	*Adults:* One tablet or 30 ml liquid 4 times daily. *Children over 6 years:* Maximum 5 mg/lb/daily.
Dyline-GG(Rx) (tablets, liquid)	Dyphylline 200 mg; guaifenesin 200 mg.	*Adults:* One tablet or 30 ml liquid 4 times daily *Children over 6 years:* Maximum 5 mg/lb/daily
Lufyllin-GG (Rx) (tablets, liquid)	Dyphylline 200 mg; guaifenesin 200 mg.	*Adults:* One tablet or 30 ml liquid 4 times daily. *Children over 6 years:* Maximum 5 mg/lb/daily.
Neothylline-GG (Rx) (tablets, liquid)	Dyphilline 200 mg; guaifenesin 200 mg.	*Adults:* One tablet or 30 ml liquid 4 times daily. *Children over 6 years:* Maximum 5 mg/lb/daily.
Primatene P (tablets)	Theophylline 130 mg; ephedrine HCl 24 mg; phenobarbital 8 mg.	*Adults:* 1-2 tablets initially, then 1 every 4 hours (up to 6 tablets) daily. *Children over 6 years:* 1/2 adult dose.
Quibron (Rx) (capsules or liquid)	Theophylline 150 mg; guaifenesin 90 mg.	*Adults:* 1-2 capsules or 1-2 tbsp every 6-8 hours. *Children 9-12 years:* 4-5 mg/kg every 6-8 hours. *Children under 9 years:* 4-6 mg/kg every 6-8 hours.
Slo-Phyllin GG (Rx)	Theophylline 150 mg; guaifenesin 90 mg.	*Adults or children 16 or or older:* 13 mg /kg/day or 900 mg daily (whichever is less) in divided doses every 6-8 hours. *Children 6 months to 9 years:* 24 mg/kg daily.

TABLE 8-5. *(Continued)*

Products (Trade Name)	Components	Dosage
		Give in divided doses every 6 hours. *Children 9-12 years:* 20 mg/kg daily. Give in divided doses every 6 hours. *Children 12-16 years:* 18 mg/kg daily. Give in divided doses every 6 hours.
Tedral (Rx), **TEP Tabs, Theocord, Theodrine, Theofedral, Theophenyllin, Theoral Theophenyllin, Theoral**	Theophylline 130 mg; ephedrine HCl 24 mg; phenobarbital 8 mg	*Adults:* 1-2 tablets every 4 hours *Children over 60 lbs:* 1/2 the adult dose

Mary Ann Bolter

DECONGESTANTS

NASAL DECONGESTANTS

ACTION OF THE DRUG: (1) The main action of the decongestants is a direct effect on the alpha receptors of blood vessels in the nasal mucosa to produce vasoconstriction. This vasopressor action reduces blood flow, fluid exudation, and mucosal edema. (2) Many agents also have a beta property which may cause rebound vasodilation.

ASSESSMENT:

INDICATIONS: Used for the relief of nasal congestion associated with allergies and upper respiratory tract infections. The drugs may also be used as adjunctive therapy for middle ear infections to decrease congestion around the eustachian tubes. Ear block and pressure pain incurred during air travel may respond to nasal inhalers.

SUBJECTIVE: History of nasal congestion, postnasal drip, nasal discharge, sneezing, sore throat, headache, itchy eyes, lacrimation, nasal polyps, earache, decreased hearing, upper respiratory infection, or allergies.

OBJECTIVE: Nasal discharge, mucosal edema, mucosal inflammation, polyps, sinus tenderness, pharynx erythematosus, exudates in pharynx, tender lymph nodes, enlarged lymph nodes, and tympanic membrane abnormalities: bulging, perforated, red, external canal inflamed and with discharge. Decreased or absent air flow through nostrils, decrease in size of nasal passages.

PLAN:

CONTRAINDICATIONS: Hypersensitivity to adrenergic agents, narrow-angle glaucoma, and concurrent MAO inhibitor or tricyclic antidepressant therapy are conditions in which decongestants should not be used. Do not use during general anesthesia with cyclopropane or halogenated hydrocarbons, or in the presence of loss of sensation in the fingers and toes.

WARNINGS: These preparations should be used cautiously in patients with hypertension, arrhythmias, heart disease, angina, hyperthyroidism, diabetes, advanced arteriosclerotic conditions, glaucoma, prostatic hypertrophy, or chronic cough because of the possibility of systemic vasoconstriction and tachycardia. Also use with caution in patients with a long history of asthma and emphysema complicated by degenerative heart disease. Excessive administration of topical decongestants may result in gastrointestinal absorption and cause systemic effects. Safety in pregnancy has not been established.

PRECAUTIONS: If headache and nervousness result from excessive administration, discontinue treatment. Frequent and continual use of the topical decongestants or at dosages greater than recommended may result in a rebound phenomenon. Topical decongestants should be used only in acute states, for no longer than 3 to 5 days, and sparingly in children and the elderly.

IMPLEMENTATION:

DRUG INTERACTIONS: Systemic effects may be potentiated by concurrent use of other sympathomimetics, MAO inhibitors, tricyclic antidepressants, antihistamines, and thyroxine. Caution should be used in stable hypertensive patients on guanethidine, bethanidine and debrisoquine sulfate. Use with high doses of digitalis, mercurial diuretics, or other drugs which may sensitize the heart to arrhythmias should be avoided as anginal pain may result when there is evidence of coronary insufficiency.

ADMINISTRATION AND DOSAGE: *Oral:* Oral decongestants are considered to be more effective than nasal preparations because they will produce effects in inaccessible parts of the convoluted mucous membrane nasal passages. The effects may be more prolonged than those achieved by topical preparations. The disadvantage of the systemic agents is that their effects may be generalized and not limited to the nasal mucosa. *Topical:* Topical application may take the form of drops, sprays, jellies, and oral inhalation. The advantage of this form of administration is rapid onset of action and direct stimulation of the nasal mucosa. Drops have a tendency to pass into the hypopharynx and then be swallowed, thus passing into the gastrointestinal tract. Sprays deliver a fine mist that is easily trapped in the upper respiratory tract and are less likely to reach the gastrointestinal tract. Topical preparations should not be used for more than 3 to 5 days because of the risk of rebound phenomenon. Oral preparations are more appropriate for long-term use. See specific products for information on exact dosages.

IMPLEMENTATION CONSIDERATIONS:

—Be alert for signs of developing systemic toxicity, and terminate the drug if signs appear.

—Drops should be instilled with the patient in the lateral head-low position to prevent swallowing of the drug.

—Solutions of topical decongestants can become contaminated with use and result in growth of bacteria and fungi.

—Prescribe topical decongestants for acute nasal congestion and limit their use to 3 to 5 days.

WHAT THE PATIENT NEEDS TO KNOW:

—To administer drops: blow the nose gently, assume a reclining position with head tipped back over the edge of the bed. Put 1-2 drops of solution on the lower nasal mucosa, breathe through the mouth, and remain in the position for 5 minutes while turning head from side to side. This will help the drops run back into your nose instead of down your throat.

—When using a spray, keep the container upright to obtain a fine mist. Gently blow the nose and squeeze the bottle firmly in each nostril. After 3-5 minutes, blow the nose again, and repeat application if congestion remains.

—Always rinse the dropper after putting drops into the nose. This will help prevent growth of bacteria and fungi.

—Use separate bottles of nasal spray for each person in the family. Do not share topical decongestants.

—Jellies are administered by putting a small amount on the finger, and applying it to the nasal mucosa, and snuffing deeply through the nose.

—Inhalers are administered by inserting the open end of the plastic tube in each nostril and inhaling two times.

—Avoid excessive use of these medicines or they will cause the symptoms which you are trying to reduce.

—Missed doses may be taken within an hour of the scheduled time and then the regular schedule may be resumed. If more time has passed, skip that dose and return to the regular schedule. Relief should be noticed within a few minutes of administration.

EVALUATION:

ADVERSE REACTIONS: *Dermatologic:* Stinging and burning secondary to mucosal dryness sometimes following topical administration may occur. Rebound congestion following prolonged use of topical agents may appear. When absorbed from the gastrointestinal tract, systemic effects such as nervousness, nausea, dizziness, CNS stimulation, tachycardia, arrhythmia, and transient increase in blood pressure may occur. Rarely, a severe shocklike syndrome with hypotension and coma has been reported in children. Psychic dependence and toxic psychoses have been reported with long-term high dose therapy.

OVERDOSAGE: The severity of overdosage varies widely, resulting in a variety of symptoms. In children, profound CNS depression has been reported. In severe overdosage CNS depression, hypertension, bradycardia, and decreased cardiac output may result. This state can be followed by rebound hypotension and cardiovascular collapse. Treatment involves referral for gastric lavage and supportive treatment.

PARAMETERS TO MONITOR: The patient should be monitored for the cessation of the following symptoms. *Nasal:* discharge, mucosal edema, inflammation, boggy membranes. *Pharynx:* inflamed throat, postnasal drip, exudates. *Glands:* swollen and/or tender. *Ear:* tympanic membrane bulging, inflamed, perforated, or with decreased hearing. *Chest:* rales. Usually, no laboratory tests are necessary. If streptococcal pharyngitis is suspected, a throat culture should be done. If allergic rhinitis needs to be confirmed, an eosinophil count or smear may be helpful.

EPHEDRINE

PRODUCTS (TRADE NAME):
Efedron Nasal (Available in 0.6% concentration in 20 gm jelly.) **Ephedrine Sulfate** (Available in 3% drops in 30 ml bottle.) **Ephedsol-1%** (Available in 1% drops in 30 ml bottle.) **Vatronol** (Available in 0.5% drops in 15 and 30 ml dropper bottle.)

DRUG SPECIFICS:
This agent produces vasoconstriction of arterioles in the nasal mucosa. It may produce burning, stinging, dryness of nasal mucosa, and sneezing.

ADMINISTRATION AND DOSAGE SPECIFICS:
Adults and children 6 years and older: 2 or 3 drops, or application of a small amount of jelly in each nostril every 3 or 4 hours. Do not use in children under 6 years of age.

EPINEPHRINE HYDROCHLORIDE

PRODUCTS (TRADE NAME):
Adrenalin Chloride (Available in 0.1% drops in 30 ml dropper bottle.)

DRUG SPECIFICS:
Epinephrine stimulates both alpha- and beta-receptors. There might be slight stinging after instillation of this drug due to the presence of sodium bisulfate, a preservative.

ADMINISTRATION AND DOSAGE SPECIFICS:
1 to 2 drops in each nostril every 4 to 6 hours.

INHALERS

PRODUCTS (TRADE NAME):
Benzedrex (Available in 250 mg prophylhexedrine inhaler.) **Vicks Inhaler** (Available in 50 mg *l*-desoxyephedrine inhaler.)
DRUG SPECIFICS:
May be used as often as needed but excessive use should be avoided. Rarely causes CNS stimulation.
ADMINISTRATION AND DOSAGE SPECIFICS:
Insert plastic tip in nostril, close other nostril, and inhale 2 times. Repeat on other side.

NAPHAZOLINE HYDROCHLORIDE

PRODUCTS (TRADE NAME):
Privine (Available in .05% spray or drops.)
DRUG SPECIFICS:
This agent has marked alpha-adrenergic effects producing vasoconstriction in the nasal arterioles which is rapid and prolonged. This drug produces CNS depression rather than stimulation when swallowed. Insomnia has not been reported when using this preparation; thus, one dose may be taken close to bedtime.
ADMINISTRATION AND DOSAGE SPECIFICS:
Adults and children 6 years and over: 2 drops in each nostril no more frequently than every 3 hours. Not recommended for use with children under 6 years of age.

OXYMETAZOLINE HYDROCHLORIDE

PRODUCTS (TRADE NAME):
Afrin (Available in 0.025% drops and 0.05% spray and drops.) **Dristan** (Available in 0.05% regular or menthol spray.) **Duramist Plus** (Available in 15 ml spray.) **Duration** (Available in 0.05% spray or mentholated vapor spray, or in 0.05% drops.) **Neo-Synephrine Twelve Hour** (Available in 0.05%, and 0.025% drops, and in 0.5% regular or mentholated spray.) **Sinex Long-Lasting** (Available in 0.05% 15

and 30 ml spray.) **Dristan Long-Lasting Nasal Spray** (Available in 0.5% 15 and 30 ml spray and with menthol.)
DRUG SPECIFICS:

This is a frequently used adrenergic topical agent sold over the counter. This preparation acts directly on alpha-receptors to produce vasoconstriction in the nasal passages. These products have the most prolonged decongestant effects. There is a tendency for patients to overuse this drug which results in rebound congestion. Thus, it should be used no longer than 3 days in succession.
ADMINISTRATION AND DOSAGE SPECIFICS:

Adults and children 6 years of age or older: 2 squeezes in each nostril twice daily, or 2 to 4 drops in each nostril twice daily.

PHENYLEPHRINE HYDROCHLORIDE

PRODUCTS (TRADE NAME):

Alconefrin (Available in 0.16, 0.25, and 0.5% drops.) **Allerest Nasal** (Available in 0.5% drops.) **Coricidin** (Available in 0.5% drops or spray.) **Duration Mild** (Available in 0.5% spray.) **Neo-Synephrine** (Available in 0.125, 0.25, 0.5 and 1% drops; and 0.5% jelly.) **Rhinall** (Available in 0.2% and 0.25% drops and spray. **Sinarest Nasal, Sinex** (Available in 0.5% spray.) **Super Anahist** (Available in 0.25% spray.) **Vacon** (Available in 0.2% spray or drops.)
DRUG SPECIFICS:

Not to be used for more than 3 days. Protect from freezing and light. Oxidation and potency loss result from exposure to air, strong light, or heat. One of the most effective topical preparations, but it may cause marked local irritation.
ADMINISTRATION AND DOSAGE SPECIFICS:

Adults: Use 0.25 to 1.0% strength, 3 to 4 drops or 1 to 2 sprays every 4 hours.
Children 6-12 years: Use 0.25%, 2 to 3 drops every 3 to 4 hours.
Children 2-6 years: Use 0.167%, 2 to 3 drops every 4 hours.
Infants: Use 0.125%. 2 to 3 drops every 3 to 4 hours.

Jelly is not widely used but has a somewhat longer action and may provide a degree of protection against irritation.

PHENYLPROPANOLAMINE HYDROCHLORIDE

PRODUCTS (TRADE NAME):

Phenylpropanolamine HCl (Available in 25 and 50 mg tablets and in 75 mg timed release capsules.) **Propagest** (Available in 25 mg tablets and 12.5 mg/5 ml syrup.) **Propadrine** (Available in 25 and 50 mg capsules and as 20 mg/5 ml elixir.) **Rhindecon** (Available in 75 mg timed release capsules.)

DRUG SPECIFICS:

This drug resembles ephedrine but has greater pressor effects and fewer CNS effects. It stimulates alpha-receptors of vascular smooth muscles resulting in vasoconstriction. This agent is also available over the counter as an anorexiant (questionable).

ADMINISTRATION AND DOSAGE SPECIFICS:

Adults: 25 mg po every four hours or 50 mg every 6 to 8 hours. Not to exceed 150 mg daily.

Children 6 to 12 years: 12.5 mg po every 4 hours or 25 mg every 8 hours.

Children 2 to 6 years: 6.25 mg po every 4 hours or 12.5 mg every 8 hours.

PSEUDOEPHEDRINE HYDROCHLORIDE (*d*-ISOEPHEDRINE HCL)

PRODUCTS (TRADE NAME):

Neofed (Available in 60 mg tablets.) **Novafed** (Available in 120 mg timed release capsules and 30 mg/5 ml liquid.) **Pseudoephedrine HCl** (Available in 30 and 60 mg tablets and 30 mg/5 ml liquid.) **Sudafed** (Available in 30 and 60 mg tablets, 120 mg timed release capsules, and 30 mg/5 ml syrup.)

DRUG SPECIFICS:

This preparation acts on sympathetic nerve endings as well as directly on smooth muscle. Fewer side effects are caused by this drug than epinephrine. It is an oral decongestant and can be given concurrently with antihistamines.

ADMINISTRATION AND DOSAGE SPECIFICS:

Adults and children 12 years and older: 60 mg po three to four times daily; or 120 mg timed release capsule can be given po every 12 hours.

Children 6-12 years: 30 mg po three to four times daily.

Children 2-3 years: 15 mg po three to four times daily.

TETRAHYDROZOLINE HYDROCHLORIDE

PRODUCTS (TRADE NAME):

Tyzine (Available in 0.05% and 0.1% drops.)

DRUG SPECIFICS:

Available by prescription only. Not for use in children under the age of 2 years. Avoid prolonged use.

ADMINISTRATION AND DOSAGE SPECIFICS:

Adults and children 6 years and older: 2 to 4 drops of 0.1% solution in each nostril as needed but no more than every 3 hours.

Children 2 to 6 years: 2 to 3 drops of O.05% solution in each nostril as needed but no more than every 3 hours.

XYLOMETAZOLINE HYDROCHLORIDE

PRODUCTS (TRADE NAME):
 Chlorohist-LA (Available in 0.1% spray.) **Corimist**(Available in 0.1% spray.) **Neo-Synephrine II Long Acting** (Available in 0.05% drops and 0.1% drops, regular and menthol spray.) **Otrivin** (Available in O.05% drops and in 0.1% drops and spray.)
DRUG SPECIFICS:
 Action lasts for 8 to 10 hours. Not to be used for more than 3 days. Overdose can cause extreme CNS depression in children.
ADMINISTRATION AND DOSAGE SPECIFICS:
 Adults: Give 2 to 3 sprays or 2 to 3 drops in each nostril every 8 to 10 hours.
 Children under 12 years: Use 2 to 3 drops of O.05% every 8 to 10 hours.

Mary R. Rapson and Irene McCrea

DECONGESTANT COMBINATIONS

DRUG SPECIFICS:
 These drugs contain a decongestant and an antihistamine or analgesic. The action of each component of the drug listed in Table 8-6 should be considered in prescribing. Products are available over the counter unless otherwise noted with "Rx".

TABLE 8-6. DECONGESTANT COMBINATIONS

Products (Trade Name)	Components	Dosage
Actifed (available tablets and liquid	*Tablet:* Pseudoephedrine HCl 60 mg, triprolidine HCl 2.5 mg; *Liquid:* Pseudoephedrine HCl 30 mg; triprolidine HCl 1.25 mg in 10 ml syrup.	1 tablet or 10 ml three or four times daily.

TABLE 8-6. *(Continued)*

Products (Trade Name)	Components	Dosage
Allerest Tablets	Phenylpropanolamine HCl 18.7 mg; chlorpheniramine maleate 2 mg	2 tablets every four hours
Allergesic Tablets	Phenylprop-anolamine HCl 18.7 mg; chlorpheniramine maleate 2 mg	2 tablets every four hours
Allerstat Capsules	Phenylpropanolamine HCl 25 mg; phenylephrine HCl 2.5 mg; pheniramine maleate 12.5 mg; pyrilamine maleate 12.5 mg	1 capsule three or four times daily
Apochist Allergy Tablets	Phenylpropanolamine HCl 25 mg;	
Chlor-Trimeton Decongestant (available in tablets)	Pseudoephedrine HCl 60 mg; chlorpheniramine maleate 4 mg.	1 every four to eight hours
Conex DA (available in timed release tablets)	Phenylpropanolamine HCl 50 mg; phenyltoloxamine citrate 50 mg.	1 every eight hours
Congespirin (available in chewable pediatric tablets)	Phenylephrine HCl 1.25 mg; aspirin 81 mg.	2 to 8 tablets every four hours for children
Covanamine (available in liquid)	Phenylpropanolamine HCl 6.25 mg; phenylephrine HCl 3.75 mg; pyrilamine maleate 6.25 mg; chlorpheniramine maleate 1 mg.	10 ml every four hours
Dimetapp (available in sustained release tablets and elixir)(Rx)	Phenylpropanolamine HCl 5 mg; brompheniramine maleate 4 mg; with 2.3% alcohol in elixir; or phenylpropanolamine HCl	5-10 ml three or four 1 tablet every 12 hours

TABLE 8-6. *(Continued)*

Products (Trade Name)	Components	Dosage
	15 mg; phenylephrine HCl 15 mg; brompheniramine maleate 12 mg.	
Dristan (available in capsules)	Phenylephrine HCl 5 mg; chlorpheniramine maleate 2 mg; aspirin 325 mg; caffeinep 16.2 mg.	1 or 2 every four hours
Drixoral (available in timed release tablets)(Rx)	Pseudoephedrine sulfate 120 mg; dexbrompheniramine maleate 6 mg.	1 every 12 hours
Endecon (available in tablets)	Phenylpropanolamine HCl 25 mg; acetaminophen 325 mg.	1 or 2 every four hours
Fedahist (available in syrup)	Pseudoephedrine HCl 30 mg; chlorpheniramine maleate 2 mg.	10 ml every six hours
Fedahist Gyrocaps (Rx) (available in capsules)	Pseudoephedrine HCl 65 mg; chlorpheniramine maleate 10 mg.	1 capsule every 12 hours
Fedrazil (available in tablets)	Pseudoephedrine HCl 30 mg; chlorcyclizine HCl 25 mg.	1 tablet three times
Naldegesic (available in tablets)	Pseudoephedrine HCl 15 mg; acetaminophen 325 mg.	2 tablets three times daily
Novafed A (available in syrup)	Pseudoephedrine HCl 30 mg; chlorpheniramine maleate 2 mg; alcohol 5%.	10 ml every four hours
Novahistine Elixir (available in syrup)	Phenylpropanolamine HCl 18.75 mg; chlorpheniramine 2 mg; alcohol 5%.	10 ml every four hours
Novahistine Cold Tablets	Phenylpropanolamine HCl 18.7 mg; chlorpheniramine maleate 2 mg.	2 tablets every four
Ornade (available in capsules)(Rx)	Phenylpropanolamine HCl 75 mg; chlorpheniramine maleate 12 mg.	1 capsule every 12

TABLE 8-6. *(Continued)*

Products (Trade Name)	Components	Dosage
PBZ with Ephedrine (Rx)(available in tablets)	Ephedrine sulfate 12 mg; tripelennamine HCl 25 mg.	1 or 2 tablets four times daily
Sinutab (available in tablets)	Phenylpropanolamine HCl 25 mg; phenyltoloxamine 22 mg; acetaminophen 325 mg.	1 tablet every four hours
Triaminic (available in tablets)	Phenylpropanolamine HCl 50 mg; pheniramine maleate 25mg; daily pyrilamine maleate 25 mg.	1 tablets three times

Irene McCrea

DECONGESTANT AND ANTIHISTAMINE COMBINATIONS MISCELLANEOUS

DRUG SPECIFICS:

Consider the need for all components of the drugs listed in Table 8-7 before prescribing. All products are available over the counter.

TABLE 8-7. MISCELLANEOUS DECONGESTANT AND ANTIHISTAMINE COMBINATIONS

Products (Trade Name)	Components	Dosage
Citra (available in capsules)	Phenylephrine HCl 10 mg; pyrilamine maleate 8.33 mg; pheniramine maleate 6.25 mg; chlorpheniramine maleate 1 mg; salicylamide 227 mg; ascorbic acid 50 mg; caffeine 30 mg.	1 capsule every four hours

TABLE 8-7. *(Continued)*

Products (Trade Name)	Components	Dosage
Coryban-D (available in capsules)	Phenylpropanolamine HCl 25 mg; chlorpheniramine maleate hours 2 mg; caffeine 30 mg.	2 capsules every four hours
Duadacin (available in capsules)	Phenylephrine HCl 12.5 mg; chlorpheniramine maleate 2 mg; acetaminophen 325 mg.	2 capsules every four hours
Duradyne Forte(available in tablets)	Phenylephrine HCl 5 mg; chlorpheniramine maleate 2 mg; salicylamide 225 mg; acetaminophen 160 mg; caffeine 30 mg.	1 tablet every four hours
Hista-Compound No. 5 (available in tablets)	Chlorpheniramine maleate 2 mg; acetaminophen 150 mg; salicylamide 175 mg.	1 or 2 tablets every hour
Pyrroxate (available in capsules)	Phenylpropanolamine HCl 25 mg; chlorpheniramine maleate 2 mg; acetaminophen 500 mg.	1 capsule every four to six hours
Sinulin (available in tablets)	Phenylpropanolamine HCl 37.5 mg; chlorpheniramine maleate 2 mg; acetamenophen 325 mg; salicylamide 250 mg; homatropine MBr 0.75 mg.	1 tablet every four hours
Super-Decon (available in capsules)	Phenylephrine HCl 5 mg; pyrilamine maleate 12.5 mg; salicylamide 250 mg; ascorbic acid 50 mg; caffeine 32 mg.	1 every 2 or 3 hours

Irene McCrea

DECONGESTANT, ANTIHISTAMINE, AND ANALGESIC COMBINATIONS

DRUG SPECIFICS:

The products in Table 8-8 contain a decongestant, an antihistamine and an analgesic. The action of each component of the drug listed should be considered when prescribing. All are available over-the-counter unless marked with "Rx". Liquid prescriptions contain alcohol.

TABLE 8-8. DECONGESTANT, ANTIHISTAMINE AND ANALGESIC COMBINATIONS

Products (Trade Name)	Components	Dosage
Codimal (available in tablets and capsules)	Pseudoephedrine HCl 30 mg; chlorpheniramine maleate 2 mg; acetaminophen 325 mg.	1 or 2 every four hours
Colrex (available in tablets) (Rx)	Phenylephrine HCl 10 mg; chlorpheniramine maleate 2 mg; acetaminophen 325 mg; codeine phosphate 16 mg.	1 or 2 three or four times a day
Conex Plus (available in tablets)	Phenylpropanolamine HCl 25 mg; phenyltoloxamine citrate 25 mg; acetaminophen 250 mg.	1 or 2 every 8 hours
Coricidin "D" (available tablets)	Phenylpropanolamine HCl 12.5 mg; chlorpheniramine maleate 2 mg; aspirin 325 mg.	2 every four hours
CoTylenol (available in tablets)	Pseudoephedrine HCl 30 mg; chlorpheniramine maleate 2 mg; acetaminophen 325 mg; 15 mg dextromethorphan HBr.	2 every six hours
Covangesic (available in tablets)	Phenylpropanolamine HCl 12.5 mg; phenylephrine HCl 7.5 mg; pyrilamine maleate 12.5 mg; chlorpheniramine maleate 2 mg; acetaminophen 275 mg; tartrazine.	1 every four to six hours
Novahistine Sinus Tablets	Pseudoephedrine HCl 30 mg; chlorpheniramine maleate 2 mg; acetaminophen 325 mg.	2 every four hours
Sinarest (available in tablets)	Phenylpropanolamine HCl 18.75 mg; chlorpheniramine maleate 2 mg; acetaminophen 325 mg.	2 every four hours

TABLE 8-8. *(Continued)*

Products (Trade Name)	Components	Dosage
Sine-Off (available in tablets)	Phenylpropanolamine HCl 18.75 mg; chlorpheniramine maleate 2 mg; acetaminophen 325 mg.	2 every six hours
Sinustat (available in tablets)	phenylpropanolamine HCl 25 mg; phenyltoloxamine citrate 22 mg; acetaminophen 325 mg.	1 every four hours
Sinutab Extra Strength (available in tablets)	Phenylpropanolamine HCl 18.75 mg; chlorpheniramine maleate 2 mg; acetaminophen 500 mg.	

Irene McCrea

DECONGESTANT, ANTIHISTAMINE, AND ANTICHOLINERGIC COMBINATIONS—SUSTAINED RELEASE

DRUG SPECIFICS:

The products in Table 8-9 contain anticholinergics which cause drying of mucus secretions. They should be avoided in those patients with asthma or chronic obstructive pulmonary disease. Products are available over the counter unless indicated by "Rx."

TABLE 8-9. SUSTAINED RELEASE DECONGESTANT, ANTIHISTAMINE, AND ANTICHOLINERGIC COMBINATIONS

Products (Trade Name)	Components	Dosage
Alersule Capsules (Rx)	Phenylephrine HCl 20 mg; chlorpheniramine maleate 8 mg; methscopolamine nitrate 2.5 mg.	1 every 12 hours

TABLE 8-9. *(Continued)*

Products (Trade Name)	Components	Dosage
Allerprop Capsules	Phenylpropanolamine HCl 50 mg; chlorpheniramine maleate 4 mg; belladonna alkaloids 0.2 mg.	1 every 8 hours
Contac (available in sustained release capsules)	Phenylpropanolamine HCl 75 mg; chlorpheniramine maleate 8 mg.	1 every 12 hours
Extendryl Sr Capsules	Phenylephrine HCl 20 mg; chlorpheniramine maleate 8 mg; methscopolamine nitrate 2.5 mg.	1 every 12 hours
Histabid (available in sustained release capsules)	Phenylpropanolamine HCl 75 mg; chlorpheniramine maleate 8 mg.	1 every 12 hours
Rhinolar-Ex (available in sustained release capsules)	Phenylpropanolamine HCl 75 mg; chlorpheniramine maleate 8 mg.	1 every 12 hours
Sinovan Timed Capsules	Phenylephrine HCl 20 mg; chlorpheniramine maleate 8 mg; methscopolamine nitrate 2.5 mg.	1 every 12 hours
Spantac (available in capsules)	Phenylpropanolamine HCl 50 mg; chlorpheniramine maleate 4 mg; belladonna alkaloids 0.2 mg.	
Supres Capsules	Phenylpropanolamine HCl 50 mg; chlorpheniramine maleate 1 mg; pheniramine maleate 12.5 mg; belladonna alkaloids 0.16 mg	

Irene McCrea

EXPECTORANTS

ACTION OF THE DRUG: All expectorant products are believed to decrease the thickness of respiratory secretions by increasing the amount of fluid in the respiratory tract. These increased liquid secretions promote ciliary action and decrease the amount of coughing while increasing the amount of sputum produced. There is a lack of objective studies to support the clinical effectiveness of these drugs.

ASSESSMENT:

INDICATIONS: These drugs are used for symptomatic treatment of nonproductive cough. These products may be useful in chronic respiratory disease when thick mucus is a complication.
SUBJECTIVE: Frequent, dry cough.
OBJECTIVE: Continuous nonproductive cough. Evidence of mucus in the respiratory tract, rhonchi, and/or rales.

PLAN:

CONTRAINDICATIONS: There are no absolute contraindications to the use of over-the-counter oral expectorants except hypersensitivity to any of their components. See specific products for relative contraindications.
PRECAUTIONS: Expectorants are not to be used in persistent cough without the advice of a health care provider. Chronic or persistent cough may be the result of a serious condition and should not be ignored.

IMPLEMENTATION:

DRUG INTERACTIONS: Guaifenesin may increase bleeding tendency, and patients on anticoagulants must be closely monitored. This drug also interferes with the results of 5-hydroxyindoleacetic acid (5-HIAA) and vanillylmandelic acid (VMA) laboratory tests.
ADMINISTRATION AND DOSAGE: Taking an increased amount of fluid each day and breathing humid air are important in liquefying secretions. Medication should be taken with at least one full glass of water.
IMPLEMENTATION CONSIDERATIONS:
—Obtain a complete health history, including the history of cough, presence of other respiratory disease, hypersensitivity, other medications which may cause drug interactions.
—Perform a thorough chest examination. Ascertain if there are adventitious lung sounds, presence of fever, or clinical signs of dehydration.
—Use of more than the recommended dose can lead to adverse reactions.

WHAT THE PATIENT NEEDS TO KNOW:
—This drug will help make your sputum more liquid. This will make it easier to bring up when you cough.

—Using a humidifier and drinking at least two quarts of water a day are advised while you are taking this product. These will aid the medication in bringing mucus up.

—Notify your health care provider if the cough is accompanied by high fever, rash or persistent headaches or if the cough returns once you feel it has been under control.

—Use this medication only in dose recommended in order to decrease chances of side effects.

EVALUATION:

ADVERSE REACTIONS: Gastrointestinal upset may occur. (See specific drug monographs on products contained in each preparation for additional specifics.)

PARAMETERS TO MONITOR: Watch vital signs, clinical state of hydration. Perform a complete ear, nose, throat, and chest examination. A chest x-ray may be indicated if there is any question of lung consolidation. Patient should be monitored for therapeutic effect: liquefication of secretions, more productive cough. Observe for adverse effects.

AMMONIUM CHLORIDE

PRODUCTS (TRADE NAME);

Amonidrin (Available in 200 mg ammonium chloride tablets with 100 mg guaifenesin.) **Ipsatol** (Available as syrup with 22 mg ammonium chloride and 0.24 mg/5 ml ipecac alkaloids.)

DRUG SPECIFICS:

This drug may cause serious illness in healthy normal individuals if more than 50 grams are ingested. In those patients with hepatic, renal, or heart disease, as little as 5 grams may cause poisoning. Use caution with these patients and with those with pulmonary insufficiency. Ammonium chloride will acidify the urine and may affect excretion of other drugs. Use of more than the recommended dosage may predispose the patient to metabolic acidosis. This is available over the counter in combination with other expectorants.

ADMINISTRATION AND DOSAGE SPECIFICS:

Adults: 1 or 2 tablets po 4 times daily, or 5-10 ml po every 3-4 hours.

GUAIFENESIN

PRODUCTS (TRADE NAME):

Anti-Tuss, Baytussin, Colrex Expectorant (Available in 100 mg/5 ml syrup.)

G-200 (Availble in 200 mg capsules.) **Gee-Gee** (Available in 200 mg tablets.) **GG-CEN** (Available in 200 mg capsules and 100 mg/5 ml syrup.) **GG-Tussin, Glyate** (Available in 100 mg/5 ml syrup.) **Glycotuss** (Available in 100 mg tablets and 100 mg/5 ml syrup.) **Glytuss** (Available in 200 mg tablets.) **Guaifenesin** (Available in 100 mg/5 ml syrup.) **Hytuss** (Available in 100 mg tablets.) **Liquitussin, Nortussin, Robitussin, 2/G** (Available 100 mg/5 ml syrup.)

DRUG SPECIFICS:

Although there is a lack of convincing evidence to document clinical efficacy, this is a widely publicized product, claimed to have expectorant action through reduction of adhesiveness and surface tension in the respiratory tract. Dry productive coughs may become more productive and less frequent. Adverse reactions include nausea, vomiting,* and occasional drowsiness. Use of more than prescribed doses can lead to an increased bleeding tendency. This drug may interfere with the results of 5-hydroxyindoleacetic acid (5-HIAA) and vanillylmandelic acid (VMA) laboratory tests. Any persistent cough should be investigated to rule out a serious condition. If cough persists longer than one week, recurs, or is accompanied by other symptoms, patient should return to the health care provider. The syrup preparations may contain alcohol. This drug is available in many over-the-counter preparations.

ADMINISTRATION AND DOSAGE SPECIFICS:

Adults: 100 to 400 mg po every 4 to 6 hours; maximum dose 2.4 gm/day.

Children 6-12 years: 50 to 100 mg po every 4 to 6 hours; maximum dose 600 mg/day.

Children 2-6 years: 50 mg po every 4 hours; maximum dose 300 mg/day.

IODINATED GLYCEROL

PRODUCTS (TRADE NAME):

Organidin (Available in 30 mg tablets, 60 mg/5 ml elixir with 23.75% alcohol, and 50 mg/ml solution with dropper.)

DRUG SPECIFICS:

This product is used in patients with bronchitis, bronchial asthma, pulmonary emphysema, cystic fibrosis, and chronic sinusitis. Contraindicated in those with significant sensitivity to inorganic iodides, in pregnancy, newborns, and nursing mothers due to the goitrogenic effect. Avoid use or use with caution in patients with thyroid disease. Patients may develop dose-related dermatitis, gastrointestinal upset, or rash. Hypersensitivity, thyroid enlargement and acute parotitis are rare. Children with cystic fibrosis are at a higher risk of developing goiter. Do not use continuously. Discontinue if rash develops. Available by prescription only.

ADMINISTRATION AND DOSAGE SPECIFICS:

One drop is approximately equal to 3 mg.

Adults: 60 mg po 4 times daily with water; one teaspoon (5 ml) elixir 4 times daily; or 20 drops of solution 4 times daily with water. May also be taken with juice or milk if diet allows.

Children: Up to 1/2 adult dose based on weight.

IODINE PRODUCTS

PRODUCTS (TRADE NAME):

Hydriodic Acid (Available in 70 mg hydrogen iodide per 5 ml syrup.) **Iodized Lime** (Available in iodine, potassium iodide and calcium carbonate tablets.) **Iodo-Niacin** (Available in tablets of 135 mg potassium iodide and 25 mg niacinamide hydroiodide.) **Pima** (Available in 325 mg potassium iodide per 5 ml syrup.) **Potassium Iodide** (Available in 300 mg enteric coated tablets, 500 mg/15 ml liquid, and 1 gm/ml saturated solution.) **SSKI** (Available in 1 gm/ml potassium iodide solution.)

DRUG SPECIFICS:

Iodine products are used in chronic pulmonary diseases but may be contraindicated in pulmonary tuberculosis. They are contraindicated for use in the presence of hypersensitivity to iodine and in hyperthyroidism. Use with caution in the presence of goiter. Do not use in pregnancy or in nursing mothers due to the goitrogenic effect.

ADVERSE REACTIONS include: *Gastrointestinal:* epigastric pain, gastrointestinal upset, metallic taste, nausea, salivary gland swelling, increased salivation, vomiting. *Other:* coryza, fever, mucous membrane ulceration, skin rash, and a rare dry fever. Notify health care provider and discontinue use if epigastric pain, skin rash, fever, metallic taste or nausea and vomiting occur. Do not use continuously since prolonged use may lead to hypothyroidism. Available by prescription only except for Hydriodic Acid.

ADMINISTRATION AND DOSAGE SPECIFICS:

Hydriodic Acid:
Adults: 1.25 to 5 ml, well diluted in water, 2-3 times daily after meals.
Children 1 year and older: 1 to 10 drops, well diluted in water 2-3 times daily after meals.
Iodized Lime:
Children over 2 years: 1 to 2 tablets with warm water.
Iodo-Niacin:
Adults: 2 tablets 3 times a day with water after meals.
Children 8 years and older: 1 tablet with water after meals.
Pima:
Adults: 5 to 10 ml every 4-6 hours.
Children: 2.5 to 5 ml every 4-6 hours.
Potassium Iodide:
Adults: 300 mg in liquid every 4-6 hours.
Children: 250 to 1000 mg daily in 2-4 divided doses.

SSKI:
Adults: 0.3 to 0.6 ml 4-12 times daily diluted in a glass of water, juice, or milk.

Irene McCrea

STEROIDS

TOPICAL NASAL STEROIDS

ACTION OF THE DRUG: The main action of topical nasal steroids is the glucocorticoid effect of decreasing local congestion through suppression of inflammatory reactions.

ASSESSMENT:

INDICATIONS: Topical nasal steroids are used in the treatment of allergic, mechanical, or chemically induced local nasal inflammation or nasal polyps only when more conventional treatment has been tried and found to be ineffective.

SUBJECTIVE: Patient may present with a history of difficulty breathing through nose, stuffy nose, sneezing, nasal discharge, and nasal polyps which may be associated with allergic states.

OBJECTIVE: Upon examination, edema and inflammation of nasal mucosa secondary to chemical, mechanical or allergic stimuli may be seen.

PLAN:

CONTRAINDICATIONS: Do not use in the presence of hypersensitivity to fluorocarbon propellants, systemic fungal infections, tuberculosis, ocular herpes simplex, or local infections from any source.

WARNINGS: Careful consideration should be given to the decision to use nasal steroid preparations during pregnancy and nursing since the drug crosses the placental barrier and appears in breast milk. The dosage of the drug should be gradually withdrawn to avoid adrenocortical insufficiency. The drug may decrease resistance to infection as well as mask some common signs of infection. Concurrent antibiotic therapy is indicated in the presence of bacterial infection. The drug may activate latent amebiasis and cause a false negative nitroblue-tetrazolium test for bacterial infection.

PRECAUTIONS: Elevation of blood pressure, retention of salt and water, and increased potassium and calcium loss may occur with large doses. This may be treated with dietary salt restriction and potassium supplementation. Smallpox vaccination and immunizations should not be given since immunological response may be depressed. In the presence of latent tuberculosis or tuberculosis reactivity, close observation and possible chemoprophylaxis may be indicated. The effects of the drug are enhanced in hypothyroidism and cirrhosis.

IMPLEMENTATION:

DRUG INTERACTIONS: Nasal steroids may interact with phenytoin, phenobarbital, ephedrine, rifampin, anticoagulants, potassium depleting diuretics, antiinflammatory agents, alcohol, digitalis preparations, aspirin, hypoglycemics, and somatotropin. (See drug monograph on systemic corticosteroids).

ADMINISTRATION AND DOSAGE: This drug should not be used in children under 6 years of age. Recommended dosage must not be exceeded. Dosage should be decreased with subjective improvement of the patient.

IMPLEMENTATION CONSIDERATIONS:

—Obtain a complete health history, including the presence of hypersensitivity, fungal infections, tuberculosis, ocular herpes simplex, local infections (especially of nose, sinus, or throat), and possibility of pregnancy.

—Determine patient's past experience and response to nasal sprays.

—Nasal dryness and irritation are side effects and do not usually necessitate discontinuing the drug.

—Corticosteroids may decrease resistance to or mask infection. Close observation is indicated.

—Loss of ability to smell, shortness of breath, unrelieved stuffy nose, chest tightness or wheezing indicates a need for health care provider intervention.

—The patient should be observed for signs of systemic absorption since fluid retention and temporary inhibition of pituitary-adrenal function may develop.

WHAT THE PATIENT NEEDS TO KNOW:

—This drug is used to relieve nasal stuffiness due to allergy, chemical or mechanical irritation.

—This drug should not be used in the presence of infection. Notify your health care provider if you develop an infection while taking this drug.

—To avoid the chances of the medication being absorbed into the general circulation, the prescribed dosage and frequency must not be exceeded.

—Dryness and irritation of the nose may occur temporarily. Notify health care provider if these problems persist.

—The drug should be used in the smallest effective dose for the shortest period of time to prevent general absorption.

—Dosage may need to be tapered slowly, and not stopped suddenly, especially if large doses have been used for long periods of time.

—The health care practitioner should be notified if symptoms do not improve or if they get worse.

EVALUATION:

ADVERSE REACTIONS: Asthma, headache, lightheadedness, loss of sense of smell, nasal irritation and dryness, nausea, nosebleeds, perforation of the nasal septum, rebound congestion, skin rash.

OVERDOSAGE: For signs and symptoms of systemic absorption, see drug monograph section on systemic corticosteroids.

PARAMETERS TO MONITOR: Evaluate for therapeutic action: reduction in nasal stuffiness, obstruction, discharge, relief of sinus headaches. Also monitor frequency of use and dosage used. Look for evidence of cracked or bleeding nasal mucosa. Watch for adverse reactions: signs of systemic absorption and fluid retention, elevated blood pressure, weight gain, ankle edema, or evidence of local infection.

BECLOMETHASONE DIPROPIONATE

PRODUCTS (TRADE NAME):

Beclovent, Vanceril Nasal Inhaler (Available in medihaler which delivers approximately 200, 42 mcg doses.)

DRUG SPECIFICS:

Use this medication for seasonal allergy symptoms only when response to other conventional therapy has been unacceptable. Symptomatic relief is not immediate, and therapy should be continued even with initial minimal response. Maximal response should be seen within 3 weeks or medication should be discontinued. Systemic absorption is minimal if used in the recommended dosages however, adrenal suppression can occur. This drug is available by prescription only.

ADMINISTRATION AND DOSAGE SPECIFICS:

Adults and children over 12 years: One inhalation in each nostril 2-4 times a day. Taper off gradually as symptomatic relief is obtained.

DEXAMETHASONE SODIUM PHOSPHATE

PRODUCTS (TRADE NAME):

Beconase Nasal Inhaler; Decadron Phosphate Turbinaire (Available as a medihaler with 174 sprays with 84 mcg per spray.)

DRUG SPECIFICS:

Use this product to obtain relief from symptoms of seasonal allergies only when response to more conventional therapy has been unacceptable. Gradually reduce dosage when there is improvement. May be able to use as little as 1 spray 2 times a day. Treatment should be discontinued as soon as possible. The maximum dosage for adults is 12 sprays a day and 8 sprays a day for children. This drug is available by prescription only.

ADMINISTRATION AND DOSAGE SPECIFICS:

Adults: 2 sprays 2 or 3 times a day.

Children 6 years or older: 1 or 2 sprays 2 times a day.

Inhaler-Adults and children over 12: One inhalation 2-4 times a day.

FLUNISOLIDE

PRODUCTS (TRADE NAME):

Nasalide (Available as spray with 200 sprays of 25 mcg per bottle).

DRUG SPECIFICS:

Use this drug to obtain relief from symptoms of seasonal allergies only when response to more conventional therapy has been unacceptable. Drug is minimally absorbed systemically when used in recommended dosages. Do not use for longer than three weeks if substantial response to the medication has not developed. Available by prescription only.

ADMINISTRATION AND DOSAGE SPECIFICS:

Adults: 2 sprays in each nostril 2 times a day; may increase to 3 times a day if warranted. Do not use more than 8 sprays/day/nostril. As symptoms decrease, off dosage. Maintenance dose may be 1 spray/day/nostril.

Children 6 to 14 years: 1 spray in each nostril 3 times a day; may give 2 sprays in each nostril 2 times/day. Maximum dose is 4 sprays/day/nostril. Taper dosage down as symptoms resolve. Maintenance dose may be 1 spray/day/nostril.

Irene McCrea and Marilyn W. Edmunds

TOPICAL PREPARATIONS

ANORECTAL PREPARATIONS

LOCAL ANESTHETIC-CONTAINING PRODUCTS

ACTION OF THE DRUG: This category of drugs includes over the counter preparations for topical anesthesia of rectal areas.

ASSESSMENT:

INDICATIONS: Used for symptomatic relief of discomfort associated with hemorrhoids. Often used for long-term relief of mild hemorrhoid discomfort. Relief is often obtained in hemorrhoids associated with pregnancy, prolonged sitting, or other temporary problems.

SUBJECTIVE: History of rectal irritation and pain from hemorrhoids.

OBJECTIVE: Edema and erythema of rectal mucosa or visible hemorrhoid tags may be present.

PLAN:

WARNINGS: Keep out of reach of children. This medication should not be swallowed.

PRECAUTIONS: Do not use near or in the eyes.

IMPLEMENTATION:

PRODUCTS (TRADE NAME):
Anusol (Available in 1% pramoxine HCl, benzyl benzoate, balsam Peru and zinc oxide ointment.) **Nupercainal** (Available in 2.5 mg dibucaine USP suppository; 1% dibucaine USP and lubricant base ointment.) **Rectal Medicone** (Available in 130 mg benzocaine, hydroxyquinoline sulfate, zinc oxide, menthol, balsam of Peru suppositories.) **Surfacaine** (Available in 10 mg cyclomethycaine sulfate suppositories.)

ADMINISTRATION AND DOSAGE: Apply ointment morning and night and after each bowel movement. For suppositories, insert one after each bowel movement. Products may be purchased over the counter.

IMPLEMENTATION CONSIDERATIONS:
—Obtain a health history, including any allergies.
—Determine severity of patient's symptoms. Is rectal bleeding present?

WHAT THE PATIENT NEEDS TO KNOW:
—Use ointment or suppository exactly as ordered.
—Avoid contact of medication with eyes.
—In the case of rectal bleeding, discontinue use and consult health care provider.

—Keep this medication out of the reach of children and others for whom it is not prescribed.

EVALUATION:

ADVERSE REACTIONS: The most frequently reported adverse effect of topical local anesthetics is sensitization. The lowest dose for effective, temporary relief of discomfort should be used to prevent and minimize the possibility of systemic toxicity.

PARAMETERS TO MONITOR: Observe for symptomatic relief with decrease in swelling and irritation of rectal mucosa.

Carol Burke

ANORECTAL PREPARATIONS WITH STEROIDS

ANUSOL-HC

ACTION OF THE DRUG: Anusol-HC is an anti-inflammatory, antipruritic and vasoconstrictive preparation which helps to relieve the discomfort of irritated anorectal tissues.

ASSESSMENT:

INDICATIONS: Used to obtain relief of local pain following anorectal surgery, pruritus ani, external and internal hemorrhoids, proctitis, papillitis, cryptitis, and anal fissures.

SUBJECTIVE: History of rectal irritation and pain from hemorrhoids prior to and following surgery.

OBJECTIVE: Edema and erythema of rectal mucosa and/or visible hemorrhoid tags may be present.

PLAN:

CONTRAINDICATIONS: History of hypersensitivity to hydrocortisone acetate, bismuth subgallate, benzyl benzoate, Peruvian balsam, zinc oxide, bismuth subiodide, or calcium phosphate.

WARNINGS: The use of topical steroids has not been proven safe during pregnancy. When clinically indicated, the product should be used sparingly and for a limited length of time.

PRECAUTIONS: If irritation develops, discontinue use and consult health care provider. If bacterial or fungal infection coexists, appropriate treatment should be initiated and corticosteroid use should be discontinued until infection is under control.

IMPLEMENTATION:

PRODUCTS (TRADE NAME):
Anugard-HC, Anusol-HC, Hemorrhoidal HC, Hemusol HC (Available in 0.5% hydrocortisone acetate cream, or 10 mg hydrocortisone acetate suppositories.)
Rectacort (Available in 10% hydrocortisone acetate suppositories.)

ADMINISTRATION AND DOSAGE:
Suppository: Insert suppository morning and bedtime for three-six days, or until inflammation subsides.
Cream: Apply to anal area and gently rub in 3-4 times each day for 3-6 days, or until inflammation subsides.

IMPLEMENTATION CONSIDERATIONS:
—Obtain a health history including allergies, possibility of pregnancy.
—Evaluate for co-existence of bacterial or fungal infections.

WHAT THE PATIENT NEEDS TO KNOW:
—This medication is for the temporary relief of rectal problems. Continued problems should be reported to your health care provider.
—Store suppositories in cool place to avoid melting.
—Product may cause staining of underclothes. Hand or machine-washing with laundry detergent will remove stains.
—If irritation develops, discontinue use and consult health care provider.
—Eat fruits and bulk producing food to prevent constipation while healing is in progress.

EVALUATION:

ADVERSE REACTIONS: increase in rectal irritation.
PARAMETERS TO MONITOR: Observe for therapeutic response with decrease in rectal discomfort. Observe for development of irritation, superinfections.

Carol Burke

CORTIFOAM

ACTION OF THE DRUG: This medication has an anti-inflammatory action.

ASSESSMENT:

INDICATIONS: Cortifoam is used as adjunctive therapy in the topical treatment of ulcerative proctitis. This medication is prescribed to clients who are unable to retain hydrocortisone or other corticosteroid enemas.

SUBJECTIVE: Rectal discomfort accompanied by the presence of mucus, blood or pus in the stool. Repeated urge to evacuate rectum.

OBJECTIVE: Inflamed mucous membranes of distal portion of rectum.

PLAN:

CONTRAINDICATIONS: Local contraindictions include abscess, obstruction, perforation, peritonitis, fistulas and sinus tracts, fresh intestinal anastomoses. Absolute contraindications are tuberculosis, ocular herpes simplex and acute psychosis. Relative contraindications are active peptic ulcer, acute glomerulonephritis, myasthenia gravis, osteoporosis, diverticulitis, thrombophlebitis, psychic disturbances, pregnancy, diabetes, hyperthyroidism, acute coronary disease, hypertension, limited cardiac reserve, and local or systemic fungal infections.

WARNINGS: Aerosol container should not be inserted into the anal canal.

PRECAUTIONS: Caution should be used when administering to clients with a history of severe ulcerative disease because of the increased risk of bowel perforation. Avoid use during immediate post-operative period following ileorectosomy.

IMPLEMENTATION:

PRODUCTS (TRADE NAME):

Cortifoam (Available in 10% hydrocortisone acetate in 20 gm aerosol. Each application delivers 80 mg hydrocortisone.)

ADMINISTRATION AND DOSAGE: Insert one applicator full rectally once or twice daily for 2-3 weeks, then every other day. As with all corticosteroid medications, therapy should be decreased gradually to allow for possible adrenal insufficiency.

IMPLEMENTATION CONSIDERATIONS:

—Obtain a complete health history: history of severe ulcerative bowel disease, recent rectal surgery, tuberculosis, ocular herpes simplex or acute psychosis.

—Product should be stored at room temperature.

—Aerosol container should not be punctured or burned.

WHAT THE PATIENT NEEDS TO KNOW:

—Instructions for use of aerosol and applicator are to be followed exactly.

—If condition worsens, contact health provider so drug can be discontinued safely.

EVALUATION:

ADVERSE REACTIONS: These are the side effects of corticosteroid therapy: *CNS:* fatigue, headaches, insomnia, increased intracranial pressure, mental symptoms, neuropathy. *Gastrointestinal:* excessive appetite, pancreatitis, peptic ulcer. *Musculoskeletal:* aseptic necrosis to hip and humerus may occur secondary to long-term catabolic effects, osteoporosis, spontaneous fractures. *Other:* abnormal fat deposits, acne, dry scaly skin, ecchymosis, increased sweating, fluid retention, moon facies, pigmentation, thinning scalp hair, decreased resistance to infection, delayed bone and wound healing, menstrual disorders, decreased glucose tolerance, adrenal insufficiency, hypertension, hypopotassemia.

PARAMETERS TO MONITOR: Observe for therapeutic effects and adverse reactions. Symptomatic improvement usually occurs within 5-7 days. In addition to client's symptomatic relief, it is recommended that sigmoidoscopy be utilized to monitor clinical course.

Carol Burke

MOUTH AND THROAT PREPARATIONS

ACTION OF THE DRUG: These miscellaneous products are used to soothe minor oral inflammation. Some release oxygen to provide cleansing while others contain an anesthetic property to reduce pain.

ASSESSMENT:

INDICATIONS: Products are indicated for minor oral inflammation such as canker sores, dental irritation, post dental procedure irritation, relief of dryness of mouth and throat, or for treatment of minor sore throat discomfort and control of coughs due to colds.

SUBJECTIVE: Patient may have undergone recent dental surgery or may present with complaints associated with minor trauma or colds.

OBJECTIVE: Tongue, buccal mucosa, gums, or throat may show evidence of bleeding, erythema, or increased vascularization. There may also be no objective findings.

PLAN:

CONTRAINDICATIONS: Products should not be used in the presence of hypersensitivity to any of the drugs or in cases of severe mouth or throat infections.

PRECAUTIONS: Patients must be educated in the intelligent use of these products to avoid delays in seeking therapy when medical attention is warranted. Lozenges should not be given to children under 3 years.

IMPLEMENTATION:

ADMINISTRATION AND DOSAGE: Products are available in mouthwashes, sprays, solutions, troches, lozenges, and discs. Patient should be taught appropriate administration technique for the relevant drug. See specific product information. Administration should not exceed 3 or 4 days for normal therapy.

IMPLEMENTATION CONSIDERATIONS:

—Obtain a complete health history, including the presence of hypersensitivity, underlying systemic disease, and concurrent use of other medications.

—Ascertain the source of the problem and verify that it is a superficial, localized, and minor problem.

—Teach patient proper method of administration: spray, mouthwash, lozenge, etc.

—Encourage patient to return for evaluation if fever, lymphadenopathy, coughing up sputum, or other untoward effect develops.

WHAT THE PATIENT NEEDS TO KNOW:

—This medication is available without a prescription and is taken to relieve a minor problem. If you begin to feel worse (develop a temperature, get swollen glands in your neck, begin coughing up sputum), or your symptoms do not decrease in a few days, return to see your health care provider.

—This medication should not be given to children under 3 years old.

—Your practitioner will explain to you exactly how you should use mouthwash, sprays, or lozenges.

—Keep this medication out of the reach of children and others for whom it is not prescribed. Lozenges are often confused with candy by young children and this may represent a hazard for them.

EVALUATION:

PARAMETERS TO MONITOR: Observe for therapeutic effects or for development of more serious or systemic problems.

CARBAMIDE PEROXIDE (UREA PEROXIDE)

PRODUCTS (TRADE NAME):

Cankaid, Gly-Oxide, Periolav (Available in 10% solution.) **Proxigel** (Available in 11% gel.)

DRUG SPECIFICS:

These products are indicated for minor oral inflammation (canker sores, dental irritation, post dental procedure irritation.) These agents release oxygen upon contact with the mouth tissues to provide cleansing effects. Carbamide peroxide is an adjunct to oral hygiene after regular brushing. If condition worsens, persists, or if irritation develops, discontinue use of this product. The gel form of carbamide peroxide is more useful in some conditions since it adheres to affected areas for longer oxygenating and debriding action.

Inform the patient that this product foams when mixed with saliva. It is best to use this product after meals and at bedtime. Do not rinse for 5 minutes after using carbamide peroxide.

ADMINISTRATION AND DOSAGE SPECIFICS:

The drug is not to be diluted. Apply directly to affected area 4 times daily. Expectorate after 2 to 3 minutes. Do not use in children who are too young to understand how to expectorate.

LOZENGES AND TROCHES

PRODUCTS (TRADE NAME):

Cepacol (Available in 27 lozenges in 3 pocket packs of 9, or 18 troches in 2 pocket packs of 9.) **Cepastat Lozenges** (Available in box of 18 with 2 pocket packs of 9.) **Children's Chloraseptic Lozenges** (Available in box of 18.) **Menthol or Cherry Chloraseptic Lozenges** (Available in boxes of 18 and 45.) **Chloraseptic Cough Control Lozenges** (Available in box of 12.) **Sucrets** (Available in regular, mentholated, and children's cherry flavored.) **Sucrets Sore Throat Lozenges, Sucrets Decongestant Lozenges, Sucrets Cough Control Lozenges** (Available in tins of 24 lozenges.)

DRUG SPECIFICS:

The active ingredient in the Sucrets throat lozenge is hexylresorcinol, 2.4 mg per lozenge. Phenylpropanolamine HCl, 25 mg per lozenge, is the active ingredient in the decongestant lozenge. The cough control lozenge contains 7.5 mg of dextromethorphan hydrobromide.

The sore throat lozenges are used for minor sore throat and mouth irritations. Do not give to children under age 3. With persistent sore throat or sore throat accompanied by a fever, headache, nausea or vomiting, seek medical advice.

The decongestant lozenges are for relief of nasal congestion. If symptoms do not improve within 1 week, or if they are accompanied by a high fever, seek medical advice. Do not take if you have high blood pressure, heart disease, diabetes, or thyroid disease. Do not take if you are currently taking an MAO inhibitor drug. Do not give to children under 12.

Cough control lozenges are used for suppression of cough and relief of minor throat irritations. Do not use for more than 2 days, and do not give to children under age 6. If cough persists or is accompanied by high fever, seek medical advice.

Cepacol throat lozenges contain cetylpyridinium chloride 1:1500, benzyl alcohol 0.3%, aromatics, and a yellow mint candy base. These stimulate salivation to provide temporary relief of dryness and minor irritation of the mouth and throat.

Cepacol anesthetic troches contain cetylpyridinium chloride 1:1500, benzocaine, aromatics, and a green citrus candy base. They stimulate salivation and have an anesthetic effect.

Lozenges and troches should not be given to children under 3 years of age. Severe sore throat, sore throat accompanied by high fever, headache, nausea, vomiting, and a sore throat lasting longer than 2 days are all symptoms for which a person should seek medical attention.

All of the Chloraseptic products, except for Children's Chloraseptic Lozenges, contain phenol, which is a topical anesthetic. The Children's Lozenges contain benzocaine for topical anesthetic action. The Cough Control Lozenges contain a therapeutic dose (10 mg) of dextromethorphan hydrobromide.

As their forms dictate, these products may be used as an antiseptic, anesthetic, or for relief of minor sore throat or discomfort due to gum or mouth irritations. They may also be used for control of coughs due to colds.

ADMINISTRATION AND DOSAGE SPECIFICS:

Children's Lozenges: Dissolve 1 lozenge in mouth up to every hour if needed. Limit is 12 lozenges daily.

Lozenges: Adults: dissolve 1 lozenge in mouth every 2 hours, with limit of 8 lozenges daily. *Children 6 to 12 years:* dissolve 1 lozenge in mouth every 3 hours, with limit of 4 lozenges daily.

Cough Control Lozenges: Adults: dissolve 1 lozenge in mouth every 2 hours with limit of 8 lozenges daily. *Children 6 to 12 years:* dissolve 1 lozenge in mouth every 4 hours, with limit of 4 lozenges daily.

Sore throat lozenges: Use as needed. Dissolve slowly.

Decongestant lozenges: Adults and children 12 and over: take 1 lozenge every 4 hours as needed. Limit 6 lozenges in 24 hours.

GARGLES, GELS, MOUTHWASHES, AND SPRAYS

PRODUCTS (TRADE NAME):

Cepacol (Available in 6, 12, 18, and 24 oz mouthwash.) **Cepastat Sore Throat Spray** (Available in 14 oz spray and gargle.) **Cherry Chloraseptic Liquid** (Available in 12 oz bottles.) **Menthol or Cherry Chloraseptic Spray** (Available in 6 oz bottle or 1.5 oz spray can.) **Chloraseptic Gel** (Available in 1/4 oz tube.) **Menthol Chloraseptic Liquid** (Available in 8 or 12 oz bottle.)

DRUG SPECIFICS:

Cepacol mouthwash/gargle contains alcohol 14%, cetylpyridinium chloride 1:2000, and phosphate buffers and aromatics. Cetylpyridinium chloride is a cationic quarternary ammonium compound which in aqueous solution has a surface tension lower than that of water. This property is the basis of the foaming and spreading action of this product.

The spray and gargle contain phenol (1.4%) and glycerin in an aqueous solution. The lozenges contain phenol (1.45%) and menthol (0.12%) in a sorbitol base. Phenol is a topical anesthetic. Glycerin provides a soothing effect and menthol provides a cooling sensation.

These products are indicated for minor discomfort or pain of sore throat, mouth, or gums. If symptoms are severe, persist for more than 2 days or are accompanied by high fever, headache, nausea, or vomiting, seek medical advice. Do not use for more than 10 consecutive days. Do not give to children under age 6 and do not exceed recommended dosage.

ADMINISTRATION AND DOSAGE SPECIFICS:

Follow directions as listed on bottle or package. There is wide variation among products.

NYSTATIN

PRODUCTS (TRADE NAME):

Mycostatin, Nilstat (Available in oral suspension with 100,000 units/ml.)

DRUG SPECIFICS:

This product has both fungistatic and fungicidal antibiotic activity against a wide variety of yeasts and yeast-like fungi. Cell membrane permeability is altered, allowing intracellular components to leak out. The drug is used for oral candidiasis. Patients may experience diarrhea, GI distress, nausea and vomiting with large doses. No adverse effects have been noted in children born to mothers treated with nystatin. Treatment should continue for at least 2 days after symptoms have decreased and/or cultures have returned to normal.

ADMINISTRATION AND DOSAGE SPECIFICS:

Adults and children: 400,000 to 600,000 units 4 times daily. Take half of each dose, hold in one side of mouth for at least two minutes and then swallow. Repeat, using rest of medication on other side of mouth.

Infants: 200,000 units 4 times daily.

Premature and low birth weight infants: 100,000 units 4 times daily.

SALIVA SUBSTITUTES

PRODUCTS (TRADE NAME):

Moi-Stir, Orex, Salivart, Zero-Lube (Available in 120 or 180 ml electrolyte solutions in a carboxymethylcellulose base.)

DRUG SPECIFICS:

These solutions are used to relieve dry mouth and throat in xerostomia. There is slight variation in the properties of the various products. All come with pump spray or spray can with carbon dioxide propellant.

ADMINISTRATION AND DOSAGE SPECIFICS:

Spray into mouth as needed to relieve dryness and irritation.

THROAT DISCS

PRODUCTS (TRADE NAME):
Throat Disc (Available in box of 60 throat lozenges.)

DRUG SPECIFICS:
Each throat disc contains capsicum, peppermint, anise, cubeb, licorice, and linseed. They are indicated for relief of minor sore throat irritations.

Do not give to children under age 3. For severe or persistent symptoms or sore throat accompanied by high fever, headache, nausea or vomiting, seek medical advice.

ADMINISTRATION AND DOSAGE SPECIFICS:
Allow lozenge to dissolve slowly. Do not use more than 4 lozenges per hour.

Mary Ann Bolter

OPHTHALMIC DRUGS

ANESTHETICS—LOCAL

ACTION OF THE DRUG: The neuronal membrane is stabilized and made less permeable by the action of these drugs. Thus, initiation and transmission of impulses is prevented.

ASSESSMENT:

INDICATIONS: These drugs are useful in procedures such as tonometry, gonioscopy, cataract surgery, and removal of foreign bodies from the cornea when use of short-acting topical anesthetics is required.

SUBJECTIVE-OBJECTIVE: Patient may present with a history of injury to eye requiring local anesthesia. Product may also be used routinely during tonometry examinations.

PLAN:

CONTRAINDICATIONS: Do not use with history of allergy to drugs of similar chemical make-up, para-aminobenzoic acid or its derivatives, or to other active ingredients.

WARNINGS: This group of medications is for topical ophthalmic use only. The use of any topical ocular anesthetic over a prolonged period may decrease wound healing or cause epithelial erosions of the cornea. Permanent opacification of the cornea has been reported.

PRECAUTIONS: Use with caution in patients with known allergies, cardiac disease, hyperthyroidism, or with abnormal or decreased levels of plasma esterases. Dosage should be adjusted according to the status of the patient. Acutely ill or debilitated patients require reduced doses. The eye should be protected during the time of anesthesia since inadvertent injury may occur from rubbing or touching the anesthetized cornea and conjunctiva.

IMPLEMENTATION:

ADMINISTRATION AND DOSAGE: The lowest dose that results in effective anesthesia should be employed.
IMPLEMENTATION CONSIDERATIONS:
—Obtain a complete health history, including presence of known allergies, cardiac disease or hyperthyroidism, abnormal or reduced levels of plasma esterases.
—Avoid prolonged use.

WHAT THE PATIENT NEEDS TO KNOW:
—Do not rub or touch eyes when medication has been instilled.
—Medication is to be used sparingly and only as directed. Prolonged use may cause delayed wound healing.
—Instillation may cause temporary stinging, burning, and tearing.

EVALUATION:

ADVERSE REACTIONS: *Dermatologic:* local temporary reactions with burning, conjunctival erythema, lacrimation, and photophobia. Stinging occurs occasionally. Erosions of the corneal epithelium, scarring, and permanent corneal opacification have been reported. Although rare, a severe, immediate hypoallergenic corneal reaction may occur with the development of diffuse keratitis and sloughing.
OVERDOSAGE: Systemic toxicity is rare. *Signs and symptoms:* CNS stimulation followed by CNS and cardiovascular depression.
PARAMETERS TO MONITOR: Preparation should produce topical anesthesia. Watch for adverse reactions.

BENOXINATE HCL AND FLUORESCEIN SODIUM

PRODUCTS (TRADE NAME):
Fluress (Available in 0.4% solution.)
DRUG SPECIFICS:
Often used when suturing of eye is required.

ADMINISTRATION AND DOSAGE SPECIFICS:
Suturing, tonometry, removal of foreign bodies: Instill 1 to 2 drops prior to procedure.
Deep ophthalmic anesthesia: Instill 2 drops in each eye at 90 second intervals for 3 doses.

PROPARACAINE HCL

PRODUCTS (TRADE NAME):
AK-Taine, Alcaine, Ophthaine, Ophthetic (Available in 0.5% solution).
DRUG SPECIFICS:
This product may be used for deep anesthesia as well as more local surgery.
ADMINISTRATION AND DOSAGE SPECIFICS:
Tonometry: Instill 1 or 2 drops immediately before measurement.
Suture removal: Instill 1 or 2 drops two or three minutes prior to suture removal.
Removal of foreign body: Instill 1 or 2 drops before starting procedure.
For deep anesthesia: Instill 1 drop every 5 to 10 minutes for a total of 5 to 7 doses.

TETRACAINE

PRODUCTS (TRADE NAME):
Anacel 1/2, Pontocaine HCl (Available in 0.5% solution.) **Pontocaine Eye** (Available in 0.5% ointment.)
DRUG SPECIFICS:
Epinephrine 1:1000 may be added to Tetracaine to produce vascular constriction. Prolonged use of tetracaine and self-medication should be avoided.
ADMINISTRATION AND DOSAGE SPECIFICS:
Solution: Instill 1 or 2 drops.
Ointment: Apply 1/2 to 1 inch of ointment topically to the lower conjunctival fornix.

Carol Burke

ANTISEPTIC OINTMENTS

SILVER NITRATE

ACTION OF THE DRUG: Silver nitrate is an anti-infective. It has germicidal and astringent properties.

ASSESSMENT:

INDICATIONS: Silver nitrate is used for the prevention of gonorrheal ophthalmia neonatorum.

SUBJECTIVE-OBJECTIVE: Medication is used prophylactically.

PLAN:

WARNINGS: Silver nitrate may irritate skin and mucous membranes. Use the medication with caution since cauterization of the cornea and blindness may result, especially with repeated use.

PRECAUTIONS: Silver nitrate should be handled carefully; it may stain the skin.

IMPLEMENTATION:

PRODUCTS (TRADE NAME):

Silver Nitrate Ophthalmic (Available in 1% solution with acetic acid and sodium acetate.)

ADMINISTRATION AND DOSAGE: Separate lids and instill 2 drops of 1% solution. Separate lids to allow solution to cover eyeball for at least 30 seconds.

IMPLEMENTATION CONSIDERATIONS:

—At birth, the baby's eyelids should be cleansed with sterile gauze and sterile water. Wash from nose outward. Then instill drops.

—Irrigation of eyes after instillation of silver nitrate solution is not recommended.

—Ampules of silver nitrate should be protected from light and stored at room temperature. Do not freeze or use when cold.

EVALUATION:

ADVERSE REACTIONS: In approximately 20% of cases a mild chemical conjunctivitis may occur.

OVERDOSAGE: Ingestion of silver nitrate is highly toxic to both the gastrointestinal tract and central nervous system. Gastric lavage should be performed with sodium chloride in case of accidental swallowing.

PARAMETERS TO MONITOR: Observe for any conjunctivitis which may develop.

Carol Burke

SILVER PROTEIN, MILD

ACTION OF THE DRUG: Mild silver protein has an antimicrobial action. It stains and coagulates mucus when used prior to ophthalmologic surgery. It is effective against gram-positive and gram-negative organisms.

ASSESSMENT:

INDICATIONS: This drug is usually used prior to eye surgery and in mild eye infections.

SUBJECTIVE-OBJECTIVE: Patient is prepared for surgery with this product, which is used prophylactically. It is also used when patient complains of tearing, conjunctival irritation, and eye appears red and inflamed.

PLAN:

CONTRAINDICATIONS: Do not use with hypersensitivity to medication.

WARNINGS: Usage in pregnancy, breast-feeding, and in childhood is not recommended.

PRECAUTIONS: Do not use over extended time period.

IMPLEMENTATION:

PRODUCTS (TRADE NAME):
Argyrol S.S. 20% (Available in 20% solution with EDTA.)
ADMINISTRATION AND DOSAGE:
Infections: Instill 1 to 3 drops in eyes every 3 to 4 hours for several days.
Preoperative usage: Instill 2 to 3 drops in eyes and rinse with a sterile irrigating solution.
IMPLEMENTATION CONSIDERATIONS:
—Obtain a complete health history, especially for drug allergies; possibility of pregnancy, or breast-feeding.
—Use of this drug should be for short-term therapy only.

WHAT THE PATIENT NEEDS TO KNOW:
—This drug causes staining of hands, clothing, and even the eyes. Care should be taken in administering the drug.
—This drug can be purchased without a prescription.

EVALUATION:

ADVERSE REACTIONS: Too frequent or prolonged use may cause permanent discoloration of the skin and conjunctiva.

PARAMETERS TO MONITOR: Observe for therapeutic effects: resolution of clinical symptoms of infection.

Carol Burke

THIOMEROSAL

ACTION OF THE DRUG: Thimerosal is an organomercurial antiseptic used in bacterial and fungal ocular infections.

ASSESSMENT:

INDICATIONS: Used in treatment of conjunctivitis and corneal ulcer and as prophylaxis following foreign body removal.
SUBJECTIVE: History of corneal abrasion or inflammation of conjunctiva.
OBJECTIVE: Injection of conjunctiva with purulent discharge, pruritus, and crusting of lids upon awakening.

PLAN:

CONTRAINDICATIONS: Do not use with known hypersensitivity to this or mercury radicals.
WARNINGS: Discontinue use if irritation persists or worsens. Medication is not to be used for prolonged periods.

IMPLEMENTATION:

PRODUCTS (TRADE NAME):
Merthiolate Ophthalmic (Available in 1:5000 ointment.)
ADMINISTRATION AND DOSAGE: Apply small amount once or twice daily to inner surface of lower eye lid.
IMPLEMENTATION CONSIDERATIONS:
—Obtain a thorough health history, including patient's drug allergies.
—It is best to use a specific antibiotic treatment for ocular infections if this is possible.

WHAT THE PATIENT NEEDS TO KNOW:
—Wash hands before applying ointment. Pull down lower eye lid with one hand and hold tube with other hand. Squeeze small amount of ointment onto lower part of lid.
—If irritation persists or worsens, discontinue and consult health care provider.

EVALUATION:

PARAMETERS TO MONITOR: Observe for therapeutic response. If irritation does not decrease promptly, another medication should be substituted.

Carol Burke

OPHTHALMIC ANTI-INFECTIVES

ACTION OF THE DRUG: Antibiotics and antifungals are used in low concentrations for treatment of common eye infections. They are bactericidal or bacteriostatic, depending upon organism and concentration. See specific antibiotics and antifungals listed in anti-infective section for greater detail.

ASSESSMENT:

INDICATIONS: These products are used for superficial infections of the eye including infections of the cornea and conjunctiva. Other indications include the presence of corneal ulcers, keratitis, blepharitis, blepharoconjunctivitis, acute meibomianitis, and dacryocystitis. These drugs may be part of systemic therapy in more severe infections. Some products are specifically used in the treatment of trachoma.

SUBJECTIVE: Patient may complain of eye pain, redness, discharge, and blurring of vision. Symptoms may be acute or chronic.

OBJECTIVE: Conjunctiva may be swollen and erythematous and demonstrate increased vascularity. There may be involvement of cornea, lens, or pupil. Discharge is often copious. Numerous white blood cells may be observed, and bacteria may be cultured from the eye. Patient may demonstrate photophobia.

PLAN:

CONTRAINDICATIONS: Do not use in the presence of hypersensitivity to the drug.

PRECAUTIONS: General guidelines have not been established for the use of some of these preparations in pregnant women, nursing mothers, or children. Consult specific product information before prescribing to these groups.

IMPLEMENTATION:

DRUG INTERACTIONS: Usually there are no drug interactions. If patient is taking other medications, consult specific product information.

ADMINISTRATION AND DOSAGE: Instill drops regularly, especially during the acute stage of the infection. Avoid contaminating uninfected eye.

IMPLEMENTATION CONSIDERATIONS:

—Obtain a complete health history, including the presence of hypersensitivity, underlying systemic disease, the concurrent use of other medications, or the possibility of pregnancy.

—Teach patient or family member proper way to instill eye drops or ointment.

—Corneal healing may be retarded with use of ophthalmic ointment, and this should be watched for in relevant cases.

—If irritation or hypersensitivity develops, discontinue the drug and initiate appropriate treatment.

—Obtain culture prior to treatment. Overgrowth of susceptible organisms is possible.

WHAT THE PATIENT NEEDS TO KNOW:

—Take this medication as instructed. Instill drops into affected eye by lying down, pulling the conjunctival sac down, and having a second person put the drops into the conjunctival sac. Do not put solution directly on cornea itself. Allow product to flood over eye by gently closing eyes. Avoid contamination of eye dropper and uninfected eye. Wash hands before and after procedure. For instilling ointment, apply 1/2 to 1 inch ribbon of ointment into lower conjunctival sac. Close eyes briefly to allow medication to spread over eye.

—A transient visual haze may occur after application, particularly with use of ointment.

—Keep your washcloth and towel separate from those of other family members. Dispose of tissues used to wipe eyes. These steps are to avoid spreading the infection to others.

—If you note any local irritation, redness, burning, or itching, discontinue product and notify your health care provider.

—If you have any discharge or crusts on your eyes, wash them away carefully before putting medicine into eyes.

—Keep this medicine out of the reach of children and all others for whom it is not prescribed.

EVALUATION:

ADVERSE REACTIONS: Observe for development of sensitivity: burning, stinging, pruritus, dermatitis and angioedema.

PARAMETERS TO MONITOR: Obtain culture prior to initiating treatment. Observe for therapeutic effects and development of adverse reactions. Reculture if necessary.

BACITRACIN

PRODUCTS (TRADE NAME):

Baciguent Ophthalmic Ointment, Bacitracin Opthalmic (Available in 500 U/gm tube.)

DRUG SPECIFICS:

Used for superficial infections of the eye. Properties may be bactericidal or bacteriostatic depending upon the concentration of the drug and the infecting organism.

Bacitracin should be used with caution in patients with history of hypersensitivity to antibiotics. Do not use in conjunction with heavy metals.

Side effects include retarded corneal healing and overgrowth of nonsusceptible organisms. As with any eye ointment, there will be a transient visual haze after use.

Eye should be cleansed prior to application. Wash hands before and after application of the ointment. Caution patient to have separate washcloth and towel to prevent infection of other family members.

If redness, itching or burning of the eye or eyelid develops, the drug should be stopped. If there is no improvement after 3 days of therapy, the health care provider should be notified.

ADMINISTRATION AND DOSAGE SPECIFICS:

Adults and children: Apply sparingly into conjunctival sac 2 to 3 times daily.

CHLORAMPHENICOL

PRODUCTS (TRADE NAME):

Antibiopto Oph (Available in 5 mg/ml solution.) **Chloromycetin Ophthalmic** (Available in 10 mg ointment and 25 mg/15 ml solution.) **Chloroptic S.O.P. Ophthalmic** (Available in 0.5% solution or 10 mg ointment.) **Econochlor Ophthalmic** (Available in 0.5% solution and 10 mg ointment.) **Ophthochlor Ophthalmic** (Available in 0.5% solution.)

DRUG SPECIFICS:

These drugs are indicated for superficial ocular infections of the conjunctiva or cornea. Chloramphenicol is contraindicated in those hypersensitive to the drug. General guidelines have not been established for use by children, pregnant women, or nursing mothers.

As with any ointment, there will be transient visual haze, and retardation of corneal wound healing may occur. Overgrowth of nonsusceptible organisms may occur. Bacteriologic studies should be done to determine the causative organisms and their sensitivity.

Adverse reactions include burning, stinging, pruritus, dermatitis, and angioedema. If any of these symptoms develop, the therapy should be discontinued. One case of bone marrow hypoplasia has been reported after prolonged use (23 months).

ADMINISTRATION AND DOSAGE SPECIFICS:

Adults: Apply small amount of ointment to the lower conjunctival sac, or instill 2 drops of solution every 3 hours for first 48 hours. Then interval may be increased. Treatment should be continued for at least 48 hours after the eye appears to be normal.

CHLORTETRACYCLONE HYDROCHLORIDE AND TETRACYCLINE HYDROCHLORIDE

PRODUCTS (TRADE NAME):

Achromycin (Available in 10 mg ointment and 10 mg/ml suspension.) **Aureomycin Ophthalmic** (Available in 10 mg ointment.)

DRUG SPECIFICS:

Aureomycin and Achromycin are used for treatment of superficial ocular infections which are susceptible to tetracycline HCl. They are also used in the treatment of trachoma (in conjunction with oral therapy). These drugs are contraindicated in those patients who have shown hypersensitivity to any of the tetracyclines.

As with any antibiotic, the overgrowth of nonsusceptible organisms is possible. Pruritus, burning, and dermatitis are adverse reactions. If any of these symptoms develop, stop the drug. With the ointment form of this drug, a transient visual haze will occur after application.

Warn patients to keep their wash cloth and towel separate from those used by other family members.

ADMINISTRATION AND DOSAGE SPECIFICS:

Ointment: Apply to affected eye every 2 hours as the severity of the infection and the degree of response dictates. Severe infections may require longer treatment and may also require oral therapy.

Suspension: Instill 1 to 2 drops two to four times daily, depending upon the severity of the infection.

Trachoma: Instill 2 drops or apply ointment two to four times daily for one to two months.

ERYTHROMYCIN

PRODUCTS (TRADE NAME):

Ilotycin Ophthalmic (Available in 5 mg ointment.)

DRUG SPECIFICS:

Ilotycin ophthalmic is indicated for superficial ocular infections involving the conjunctiva and/or cornea. Use this only if sensitivity studies have shown that the organism is susceptible to erythromycin.

Its use is contraindicated in those patients with hypersensitivity to erythromycin. General guidelines have not been established for children and pregnant and nursing mothers.

Overgrowth of nonsusceptible organisms is possible. Retarded corneal healing and a transient visual haze may occur. Signs of hypersensitivity include pruritic and burning eye, dermatitis, angioedema, and urticaria.

As with any eye infection, caution patients not to let others use their wash cloth and towel.

ADMINISTRATION AND DOSAGE SPECIFICS:

Adults: Apply to affected eye daily or more often if severity of infection warrants it.

GENTAMICIN SULFATE

PRODUCTS (TRADE NAME):

Garamycin Ophthalmic, Genoptic Ophthalmic (Available in 0.3% solution and 3 mg ointment.)

DRUG SPECIFICS:

Gentamicin Sulfate is indicated in the treatment of infections of the external eye and its adnexa caused by susceptible organisms. Such infections include: conjunctivitis, corneal ulcers, keratitis, blepharitis, blepharoconjunctivitis, acute meibomianitis, and dacryocystitis.

This drug should not be used in those who have known hypersensitivity to any of the drug components.

Never inject the solution subconjunctivally or introduce directly into the anterior chamber. With prolonged use, overgrowth of nonsusceptible organisms may occur. If irritation or hypersensitivity develop, discontinue the drug and initiate appropriate treatment.

As with any ophthalmic ointment, corneal healing may be retarded and a transient visual may haze occur after applications. A culture should be taken prior to initiating therapy.

Tell the patient to keep his or her wash cloth and towel separate from those used by other family members.

ADMINISTRATION AND DOSAGE SPECIFICS:

Adults and children: Instill 1 to 2 drops into affected eye every 4 hours. In severe infections, dosage may be increased to as much as 2 drops hourly. Ointment may be applied sparingly to lower conjunctival sac two to three times daily.

NEOMYCIN SULFATE

PRODUCTS (TRADE NAME):

Myciguent Ophthalmic (Available in 3.5 mg neomycin ointment.)

DRUG SPECIFICS:

Neomycin sulfate may be used alone or as an adjunct with other antibiotic therapy for superficial ocular infections involving the conjunctiva or cornea. This drug is effective against both gram-positive and gram-negative organisms.

Use of this product is contraindicated in those patients hypersensitive to aminoglycosides. Local dermatitis, pruritus, and burning are signs of hypersensitivity to neomycin sulfate, and the drug should be stopped. Overgrowth of non-susceptible organisms is possible. As with any ophthalmic ointment, retarded corneal healing and a transient visual haze after application of drug are possible.

Patient should keep his or her wash cloth and towel separate from those used by other family members.

ADMINISTRATION AND DOSAGE SPECIFICS:
Adults and children: Apply to lower conjunctival sac 1 to 3 times daily.

POLYMYXIN B SULFATE

PRODUCTS (TRADE NAME):
Aerosporin, Polymyxin B Sulfate Sterile (Available in a powder form reconstituted to 0.1% and 0.25% drops with 500,000 units.)
DRUG SPECIFICS:
Polymyxin B sulfate may be used alone or as an adjunct with other agents for treating corneal ulcers resulting from infections caused by gram-negative organisms, especially *Pseudomonas*. It is often used with neomycin sulfate.

Obtain culture prior to treatment with this drug. Overgrowth of nonsusceptible organisms is possible. Local irritation, burning, and pruritus are signs of sensitivity.

Tell the patient to keep his or her wash cloth and towel separate from those of other family members.

This product is not available commercially. The powder must be reconstituted with sterile water for injection or normal saline solution.
ADMINISTRATION AND DOSAGE SPECIFICS:
Adults and children: Instill 1 to 2 drops of 0.1% to 0.25% every hour. May increase interval according to patient's response.

SULFACETAMIDE SODIUM, SULFISOXAZOLE DIOLAMINE

PRODUCTS (TRADE NAME):
AK-Sulf (Available in 10% and 30% solution.) **Bleph 10 Liquifilm** (Available in 10% sulfacetamide sodium solution.) **Cetamide Ophthalmic** (Available in 10% sulfacetamide sodium solution or ointment.) **Gantrisin Ophthalmic** (Available in 4% sulfisoxazole diolamine solution or ointment.) **Isopto Cetamide Ophthalmic** (Available in 15% sulfacetamide sodium solution). **Opthacet** (Available in 10% sulfacetamide sodium solution.) **Sodium Sulamyd Ophthalmic** (Available in 10% or 30% sulfacetamide sodium solution or ointment.) **Sodium Sulfacetamide** (Available in 10% or 30% sulfacetamide sodium solution or ointment.) **Sulf-10** (Available in 10% sulfacetamide sodium solution.) **Sulfacel-15** (Available in 15% sulfacetamide sodium solution.)

DRUG SPECIFICS:

Sulfonamides are appropriate for the treatment of bacterial conjunctivitis, corneal ulcers, and other superficial ocular infections due to susceptible organisms. They are also used as an adjunct in systemic sulfonamide therapy of trachoma.

These drugs are contraindicated in those patients who have shown hypersensitivity to sulfonamide preparations. As with all forms of this drug, severe allergic reactions have been identified in individuals with no prior history of sulfonamide hypersensitivity. Redness, pruritus, and burning are symptoms of sensitivity, and the drug should be discontinued.

The ointments cause a transient visual haze after application and may also retard corneal wound healing. With use of the solution there may be transient stinging or burning.

As with all antibiotics, there may be overgrowth of nonsusceptible organisms. If purulent exudates are present, obtain culture prior to initiating therapy. These exudates should be removed prior to instilling medicine as they will inactivate sulfonamides. Local anesthetics will decrease sulfonamide action. Silver preparations are incompatible with these drugs.

Warn patient not to use the ophthalmic solution if it is discolored. Patient should keep his or her wash cloth and towel separate from those used by other family members.

ADMINISTRATION AND DOSAGE SPECIFICS:

Adults and children:

Sulfacetamide Sodium 10%: Instill 1 to 2 drops into lower conjunctival sac every 2 to 3 hours during the day and less at night.

Cetamide ointment: Apply 1/2 to 1 inch ribbon in lower conjunctival sac at night in conjunction with the use of drops during the day, or before eye is patched.

Sodium Sulamyd Ophthalmic: Apply small amount four times daily and at bedtime. The ointment may be used as adjunct with solution.

Sulfacetamide Sodium 15% with Isopto Cetamide: Instill 1 to 2 drops in the lower conjunctival sac every 1 to 2 hours initially. May increase time interval as condition improves.

Sulfacetamide Sodium 30%: For conjunctivitis or corneal ulcer, instill 1 drop into lower conjunctival sac every 2 hours, or less frequently depending upon the severity of infection. For trachoma, 2 drops every 2 hours; concomitant systemic sulfonamide therapy is needed.

Sulfisoxazole diolamine: Use 1 to 2 drops of solution every 4 hours. In severe infections, dosage may be increased to 2 drops every hour. For ointment, apply sparingly 2 to 3 times daily.

Mary Ann Bolter

ANTIVIRAL AGENTS

ACTION OF THE DRUG: Agents are used to interfere with DNA synthesis in Herpes simplex virus type I.

ASSESSMENT:

INDICATIONS: Vidarabine is indicated for acute keratoconjunctivitis, recurrent epithelial keratitis caused by herpes simplex virus types 1 and 2, and superficial herpes simplex keratitis which is resistant to idoxuridine or if toxic or hypersensitivity reactions to idoxuridine have developed.

Trifluridine is used primarily for the treatment of keratoconjunctivitis and recurrent epithelial keratitis resulting from herpes simplex virus, types 1 and 2. It is generally used in cases which have not responded to therapy with idoxuridine or vidarabine.

SUBJECTIVE-OBJECTIVE: Patient presents with cutaneous lesions which are painful. Lesions are most commonly found on the genitalia, buccal-lingual areas or lips. Diagnosis should be confirmed through positive cultures for herpes simplex virus, and the finding of multinucleated giant cells in smears prepared from lesion exudate or scrapings. Differentiation between herpes simplex types 1 and 2 is not possible clinically, but may be made by fluorescein dyes.

PLAN:

COMPLICATIONS: Do not give to patients with known hypersensitivity to components of the drug.

WARNINGS: Safety for use in pregnant or breast-feeding women has not been established.

PRECAUTIONS: Do not exceed recommended dosage or length of treatment schedules.

IMPLEMENTATION:

DRUG INTERACTIONS: Allopurinol may interfere with vidarabine metabolism. Use caution when administering with CNS stimulants or anticholinergic drugs.

ADMINISTRATION AND DOSAGE: Care should be used during application in order to avoid spread of infection to other body sites and spread of infection to others. Therapy should be started as soon as signs and symptoms develop.

IMPLEMENTATION CONSIDERATIONS:

—Take a complete health history, including the contact, course of the disease, allergies, presence of other systemic illnesses, and possibility of pregnancy.

—Begin therapy as soon as possible once diagnosis has been made.

—Give emotional support and counseling regarding this new and at present incurable disease.

—Evaluate patient for presence of other sexually transmitted diseases.

—Report disease to county health department and comply with standard protocols for followup and monitoring of contacts.

—Product does not appear to be absorbed systemically.

WHAT THE PATIENT NEEDS TO KNOW:

—Take medication as instructed by your health care provider.

—Medication will not cure Herpes, but may help to speed healing. This medication will not prevent further outbreaks of Herpes, and should not be taken prophylactically.

—While you have open sores you should avoid intimate contact with others since you may infection them. You should be careful about handling your personal towel and wash cloths, keeping them away from others. Wash your hands carefully.

EVALUATION:

ADVERSE REACTIONS: See individual drug writeups.
PARAMETERS TO MONITOR: Watch for development of sensitivity and monitor therapeutic effects. Give patient emotional support and counseling.

IDOXURIDINE (IDU)

PRODUCTS (TRADE NAME):

Dendrid (Available in 0.1% ophthalmic solution.) **Herplex Liquifilm Ophthalmic** (Available in 0.1% solution). **Stoxil Ophthalmic** (Available in 0.1% solution and 0.5% ointment (5 mg/gm.)

DRUG SPECIFICS:

Idoxuridine is to be used only for the treatment of keratitis caused by the virus of herpes simplex. Its use is contraindicated if there is hypersensitivity to any component of the preparation.

Idoxuridine has teratogenic effects when instilled into the eyes of animals. Consider risk-benefit ratio in pregnant women or women of childbearing age. Whether idoxuridine appears in breast milk is unknown; in general, nursing should not be done during therapy.

Some forms of the herpes simplex virus appear to be resistant to idoxuridine. If there is no improvement (lessening of fluorescein staining) within 14 days of Herpex Liquifilm treatment, or within 7 to 8 days after using Stoxil, an alternative therapy should be used. After healing of the lesion, the medicine should be continued for 5 to 7 days to prevent recurrence. Use of corticosteroids is usually contraindicated in viral infections. Concomitant use of boric acid may cause irritation.

Adverse reactions to idoxuridine may include pain, pruritus, inflammation, edema of the eyes or eyelids, and photophobia. Occasionally corneal clouding, stippling, and punctate defects of the epithelium have been reported.

Tell the patient to keep his or her towel and wash cloth separate from those used by other family members.

ADMINISTRATION AND DOSAGE SPECIFICS:

Herpex Liquifilm: Saturate the tissue for the best results. Use one of these methods: (1) Instill 1 drop in the infected eye(s) every hour during the day. At night, instill 1 drop every other hour. (2) Instill 1 drop every minute for 5 minutes. Repeat this every 4 hours, day and night.

Stoxil Solution: Initially place 1 drop in the affected eye(s) every hour during the day and every 2 hours at night. After improvement, instill 1 drop every 2 hours during the day and every 4 hours at night.

Stoxil Ointment: Apply 5 times daily. Give approximately every 4 hours, with the last application at bedtime.

TRIFLURIDINE

PRODUCTS (TRADE NAME):
Viroptic (Available in 1% ophthalmic drops.)
DRUG SPECIFICS:

Trifluridine is used primarily for the treatment of keratoconjunctivitis and recurrent epithelial keratitis resulting from herpes simplex virus, types 1 and 2. It is generally used in cases which have not responded to therapy with idoxuridine or vidarabine. This product is not effective against bacterial, fungal or chlamydial infections of the cornea or nonviral trophic lesions. Safety for use in pregnancy and breast-feeding women has not been demonstrated. product is known to be teratogenic in larger doses in animals. Product may also have mutagenic effects which could cause genetic damage in humans.

Product may produce mild local but usually transient irritation of the cornea and conjunctiva following instillation. Do not exceed the dosage or frequency of adminstration. Increased ocular pressure and hypersensitivity reactions may also be found in some patients.

Patients should notify health care provider if condition does not improve within seven days of beginning therapy. If no improvement is found after 14 days, consider other forms of therapy. Do not continue therapy for more than 21 days because of potential for ocular toxicity.

Refrigerate drug since heat will accelerate its decomposition.
ADMINSTRATION AND DOSAGE SPECIFICS:

Corneal ulcers: Instill 1 drop onto the cornea of the effected eye every 2 hours while awake to a maximum of 9 drops/day. Continue this course until reepithelialization, then continue for 7 more days with one drop every 4 hours while awake, with a minimum of 5 drops/day.

VIDARABINE (ADENINE ARABINOSIDE, ARA-A)

PRODUCTS (TRADE NAME):
Vira-A 3% Ophthalmic (Available in 3% ointment.)

DRUG SPECIFICS:

This drug is contraindicated in those who develop hypersensitivity reactions to it.

Vidarabine has mutagenic and oncogenic potential. The recommended frequency and duration of therapy should not be exceeded. This drug has also been found to be teratogenic in laboratory animals. Consider risk-benefit ratio in pregnant women. Nursing mothers should not take this drug.

Adverse reactions to vidarabine include foreign body sensation, lacrimation, burning, irritation, conjunctival injection, pain, photophobia, superficial punctate keratitis, punctal occlusion and sensitivity. As with any ophthalmic ointment, there is transient blurring of vision following application.

Some topical antibiotics (gentamicin, erythromycin, chloramphenicol) and topical steroids (prednisolone or dexamethasone) have been given concurrently with vidarabine without any increase in untoward effects.

If after 7 days of therapy there are no signs of improvement, or after 21 days complete reepithelialization has not occurred, another form of therapy should be considered. After reepithelialization has occurred, reduced dosage (twice daily) is recommended for an additional week.

ADMINISTRATION AND DOSAGE SPECIFICS:

Apply 1/2 inch of ointment to the lower conjunctival sac 5 times daily at 3-hour intervals.

Mary Ann Bolter

ARTIFICIAL TEARS

ACTION OF THE DRUG: Artificial tear solutions are composed of a variety of wetting agents and lubricants which are used to substitute for inadequate aqueous or mucin components of the precorneal tear film. They lubricate and smooth irritated ocular tissue and are particularly useful for irritation due to hard contact lenses.

ASSESSMENT:

INDICATIONS: These solutions provide tear-like lubrication for the relief of dry eyes and eye irritation secondary to deficient tear production. The condition known as dry eyes is most often due to conjunctival cicatrization (the formation of a permanent fibrous tissue as a result of healing from inflammatory conditions) which occludes the openings of the lacrimal glands. Dry eyes are often a symptom of a systemic condition such as Sjogren's disease, amyotropic lateral sclerosis, keratitis sicca, Reiter's syndrome, Stevens-Johnson syndrome, trachoma, chemical and radiation burns of the conjunctiva, and arthritis. The incidence of dry eyes is higher in menopausal women. Some artificial tear products may also be used for lubrication with prostheses, after tonometry, and in other eye conditions such as band-shaped keratitis, corneal dystrophies, and healed pannus. Keratoconjunctivitis sicca is the most common aqueous deficient dry eye condition seen in the United States.

SUBJECTIVE: Complaints of dry scratchy eyes and irritation. No complaints of drainage of purulent material. Scratchy, foreign body sensation is often evident. Contact lens wearers may complain of inability to wear lenses. Problem may be increased if patient has seasonal allergies which affect the eyes, and for which he or she may be taking antihistamines.

OBJECTIVE: Deficient tear production, with increased redness and vascularity of the conjunctivial tissue. This can be seen by Schirmer and fluorescein tests.

PLAN:

CONTRAINDICATIONS: Most artificial tear solutions are contraindicated for use with soft contact lenses. Patients who wear soft contact lenses should be instructed to carefully read labels of all ophthalmic over the counter preparations prior to their use or purchase.

PRECAUTIONS: Maintain sterility of dropper tip to prevent contamination of solution.

IMPLEMENTATION:

PRODUCTS (TRADE NAME):
Isopto Alkaline (Available in 1% hydroxypropyl methylcellulose with 0.1 % benzalkonium chloride.) **Lacril** (Available in 0.5% hydroxypropyl methylcellulose, 0.01% gelatin A and 0.5% chlorobutanol).**Liquifilm Forte** (Available in 3% polyvinyl alcohol with 0.002% thimerosol and EDTA.) **Methopto Forte** (Available in 0.5% or 1% methylcellulose with 0.004% benzalkonium chloride solution.) **NuTears, Tears Plus** (Available in 1.4% polyvinyl alcohol povidone with 0.5% chlorobutanol.) **Tearisol** (Available in 0.5% hydroxypropyl methylcellulose with 0.01% benzalkonium chloride and 0.01% EDTA). **Ultra-Tears** (Available in 1% hydroxypropyl methylcellulose and 0.01% benzalkonium chloride.)

ADMINISTRATION AND DOSAGE: For these artificial tear solutions, 1 to 3 drops may be instilled in eye(s) 3 to 4 times daily or as needed. Tearisol is not for use with soft contact lenses.

IMPLEMENTATION CONSIDERATIONS:
—Obtain complete health history regarding the problem.
—Determine if patient wears contact lenses, and whether they are hard or soft lenses.
—Rule out a possible infectious case of patient's symptoms: i.e., viral or bacterial infectious process.
—Determine if patient is exposed to fumes or toxic products which could be responsible for symptoms.
—Determine if there is a systemic cause for dry eye symptoms.

WHAT THE PATIENT NEEDS TO KNOW:
—Do not touch dropper tip to any surface. Solution must remain sterile.
Using clean hands, pull down the lower eyelid and put drops into conjunctival

sac. Do not put medication directly on cornea. Shut eyes and let medication cover eyes.

—If eye irritation persists or worsens, consult health care provider.

—Soft contact lens wearers should not use artifical tear solutions. If you are using hard contact lenses, be careful not to use medication so that eyes are abused.

—Avoid hot, dry environment or exposure to toxic fumes.

EVALUATION:

PARAMETERS TO MONITOR: Assess for primary cause of dry eye syndrome to rule out systemic causes. Monitor for therapeutic effects. Watch for decreased dryness of the eyes and relief of symptoms of irritation. Individuals using artificial tear solutions for relief of irritation due to hard contact lenses should be assessed to rule out improper wearing habits or techniques.

Carol Burke and Geraldine Polly Bednash

CARBONIC ANHYDRASE INHIBITORS

ACTION OF THE DRUG: This category of drugs is made up of sulfonamide diuretics which inhibit the action of carbonic anhydrase. The diuretic action has limited use, but ability of these drugs to reduce aqueous humor secretion by 40-60% has led to their utilization as an antiglaucoma agent. The bicarbonate ion secretion into the posterior chamber is inhibited, decreasing the osmotic pressure in this chamber. The result is a decrease in water drawn into this compartment. Outflow of aqueous humor remains constant, resulting in a decrease in intraocular pressure.

ASSESSMENT:

INDICATIONS: May be used for acute attacks of angle-closure glaucoma in conjunction with other agents for rapid reduction of intraocular pressure. It may be used in conjunction with local agents for long term treatment of open-angle glaucoma. Also indicated for use in short term therapy of secondary glaucomas as preparation for surgical intervention.

SUBJECTIVE: *Open-angle glaucoma:* Patient is usually devoid of subjective symptoms. However, open-angle glaucoma is a genetically inherited disease. A history of this disease occurring in the patient's family should lead the health care provider to more closely examine for objective findings which accompany this problem.

OBJECTIVE: *Open-angle glaucoma:* Funduscopic examination may reveal increased size and depth of the physiologic cup, nasal displacement of the blood vessels, or optic atrophy. Tonometry measurements of greater than 25 mm Hg occur with this illness.

PLAN:

CONTRAINDICATIONS: Do not use in individuals with hypersensitivity to sulfonamides. Also contraindicated in adrenocortical insufficiency, hypokalemia, hyponatremia, hepatic insufficiency, and renal insufficiency. The use of carbonic anhydrase inhibitors in pregnancy should be avoided. Animal studies have indicated possible teratogenic effects although this has not been shown in humans. Due to their ability to increase renal HCO_3 secretion, these drugs should not be used in acidotic individuals. Not recommended for use in chronic noncongestive angle-closure glaucoma.

PRECAUTIONS: Individuals with compromised hepatic function may develop hepatic coma due to hypokalemia. These drugs should also be used with caution in individuals on steroid therapy. Diuresis is not promoted by dosages above recommended levels and may result in an increased incidence of paresthesias. These products should be used with caution in individuals with chronic respiratory problems which result in acid-base imbalance.

IMPLEMENTATION:

DRUG INTERACTIONS: Carbonic anhydrase inhibitors interfere with the action of the urinary antiseptic methenamine. Drug-induced osteomalacia has been reported when used with phenytoin.

ADMINISTRATION AND DOSAGE: May be administered orally or parenterally. Parenteral administration is limited to acute angle-closure attacks. Dosage varies with preparation used. See individual product listings.

IMPLEMENTATION CONSIDERATIONS:

—Obtain a complete health history, including presence of renal, hepatic, or respiratory insufficiency, hypersensitivity to sulfonamides or carbonic anhydrase inhibitors,and possibility of pregnancy.

—Obtain baseline electrolyte studies, complete blood count and urinalysis prior to initiating therapy. These should be assessed frequently with a patient on long-term therapy.

—Determine baseline weight, especially in children. The most frequently experienced side effect in children is weight loss.

—Do complete funduscopic examination and tonometry measurements.

—A slight metabolic acidosis may occur with chronic use and may be overcome with bicarbonate administration.

WHAT THE PATIENT NEEDS TO KNOW:

—This medication should be taken exactly as ordered.

—This drug may make you urinate more for a short period of time, but this effect should decrease with continued use.

—Potassium will be lost in the urine, so dietary supplementation with foods rich in potassium is important. Recommended foods are bananas, citrus fruits, and dried fruits. Your health care provider can give you a list of foods rich in potassium.

—If you notice any hearing loss, stop taking your medicine, and report to your health care provider immediately.

—Some people experience side effects in taking this drug. The most frequently encountered symptoms are: drowsiness, nausea, numbness and tingling of fingers, toes, lips, and anus, diarrhea, headaches, changes in smell and taste, loss of appetite, and lethargy. These side effects last only briefly and should be reported to the health care provider if they persist.

—If you develop a rash and fever, do not take any more medicine, and contact your health care provider immediately.

EVALUATION:

ADVERSE REACTIONS: Common side effects include: altered taste and smell, anorexia, depression, headache, paresthesias, tiredness, weight loss in children. *Other:* acidosis, ataxia (rare), bone marrow depression, disorientation (rare), exanthema, fever, globus hystericus (rare), hepatic coma if previous compromised hepatic function, leukopenia, pancytopenia, rash, renal calculi, Stevens-Johnson syndrome, thrombocytopenic purpura.

PARAMETERS TO MONITOR: Electrolyte studies, complete blood count and urinalysis should be done every two months after baseline studies have been completed. Signs and symptoms of hypokalemia and hyponatremia should be assessed. Complete funduscopic examination and intraocular pressure recordings should be done each visit to determine if disease progression and damage has occurred.

Depression is a side effect often overlooked. Psychosocial assessment of the patient should be done to determine if changes have occurred which may be attributable to the use of carbonic anhydrase inhibitors. Continued use of these medications should then be reassessed with the patient.

ACETAZOLAMIDE

PRODUCTS (TRADE NAME):

Acetazolamide, Ak-Zol, Cetazol (Available in 250 mg capsules.) **Diamox** (Available in 125 and 250 mg capsules and 500 mg/vial injection.) **Diamox Sequels** (Available in 500 mg sustained release capsules.)

DRUG SPECIFICS:
Effective duration of these drugs is short and they must be given around-the-clock to provide controlled decrease of intraocular pressure. Additive effects are found to occur when the drug is used in combination with epinephrine. Side effects are dose-related.

ADMINISTRATION AND DOSAGE SPECIFICS:
Chronic open-angle glaucoma:
Adults: Give 250 mg to 1 gm po per day in divided doses.
Sequels: Take one tablet every 12 hours.
Acute-angle closure:
Adults: Give 250 mg po every four hours. Initial loading dose of 500 mg may be given. Drug may also be administered intravenously.
Children: Use 5-10 mg/kg po every four to six hours.

DICHLORPHENAMIDE

PRODUCTS (TRADE NAME):
Daranide, Oratrol (Available in 50 mg tablets).
DRUG SPECIFICS:
These products cause greater incidence of hypokalemia. The most common side effects are anorexia, ataxia, tremor, depression and paresthesia. Used orally only.
ADMINISTRATION AND DOSAGE SPECIFICS:
Adults: A priming dose of 100 mg to 200 mg po is given. This is followed by 100 mg every 12 hours until desired response is obtained. Maintenance dose is 25 mg to 50 mg two to four times daily.

METHAZOLAMIDE

PRODUCTS (TRADE NAME):
Neptazane (Available in 50 mg tablets.)
DRUG SPECIFICS:
The incidence of renal calculi is less with methazolamide than with acetazolamide. Marked malaise may be experienced with use of this drug. Available for oral use only.
ADMINISTRATION AND DOSAGE SPECIFICS:
Adults: 50-100 mg po two to four times daily.

Geraldine Polly Bednash

CHOLINERGIC BLOCKING AGENTS

MYDRIATIC-CYCLOPEGICS

ACTION OF THE DRUG: These drugs block the action of acetylcholine or other cholinergic agonists. The sphincter of the iris is paralyzed, causing mydriasis, and the ciliary muscles are paralyzed, blocking accommodation. Atropine and scopolamine are long-acting agents that produce complete cycloplegia. Homatropine, cyclopentolate and tropicamide have shorter durations of action and are most useful for diagnostic procedures.

ASSESSMENT:

INDICATIONS: The longer-acting cycloplegic mydriatics are used for prevention of posterior synechiae (adhesions of the iris to the lens) as a result of inflammation due to iritis, iridocyclitis, anterior uveitis or keratitis. The mydriasis that occurs prevents the development of adhesions. Occasionally, atropine or scoplamine will be alternated with miotic agents such as pilocarpine to break adhesions between the lens and iris.

SUBJECTIVE: Photophobia, visual loss, excessive lacrimation and eye pain are often present.

OBJECTIVE: Ciliary injection, cloudy anterior chamber and distortion of the iris size and shape may be observed.

PLAN:

CONTRAINDICATIONS: These drugs should not be administered to individuals with narrow anterior angle chamber or acute angle-closure glaucoma, nor should they be given to individuals with known sensitivity to any component of the drug solution.

PRECAUTIONS: A gonioscopic examination should be done prior to administration of this medication. The risk-benefit ratio should be assessed before considering long-term use in pregnant or breast-feeding women. Increased susceptibility to toxic effects has been reported in children with brain damage, Down's syndrome or spastic paralysis. This has also been reported in blondes and infants. Extreme caution should be used when prescribing or administering this drug to these individuals.

IMPLEMENTATION:

ADMINISTRATION AND DOSAGE: The frequency and dosage varies with purpose and type of medication used. See individual product listing. A summary of the peak and duration of action drugs included in this category is found in Table 9-1.

TABLE 9-1. PEAK AND DURATION OF CYCLOPEGIA AND MYDRIATIC DRUGS

Drug	Mydriasis		Cyclopegia	
	Peak	Duration	Peak	Duration
Atropine	30-40 minutes	10 days	1-3 hours	14 days
Cyclopentolate	½-1 hour	1 day	1 hour	24 hours
Homatropine	1 hour	3 days	1 hour	24 hours
Scopolamine	20-30 minutes	7 days	½-1 hour	7 days
Tropicamide	20-40 minutes	6 hour	30 minutes	4-6 hour

IMPLEMENTATION CONSIDERATIONS:

—Obtain a complete health history, including history of untoward response to drugs in this category, history of narrow anterior angle chamber, acute angle-closure glaucoma and possibility of pregnancy or breast-feeding.

—Individuals with brown or hazel irides may require stronger concentrations of these drugs than individuals with green or blue irides.

—Physostigmine is the accepted antidote for toxic response to all of these drugs.

—Atropine may cause an allergic conjunctivitis, which can be controlled by use of topical antihistaminic agents.

—Slit lamp examination and gonioscopic measurement must be done prior to prescribing or administering any of these drugs to avoid the occurrence of acute angle-closure glaucoma attacks.

—Psychotic reactions, behavioral disturbances and convulsions have occurred in children after administration of cyclopentolate, especially in higher concentrations (i.e., 2%).

WHAT THE PATIENT NEEDS TO KNOW:

—Use proper technique for putting medication into eyes. With clean hands, pull down the lower eyelid and put drops into conjunctival sac. Do not put medication directly on cornea. Shut eyes and allow medication to cover eyes. At the same time apply pressure at nasolacrimal ducts for 1-2 minutes after instillation to decrease chances of systemic response.

—If a dose is missed, take the missed dose as close as possible to the regularly scheduled dose. If the time for the next dose is very close, do not take the missed dose but instead resume the regular schedule.

—Using any of these drugs will make the eyes extremely sensitivity to bright light. It may be necessary to wear sunglasses for all outdoor activities. This effect will persist for several days after stopping the medicine (see Table 9-1).

—If signs of systemic absorption occur, the drug should be stopped and your health care provider should be contacted immediately.

—Take care to read labels on over-the-counter preparations such as cold, cough or sleeping preparations to avoid atropine or atropine-like substances that could have additive effects.

—Elderly patients should be cautioned that blurred vision may increase their chance of falls. Precautions should be taken to avoid this danger.

EVALUATION:

ADVERSE REACTIONS: *Local:* chronic conjunctivitis (following long-term use of atropine), photophobia, swelling of the eyelids. *Systemic:* confusion, dermatitis, fever, hallucinations, increased thirst, lethargy, psychotic reactions (in children), slurred speech, tachycardia.

OVERDOSAGE: Atropine and scopolamine have a higher incidence of toxic reactions than the synthetic colinergic blocking agents, especially when used in children. The most frequently seen toxic symptoms are a rash over the head and upper trunk, hot dry flushed skin, extreme thirst and tachycardia. These reverse rapidly with cessation of the drug.

PARAMETERS TO MONITOR: The anterior chamber angle must be measured prior to administration of any of these drugs. When these drugs are used for diagnostic purposes, the patient must be carefully assessed to rule out the possibility of adverse responses before going home. Blood pressure, pulse and respiration should be measured before and after administration. The patient should be questioned carefully about the presence of subjective symptoms such as anxiety or excitability to determine if behavioral disturbances have been precipitated by drug used. Patients with long-term use of the cyclopegic-mydriatics should be frequently reassessed. They should be seen for slit-lamp examination and assessment of infectious process to determine response to therapy and possible termination of therapy.

ATROPINE SULFATE

PRODUCTS (TRADE NAME):
Atropine Care, Atropine Sulfate Sterile Opthalmic Solution and Ointment) (Available in 0.125% to 3% solutions). **Atropisol** (Available in 0.5% to 3% solutions). **Bufopto Atropine** (Available in 0.5% and 1% solutions). **Isopto Atropine, Murocoll Atropine** (Available in 0.5% to 3% solutions).

DRUG SPECIFICS:
Atropine sulfate is useful for producing cyclopegia and mydriasis. It is used in refraction and in inflammatory conditions involving the uveal tract and iris. There is a wide range of prices for this drug.

ADMINISTRATION AND DOSAGE SPECIFICS:
Adults: One drop of 0.5% or 1% solution one to three times a day, or 0.3 cm to 0.5 cm of 1% ointment one to three times a day.

Children: One drop of 0.125% to 1% solution one to three times a day, or 0.3 cm to 0.5 cm of 0.5% or 1% ointment one to three times a day.

Uveitis: One drop of 1% or 2% solution two to three times a day.

CYCLOPENTOLATE HCl

PRODUCTS (TRADE NAME):

Ak-Pentolate (Available in 1% solution). **Cyclogic** (Available in 0.5% to 2% solutions). **Cyclomydril** (Available in 1% phenylephrine and 0.2% cyclopentolate solutions).

DRUG SPECIFICS:

This drug is used for producing mydriasis and cyclopegia primarily during diagnostic procedures.

ADMINISTRATION AND DOSAGE SPECIFICS:

Adults: One drop of a 1% or 2% solution; repeat in 5 minutes. Ophthalmoscopy can occur immediately. Refraction can occur in 40-50 minutes.

Children:

Mydriasis: One drop of 0.5% or 1% solution.

Refraction: One drop of 1% or 2% solution; repeat in 5 minutes. Refraction can occur in 40-50 minutes.

HOMATROPINE HYDROBROMIDE

PRODUCTS (TRADE NAME):

Homatrocel (Available in 2% or 5% solutions). **Homatropine Hydrobromide Ophthalmic Solution, Isopto Homatropine, Murocoll Homatropine** (Available in 1% to 5 % solutions).

DRUG SPECIFICS:

This product is used primarily for refraction. It is a moderately long-acting mydriatic and cyclopegic. It is sometimes used in treatment of inflammatory conditions of the uveal tract.

ADMINISTRATION AND DOSAGE SPECIFICS:

Adults:

Refraction: One drop of 2% or 5% solution; repeat two to five times until desired results.

Uveitis: One drop of 2% or 5% solution two to three times a day.

Children:

Refraction: One drop of 1% or 2% solution every 10 minutes two to five times.

SCOPOLAMINE HYDROBROMIDE

PRODUCTS (TRADE NAME):
Isopto Hyoscine (Available in 0.25% solution). **Murocoll #2** (Available with phenylephrine 10% and scopolamine in 0.3% solution). **Murocoll #19** (Available in 0.2% to 0.25% solutions). **Scopolamine S.O.P.** (Available in 0.2% to 0.25% solutions).

DRUG SPECIFICS:
This is a parasympatholytic agent used in cycloplegic refraction or for pupil dilation in acute inflammatory conditions of the uveal tract and iris.

ADMINISTRATION AND DOSAGE SPECIFICS:
Adults:
Uveitis: One drop of 0.25% solution one to three times a day.
Children:
Refraction: One drop of 0.2% or 0.25% solution two times a day for 2 days prior to refraction.
Uveitis: One drop of 0.2% or 0.25% solution one to three times a day.

TROPICAMIDE

PRODUCTS (TRADE NAME):
Mydriacyl (Available in 0.5% and 1% solutions).

DRUG SPECIFICS:
Tropacamide is used for diagnostic purposes requiring mydriasis and cycloplegia.

ADMINISTRATION AND DOSAGE SPECIFICS:
Adult diagnostic: One drop of 1% solution; repeat in 5 minutes.
Children diagnostic: One drop of 0.5% solution; repeat in 5 minutes.

Geraldine Polly Bednash

DIAGNOSTIC PRODUCTS

FLUORESCEIN SODIUM, TOPICAL

ACTION OF THE DRUG: Fluorescein sodium causes ulcerated areas to stain green by ordinary light or bright yellow if a cobalt blue filter is used. Surface irregularities of the conjunctiva appear bright orange-yellow in ordinary light.

ASSESSMENT:

INDICATIONS: This product is used in the diagnosis of external ocular disorders, including defects in corneal epithelium, conjunctiva, and patency of lacrimal apparatus. Fluorescein has also been used recently in the fitting of contact lenses.

SUBJECTIVE-OBJECTIVE: Patient may present with a history of eye pain and irritation. Use of fluorescein may allow corneal scratches to become visible.

PLAN:

CONTRAINDICATIONS: Do not use when known hypersensitivity to ingredients exists.

WARNINGS: For topical ophthalmic use only.

PRECAUTIONS: Maintain sterility of the product. Keep bottle tightly closed and avoid contamination of dropper tip.

IMPLEMENTATION:

PRODUCTS (TRADE NAME):

Fluorescein Sodium, Flurasceptic (Available in 2% solution.) **Flur-I-Strip**(Available in 9 mg strips.) **Flur-I-Strip-A.T.** (Available in 1 mg strip.) **FluGlo** (Available in 0.6 mg strips.)

ADMINISTRATION AND DOSAGE: For examination of corneal and conjunctival epithelium, instill 1 drop and close lid for 60 seconds. Following diagnostic examination, eye may be irrigated with sterile normal saline.

IMPLEMENTATION CONSIDERATIONS:

—Obtain a complete health history, including presence of allergies.

—Use care to maintain the sterility of the solution and dropper.

WHAT THE PATIENT NEEDS TO KNOW:

—Solution is a temporary stain and discoloration is easily flushed with irrigation of normal saline.

EVALUATION:

ADVERSE REACTIONS: local irritation.

PARAMETERS TO MONITOR: Check for local irritation. Corneal irregularities should be visualized if present.

Carol Burke

LONG-ACTING CHOLINESTERASE INHIBITORS

MIOTIC-ANTIGLAUCOMA AGENTS

ACTION OF THE DRUG: Drugs in this category are long-acting organophosphorous compounds which inactivate acetylcholinesterase to provide iris sphincter contraction leading to miosis, ciliary muscle constriction which increases accommodation and increased aqueous humor outflow. Usefulness in open-angle glaucoma is believed to be due to the ciliary muscle constriction which opens the trabecular meshwork and increases aqueous humor outflow. The organophosphorous cholinesterase inhibitors also cause extreme dilatation of the intraocular vascular supply.

ASSESSMENT:

INDICATIONS: This drug is indicated for severe open-angle glaucoma which is resistant to therapy with other more commonly applied drugs such as pilocarpine, epinephrine, or timolol. The decision to use long-acting cholinesterase inhibitors, which are extremely toxic and have severe side effects, is usually based upon treatment failure with safer, less toxic drugs and progressive irreversible ocular damage due to the glaucoma. Although it is unlikely that nurse practitioners would prescribe the long-acting anticholinesterase agents, it is likely that they might be caring for individuals who may be using these drugs.

These drugs are also used for the individual with accommodative esotropia. The increased accommodation provided by these drugs decreases nerve impulses to the medial recti muscles and less convergence occurs during accommodation. These drugs are used in combination with bifocal correction for accommodative esotropia.

SUBJECTIVE: In open-angle glaucoma, the patient is usually devoid of subjective symptoms. However, open-angle glaucoma is a genetically inherited disease. A history of this disease occurring in the patient's family should lead the health care provider to more closely examine for objective findings which accompany this problem.

OBJECTIVE: Fundoscopic examination may reveal increased size and depth of the physiologic cup, nasal displacement of the blood vessels, or optic atrophy. Tonometry measurements of greater than 25 mg Hg occur with this illness.

PLAN:

CONTRAINDICATIONS: These products should not be administered to individuals with active uveitis, or to persons with known sensitivity to any component of the drug. Long-acting cholinesterase inhibitors are used in angle-closure glaucoma only after iridectomy has been performed.

PRECAUTIONS: Long-acting cholinesterase inhibitors should be used with extreme caution in individuals with asthma, bradycardia, hypotension, epilepsy, spasm of the gastrointestinal system, recent myocardial infarction, parkinsonism, peptic ulcer disease, history of retinal detachment, marked vagotonia or Down's syndrome. If used in pregnant or breast-feeding women, risks must be weighed against benefits. These products should be discontinued 4 weeks prior to ocular surgery due to increased risk of hyphema which occurs with extreme vasodilatation caused by these drugs.

IMPLEMENTATION:

DRUG INTERACTIONS: The use of succinylcholine in individuals who are receiving long-acting cholinesterase inhibitors will lead to a prolonged action of the succinylcholine. Use of systemic cholinesterase inhibitors in individuals using ophthalmic cholinesterase inhibitors can have additive effects leading to toxicity.

Many organic pesticides used for home and garden, community spraying, and farms are cholinesterase inhibitors and have additive effects on the individual using these in ophthalmic form. Patients should be cautioned to avoid exposure to these agents through either personal use or exposure in the community. Some commonly seen insecticides with this action are (trade name in parentheses): carbaryl (Sevin), demeton (Systox), diazinon, malathion, parathion, ronnel (Trolene.)

Use of physostigmine ophthalmic solution prior to instilling echothiophate or isoflurophate will inactivate the latter two drugs.

ADMINISTRATION AND DOSAGE: The dose and concentration used varies with preparation and desired response. See individual product information.

IMPLEMENTATION CONSIDERATIONS:

—Obtain a complete health history of glaucoma and response to other therapy, presence of myocardial infarction, parkinsonism, peptic ulcer disease, retinal detachment, epilepsy, bradycardia, severe hypotension, marked vagotonia, or asthma, as well as possibility of pregnancy or breast-feeding.

—Perform funduscopic examination and assessment of ocular damage due to glaucoma.

—Determine anterior angle measurements with gonioscopy.

—Individuals with hazel or brown irises may require stronger concentrations of medicine than those with green or blue irises.

—Tolerance may develop with prolonged use. Usefulness may be restored by substitution of other miotics for a short period of time.

—Atropine sulfate is the antidote for long-acting cholinesterase inhibitors. Pralidoxime may be used in conjunction with, but not as a substitute for, atropine.

—Iris cyst formation may occur with prolonged use. This may be decreased by concurrent use of phenylephrine.

—Nasolacrimal obstruction and conjunctival thickening may occur with prolonged use.

—Frequent assessment of the drug's efficacy and possible systemic response must be done.

—Lens opacities have been reported with long-term use of ophthalmic cholinesterase inhibitors.

—Local side effects tend to decrease with continued therapy, although some other problems only develop after prolonged treatment. If a patient develops any systemic reactions to the drug, which is infrequent, reevaluate whether proper technique and dosage is being followed.

WHAT THE PATIENT NEEDS TO KNOW:

—Medication should be taken exactly as prescribed.

—If a daily dose is missed, it should be administered as close to the regularly scheduled time as possible. If the missed dose is not remembered until the next day, do not apply two doses. Resume regular schedule of doses. If the medication is prescribed more frequently than once daily, missed doses should not be taken if the error is realized close to the next dose.

—Use the proper technique for putting in eye drops. Using clean hands, pull down the lower eyelid and put the drops into the conjunctival sac. Do not put medication directly on cornea. Shut eyes and let medication cover the eye. At the same time, apply pressure over the lacrimal puncta to decrease systemic absorption of the drug. Compression should be done for one to two minutes.

—Many common organic pesticides contain cholinesterase inhibitors which would be additive to the medication you are already taking. You should read labels of insecticides you are working with, and stay out of the way of spraying which is going on in the community.

—A Medic-Alert bracelet or other identifying information should be carried specifying this drug is part of your therapy.

—Inform your health care provider of possible pregnancy.

—Some people experience side effects as a result of this drug. Be certain to report any new or uncomfortable symptoms promptly to your health care provider.

—Wash hands thoroughly after putting in eye drops in order to avoid accidentally swallowing any medication.

—Use extreme care when working or sitting in areas with poor lighting since drugs may cause extreme miosis in these situations.

EVALUATION:

ADVERSE REACTIONS: brow ache, burning, conjunctival and ciliary injection, eye ache, headache, lid twitching, stinging, tearing, visual blurring. Iris cysts have occurred with long-term use, especially in children. Occasionally they may enlarge and obscure vision or break free to float in the aqueous humor. These cysts should recede with discontinuation of therapy. Conjunctival thickening, lens opacities, nasolacrimal duct obstruction, and retinal detachment also have been reported to occur with long-term use. *Systemic response:* bradycardia, chest tightness, diarrhea, increased salivation, lethargy, loss of bladder control, muscle weakness, nausea, profuse perspiration, shortness of breath, stomach cramps, urinary frequency, vomiting. If systemic side effects occur, the drug should be discontinued and the patient must be assessed.

PARAMETERS TO MONITOR: Frequent tonometry and slit lamp exams should be done to determine presence of undesirable effects. Complete funduscopic exam should determine progression of ocular damage. The patient should be thoroughly questioned about systemic response and undesirable local effects. Sudden changes or blurring of vision should be assessed thoroughly for possible retinal detachment. Blood pressure, pulse, and respiratory status should be monitored to determine if systemic symptoms are present.

DEMECARIUM BROMIDE

PRODUCTS (TRADE NAME):
   Humorsol Ophthalmic (Available in 0.125% and 0.25% solution.)
DRUG SPECIFICS:
   Should be stored in tightly sealed, light-resistant container in a cool location. Miosis occurs in 15-60 minutes and peaks within 4 hours. Miosis lasts 3-10 days.
ADMINISTRATION AND DOSAGE SPECIFICS:
   Antiglaucoma agent: Use one drop of 0.125% or 0.25% solution one to two times a day. Intraocular pressure reduction peaks in 24 hours and lasts approximately 9 days.
   For accommodative esotropia: Use one drop of 0.125% or 0.25% solution daily for 2-3 weeks, then one drop every two days for 3-4 weeks. This is then decreased to one drop one or two times a week based upon response to the drug. Drug is discontinued if one drop every two days is still needed after four months.

ECHOTHIOPHATE IODIDE

PRODUCTS (TRADE NAME):
   Echodide, Phospholine Iodide (Available in 0.03% to 0.25% powder for reconstitution.)
DRUG SPECIFICS:
   Miosis occurs rapidly, in 10-30 minutes and lasts one to four weeks. Medication may be stored at room temperature for up to one month or refrigerated for 4-12 months.
ADMINISTRATION AND DOSAGE SPECIFICS:
   Antiglaucoma: Use one drop of 0.03% to 0.25% solution, one to two times a day. Reduction in intraocular pressure peaks in 24 hours and lasts up to 28 days.
   Accommodative strabismus: Use one drop of 0.03% to 0.125% solution once a day or every two days.

ISOFLUROPHATE

PRODUCTS (TRADE NAME):
Floropryl OpHthalmic Ointment (Available in 0.025% ointment.)
DRUG SPECIFICS:
  Isoflurophate must be protected from moisture and stored in a cool location. Systemic side effects are less frequent with isoflurophate than with demecarium or echothiophate.
ADMINISTRATION AND DOSAGE SPECIFICS:
  Antiglaucoma: Use 0.5 cm strip of 0.025% ointment. Frequency can range from every three days to three times daily.
  Accommodative esotropia: Use 0.5 cm strip of 0.025% ointment at bedtime for two weeks. Then decrease to every two days and gradually decrease to every week for a two-month period.

Geraldine Polly Bednash

PARASYMPATHOMIMETIC OPHTHALMIC DRUGS— MIOTICS

CARBACHOL

ACTION OF THE DRUG: Carbachol is a parasympathomimetic which acts as a cholinergic agonist. Its action in reducing intraocular pressure is similar to that of pilocarpine. It produces miosis as a result of iris sphincter contraction. Miosis increases outflow of aqueous humor through the trabecular meshwork by opening up the anterior chamber angle. The miosis produced is similar to pilocarpine, but lasts three times as long.

ASSESSMENT:

INDICATIONS: Carbachol is a potent miotic which is used as an alternative to pilocarpine when drug tolerance has developed in the individual who has open-angle glaucoma. A short period of carbachol use will allow pilocarpine to regain its usefulness in lowering intraocular pressure. It is also used in its intraocular form for injection to produce miosis necessary for surgical procedures. Controversy exists concerning the usefulness of this drug in acute-angle closure glaucoma attacks due to its ability to increase circulation in the vessels of the iris and the ciliary body. Tolerance to carbachol may occur with prolonged use.
  SUBJECTIVE: *Open-angle glaucoma:* Usually there are no subjective symptoms. However, open-angle glaucoma is a genetically inherited disease. A history

of this disease occurring in the patient's family should lead the health care provider to more closely examine for objective findings which accompany this problem. *Angle-closure glaucoma:* History of eye pain after sitting in darkened theater or room for several hours, which may be relieved by bright light. Intense stabbing pain in affected eye may occur. This may also be accompanied by nausea and vomiting. Profuse perspiration, halo vision, and bradycardia may also accompany this pain.

OBJECTIVE: *Open-angle glaucoma:* Funduscopic examination may reveal increased size and depth of the physiologic cup, nasal displacement of the blood vessels, or optic atrophy. Tonometry measurements of greater than 25 mm Hg occur with this problem. *Angle-closure glaucoma:* Ciliary injection, semidilated pupil which may be nonreactive to light, and cloudy anterior chamber may be present. Hyperemia of optic nerve head with edema may occur, and there may be corneal edema.

PLAN:

CONTRAINDICATIONS: Carbachol should not be used in acute iritis where adhesions of the iris may occur with prolonged miosis. Also contraindicated in individuals with known hypersensitivity to the drug or any of its components.

PRECAUTIONS: Use of carbachol in individuals who have corneal abrasions will allow excessive absorption leading to systemic response. It should be used with caution in individuals who have asthma, cardiac failure, gastrointestinal spasm or hypermotility, active peptic ulcer, hyperthyroidism, urinary tract obstruction, or Parkinson's disease. Individuals who have a history of retinal detachment may be predisposed to a reoccurrence of this with the use of potent miotics such as carbachol. Risks-benefit ratio should be assessed if individual is pregnant or breast-feeding.

IMPLEMENTATION:

ADMINISTRATION AND DOSAGE: Carbachol is administered topically to the conjunctiva, one drop two to four times a day. It is available in solutions of 0.75% to 3% for titration to individual patient needs. Onset of miosis is within 10-20 minutes and lasts 4-8 hours. Intraocular pressure reduction occurs within 4 hours and lasts 8 hours.

Carbachol is also used for intraocular injection to provide long-lasting miosis for surgical procedures. When injected in this manner onset of action is 5 minutes and lasts 24 hours.

IMPLEMENTATION CONSIDERATIONS:

—Obtain a complete health history, including the presence of family history of glaucoma, previous intraocular pressure readings, presence or history of retinal detachment, asthma, cardiac failure, active peptic ulcer disease, gastrointestinal spasm or hypermotility, hyperthyroidism, urinary tract obstruction, or Parkinson's disease. Also determine possibility of pregnancy or breast-feeding.

—Determine if patient has iritis or corneal abrasion. Medication should not be used immediately following tonometry or invasive procedures involving the cornea in order to avoid systemic absorption of the drug.

—Atropine is the accepted antidote for overdosage or toxic response to carbachol.

—Carbachol produces more severe headaches and accommodative spasms than pilocarpine, but these will usually decrease after several days' use of the drug.

—Individuals with brown or hazel irides may require higher concentration of carbachol than those with blue or green irides.

WHAT THE PATIENT NEEDS TO KNOW:

—Glaucoma is a chronic disease which will require lifelong treatment.

—Carbachol should be taken only as prescribed.

—If a dose is missed, take it as soon as possible after the missed dose was due. If the next dose is due shortly, do not take the missed dose but instead resume the regular dosage schedule.

—If irritation in the eye develops or the eye has been injured by a foreign body, do not use the drug. Instead, consult with your health care provider immediately.

—If you develop diarrhea, vomiting, cramps, flushing, or excess perspiration, shortness of breath, wheezing, increased salivation or urinary frequency, the drug should be stopped and your health care provider contacted immediately.

—Night vision or the ability to see in low light will be decreased due to pupillary constriction and inability of the pupil to dilate.

—Use the proper technique in instilling eye drops. Using clean hands, pull down the lower lid of the eye and put drops into conjunctival sac. Do not put medication directly on cornea. Close eye and let medication cover eye. Place pressure at the lacrimal puncta for one to two minutes after putting in eye drops in order to decrease systemic absorption.

—You may note some irritation and spasm of the eye when you begin using these drops. These local effects usually decrease in frequency and intensity with continued use of the drug.

EVALUATION:

ADVERSE REACTIONS: blurred vision, eye pain (due to accomodative spasm), headache, irritation of the eyes, twitching of the eyelids. *Systemic response:* asthma, cardiac arrhythmias, diarrhea, excess perspiration, excessive salivation, flushing, gastrointestinal cramping, shortness of breath, syncope, vomiting, wheezing. The drug should be immediately stopped if a systemic response occurs and the patient should be assessed for toxicity.

PARAMETERS TO MONITOR: If carbachol is prescribed to overcome a tolerance which has developed to pilocarpine, the patient should be returned to the original treatment regimen after several weeks of carbachol therapy. Patient should be assessed at regular intervals during the carbachol therapy to ensure that intraocular pressure has decreased and that ocular damage is not progressing. After return to the original therapeutic regimen, the patient should be assessed at regular intervals to determine intraocular pressure and therapeutic response.

CARBACHOL

PRODUCTS (TRADE NAME):
   Carbacel Ophthalmic (Available in 0.75%, 1.5% and 3% solution.) **Isopto Carbachol Ophthalmic** (Available in 0.75%, 1.5%, 2.25% and 3% solution.)
DRUG SPECIFICS:
   This medication is particularly useful for patients who have become resistant to pilocarpine or who have developed irritation from its use.
ADMINISTRATION AND DOSAGE SPECIFICS:
   Use one to two drops in each eye two to three times a day. Concentration of solution and frequency of administration are titrated to individual patient status.

CARBACHOL INTRAOCULAR SOLUTION

PRODUCTS (TRADE NAME):
   Miostat Intraocular (Available in 0.01% solution.)
DRUG SPECIFICS:
   This drug is used most frequently to obtain miosis during surgery.
ADMINISTRATION AND DOSAGE SPECIFICS:
   This is for intraocular irrigation. Instill 0.5 ml of a 0.01% solution into the anterior chamber. Remainder of solution should be discarded.

Geraldine Polly Bednash

CHOLINESTERASE INHIBITORS

PHYSOSTIGMINE SALICYLATE

ACTION OF THE DRUG: Physostigmine temporarily inactivates acetylcholinesterase to allow increased parasympathetic tone from accumulation of endogenous acetylcholine. This causes iris sphincter contraction resulting in miosis and increased ciliary muscle constriction which produces increased accommodation. Intraocular pressure is reduced due to the decreased resistance to aqueous humor flow into the anterior chamber through the trabecular meshwork.

ASSESSMENT:

INDICATIONS: Physostigmine is a potent miotic which is useful in open-angle glaucoma for the reduction of intraocular pressure. Physostigmine is not considered a first choice drug for this disase and is used only if treatment failure has occurred with other drugs. Physostigmine is also useful as a substitute miotic when tolerance to other agents, such as pilocarpine or carbachol has developed. A short term of therapy with physostigmine will allow the previously used agent to regain its usefulness for the patient.

Controversy exists concerning the use of physostigmine in acute angle-closure glaucoma. Its rapid miotic action allows increased outflow of aqueous humor through the trabecular meshwork, providing a rapid reduction in intraocular pressure. For this reason, physostigmine, in combination with pilocarpine, is recommended by some ophthalmologists for use in attacks of angle-closure glaucoma. However, physostigmine also causes dilatation of intraocular vessels, which increases ocular congestion. It is this action which causes some ophthalmologists to disallow its usefulness as an agent for acute angle-closure attacks.

SUBJECTIVE: *Open-angle glaucoma:* Patient is usually devoid of subjective symptoms. However, open-angle glaucoma is a genetically inherited disease. A history of this disease occurring in the patient's family should lead the health care provider to more closely examine for objective findings which accompany this problem. *Angle-closure glaucoma:* History of eye pain after sitting in a darkened theater or room for several hours and which may be relieved by bright light. Intense stabbing pain in affected eye; sometimes accompanied by nausea and vomiting. Profuse perspiration, halo vision, and bradycardia may also be present with pain.

OBJECTIVE: *Open-angle glaucoma:* Funduscopic examination may reveal increased size and depth of the physiologic cup, nasal displacement of the blood vessels, or optic atrophy. Tonometry measurements of greater than 25 mm Hg occur with this illness. *Angle-closure glaucoma:* Ciliary injection, semidilated pupil which is nonreactive to light, and a cloudy anterior chamber may be present. Hyperemia of optic nerve head with edema is seen. Corneal edema may also be noted.

PLAN:

PRECAUTIONS: Physostigmine should be used with caution in individuals with corneal injury or active uveitis. Risks-benefit ratio should be carefully assessed before prescribing physostigmine to pregnant or breast feeding women. It should be used with caution in individuals who have asthma, heart block greater than first degree, or heart failure.

IMPLEMENTATION:

DRUG INTERACTIONS: Instillation of physostigmine prior to using echothiophate or isoflurophate may cause inactivation of the latter two drugs.

PRODUCTS (TRADE NAME):
Eserine Sulfate (Available in 0.25% ointment.) **Isopto Eserine** (Available in 0.5% solutions.) **Isopto P-ES** (Available in physostigmine 0.25% and pilocarpine 2% solutions.) **Miocel** (Available in physostigmine 0.125% and pilocarpine 2% solutions.)

ADMINISTRATION AND DOSAGE: Physostigmine is applied as a solution or ointment topically to the conjunctival sac. The usual dose is one drop of either 0.25% or 0.5% solution, two to three times a day. Use of ointment allows more prolonged release of physostigmine and is recommended for bedtime application.

Squeeze 1 cm strip of 0.25% physostigmine into conjunctival sac. Miosis occurs rapidly, reaching its peak within 30 minutes, and lasts for several days. Reduction of intraocular pressure lasts 4-6 hours. Combination products are used according to individual patient needs.

IMPLEMENTATION CONSIDERATIONS:

—Obtain a complete health history, including history of glaucoma, previous treatment, intraocular pressure readings, presence of asthma, cardiac failure or greater than first-degree heart block, and possibility of pregnancy or breast-feeding.

—A complete funduscopic examination should be done, including tonometry measurements, and a detailed examination should be made of the ocular damage which may have previously occurred. Information should be compared to previous findings in order to determine need for alternative therapy.

—Determine if the patient has iritis or corneal abrasion. This drug should not be used if active iritis exists, due to its ability to cause posterior synechiae (adhesions between the lens and iris.)

—Individuals with brown or hazel irises may require stronger concentrations of the drug than those with green or blue irises.

—Tolerance to physostigmine may develop with prolonged use and can be overcome by switching to another miotic for short-term therapy.

—Exposure to light and heat will cause the solution to turn red and form crystals. Drug should be discarded if this occurs. Drug should be stored in light-resistant bottle in a cool location.

—Local irritations to eye as a result of using the drug will usually decrease with continued use. Systemic responses to the drug are infrequent; however, their presence is an indication for discontinuing the medication and reevaluating the patient's status.

WHAT THE PATIENT NEEDS TO KNOW:

—Glaucoma is a chronic disease which will require lifelong treatment.

—Physostigmine should be taken only as prescribed.

—If a dose is missed, take it as soon as possible after the missed dose was due. If the next dose is due shortly, do not take the missed dose, but instead resume the regular dosage schedule.

—If irritation in the eye develops or the eye has been injured by a foreign body, do not use the drug. Instead, consult with your health care provider immediately.

—Blurred vision, headache, eye pain, and twitching of the eyelids occasionally occur and should decrease with continued use of the drug.

—Night vision or the ability to see in low light will be decreased due to pupillary constriction and inability of the pupil to dilate.

—Use the proper technique to put in eye drops. Using clean hands, pull down the lower eyelid, and put drops into conjunctival sac. Do not put medicine directly on cornea. Shut eyes and allow medicine to cover eye. At the same time, apply pressure at the lacrimal puncta for one to two minutes in order to avoid systemic absorption of the drug.

EVALUATION:

ADVERSE REACTIONS: blurring of vision, brow ache, burning or irritation after instillation of drops, excessive tearing of eyes, eye pain (due to spasm of accommodation), headache, irritation of eyes, twitching of eye lids. Long-term use may also cause follicular hypertrophy of the tarsal conjunctiva. *Systemic response:* bradycardia, diarrhea, dyspnea, excessive perspiration or salivation, gastrointestinal spasm, loss of bladder control, muscle weakness, nausea, urinary frequency, vomiting.

PARAMETERS TO MONITOR: As with other antiglaucoma drugs, regular intraocular pressure determinations should be done to assess the utility of the drug in lowering intraocular pressure. Complete funduscopic exams should be done at every visit to determine if ocular damage is progressing. The patient should be questioned about undesirable effects and compliance with the drug. Pupillary size and response to light should be used as indicators of compliance to the dosage regimen. The undesirable local effects of the drug will often decrease willingness of the patient to continue physostigmine therapy. Education about treatment and reduction of side effects with prolonged use should be done at each visit.

Geraldine Polly Bednash

PILOCARPINE

ACTION OF THE DRUG: Pilocarpine is a cholinergic agonist which produces miosis and increased accommodation. Intraocular pressure is reduced due to increased facility of outflow of aqueous humor through the trabecular meshwork. Contraction of the ciliary muscle also allows opening of the anterior angle by pulling the iris away from the trabecular meshwork. This action allows increased flow of aqueous humor in narrow-angle glaucoma, acute angle-closure glaucoma, or open-angle glaucoma.

ASSESSMENT:

INDICATIONS: This is a primary drug for the treatment of chronic open angle glaucoma and for attacks of acute angle-closure edema. It is also used to counteract effects of mydriatics such as atropine. It may be administered alternately with mydriatics to prevent adhesions of iris and lens in attacks of uveitis.

SUBJECTIVE: *Open-angle glaucoma:* Patient is usually devoid of subjective symptoms. However, open-angle glaucoma is a genetically inherited disease. A history of this disease occurring in the patient's family should lead the health care provider to more closely examine for objective findings which accompany this problem. *Angle-closure glaucoma:* History of eye pain after sitting in darkened theater or room for several hours and which may be relieved by bright light. Intense stabbing pain in affected eye; sometimes accompanied by nausea and vomiting. Profuse perspiration, halo vision, and bradycardia may also be present with pain.

OBJECTIVE: *Open-angle glaucoma:* Funduscopic examination may reveal increased size and depth of the physiologic cup, nasal displacement of the blood vessels, or optic atrophy. Tonometry measurements of greater than 25 mm Hg occur with this illness. *Angle-closure glaucoma:* Ciliary injection, semidilated pupil which is nonreactive to light, and a cloudy anterior chamber may be present. Hyperemia of optic nerve head with edema is seen. Corneal edema may also be noted.

PLAN:

CONTRAINDICATIONS: This drug should not be used for individuals with known sensitivity to any component of the drug.

PRECAUTIONS: Pilocarpine should be used with caution in individuals with asthma, iritis, chronic conjunctivitis, or keratitis. Also, it should be used with caution in individuals with a history of retinal detachment. Risks versus benefit ratio must be considered when prescribing this medication for pregnant or breast feeding women.

IMPLEMENTATION:

ADMINISTRATION AND DOSAGE: Pilocarpine is available in a variety of forms for alternative administration regimens. Pilocarpine HCl is available in solutions ranging from 0.25% to 10%. Pilocarpine nitrate is available in solutions ranging from 0.25% to 6%. Pilocarpine is also available in combination with physostigmine or epinephrine. A newer form of pilocarpine administration is Ocusert, a slow-release ocular insert system which lasts for 7 days.

When prescribing pilocarpine solutions for open-angle glaucoma, dosages will be titrated relative to patient's response and ability to comply with dosing regimen. Use of topical pilocarpine solution results in miosis within 10-30 minutes, and may last 4-8 hours. Reduction in intraocular pressure occurs within 4 hours and may last up to 14 hours. Pilocarpine topical solution is administered four times a day in dosages ranging from 1% to 4%.

The ocular timed release system, Ocusert, is available in 20 mcg and 40 mcg form and is inserted once a week. Steady state miosis and accommodative response occurs within several hours after insertion of this system and is maintained for a period of 7 days.

IMPLEMENTATION CONSIDERATIONS:

—Obtain a complete health history, including previous intraocular pressure readings, history of asthma, chronic iritis, chronic conjunctivitis, keratitis, retinal detachment, possibility of pregnancy, or breast-feeding.

—Perform complete funduscopic examination, including tonometry measurements for baseline information and to assess efficacy of therapy.

—An individual who has ocular damage and intraocular pressure recordings consistently above 30 mm Hg may be tried on a therapeutic trial of pilocarpine. If the pressure in the treated eye is lowered and undesirable effects do not occur, the patient should begin treatment with pilocarpine.

—Tolerance to pilocarpine may develop with long-term use. This may be overcome by using other miotics for a short period of time and then returning to pilocarpine.

—Compliance in use of prescribed drugs will increase as length of time between doses is increased. Compliance therefore should be greater with ocular insert systems. However, some individuals are unable to tolerate the foreign body sensation which this produces, and are unable to use this form of the medication.

—The more controlled steady state myopia produced by ocular insert systems allows use of contact lenses to correct visual distortion.

—If the ocular insert system is to be used, chronic conjunctivitis or keratitis must be ruled out.

—In acute angle-closure glaucoma attack, the abnormality leading to this is usually bilateral. Prophylactic treatment of the unaffected eye should be given to avoid attack in this eye.

WHAT THE PATIENT NEEDS TO KNOW:

—Glaucoma is a chronic disease which will need lifelong treatment.

—Drugs prescribed should be used only in doses prescribed.

—Headaches and problems with accommodation are side effects which can occur with pilocarpine but will diminish significantly with continued use.

—If tremors, nausea, shortness of breath, increased salivation, or increased perspiration occur, these should be immediately reported to your health care provider. However, adverse effects and systemic side effects with pilocarpine use are rare.

—Use the proper technique for putting in eye drops. Using clean hands, pull down the lower lid of one eye, and put the drops into the conjunctival sac. Do not put drops directly on cornea. Shut the eye and allow the medication to cover the eye. Avoid systemic absorption by applying pressure at the lacrimal puncta for one to two minutes after putting in eye drops.

—Pilocarpine may cause difficulty with night vision due to decreased dilatation which pilocarpine produces. Take extra precautions when doing activities at night and use extreme caution if driving.

—If a dose of pilocarpine is missed, apply the missed dose as soon as possible after the regularly scheduled time. If it is almost time for the next dose, do not apply the missed dose, but instead resume the regular schedule of dosages.

—Pilocarpine ophthalmic solution should be tightly sealed and stored in a cool location.

—If using the Ocusert system:

a. Your health care provider will teach you how to insert the Ocusert system.

b. You will be given the package information for home reference. Read this thoroughly and ask your health care provider about any questions you may have.

c. Ocusert system can produce a sudden burst of pilocarpine when first introduced into the eye. Ocusert should be put in before bedtime to diminish the response to this sudden release of drug.

d. If the Ocusert appears damaged, do not use it.

e. Ocusert should be stored in the refrigerator.

f. The foreign body sensation which occurs with these systems should diminish greatly over the first week and may be unnoticeable after this period of time.

g. Ocusert may be used with hard contact lenses only.

EVALUATION:

ADVERSE REACTIONS: blurred vision, eye pain (due to spasm of accommodation), headache, irritation of the conjunctiva, twitching of the eyelids. *Systemic Response* (rare): diarrhea, increased salivation, nausea, tremors, unusual perspiration, vomiting, wheezing.

PARAMETERS TO MONITOR: Regular complete ophthalmic examinations and intraocular pressure measurements should be done to assess efficacy of the therapeutic regimen. This should include size of disc and physiologic cupping. Visual field changes should be measured to determine if ocular damage has progressed. Therapy for open-angle glaucoma should begin with 1%-2% pilocarpine. If titration to 4% does not control intraocular pressure, the addition of epinephrine should be considered. Open-angle glaucoma is a symptom-free disease until extensive damage has occurred. Frequent education and monitoring of the therapeutic response are necessary to determine if disease-related ocular damage is progressing.

PILOCARPINE HYDROCHLORIDE

PRODUCTS (TRADE NAME):

Adsorbocarpine (Available in 1%, 2% and 4% solution.) **Akarpine** (Available in 1%, 2% and 4% solutions.) **Almocarpine** (Available in 1%, 2% and 4% solutions.) **Isopto Carpine** (Available in 0.25%, 0.5%, 1%, 1.5%, 2%, 3%, 4%, 5%, 6%, 8% and 10% solutions.) **Pilocar** (Available in 0.5%, 1%, 2%, 3%, 4%, and 6% solutions.) **Pilocel** (Available in 0.25% , 1%, 1.5%, 2%, 3%, 4%, 5%, and 6% solutions.) **Pilomiotin** (Available in 1%, 2% and 4% solutions.) *Combinations:* **E-Carpine, E-Pilo, PE** (Available in 1%, 2%, 3%, 4%,6% pilocarpine and 1% epinephrine bitartrate solutions.) **Isopto-P-ES** (Available in 2% pilocarpine and 0.25% physostigmine solutions.) **Miocel** (Available in 2% pilocarpine with 0.125% physostigmine solution.)

DRUG SPECIFICS:

Administration of drugs containing a combination of products should be based upon individual needs of patient.

ADMINISTRATION AND DOSAGE SPECIFICS:

Acute-angle closure: One drop of 1% or 2% solution every five to ten minutes for three to six doses until pressure is reduced. Then one drop every hour until stabilization has occurred. Chronic miosis is then maintained with doses four times a day until surgery. Prophylaxis in unaffected eye is desirable. This is done with one drop of 1 or 2% solution four times a day until surgery.

PILOCARPINE NITRATE

PRODUCTS (TRADE NAME):
  P.V. Carpine Liquifilm (Available in 0.5%, 1%, 2%, 3%, 4%, and 6% solutions.)
DRUG SPECIFICS:
  If patients do not tolerate Pilocarpine HCl, they may be tried on this product, which is similar in most respects.
ADMINISTRATION AND DOSAGE SPECIFICS:
  Concentration and frequency will vary relative to patient response to drug. Usual frequency is four times a day of 1% to 4% solution.

PILOCARPINE OCULAR RELEASE SYSTEM

PRODUCTS (TRADE NAME):
  Ocusert Pilo 20, Ocusert Pilo 40 (Available in 20 mcg and 40 mcg systems.)
DRUG SPECIFICS:
  See general statement for patient instructions regarding this product.
ADMINISTRATION AND DOSAGE SPECIFICS:
  Use one ocular insert at bedtime every 7 days. Insert into the conjunctival sac. It delivers 20 or 40 mcg every hour.

Geraldine Polly Bednash

BETA-BLOCKERS—ANTIGLAUCOMA AGENTS

TIMOLOL MALEATE

ACTION OF THE DRUG: Timolol is a nonselective beta-adrenergic blocking agent which has been shown to significantly lower intraocular pressure. The exact mechanism for this result is unclear. Pupillary size or response is not affected by timolol. Aqueous humor production is thought to be decreased by this preparation, resulting in a drop in intraocular pressure. Tolerance to the drug has not been shown to occur in individuals who have used it for as long as three years.

ASSESSMENT:

INDICATIONS: Timolol is an effective agent for the lowering of intraocular pressure in open-angle glaucoma. It has been shown to be equal to pilocarpine in its ability to reduce intraocular pressure. Few visual disturbances are experienced by the patient using this drug due to its lack of pupillary effects. This factor also makes timolol a particularly good choice for the patient with lenticular opacities in whom miosis would further constrict the visual field. The addition of timolol to a multi-drug therapeutic regimen has been shown to reduce intraocular pressure in individuals whose glaucoma has been resistant to treatment.

SUBJECTIVE: Open angle glaucoma is usually devoid of subjective symptoms. However, open-angle glaucoma is a genetically inherited disease, so a history of this disease occurring in the patient's family should lead the health care provider to examine more closely for the objective findings which accompany this disease.

OBJECTIVE: Funduscopic examination may reveal increased size and depth of the physiologic cup, nasal displacement of the blood vessels, or optic atrophy. Tonometry measurements of greater than 25 mm Hg occur with this problem.

PLAN:

CONTRAINDICATIONS: Timolol is contraindicated for use in individuals who have shown sensitivity to any component of the product. Timolol has not been approved for use in children.

PRECAUTIONS: This drug should be used with caution in individuals with asthma, cardiac failure, chronic lung disease, myasthenia gravis, or greater than first degree heart block. Systemic absorption of the drug has been shown to occur. Timolol ophthalmic solution should also be used cautiously in individuals who are receiving other adrenergic blocking agents to assess the likelihood of additive effects. Use of timolol in pregnant or breast-feeding women should be weighed against possible risks since systemic absorption is likely to occur.

IMPLEMENTATION:

PRODUCTS (TRADE NAME):
Timoptic (Available in 0.25% and 0.5% solution.)
ADMINISTRATION AND DOSAGE:
For glaucoma patients wearing contacts, timoptic has been approved for use with hard (PMMA) contact lenses. Apply one drop to conjunctival sac one to two times a day. Onset of action occurs within 1/2 hour and lasts 24 hours, with peak action within two hours.
IMPLEMENTATION CONSIDERATIONS:
—Obtain a complete health history, including history of glaucoma in family, patient's previous intraocular pressure levels, adverse reactions to timolol or other adrenergic blocking agents, history of asthma or other respiratory diseases, cardiac failure, heart block, myasthenia gravis, diabetes, or other drugs taken concurrently which may cause drug interactions, and possibility of pregnancy.
—Perform a complete funduscopic examination, including tonometry measurements, with appropriate recording of findings for use as baseline data or measurement of the medication's effectiveness.

WHAT THE PATIENT NEEDS TO KNOW:
—Glaucoma is a chronic disease and will require lifelong treatment.

—Use proper technique in instilling eye drops. With clean hands pull down the lower eyelid and drop the medication into the conjunctival sac. Do not put medicine directly onto cornea. Shut the eye and let the medicine cover the eye. Apply pressure at the lacrimal puncta for one to two minutes after putting in drops to avoid systemic absorption.

—Drug should be used only as prescribed. Do not use more or less than ordered.

—If a daily dose is missed, take it as soon as possible after realizing the dose was not taken. Do not administer a double dose if an entire day has passed. If the medicine is prescribed to be taken twice a day, take the missed dose as close to the regular time as possible but do not take the missed dose if the next dose time is very close.

—Inform health care provider if you become pregnant or decide to breast-feed.

—Report any signs of systemic response such as mental confusion, lethargy, slow pulse, respiratory distress, or shortness of breath.

EVALUATION:

ADVERSE REACTIONS: *Local:* irritation of conjunctiva. *Systemic* response: mental confusion, depression, dyspnea, shortness of breath, bradycardia, wheezing, lethargy, hypotension. Anorexia and nausea have occurred rarely.

PARAMETERS TO MONITOR: Regular tonometry measurements or intraocular pressure readings should be done to determine effectiveness of timolol. Response may take up to 4 weeks. Reevaluation four weeks after beginning timolol therapy will identify the need to maintain or increase the dosage. Titration of dosage to higher concentrations or increased frequency of administration should be done based upon the patient's response to the drug and ability to comply with more frequent administration. Indices of systemic response which should be evaluated are blood pressure, heart rate, and respiratory status. If the patient shows signs of developing bradycardia, hypotension, or compromised respiratory status, the therapeutic regimen should be reassessed for possible alternative agents.

Geraldine Polly Bednash

SYMPATHOMIMETIC OPHTHALMIC DRUGS
ANTIGLAUCOMA AGENTS

EPINEPHRINE

ACTION OF THE DRUG: Alpha-adrenergic agonist action of epinephrine produces vasoconstriction and decreases intraocular pressure in open-angle glaucoma.

The mechanism by which this occurs is not known, but it is thought to be due to a decrease in aqueous humor production secondary to the vasoconstriction and an increase in outflow of aqueous humor through the trabecular meshwork. Epinephrine causes mild mydriasis through stimulation of the dilator muscle of the iris.

ASSESSMENT:

INDICATIONS: Epinephrine is used in the treatment of open-angle glaucoma, usually in combination with cholinergic agents.

SUBJECTIVE: Open-angle glaucoma is usually devoid of subjective symptoms. However, open-angle glaucoma is a genetically inherited disease so a history of this disease occurring in the patient's family should lead the health care provider to look more closely for the objective findings which accompany this disease.

OBJECTIVE: Examination of the fundus may reveal increased size and depth of the physiologic cup, nasal displacement of the blood vessels, or optic atrophy. Tonometry measurements of greater than 25 mm Hg occur with this problem.

PLAN:

CONTRAINDICATIONS: Epinephrine should not be administered in the presence of angle-closure glaucoma or if a narrow anterior chamber angle exists.

PRECAUTIONS: Epinephrine should be administered with caution to individuals with cardiac or cerebral arteriosclerosis, diabetes mellitus, hypertension, hyperthyroidism, or aphakia. Ophthalmic use of epinephrine does not rule out the possibility of a systemic response.

IMPLEMENTATION:

DRUG INTERACTIONS: Use of epinephrine with halogenated anesthetics may lead to ventricular fibrillation. Use of tricyclic antidepressants in conjunction with epinephrine may increase the likelihood of cardiovascular effects. Should be used with caution in patients receiving digitalis preparations which increase myocardial response to epinephrine.

ADMINISTRATION AND DOSAGE: Available in preparations of 0.25% to 2%. A solution of 1% or greater is necessary to cause pupillary dilatation. The usual dosage is two drops of 0.5-2% solution two times a day. Titration of dosage is necessary to determine the frequency and strength of solutions which are therapeutic for the individual. Decrease in aqueous humor pressure occurs within one hour and generally lasts 4-8 hours, but may last aslong as 24 hours. Vasoconstriction occurs rapidly, usually within a few minutes and ends within 1 hour. Epinephrine is available as epinephrine hydrochloride, epinephrine bitartrate, and epinephrine borate ophthalmic solutions. It is also available in combination with cholinergic drugs such as pilocarpine.

IMPLEMENTATION CONSIDERATIONS:

—Obtain a complete health history, including family history of glaucoma, previous history of cerebral or cardiac arteriosclerosis, hypertension, hyperthyroidism, diabetes mellitus, or aphakia; and other medications taken concurrently which may produce drug interactions.

—Perform complete fundoscopic examination with appropriate recording of findings for use as baseline data or as measurement of the medications' effectiveness.

—Perform regular tests of intraocular pressure to determine if the dose prescribed is adequate. Aqueous humor outflow may not be increased for two to three months, however, and treatment with epinephrine should be continued for at least this period of time before concluding that the drug is not useful for a particular patient.

—Should be administered to individuals with aphakia (absence of a crystalline lens) with caution. The incidence of macular edema in aphakic individuals treated with epinephrine has been reported to be as high as 30%.

WHAT THE PATIENT NEEDS TO KNOW:
—Glaucoma is a chronic disease which will require lifelong treatment.

—Topical instillation of epinephrine may cause stinging or burning of eyes, but this should decrease with continued use.

—To apply eye drops, pull down the lower eyelid and instill drops into the conjunctival sac below the eye. Do not put drops directly on cornea. Shut eye briefly and let medication cover eye. Apply pressure at the lacrimal puncta for one or two minutes after putting in medication to avoid systemic (throughout the body) absorption of the drug. Your health provider will demonstrate how this should be done.

—Epinephrine is an unstable solution and should be stored in a light-resistant container which should be kept tightly sealed kept and in a cool location.

—If solution turns brown, pinkish, or forms precipitates (particles on the bottom), it should be discarded.

—If a dose of medicine is missed, it should be taken as soon after the regularly scheduled time as possible. If the missed dose is remembered close to the time for the next dose, do not take the missed dose.

—If you experience rapid heartbeat, shakiness, paleness, faint feeling or unusual perspiration after taking epinephrine, the medicine should be stopped and the health care provider notified promptly.

—Patients often experience side effects to drugs. If you note anything new or uncomfortable, do not hesitate to notify your health care provider. Patients often experience headache, browache, eye pain, blurred vision, or irritation of the eyes, but this should decrease with continued use.

EVALUATION:

ADVERSE REACTIONS: Headache, brow ache, irritation or excessive tearing of eyes. Signs of systemic response to opthalmic epinephrine are palpitations, increased perspiration, tremors, paleness, lightheadedness, or feeling of faintness.

PARAMETERS TO MONITOR: Intraocular pressure determinations should be done both prior to initiating therapy and monthly while titrating dosages for the individual patient. If eye pain and blurred vision do not decrease with continued use, the patient should be assessed for possible macular edema. After stabilization of intraocular pressure, the patient should be seen on a regular basis for evaluation of the drug's efficacy. Routine follow-up examinations should include complete funduscopic exam to determine if damage due to disease progression has occurred. Subjective complaints indicating systemic response to the drug should be assessed to determine if patient's technique for instillation of drug is appropriate.

EPINEPHRINE BITARTRATE OPHTHALMIC SOLUTION

PRODUCTS (TRADE NAME):

E-Carpine, E-Pilo (Available in solutions of 1% epinephrine bitartrate and 1%, 2%, 3%, 4% or 6% pilocarpine.) **Epitrate** (Available in 1% solution as1.82% bitartrate.) **Murocoll** (Available in 1% solution with 1.82% bitartrate or in 2% solution with 3.64% bitartrate.) **Mytrate** (Available in 0.5% solution with 1% bitartrate or 1% solution with 2% bitartrate.)

DRUG SPECIFICS:

E-Carpine and E-Pilo are combination products which include pilocarpine and epinephrine bitartrate. The epinephrine concentration is held constant while the pilocarpine varies. When used, together they have additive effects in lowering intraocular pressure while decreasing the pupillary dilatation or constriction. Fixed combinations do not allow flexibility in dosage adjustment.

ADMINISTRATION AND DOSAGE SPECIFICS:

Antiglaucoma agent: Use one drop of 0.5% to 2% solution twice a day as required for individual patient.

EPINEPHRINE BORATE OPHTHALMIC SOLUTION

PRODUCTS (TRADE NAME):

Epinal (Available in 0.25%, 0.5% and 1% solutions.) **Eppy/N** (Available in 0.5% and 1% solutions.)

DRUG SPECIFICS:

Epinephrine borate causes less stinging than epinephrine hydrochloride but is less stable and oxidizes rapidly.

ADMINISTRATION AND DOSAGE SPECIFICS:

Antiglaucoma agent: Use one drop of 0.5% to 1% solution topically on conjunctiva twice a day.

EPINEPHRINE HYDROCHLORIDE OPHTHALMIC SOLUTION

PRODUCTS (TRADE NAME):
Epifrin (Available in 0.25%, 0.5%, 1% and 2% solutions.) **Glaucon** (Available in 0.5%, 1% and 2% solutions.)
DRUG SPECIFICS:
Choice of epinephrine solution may depend upon patient's reaction. If patient is irritated by one epinephrine product, switch to another.
ADMINISTRATION AND DOSAGE SPECIFICS:
Antiglaucoma agent: Use topically: one drop in conjunctival sac twice daily. Concentration varies with individual needs.
Vasoconstrictor: Use 0.1% applied two to three times until desired mydriasis is achieved, or for control of bleeding during ocular surgery.

DIPIVEFRIN HYDROCHLORIDE

PRODUCTS (TRADE NAME):
Propine (Available in 0.1% solution.)
DRUG SPECIFICS:
Dipivefrin hydrochloride is a member of a new class of drugs called prodrugs. Prodrugs are precursors of drugs which are biochemically transformed to an active form after administration. Dipivefrin is biotransformed to epinephrine after instillation in the conjunctival sac. As such it is not really an epinephrine product but is placed in this category because once it is transformed into epinephrine, all actions are the same. Onset of action occurs in 30 minutes and peaks within one hour.

Considerations for using dipivefrin are similar to those for epinephrine ophthalmic use. If dipivefrin is used to replace epinephrine ophthalmic solution, the epinephrine should be discontinued when dipivefrin therapy is begun. If dipivefrin is used to replace an agent other than epinephrine, the other drug should not be discontinued until dipivefrin has been used for one day. Dipivefrin has not been approved for pediatric use.
ADMINISTRATION AND DOSAGE SPECIFICS:
Antiglaucoma agent: Use one drop of 0.1% solution every twelve hours.

Geraldine Polly Bednash

MYDRIATICS

PHENYLEPHRINE HCL AND HYDROXYAMPHETAMINE HBR

ACTION OF THE DRUG: These mydriatic drugs are alpha-adrenergic agonists which cause contraction of the dilator muscles of the pupil, leading to mydriasis and vasoconstriction of the arterioles of the conjunctiva.

ASSESSMENT:

INDICATIONS: Phenylephrine and hydroxamphetamine are used primarily as mydriatics, allowing complete visualization of the ocular fundus. They may be used as an antiglaucoma agent although they are not the preferred agent for this disease due to their increased incidence of systemic effects with the 10% solution necessary to control open-angle glaucoma. Phenylephrine is used after ocular surgery for mydriatic response. Solutions of 0.15% or less are useful for conjunctival hyperemia secondary to dust, smoke, or chemical fumes.

SUBJECTIVE: Open-angle glaucoma is usually devoid of subjective symptoms. However, open-angle glaucoma is a genetically inherited disease so a history of this disease occurring in the patient's family should lead the health care provider to more closely examine for the objective findings which accompany this disease. The health care provider should also ask about complaints of redness, itching, or irritation due to allergy, smoke, or dust fumes.

OBJECTIVE: Inability to do a funduscopic exam due to extreme miotic response to examination light. Presence of open angle of anterior chamber. Conjunctival injection and tearing without signs of infectious process.

PLAN:

CONTRAINDICATIONS: This drug should not be administered in the presence of narrow anterior chamber angle or in the event of an acute angle-closure attack. Also it should not be administered within 21 days of taking a monoamine oxidase inhibitor.

PRECAUTIONS: These products should be administered with caution to individuals with cardiac or cerebral arteriosclerosis, diabetes mellitus, hypertension, hyperthyroidism, or aphakia.

IMPLEMENTATION:

DRUG INTERACTIONS: Use of these solutions in individuals who are using sympathetic denervation agents can lead to severe vascular hypertensive response to mydriatic drugs. Use with tricyclic antidepressants may also potentiate the hypertensive effects of phenylephrine.

ADMINISTRATION AND DOSAGE: Mydriasis usually occurs within one hour and is easily neutralized with cholinergic agents. The mydriatic effect will recede within 6 hours of administration.

IMPLEMENTATION CONSIDERATIONS:

—Obtain a complete health history, including family history of glaucoma, presence of cerebral or cardiac arteriosclerosis, hypertension, hyperthyroidism, diabetes mellitus or aphakia, as well as other drugs taken concurrently which may produce drug interactions.

—Perform complete funduscopic examination with appropriate recording of findings for use as baseline data.

—Should be administered with caution to patient with aphakia (absence of a crystalline lens) since macular edema may occur.

—This drug is not often used in treatment of open-angle glaucoma so the need to be concerned about chronic use-induced maculopathy is decreased.

WHAT THE PATIENT NEEDS TO KNOW:

—Topical instillation of phenylephrine may cause stinging or burning of eyes, but this should decrease with continued use.

—Use proper technique in instilling eye drops. Pull the lower lid of the eye down and drop the medicine into the conjunctival sac. Do not put medicine directly on the cornea. Shut eyes and allow medicine to cover eye. Apply pressure at the lacrimal puncta for one to two minutes after instilling medication to avoid systemic absorption.

—This medicine is an unstable solution and should be stored in a lightresistant container which should be kept tightly sealed and kept in a cool location.

—If solution turns brown, pinkish, or forms precipitates (particles on the bottom), it should be discarded.

—If a dose of medicine is missed, it should be taken soon after the regularly scheduled time as possible. If the missed dose is remembered close to the time for the next dose, do not take the missed dose.

—If you experience rapid heart beat, shakiness, paleness, a faint feeling, or unusual perspiration after taking this medicine, the medicine should be stopped and the health care provider should be notified.

—You may experience slight headache, brow ache, eye pain, blurred vision, or irritation of the eyes, but this should decrease with continued use.

—Avoid concurrent use of phenylephrine and any of the following: guanethidine, tricyclic antidepressants, or monoamine oxidase (MAO) inhibitors. Many over-the-counter preparations contain phenylephrine so labels should be carefully read when taking any drugs.

—Use dark glasses if light sensitivity occurs after taking this drug.

—Phenylephrine should only be used in prescribed doses to avoid the likelihood of unfavorable responses.

EVALUATION:

ADVERSE REACTIONS: Brow ache, headache, increased sensitivity to light, watering of eyes. Signs of systemic response are dizziness, tremors, unusual perspiration, paleness, and palpitations. The incidence of systemic response increases with increased strength of the solution used. Systemic reactions are rare with 2.5% solutions and infrequent with 10% solutions.

PARAMETERS TO MONITOR: Monitor for therapeutic effects and side effects. Subjective complaints of irritation should decrease with use of this drug. If drug is prescribed for chronic mydriatic response, pupil size should be assessed to determine if chronic use has resulted in an undesired rebound miosis. Signs of systemic response should be ruled out, and patient should be questioned regarding the occurrence of these symptoms. Blood pressure determinations should be done at each visit to ensure that the patient is not having hypertensive response. Patient should be questioned frequently about other medications to rule out undesired interactions.

PHENYLEPHRINE HCL

PRODUCTS (TRADE NAME):

Ak-Dilate (Available in 2.5% solutions.) **Efricel** (Available in 2.5% and 10% solutions.) **Mydfrin** (Available in 2.5% solutions.) **Neo-Synephrine** (Available in 2.5% and 10% solutions.) **Phenoptic** (Available in 2.5% and 10% solutions.) **Phenylephrine HCl Ophth** (Available in 10% solutions.)

Combination solutions: **Ak-Cide, Blephamide, Sulphrine, Vasocidin Solution and Vasocidin ointment** (Available in steroid, antibiotic, and 0.12% phenylephrine combinations for nonpurulent keratitis or conjunctivitis.) **Cyclomydril** (Available in cyclopentolate and 0.2% phenylephrine solution for mydriasis.) **Murocoll #2** (Available in scopolamine and 10% phenylephrine solutions for cycloplegia and mydriasis.) **Prefrin-A** (Available in pyrilamine maleate and 0.12% phenylephrine for allergic conjunctivitis.) **Prefrin-Z Liquifilm** (Available in zinc sulfate and 0.12% phenylephrine solution for artificial tears and eye whitening.) **Vasocon A** (Available in 0.05% naphazoline HCl and 0.5% antazoline phosphate solution.) **Vasosulf** (Available in sodium sulfacetamide and 0.125% phenylephrine solutions for conjunctivitis.) **Vernacel** (Available in pheniramine maleate and 0.125% phenylephrine solutions for allergic conjunctivitis.)

Nonprescription drugs containing phenylephrine: **Eye Cool, Isopto Frin, Neozin, Optised, Phenylzin, Prefrin Liquifilm, Tear-Efrin, Zincfrin** (Available in 0.12% solution.)

DRUG SPECIFICS:

Consult individual ingredients for drug contraindications and usage.

ADMINISTRATION AND DOSAGE SPECIFICS:

Mydriasis: One drop of 2.5% to 10% solution topically on conjunctiva. Repeat in 5 minutes if effect is inadequate.

Chronic mydriasis: One drop of 2.5% or 10% solution topically on conjunctiva two to three times a day.

Vasoconstriction: One drop of 0.02% to 0.15% solutions topically to conjunctiva three to four times a day as needed.

Conjunctivitis: One or two drops every hour until condition improves and then one drop three to four times a day. For ointment, use one strip in conjunctival sac four times a day. In allergic conditions, use one to two drops every three to four hours prn.

Artificial tears: Use one to two drops every 3-4 hours prn.

HYDROXYAMPHETAMINE HYDROBROMIDE

PRODUCTS (TRADE NAME):
   Paradrine (Available in 1% ophthalmic solutions.)
DRUG SPECIFICS:
   This product causes pupillary dilatation when instilled into the conjunctival sac. It is similar to phenylephrine in action although dilatation capabilities are less. Its main use is as an aid to complete fundoscopic exam. Nursing actions and implications are similar to those for phenylephrine.
ADMINISTRATION AND DOSAGE SPECIFICS:
   Instill one or two drops into conjunctival sac.

Geraldine Polly Bednash

VASOCONSTRICTORS
NAPHAZOLINE HYDROCHLORIDE

ACTION OF THE DRUG: This product causes direct stimulation of alpha receptors of vascular smooth muscle, leading to vasoconstriction. The action lasts for several hours.

ASSESSMENT:

INDICATIONS: Although this drug is similar to other sympathomimetics in its action, its primary vasoconstrictive properties have led to the use of this drug to decrease conjunctival injection due to irritation from smoke, fumes, hard contact lenses, and allergens.

SUBJECTIVE/OBJECTIVE: Rule out the possibility of an infectious process as the causative agent in the patient's complaints of reddened, watery eyes.

PLAN:

PRECAUTIONS: This drug should be avoided by individuals using MAO inhibitors. The presence of angle-closure glaucoma or a narrow anterior chamber angle precludes the use of this drug. Naphazoline may cause adverse reactions in individuals with cerebral or cardiac arteriosclerosis, hypertension, or diabetes mellitus. This drug is a component of many over-the-counter ophthalmic preparations used to whiten eyes, so patients in any of the above situations should be cautioned to carefully read labels for contents and precautions.

IMPLEMENTATION:

DRUG INTERACTIONS: Use of these solutions in individuals who are using sympathetic denervation agents can lead to severe vascular hypertensive response to mydriatic drugs. Use with tricyclic antidepressants may also potentiate the hypertensive effects of this drug.

PRODUCTS (TRADE NAME):

Ak-Con (Available in 0.1% solutions.) **Albalon Liquifilm** (Available in 0.1% solutions.) **Allerest, Clear Eyes, Degest 2, Naphcon** (Available in O.01% solutions.) **Naphcon Forte** (Available in 0.1% solutions.) **Vaso Clear** (Available in 0.02% solutions.) **Vasocon Regular.** (Available in 0.1% solutions.)

Combination naphazoline HCl and antihistamine: **Albalon-A** (Available in 0.1% naphazoline solutions.) **Naphcon-A** (Available in 0.025% nephazoline solutions.) **Vasocon-A** (Available in 0.05% naphazoline solutions.)

ADMINISTRATION AND DOSAGE: Mydriasis usually occurs within one hour and is easily neutralized with cholinergic agents. The mydriatic effect will recede within 6 hours of administration. The products listed all require prescription. The combination drugs with antihistamine have been classified as "possibly effective" by the National Academy of Sciences National Research Council. This classification requires further investigation of the drugs usefulness.

Use one or two drops two to three times a day as needed to relieve irritation or redness.

IMPLEMENTATION CONSIDERATIONS:

—Obtain a complete health history, including family history of glaucoma, presence of cerebral or cardiac arteriosclerosis, hypertension, hyperthyroidism, diabetes mellitus or aphakia, as well as other drugs taken concurrently which may produce drug interactions.

—Perform complete funduscopic examination with appropriate recording of findings for use as baseline data.

—Should be administered with caution to patient with aphakia (absence of a crystalline lens) since macular edema may occur.

—This drug is not often used in treatment of open-angle glaucoma so the need to be concerned about chronic use-induced maculopathy is decreased.

WHAT THE PATIENT NEEDS TO KNOW:

—Topical instillation of medication may cause stinging or burning of eyes, but this should decrease with continued use.

—Use proper technique in instilling eye drops. Pull the lower lid of the eye down and drop the medicine into the conjunctival sac. Do not put medicine directly on the cornea. Shut eyes and allow medicine to cover eye. Apply pressure at the lacrimal puncta for one to two minutes after instilling medication to avoid systemic absorption.

—This medicine is an unstable solution and should be stored in a light-resistant container which should be kept tightly sealed and kept in a cool location.

—If solution turns brown, pinkish, or forms precipitates (particles on the bottom), it should be discarded.

—If a dose of medicine is missed, it should be taken soon after the regularly scheduled time as possible. If the missed dose is remembered close to the time for the next dose, do not take the missed dose.

—If you experience rapid heart beat, shakiness, paleness, a faint feeling, or unusual perspiration after taking this medicine, the medicine should be stopped and the health care provider should be notified.

—You may experience slight headache, browache, eye pain, blurred vision, or irritation of the eyes, but this should decrease with continued use.

—Avoid concurrent use of this medication and any of the following: guanethidine, tricyclic antidepressants, or monoamine oxidase (MAO) inhibitors. Many over-the-counter preparations contain similar chemicals so labels should be carefully read when taking any drugs.

—Use dark glasses if light sensitivity occurs after taking this drug.

—This medicine should only be used in prescribed doses to avoid the likelihood of unfavorable responses.

EVALUATION:

ADVERSE REACTIONS: Brow ache, headache, increased sensitivity to light, watering of eyes. Signs of systemic response are dizziness, tremors, unusual perspiration, paleness, and palpitations. The incidence of systemic response increases with increased strength of the solution used. Systemic reactions are rare with 2.5% solutions and infrequent with 10% solutions.

PARAMETERS TO MONITOR: Monitor for therapeutic effects and side effects. Subjective complaints of irritation should decrease with use of this drug. If drug is prescribed for chronic mydriatic response, pupil size should be assessed to determine if chronic use has resulted in an undesired rebound miosis. Signs of systemic response should be ruled out, and patient should be questioned regarding the occurrence of these symptoms. Blood pressure determinations should be done at each visit to assure that the patient is not having hypertensive response. Patient should be questioned frequently about other medications to rule out undesired interactions.

Geraldine Polly Bednash

TETRAHYDROZOLINE HYDROCHLORIDE

ACTION OF THE DRUG: Tetrahydrozoline is a member of the imidazoline class of sympathomimetics which includes naphazoline hydrochloride. This drug's major action is to cause vasoconstriction of the conjunctival arterial smooth muscle. Tetrahydrozoline is the major ingredient in many nonprescription ophthalmic solutions which are available to relieve conjunctival edema or hyperemia secondary to allergens or irritants.

ASSESSMENT:

INDICATIONS: Although this drug is similar to other sympathomimetics in its action, its primary vasoconstrictive properties have led to the use of this drug to decrease conjunctival injection due to irritation from smoke, fumes, hard contact lenses, and allergens.

SUBJECTIVE: Look for history of allergic reactions or exposure to eye irritants.

OBJECTIVE: Conjunctival edema or hyperemia.

PLAN:

PRECAUTIONS: As with other sympathomimetics, precautions concerning its use in narrow-angle glaucoma, hypertension, hyperthyroidism, and cerebral or cardiac arteriosclerosis should be discussed with the patient. Patients should be cautioned to thoroughly read labels if any of the above conditions exist.

These are all over-the-counter preparations and are less expensive than prescription items.

IMPLEMENTATION:

DRUG INTERACTIONS: Use of these solutions in individuals who are using sympathetic denervation agents can lead to severe vascular hypertensive response to mydriatic drugs. Use with tricyclic antidepressants may also potentiate the hypertensive effects of this drug.

PRODUCTS (TRADE NAME):
Clear and Brite, Murine Plus, Opt-Ease, Tetracon, Tetrasine, Visine Eye Drops.

ADMINISTRATION AND DOSAGE: Mydriasis usually occurs within one hour and is easily neutralized with cholinergic agents. The mydriatic effect will recede within 6 hours of administration. The products listed all require prescription. The combination drugs with antihistamine have been classified as "possibly effective" by the National Academy of Sciences National Research Council. This classification requires further investigation of the drugs' usefulness.

Use one or two drops in each eye two to three times daily as needed.

IMPLEMENTATION CONSIDERATIONS:
—Obtain a complete health history, including family history of glaucoma, pres-

ence of cerebral or cardiac arteriosclerosis, hypertension, hyperthyroidism, diabetes mellitus or aphakia, as well as other drugs taken concurrently which may produce drug interactions.

—Perform complete funduscopic examination with appropriate recording of findings for use as baseline data.

—Should be administered with caution to patient with aphakia (absence of a crystalline lens) since macular edema may occur.

—This drug is not often used in treatment of open-angle glaucoma so the need to be concerned about chronic use-induced maculopathy is decreased.

WHAT THE PATIENT NEEDS TO KNOW:

—Topical instillation of medication may cause stinging or burning of eyes, but this should decrease with continued use.

—Use proper technique in instilling eye drops. Pull the lower lid of the eye down and drop the medicine into the conjunctival sac. Do not put medicine directly on the cornea. Shut eyes and allow medicine to cover eye. Apply pressure at the lacrimal puncta for one to two minutes after instilling medication to avoid systemic absorption.

—This medicine is an unstable solution and should be stored in a light-resistant container which should be kept tightly sealed and kept in a cool location.

—If solution turns brown, pinkish, or forms precipitates (particles on the bottom), it should be discarded.

—If a dose of medicine is missed, it should be taken soon after the regularly scheduled time as possible. If the missed dose is remembered close to the time for the next dose, do not take the missed dose.

—If you experience rapid heart beat, shakiness, paleness, a faint feeling, or unusual perspiration after taking this medicine, the medicine should be stopped and the health care provider should be notified.

—You may experience slight headache, browache, eye pain, blurred vision, or irritation of the eyes, but this should decrease with continued use.

—Avoid concurrent use of this medication and any of the following: guanethidine, tricyclic antidepressants, or monoamine oxidase (MAO) inhibitors. Many over-the-counter preparations contain similar chemicals so labels should be carefully read when taking any drugs.

—Use dark glasses if light sensitivity occurs after taking this drug.

—This medicine should only be used in prescribed doses to avoid the likelihood of unfavorable responses.

EVALUATION:

ADVERSE REACTIONS: Brow ache, headache, increased sensitivity to light, watering of eyes. Signs of systemic response are dizziness, tremors, unusual perspiration, paleness, and palpitations. The incidence of systemic response increases with increased strength of the solution used. Systemic reactions are rare with 2.5% solutions and infrequent with 10% solutions.

PARAMETERS TO MONITOR: Monitor for therapeutic effects and side effects. Subjective complaints of irritation should decrease with use of this drug. If drug is prescribed for chronic mydriatic response, pupil size should be assessed to determine if chronic use has resulted in an undesired rebound miosis. Signs of systemic response should be ruled out, and patient should be questioned regarding the occurrence of these symptoms. Blood pressure determinations should be done at each visit to assure that the patient is not having hypertensive response. Patient should be questioned frequently about other medications to rule out undesired interactions.

Geraldine Polly Bednash

OTIC PREPARATIONS

ACTION OF THE DRUG: Topical antibiotics are used to control superficial infections of the ear through bactericidal or bacteriostatic mechanisms. Other products may be used in prophylaxis of infections for swimmers, and for removing ceruminous accumulations. See sections on anti-infectives and steroids for additional information about ear products.

ASSESSMENT:

INDICATIONS: Antibiotics are used primarily for treatment of otitis externa and otitis media as either the sole therapy or as adjunctive systemic therapy. Some products are also used in the treatment of superficial canal infections, including swimmer's ear. In patients with history of ceruminous occlusion, some products may be used to increase the effects of irrigation.

SUBJECTIVE: Parents may observe infants pulling at their ear, along with a picture of crying and general irritability. Older patients may complain of earache, and may have accompanying signs of fever, headache, neck muscle stiffness, and nasal congestion. There may be a history of prolonged exposure to water by swimmers. Some patients may complain of a gradual loss of hearing without other symptoms.

OBJECTIVE: There may be loss of hearing, tenderness on movement of the pinnea, erythema of the external ear canal, discharge, bulging or retracted tympanic membrane with evidence of fluid or air bubbles in the middle ear. Lymphadenopathy may also be present. There may also be evidence of infection in nasal and oral passages. In patients without infection, the external canal may be completely occluded by cerumen, dust, and sometimes foreign particles.

PLAN:

CONTRAINDICATIONS: Do not give in the presence of hypersensitivity to the drug. Consult individual products for specific contraindications.

PRECAUTIONS: If discharge is present, culture should be taken. If infection does not respond within several days, reconsider drug being used.

IMPLEMENTATION:

DRUG INTERACTIONS: Consult individual products for specific interactions.

ADMINISTRATION AND DOSAGE: Antibiotics should be administered to the patient by a second individual. Patient should lie down on a pillow, with the affected ear up. The medication should be dropped into the ear canal, taking care not to touch the dropper to the ear. The patient should remain lying down for at least 5 minutes following administration of the drops. A cotton ball may be inserted into the outside if ear seems unusually sensitive to cold.

Some infections seem to respond well to cotton pulled into a wisp and soaked well in the antibiotic and inserted into the ear canal as a wick. This can be left in place for several hours.

If the ear is occluded with cerumen, manual cleaning with cotton-tipped applicators or other instruments is to be avoided. (This often just pushes wax back against the tympanic membrane). Cerumenex should be used to loosen secretions, which then can be washed out by normal saline irrigation.

IMPLEMENTATION CONSIDERATIONS:

—Obtain a complete health history, including the presence of hypersensitivity, underlying systemic disease, past history of ear infections or trauma, and concurrent use of medications.

—Teach patient or family proper way to instill ear drops.

—If patient does not respond promptly to therapy, reevaluate diagnosis and drug choice.

—Systemic therapy may be required in addition to topical preparations.

—Teach patient or family about proper cleansing of ears and to avoid digging in ears with cotton-tipped applicators, bobby pins, toothpicks, and other instruments.

WHAT THE PATIENT NEEDS TO KNOW:

—Take this medication exactly as ordered. Try to not miss any doses, especially during the first 3 days of therapy. If there is an increase in symptoms, or you do not feel better in 48 hours, return to your health practitioner.

—To take ear drops, patient should lie down with the head on a pillow with the affected ear up. A second individual should put the appropriate number of drops into the ear, dropping them so they will run down into the ear canal, but taking care not to touch the ear with the dropper. The patient should

remain lying down for at least 5 minutes following administration of ear drops.
—Keep this medicine out of the reach of children and all others for whom it is not prescribed.
—If you notice development of a fever, swollen neck glands, increased pain or loss of hearing, itching or redness of your ear, return to your health provider.

EVALUATION:

ADVERSE REACTIONS: Watch for signs of drug sensitization. Consult individual products for adverse reactions specific to the drug.

PARAMETERS TO MONITOR: Monitor for therapeutic effects and development of adverse reactions. Obtain baseline physical examination of mouth, throat, neck and ears, and repeat when therapy is concluded.

ACETIC ACID

PRODUCTS (TRADE NAME):
Domeboro Otic, Vo-Sol Otic (Available in 2% solutions.)
DRUG SPECIFICS:
These products are used for external ear infections and prophylaxis of swimmer's ear. Do not use in the presence of perforated tympanic membrane or if hypersensitivity exists.

Acetic acid has antipruritic, anti-inflammatory and anti-infective properties. *Pseudomonas aeruginosa* is especially sensitive to this drug. As with any antibiotic, there may be an overgrowth of nonsusceptible organisms. If drainage persists, reculture.

Irritation, pruritus, and urticaria are signs of sensitivity to the drug, and therapy should be discontinued if these symptoms appear.

ADMINISTRATION AND DOSAGE SPECIFICS:
External ear canal infections: Insert saturated wick into ear and keep moist for 24 hours by occasionally adding a few drops of solution. Remove wick after 24 hours and instill 5 drops, three to four times daily.

Prophylaxis of swimmer's ear: Instill 2 drops in ear, morning and evening.

BENZOCAINE

PRODUCTS (TRADE NAME):
Americaine-Otic (Available in 20% benzocaine solution.) **Auralgan otic, Auromid** (Available in 1.4% benzocaine and 5.4% antipyrine solution.) **ERO Forte**

Otic (Available in 20% benzocaine solution.) **Oto Ear Drop** (Available in 1.4% benzocaine and 5.4% antipyrine.)

DRUG SPECIFICS:

This product is used for the relief of pain and itching in acute congestive and serous otitis media, acute swimmer's ear, and otitis externa.

Do not use in infants under the age of one year. Discontinue drug if sensitivity develops. Indiscriminate use of anesthetic drops could mask symptoms of fulminating infection of the middle ear.

ADMINISTRATION AND DOSAGE SPECIFICS:

Lay patient on side with affected ear up. Swab ear with otic solution. Instill 4 to 5 drops of warmed solution. Insert cotton pledget in meatus. Patient should remain on side for a few minutes.

CARBAMIDE PEROXIDE

PRODUCTS (TRADE NAME):

Auro Ear Drops, Benadyne Ear Drops, Debrox, Murine Ear Drops, Oxy-Otic Antiseptic (Available in 6.5% solution.)

DRUG SPECIFICS:

This drug provides a safe, nonirritating means of removing ear wax. Also, it aids in the prevention of ceruminosis. Do not use if eardrum is perforated.

Tell patient to contact health care provider if irritation, pain, swelling or redness persists or increases. No drug interactions or side effects have been reported.

ADMINISTRATION AND DOSAGE SPECIFICS:

Adults and children: Tilt head so that affected ear is up. Instill 5 to 10 drops, keeping head tilted so that solution stays in ear. Maintain position for a few minutes. Repeat twice daily for 3 to 4 days. Any remaining wax may be removed by flushing with warm water using a bulb syringe.

CHLORAMPHENICOL

PRODUCTS (TRADE NAME):

Chloromycetin Otic (Available in .5% solution with dropper.)

DRUG SPECIFICS:

Chloramphenicol is used for superficial infections of the external auditory canal caused by susceptible strains of various gram-positive and gram-negative organisms. Susceptible organisms include: *Staphylococcus aureus, Escherichia coli, Haemophilus influenzae, Pseudomonas aeruginosa, Aerobacter aerogenes, Klebsiella pneumoniae* and *Proteus* species. A culture of exudates should be obtained prior to drug therapy.

This product should not be used in persons sensitive to chloramphenicol. Bone marrow hypoplasia, including aplastic anemia and death, have been reported with the topical preparation of this drug. Extended use of this drug may result in the overgrowth of nonsusceptible organisms.

Unless the infection is extremely superficial, the topical treatment should be supplemented by appropriate systemic therapy.

Pruritus, burning, angioneurotic edema, urticaria, and vesicular and maculo-papular dermatitis are signs of sensitivity to the drug, and therapy with chloramphenicol should be stopped.

Avoid prolonged use of this product. If infection persists, reculture exudates.

ADMINISTRATION AND DOSAGE SPECIFICS:

Adults and children: Instill 2 to 3 drops into the ear three times daily.

DESONIDE ACETIC ACID

PRODUCTS (TRADE NAME):

Tridesilon Otic Solution (Available in 0.05% desonide and 2% acetic acid solution in 10 ml bottle).

DRUG SPECIFICS:

This product is useful for superficial infections of the external auditory canal which are accompanied by inflammation. It is contraindicated in perforated tympanic membranes and hypersensitivity. Consider risk-benefit ratio in pregnant women.

As with any antibiotic, overgrowth of nonsusceptible organisms may occur. Reculture and institute appropriate therapy as needed. If problems persist, discontinue use of corticosteroid until infection is controlled. Adverse reactions could be any of those associated with topical corticosteroids (pruritus, irritation, dryness, folliculitis, hypertrichosis, hypopigmentation, allergic contact dermatitis, maceration, secondary infection, atrophy of the skin, or burning sensation).

ADMINISTRATION AND DOSAGE SPECIFICS:

Instill 3 to 4 drops into affected ear three to four times daily.

POLYMYXIN B SULFATE

PRODUCTS (TRADE NAME):

Aerosporin Otic (Available in 10,000 U/ml solution with dropper.) **Lidosporin Otic** (Available in 10,000 U/ml with 50 mg Lidocaine HCl/ml.)

DRUG SPECIFICS:

Polymyxin B sulfate is used for acute and chronic otitis externa, otitis media (if tympanic membrane is perforated), and postoperative aural cavities. It is possibly effective in otomycosis.

Do not prescribe for those allergic to Polymyxin B. Pruritus, irritation, and urticaria are signs of sensitivity, and drug should be discontinued if they develop.

If drainage is persistent, reculture. As with any antibiotic, overgrowth of non-susceptible organisms is possible. Polymyxin B sulfate is often used in combination with other antibiotics.

Some patients prefer to warm the medicine prior to use. This procedure should be done with care since the antibiotic loses its potency if heated above room temperature.

ADMINISTRATION AND DOSAGE SPECIFICS:

Adults: Instill 3 to 4 drops, three to four times daily.

Children: Instill 2 to 3 drops, three to four times daily.

TRIETHANOLAMINE POLYPEPTIDE OLEATECONDENSATE

PRODUCTS (TRADE NAME):

Cerumenex (Available in 10% solution.)

DRUG SPECIFICS:

This is a cerumenolytic agent. Its use is contraindicated in the case of hypersensitivity or a positive patch test. Patients with dermatologic idiosyncrasies or history of allergic reactions in general should have this test. To test, place one drop of cerumenex on flexor surface of forearm; cover with small adhesive bandage. Results are read in 24 hours. A positive reaction indicates the probability of an allergic reaction after instillation of the drug into the ear.

It is recommended that exposure of the ear canal to Cerumenex be limited to 15 to 30 minutes. Avoid contact with periaural skin. If contact occurs, wash area with soap and water.

The presence of perforated tympanic membrane or otitis media is a relative contraindication to use of this product. If otitis externa is present, use drug with caution.

One percent of patients receiving this therapy will develop local reactions. The reaction usually lasts 2 to 10 days and resolves with no residual complications. Treatment is symptomatic. Anti-inflammatory agents may be needed.

ADMINISTRATION AND DOSAGE SPECIFICS:

Adults and children: Tilt patient's head to 45-degree angle and fill ear canal with solution. Insert cotton plug for 30 minutes. Gently flush ear with warm water using a soft, rubber syringe. Procedure may be repeated for unusually hard impactions.

Mary Ann Bolter

TOPICAL SKIN PREPARATIONS
ACNE PRODUCTS

BENZOYL PEROXIDE

ACTION OF THE DRUG: Benzoyl peroxide is a bacteriostatic and comedolytic agent. It has antiseptic and drying actions.

ASSESSMENT:

INDICATIONS: Topical application for the treatment of mild to moderate acne vulgaris.

SUBJECTIVE: History of intermittent or chronic skin eruptions. Areas may be tender and drain purulent and/or bloody, odorless discharge.

OBJECTIVE: Comedones, erythematous papules, pustules seen primarily on face, but also on neck, chest, shoulders, and back may be involved. Skin, scalp, and hair are frequently very oily.

PLAN:

CONTRAINDICATIONS: Hypersensitivity to benzoyl peroxide. Not to be used on eyelids, mucous membranes, or inflamed or sensitive skin.

WARNINGS: For external use only. Discontinue use if undue irritation develops.

PRECAUTIONS: Avoid contact with hair and colored fabric.

IMPLEMENTATION:

PRODUCTS (TRADE NAME):
Benzoyl Peroxide Cleanser, Desquam-X Wash (Available in 4% liquid.) **Benoxyl 5, Benoxyl 10** (Available in 5% and 10% lotion.) **Xerac BP5, Xerac BP10**(Available in 5% and 10% gel with Laureth-4.)

ADMINISTRATION AND DOSAGE: Apply once daily to affected areas after cleansing skin. After 3-4 days, if redness, dryness and peeling do not occur, increase application to twice daily. Amount of drying and peeling may be modified by changing frequency of use. Medication may be used alone, under makeup, or allowed to remain on skin overnight.

IMPLEMENTATION CONSIDERATIONS:

—Obtain complete health history: concurrent use of any topical acne medications, previous course of acne, presence of allergies, or sensitivity.

—Benoxyl 5 and 10 are over the counter drugs.

WHAT THE PATIENT NEEDS TO KNOW:
—Keep medication away from eyes, mucous membranes, mouth, angles of nose, hair and colored fabric.
—Medication often causes temporary sensation of warmth or slight stinging and promotes dryness and peeling of the skin.
—Decrease frequency of use or discontinue temporarily if undue redness or discomfort occurs.
—Medication may be used alone, under makeup, or allowed to remain on skin overnight.

EVALUATION:

ADVERSE REACTIONS: Excessive dryness, erythema, and peeling of the skin.
PARAMETERS TO MONITOR: Monitor for improvement in clinical picture: mild dryness and peeling of skin, decreased numbers of comedones and papules.

Carol Burke

MEDICATED BAR SOAPS AND FOAMS

PRODUCTS (TRADE NAME):
Acne-Aid Cream or Bar (Available in 6.3% sulfated surfactant blend.) **Aveenobar Medicated** (Available in 2% sulfur, 2% salicylic acid, and 50% colloidal oatmeal.) **BUF Acne Cleansing Bar** (Available in 1% sulfur and 1% salicylic acid.) **Clearasil** (Available in 0.75% stick or soap.) **Triclosan, Fostex Cleaner** (Available in 2% sulfur and 2% salicylic acid.) **Ionax** (Available in 0.2% benzalkonium chloride and polyoxyethylene ethers in a non-ionic/cationic foam base; skin cleanser, or cream.) **Salicylic Acid and Sulfur Bars** (Available in 10% precipitated sulfur and 3% salicylic acid.) **Sulfur Soap** (Available in 10% precipitated sulfur bars.)

DRUG SPECIFICS:
These products are for external use only. Avoid contact with eyes. If undue skin irritation develops, discontinue use and consult with health care provider. All of these products may be purchased over the counter.

ADMINISTRATION AND DOSAGE SPECIFICS:
Used instead of soap, these products promote drying and provide a gently abrasive action when applied to the skin.

Carol Burke

SULFUR PREPARATIONS

ACTION OF THE DRUG: Sulfur preparations promote peeling and drying of the skin.

ASSESSMENT:

INDICATIONS: Used for the treatment of oily skin and mild acne.
SUBJECTIVE: Oily skin with history of intermittent or chronic skin eruptions.
OBJECTIVE: Presence of comedones, erythematous papules and/or pustules.

PLAN:

WARNINGS: Keep away from eyes. For external use only.
PRECAUTIONS: Discontinue use if severe irritation of the skin occurs.

IMPLEMENTATION:

PRODUCTS (TRADE NAME):
Xerac (Available in 4% microcrystalline sulfur and 44% isopropyl alcohol gel.) **Acne-Aid** (Available in 10% sulfur and 10% alcohol lotion.) **Transact** (Available in 2% sulfur, 6% laureth-4, and 37% alcohol gel with a greaseless base.) **Fostex CM** (Available in 2% sulfur cream.) **Liquimat** (Available in 5% sulfur and 22% alcohol.)
ADMINISTRATION AND DOSAGE: Thin film of medication should be applied once or twice a day to clean skin.
IMPLEMENTATION CONSIDERATIONS:
—Obtain a health history: presence of allergies, sensitivities, concurrent use of other acne products.
—Teach patient about proper cleansing of skin; keeping hands off irritated areas.

WHAT THE PATIENT NEEDS TO KNOW:
—Apply a thin film of medication to affected areas once or twice daily. Apply only to clean skin.
—Avoid contact of medication with eyes.
—Reddening and scaling of the skin are to be expected; however, if undue irritation develops, discontinue use and notify health care provider.

EVALUATION:

ADVERSE REACTIONS: Severe irritation of skin with erythema and peeling may occur.

PARAMETERS TO MONITOR: Monitor for clinical improvement: decreased oiliness of skin, fewer comedones and papules.

Carol Burke

TETRACYCLINE HCL—TOPICAL

ACTION OF THE DRUG: Mechanism of action is not known, but tetracycline works at the level of pilosebaceous apparatus and surrounding tissues.

ASSESSMENT:

INDICATIONS: Used in topical treatment of acne vulgaris.

SUBJECTIVE: History of intermittent or chronic skin eruptions. Areas may be tender and drain purulent and/or bloody, odorless discharge.

OBJECTIVE: Comedones, erythematous papules, pustules seen primarily on face, but also on the neck, chest, shoulders and back. Skin, scalp, and hair are frequently very oily.

PLAN:

CONTRAINDICATIONS: Allergy to other tetracyclines.

WARNINGS: Safe use during pregnancy and lactation has not been proven. Use with caution in patients with known hepatic or renal dysfunction since absorption may occur with prolonged use.

PRECAUTIONS: This medication is for external use only. Avoid contact with eyes, nose, and mouth.

IMPLEMENTATION:

PRODUCTS (TRADE NAME):
Topicycline (Available in 2.2 mg/ml in 70 ml solution.)

ADMINISTRATION AND DOSAGE: Apply generous amount to affected areas twice daily. Adjust frequency of application depending on clinical response.

IMPLEMENTATION CONSIDERATIONS:

—Obtain complete health history: drug allergies, history of liver or kidney disease, possibility of pregnancy, or breast-feeding.

—Patient may experience transient feeling of stinging or burning with application.

WHAT THE PATIENT NEEDS TO KNOW:

—Apply medication once or twice daily to clean skin.

—You may experience a brief sensation of stinging or burning when you put medication on.

—You may notice a slight yellowing of skin, especially if complexion is light. This is easily removed by washing.

—Areas of skin treated with tetracycline will fluoresce under ultraviolet light.

—Avoid eyes, mouth, and nose when applying medication.

EVALUATION:

PARAMETERS TO MONITOR: Observe for clinical signs of improvement of acne.

Carol Burke

TRETINOIN
(RETINOIC ACID, VITAMIN A ACID)

ACTION OF THE DRUG: Tretinoin (1) inhibits the formation of comedones causing loosening or ejection of existing comedomes by increasing epidermal cell turn-over and decreasing the cohesiveness of horney cells. (2) It also causes changes in follicular keratinization. (3) The decrease in the normal cell layers may promote better penetration of other topical preparations.

ASSESSMENT:

INDICATIONS: Topical applications are used for the treatment of acne vulgaris with mild to moderate involvement (many comedones, some papules and/or pustules). It is not effective in severe pustular and deep cystic acne.

SUBJECTIVE: History of intermittent or chronic skin eruptions.

OBJECTIVE: Comedones, erythematous papules, pustules seen primarily on face, but also on neck, chest, shoulders and back. Skin, scalp, and hair are frequently very oily. Areas may be tender and drain purulent and/or bloody, odorless discharge.

PLAN:

WARNINGS: Avoid contact with eyes, angles of the nose, mouth, mucous membranes, and open wounds.

PRECAUTIONS: While using this medication, do not use medicated soaps, abrasive cleansers, or cosmetics which contain alcohol, astringents, spices, or limes. Exposure to sunlight, including sunlamps, should be minimized.

IMPLEMENTATION:

DRUG INTERACTIONS: Do not use with other topical medications that contain peeling agents (sulfur, resorcinol, benzoyl peroxide, salicylic acid).

PRODUCTS (TRADE NAME):
Retin-A (Available in 0.025% and 0.01% gel, 0.05% and 0.1% cream, and 0.05% liquid.)
ADMINISTRATION AND DOSAGE: Apply to affected area once a day at bedtime. Fair-complexioned patients with easily irritated skin should start with 0.05% cream or gel.
IMPLEMENTATION CONSIDERATIONS:
—Obtain a thorough health history: other medications which may cause acne (oral contraceptives, corticosteroids, ACTH, androgens, iodides, bromides), or other stimulating chemicals: trimethadione, dilantin, INH, lithium, halothane, cobalt irradiation, and hyperalimentation therapy; occupation requiring considerable sun exposure or contact with heavy oils, greases or tars, and diet history.
—If patient is sunburned, do not start using medication until sunburn has resolved.

WHAT THE PATIENT NEEDS TO KNOW:
—During initial treatment acne may seem to worsen (first 4-6 weeks). Improvement in inflammatory areas is expected within 8 weeks. Maximum results usually require 12 weeks of therapy.
—Attempt to stay out of direct sunlight, wind, and cold weather.
—Apply medication to skin that has been thoroughly cleansed with soap and water. Apply only to affected areas, avoiding eyes, angles of the nose, mouth and mucous membranes.
—Contact health care provider if excessive irritation, redness, or blisters develop.
—Continue application of medication after lesions have cleared.
—Water-based cosmetics may be used.

EVALUATION:

ADVERSE REACTIONS: *Local:* erythema, warmth, stinging sensation, hypopigmentation or hyperpigmentation.
OVERDOSAGE: Severe dryness and excessive irritation.
PARAMETERS TO MONITOR: Observe for clinical improvement of inflammatory lesions and decrease in papules, pustules, and comedones. Erythema and peeling of the skin normally occur. Severe dryness and excessive irritation are to be avoided.

Carol Burke

COMBINATION PRODUCTS

PRODUCTS (TRADE NAME):
Fostril (Available in 2% sulfur and 6% laureth-4 lotion in a greaseless base

with zinc oxide and talc.) **Acnederm** (Available in 5% sulfur, 1% zinc sulfate and 10% zinc oxide with 21% isopropyl alcohol lotion in a greaseless water washable base.) **Acnophill** (Available in 5% sulfur, 10% zinc oxide, 5% potassium and zinc sulfides-polysulfides in a water washable ointment base cream.) **Acnomel** (Available in 4% sulfur and 1% resorcinol cake or cream or lotion.) **Xerac A C** (Available in 6.25% aluminum chloride hexahydrate in 96% anhydrous ethyl alcohol.)

DRUG SPECIFICS:

If excessive skin irritation develops, discontinue use. These products are for external use only. Keep away from eyes. Xerac A C is the only preparation requiring a prescription.

ADMINISTRATION AND DOSAGE SPECIFICS:

These products contain astringents and keratolytics. Sulfur, salicylic acid, and resorcinol are keratolytics. Alcohol and acetone are defatting agents. Zinc oxide and zinc sulfate are used because of their astringent properties. Some products also have organic solvent bases.

Carol Burke

ADRENOCORTICAL STEROIDS

GLUCOCORTICOIDS

ACTION OF THE DRUG (1) The major action of the glucocorticoids is the stimulation of protein synthesis of enzymes responsible for three systemic effects: antiinflammatory, immunosuppressant, and metabolic. The latter action causes the catabolism of protein fats and carbohydrates into glucagon and ultimately raises the serum glucose level. (2) Naturally occurring glucocorticoids (cortisone and hydrocortisone) also have moderate mineralocorticoid activity which causes reabsorption of sodium and excretion of potassium.

ASSESSMENT:

INDICATIONS: *Acute and chronic dermatoses:* angiogenital pruritus; atopic, seborrheic, and some types of chronic eczematous dermatitis; cutaneous manifestations of systemic collagen diseases (lupus dermatomyositis, pemphigus), infantile eczema, intertriginous psoriasis, neurodermatitis.

Rectum: ulcerative colitis, proctitis, sigmoiditis, other inflammatory conditions of the distal intestine.

SUBJECTIVE-OBJECTIVE: Patient may present with pre-existing disease or with signs and symptoms of pruritus, erythema, excoriations secondary to scratching of the skin. Bowel problems may be detected following an evaluation of change in bowel habits, especially episodes of diarrhea with mucus or blood. Nocturnal diarrhea is especially significant. Sigmoidoscopy and proctoscopy with biopsy may help in specific diagnosis.

PLAN:

CONTRAINDICATIONS: Do not give in tuberculosis of the skin, herpes simplex, vaccinia, and infections (in the absence of anti-infective agents), when circulation to the skin is markedly impaired. *Rectal:* Do not give with obstruction, abscess, perforation, peritonitis, fresh intestinal surgery, extensive fistulas, and/or sinus tracts.

WARNINGS: Although glucocorticoids are exceptionally potent drugs, short-term administration of even extremely large doses is not likely to net long-term sequelae. However, moderate and long-term administration (longer than six days systemic treatment) places the patient at high risk to a large number of serious adverse effects and the risk/benefit ratio must be carefully considered. (See adverse effects.) The immediate and long-term effects of the drug are exceedingly variable and depend on the individual disease, route of administration, dose, frequency, duration, and time of administration.

Corticosteroid drugs cannot be withdrawn without gradual weaning. Sudden withdrawal leads to steroid withdrawal syndrome (anorexia, nausea and vomiting, lethargy, headache, fever, joint pain, desquamation, myalgia, weight loss and hypotension). Abrupt cessation may also result in rebound of the condition being treated.

When the drug is administered for longer than one to two weeks at phemarcological doses, pituitary release of ACTH is suppressed, producing secondary adrenocortical insufficiency. Patients undergoing physiological, emotional, or psychological stress may need support via additional amounts of steroids. This suppression may last up to two years following discontinuation of the drug.

Normal or large doses, especially of cortisone and hydrocortisone, can cause hypertension, sodium and water retention, and potassium loss. All corticosteroids promote calcium excretion.

Corticosteroids mask infection and increase the patient's susceptibility to them. Corticosteroids are particularly dangerous to use in patients with a history of tuberculosis. The disease can be reactivated; therefore, administer chemoprophylaxis in these patients. In patients with active fulminating or disseminated tuberculosis, or any infection, use steroids only in conjunction with a total anti-infective regimen. Due to the altered antibody response, patients receiving corticosteroid should not be immunized against smallpox or other disease.

Although corticosteroids do cross the placental barrier, there is no research to document problems in humans. Fetal abnormalities have been noted in animal studies. Ratio of benefits to risks should be weighed. Mother and infant should be closely monitored for hypoadrenalism at the time and following birth if steroid therapy has been administered.

There have been no documented problems in steroid use with nursing mothers. However, high dose steroid consumption in the mother may result in growth suppression of the infant.

PRECAUTIONS: Significant systemic absorption may occur if (1) extensive areas are treated, (2) denuded areas are treated, or (3) if the occlusive technique is used. If infection is present, use appropriate anti-fungal or antibiotic with the corticosteroid. If a favorable response is not present within several days, discontinue the corticosteroid until the infection has begun to resolve. Use caution in pregnant women when extensive amounts, large areas, or prolonged treatment are indicated.

IMPLEMENTATION:

DRUG INTERACTIONS: Corticosteroids increase the effects of: barbiturates, sedatives, narcotics, and anticoagulants. They decrease the effects of insulin and oral hypoglycemics, coumarin anticoagulants, choline-like drugs (effectiveness reduced in treatment of glaucoma), aspirin (higher doses necessary which has led to salicylism after discontinuation of steroids), and broad spectrum antibiotics (may result in resistant strains). Drugs which increase the effects of steroids are indomethacin, aspirin, and oral contraceptives, especially estrogen (estrogen increases the anti-inflammatory effect of hydrocortisone by slowing its breakdown in the liver). Drugs which decrease the effects of steroids include barbiturates, phenytoin, antihistamines, chloral hydrate, glutethimide, phenylbutazone (increases effect and then reduces it), and propranolol.

Some drugs produce exaggerated side effects when given with steroids. These include: alcohol, aspirin and anti-inflammatory drugs (ulcerogenic); thiazides and other potassium-wasting diuretics (excessive potassium loss); stimulants such as epinephrine, amphetamines and ephedrine, and anticholinergics (increased intraocular pressure); and cardiac glycosides (enhances possibility of arrhythmias and digitalis toxicity).

Steroids also increase the laboratory serum levels of amylase, CO_2, glucose, and sodium. They decrease the laboratory levels of serum calcium, potassium and platelets.

ADMINISTRATION AND DOSAGE: Dosages vary radically; they are individualized by the diagnosis, severity, prognosis, probable duration of the disease, and patient response and tolerance. Individuals may respond better to one form than another in a somewhat unpredictable manner. The general rule, regardless of route of administration, is to initially prescribe as high a dose as necessary to obain a favorable response and then decrease the amount gradually to the lowest level that will maintain the therapeutic effect and yet minimize complications.

The topical route circumvents most side effects of systemic treatment and is more effective in treating some problems. The appropriate drug is selected on the basis of patient skin hydration, site, severity, age, whether the lesion is moist or dry, potency and strength of the product, and the method of application (open vs occlusive).

Topical corticosteroids are metabolized in the skin. Fluorinated compounds are generally more potent and more prone to cause side effects since they are more slowly metabolized and thus are systemically absorbed in higher amounts.

The risk of side effects is also enhanced by repeated or long term applications. This leads to a cumulative effect with prolonged duration of action and greater systemic absorption. Again, the possibility of hypothalamic-pituitary-adrenal axis suppression and adverse effects must not be ignored.

There are a large number of available preparations. See Table 9-2. Generally, the practitioner uses the lowest potency which will control the symptoms. Preparations which contain a free 17-hydroxy ion and are *not* fluorinated are also considered less likely to cause side effects and may be the most appropriate form for less severe problems. Children generally should be given low potency, nonfluorinated, free 17-hydroxy forms such as hydrocortisone, hydrocortisone acetate, or prednisolone whenever possible.

Many steroids are available as lotion, cream, or ointment. Select a lotion to treat weeping lesions, particularly in intertriginous areas prone to chafing (axilla, groin, feet). A cream is appropriate for moist lesions, and an ointment, with its petrolatum base, is recommended for dry, scaling lesions. Foams, gels and aerosols usually contain alcohol and thus are also indicated for moist skin eruptions. The cream should be rubbed gently into the skin. The ointment should be applied in a thin coat over the indicated area. The general regimen is to apply sparingly two to four times per day.

If the patient has been treated for two weeks without substantial improvement, particularly if lesions cover more than 5% of body surface, refer patient to a dermatologist.

Greater absorption and hydration can be achieved by using the occlusive technique. The steroid is rubbed into clean skin and an additional layer of the preparation may be added. This is covered with a plastic film such as Saran Wrap. (Plastic gloves may be used for hand dressings; garment bags have been used successfully over the buttocks and trunk; a tight shower cap is used over the scalp.) Be aware of the danger of suffocation when using plastic dressings on small children. If the dermatosis is dry, make the dressing airtight and watertight with tape. Added moisture to the skin may be achieved by placing a damp cloth or gauze over the ointment or cream. Most lesions need not be sealed. Dressing changes are determined on an individual basis ranging from every 12 hours to every 4 days in very resistant cases. Note that the longer the patient is treated with occlusive dressings, the more rapid the response. To minimize adverse reactions, the occlusive technique is used intermittently. Often, patients can remove the dressing in the morning, use the prescribed preparation alone in the daytime, and reapply it occlusively at night. The lesion should be inspected carefully for infection between dressings. If an infection develops, the steroid treatment should be held until the infection is controlled.

TABLE 9-2—CLASSIFICATION OF TOPICAL STEROIDS

Low Potency %	Intermediate Potency %	High Potency %
Hydrocortisone Acetate 0.5%, 1%, 2.5%[x$$$]	Betamethasone 0.2%[x*]	Betamethasone Diproprionate 0.05%, 0.1% [*$$$]
Hydrocortisone 0.125% 1%, 2.5%[X$]	Hydrocortisone Acetate 5%	Fluocinolone Acetonide 0.2% [*]
	Dexamethasone 0.1%[*$$]	
Dexamethasone NaPO$_4$ 1%[x*]	Betamethasone Valerate 0.1% 0.15%[*$$]	Fluocinonide 0.05% Desoximetasone 0.25%[*$$]

TABLE 9-2—Continued

Low Potency %	Intermediate Potency %	High Potency %
Dexamethasone 0.01%, .04%ˣ*	Betamethasone Benzocate 0.025%*	Flurandrenolide 4 mcg 0.004 mg/cm² *
Flurandrenolide 0.025%*	Flumethesone Pivalate 0.03%ˣ*	Halcinonide 0.1% *$$ Triamcinalone Acetonide 0.5%*
Methylprednisolone Acetate 0.25%, 1.0%*	Fluocinolone Acetonide .01%, .025%*$$	
Prednisolone 0.033%, 0.5%ˣ	Desoximetasone 0.05%* Flurandrenolide 0.05%*$$	
Triamcinolone Acetonide 0.015%, 0.025%*$$	Fluorometholone 0.025%*ˣ Halcinonide 0.025%* Triamcinolone Acetonide 0.1%	

* = fluorinated
x = contains free 17-hydroxy ion
Drugs most likely to be available at local pharmacies:
$ = inexpensive
$$ = moderately priced
$$$ = most expensive

IMPLEMENTATION CONSIDERATIONS:

—Obtain a complete health history, including history of infection (especially systemic fungal infections), positive tuberculin test or tuberculosis, hypersensitivity, underlying medical diseases, medications taken concurrently which may produce drug interactions, and possibility of pregnancy.

—Doses are quite variable, and patients must be closely observed for response in order to make dosage adjustments.

—Generic forms of the drugs are considerably less expensive.

—All patients on corticosteroids should be monitored often and the dose adjusted to reflect remissions, exacerbations, individual response, or occurrence of stress (injury, infection, surgery, emotional crisis, etc.). Patients should be monitored for one or two years following high doses or long-term treatment.

—Patient on steroids should be given prescriptions which cannot be refilled in order to prevent unmonitored steroid consumption.

—Review information under Administration and Dosage regarding specific steps to follow in using corticosteroids for topical applications.

WHAT THE PATIENT NEEDS TO KNOW:
—Do not put a bandage over open sores and topical medicine unless directed to do so by your health care provider.
—Avoid tight diapers and rubber pants with infants using topical steroids.
—Preparations containing alcohol may normally sting for a short time following application.
—Overuse on thin skin may lead to thinning and stretch marks.
—The skin must be extremely clean to avoid infection. Any signs of redness, tenderness, or fever should be immediately reported to your health care provider.
—On sites with hair, part the hair and apply medicine directly to the sore or lesion.
—In using dressings which cover a sore (occlusive dressings), if irritation develops at the tape site, the dressing can be held in place with gauze, stockingette, stockings, or Ace bandages.
—Use the steroid topical preparation for a few days after the lesions or sores clear to prevent recurrences.

EVALUATION:

ADVERSE REACTIONS: Small physiologic doses or short-term emergency pharmacologic doses generally do not cause adverse effects.
OVERDOSAGE: Particularly in areas of thin skin (the face, groin, axilla) overdosage may result in thinning and development of striae. *Treatment:* Decrease or diminish the dose.
PARAMETERS TO MONITOR: Before beginning therapy, obtain baseline history and physical examination, documenting current patient status. On each visit monitor for the resolution of underlying problem and for occurrence of adverse effects. Hypothalamic-pituitary-adrenal axis suppression should be monitored, particularly following withdrawal of high doses or long-term treatment.

CORTICOSTEROIDS—TOPICAL

BETAMETHASONE

PRODUCTS (TRADE NAME):
Celestone (Available in 0.2% cream.)
DRUG SPECIFICS:
Cream available in a water miscible base. Fairly expensive compared to other products.

ADMINISTRATION AND DOSAGE SPECIFICS:
Apply gently one to three times per day, more if condition warrants.

BETAMETHASONE BENZOATE

PRODUCTS (TRADE NAME):
Benisone, Uticort (Available in 0.025% ointment, cream, lotion and gel.)
DRUG SPECIFICS:
This is a synthetic fluorinated corticosteroid topical preparation of the intermediate class of potency. Avoid application near the eyes. This preparation may be covered and used occlusively.
ADMINISTRATION AND DOSAGE SPECIFICS:
Adults: Apply gently one to three times per day, more if condition warrants.
Children: Apply daily.

BETAMETHASONE DIPROPIONATE

PRODUCTS (TRADE NAME):
Diprosone (Available in 0.05% cream, lotion, or ointment, or in 0.1% topical aerosol.)
DRUG SPECIFICS:
This is a highly potent synthetic fluorinated corticosteroid and is one of the more expensive preparations. It is used for dermatoses needing anti-inflammatory and antipruritic medication. It is also used occlusively (as a covered dressing) for management of refractory psoriasis and other intractable dermatoses. It is not for ophthalmic use.

The aerosol form is effective mainly for contact dermatitis and is not appropriate for an occlusive dressing.
ADMINISTRATION AND DOSAGE SPECIFICS:
The *cream* should be rubbed gently into affected areas that have been cleansed. Adults should use it twice a day; children, once a day.

For *lotion*, apply a few drops to affected area daily.

For *ointment*, apply sparingly. Adults should use it twice a day; children, once a day.

Topical aerosol: apply for 3 seconds, holding can six inches away from affected area. Adults should use it three times a day; children, once a day.

BETAMETHASONE VALERATE

PRODUCTS (TRADE NAME):
  Beta-Val (Available in 0.1% cream.) **Valisone** (Available in 0.01%, reduced strength, and 0.1% cream, 0.1% lotion, and 0.1% ointment.)

DRUG SPECIFICS:
  This product is an intermediate fluorinated preparation indicated for dermatoses with inflammatory manifestations known to respond to corticosteroids. All forms may be used with occlusive dressings. They are not for ophthalmic use. Lotion must be shaken well.

ADMINISTRATION AND DOSAGE SPECIFICS:
  Cream: Gently rub in reduced strength medication 1-4 times a day, or more often if indicated. Use 0.01% cream one to four times/day; use 0.1% cream once a day.
  Lotion: Apply two drops 1-2 times/day for adults; once a day for children.
  Ointment: Apply sparingly 1-3 times/day for adults; once a day for children.

DESONIDE

PRODUCTS (TRADE NAME):
  Tridesilon (Available in 0.05% cream and ointment.)

DRUG SPECIFICS:
  This product is moderately priced.

ADMINISTRATION AND DOSAGE SPECIFICS:
  Gently rub in medication 2 to 4 times/day.

DESOXIMETASONE

PRODUCTS (TRADE NAME):
  Topicort (Available in 0.05% and 0.25% cream or 0.05% gel.)

DRUG SPECIFICS:
  Do not use near the eyes. Store in collapsible tubes.

ADMINISTRATION AND DOSAGE SPECIFICS:
  For corticosteroid responsive dermatoses:
  Adults: Apply sparingly twice a day.
  Children: Apply sparingly once a day.

FLUMETHASONE PIVALATE

PRODUCTS (TRADE NAME):
Locorten (Available in 0.03% cream.)
DRUG SPECIFICS:
This is an intermediate potency, fluorinated, synthetic steroid. It is not for ophthalmic use. Store in collapsible tube. It is suitable for occlusive dressings.
ADMINISTRATION AND DOSAGE SPECIFICS:
For steroid-responsive dermatoses:
Adults: Apply sparingly three to four times a day.
Children: Apply sparingly one to two times a day.

FLUOCINOLONE ACETONIDE

PRODUCTS (TRADE NAME):
Fluocinolone Acetonide (Available in 0.01% and 0.025% cream and 0.01% solution.) **Fluonid** (Available in 0.025% ointment, 0.01% and 0.025% cream, and 0.01% solution.) **Flurosyn** (Available in 0.025% cream.) **Synalar** (Available in 0.025%, 0.01%, 0.2, 0.25% cream; 0.025% ointment, and 0.01% solution.) **Synemol Cream** (Available in 0.025% cream.)
DRUG SPECIFICS:
Do not use ophthalmologically. Store in an air tight container without freezing. Treat multiple or extensive eruptions sequentially. Apply only to small areas at a time. Fluonid solution on dry lesions may increase the dryness, scaling or itching; on denuded areas it may cause stinging or burning. If this persists, discontinue solution. Do not exceed application of two grams of Synalar high potency cream per day or use it for prolonged periods of time.
ADMINISTRATION AND DOSAGE SPECIFICS:
For dermatoses:
Cream: Rub in gently, apply sparingly.
Adults: Apply topically two to four times a day.
Children: Use 0.1% potency one to two times a day or O.025% once daily. high potency is not recommended for children under two years.
Cream:
Adults: Apply sparingly two to four times a day.
Children: Apply sparingly once a day.
Solution:
Adults: Apply two to four times a day.
Children: Apply one to two times a day.

FLUOCINONIDE

PRODUCTS (TRADE NAME):
Lidex (Available in 0.05% cream and ointment.) **Topsyn** (Available in 0.05% gel.)

DRUG SPECIFICS:
Product comes in water miscible, greaseless base, or as an emollient base for use occlusively.

ADMINISTRATION AND DOSAGE SPECIFICS:
For dermatoses: Apply topical preparation sparingly.
Cream or gel:
Adults: Apply three to four times a day.
Children: Apply once a day.
Ointment:
Adults: Apply either strength two to three times a day.
Children: Apply once a day.

FLUOROMETHOLONE

PRODUCTS (TRADE NAME):
Oxylone (Available in 0.025% cream.)

DRUG SPECIFICS:
Indicated for susceptible skin diseases such as psoriasis and chronic neurodermatitis. Apply to cleansed skin.

ADMINISTRATION AND DOSAGE SPECIFICS:
Adults: Apply cream one to three times a day.
Children: Apply once a day.

FLURANDRENOLIDE

PRODUCTS (TRADE NAME):
Cordran (Available in 0.025%, 0.05% ointment and cream and in 0.05% lotion.) **Cordran Tape** (Available in 4 mcg/sq cm tape.) **Flurandrenolide** (Available in 0.5% lotion.)

DRUG SPECIFICS:
Shake lotion well; protect from light, heat, and freezing. Cordran Tape is a polyethylene film impregnated with flurandrenolide which acts as an occlusive dressing. It is not to be used in intertriginous areas or on exudative eruptions. To use: cleanse the skin, remove scales, crusts, etc.; allow to dry exposed for one hour.

Shave or clip hair for good contact and comfortable removal. Apply tape. If ends loosen prematurely, trim and replace with new tape. The lowest incidence of side effects is when the tape is changed every twelve hours, but it may be left on for twenty-four hours if well tolerated. Reported adverse effects include purpura, striping of epidermis, and furunculosis.

ADMINISTRATION AND DOSAGE SPECIFICS:

Cream:

Adults: Apply sparingly two or three times a day.

Children: Use 0.025% and apply sparingly twice a day; or use 0.05% and apply once a day.

Lotion:

Adults: Apply two or three times a day.

Children: Apply once a day.

Tape:

Adults: Apply once or twice a day for twelve hours.

Children: Apply once a day for twelve hours.

HALCINONIDE

PRODUCTS (TRADE NAME):

Halog (Available in 0.025%, 0.1% cream and ointment and in 0.1% solution.) **Halog-E** (Available in 0.1% cream.)

DRUG SPECIFICS:

Protect cream and ointment from freezing and store in tight containers. Keep ointment protected from light. Can be used as an occlusive dressing at night. Use without occlusion in the daytime. Occlude one part of the body at a time.

ADMINISTRATION AND DOSAGE SPECIFICS:

Cream:

Adults: Apply gently two to three times a day.

Children: Rub in gently once a day.

Ointment:

Adults: Apply sparingly two or three times a day.

Children: Apply sparingly once a day.

Solution:

Adults: Apply a few drops two or three times a day.

Children: Apply a few drops once a day.

HYDROCORTISONE

PRODUCTS (TRADE NAME):

Cort-Dome (Available in 1% cream and in 0.125, 0.25%, 0.5% and 1% lotion.)

Cortril (Available in 0.5% cream and 1% ointment.) **Hydrocortisone** (Available in 0.5%, 1%, 2.5% cream and 0.5%, 0.1% lotion and ointment.) **Hytone** (Available in 1%, 2.5% cream and 0.5%, 1% and 2.5% ointment.) **Texacort Scalp Lotion** (Available in 1% lotion.) **Ulcort** (Available in 1% cream and 0.5% and 1% lotion.) **Wellcortin** (Available in 0.5% ointment.)

DRUG SPECIFICS:

This preparation is one of the few steroids that can be used safely on the face, axilla, groin, under the breasts, and in other intertriginous areas. It is generally indicated for the gamut of mild to moderate steroid-responsive dermatoses including seborrheic dermatitis. The 0.5% strength is available without a prescription. Use lowest dosage in mild and recent lesions, saving the 5% dosage for severe and chronic lesions.

ADMINISTRATION AND DOSAGE SPECIFICS:

Ointment or cream: Apply a thin coat.

Adults: 0.125% to 2.5%, depending on severity. Apply one to four times a day.

Children: Apply 0.25% to 1% one to two times a day; 2.5% ointment one time per day.

Lotion: Shake bottle well.

Adults: Apply appropriate strength three to four times a day.

Children: Apply appropriate strength one to two times a day. Gradually reduce after a favorable response is obtained.

HYDROCORTISONE ACETATE

PRODUCTS (TRADE NAME):

CaldeCort Rectal-Itch (Available in 0.5% cream or ointment.) **Cortaid** (Available in 0.5% cream or ointment.) **Cortef Acetate** (Available in 0.5% and 5% ointment.) **Gynecort** (Available in 0.5% cream.) **Hydrocortone Acetate** (Available in 1% ointment.) **Lanacort** (Available in 0.5% cream.) **Pharm-Cort** (Available in 0.5% cream.) **Resicort** (Available in 0.5% cream.) **Rhulicort** (Available in 0.5% lotion and cream.)

DRUG SPECIFICS:

The concentration selected is dependent on the severity of the dermatosis. Use 0.5% for the mildest problems and 2.5% for the most severe. The 0.5% strength of hydrocortisone acetate is available without prescription. This form is more expensive than hydrocortisone. Not for ophthalmic use.

ADMINISTRATION AND DOSAGE SPECIFICS:

Apply a thin coat of ointment or apply the cream gently and sparingly.

Adults: Apply one to four times a day.

Children: Apply 0.5% or 1% once or twice a day; apply 2.5% strength preparation once a day.

CORTICOSTEROIDS—RECTAL

HYDROCORTISONE OR METHYLPREDNISOLONE RETENTION ENEMAS

PRODUCTS (TRADE NAME):

Cortenema Retention Enemas (Available in 100 mg/60 ml hydrocortisone enemas.) **Medrol Enpak** (Available in 40 mg/bottle methylprednisolone retention enema.)

DRUG SPECIFICS:

These preparations are useful for anti-inflammatory treatment of ulcerative proctitis and distal ulcerative colitis. (The adjunctive therapy should include diet therapy, sedatives, antidiarrheals, antibiotics and/or other indicated therapeutics.) This medication is contraindicated in systemic fungal infections and in ileocolostomy during the immediate postoperative period. It must be used with caution in cases of potential perforation, abscess, or pyogenic infection. In severe ulcerative pathology, do not postpone needed surgery to await medical response.

Hydrocortisone is absorbed efficiently from the colon (up to 50% of the dose may be absorbed). Consequently, prolonged use is likely to cause some systemic reaction.

It is prudent to perform a rectal or proctoscopic examination before beginning treatment. Shake Medrol Enpak well before and every half hour during administration. Carefully instruct patients on proper self-administration. Damage to the rectal wall can result from improper insertion. Best results are obtained if enema is administered after a bowel movement. Patient should lie on his or her left side for a minimum of 30 minutes and optimally should retain enema all night. See anorectal drug section for additional details.

ADMINISTRATION AND DOSAGE SPECIFICS:

Adjunctive treatment of colitis and proctitis:

Adults: 100 mg (one container) as retention enema before bed for 21 days or until clinical and proctological signs and symptoms have responded. Difficult cases may require nightly applications for two to three months. Withdraw the use of the drug gradually if administered longer than 21 days. Use one administration every other night for two to three weeks.

HYDROCORTISONE FOAM

PRODUCTS (TRADE NAME):

Cortifoam (Available as 10% hydrocortisone aerosol; one dose contains 80 mg hydrocortisone.) **Epifoam** (Available in 1% aerosol of hydrocortisone acetate.)

DRUG SPECIFICS:

This preparation is useful for anti-inflammatory treatment of ulcerative proctitis and distal ulceraive colitis for patients who cannot retain an enema. (It should be considered adjunctive treatment along with diet therapy, sedatives, antidiarrheals, antibiotics and/or other indicated therapeutics.) It is contraindicated in systemic fungal infections and in ileocolostomy during the immediate postoperative period. It must be used with caution in cases of potential perforation, abscess, or pyogenic infection. In severe ulcerative pathology, do not postpone needed surgery to await medical response.

Hydrocortisone is absorbed efficiently from the colon (up to 50% of the dose may be absorbed). Consequently, prolonged use is likely to cause some systemic reaction. Patients should be told not to insert any portion of the aerosol container into the rectum but to use the applicator. If there is no clinical or cytologic improvement within 2 to 3 weeks, gradually discontinue the drug. Improvement should occur within 5-7 days. Follow progress with proctological exams. See anorectal drug section for more details.

ADMINISTRATION AND DOSAGE SPECIFICS:

Give one applicatorful, 1 to 2 times per day for two to three weeks, then once every two days.

METHYLPREDNISOLONE ACETATE

PRODUCTS (TRADE NAME):

Medrol Acetate (Available in 0.25% and 1% ointment.)

DRUG SPECIFICS:

1% concentration is usually very expensive.

ADMINISTRATION AND DOSAGE SPECIFICS:

Inflammation secondary to corticosteroid-responsive dermatoses:
Adults: Apply one to four times daily.
Children: Apply one to two times daily.

PREDNISOLONE

PRODUCTS (TRADE NAME):

MetiDerm (Available in 0.5% cream.)

DRUG SPECIFICS:

Prednisolone is five times more potent than cortisone. Not for ophthalmological use. Keep the cream in airtight containers or collapsible tubes.

ADMINISTRATION AND DOSAGE SPECIFICS:
Adults: Apply 3 to 4 times a day.
Children: Apply 1 to 2 times a day.

TRIAMCINOLONE ACETONIDE

PRODUCTS (TRADE NAME):
Aristocort (Available in 0.1%, 0.5%, 0.025% ointment and 0.1% and 0.5% cream.) **Aristocort A** (Available in 0.1%, 0.5%, 0.025% ointment and 0.1% and 0.5% cream.) **Kenalog** (Available in 0.025% and 0.1% ointment, cream, and lotion, and 0.5 mg ointment and cream and 0.2 mg aerosol.) **Triamcinolone Acetonide** (Available in 0.025%, 0.1% ointment and 0.5% cream.)

DRUG SPECIFICS:
This is a fluorinated steroid which is considered high potency in its highest strength. It is not to be used on the face since it has caused a paradoxical skin reaction in long-term use, nor is it to be used ophthalmologically. Use particular caution in administering this preparation to patients with decreased renal function. See triamcinolone—systemic section also.

ADMINISTRATION AND DOSAGE SPECIFICS:
Adults: Apply to the affected area 2 to 4 times a day.
Children: Use weaker strengths and apply 1 to 2 times a day.

GLUCOCORTICOID—ANTIBIOTIC TOPICAL PREPARATIONS

HYDROCORTISONE PLUS ANTIBIOTICS

PRODUCTS (TRADE NAME):
Cortisporin Ointment (Available with neomycine sulfate, polymixin B 0.5%, hydrocortisone.) **Neo-Cortef** (Available with neomycin sulfate, 1% hydrocortisone.) **Neo-Cort-Dome** (Available with neomycin plus hydrocortisone 1 or 2.5% as a cream.)

DRUG SPECIFICS:
Combinations of antibiotics and steroids are considered by the Food and Drug Administration to be "possibly effective" in treating bacterial inflammatory skin conditions. This medication may be used occlusively.

ADMINISTRATION AND DOSAGE SPECIFICS:
Adults and children: Apply to affected area 2 to 3 times a day. Withdraw gradually if medication has been used chronically.

GLUCOCORTICOIDS—ANTIBACTERIAL TOPICAL COMBINATIONS

HYDROCORTISONE PLUS IODOCHLORHYDROXYQUIN

PRODUCTS (TRADE NAME):
Domeform-HC, Hydrocortisone with Iodochlorhydroxyquin, Vioform-Hydrocortisone, Vytone (Available in 3% iodo with 0.5% hydrocortisone, or 3% iodo with 1% hydrocortisone, cream, lotion and ointment.)

DRUG SPECIFICS:
This combination is possibly useful in eczema, cutaneous or mucocutaneous *Candida* infections, and other inflammatory skin conditions. Note: Patients sensitive to iodine preparations may show reactions to this drug. Use with caution in herpes simplex, TB, and viral infections. Warn the patient that this preparation may stain fabric, nails, hair, and skin. If ointment is used occlusively, the medication may cause increased steroid absorption. See hydrocortisone plus specific antibacterials for additional information.

ADMINISTRATION AND DOSAGE SPECIFICS:
Adults and children:
Cream: Use for moist, weepy lesions. The dosage with the least hydrocortisone is the best for extensive use. Apply 2 to 4 times per day.
Lotion: For intertriginous use. Shake well. Apply as for cream.
Ointment: For dry, scaling lesions. Apply as for cream.

TRIAMCINOLONE PLUS ANTIFUNGALS

PRODUCTS (TRADE NAME):
Mycolog, MycoTriacet, Mytrex (Contains 100,000 U nystatin, 0.25% neomycin, 0.25 mg gramcidin, and 0.1% triamcinolone/gm in cream and ointment.)

DRUG SPECIFICS:
The Food and Drug Administration considers this preparation "possibly effective" against an infection sensitive to the antifungal when an anti-inflammatory agent is also indicated. Use with caution in any fungal infection except candidiasis. See hydrocortisone plus antibiotics for additional information.
Caution: Ototoxicity and nephrotoxicity have been reported if this preparation has been overused or applied to a large area of denuded skin. It may be used occlusively.

ADMINISTRATION AND DOSAGE SPECIFICS:
Adults and children: Apply to affected areas 2 to 3 times a day.

TOPICAL ANORECTAL HYDROCORTISONE EMOLLIENTS

PRODUCTS (TRADE NAME):

Anugard-HC, Anusol-HC, Hemorrhoidal HC, Hemacetate/HC, Rectacort (Available with hydrocortisone 5 mg/gm, bismuth subgallate, benzyl benzoate, Peruvian balsam, and zinc oxide in a cream; and in 10 mg hydrocortisone suppositories.)

DRUG SPECIFICS:

This is a glucocorticoid emollient for treatment of pain, itching, or discomfort from hemorrhoids, pruritus ani, proctitis, and other miscellaneous problems. This is not an antibacterial preparation and thus is not to be used solely in rectal infections. Stains on clothing may be removed with household detergent.

ADMINISTRATION AND DOSAGE SPECIFICS:

Adults:

Cream: Apply to the exterior anorectal area and gently rub in. Apply internally with special applicator. Apply 3 to 4 times a day for 3 to 5 days or until the infection subsides.

Suppository: Insert one suppository in the morning and one before bedtime.

TOPICAL COMBINATIONS—MISCELLANEOUS

PRODUCTS (TRADE NAME):

Cordran-N (Available with 0.5% neomycin sulfate and fluradrenolide 0.05%.) **NeoDecadron** (Available with 0.5% neomycin sulfate and 0.1% dexamethasone phosphate in cream.) **Neo-Synalar** (Available with 0.5% neomycin sulfate and 0.025% fluocinolone acetonide in cream.)

DRUG SPECIFICS:

See hydrocortisone plus specific antibiotics for additional information.

ADMINISTRATION AND DOSAGE SPECIFICS:

Cream: Rub in scant amount 2 to 3 times a day.

Ointment: Apply a thin film 2 to 3 times a day.

Molly Craig Billingsley

ANESTHETICS FOR MUCOUS MEMBRANES AND SKIN

ACTION OF THE DRUG: These products act by inhibiting conduction of nerve impulses from sensory nerves by altering permeability of the cell membrane to ions.

They are readily absorbed from mucous membranes, thus increasing their effectiveness in traumatized tissue.

ASSESSMENT:

INDICATIONS: These products are used primarily in treatment of local skin disorders such as pruritus, pain, and discomfort due to fungus infections, skin burns and scalds, wounds, bruises, sunburn, insect bites, episiotomy, eczema, diaper rash, prickly heat, and dermatological irritation due to plant toxins. They may also be used for local anesthesia prior to surgery on mucous membranes throughout the body.

SUBJECTIVE-OBJECTIVE: Patient may present with complaints of trauma, or exposure to irritating substances such as sun, insects, or poisonous plants. Area affected may be abraded, or may have indications of erythema and swelling.

PLAN:

CONTRAINDICATIONS: Do not give to individuals with hypersensitivity to any of the products. These products should not be used in the presence of secondary infection to the area. These medications are not indicated for ophthalmic use.

WARNINGS: Significant systemic absorption may take place if extensive areas are treated. Exercise caution in persistent, severe, or extensive skin disorders. Safety for use in pregnancy has not been demonstrated.

PRECAUTIONS: Use minimum dosage possible of all local anesthestics. Lidocaine should be used in patients with heart block or who have potential for severe shock. Topical use of anesthetics in the mouth may interfere with swallowing, and thus may pose a danger for small children. Food should not be taken within 60 minutes of the medication in order to reduce chances of aspiration.

IMPLEMENTATION:

DRUG INTERACTIONS: None anticipated in normal dosage.

ADMINISTRATION AND DOSAGE: Preparations come in gel, spray, ointment or liquid for topical application, or may come in parenteral form for local injection.

IMPLEMENTATION CONSIDERATIONS:
—Obtain a complete health history regarding the nature of the problem.
—Use the smallest amount possible in order to minimize systemic effects.

WHAT THE PATIENT NEEDS TO KNOW:
—This medication is to help reduce pain temporarily. You may feel numbness at the site for a short time, with feeling gradually returning to the area.
—Report any new or troubling sensations in this area to your health care provider.
—If you are taking this medication as a gargle or mouth medication, do

not eat at least 60 minutes after using medication since swallowing may be difficult. Food and gum should be avoided while mouth is anesthetized, since biting of tongue or buccal mucosa may occur.

EVALUATION:

ADVERSE REACTIONS: Most reactions to these products represent allergic processes demonstrated by urticaria, pruritus, edema, contact dermatitis, and cutaneous lesions. Rare anaphylactoid reactions with fatalities have been reported. Burning, stinging, swelling, erythema, tenderness, and tissue irritation with occasional necrosis and sloughing may rarely be seen. Urethritis with and without bleeding has also been occasionally found.

OVERDOSAGE: Effects result from high plasma levels due to excessive dosage or rapid absorption. Oral lidocaine has promoted seizures in some children. Methemoglobinemia has been noted following topical applications of benzocaine or lidocaine for teething discomfort and as a laryngeal anesthetic.

PARAMETERS TO MONITOR: Check site of injury. Monitor for any adverse effects.

BENZOCAINE (ETHYL AMINOBENZOATE)

PRODUCTS (TRADE NAME):
Ambesol (Available in 6.3% liquid.) **Americaine** (Available in 20% ointment, aerosol or gel.) **Benzocaine Topical** (Available in 5% cream and ointment.) **Burntame** (Available in 20% aerosol.) **Cetacin** (Available in ointment, liquid, spray or gel.) **Derma Medicone** (Available in ointment.) **Dermoplast** (Available in 20% aerosol.) **Foille** (Available in 2% ointment or liquid.) **Hurricaine** (Available in 20% liquid, gel or spray.) **Medicone Dressing** (Available in cream.) **San Cura** (Available in ointment.) **Solarcaine** (Available in 1% cream, .5% lotion, 0.4% aerosol.) **Unguentine** (Available in 3% aerosol.)

DRUG SPECIFICS:
Benzocaine gel is indicated for the relief of toothaches. The solution and gel are indicated for the treatment of wounds, ulcers, lesions, and other disorders of the oral mucosa. Any form of benzocaine is used for the relief of pruritus, pain and inflammation of the skin. Benzocaine rectal ointment is used for hemorrhoids or rectal irritation.

The use of this product is contraindicated if the patient is hypersensitive to procaine or other para-aminobenzoic acid derivatives. Problems with benzocaine and pregnant women or nursing mothers have not been documented. However, one should always consider the risk-benefit ratio. Cautious use of benzocaine is necessary with infants as methemoglobinemia may develop from increased absorption. Carefully consider use of this product in the presence of bleeding hemorrhoids, secondary bacterial infections, sepsis, or severe traumatized mucosa in the treatment area, or severe and extensive skin disorders.

Discontinue this product if redness, rash, or pruritus develops. Avoid contact of benzocaine with the eyes.

ADMINISTRATION AND DOSAGE SPECIFICS:

Benzocaine topical aerosol solution:
Adults and children 2 years and older: Apply 20% aerosol to affected area 2 to 3 times daily.

Benzocaine gel:
Adults: Apply 20% gel to gums or oral cavity as needed.
Children: Apply 5% gel sparingly to gums as needed.

BUTAMBEN PICRATE

PRODUCTS (TRADE NAME):
Butesin Picrate (Available in 1% ointment.)

DRUG SPECIFICS:

Butesin picrate is indicated for the temporary relief of pain caused by minor burns. This product should not be applied repeatedly to large surfaces. If a rash or other irritation develops, discontinue use of drug. This drug stains and cannot be removed from animal fibers (silk, wool or hair.)

ADMINISTRATION AND DOSAGE SPECIFICS:

Apply sparingly to small areas as needed.

COCAINE ALKALOID, COCAINE HYDROCHLORIDE

PRODUCTS (TRADE NAME):
Cocaine HCL Solvets (Available in 135 mg soluble tablets.) **Cocaine HCl U.S.P.** (Supplied in bulk powder of 2 and 4 ounces.) Not available commercially.

DRUG SPECIFICS:

Topical application of cocaine blocks nerve conduction and produces surface anesthesia and local vasoconstriction. This product is now primarily used for nasal or throat procedures. Cocaine is contraindicated for systemic or ophthalmic use or with sepsis in the area to be treated. Use with caution in those with a history of drug sensitivities or drug abuse.

When used in the throat, give the patient nothing to drink until sensation returns. Systemic absorption can produce euphoria, excitement, restlessness, tremors, convulsions, nausea, vomiting, chills, fever, abdominal pain, elevated blood pressure, tachycardia, tachypnea, ventricular fibrillation or respiratory failure. Continued use of this product can result in addiction and tolerance.

ADMINISTRATION AND DOSAGE SPECIFICS:
Used topically as a 1% or 2% solution at the discretion of the physician.

CYCLOMETHYCAINE SULFATE

PRODUCTS (TRADE NAME):
Surfacaine (Available in 0.5% cream, 1% ointment and 0.75% jelly.)
DRUG SPECIFICS:
Surfacaine is used as a topical anesthetic and lubricant on nontraumatized, accessible mucous membranes prior to examination and instrumentation. The use of this product is contraindicated in the presence of hypersensitivity. Do not use in the eyes. Discontinue use of Surfacaine if irritation develops. A brief burning or stinging sensation may be felt prior to the anesthetic effect.
ADMINISTRATION AND DOSAGE SPECIFICS:
At the discretion of the practitioner. Limit is 30 ml/12 hrs.

DIBUCAINE HYDROCHLORIDE

PRODUCTS (TRADE NAME):
D-Caine, Dibucaine HCl (Available in 1% ointment.) **Nupercainal** (Available in 1% or 0.5% cream.)
DRUG SPECIFICS:
This product is used for painful skin conditions such as abrasions, minor burns, and sunburn. It is also used to provide relief from the discomfort of hemorrhoids.
Do not use Nupercainal ointment or cream in or near eyes. Discontinue use if irritation develops. Cleanse surface to be treated prior to application of the drug.
ADMINISTRATION AND DOSAGE SPECIFICS:
Adults and children: Apply *ointment or cream* sparingly to affected area 2 to 3 times daily.
Suppositories: Insert one suppository rectally in the morning, evening and after each bowel movement. Limit 6 in 24 hours.

DYCLONINE HYDROCHLORIDE

PRODUCTS (TRADE NAME):
Dyclone (Available in 0.5% and 1% solution.)

DRUG SPECIFICS:

Dyclonine 0.5% solution is indicated for the anesthetizing of wounds, lesions, ulcers of the oral mucosa, for the suppression of the gag reflex during dental or other types of oral surgery, and for relief of pain associated with anogenital lesions. Dyclonine is also used to anesthetize mucous membranes prior to endoscopic procedures and instrumentation of the urethra and urinary tract.

As this drug is a ketone, there is less probability of a hypersensitive reaction. Do not use for extended periods in patients with chronic conditions.

Dyclonine reacts with iodine-containing contrast agents used in pyelography. If using dyclonine prior to cystoscopic procedures but following pyelography, there will be interference with visualization due to the precipitation of iodine.

ADMINISTRATION AND DOSAGE SPECIFICS:

Mucous membrane anesthesia: 40 to 200 mg topical as a 0.5% or 1% solution. Limit is 200 mg.

HEXYLCAINE HYDROCHLORIDE

PRODUCTS (TRADE NAME):

Cyclaine (Available in 5% (50 mg/ml) solution.)

DRUG SPECIFICS:

Hexylcaine is indicated as a topical anesthetic to prevent and control pain during endoscopic procedures and instrumentation of the urinary tract. It is also used on the mucous membranes of the respiratory tract prior to endoscopy, intubation or other procedures.

The onset of action of this drug is 5 minutes and duration of action is approximately 30 minutes.

As with any drug, hypersensitivity is possible. If untoward reactions occur, discontinue use of this product and treat symptomatically.

ADMINISTRATION AND DOSAGE SPECIFICS:

Not to exceed 500 mg.

LIDOCAINE

PRODUCTS (TRADE NAME):

Anestacon (Available in 2% solutions.) **Lida-Mantle Cream** (Available in 3% cream.) **Lidocaine HCl** (Available in 5% ointment.) **Ungentine Plus** (Available in 2% cream). **Xylocaine** (Available in 2% jelly, 2.5 and 5% ointment, 4% solution, 2% viscous solution, and 2% and 4% spray solutions.)

DRUG SPECIFICS:

Lidocaine ointment and jelly are used as dental anesthetics. Lidocaine jelly is used to prevent and control pain during endoscopic procedures and instrumentation of the urinary tract. Lidocaine (excluding aerosols and creams) is used for anesthesia of respiratory tract mucous membranes prior to endoscopy. The ointment form of this drug is also indicated for the relief of inflammation, pruritus and pain of skin disorders.

As with any topical drug, absorption is increased with traumatized skin or mucous membranes. The duration of action of topical lidocaine is approximately 45 minutes.

If the gag reflex has been suppressed, monitor patient to avoid aspiration. Should hypersensitivity develop, discontinue the drug and treat symptomatically.

ADMINISTRATION AND DOSAGE SPECIFICS:

Dosage listed is for adults. Dosage must be individualized for children.

Ointment: Apply 5% to oropharyngeal mucosa as needed. Apply 2.5% to skin as needed. Limit is 35 grams daily.

Jelly: Apply small amount to catheter prior to intubation of esophagus, larynx, or trachea. Limit is 30 ml/12 hours.

Viscous solution: Use 300 mg (15 ml) swished in mouth and swallowed every 3 hours as needed. Limit is 8 doses (2.4 gm) in 24 hours.

Solution: Use 40 to 200 mg as a 4% solution to mucous membranes prior to endoscopy.

Spray solution: Use 20 to 200 mg (0.5 to 5 ml) as a 2 or 4% solution to pharynx or larynx prior to endoscopy. Limit is 3.0 mg/kg.

PRAMOXINE HYDROCHLORIDE

PRODUCTS (TRADE NAME):

ProctoFoam 1% (Available in 1% nonsteroidal aerosol.) **Tronothane** 1% (Available in 1% cream.)

DRUG SPECIFICS:

ProctoFoam is indicated for anorectal inflammation, pruritus, and pain associated with hemorrhoids, proctitis, cryptitis, fissures, and surgery. Tronothane is indicated for pain and pruritus associated with dermatoses, minor burns, hemorrhoids, anal fissures.

These products are contraindicated in persons hypersensitive to any of the ingredients. They are not for prolonged use. Do not use in the eyes or nose. Do not apply to large surface areas. Discontinue use if pain, swelling, redness or other irritation develops. Cleanse area to be treated prior to application.

ADMINISTRATION AND DOSAGE SPECIFICS:

Tronothane: Apply sparingly every 3 to 4 hours as needed.

ProctoFoam: One applicatorful rectally 2 to 3 times daily and after each bowel movement.

TETRACAINE HYDROCHLORIDE

PRODUCTS (TRADE NAME):
Pontocaine (Available in 1% cream, 2% solution and 0.5% ointment.)

DRUG SPECIFICS:
Pontocaine is indicated for the relief of discomfort from hemorrhoids and minor skin disorders (contact dermatitis, sunburn.) It is contraindicated in those with hypersensitivity to procaine or other para-aminobenzoic acid derivatives. Should irritation develop from use of Pontocaine, discontinue this product. Cleanse area to be treated prior to application of the drug.

ADMINISTRATION AND DOSAGE SPECIFICS:
Adults and children: Apply sparingly to affected areas 3 to 4 times daily. Limit for adult is 28 gm in 24 hours; limit for children is 7 gm in 24 hours.

Mary Ann Bolter

ANTI-INFECTIVES AND ANTIFUNGALS—TOPICAL

ACTION OF THE DRUG: Antibiotics and antifungals are used in low concentrations on the skin for bactericidal, bacteriostatic or fungicidal effects.

ASSESSMENT:

INDICATIONS: Antibiotics and antifungal products may be used on the skin to prevent and control superficial infections which develop from minor trauma or injury.

SUBJECTIVE: Patient may complain of localized itching, burning, soreness, or irritation. Patient may also present with skin wounds or sores that may not heal.

OBJECTIVE: Superficial and well-localized evidence of trauma, erythema, swelling may be present. Small open lesions or wounds may also be apparent. In complaints of hemorrhoids, small external tags may be documented.

PLAN:

CONTRAINDICATIONS: Do not use in the presence of hypersensitivity.

PRECAUTIONS: Carefully consider use of these preparations where active bleeding is present, in secondary bacterial infections, sepsis, severely traumatized mucosa in the treatment area, or severe and extensive skin disorders. Consult specific product information for other relevant contraindications.

IMPLEMENTATION:

ADMINISTRATION AND DOSAGE: These topical preparations should be used sparingly on small areas. Large open wounds are to be avoided. Usually area is not occluded with a dressing after application.

IMPLEMENTATION CONSIDERATIONS:

—Obtain a complete health history, including the presence of hypersensitivity, underlying systemic disease and concurrent use of other medications.

—If the condition worsens or does not improve, stop the drug and re-evaluate.

—As with any antibiotic, overgrowth of non-susceptible organisms may develop. This usually occurs with prolonged use of the drug.

—Allergic contact sensitivity to these topical agents is rare with the exception of neomycin.

WHAT THE PATIENT NEEDS TO KNOW:

—Apply this preparation as directed by your health care provider. If the condition worsens, or does not improve, return to your health care provider.

—This product is to be applied sparingly and frequently. The area to be treated should be cleansed of adherent crusts or particles. Do not cover with a dressing.

—Do not use in eyes or on large surface areas.

—Watch for signs of local irritation or renewed signs of infection.

—Some products may stain clothing and skin.

EVALUATION:

ADVERSE REACTIONS: Watch for local sensitivity or overgrowth of infection.

PARAMETERS TO MONITOR: Evaluate for therapeutic effects and development of adverse reactions.

ANTIBIOTICS

PRODUCTS: (See Table 9-3.)

DRUG SPECIFICS:

These products are indicated for superficial infections of the skin caused by susceptible organisms, minor wounds, and burns and abrasions. Allergic contact sensitivity to these topical agents is rare with the exception of neomycin. However, if sensitivity is known to exist (or develops), do not use the product. As with any antibiotic, overgrowth of nonsusceptible organisms may develop. This usually occurs with prolonged use of the drug.

Do not use these products on large surface areas. Do not use in the eyes. If the condition worsens or does not improve, stop the drug and reevaluate. These products are to be applied frequently. The area to be treated should be cleansed of adherent crusts and debris. Do not apply under occlusive dressings. (See section on antibiotics for more information).

ADMINISTRATION AND DOSAGE SPECIFICS:
Adults and children: Apply sparingly 3 to 6 times daily, as needed.

TABLE 9-3. ANTIBIOTICS

Generic Name	Trade Name	Strength
Bacitracin	Baciguent, Bacitin	1/2 oz tube, 500 U/gm ointment
Chloramphenicol	Chloromycetin 1%	1 oz tube ointment
Chlortetracycline HCl	Aureomycin 3%	1/2 and 1 oz tube ointment
Erythromycin	Ilotycin	1/2 and 1 oz tube ointment
		1 lb jar 10 mg/gm
Gentamicin	Garamycin 0.1%	15 mg tube ointment
	Gentamicin 0.1%	or cream
Neomycin sulfate	Myciguent, Neomycin	1/2 , 1 and 4 oz tube

ANTIBIOTIC COMBINATIONS

PRODUCTS (TRADE NAME):
Neo-Polycin Ointment, Neosporin (Available in 5000 U Polymyxin B sulfate and 3.5 mg neomycin and 400 U zinc bacitricin/gm.) **Polysporin Ointment** (Available in 10,000 U Polymyxin B sulfate and 500 U zinc bacitracin/gm.)

DRUG SPECIFICS:
These products are indicated for topical infections (primary or secondary) caused by susceptible organisms. The use of antibiotic mixtures is justified due to the difficulty in fast identification of the causative organism, the frequent presence of more than one pathogen, and the relative safety of these drugs when used topically.

Contact dermatitis with topical antibiotics is rare, except for neomycin. Polysporin contains no neomycin. These multiple antibiotics contain bacitracin and polymyxin B. Neosporin and Neo-Polycin also contain neomycin.

These products are contraindicated in the presence of hypersensitivity. If sensitivity develops, discontinue use of the product. Do not use in the eyes. Do not use on large surface areas.

As with any antibiotic, prolonged use may result in overgrowth of nonsusceptible organisms. If the condition worsens or does not improve, stop treatment and reevaluate. This product is to be applied frequently. The area to be treated should be cleansed of adherent crusts and debris. Do not apply under occlusive dressings. (See section on antibiotics for more information).

ADMINISTRATION AND DOSAGE SPECIFICS:
Adults and children: Apply sparingly 3 to 6 times daily, as needed.

ANTI-INFECTIVE ANTI-FUNGALS—TOPICAL

PRODUCTS:(See Table 9-4.)

TABLE 9-4. ANTIFUNGALS

Generic Name	Trade Name	Strength
Acrisorcin	Akrinol Cream	2 mg/gm cream
Ciclopiroxolamine	Loprox	1% cream
Clotrimazole	Lotrimin	1% cream in 15, 30, 45 gm tube; 1% solution in 10 and 30 ml
Econazole nitrate	Spectazole	1% cream
Haloprogin	Halotex	1% cream in 15, 30 gm tube; 1% solution in 15 and 30 ml
Iodochlorhydroxyquin	Iodochlor	3% cream or ointment
	Quin III	3% cream or ointment
	Torofor	3% cream or ointment
	Vioform	3% cream or ointment in 1 oz tube.
Miconazole nitrate	MicaTin	2% cream in 15 gm; 1 and 3 oz tube;
	Monistat-Derm	2% lotion 12 and 30 ml
Tolnaftate	Aftate Tinactin	1% cream in 15 gm tube and 10 ml solution, 45 gm powder or 100 gm powder aerosol
Triacetin	Enzactin	Cream in 1 oz tube
Undecylenic acid	Cruex	Cream in 0.5 oz tube; powder in 1.8, 3.5, or 5.5 oz aerosol and 1.5 oz squeeze bottle

TABLE 9-4—Continued

Generic Name	Trade Name	Strength
	Desenex	Spray-on powder (2.7, 5.5 oz aerosol); powder (1.5 and 3 oz) tube); liquid (1.5 oz pump spray); penetrating foam (1.5 oz aerosol); and soap (3.25 oz bar).

DRUG SPECIFICS:

As a group, these drugs are used to treat tinea pedis, tinea cruris, tinea corporis and tinea versicolea Halotex and Tinactin are also used for tinea manuum.

Use of these products is contraindicated in the presence of hypersensitivity. The safe use of these topical antifungal agents has not been established for pregnant women and nursing mothers. These products are not to be used in the eyes.

Irritation or sensitivity may develop. If this occurs, discontinue use of the product. Fungal infections may take longer than other infections to respond to treatment. However, if there has been no response within 4 weeks of therapy, reevaluate the diagnosis.

Development of fungal infections is enhanced by heat, moisture, and maceration. If these factors cannot be changed, probabilities of cure are less. Intertriginous or interdigital areas should be thoroughly dried after bathing or showering. (See section on antifungals for more information).

ADMINISTRATION AND DOSAGE SPECIFICS:

Product should be continued for full treatment period even if improvement is noted.

Adults and children: Apply sparingly to affected area once in the morning and once in the evening.

Mary Ann Bolter

ANTIPSORIATICS

AMMONIATED MERCURY

ACTION OF THE DRUG: Ammoniated mercury has an antiseptic action on the skin. It accelerates the scaling and healing of dry lesions in chronic psoriasis.

ASSESSMENT:

INDICATIONS: Used in psoriasis and seborrheic dermatitis.

SUBJECTIVE: History of plaques with scaling of skin (particularly elbows, knees, scalp, genitalia, and upper gluteal fold).

OBJECTIVE: Psoriasis consists of erythematous, well-circumscribed plaques covered by silvery scales. Most lesions are asymptomatic; however, pruritus has been reported in approximately 20 percent of patients.

PLAN:

CONTRAINDICATIONS: Do not use if known hypersensitivity to ammoniated mercury exists.

WARNINGS: Continued use in infants and young children is contraindicated since toxic amounts of mercury may be absorbed through skin in some rare circumstances.

PRECAUTIONS: Product is for external use only. It may cause skin irritation. Do not apply to large areas of the body, sunburned or inflamed skin, or open wounds. Discontinue use if redness or swelling develops or signs of infection or rash appear.

IMPLEMENTATION:

DRUG INTERACTIONS: Do not use in conjunction with topical iodine or sulfur-containing products.

PRODUCTS (TRADE NAME):

Ammoniated Mercury (Available in a 5% or 10% ointment.) **Emersal** (Available in 5% lotion with 2.5% salicylic acid.)

ADMINISTRATION AND DOSAGE: Apply 1 or 2 times daily.

IMPLEMENTATION CONSIDERATIONS:

—This product must not be applied to extensive areas of the skin, open wound, or inflamed skin.

—Consider other skin medications patient may be using to make certain there will be no drug interactions.

WHAT THE PATIENT NEEDS TO KNOW:

—Avoid use of topical iodine or sulfur-containing products while using this drug.

—This product may cause local allergic reactions. If rash or irritation occurs, discontinue use and consult your health care provider.

EVALUATION:

ADVERSE REACTIONS: Since ammoniated mercury is a potential sensitizer, allergic reaction may occur following application.

PARAMETERS TO MONITOR: Observe for therapeutic effect and signs of clinical improvement.

Carol Burke

ANTHRALIN (DITHRANOL)

ACTION OF THE DRUG: Anthralin inhibits enzyme metabolism and reduces epidermal mitotic activity.

ASSESSMENT:

INDICATIONS: Used in the treatment of severe or widespread psoriatic lesions.

SUBJECTIVE: History of plaques with scaling of skin (particularly elbows, knees, scalp, genitalia, upper gluteal fold).

OBJECTIVE: Erythematous, well-circumscribed plaques covered by silvery scales. Most lesions are asymptomatic; however, pruritus has been reported in approximately 20 percent of patients. Punctate pitting of nails or collections of subungual keratotic material are also characteristic.

PLAN:

CONTRAINDICATIONS: Do not use if there is a history of renal impairment or known hypersensitivity to drug.

WARNINGS: Do not use near eyes. Do not apply to face, genitalia, or intertriginous skin areas.

PRECAUTIONS: Safe use of this drug during pregnancy and lactation has not been established. Anthralin was shown to have some co-carcinogenic and tumorigenic activity in long-term studies using mice.

IMPLEMENTATION:

PRODUCTS (TRADE NAME):
Anthra-Derm (Available in 0.1%, 0.25%, 0.5%, 1.0% Ointment). **Drithocreme** (Available in 0.1%, 0.25%, and 0.5% cream). **Lasan Unguent** (Available in 0.4% ointment.)

ADMINISTRATION AND DOSAGE: Apply a thin layer of 0.1% ointment once or twice a day for two weeks. It may be applied at bedtime without a dressing. May increase to 0.25% if adjacent normal skin does not become erythematous or hyperpigmented. If necessary, after using 0.25% for an additional two to three weeks, may prescribe 0.5%. It is necessary in some cases to use 1.0%.

With Lasan Unguent, apply at bedtime and remove in morning with warm liquid petrolatum followed by a bath. For scalp, massage into affected areas, avoiding scalp margins. Shampoo in the morning.

IMPLEMENTATION CONSIDERATIONS:
—Obtain a complete health history, including history of renal disease and possibility of pregnancy or breast-feeding.
—Observe for signs of further irritation.

WHAT THE PATIENT NEEDS TO KNOW:
—Follow directions for use carefully.
—Medication causes urine color to change to red.
—Keep away from eyes. Anthralin may cause severe irritation if accidentaly rubbed into eyes. Notify health care provider at once if this happens.
—Use medication only on chronic psoriasis patches. Avoid contact with normal skin and inflamed lesions.
—A protective film of petrolatum applied to areas surrounding plaques may prevent irritation of normal skin.
—Anthralin stains clothing and skin and may temporarily discolor grey or white hair. Use special pillowcases or bedding when using medication overnight.

EVALUATION:

ADVERSE REACTIONS: *Dermatologic:* pustular folliculitis. *Renal:* albuminuria, casts.

PARAMETERS TO MONITOR: Monitor for therapeutic effect and development of adverse reactions. Weekly urinalysis with microscopic examination to look for casts should be performed.

Carol Burke

ANTISEBORRHEIC PRODUCTS

ANTISEBORRHEIC SHAMPOOS

ACTION OF THE DRUG: Salicylic acid and sulfur are used in combination because salicylic acid promotes shedding and softening of the horny cell layer while sulfur inhibits the growth of microorganisms. Tar preparations are used for their antipruritic, antiseborrheic, and antibacterial effects.

ASSESSMENT:

INDICATIONS: Used for the treatment of itching and scaling of the scalp associated with seborrhea and dandruff.

SUBJECTIVE: History of pruritus and flaking of the scalp.

OBJECTIVE: Profuse, dry, powdery scales distributed over scalp.

PLAN:

PRECAUTIONS: Avoid contact with eyes. If signs of irritation develop, temporarily discontinue use.

IMPLEMENTATION:

PRODUCTS (TRADE NAME):
Capitrol (Available in 2% chloroxine shampoo.) **Danex** (Available in 1% pyrithione zinc shampoo.) **Fostex** (Available with 2% sulfur and 2% salicylic acid as a cream or liquid shampoo.) **DHS Zinc** (Available in 2% pyrithione zinc shampoo.) **Head and Shoulders** (Available in 2% pyrithione zinc shampoo.) **Metasep, nu-FLOW** (Available in 2% parachlorometaxylenol shampoo.) **Sebex** (Available as 2% colloidal sulfur and 2% salicylic acid shampoo.) **Sebulex** (Available with 2% sulfur and 2% salicylic acid as a cream or lotion shampoo.) **Sebisol** (Available with 2% salicylic acid, 0.1% orthobenzylparachlorophenol and 1% betanaphthol shampoo.) **Sebutone** (Available with 0.5% coal tar, 2% sulfur and 2% salicylic acid as a liquid shampoo or cream.) **Xseb** (Available in 4% salicylic acid with surfactants shampoo.) **Zincon** (Available in 1% pyrithione zinc shampoo.)

ADMINISTRATION AND DOSAGE: Massage into wet scalp for five minutes. Rinse and repeat. Rinse thoroughly. May use daily. Decrease to once or twice weekly as symptoms abate.

IMPLEMENTATION CONSIDERATIONS:
—Tolerance often develops to these preparations after a short time. It may be necessary to prescribe several shampoos and switch from one to another when one ceases to be effective.

—Prescription required for Sebutone.

WHAT THE PATIENT NEEDS TO KNOW:
—Avoid getting shampoo in eyes.

—If irritation develops, or if medication seems to stop working, temporarily discontinue medication and notify health care provider.

—With Sebutone, temporary discoloration of white, blond, bleached or tinted hair may occur although this is rare.

EVALUATION:

ADVERSE REACTIONS: localized skin irritation.

PARAMETERS TO MONITOR: Monitor for therapeutic effects and symptomatic relief of scaling and pruritus of scalp.

Carol Burke

POVIDONE-IODINE SHAMPOO

ACTION OF THE DRUG: Povidone-iodine is a broad-spectrum antimicrobial product.

ASSESSMENT:

INDICATIONS: This medication provides temporary relief of itching and scaling of the scalp. Used for treatment of dandruff.
SUBJECTIVE: History of pruritus and flaking of the scalp.
OBJECTIVE: Profuse, dry, powdery scales distributed over scalp.

PLAN:

PRECAUTIONS: Avoid contact with eyes. If signs of irritation develop, temporarily discontinue use.

IMPLEMENTATION:

PRODUCTS (TRADE NAME):
Betadine (Available in 7.5% shampoo).
ADMINISTRATION AND DOSAGE: Apply 2 tsp to hair and scalp. Lather with warm water and rinse. Repeat application and allow to remain on scalp five minutes. Rinse thoroughly. Use twice weekly until improvement is noted, and then decrease to weekly application.
IMPLEMENTATION CONSIDERATIONS:
—Patients often need to switch from one antiseborrheic product to another as tolerance to products develop.

WHAT THE PATIENT NEEDS TO KNOW:
—Avoid contact with eyes.
—If irritation to scalp develops, discontinue use.

EVALUATION:

PARAMETERS TO MONITOR: Monitor for therapeutic effects: decrease in scaling and pruritus of scalp.

Carol Burke

SELENIUM SULFIDE

ACTION OF THE DRUG: Selenium sulfide acts by decreasing epidermal proliferation and inhibiting mitotic activity. This medication is used to control mild to moderately severe seborrheic dermatitis.

ASSESSMENT:

INDICATIONS: Used for the treatment of chronic seborrhea.
SUBJECTIVE: History of pruritus and flaking of the scalp.
OBJECTIVE: Profuse, dry, powdery scales distributed over scalp.

PLAN:

CONTRAINDICATIONS: Do not use if scalp is cut or scratched or in the presence of acute inflammatory lesions.
WARNINGS: If swallowed, induce vomiting and contact health care provider. Do not use medication more than is recommended. Safety for use in infants has not been established.
PRECAUTIONS: Avoid contact with eyes. If medication gets into eyes, it is important to rinse with clear water for several minutes. Medication is to be used on hair and scalp only.

IMPLEMENTATION:

PRODUCTS (TRADE NAME):
Exsek (Available in 2.5% lotion shampoo.) **Selenium Sulfide, Selsun, Selsun Blue** (Available in 1% and 2.5% lotion shampoo.)
ADMINISTRATION AND DOSAGE: Medication should be stored in original container, closed tightly and away from heat.
Massage 1 or 2 teaspoonsful into wet scalp. Allow medicated shampoo to remain on scalp for 2 to 3 minutes. Rinse thoroughly. Repeat application and rinse thoroughly. Use two applications each week for two weeks, then weekly for two weeks, or even every 3 or 4 weeks depending upon control of symptoms.
IMPLEMENTATION CONSIDERATIONS:
—Obtain a complete health history, including history of skin/scalp problems, existence of any acute inflammatory lesions, drug allergies or sensitivities, medications which have been used in the past and patient response to these treatment.
—Prescription required for selenium sulfide.

WHAT THE PATIENT NEEDS TO KNOW:
—Use medication on hair and scalp only. Follow instructions on bottle. Avoid contact with eyes.

—In order to prevent possible discoloration of bleached, tinted, or permed hair, it is suggested that hair be thoroughly rinsed with cool water for at least five minutes after each treatment.
—Notify health care provider if undue scalp irritation develops.

EVALUATION:

ADVERSE REACTIONS: Dryness or oiliness of the hair and scalp, increased hair loss, discoloration of hair.
OVERDOSAGE: Systemic absorption of selenium sulfide from the scalp is unlikely; however, the drug is toxic if taken internally.
PARAMETERS TO MONITOR: Monitor therapeutic response, i.e. decrease in scaling and flaking of scalp.

Carol Burke

SULFACETAMIDE SODIUM

ACTION OF THE DRUG: Sulfacetamide sodium is bacteriostatic against organisms commonly involved in cutaneous infections.

ASSESSMENT:

INDICATIONS: Mild seborrheic dermatitis.
SUBJECTIVE: History of pruritus and flaking of the scalp.
OBJECTIVE: Profuse, dry, powdery scales distributed over scalp.

PLAN:

CONTRAINDICATIONS: History of topical sensitivity to sulfonamides.
WARNINGS: Discontinue use if irritation develops.

IMPLEMENTATION:

DRUG INTERACTIONS: This product is incompatible with silver preparations.
PRODUCTS (TRADE NAME):
Sebizon (Available in 10% lotion.)
ADMINISTRATION AND DOSAGE: Apply at bedtime and allow to remain on scalp overnight. Prior to application, shampoo hair and scalp with nonirritating shampoo. In severe cases with crusting and inflammation, apply twice a day.
IMPLEMENTATION CONSIDERATIONS:
—Obtain a complete health history, including allergies to sulfa preparations, or concurrent use of any silver preparations.
—Prescription is required for this product.

WHAT THE PATIENT NEEDS TO KNOW:
—Do not use in combination with any silver products.
—Use cautiously on areas where skin is denuded or abraded.
—If irritation develops, discontinue use and consult health care provider.

EVALUATION:

PARAMETERS TO MONITOR: Observe for therapeutic effect and symptomatic relief of symptoms.

Carol Burke

ANTIVIRAL AGENTS—TOPICAL

ACYCLOVIR

ACTION OF THE DRUG: Acyclovir interferes with herpes simplex virus DNA polymerase and the viral DNA replication is terminated.

ASSESSMENT:

INDICATIONS: This product is used for treating the lesions in the initial episodes of herpes genitalis and in limited non-life-threatening situations for mucocutaneous herpes simplex virus infections in immunocompromised patients. It is used to decrease healing time, and in some cases to decrease duration pf viral shedding and pain. There is no evidence of clinical benefit in recurrent herpes genitalis and of herpes labialis in non-immunocompromised patients, although there may be some decrease in the duration of viral shedding. Will not prevent transmission of infection to other persons or prevent recurrent infections when used in the absence of signs and symptoms.

SUBJECTIVE-OBJECTIVE: Patient presents with cutaneous lesions which are painful. Lesions are most common found on the genitalia, buccal-lingual areas or lips. Diagnosis should be confirmed through positive cultures for herpes simplex virus, and the finding of multinucleated giant cells in smears prepared from lesion exudate or scrapings. Differentiation between herpes simplex types 1 and 2 is not possible clinically, but may be made by fluorescein dyes.

PLAN:

COMPLICATIONS: Do not give to patients with known hypersensitivity to components of the drug.

WARNINGS: Do not use this product for ophthalmic lesions. Safety for use in pregnant or breast-feeding women has not been established.

PRECAUTIONS: Do not exceed recommended dosage or length of treatment schedules.

IMPLEMENTATION:

DRUG INTERACTIONS: None reported at present.

PRODUCTS (TRADE NAME):

Zovirax 15% (Available in 15 gm tubes with 50 mg/gm).

ADMINISTRATION AND DOSAGE: A finger cot or rubber glove should be used during application in order to avoid spread of infection to other body sites and spread of infection to others. Therapy should be started as soon as signs and symptoms develop.

Cover all lesions every 3 hours, 6 times a day for 6 days. Approximately one-half inch ribbon of ointment per 4 square inches of surface area should be used.

IMPLEMENTATION CONSIDERATIONS:

—Take a complete health history, including the contact, course of the disease, allergies, presence of other systemic illnesses, and possibility of pregnancy.

—Begin therapy as soon as possible once diagnosis has been made.

—Give emotional support and counseling regarding this new and at present incurable disease.

—Evaluate patient for presence of other sexually transmitted diseases.

—Report disease to county health department and comply with standard protocols for follow-up and monitoring of contacts.

—Product does not appear to be absorbed systemically.

WHAT THE PATIENT NEEDS TO KNOW:

—Use this ointment on the sores as instructed by your health care provider. It should be applied to all sores every 3 hours, 6 times daily.

—Do not use near eyes.

—Use gloves or plastic to cover hands when putting medication on sores. This should help prevent the spread of infection.

—Medication will not cure herpes, but may help to speed healing of the first infection. The average length of time for the first infection is 12 days. Recurrent problems generally last only 4-6 days. This medication will not prevent further outbreaks of herpes, and should not be taken prophylactically.

—While you have open sores you should avoid intimate contact with others since you may infection them. You should be careful about handling your personal towel and washcloths, keeping them away from others. Wash your hands carefully after going to the bathroom. If you have sores on your lips or in your mouth, use care in eating around others, using your toothbrush, and avoid kissing or close contact with others.

—Occasionally patients will note briefly stinging, burning, itching, or a rash when ointment is applied. Notify your health care provider if any of these symptoms become a problem.

EVALUATION:

ADVERSE REACTIONS: Mild pain, pruritus, vulvitis, and rash may be present.

PARAMETERS TO MONITOR: Watch for development of sensitivity and monitor therapeutic effects. Give patient emotional support and counseling, and refer to community groups organized for victims of herpes.

Marilyn W. Edmunds

BURN PREPARATIONS

MAFENIDE

ACTION OF THE DRUG: Mafenide is a synthetic antibacterial that appears to interfere with bacterial cellular metabolism. It is bacteriostatic against many gram-positive and gram-negative organisms, including staphylococci, streptococci, and *Pseudomonas* species. The medication is active in the presence of pus and serum.

ASSESSMENT:

INDICATIONS: This drug is used as adjunctive therapy in patients with second and third degree burn wounds.

SUBJECTIVE: History of burns or large open wounds.

OBJECTIVE: Erythema with blistering of skin. With third degree burns, skin may have brownish, leathery appearance.

PLAN:

CONTRAINDICATIONS: Do not use in presence of known hypersensitivity to mafenide.

WARNINGS: Safety of use during pregnancy has not been established. Because of long-term effects, it is not recommended for use in women of childbearing potential unless burned area covers more than 20% of the total body surface or need exceeds possible risks to any future fetus.

PRECAUTIONS: Mafenide acts as a weak carbonic anhydrase inhibitor and may cause systemic acidosis. Use with caution in patients with acute renal failure or pulmonary dysfunction.

IMPLEMENTATION:

PRODUCTS (TRADE NAME):
Sulfamylon (Available in 85 mg/gm cream.)
ADMINISTRATION AND DOSAGE: Burns should be cleansed and debrided prior to application of medication with sterile gloved hand. Apply once or twice daily to a thickness of approximately 1/16 inch. No dressing is required, but burned areas should remain covered with mafenide. Therapy should continue until burn site is ready for grafting or is healing well.

IMPLEMENTATION CONSIDERATIONS:
—Obtain thorough health history, including history of drug allergies, presence of pulmonary or renal impairment, and possibility of pregnancy.
—Observe for adverse effects. It is difficult to distinguish between the effect of a severe burn and a reaction to this medication.

WHAT THE PATIENT NEEDS TO KNOW:
—Application of medication may cause a burning sensation.
—Report any new or uncomfortable symptoms to health care provider.

EVALUATION:

ADVERSE REACTIONS: *Dermatologic:* burning sensation or pain upon application. *Hypersensitivity:* blisters, edema, eosinophilia, erythema, facial edema, hives, pruritus, rash. *Other:* acidosis, bone marrow depression (rare), elevations in serum chloride, excoriations and bleeding of skin, fatal hemolytic anemia (rare), lowered arterial carbon dioxide pressure, porphyria (rare), tachypnea.

PARAMETERS TO MONITOR: Monitor for therapeutic effects and development of adverse reactions. Close monitoring of acid-base balance is required, especially when there are extensive second degree or partial thickness burns and in patients with compromised respiratory and/or renal function.

Carol Burke

NITROFURAZONE

ACTION OF THE DRUG: Nitrofurazone is bactericidal against most bacteria commonly involved in surface infections. It inhibits enzymes required for carbohydrate metabolism.

ASSESSMENT:

INDICATIONS: Nitrofurazone is used topically on second and third degree burns when bacterial resistance poses a potential threat and in skin grafting where there is a possibility of graft rejection and/or infection of the donor site because of contamination. It can be used for prophylaxis and treatment of infections of the skin.

SUBJECTIVE: History of burn or skin wound.

OBJECTIVE: Erythema with blistering of skin. With third degree burn, skin may have brownish, leathery appearance.

PLAN:

CONTRAINDICATIONS: Do not use if there is known hypersensitivity to nitrofurazone.

WARNINGS: Safe use during pregnancy has not been established. It is also not recommended for use in women of childbearing potential unless the need outweighs the possible risk. Mammary tumors have been produced in female rats when fed high doses of this medication; however, it is not known if this finding has any relevance to the topical administration of nitrofurazone in humans.

PRECAUTIONS: This drug should be used with caution in patients with G-6-PD deficiency. The use of this medication may lead to overgrowth of nonsusceptible bacterial or fungal organisms.

IMPLEMENTATION:

PRODUCTS (TRADE NAME):
Furacin (Available in 0.2% soluble dressing or 0.2% topical cream.) **Nitrofurazone** (Available in 0.2% soluble dressing.)

ADMINISTRATION AND DOSAGE:
Soluble dressing: Apply 0.2% solution directly to lesion. Reapply once daily or weekly.

Topical Cream: Apply 0.2% cream directly to lesion once daily or every few days.

IMPLEMENTATION CONSIDERATIONS:
—Obtain a thorough health history, including presence of drug allergies, G-6-PD deficiency, and possibility of pregnancy.
—Watch for overgrowth of nonsusceptible bacterial or fungal organisms.

WHAT THE PATIENT NEEDS TO KNOW:
—Apply this medication exactly as shown by your health care provider.
—Medication may be put directly on burned area, or may be placed first on a gauze pad.
—Contact dermatitis and sensitivity may occur. If irritation occurs, contact health care provider.

EVALUATION:

ADVERSE REACTIONS: Local sensitivity or contact dermatitis may occur.

In rare instances of severe contact dermatitis, steroid administration may be indicated.

OVERDOSAGE: No significant toxicity with topical applications.

PARAMETERS TO MONITOR: Observe for therapeutic effects and appearance of local sensitivity reactions or overgrowth of nonsusceptible organisms.

Carol Burke

SILVER NITRATE

ACTION OF THE DRUG: Silver nitrate establishes an antibacterial environment for epithelialization and tissue graft proliferation.

ASSESSMENT:

INDICATIONS: Used to maintain wet, bacteriostatic wound dressing for burns.

SUBJECTIVE: History of burns.

OBJECTIVE: Erythema, blistering of skin. With third degree burns, skin may have brownish, leathery appearance.

PLAN:

WARNINGS: Silver nitrate is for external use only. It may cause burns itself if applied directly to skin. Methemoglobinemia has caused fatality during therapy with 0.5% silver nitrate solution. The presence of cyanosis or brownish discoloration of fresh blood sample is indicative of possible methemoglobinemia and necessitate discontinuance of preparation.

PRECAUTIONS: Serum electrolytes need to be monitored and replaced as necessary if burn is extensive. Since electrolyte losses may be more severe in infants and children, more frequent monitoring may be necessary for this population.

IMPLEMENTATION:

PRODUCTS (TRADE NAME):

Silver Nitrate (Available in wax ampules No. 146.)

ADMINISTRATION AND DOSAGE: Dressing should be saturated with warmed solution and applied to burn wound. Mold dressing to body surface and cover with dry dressing. Reapply solution every two hours. Dressings should be changed at least once daily initially, and should be changed more often when wound drainage increases.

IMPLEMENTATION CONSIDERATIONS:

—Medication is for external use only. Any contact with eyes or skin necessitates flushing with water for at least 15 minutes.

—Medication should be applied to well-cleansed wounds to promote penetration into tissues.

—Patient's electrolyte balance needs to be monitored closely.

—Observe for signs of brownish discoloration of fresh blood samples or cyanosis.

WHAT THE PATIENT NEEDS TO KNOW:

—Avoid direct contact of skin and eyes with solution since medication is very strong. If skin or eyes accidentally come in contact with medication, flush with water for at least 15 minutes and notify health care provider.

EVALUATION:

ADVERSE REACTIONS: Burning of skin from direct contact with medication.

PARAMETERS TO MONITOR: Observe condition of skin; watch for signs of healing, infection, sloughing of tissue. Serum electrolytes should be monitored.

Carol Burke

SILVER SULFADIAZINE

ACTION OF THE DRUG: Silver sulfadiazine acts only on the cell membrane and cell wall to produce a bactericidal effect against many gram-positive and gram-negative bacteria as well as *C. albicans, Pseudomonas aeruginosa and S. aureus.*

ASSESSMENT:

INDICATIONS: Used for the prevention and treatment of wound sepsis.

SUBJECTIVE: History of burns or large open wounds.

OBJECTIVE: Erythema with blistering of skin. Skin may have brownish, leathery appearance in third degree burns.

PLAN:

CONTRAINDICATIONS: Do not use in pregnancy at term or on premature or newborn infants. The existence of cross-sensitivity to other sulfonamides is not known.

WARNINGS: Administer with caution if history of hypersensitivity exists. Hemolysis may occur if used in individuals with G-6-PD deficiency. Safe use during pregnancy has not been established. Concomitant fungal infections may develop. If a large percentage of total body surface is being treated topically, serum sulfa concentrations should be monitored. Renal function should also be monitored, along with checking urine for sulfa crystals.

PRECAUTIONS: Use caution when giving to patients with hepatic or renal impairment since accumulation of drug may occur.

IMPLEMENTATION:

DRUG INTERACTIONS: Silver may inactivate enzymes if proteolytic enzymes are used topically in conjunction with silver sulfadiazine therapy.

PRODUCTS (TRADE NAME):
Silvadene, Silver Sulfadiazine (Available in 10 mg/gm cream.)

ADMINISTRATION AND DOSAGE: Store medication at room temperature. Burned areas should be cleansed and debrided prior to application of medication with a sterile, gloved hand. It should be applied once or twice daily to a thickness of approximately 1/16 inch. Dressings are not required, but burned areas should remain covered with medication. Treatment should be continued until healing has progressed and/or burn site is ready for grafting.

IMPEMENTATION CONSIDERATIONS:

—Obtain a complete health history, including hypersensitivity to silver sulfadiazine or sulfonamides, presence of renal or hepatic dysfunction, and possibility of pregnancy.

—Watch for adverse reactions.

WHAT THE PATIENT NEEDS TO KNOW:

—A stinging sensation may be felt when you apply the medication.

—If rash or irritation develops from using this medication, consult health care provider.

—Medication does not stain clothing.

—Drink at least 8 glasses of water per day while on this medication unless this is restricted by your health care provider.

EVALUATION:

ADVERSE REACTIONS: If significant quantities of medication are absorbed, adverse reactions attributable to sulfonamides may occur.

PARAMETERS TO MONITOR: Observe for therapeutic effect, signs of healing, and adverse effects. During extensive use of medication, serum sulfa concentrations should be monitored. Urine should be checked for sulfa crystals and renal function evaluated.

Carol Burke

SCABICIDES/PEDICULOCIDES

GAMMA BENZENE HEXACHLORIDE (LINDANE) AND MALATHION

ACTION OF THE DRUG: These products are ectoparasiticides and ovicides.

ASSESSMENT:

INDICATIONS: Used in the treatment of scabies and pediculosis.
SUBJECTIVE: History of scabies or pediculosis in home or school, itching.
OBJECTIVE: Nits in hair, excoriations in skin secondary to scratching. Microscopic evidence of scabies from scrapings. Patterns of scabies burrowing in interphalangeal areas.

PLAN:

CONTRAINDICATIONS: Hypersensitivity to this category of drugs.
WARNINGS: Should be used with caution on infants, children, and pregnant women. Do not put on face. Concomitant use of other creams or ointments may potentiate the effects of this drug. Do not exceed recommended dosage. Drugs are only for external use. Malathion is flammable and should not be used near hair dryers. Do not use in pregnant or breast-feeding women.
PRECAUTIONS: If accidental ingestion occurs, referral for prompt gastric lavage and also a saline cathartic for intestinal evacuation is indicated. If there is accidental contact with the eyes, flush with water immediately. Do not apply to open surfaces.

IMPLEMENTATION:

DRUG INTERACTIONS: Other skin preparations such as lotions, ointments or oils, if applied simultaneously can increase the absorption of this drug through the skin.
ADMINISTRATION AND DOSAGE: This drug is absorbed through the skin; therefore, a potential for central nervous system toxicity exists. Do not use in a concentration greater than 1%. Drug is for external use only. Careful instructions are needed regarding application and dosage. To prevent reinfection or spreading, all clothing, bed linens, and towels should be washed in very hot water or dry cleaned.
IMPLEMENTATION CONSIDERATIONS:
—Take a complete history regarding medication sensitivities.
—Discover through history the source of initial infection.
—Treatment may be needed for other members in the household.

—If patient is using medication for pubic lice, the sexual partner should also be treated.

—Experiment personally with the methods of application so you can explain them.

—Caution patient against using other skin preparations at the same time.

WHAT THE PATIENT NEEDS TO KNOW:

—Use the medicine only as directed by your health care provider. For malathion, do not use near hair dryers as product is flammable.

—Keep this medicine away from your eyes, mouth and mucous membranes.

—Medicine is for external use only.

—Do not apply to areas of broken skin or open wounds.

—Do not use any other lotions or creams on your skin at the same time with this medicine.

—Do not use if you are pregnant or breast-feeding.

—If itching continues more than one week after using medication, consult your health care provider again.

EVALUATION:

ADVERSE REACTIONS: *Cardiovascular:* unusually fast heart rate. *CNS:* convulsions, clumsiness or unsteadiness, unusual nervousness, restlessness or irritability. *Gastrointestinal:* vomiting. *Integumentary:* irritation of skin, itching of skin, skin rash. *Other:* muscle cramps.

OVERDOSAGE: Lindane may cause amblyopia, coma, convulsions, insomnia, irritability, stupor, and vertigo following excessive cutaneous application. Malathion may cause symptoms of cholinesterase depletion if taken in oral doses. Patient should have immediate stimulius to vomiting and gastric gavage, followed by supportive therapy.

PARAMETERS TO MONITOR: Someone at home should check patient for head lice after treatment has started and report back to health care provider. Patient should return to health care provider if itching continues. Health care provider should make certain that the patient is using the medication as directed if resolution of itching is not prompt.

CROTAMITON

PRODUCTS (TRADE NAME):

Eurax (Available as 10% cream or 10% lotion.)

DRUG SPECIFICS:

Used for eradication of scabies and the symptomatic treatment of most pruritic skin conditions. Irritating if applied to denuded areas.

ADMINISTRATION AND DOSAGE SPECIFICS:

Scabies: Thoroughly massage into the skin of the whole body, making sure the creases and folds are covered. Twenty-four hours later, apply a second coat. Clothing and bed linen should be changed after 24 hours. A bath should be taken 48 hours after the last application.

GAMMA BENZENE HEXACHLORIDE

PRODUCTS (TRADE NAME):

Kwell (Available as 1% cream, lotion and shampoo.) **Lindane** (Available as 1% lotion and shampoo.)

DRUG SPECIFICS:

Creams or lotions should be applied in a thin layer over skin and not removed for 24 hours. Store product in a tightly sealed container and protect from freezing. Do not use in concentrations greater than 1%. Use only as directed. For the shampoo, shake well before using. Note that Kwell shampoo is not used as a routine shampoo. Another treatment for pediculosis capitis and pubis may be indicated after seven days if reinfestation appears.

ADMINISTRATION AND DOSAGE SPECIFICS:

Scabies Treatment: Should be applied to dry skin in a thin layer and rubbed in thoroughly. If warm bath is taken before application, allow skin to cool and dry. Usually one ounce is sufficient for an adult. Application should be made over total body. Leave on for 8 12 hours, then remove with shower or bath.

Pediculosis Capitis: Cream and lotion can be rubbed into the scalp and hair and left in place for 12 hours, then removed in a bath or shower. Retreatment is usually not necessary. Use shampoo for both pediculosis capitis and pediculosis pubis: apply sufficient quantity of shampoo to thoroughly wet the hair and skin of the infested and adjacent hairy areas. After the hair and skin are thoroughly wet with the shampoo, add small quantities of water, working the shampoo into the hair and skin until a good lather forms. Continue this for 4 minutes. Rinse thoroughly; towel briskly. For head lice, comb the hair with a fine-toothed comb when the hair is dry to remove any remaining nits.

Pediculosis pubis: Apply a sufficient quantity only to cover thinly the hair and skin of the pubic area and, if infested, the thighs, trunk and axillary areas. The medicine should be rubbed into the skin and hair and left in place for 12 hours, then removed in a shower or bath.

MALATHION

PRODUCTS (TRADE NAME):

Prioderm (Available in 0.5% lotion.)

DRUG SPECIFICS:

This product is a weak cholinesterase inhibitor and therefore safer than other organophosphates. Evaluate other family members for infestation and treat as necessary.

ADMINISTRATION AND DOSAGE SPECIFICS:

In the evening, sprinkle malathion on the hair and gently rub until scalp is uniformly wet. Allow hair to dry without covering or using heat. In the morning shampoo hair. Rinse hair well and use a fine-tooth-comb to remove all dead lice and eggs. Repeat in 7 to 9 days if needed.

Linda Ross

TOPICAL SKIN PREPARATIONS—MISCELLANEOUS

CAUTERIZING AGENTS, EMOLLIENTS, KERATOLYTICS, AND WET DRESSINGS AND SOAKS

ACTION OF THE DRUG: Topical preparations may be applied to skin for protection, or a debriding aid, or as a moisturizing technique. The individual use depends upon the underlying need. Wet dressings and soaks are used primarily to produce local vasoconstriction. The dressings themselves aid in cleansing the skin of crusts, exudates and debris and promote drainage of infected areas. Keratolytics cause shedding and softening of the horny layer of the skin.

ASSESSMENT:

INDICATIONS: Emollients are used primarily to relieve pruritus, and to aid in healing of skin lesions by stimulating granulation and epithelization. Wet soaks and dressings are used for inflammatory conditions of the skin such as insect bites, contact dermatitis, swellings, bruises, and athlete's foot. Keratolytics are used for acne, calluses, hyperkeratosis, seborrheic dermatitis, psoriasis and other scaling dermatoses, superficial fungal infections, and warts. Silver nitrate is used in ophthalmic solutions to prevent and treat ophthalmic neonatorum. Stronger solutions and toughened silver nitrate are used to cauterize mucous membranes, fissures, granulomatous tissue, and warts.

SUBJECTIVE: Patient may complain of itching, erythema, flaking, or thickening of skin.

OBJECTIVE: There may be open lesions or areas of erythema, flaking, and crusting. Patient may also present with obvious insect bites, warts, or eruptions of acne.

PLAN:

CONTRAINDICATIONS: Do not use these preparations in the presence of hypersensitivity. Avoid contact of these solutions with face or eyes. See specific product information.

PRECAUTIONS: Some solutions may irritate the skin. If erythema, pruritus or swelling develops, first check the concentration of the solution. Discontinue use if solution is of correct concentration. Oatmeal baths are not for ingestion. Silver nitrate may cause burns and permanent stains on clothing and skin.

IMPLEMENTATION:

ADMINISTRATION AND DOSAGE: Lowest dosage or concentration possible should be used. Avoid prolonged exposure to skin and avoid using medication on healthy tissue. See individual product information for detailed information on using each preparation.

IMPLEMENTATION CONSIDERATIONS:

—Obtain a complete health history, including the presence of hypersensitivity, underlying systemic disease (such as diabetes or other causes of poor circulation), and concurrent use of other medications.

—Remember that success in using these medications will come through patient teaching. The patient must know what to do and when to return for assistance if problems develop or improvement is not seen.

WHAT THE PATIENT NEEDS TO KNOW:

—Your health care provider will give you detailed instructions on how to use these products. You must follow them exactly as prescribed. It is important to administer the appropriate number of treatments each day in order to control the problem.

—If you note any new or troublesome symptoms while carrying out this procedure, notify your health care practitioner so that they may be evaluated.

—If the problem does not improve after careful treatment, return for reevaluation.

—These products may be very potent. Avoid contact of the solutions with your face and eyes. Wash hands after procedure is completed. Avoid prolonged exposure to the chemicals.

—Keep all drugs out of the reach of children and all others for whom they are not prescribed.

—Remove all evidence of previous applications from area before applying new medicine.

EVALUATION:

ADVERSE REACTIONS: Observe for sensitization: erythema, swelling, pruritus. Consult specific product information for other reactions.

PARAMETERS TO MONITOR: Observe for therapeutic effect and development of adverse reactions.

CAUTERIZING AGENTS

ACTION OF THE DRUG: These products are strong caustic drugs which penetrate and cauterize skin, keratin and other tissues.

ASSESSMENT:

INDICATIONS: These products are used in the removal of verrucae (warts), calluses, hard and soft corns, seborrheic keratoses, ingrown nails, cysts and benign erosion of the cervix. They may also be used to stop epistaxis.

SUBJECTIVE-OBJECTIVE: Patient may complain of lesion and request removal. Lesions should be well demarcated and have easy access to base.

PLAN:

CONTRAINDICATIONS: Do not use in the presence of hypersensitivity, or to open wounds, cuts or broken skin.

PRECAUTIONS: Apply only to lesion being treated. Solution may cause severe burning, inflammation or tenderness of skin. Perform biopsy of suspicious cervical lesions to make certain cauterization is indicated.

IMPLEMENTATION:

ADMINISTRATION AND DOSAGE: Consult manufacturers' instructions. Administration technique may differ depending upon type and location of tissue being removed.

IMPLEMENTATION CONSIDERATIONS:

—Obtain complete health history regarding nature of problem.

—A thin layer of petroleum may be applied to the normal tissue surrounding the area to be treated to help protect normal tissues from the caustic solution.

WHAT THE PATIENT NEEDS TO KNOW:

—This medication is used to help remove unwanted skin tissue.

—Keep area dry and covered with an adhesive bandage for 4 to 6 days.

—Treated skin area will gradually peel off.

—More than one application may be necessary before all unwanted tissue is removed.

EVALUATION:

ADVERSE REACTIONS: Observe for redness or irritation of skin, or damage to tissue adjacent to treated area.

PARAMETERS TO MONITOR: Evaluate both treated area and adjacent tissue to determine status. Retreatment may be required to obtain full removal of skin.

DICHLOROACETIC ACID

PRODUCTS (TRADE NAME):

Bichloracetic Acid (Available in kit with 10 ml solution, petrolatum, and all equipment for administration.)

DRUG SPECIFICS:

Apply petrolatum to tissue surrounding area to be treated. Solution should then be carefully applied to lesion, using the equipment provided in the kit. Manufacturer's instructions are detailed and specific.

ADMINISTRATION AND DOSAGE SPECIFICS:

Amount to be used, and technique for application depend upon the nature of the lesion.

MONOCHLORACETIC ACID

PRODUCTS (TRADE NAME):

Monocete Solution (Available in 80% solution.)

DRUG SPECIFICS:

This product is used for the removal of verrucae. Do not drip solution on normal tissue or mucous membranes.

ADMINISTRATION AND DOSAGE SPECIFICS:

Remove callus tissue and apply to verruca with cotton tip applicator or capillary tube. Cover with bandage and allow to remain in place for 4 to 6 days. May require more than one application.

SILVER NITRATE

PRODUCTS (TRADE NAME):

Silver Nitrate Solution (Available in 10%, 25%, 50% solutions.) **Applicators, Toughened Sticks** (Available in 1 inch or 6 inches.)

DRUG SPECIFICS:
Silver nitrate (0.1% to 0.5%) is used as a germicide and astringent. In solid form or in solutions stronger than 5%, it is a caustic. Silver nitrate ophthalmic solution (1%) is used to prevent and treat ophthalmic neonatorum. Strong solutions and toughened silver nitrate are used to cauterize mucous membranes, fissures, granulomatous tissue and warts.

Toughened silver nitrate (sticks, pencils) must be dipped in water prior to use.

Argyria (silver discoloration of skin) may develop with prolonged use and is usually permanent. It is aggravated by exposure to sunlight.

Silver nitrate will stain clothing and skin. It may cause burns. Seek immediate medical care if accidental contact of drug occurs with eyes and skin. Ingestion may prove fatal.

ADMINISTRATION AND DOSAGE SPECIFICS:
Apply to local area as needed by qualified practitioner.

Mary Ann Bolter

EMOLLIENTS

DEXPANTHENOL

PRODUCTS (TRADE NAME):
Panthoderm (Available in 2% cream or lotion.)

DRUG SPECIFICS:
By stimulating epithelization and granulation, this product may aid in the healing of skin lesions. It also relieves pruritus.

There are no significant side effects or drug interactions with the topical use of this drug. Dexpanthenol is contraindicated in lesions of hemophilia patients. Oozing lesions do not respond as well to this therapy as dry lesions.

ADMINISTRATION AND DOSAGE SPECIFICS:
Prior to application of dexpanthenol, all traces of previous application should be removed.

Adults and children: Apply directly to affected area once or twice daily (may use more often if needed.)

UREA (CARBAMIDE)

PRODUCTS (TRADE NAME):
Aquacare (Available in 2%, 10% cream or lotion.) **Carmol-20** (Available in

20% cream and 10% lotion.) **Nutraplus** (Available in 10% cream and lotion.) **ReaLo** (Available in 15% lotion and 30% cream.) **Ultra Mide** (Available in 25% lotion.)

DRUG SPECIFICS:

Most of these preparations are available without prescription. These urea-containing creams or lotions provide excellent hydration, and they aid in removing scales and crusts (keratolytic.)

Use of these products is contraindicated in patients with impaired circulation or viral skin disorders. Their use is not recommended for children.

There are no significant interactions with other drugs. If the skin is broken or irritated, application of this drug may cause stinging.

ADMINISTRATION AND DOSAGE SPECIFICS:

Prior to application of urea products, all traces of previous application should be removed.

Adults: Apply to affected area two to three times daily.

COLLOIDAL ADDITIVES AND BATH OILS

PRODUCTS (TRADE NAME):

Alpha Keri Therapeutic Bath Oil, Aveeno Colloidal Oatmeal, Aveeno Oilated Bath, Lubrasol Bath Oil, Nutraderm Bath Oil (The oils are supplied in 4, 8, and 16 oz bottles; the colloidal is available in single packets or multipackets.)

DRUG SPECIFICS:

These preparations are available without prescription. For treating widespread eruptions, the solution added to baths is very useful. The medicated bath may be soothing, antipruritic and anti-inflammatory. The bath should be limited to 30 minutes. The patient should be cautious, for most of the oils make the tub very slippery. The patient must avoid getting these products in the eyes. If this occurs, flush the eyes with water. Oatmeal is comprised of 50% starch, approximately 25% protein, and 9% oil. The colloidal oatmeal is not to be confused with food. This product is not for ingestion. The bath oils are used to prevent drying of the skin. Usually, they contain a vegetable or mineral oil and a surfactant.

ADMINISTRATION AND DOSAGE SPECIFICS:

Aveeno Colloidal Oatmeal, Aveeno Oilated Bath:
Adults: One packet in half-full tub of warm water.
Children: One to two heaping tablespoonfuls in 3 to 4 inches of warm water.
Infants: Two to three level teaspoonfuls in small tub of warm water.
Alpha Keri Therapeutic Bath Oil, Lubriderm Bath Oil: These should always be used with water. They may be poured into the tub or rubbed onto wet skin. See label on product for specific amount to use. Measurements are given in number of capfuls, to use and this varies according to the size of the container.

Mary Ann Bolter

KERATOLYTICS

SALICYLIC ACID

PRODUCTS (TRADE NAME):
  Calicylic Creme (Available in 10% cream.) **Hydrisalic** (Available in 6% gel.) **Keralyt Gel** (Available in 6% salicylic acid.) **Mediplast** (Available as salicylic acid 40% in a package of 25 individually wrapped plasters). **Off-Ezy** (Available in 17% liquid.) **Salacid** (Available in 25 and 60% ointment.) **Salonil** (Available as 40% salicylic acid ointment.) **Salicylic Acid Cream** (Available as 25% cream.) **Wart-Off** (Available in 17% liquid.)

DRUG SPECIFICS:
  Salicylic acid is a keratolytic. At concentrations between 3 and 6% it causes shedding and softening of scaling of the horny layer of the skin. In concentrations of greater than 6%, it is destructive to tissue.

  These products are used for acne, calluses, hyperkeratosis, seborrheic dermatitis, psoriasis and other scaling dermatoses, superficial fungal infections and warts.

  Use with caution in patients with diabetes or with circulatory impairments or children under 2 years of age. Because of tetratogenicity in laboratory animals, use in pregnant women only if potential benefit exceeds the risk to the fetus. Use care not to allow product to contact eye and mucous membranes. Do not apply this drug to healthy tissue. Do not use on inflamed areas or where skin is not intact. Prolonged use over large areas could lead to salicylate toxicity, especially in children and patients with impaired renal or hepatic function. Watch for nausea, vomiting, tinnitus, diarrhea, hyperpnea, dizziness, or psychic disturbances.

  The most common side effect is drying of the skin. However, irritation can develop. Do not use on large areas for a prolonged period of time since this could result in salicylism. Signs of salicylate toxicity are nausea, vomiting, dizziness, psychic disturbances, diarrhea, loss of hearing, tinnitus, and lethargy.

ADMINISTRATION AND DOSAGE SPECIFICS:
  Creams: Do not apply to moles, birthmarks. Use only for corns and calluses. Cleanse and dry area to be treated. Apply cream directly on area once daily for 2 weeks.

  Keralyt Gel: Hydrate skin for 5 minutes prior to application. Apply gel to affected areas and occlude the areas. Preferably, this is done at night and washed off in the morning. Unless the hands are being treated, they should be thoroughly washed after application.

  Mediplast: Cut out piece of plaster to fit the callus. Remove backing paper and apply. Do not wear for more than 24 hours. If reapplication is needed, allow some time between applications. Discontinue if irritation develops.

Mary Ann Bolter

WET DRESSINGS AND SOAKS

BUROW'S SOLUTION (ALUMINUM ACETATE SOLUTION)

PRODUCTS (TRADE NAME):

AluWets Wet Dressing Crystals (Available in 2% aluminium chloride hexahydrate.) **Bluboro Powder, Buro-Sol Powder, Burow's Solution, Domeboro Powder and Tablets, Pedi-Boro Soak Paks** (Available in packets or tablets of aluminium acetate.)

DRUG SPECIFICS:

These products are used for open wet dressings. They cool and dry through evaporation, which causes local vasoconstriction. Wet dressings cleanse the skin of crusts, exudates, and debris and promote drainage of infected areas. These products are used for inflammatory conditions of the skin such as insect bites, contact dermatitis, swellings and bruises, and athlete's foot.

These solutions may cause irritation. If this occurs, the problem may be that the solution is evaporating to a concentration that is irritating because it is too strong. If evaporation is not the source of the irritation, the patient may be sensitive to the solution and it should be discontinued.

Caution patient to avoid contact of solution with eyes or mucous membranes. Prepared solution may be stored at room temperature for 7 days.

ADMINISTRATION AND DOSAGE SPECIFICS:

The patient should be in a comfortable position with an impermeable material under the area to be treated. The dressings need not be sterile (may use soft gauze, old, clean sheeting, or handkerchiefs). Moisten the dressings and apply multiple layers (6 to 8) to prevent rapid drying and cooling. Every 15 to 30 minutes, the dressing should be checked and moistened if needed. Continue this for 4 to 8 hours or as indicated. Consult the packet of the product for specifics regarding the preparation of the solution.

Mary Ann Bolter

VAGINAL PREPARATIONS

ANTI-INFECTIVES

ACTION OF THE DRUG: Medications are taken vaginally as bacteriocidal, fungicidal, fungostatic, or bacteriostatic mechanisms or as spermicides in regular contraceptive therapy.

ASSESSMENT:

INDICATIONS: Vaginal contraceptives are used in conjunction with a diaphragm or condoms in order to increase the degree of protection. Vaginal anti-infectives are used in the treatment of vaginitis caused by fungal infections involving *Candida albicans*, other *Candida* species, *Trichomonas vaginitis*, vulvovaginal moniliasis, and pathogenic yeasts.

SUBJECTIVE: In vaginal infections the patient may complain of vaginal itching, odor, discharge, and general irritation. If infection is severe, dysuria may be produced. Some infections present asymptomatically.

OBJECTIVE: Erythema and evidence of scratching may be seen on examination of vulva. Vaginal canal and vault may be swollen, erythematous, and with copious amounts of discharge. An obvious odor may be present. Examination of vaginal pool discharge in sterile saline or KOH may reveal Monilia or Trichomonas. At times there may be no obvious symptoms, but Pap smear reports document the presence of infection.

PLAN:

CONTRAINDICATIONS: Do not use in the presence of hypersensitivity. Consult individual products for chemical listings. Some vaginal tablets and applicators may be contraindicated in pregnant patients.

PRECAUTIONS: Use of some of these products during the first trimester of pregnancy has not been studied and therefore should be undertaken cautiously.

IMPLEMENTATION:

DRUG INTERACTIONS: Generally there are no drug interactions. However, consult individual preparation for additional information.

ADMINISTRATION AND DOSAGE: Contraceptive foams may be slightly more effective than creams or jellies since they disperse more readily throughout the vagina. Vaginal suppositories should be inserted at least 10 minutes prior to intercourse to allow time for dispersion.

Vaginal anti-infectives should be used as a specified course of therapy. The patient should be urged to continue with the complete 7 to 14 day therapy even after symptoms disappear. Use of applicator should be demonstrated.

IMPLEMENTATION CONSIDERATIONS:

—Obtain a complete health history, including the presence of hypersensitivity (especially to specific antibiotics and iodine), underlying systemic disease, and concurrent use of other medications.

—Discuss the cause of vaginal infections with patient and clarify that this does not represent a venereal disease.

—Explain the importance of taking the full course of treatment and having the sexual partner use a condom during therapy to aid in protecting against reinfection.

WHAT THE PATIENT NEEDS TO KNOW:
—Use this medication as instructed by your health care provider. Be certain to use all the medication even if your symptoms disappear and you feel better.
—During the course of therapy for a vaginal infection, avoid having intercourse, or have sexual partner use a condom in order to avoid reinfection.
—When pregnancy is contraindicated, discuss the method of birth control with the health care provider. There are alternative methods of contraception which are more reliable.
—Vaginal contraceptives are more effective as protection when used with a diaphragm or condom.
—No contraceptive can guarantee 100% effectiveness. For reliable protection read and follow the directions carefully on the product you are currently using.
—If you develop any irritation, itching, or increase in vaginal discharge return to your health care provider for evaluation.

EVALUATION:

ADVERSE REACTIONS: Localized irritation or hypersensitivity to drug.
PARAMETERS TO MONITOR: Reexamine patients who are treated for vaginal infection after the course of therapy has ended. Evaluate for therapeutic effects and development of adverse effects. For patients on contraceptive therapy, see at least yearly to discuss problems with contraception or change in protection requirements.

BENZALKONIUM CHLORIDE

PRODUCTS (TRADE NAME):
Nonsul Jelly (Available in 1:2000 vaginal gel with applicator.)
DRUG SPECIFICS:
This product is a quaternary ammonium cationic surface-active agent with germicidal activity against bacteria, fungi, protozoa and some viruses. It is used in the treatment of Trichomonis, Monilias, and non-sporulating bacteria or non-specific aginal infections. It may be used to prevent secondary infections following cauterizations or conizations. Sexual relations are contraindicated during the first ten days of therapy. Pruritus may be relieved by applying ice packs to vaginal area. Localized burning sensation is sometimes reported. Medication should be inserted high into the vagina and used for the full course of therapy. Do not douche with solutions containing soap, which may inactivate the medication.
ADMINISTRATION AND DOSAGE SPECIFICS:
Use 1/2 applicator (approximately 4 gm) and insert high into the vagina at

bedtime for 24 days. Alternate format may be to use twice daily for 12 days. Medication may be continued longer for resistant cases. During next 3 menstrual cycles, use medication the last three days of the menstrual period and two days following menses.

CANDICIDIN

PRODUCTS (TRADE NAME):
  Vanobid (Available in 0.6 mg vaginal ointment or 3 mg vaginal tablets.)
DRUG SPECIFICS:
  Vanobid is an antifungal antibiotic similar chemically and in spectrum to amphotericin B. It is specific for treatment of vaginitis caused by *Candida albicans* and other *Candida species.* Appropriate tests should confirm diagnosis before treatment. The vaginal tablets are more suitable for gravid patients.
  This drug is contraindicated for those sensitive to any of the components of the ointment or vaginal tablets. The use of an applicator may be contraindicated for gravid patients. It may be preferred that these patients insert the tablet manually.
  During treatment it is recommended that the patient refrain from sexual intercourse or that her partner wear a condom to prevent reinfection. Those patients using a diaphragm should be advised to use another form of contraception during treatment with Vanobid vaginal ointment; the diaphragm may deteriorate during prolonged contact with petroleum-based products.
  Adverse reactions to Vanobid may be sensitization or temporary irritation. However, such reactions are rare.
  Treat for two weeks. Repeat treatment if symptoms persist or reappear.
ADMINISTRATION AND DOSAGE SPECIFICS:
  One applicatorful of ointment or one vaginal tablet inserted high in the vagina twice daily: once in the morning and once at bedtime. The use of an applicator may be contraindicated during pregnancy.

CLOTRIMAZOLE

PRODUCTS (TRADE NAME):
  Gyne-Lotrimin, Mycelex-G (Available as 1% cream in 45 gm tube with applicator for 7 day treatment, box of 2 for 14-day treatment, or in 100 mg vaginal tablets in carton of 6 tablets for 3-day treatment; carton of 7 tablets for 7 day treatment).
DRUG SPECIFICS:
  Clotrimazole is a broad-spectrum antifungal agent which inhibits the growth of pathogenic yeasts. It is fungicidal against *Candida albicans* and other Candida

species. This drug is indicated for the treatment of vulvovaginial candidiasis. The diagnosis should be confirmed by KOH smears and/or cultures.

Clotrimazole is contraindicated in those hypersensitive to any component in the preparation. Use of this drug in the first trimester of pregnancy has not been studied. Use after the first trimester has not been associated with adverse effects. The use of an applicator may be contraindicated in gravid patients.

Possible side effects of clotrimazole include irritation, rash, and erythema.

Patients using the vaginal cream have a higher cure rate if they are treated for 14 days. Those using the tablets are treated for 3 to 7 days. Should the patient be unresponsive to therapy, recheck the causative pathogen with appropriate tests.

ADMINISTRATION AND DOSAGE SPECIFICS:

Gyne-Lotrimin Cream: One applicatorful intravaginally, preferably at bedtime, for 7 to 14 days.

Gyne-Lotrimin, Mycelex-G Tablets: 2 tablets intravaginally at bedtime for 3 nights or 1 tablet intravaginally at bedtime for 7 nights. In pregnant patient, 1 tablet intravaginally at bedtime for 7 nights.

GENTIAN VIOLET

PRODUCTS (TRADE NAME):

Genapax (Available in 5 mg tampons in packs of 12.) **Hyva** (Available in 2 mg vaginal tablets in packs of 14 or 28 with applicator.)

DRUG SPECIFICS:

This rosaniline dye is bacteriostatic and bactericidal against some gram positive bacteria and many fungi. It is effective for many strains of Candida. The product is a dye and will stain skin and clothing. Wearing of a sanitary napkin may reduce the staining of clothing. Chemical vulvovaginitis may sometimes be provoked by this product. Patients who do not respond to therapy should be evaluated for sources of reinfection, as well as unrecognized diabetes mellitus. Medication should be inserted high into vagina with applicator and used for the full course of time. Sexual relations should be avoided, or partner should wear a condom to prevent reinfection.

ADMINISTRATION AND DOSAGE SPECIFICS:

Insert 1 or 2 times nightly until signs and symptoms disappear. Continue treatment until cultures are negative.

MICONAZOLE NITRATE

PRODUCTS (TRADE NAME):

Monistat 7 (Available in 2% cream with applicator.)

DRUG SPECIFICS:

Miconazole nitrate is fungicidal against species of the genus *Candida*. It is indicated for the local treatment of vulvovaginal moniliasis. Diagnosis should be ascertained by KOH smears and/or cultures.

Use of this drug is contraindicated in those known to be hypersensitive to it. Stop the use of miconazole nitrate if sensitization develops. Vulvovaginal burning, pruritus, and irritation have been reported with use of this drug.

Use this drug in the first trimester of pregnancy only if it is considered essential. If the condition does not respond to therapy, repeat appropriate tests to confirm the diagnosis and to rule out other pathogens. Course of therapy may be repeated if indicated.

ADMINISTRATION AND DOSAGE SPECIFICS:

One applicatorful intravaginally at bedtime for seven days.

NYSTATIN

PRODUCTS (TRADE NAME):

Korostatin, Mycostatin, Nystatin (Available in 100,000 unit vaginal tablets.) **O-V Statin** (Available in 21 oral tablets with 500,000 units nystatin, and 14 vaginal tablets with 100,000 units nystatin.)

DRUG SPECIFICS:

This product is an antifungal antibiotic with both fungistatic and fungicidal activity. It is used primarily for the treatment of moniliasis (vulvovaginal candidiasis) which is documented by KOH smears and/or cultures. If there is no clinical response to therapy, reexamine patient to rule out presence of other pathogens. Tablets should be inserted high into the vagina and used continuously, even during the menstrual period. Partner should use condom to avoid reinfection.

ADMINISTRATION AND DOSAGE SPECIFICS:

Use 1 tablet (100,000) intravaginally daily for 2 weeks.

PROPIONATE COMPOUND

PRODUCTS (TRADE NAME):

Propion (Available in vaginal gel with applicator.)

DRUG SPECIFICS:

This product has fungicidal and fungistatic action against fungi, including *Candida albicans*. It is used in the treatment of vaginal *moniliasis*. Insert gel high into vagina with applicator. At beginning of therapy, use a warm water or weak vinegar douche; do not douche during the rest of therapy. Do not use after the seventh month of pregnancy.

ADMINISTRATION AND DOSAGE SPECIFICS:

Insert applicator high into vagina morning and evening. Apply a small amount of the gel also to the external genitalia. The gel may be reduced for the first few applicators with equal amounts of water if labia are raw or inflamed.

POVIDONE-IODINE

PRODUCTS (TRADE NAME):
Betadine (Available in 10 mg vaginal gel with applicator.)
DRUG SPECIFICS:
Betadine is indicated for the treatment of trichomoniasis vaginalis vaginitis, monilial vaginitis, and nonspecific vaginitis. (Classified by the FDA as "possibly effective" against these problems.)

This product is contraindicated in those with hypersensitivity to any of the components of the drug. Be aware that those with history of iodine sensitization should not use this product. If irritation, redness or swelling develops, stop the use of this drug.

Appropriate tests should be made to confirm vaginitis. If there is a lack of response to treatment, reevaluate. Treatment usually spans one menstrual cycle. Patient should be rechecked two weeks after therapy.

During the course of therapy, the patient should refrain from sexual intercourse or her partner should use a condom to prevent reinfection.
ADMINISTRATION AND DOSAGE SPECIFICS:
One applicatorful of gel at night followed by morning douche (with 2 tbsp to 1 quart warm water) for one menstrual cycle, including days of menses.

CONTRACEPTIVES—SPERMICIDES

PRODUCTS (TRADE NAME):
Because Foam (Available in portable 6 use combination foam/applicator unit). Conceptrol Cream (Available in 2.46 oz tube). Delfen Contraceptive Foam (Available in 0.70, 1.75 oz vials). Emko Vaginal Contraceptive Foam (Available in 40 and 90 gm can). Emko Pre-Fil Vaginal Contraceptive Foam (Available in 30 and 60 gm can). Encare Vaginal Contraceptive Insert (Available in box of 12). Gynol II Contraceptive Jelly (Available in 81 and 126 gm tube). Intercept Contraceptive Inserts (Available in box of 12). Koromex Contraceptive Foam (Available in 22 and 55 gm can). Koromex II Contraceptive Cream (Available in 75 and 128 gm tube). Koromex II A Contraceptive (Available in 81 and 135 gm tube jelly or cream or 12.5% foam). Ortho-Gynol Contraceptive Jelly (Available in 2.85 and 4.44 oz tube).

DRUG SPECIFICS:

These vaginal contraceptives are a chemical method of contraception. These products kill sperm upon contact. This method is more effective if used in conjunction with a diaphragm or condom.

Foams may be slightly more effective than creams or jellies since they disperse more readily throughout the vagina. Suppositories should be inserted at least 10 minutes prior to intercourse to allow time for dispersion.

It is important to remember to insert the product prior to each act of intercourse. If a douche is used, wait at least 6 hours after intercourse.

Occasional burning or irritation of the vagina or penis has been reported. If these symptoms develop, discontinue use of the product and switch to another brand of foam, or to an alternate form of birth control. The suppositories may produce a sensation of warmth as they dissolve.

When pregnancy is contraindicated, the patient should discuss the method of contraception with a health care provider. There are alternative methods of contraception which are more reliable. The major advantage of the chemical contraceptives is that they are available without prescription or a medical examination.

ADMINISTRATION AND DOSAGE SPECIFICS:

Although no contraceptive can guarantee 100% effectiveness, the best protection may be obtained by reading and following the directions on the product carefully. These products may differ slightly, so be sure to read the instructions on the product you are currently using.

Mary Ann Bolter

10

URINARY TRACT PRODUCTS

ACIDIFIERS (ORAL)

ACTION OF THE DRUG: Free hydrogen ion concentration is increased by acidifiers. These drugs may act by increasing the solubility of calcium to prevent formation of calculi. Acid ash or a low calcium and low vitamin D diet may be necessary with some drugs.

ASSESSMENT:

INDICATIONS: Acidifiers help to prevent calcification, control infection, or control odor-turbidity of urine.

SUBJECTIVE: History of recurrent calcium oxalate calculi may be found. Patient may currently be using antibacterial therapy (methenamine mandelate, methenamine hippurate) which is more effective in acid urine.

OBJECTIVE: Alkaline urine may be documented.

PLAN:

CONTRAINDICATIONS: Ammonium chloride should not be used in patients with marked renal dysfunction or severe hepatic failure. K-Phos M.F. (modified formula) should not be used in cases of renal insufficiency, severe hepatic disease, Addison's disease, or hyperkalemia.

WARNINGS: Consider risk-benefit ratio in pregnant women and nursing mothers.

PRECAUTIONS: Use with caution if the patient is on a sodium-restricted diet. PHos-pHaid should be used with care in patients with severe renal damage.

IMPLEMENTATION:

DRUG INTERACTIONS: Ammonium chloride and concurrent use of spironolactone could lead to systemic acidosis.

ADMINISTRATION AND DOSAGE: Increase fluid intake while on this therapy. Excessive dosage may cause diarrhea, and dosage should be reduced until symptoms disappear.

IMPLEMENTATION CONSIDERATIONS:

—Obtain a complete health history, including the presence of hypersensitivity, underlying systemic disease (such as renal or hepatic disorders, Addison's disease, hyperkalemia), concurrent use of spironolactone, or possibility of pregnancy.

—K-Phos and pHos-pHaid are at times used in conjunction with specific diets to prevent formation of calculi.

—If taking ammonium chloride, diuresis is normal for the first few days.

—Do not use in patients with hyperuricemia as acidification of the urine will cause stone formation.

WHAT THE PATIENT NEEDS TO KNOW:

—Take this medication exactly as ordered. Do not double up on doses. If you miss a dose, take it as soon as possible, unless it is close to the next scheduled time.

—If you are placed on a special diet, this is as important as the drug therapy.

—You will need to have regular health checkups if you are taking this drug as a part of long-term therapy.

—Drink at least two quarts of liquid (especially water) per day while taking this drug. This is important in helping the drug to work and in maintaining urinary output.

—Take the drug after meals to reduce gastrointestinal side effects.

—You may notice an increase in the number of times you go to the bathroom and an increase in the quantity of urine in the first few days of therapy.

—If you develop diarrhea, notify your health care provider.

EVALUATION:

ADVERSE REACTIONS: *Gastrointestinal:* diarrhea, gastric discomfort, nausea. *Other:* acidosis (with prolonged, excessive dosage.)

OVERDOSAGE: *Signs and symptoms:* Diarrhea may occur with excessive dosage. *Treatment:* Reduction of the dosage will usually correct the problem. If diarrhea persists, discontinue the therapy.

PARAMETERS TO MONITOR: Urinary pH determinations are needed before initiating therapy and at periodic intervals to ascertain that the therapeutic response is being maintained. Monitor degree of adverse reactions.

AMMONIUM BIPHOSPHATE, SODIUM BIPHOSPHATE AND SODIUM ACID PYROPHOSPHATE

PRODUCTS (TRADE NAME):
 pHos-pHaid (Available in 0.25 gm and .5 gm tablets.)

DRUG SPECIFICS:
 Enteric-coated tablets are available for patients who experience gastrointestinal side effects. Drug is taken in conjunction with an acidifying diet.

ADMINISTRATION AND DOSAGE SPECIFICS:
 Adult: 1 gm po followed by a glass of water three times daily.

AMMONIUM CHLORIDE

PRODUCTS (TRADE NAME):
 Ammonium Chloride (Available in 325 mg, 500 mg, 1 gm plain or enteric coated tablets.)

DRUG SPECIFICS:

Enteric-coated tablets are available to minimize gastric side effects, but they are absorbed erratically.

ADMINISTRATION AND DOSAGE SPECIFICS:

Adult: 4 to 12 gm po daily in divided doses.

POTASSIUM ACID PHOSPHATE

PRODUCTS (TRADE NAME):

K-Phos M.F. (Available in tablets containing potassium acid phosphate 155 mg and sodium acid phosphate, anhydrous 350 mg.) **K-Phos No. 2** (Available in 305 mg potassium acid phosphate and 700 mg sodium acid phosphate tablets.) **KPhos Original** (Available in 500 mg sodium free tablets.)

DRUG SPECIFICS:

This drug is not available in enteric-coated form. If used to lower calcium levels, it must be given in conjunction with a low calcium, low vitamin D diet.

ADMINISTRATION AND DOSAGE SPECIFICS:

Adults: 2 tablets followed by a glass of water four times daily.

Mary Ann Bolter

ALKALINIZERS (ORAL)

ACTION OF THE DRUG: Alkalinizers increase the excretion of free bicarbonate ions in the urine, raising the urinary pH. Dissolution of uric acid stones may be accomplished through maintaining an alkaline urine.

ASSESSMENT:

INDICATIONS: Urinary tract alkalinizers are indicated to correct acidosis in renal tubular disorders. They are also used to decrease uric acid crystallization. They are used as adjunctive therapy with aminoglycosides to increase antimicrobial effectiveness, and with sulfonamides to enhance sulfonamide solubility, thus preventing crystallization and possible renal damage.

SUBJECTIVE: Patient may present with a history of uric acid calculi of the urinary tract. There may be current use of uricosuric agents for gout therapy, or antimicrobial therapy with aminoglycosides or sulfonamides.

OBJECTIVE: Acidic urine may be documented.

PLAN:

WARNINGS: Chronic use of alkalinizers may lead to systemic alkalosis. Sodium in some products may cause weight gain and edema.

PRECAUTIONS: Risk-benefit ratio must be considered in pregnant women and nursing mothers.

IMPLEMENTATION:

DRUG INTERACTIONS: Urinary excretion of salicylates is increased; urinary excretion of quinidine and amphetamines are decreased.

ADMINISTRATION AND DOSAGE: Extended sodium bicarbonate therapy is not recommended due to the high risk of causing metabolic alkalosis or sodium overload. Do not take other oral medications within one to two hours of sodium bicarbonate.

IMPLEMENTATION CONSIDERATIONS:

—Obtain a complete health history, including the presence of hypersensitivity, fluid and electrolyte imbalance, underlying systemic disease (especially gout, hypertension, congestive heart failure, renal dysfunction, cancer), concurrent use of other medications (especially uricosuric agents), and possibility of pregnancy.

—Obtain baseline weight in patients. Evaluate whether patient can tolerate increased sodium intake.

—Drug should not be taken with milk or milk products. Milk-alkali syndrome may result from concurrent and prolonged use.

—Patients over 60 years old usually need a decreased dosage.

—Patient may be started on alkaline ash diet to supplement the alkalinizing influence of the drug.

WHAT THE PATIENT NEEDS TO KNOW:

—Take this medication exactly as ordered by your practitioner. Because sodium bicarbonate is available without a prescription, there will be some instructions for use included when you purchase the drug.

—If you are taking this drug on a regular basis and a dose is missed, take the dose as soon as possible. Do not take it if it is almost time for the next dose. Do not double doses.

—You will need to have regular health checkups if you are taking this drug as part of long-term therapy.

—Do not take sodium bicarbonate within one to two hours of other oral medications.

—Do not take this drug with milk or milk products. It may be taken with juice, water or food.

EVALUATION:

ADVERSE REACTIONS: *Gastrointestinal:* belching, flatulence, gastric distention, stomach cramps. *Other:* milk-alkali syndrome, unusual increase in thirst.

OVERDOSAGE: *Signs and symptoms:* Watch for signs of nausea, vomiting, anorexia, headache, mental confusion, weakness, polydipsia, or polyuria. Overdosage may lead to nephrocalcinosis and progressive deterioration of renal function. *Treatment:* Patient should stop taking the drug, milk, and milk products. Chemical abnormalities then usually can be corrected. Adequate fluid intake should be maintained.

PARAMETERS TO MONITOR: Monitor patient's weight to ascertain if weight gain is developing due to sodium influence. Check for signs of edema. Urinary pH determinations must be monitored to assure that therapeutic response is maintained. Renal function tests are needed at periodic intervals with the long-term use of frequent, repeated dosage.

POTASSIUM CITRATE AND CITRIC ACID

PRODUCTS (TRADE NAME):
Polycitra K (Available in syrup, each ml containing 2 mEq potassium.)
DRUG SPECIFICS:
Useful when the administration of sodium salts is undesirable. Contraindicated in patients with severe renal dysfunction with oliguria or azotemia, untreated Addison's disease, severe myocardial damage.
ADMINISTRATION AND DOSAGE SPECIFICS:
Adults: 15 to 30 ml diluted in water, after meals and at bedtime.
Children: 5 to 15 ml diluted in water, after meals and at bedtime.

POTASSIUM CITRATE, SODIUM CITRATE AND CITRIC ACID

PRODUCTS (TRADE NAME):
Citrolith (Available in 50 mg potassium citrate and 950 mg sodium citric tablets.) **Polycitra, Polycitra-LC** (Available in syrup with each ml containing 1 mEq potassium, 1 mEq sodium, and equivalent to 2 mEq bicarbonate. Polycitra-LC is sugar free).
DRUG SPECIFICS:
Useful when the administration of sodium salts is undesirable. Contraindicated in patients with severe renal dysfunction with oliguria or azotemia, untreated Addison's disease, or severe myocardial damage.
ADMINISTRATION AND DOSAGE SPECIFICS:
Adults: 15 to 30 ml diluted in water, after meals and at bedtime.
Children: 5 to 15 ml diluted in water, after meals and at bedtime.

SODIUM BICARBONATE

PRODUCTS (TRADE NAME):
   Sodium Bicarbonate (Available in 325 and 650 mg tablets, or as powder with 1/2 tsp containing 20.9 mEq (476 mg) sodium).
DRUG SPECIFICS:
   The maximum daily dosage of sodium is 200 mEq (16.6 gm) in patients less than 60 years old; 100 mEq (8.3 gm) for those age 60 or above.
ADMINISTRATION AND DOSAGE SPECIFICS:
   Adults: 4 gm po initially, then 1 to 2 gms po every 4 hours. For solution use one tsp in a glass of water every 4 hours, adjusting dosage as necessary.
   Children: 1 to 10 mEq (23 to 230 mg) per kg of body weight daily in divided doses, adjusting dosage as needed. Solution dosage not established.

SODIUM CITRATE AND CITRIC ACID

PRODUCTS (TRADE NAME):
   Bicitra (Available in solution with each ml containing 1 mEq sodium and equivalent to 1 mEq bicarbonate).
DRUG SPECIFICS:
   Useful when the administration of potassium salts is undesirable. Contraindicated for patients on sodium-restricted diets or with severe renal dysfunction. Use with caution if patient has low urinary output. Dilute with water and take after meals to avoid laxative effect. Chilling solution before taking enhances palatability. This product is sugar free.
ADMINISTRATION AND DOSAGE SPECIFICS:
   Adults: 10 to 30 ml diluted in 1 to 3 oz water, after meals and at bedtime.
   Children: 5 to 15 ml diluted in 1 to 3 oz water, after meals and at bedtime.

Mary Ann Bolter

ANALGESICS (ORAL)

ACTION OF THE DRUG: Analgesics exert a local anesthetic or topical analgesic effect on the urinary tract mucosa. The exact mechanism of action is not known.

ASSESSMENT:

INDICATIONS: Used for the relief of pain, burning, or other discomforts associated with lower urinary tract infections or irritation.

SUBJECTIVE: Patient may complain of burning, pain, frequency, urgency or other discomforts of the lower urinary tract.

OBJECTIVE: Practitioner may observe inflammation of urinary meatus. Urinalysis may show white blood cells, red blood cells, and bacteria, indicating infection.

PLAN:

CONTRAINDICATIONS: Do not give in the presence of hypersensitivity to the drug. Ethoxazene HCl should not be given to patients with severe renal or hepatic disease. Phenazopyridine HCl is contraindicated in renal insufficiency.

WARNINGS: Consider risk-benefit ratio in prescribing this drug to pregnant women or nursing mothers. A yellowish tinge of the sclerae or skin could indicate excessive accumulation of phenazopyridine HCl and this therapy should be stopped.

PRECAUTIONS: These drugs do not treat infections which might be the cause of symptoms. If infection is present, treat appropriately with antibacterials. Use ethoxazene HCl cautiously in patients with gastrointestinal conditions.

IMPLEMENTATION:

DRUG INTERACTIONS: No significant interactions reported.

ADMINISTRATION AND DOSAGE: The dosages of these drugs are similar. Time of administration is different. Ethoxazene HCl is given before meals; phenazopyridine HCl is given with or after meals. If the reason for therapy is a urinary tract infection, this drug can usually be discontinued after about 3 days of antibiotic therapy.

IMPLEMENTATION CONSIDERATIONS:

—Obtain a complete health history, including the presence of hypersensitivity, underlying systemic disease (especially liver, gastrointestinal, or kidney dysfunction), concurrent use of medications, and possibility of pregnancy.

—Obtain urinalysis and urine culture. Therapy may be prescribed while awaiting the results of the culture.

—Fluid intake should be increased.

—These drugs cause harmless discoloration of the urine.

—Patient will need follow-up evaluation. If antibiotic is prescribed, repeat urinalysis, and urine culture should be obtained 2 to 3 days after completion of antibiotic course.

WHAT THE PATIENT NEEDS TO KNOW:

—Take this medication as prescribed. Do not double up doses.

—This drug will cause a harmless red or orange discoloration of the urine. It will stain clothing.

—If patient is a diabetic, phenazopyridine HCl may cause false urine sugar and ketone test results.

—It is important to return to your health care provider for a follow-up check after you are feeling better. This is to make certain the problem is resolved.

—Contact your health care provider if symptoms increase or if new symptoms appear.

EVALUATION:

ADVERSE REACTIONS: Ethoxazene HCl: *Gastrointestinal:* nausea, vomiting.

Phenazopyridine HCl: *CNS:* dizziness, headache. *Gastrointestinal:* abdominal cramps or pain, indigestion.

OVERDOSAGE: *Signs and symptoms:* For signs of ethoxazene HCl overdosage, consult the pharmaceutical company (Squibb). For phenazopyridine HCl, methemoglobinemia (blue or bluish-purple skin color), hemolytic anemia (unusual tiredness or weakness), impaired renal excretion or hepatotoxicity (yellow skin or sclerae) may develop. *Treatment:* 1 to 2 mg per kg of body weight of methylene blue given intravenously or 100 to 200 mg of ascorbic acid given orally is the treatment for methemoglobinemia.

PARAMETERS TO MONITOR: If patient has hepatic or renal disorders, obtain liver and kidney function tests as appropriate. Monitor for therapeutic effect, evidenced by decline or disappearance of symptoms. If infection was the etiology of symptoms, obtain follow-up urinalysis and culture 2 to 3 days after antibiotic course is completed.

ETHOXAZENE HYDROCHLORIDE

PRODUCTS (TRADE NAME):
Serenium (Available in 100 mg tablets,)

DRUG SPECIFICS:
This drug may cause interference with BSP or PSP excretion tests and urine bilirubin determinations.

ADMINISTRATION AND DOSAGE SPECIFICS:
Adults: 100 mg (before meals) po three times daily.

PHENAZOPYRIDINE HYDROCHLORIDE

PRODUCTS (TRADE NAME):
Azodine, AZO-Standard, Baridium, Di-Azo, Diamino Pyridine HCl, Phen-

ylazo, Phenazodine, Phenaopyridine HCl, Pyridiate, Pyridium, Urodine (Available in 100 and 200 mg tablets.)

DRUG SPECIFICS:

Use Clinitest for accurate urine sugar tests in diabetic patients receiving these drugs as they may change Clinistix or Tes-Tape results.

ADMINISTRATION AND DOSAGE SPECIFICS:

Adult: 100 to 200 mg po (after meals) three times daily.

COMBINATION PRODUCTS

PRODUCTS (TRADE NAME):

Pyridium Plus (Available in 150 mg phenazopyridine HCl, 0.3 mg hyoscyamine HBr and 15 mg butabarbital tablets.) **Urogesic** (Available in 100 mg phenazopyridine HCl, O.08 mg atropine sulfate, O.003 mg scopolamine HBr and 0.12 mg hyoscyamine HBr tablets.)

DRUG SPECIFICS:

These products contain antispasmodics and phenazopyridine HCl in combination.

ADMINISTRATION AND DOSAGE SPECIFICS:

Pyridium Plus: Adults: Take one tablet 4 times daily after meals and at bedtime.
Urogesic: Adults: Take one or two tablets 3 times daily before meals.

Mary Ann Bolter

ANTI-INFECTIVES

ACETOHYDROXAMIC ACID (AHA)

ACTION OF THE DRUG: This product inhibits the bacterial enzyme urease. The production of ammonia in urine is therefore decreased which is helpful when infections with urea-splitting organisms are present. The reduced pH and ammonia levels allow antimicrobial agents taken concomittantly to be more effective, thus enhancing infection cure rates.

ASSESSMENT:

INDICATIONS: Used as adjunctive therapy in chronic urea-splitting urinary tract infections. Long-term therapy may be indicated in some cases.

SUBJECTIVE-OBJECTIVE: Complaints of fever, chills, suprapubic tenderness, dysuria, frequency, and urgency should alert the practitioner to the presence of infection. Previous history of urinary tract infections may also be present. Urinalysis may show organisms and white blood cells, while culture will indicate nature of organisms and antibiotic sensitivity. Documentation that organism is urea splitting should be made before medication is started.

PLAN:

CONTRAINDICATIONS: Do not use this product if patient has poor renal function (serum creatinine more than 2.5 mg/dl and/or creatinine clearance less than 20 ml/min.), if organisms are non-urease producing, in patients whose problem requires surgical intervention, or when disease could be treated adequately by antibiotics alone. Do not use in women who do not have adequate contraception since product may cause fetal harm.

WARNINGS: Safety for use in breast-feeding women and children has not been demonstrated. A reversible Coombs' negative hemolytic anemia test has occurred in some patients taking this product, requiring close monitoring of blood work.

PRECAUTIONS: In animals, inhibition of DNA synthesis has lead to bone marrow depression. Depletion of iron stores also may develop. Hemolysis with decrease in circulating RBCs, Hgb and HCT have been seen clinically. In patients with renal impairment, reduced dosages and close monitoring is essential to prevent excessive drug accumulation. Laboratory studies also indicate caution should be taken until further issues concerning carcinogenesis, mutagenesis and impairment of fertility are more fully investigated.

IMPLEMENTATION:

DRUG INTERACTIONS: Acetohydroxamic acid should not be given concomitantly with iron, as it has the capacity to chelate heavy metal. Alcoholic beverages taken with this drug have produced a rash.

PRODUCTS (TRADE NAME):
Lithostat (Available in 250 mg scored tablets.)

ADMINISTRATION AND DOSAGE:
Adults: Take 250 mg three to four times daily in a total dose of 10 to 15 mg/kg/day. The recommended starting dose is 12 mg/kg/day at 6 to 8 hour intervals on an empty stomach. Do not exceed 1.5 gm daily.

Children: Take 10 mg/kg/day initially. Monitor clinical condition and laboratory tests. Titrate dosage as required.

Patients with reduced renal functions: Do not take more than 1.0 gm/day, dosed at 12-hour intervals if serum creatinine is greater than 1.8 mg/dl. Do not give to patients with severe renal insufficiency.

IMPLEMENTATION CONSIDERATIONS:
—Obtain a complete health history, including the presence of systemic disease, possibility of pregnancy, and nature and course of urinary tract infection. Review all relevant laboratory findings.

—All patients receiving this drug must have adequate hematologic monitoring at regular intervals. Any reticulocytosis should be closely evaluated.

—Approximately 30% of the patients taking this drug experience some sort of adverse reaction. Because this is a relatively new drug, there is still much to be learned about its actions. Patients should be encouraged to report any adverse reactions promptly for evaluation.

—Adverse reactions appear to be more likely in patients with preexisting thrombophlebitis, phlebothrombosis or advanced degrees of renal insufficiency.

—Mild headaches are common in about 30% of patients. These headaches usually respond to salicylate analgesics.

WHAT THE PATIENT NEEDS TO KNOW:

—Take this medication exactly as ordered by your health care provider. It is best taken on an empty stomach. This is a medication designed to help antibiotics become more effective in curing your infection.

—Keep medication out of the reach of children or others for whom medication is not prescribed.

—You should not drink alcohol while taking this product.

—Report any new or unusual symptoms to your health care provider. Particularly note any headaches, nausea, vomiting, tiredness, appetite changes, or nervousness.

EVALUATION:

ADVERSE REACTIONS: *Cardiovascular:* thrombophlebitis. *CNS:* anxiety, depression, headaches, nervousness, tremulousness. *Dermatologic:* alopecia, non-pruritic, macular skin rash on face and in upper extremities, which resolves spontaneously. *Gastrointestinal:* anorexia, malaise, nausea, vomiting. *Hematologic:* hemolytic anemia, mild reticulocytosis accompanying symptoms of malaise, lethargy, fatigue, and gastrointestinal symptoms.

OVERDOSAGE: Mild overdosages have produced hemolysis. These are most often seen in patients with reduced renal function. Symptomatic treatment is indicated.

PARAMETERS TO MONITOR: Obtain a complete history and physical examination, including blood studies to serve as baseline indicators. A complete blood count, including a reticulocyte count is recommended two weeks after beginning therapy. If the reticulocyte count exceeds 6%, the dosage should be reduced. Complete blood studies, Coombs' test and reticulocyte count should be done at three month intervals while patient is taking medication. Watch especially for signs of hemolysis, although platelet and white cell counts should also be monitored.

Marilyn W. Edmunds

METHENAMINE AND METHENAMINE SALTS

ACTION OF THE DRUG: Methenamine is a urinary tract antiseptic. In acid urine it is hydrolyzed to ammonia and formaldehyde. Formaldehyde is bactericidal or bacteriostatic depending upon the amount released by hydrolysis; it apparently acts by denaturing protein.

ASSESSMENT:

INDICATIONS: Methenamine and its salts are indicated for long-term prophylaxis or suppression of chronic urinary tract infections, and for infected residual urine that may accompany neurologic diseases, anatomical abnormalities of the urinary tract, and indwelling catheters.

SUBJECTIVE: *Lower urinary tract:* Patient may be asymptomatic or complain of sudden or gradual onset of burning pain on urination, frequency, urgency to void, suprapubic pain, and/or low back pain. Urine may be described as cloudy, dark, bloody and/or malodorous. *Upper urinary tract:* Patient may be asymptomatic; may or may not demonstrate lower urinary tract symptoms; and may or may not complain of headache, malaise, fever, chills, nausea, vomiting, anorexia, flank pain, and/or abdominal pain.

OBJECTIVE: *Lower urinary tract:* Physical exam: May not be significant, or may have suprapubic tenderness and/or erythema and tenderness of the urethra. Laboratory tests show significant bacteriuria (one to two organisms per high-power field in unspun urine) which may be accompanied by pyuria, and/or hematuria. Urine culture and prostatic secretion cultures demonstrate significant bacteriuria (100,000 or more organisms per ml). *Upper urinary tract:* Physical exam may not be significant or there may be fever greater than 101 degrees F. and/or CVA tenderness. Laboratory tests show significant bacteriuria which may be accompanied by pyuria, proteinuria, and/or hematuria. Urine culture should demonstrate significant bacteriuria.

PLAN:

CONTRAINDICATIONS: Do not use with hypersensitivity, renal insufficiency, severe dehydration, severe hepatic disease, or with markedly decreased urine output. Methenamine sulfosalicylate is contraindicated in patients with salicylate sensitivity.

WARNINGS: Safety of use during pregnancy has not been established. Methenamine and its salts should not be used alone in treatment of acute infections or in infections with parenchymal involvement causing systemic symptoms such as chills and fever. They should not be used if the urine cannot or should not be acidified.

PRECAUTIONS: Methenamine and its salts require an acid urine to be therapeutically effective. Its effectiveness may be decreased when treating ureasplitting organisms that increase the urinary pH, such as *Proteus* and strains of *Pseudomonas*. Large doses may cause dysuria, proteinuria, and hematuria; dosage and acidification of the urine should be reduced. Caution should be used when administering methenamine oral suspensions to the elderly and debilitated as lipid pneumonia may occur. Methenamine salts may precipitate urate crystals in the urine in patients with a history of gout. Liver function studies should be done periodically on patients receiving methenamine hippurate.

IMPLEMENTATION:

DRUG INTERACTIONS: Methenamine and its salts when taken concurrently with sulfonamides may form insoluble precipitates (crystalluria) in the urine. The concurrent use of these two drugs should be avoided. Urine alkalinizing drugs such as acetazolamide, sodium bicarbonate, and thiazide diuretics decrease the effectiveness of methenamine and its salts. Methenamine inhibits amphetamines by increasing their urinary excretion rate.

ADMINISTRATION AND DOSAGE: Methenamine and its salts are readily absorbed from the gastrointestinal tract. Antibacterial activity is found only in the urine. Maximum therapeutic effect occurs when the urine pH is 5.5 or less. Methenamine's acid salts help to maintain a low urine pH. Low urinary pH alone exerts a bacteriostatic effect. Dysuria may occur on doses of 4 gm to 8 gm/day given for longer than three to four weeks. Once sterile urine is obtained, high doses should be reduced. Methenamine and its salts should be taken at equally spaced time intervals.

IMPLEMENTATION CONSIDERATIONS:

—Obtain a complete health history: history of hypersensitivity, renal insufficiency, severe hepatic disease, gout, salicylate sensitivity, concurrent use of any drugs which may cause drug interactions, presence of dehydration, markedly low urinary output, or pregnancy.

—Obtain baseline urine pH. Urine pH should be maintained at 5.5 or less.

—Obtain baseline renal function studies (and hepatic function studies if prescribing methenamine hippurate).

—Discontinue the drug if a skin rash occurs.

—Urine acidification and/or methenamine dosage should be reduced if bladder irritation occurs.

—Compliance may be poor due to the number of pills required with some products.

—*Proteus* and *Pseudomonas* may raise the urine pH; urinary acidifiers will probably be required when treating infections caused by these organisms.

—Gastrointestinal distress may occur even when enteric-coated tablets are used; the drug should therefore be given after meals.

—Increased urine volume due to either increased fluid intake or diuretic therapy may significantly decrease the formaldehyde concentration in the urine and thus decrease the effectiveness of the drug. Optimal daily fluid intake is 1500 to 2000 ml/day.

—Supplementary acidification of the urine may be required to reduce pH to 5.5 or less. This may be achieved by limiting alkalinizing foods and encouraging acidifying foods. Alkalinizing foods are: milk, peanuts, vegetables, fruits and fruit juice. Acidifying foods are: meats, eggs, cheese, corn, lentils, cranberries, plums, prunes, breads and bread products.

—Ascorbic acid 4 to 12 gm/day given in divided doses may also be used to acidify the urine.

WHAT THE PATIENT NEEDS TO KNOW:

—Take this medication exactly as ordered as a way of ensuring its effectiveness.

—Drink eight to ten glasses of water every day.

—Test your urine pH on a regular basis. The pH should be at 5.5 or less.

—Foods which will help acidify your urine are: meats, eggs, cheese, corn, lentils, cranberries, plums, prunes, breads and bread products. Avoid an oversupply of milk, peanuts, vegetables, fruits and fruit juices.

—Beneficial effects from this drug will require continuous long-term therapy. The minimum trial period is forty-five days.

—Methenamine should be taken after meals or with food to minimize its possible stomach irritation. Antacids and sodium bicarbonate should be avoided.

—Notify the health provider if skin rash, painful or bloody urine, or severe abdominal distress occurs.

—The oral suspension should be shaken before taking each dose.

EVALUATION:

ADVERSE REACTIONS: *Dermatologic:* skin rash. *Gastrointestinal:* abdominal discomfort, elevated liver enzymes, nausea, vomiting. *Genitourinary:* albuminuria, crystalluria, dysuria, frequency, hematuria, proteinuria, urinary tract irritation with high doses.

OVERDOSAGE: Moderate: gastric irritation, nausea, vomiting, frequent and painful urination. Severe: severe irritation of the bladder with hematuria, decreased urinary output, impaired kidney function, weakness, deep breathing, stupor, coma.

PARAMETERS TO MONITOR: Observe for therapeutic effects and development of adverse reactions. Periodically while the patient is on long-term therapy, hepatic and renal function should be evaluated. Periodic bacteriological exam of the urine should be performed to monitor the effectiveness of therapy. Urinalysis should be done also to detect hematuria which may be indicative of drug irritation of the bladder. The client should be questioned on his monitoring of his urine pH, pill ingestion, and fluid intake and urinary output. Signs and symptoms of toxicity should also be monitored.

METHENAMINE

PRODUCTS (TRADE NAME):
Methenamine (Available in 0.5 gm tablets.)
DRUG SPECIFICS:
Inexpensive medication. Take with food to minimize gastric upset. Force fluids while taking medication.
ADMINISTRATION AND DOSAGE SPECIFICS:
Adult: One gram po four times a day.
Children 6 to 12 years: 500 mg po four times a day.
Children under 6 years: 50 mg/kg/day po divided into three doses.

METHENAMINE HIPPURATE

PRODUCTS (TRADE NAME):
   Hiprex, Urex (Available in one gram tablets.)
DRUG SPECIFICS:
   Take at evenly spaced intervals both night and day. Complete full course of medication. Force fluids while taking medication.
ADMINISTRATION AND DOSAGE SPECIFICS:
   Adult: 1 gm po twice a day.
   Children 6 to 12 years: 500 mg to 1 gm po twice a day.

METHENAMINE MANDELATE

PRODUCTS (TRADE NAME):
   Methenamine Mandelate (Available in 0.25, 0.5 and 1 gm plain or enteric-coated tablets; 0.25 gm/5 ml, 0.5 gm/5 ml oral suspension). **Mandelamine** (Available in 0.5 gm, 1 gm plain or enteric-coated tablets; 0.25 gm/5 ml, 0.5 gm/5 ml oral suspension, and 0.5 gm, 1 gm packets of granules).
DRUG SPECIFICS:
   Products come in a variety of doses and preparations. Granules and suspensions tend to be the most expensive.
ADMINISTRATION AND DOSAGE SPECIFICS:
   Adult: One gram po four times per day, taken after meals and at bedtime.
   Children 6 to 12 years: 500 mg po four times per day, taken after meals and at bedtime.
   Children under 6 years: 0.25 gm/14 kg/day divided into four doses, given after meals and at bedtime.

Marna J. Ross

METHYLENE BLUE

ACTION OF THE DRUG: Methylene blue is a bacteriostatic dye. In high concentrations it produces methemoglobin by oxidizing ferrous iron to the ferric form.

ASSESSMENT:

INDICATIONS: Methylene blue is indicated for use as a mild urinary antiseptic for cystitis and urethritis. It is also indicated in the treatment of idiopathic and drug-induced methemoglobinemia and as an antidote for cyanide poisoning.

SUBJECTIVE: *Lower urinary tract:* Patient may be asymptomatic or may complain of sudden or gradual onset of burning pain on urination, frequency, urgency to void, suprapubic pain, and/or low back pain. Urine may be described as cloudy, dark, bloody and/or malodorous. *Upper urinary tract:* Patient may be asymptomatic; may or may not demonstrate lower urinary tract symptoms; and may or may not complain of headache, malaise, fever, chills, nausea, vomiting, anorexia, flank pain, and/or abdominal pain.

OBJECTIVE: *Lower urinary tract:* Physical exam may not be significant, or there may be suprapubic tenderness and/or erythema and tenderness of the urethera. Laboratory tests show significant bacteriuria (one to two organisms per high-power field on unspun urine) which may be accompanied by pyuria, and/or hematuria. Urine culture and prostatic secretion culture demonstrate significant bacteriuria (100,000 or more organisms per ml). *Upper urinary tract:* Physical exam may not be significant or may show fever greater than 101 degrees F. and/or CVA tenderness. Laboratory shows significant bacteriuria which may be accompanied by pyuria, proteinuria, and/or hematuria. Urine culture should demonstrate significant bacteriuria.

PLAN:

CONTRAINDICATIONS: Do not use in the presence of hypersensitivity, or renal insufficiency.

PRECAUTIONS: Methylene blue may be ineffective in patients with G-6-PD deficiency. It may also induce hemolysis in these patients. Long-term therapy may cause anemia due to the destruction of erythrocytes. Cyanosis and cardiovascular abnormalities have been reported.

IMPLEMENTATION:

PRODUCTS (TRADE NAME):
Methylene Blue, Urolene Blue (Available in 65 mg tablet.)
ADMINISTRATION AND DOSAGE: Methylene blue is poorly absorbed from the gastrointestinal tract. It is excreted in the urine, bile and feces. Methylene blue is seldom used as a urinary tract antiseptic. However, it is found in multiple combination urinary anti-infective agents.

Cystitis, urethritis:
Adult: 65 mg po three times per day after meals, with a full glass of water.
IMPLEMENTATION CONSIDERATIONS:
—Obtain a complete health history: history of hypersensitivity, or renal insufficiency.
—Baseline CBC should be obtained, and hemoglobin monitored periodically.
—Methylene blue stain may be removed with hypochlorite solutions.

WHAT THE PATIENT NEEDS TO KNOW:

—Each dose should be taken with a full glass of water after eating. Drink at least 8 glasses of water per day.

—Methylene blue may cause urine and feces to turn blue-green in color.

—Report any new or uncomfortable symptoms to your health provider.

—This dye may stain clothing blue. This stain can be removed by hypochlorite solutions.

EVALUATION:

ADVERSE REACTIONS: *Gastrointestinal:* diarrhea, nausea, vomiting. *Genitourinary:* bladder irritation, dysuria. *Hematopoietic:* anemia with long-term use. *Other:* large doses may cause fever, methemoglobinemia, and cardiovascular abnormalities.

PARAMETERS TO MONITOR: Evaluate for therapeutic effects and development of adverse reactions. The patient's hemoglobin should be monitored regularly. Intake should be assessed to ensure that the patient is drinking at least 2,000 cc of water per day.

Marna J. Ross

NALIDIXIC ACID

ACTION OF THE DRUG: Nalidixic acid is bactericidal against most of the common gram-negative bacteria which cause urinary tract infections. Its mode of action apparently is to inhibit DNA synthesis.

ASSESSMENT:

INDICATIONS: Nalidixic acid is indicated for the treatment of acute and chronic urinary tract infections caused by susceptible strains of *Escherichia coli, Proteus, Klebsiella* and *Enterobacter.*

SUBJECTIVE: *Lower urinary tract:* Patient may be asymptomatic or complain of sudden or gradual onset of burning pain on urination, frequency, urgency to void, suprapubic pain and/or low back pain. Urine may be described as cloudy, dark, bloody and/or malodorous. *Upper urinary tract:* Patient may be asymptomatic; may or may not demonstrate lower urinary tract symptoms; and may or may not complain of headache, malaise, fever, chills, nausea, vomiting, anorexia, flank pain, and/or abdominal pain.

OBJECTIVE: *Lower urinary tract:* Physical examination may not be significant. There may be suprapubic tenderness and/or erythema and tenderness of the urethra. Laboratory tests show significant bacteriuria. Unspun urine may show one to two organisms per high power field, which may be accompanied by pyuria and/or hematuria. Urine culture and prostatic secretion culture demonstrate significant bacteriuria (100,000 or more organisms/ml). *Upper urinary tract:* Physical examination may not be significant. May have fever greater than 101 m degrees F. and/or CVA tenderness. Laboratory tests show significant bacteriuria which may be accompanied by pyuria, proteinuria, and/or hematuria. Urine culture should demonstrate significant bacteriuria.

PLAN:

CONTRAINDICATIONS: Do not use with hypersensitivity to nalidixic acid; history of convulsive disorders; infants under three months of age.

WARNINGS: Safe use during the first trimester of pregnancy has not been established. Rare CNS side effects including convulsions, increased intracranial pressure, and toxic psychosis have been reported in infants, children, and geriatric patients. They have occurred usually from overdosage or in patients with predisposing factors. Side effects disappeared rapidly upon discontinuation of the drug. Hemolysis has occurred in patients with G-6-PD deficiency.

PRECAUTIONS: Caution should be used when administering this drug during the last two trimesters of pregnancy. Caution should be used when administering this drug to patients with a history of impaired hepatic or renal function, severe cerebral arteriosclerosis, or epilepsy. Nalidixic acid may cause photosensitivity and should be discontinued if this occurs. Cross-resistance between nalidixic acid and oxolinic acid has been reported.

IMPLEMENTATION:

DRUG INTERACTIONS: Nalidixic acid may increase the effects of dicumarol and warfarin. Nitrofurantoin may antagonize the effect of nalidixic acid. Urinary acidifiers such as ascorbic acid and cranberry juice may enhance the antibacterial effect of nalidixic acid by decreasing its excretion rate. Urinary alkalinizing agents inhibit nalidixic acid by increasing its urinary excretion rate. Antacids may decrease the absorption of nalidixic acid. Alertness, judgment, and motor coordination may be decreased when nalidixic acid is taken in combination with alcohol.

PRODUCTS (TRADE NAME):

NegGram (Available in 250 mg, 500 mg and 1 gm caplets; and 250 mg/5 ml suspension.)

ADMINISTRATION AND DOSAGE: Nalidixic acid is readily absorbed from the gastrointestinal tract. Peak serum levels occur in one to two hours. It is important to avoid underdosage during the initial treatment period as bacterial resistance may occur. In prolonged therapy, the daily dose is reduced after the initial treatment period is completed. If bacterial resistance occurs, it usually develops within the first forty-eight hours of treatment. High concentrations of nalidixic acid and its metabolites are found in the urine. Antibacterial activity is not found in prostatic fluid. Nalidixic acid is not effective against Pseudomonas species.

Adult: Initial therapy: one gram po four times per day for one to two weeks.

Prolonged therapy: reduce dosage to two grams per day after the initial treatment period is completed.

Children 3 months to 12 years: Initial therapy: 55 mg/kg/day po given in four equally divided doses. Prolonged therapy: reduce dosage to 33 mg/kg/day po.

IMPLEMENTATION CONSIDERATIONS:

—Obtain a complete health history: history of hypersensitivity, seizure disorders, Parkinson's disease, kidney or liver disease, or severe cerebral arteriosclerosis; drugs taken concurrently which may cause drug interactions; possibility of pregnancy, or breast feeding.

—Obtain baseline CBC, liver and renal function studies if the patient will be on long-term therapy. Obtain a baseline urinalysis and culture and sensitivity test with a clean catch midstream urine specimen.

—Patients over sixty may require reduced dosages and lengthening of dosage intervals. Dosages may be determined by renal function studies.

—If visual disturbances occur they will usually disappear with reduced dosages.

—CNS side effects usually occur thirty minutes after the first dose or after the second or third dose.

—Asymptomatic bacteriuria is usually not treated. Exceptions are in cases of pregnancy and in patients undergoing genitourinary instrumentation.

—Analgesics such as phenazopyridine or aspirin may be prescribed for the first twenty-four to forty-eight hours to relieve pain.

—Identify predisposing factors to infection and initiate patient education and appropriate physician referral as indicated.

—Ninety percent of initial urinary tract infections are caused by *Escherichia coli. Klebsiella* and *Proteus* are the next most frequent causes.

—Relapse may occur up to fourteen days after treatment has been completed. The causative organism is the same. A relapse may indicate upper urinary tract involvement.

—Reinfection may occur weeks to months after treatment has been completed, and may be caused by a different strain.

—Female patients with two to three successive well-documented and treated infections should be referred for further medical evaluation. Men should be referred if they have more than one well-documented infection.

—Patients with recurrent infections which cannot be attributed to obstructive uropathy or renal disease may require low-dose, long-term therapy.

WHAT THE PATIENT NEEDS TO KNOW:

—Take this medication exactly as prescribed in order to avoid developing resistance to the drug. Symptoms usually disappear after two or three days; however, bacteria may still be present in the urine. It is therefore very important to take all the medicine prescribed.

—Some patients experience side effects while taking this drug. Report any new or troublesome symptoms to your health provider for evaluation. Particularly watch for marked irritability, vomiting, headache, excitement, and/or vertigo.

—Do not perform activities requiring alertness until the effects of this drug on your body are known. It may cause drowsiness, dizziness, or visual disturbances.

—You should avoid exposure to direct sunlight for more than short periods while taking this drug.

—Nalidixic acid may cause gastric upset and should be taken with food. It should not be taken with antacids as these may decrease its absorption.

—If you are a diabetic, this drug may cause false positive results when testing for urine glucose with Benedict's solution, Fehling's solution, and Clinitest tablets. Clinistix or Tes-Tape should be used instead.

—Fluid intake should be increased to at least ten to fifteen glasses of water per day during and after therapy.

—Eliminate coffee, tea, alcohol, chocolate and/or spicy foods from your diet during therapy as they may be irritating to the urinary tract.

—Return for a follow-up urinalysis and/or urine culture one week after therapy is completed to determine if a cure has been obtained.

—Bathe daily, wear cotton underwear, urinate regularly, and avoid tight fitting clothing if you are a female patient.

—Sexually active patients and their partners should wash before sexual intercourse. Female patients should urinate shortly before and after intercourse. Care should be taken not to spread rectal bacteria near the vulvar area.

—Oral contraceptives, diaphragms, tampons, douching, bubble baths, and increased frequency of intercourse may all contribute to having recurrent urinary tract infections for female patients.

EVALUATION:

ADVERSE REACTIONS: *CNS:* blurred vision, change in color perception, convulsions, diplopia, dizziness, drowsiness, headache, intracranial hypertension, papilledema, sensitivity to light, toxic psychosis (rare), vertigo, weakness. *Gastrointestinal:* abdominal pain, diarrhea, nausea, vomiting. *Hematopoietic:* eosinophilia. *Hypersensitivity:* angioedema, arthralgia with joint swelling, anaphylactoid reaction (rare), eosinophilia, fever, photosensitivity, pruritus, rash, urticaria. *Other:* cholestasis, hemolytic anemia which may be associated with G-6-PD deficiency, leukopenia, metabolic acidosis, paresthesias, thrombocytopenia.

OVERDOSAGE: *Symptoms:* moderate: nausea, vomiting, lethargy. Severe: toxic psychosis, convulsions, increased intracranial pressure, metabolic acidosis. *Treatment:* Nalidixic acid is excreted rapidly. Reactions usually last two to three hours. Gastric lavage and supportive measures should be implemented.

PARAMETERS TO MONITOR: Monitor clinical response to therapy. If it is unsatisfactory, culture and sensitivity tests should be repeated and the drug may need to be changed. Monitor for signs and symptoms of toxicity. Therapy which lasts longer than two weeks should include periodic monitoring of liver and renal function studies and CBC. Initial culture should be checked to determine presence of significant bacteria indicating urethritis, cystitis, prostatitis, or pyelonephritis as opposed to urethral syndrome. Sterilization of the urine should occur in approximately 48 hours after the initiation of therapy. The provider may wish to examine and culture the urine at this time. If there is no bacteria found, the patient should continue the therapy. Presence of bacteria, however, may indicate an upper urinary tract infection, complications or drug resistance and should be investigated further. All patients should have a follow-up urine culture one week after therapy has been completed to determine if a cure has been obtained. If bacteriuria remains, sensitivity testing should be done to direct the choice of drug therapy.

Marna J. Ross

NITROFURANTOIN

ACTION OF THE DRUG: Nitrofurantoin is an antibacterial agent for urinary tract infections. Its mode of action is to interfere with bacterial enzyme systems. It is active against most gram-negative bacilli and gram-positive cocci associated with urinary tract infections.

ASSESSMENT:

INDICATIONS: Nitrofurantoin is indicated in the treatment of pyelonephritis, pyelitis, and cystitis due to susceptible organisms: *E. Coli, S. aureus,* enterococci and certain strains of *Klebsiella, Enterobacter,* and *Proteus.* It is not indicated for treatment of associated renal cortical or perinephric abscesses. It is indicated in short-term prophylaxis or long-term suppressive therapy of chronic urinary tract infections.

SUBJECTIVE: *Lower urinary tract:* Patient may be asymptomatic or complain of sudden or gradual onset of burning pain on urination, frequency, urgency to void, suprapubic pain, and/or low back pain. Urine may be described as cloudy, dark, bloody, and/or malodorous. *Upper urinary tract:* Patient may be asymptomatic; may or may not demonstrate lower urinary tract symptoms; and may or may not complain of headache, malaise, fever, chills, nausea, vomiting, anorexia, flank pain, and/or abdominal pain.

OBJECTIVE: *Lower urinary tract:* Physical exam may not be significant, or suprapubic tenderness and/or erythema and tenderness of the urethra may be present. Laboratory may show significant bacteriuria (one to two organisms per high power field of unspun urine), which may be accompanied by pyuria, and/or hematuria. Urine culture and prostatic secretion culture demonstrate significant bacteriuria (100,000 or more organisms per ml.) *Upper urinary tract:* Physical exam may not be significant, or show fever greater than 101 degrees F. and/or CVA tenderness. Laboratory shows significant bacteriuria which may be accompanied by pyuria, proteinuria, and/or hematuria. Urine culture should demonstrate significant bacteriuria.

PLAN:

CONTRAINDICATIONS: Do not give with hypersensitivity to nitrofurantoin preparations, moderate to severe renal impairment, anuria, oliguria, creatinine clearance under 40 ml/min; G-6-PD deficiency; pregnant patients at term, or infants under one month of age.

WARNINGS: Acute, subacute, and chronic pulmonary reactions have been reported. If these occur, the drug should be discontinued immediately and appropriate therapy instituted. Insidious onset of pulmonary reactions may occur during long-term therapy. The patient should be monitored closely if these reactions occur. Deaths have been reported in relation to pulmonary reactions. Hemolysis has been reported. The drug should be withdrawn if any signs of hemolysis occur. The safety of nitrofurantoin during pregnancy and lactation has not been established. *Pseudomonas* is the organism most commonly associated with superinfections.

PRECAUTIONS: Peripheral neuropathy may occur; deaths have been reported. Nitrofurantoin should be used with caution in patients with anemia, diabetes, electrolyte imbalance, vitamin B deficiency, renal impairment, and debilitating diseases as these may predispose the patient to severe or irreversible peripheral neuropathies. Caution should be used if the patient has a history of asthma. Patients over 60 may require dosage reduction and lengthening of dosage intervals.

IMPLEMENTATION:

DRUG INTERACTIONS: The effects of nitrofurantoin may be increased by urine acidifying agents and probenecid. The effects may be decreased by antacids, alkalinizing agents, acetazolamide, phenobarbital, nalidixic acid, and magnesium trisilicate. Nitrofurantoin when taken with alcohol may cause a disulfiram-like reaction. Nitrofurantoin may cause false positive test results for serum glucose, bilirubin, alkaline phosphatase and blood urea nitrogen. False positive urine glucose determinations may occur when Benedict's solution or Clinitest is used.

ADMINISTRATION AND DOSAGE: Nitrofuratoin is well absorbed from the gastrointestinal tract. The macrocrystalline form appears to cause less gastric distress than the conventional tablets. Nitrofuratoin does not achieve antibacterial concentrations in the plasma because it is rapidly eliminated. In patients with normal renal function the average dose yields concentrations of approximately 200 micrograms/ml in the urine. Alkalinized urine may inhibit nitrofurantoin's antimicrobial activity. In patients with impaired renal function, nitrofurantoin may accumulate to toxic levels in the serum. Individuals with creatinine clearance below 40 ml/min will not achieve therapeutic levels of the drug in the urine. Nitrofurantoin should be given at equally spaced time intervals to maintain therapeutic urinary drug levels, usually every six hours. Therapy should last for ten to fourteen days when treating acute infections. Bacterial resistance develops slowly and cross-resistance and sensitization occur infrequently.

IMPLEMENTATION CONSIDERATIONS:

—Obtain a complete health history: concurrent use of medications which may produce drug interactions, contraindications to drug, possibility of pregnancy or breast-feeding.

—Blacks and ethnic groups from Mediterranean and Near Eastern areas may be predisposed to develop anemia.

—Pulmonary sensitivity reactions usually occur during the first week of therapy.

—Therapy should continue for at least three days after sterile urine specimens are obtained.

—Intramuscular injections are very painful. This method of administration should not be used for more than five days.

—Identify predisposing factors to infection and initiate patient education and appropriate physician referral as indicated.

—Ninety percent of initial urinary tract infections are caused by *Escherichia coli. Klebsiella* and *Proteus* are the next most frequent causes.

—Relapse may occur up to fourteen days after treatment has been completed. The causative organism is the same. A relapse may indicate upper urinary tract involvement.

—Reinfection may occur weeks to months after treatment has been completed, and may be caused by a different strain.

—Female patients with two to three successive well-documented and treated infections should be referred for further medical evaluation. Men should be referred if they have more than one infection.

—Patients with recurrent infections which cannot be attributed to obstructive uropathy or renal disease may require low-dose, long-term therapy.

WHAT THE PATIENT NEEDS TO KNOW:

—Take this medication exactly as prescribed. Symptoms usually disappear after two to three days; however, bacteria may still be present in the urine. It is therefore very important to take all the medicine prescribed.

—This drug sometimes produces side effects. It is important to notify your health provider if you have any new or uncomfortable symptoms. Note particularly any numbness or tingling of the arms or legs; flu-like syndrome; cough, or shortness of breath.

—This drug may cause stomach upset and therefore should be taken with meals. Notify the health provider if nausea or stomach distress is a problem.

—This drug must be taken at evenly spaced intervals to maximize its effectiveness.

—Nitrofurantoin may cause the urine to turn brown.

—Nitrofurantoin may stain the teeth. Avoid crushing tablets and dilute oral suspensions to avoid this problem.

—Notify the health provider if urinary output decreases or stops, if urine turns milky, foul-smelling, and if irritation and painful urination occur. These may be symptoms of another infection.

—Fluid intake should be increased to at least ten to fifteen glasses of water per day during and after therapy.

—Eliminate coffee, tea, alcohol, chocolate, and/or spicy foods from your diet during therapy as they may be irritating to the urinary tract.

—Return for a follow-up urinalysis and/or urine culture one week after therapy is completed to detemine if a cure has been obtained.

—Sexually active patients and their partners should wash before sexual intercourse. The female patient should urinate shortly before and after intercourse. Care should be taken not to spread rectal bacteria to the vulvar area.

—Oral contraceptives, diaphragms, tampons, douching, bubble baths, and increased frequency of intercourse may contribute to the patient having recurrent urinary tract infections.

EVALUATION:

ADVERSE REACTIONS: *CNS:* ascending polyneuropathy with high doses or renal impairment, dizziness, drowsiness, headache, peripheral neuropathy, nystagmus, vertigo. *Dermatologic:* angioedema, erythematous, maculopapular or eczematous rash, pruritus, urticaria. *Gastrointestinal:* anorexia, abdominal pain, diarrhea, hepatitis (rare), nausea, vomiting. *Hematopoietic:* eosinophilia, granulocytopenia, hemolysis in patients with G-6-PD deficiency (rare), leukopenia, megaloblastic anemia. *Hypersensitivity:* pulmonary hypersensitivity reactions associated with short and long-term therapy: fever, chills, cough, chest pain, dyspnea, pulmonary infiltration with consolidation or effusion, eosinophilia, anaphylaxis; asthmatic attack in patients with a history of asthma, drug fever, arthralgia. *Other:* hypotension, superinfection of the urinary tract, transient alopecia.

OVERDOSAGE: Nausea, vomiting, abdominal pain and diarrhea.

PARAMETERS TO MONITOR: The patient should be monitored for therapeutic effects and adverse reactions. Watch for signs of pulmonary sensitivity, peripheral neuropathies, superinfection of the urinary tract, hemolysis, and toxicity. During prolonged therapy, monitoring of CBC, liver function, and chest x-rays is advisable.

NITROFURANTOIN

PRODUCTS (TRADE NAME):

Furadantin (Available in 50 and 100 mg tablets or capsules; 25 mg/5 ml oral suspension.) **Furalan, Furan, Furatoin** (Available in 50 and 100 mg tablets.) **Ivadantin** (Available in powder for injection: 180 mg/vial, 20 ml size.) **Nitrex** (Available in 50 and 100 mg tablets.) **Nitrofan** (Available in 50 and 100 mg capsules.) **Nitrofurantoin** (Available in 50 and 100 mg tablets or capsules.)

DRUG SPECIFICS:

For maximum effectiveness, nitrofurantoin should be given at equally spaced time intervals, preferably every six hours. IM injections are very painful. Injections should not be given for more than five days.

ADMINISTRATION AND DOSAGE SPECIFICS:

Adult: 50 to 100 mg po four times per day with meals. Long term therapy: 25 to 50 mg po four times per day; or parenterally, 180 mg IM two times per day if patient weighs more thanb 120 lbs, or 3 mg/lb/day IM in two equally divided doses if patient weighs less than 120 lbs.

Children one month to twelve years: 5 to 7 mg/kg/day po given in four divided doses. Parenteral use: safety not established in children under twelve. *Long term therapy:* 1 mg/kg/24 hours given in 1 or 2 doses.

NITROFURANTOIN MACROCRYSTALS

PRODUCT (TRADE NAME):

Macrodantin (Available in 25, 50 and 100 mg capsules.)

DRUG SPECIFICS:

Macrocrystals are less likely to cause gastric distress than the conventional tablets and capsules. Efficacy is the same.

ADMINISTRATION AND DOSAGE SPECIFICS:

Adult: 50 to 100 mg po four times a day.

Children one month to twelve years: 5 to 7 mg/kg/day po. Give in divided doses four times per day.

Marna J. Ross

TRIMETHOPRIM

ACTION OF THE DRUG: Trimethoprim is a synthetic antibacterial agent which interferes with the bacterial biosynthesis of nucleic acids and proteins. Its spectrum of activity includes the common urinary tract pathogens with the exception of *Pseudomonas aeruginosa.*

ASSESSMENT:

INDICATIONS: Trimethoprim is indicated in the treatment of initial episodes of uncomplicated urinary tract infections caused by susceptible strains of *Escherichia coli, Proteus mirabilis, Klebsiella pneumoniae,* and *Enterobacter* species. It also reduces or eliminates these microorganisms from the vaginal and fecal flora.

SUBJECTIVE: *Lower urinary tract:* Patient may be asymptomatic or complain of sudden or gradual onset of burning pain on urination, frequency, urgency to void, suprapubic pain and/or low back pain. Urine may be described as cloudy, dark, bloody and/or malodorous. *Upper urinary tract:* Patient may be asymptomatic; may or may not demonstrate lower urinary tract symptoms; and may or may not complain of headache, malaise, fever, chills, nausea, vomiting, anorexia, flank pain and/or abdominal pain.

OBJECTIVE: *Lower urinary tract:* Physical exam may not be significant or suprapubic tenderness and/or erythema and tenderness of the urethra may be present. Laboratory shows significant bacteriuria (one to two organisms per high power field on unspun urine) which may be accompanied by pyuria, and/or hematuria. Urine culture and prostatic secretion culture demonstrate significant bacteriuria (100,000 or more organisms per ml). *Upper urinary tract:* Physical exam may not be significant or may reveal a fever greater than 101 degrees F., and/or CVA tenderness. Laboratory tests show significant bacteriuria which may be accompanied by pyuria, proteinuria, and/or hematuria. Urine culture should demonstrate significant bacteriuria.

PLAN:

CONTRAINDICATIONS: Do not use with hypersensitivity to trimethoprim; or with megaloblastic anemia due to folate deficiency.

WARNINGS: Prolonged therapy with trimethoprim at high doses may cause bone marrow depression. Trimethoprim should be discontinued if there is a significant reduction in the count of any formed blood element. Trimethoprim may interfere with folic acid metabolism. It should only be used in pregnancy when the potential benefit justifies the potential risk to the fetus. Safety for use in infants under two months of age has not been established.

PRECAUTIONS: The efficacy for use in children under twelve has not been established. Trimethoprim should be used with caution in patients with folic acid deficiency and impaired renal or hepatic function. Trimethoprim is excreted in human milk and thus should be given with caution to nursing mothers. Due to the natural decline in liver and kidney function in elderly patients, trimethoprim should be given with caution; dosages may need to be reduced and dosage intervals may need to be lengthened. Elderly patients may also be more susceptible to bone marrow depression.

IMPLEMENTATION:

DRUG INTERACTIONS: Trimethoprim increases the effects of sulfamethoxazole. Unusual bleeding or bruising may occur when trimethoprim is taken concurrently with thiazide diuretics.

PRODUCTS (TRADE NAME):
Proloprim, (Available in 100 and 200 mg tablets). **Trimethoprim, Trimpex** (Available in 100 mg tablets).

ADMINISTRATION AND DOSAGE: Trimethoprim is readily absorbed from the gastrointestinal tract. Peak serum levels occur in one to four hours. Urine concentrations are considerably higher than serum concentrations. Trimethoprim should not be used in patients with a creatinine clearance of less than 15 ml/min. Patients with creatinine clearances of 15-30 ml/min will require reduced dosages.

Adult: 100 mg po every 12 hours for ten days, or 200 mg every 24 hours.

Adults with creatinine clearance of 15-30 ml/min: 50 mg po every 12 hours.

IMPLEMENTATION CONSIDERATIONS:

—Obtain a complete health history: hypersensitivity to drug, impaired renal or hepatic function, folic acid deficiency, possibility of pregnancy, or breast-feeding.

—Folate may be given with the drug without it interferring with trimethoprim's antibacterial action.

—Watch for signs of bone marrow depression: sore throat, fever, pallor, or purpura may be early indications of serious blood disorders. Complete blood counts should be done routinely, and if any of these signs occur.

—Trimethoprim should be discontinued if there is a significant reduction in the count of any formed blood element.

—Obtain baseline CBC, renal and hepatic function studies, and culture and sensitivity tests.

WHAT THE PATIENT NEEDS TO KNOW:

—Take this medication exactly as ordered. The full course of therapy must be taken in order for the drug to be effective.

—Some people experience side effects while taking this product. While most symptoms are mild, they should be evaluated by your health provider. Notify the health provider immediately if you note any sore throat, fever, pallor, unusual bleeding or bruising, itching or skin rash.

EVALUATION:

ADVERSE REACTIONS: *Dermatologic:* exfoliative dermatitis, pruritus, rash. *Gastrointestinal:* epigastric distress, glossitis, nausea, vomiting. *Hematopoietic:* leukopenia, megaloblastic anemia, methemoglobinemia, neutropenia, thrombocytopenia. *Other:* fever, elevated serum transaminase and bilirubin levels, increased BUN and creatinine levels.

OVERDOSAGE: *Signs and symptoms:* Signs of acute overdosage may appear after ingestion of one gram. Acute: nausea, vomiting, dizziness, headaches, mental depression, confusion, bone marrow depression. *Treatment:* referral for gastric lavage and supportive treatment. Signs of chronic overdosage occur after high doses or long-term therapy. Chronic: bone marrow depression (thrombocytopenia, leukopenia, megaloblastic anemia). *Treatment:* discontinue drug. Leucovorin intramuscularly may be given to restore normal hematopoiesis.

PARAMETERS TO MONITOR: Observe for therapeutic and adverse reactions. Complete blood counts should be monitored routinely on all patients.

Marna J. Ross

COMBINATION DRUGS

METHENAMINE, METHYLENE BLUE, ATROPINE SULFATE

PRODUCTS (TRADE NAME):
Dolsed, Hexalol, Prosed, Trac Tabs, U.B., Uramine, Uridon Modified, Urised, Urisep, Uritab, Urithol, Uritin Formula, Uroblue, Uro-Ves (Each tablet contains the following: methenamine 40.8 mg; atropine sulfate 0.03 mg; hyoscyamine 0.03 mg; methylene blue 5.4 mg; phenyl salicylate 18.1 mg; and benzoic acid 4.5 mg.)

DRUG SPECIFICS:
Indicated for the treatment of cystitis, urethritis, and trigonitis caused by susceptible organisms, and the relief of lower urinary tract discomfort caused by hypermotility.

ADMINISTRATION AND DOSAGE SPECIFICS:
Adult: Two tablets po four times per day. Take with one full glass of water.

METHENAMINE AND SODIUM BIPHOSPHATE

PRODUCTS (TRADE NAME):
Methenamine and Sodium Biphosphate (Available in 325 mg methenamine and 325 mg sodium phosphate tablets.)

DRUG SPECIFICS:
Sodium biphosphate is added to provide an acid urine.

ADMINISTRATION AND DOSAGE SPECIFICS:
Adult: three tablets po 4 times daily.

OXYTETRACYCLINE HCL, SULFAMETHIZOLE, PHENAZOPYRIDINE HCL

PRODUCTS (TRADE NAME):
Urobiotic-250 (Available in Oxytetracycline HCl 250 mg; sulfamethizole 250 mg; phenazopyridine HCl 50 mg per capsule.)

DRUG SPECIFICS:
Indicated for the treatment of genitourinary infections caused by susceptible organisms. Agents which contain phenazopyridine are not suitable for longterm therapy. Take medicine with a full glass of water on an empty stomach. Therapy

should continue for at least seven days.

ADMINISTRATION AND DOSAGE SPECIFICS:

Adults only: One capsule four times per day. In refractory cases, use two capsules four times per day.

SULFAMETHOXAZOLE AND PHENAZOPYRIDINE HCL

PRODUCTS (TRADE NAME):

Azo-Gantanol (Available in 0.5 gm sulfamethoxazole and 100 mg phenazopyridine HCl.)

DRUG SPECIFICS:

Indicated only for the acute, painful phase of urinary tract infections. After relief of pain has been obtained, therapy should continue with a drug which does not contain phenazopyridine, such as sulfamethoxazole. Colors urine red.

ADMINISTRATION AND DOSAGE SPECIFICS:

Adult: Four tablets initially, followed by two tablets twice a day for up to three days.

SULFISOXAZOLE AND PHENAZOPYRIDINE HCL

PRODUCTS (TRADE NAME):

Azo-Gantrisin, Azo-Sulfisoxazole, Azo-Sulfizin, Suldiazo (Available in 0.5 gm sulfisoxazole and 50 mg phenazopyridine HCl.)

DRUG SPECIFICS:

Indicated for the acute, painful phase of urinary tract infections due to susceptible organisms. After relief of pain has been obtained, therapy should continue with a drug which does not contain phenazopyridine HCl, such as sulfisoxazole.

ADMINISTRATION AND DOSAGE SPECIFICS:

Adult: Four to six tablets po initially, followed by two tablets four times per day for up to three days.

Marna J. Ross

ANTISPASMODICS

ACTION OF THE DRUG: Antispasmodics counteract smooth muscle spasm of the urinary tract directly or inhibit the muscarinic action of acetylcholine on smooth muscle.

ASSESSMENT:

INDICATIONS: Flavoxate HCl is indicated for symptomatic relief of dysuria, urgency, nocturia, suprapubic discomfort, frequency, and incontinence. Oxybutynin chloride is used for the relief of symptoms associated with voiding in patients with uninhibited neurogenic and reflex neurogenic bladder.

SUBJECTIVE: Patient may present with complaints of dysuria, urgency, frequency, suprapubic discomfort, nocturia or incontinence.

OBJECTIVE: Cystometric or other studies may confirm presence of neurogenic bladder, cystitis, prostatitis, urethritis, and/or urethrotrigonitis.

PLAN:

CONTRAINDICATIONS: Flavoxate HCl should not be used in any of the following obstructive conditions: pyloric or duodenal obstruction, obstructive intestinal lesions or ileus, achalasia, obstructive uropathy of the lower urinary tract, or gastrointestinal hemorrhage.

Oxybutynin chloride should not be used in patients with partial or complete obstruction of the intestinal tract, intestinal atony of the elderly or debilitated, megacolon, severe colitis, myasthenia gravis, obstructive uropathy, unstable cardiovascular status in acute hemorrhage, and glaucoma.

WARNINGS: Flavoxate HCl should be given cautiously in patients with suspected glaucoma. Do not give to children under the age of 12. Consider risk-benefit ratio in women who are or may become pregnant.

Oxybutynin chloride may cause heat prostration when given in the presence of high environmental temperature. It may also produce drowsiness or blurred vision. Caution should be used in performing activities requiring mental alertness. Do not give to children under the age of 5. Consider risk-benefit ratio in pregnant women.

PRECAUTIONS: Flavoxate HCl may produce drowsiness and blurred vision. Patients should not drive, operate machinery, or perform other hazardous activities requiring mental alertness.

Oxybutynin chloride should be used cautiously in patients with autonomic neuropathy, or hepatic or renal disease. Use with care in the elderly patient. Symptoms of hyperthyroidism, coronary heart disease, congestive heart failure, cardiac arrhythmias, tachycardia, hypertension, prostatic hypertrophy, and hiatal hernia with reflux esophagitis may be aggravated. Large doses in patients with ulcerative colitis may cause paralytic ileus or precipitate or aggravate toxic megacolon.

IMPLEMENTATION:

Both types of antispasmodics increase serum digoxin levels in those patients taking digoxin and increase cholinergic blockade when given with anticholinergic agents, antidepressants (tricyclic), antihistamines, belladonna alkaloids, phenothiazines, procainamide, and quinidine.

ADMINISTRATION AND DOSAGE: These drugs are for the symptomatic relief of urinary complaints. They are compatible with drugs used for treatment of urinary tract infections.

IMPLEMENTATION CONSIDERATIONS:

—Obtain a complete health history, including the presence of hypersensitivity, underlying systemic disease (especially achalasia, obstructive uropathy of lower urinary tract, pyloric or duodenal obstruction, gastrointestinal hemorrhage, glaucoma, intestinal atony in elderly or debilitated patients, megacolon, myasthenia gravis, gastrointestinal obstruction, paralytic ileus, severe colitis, or unstable cardiovascular status in acute hemorrhage), concurrent use of medications, and possibility of pregnancy.

—Oxybutynin Cl suppresses sweating and could precipitate fever or heat stroke in hot weather.

—Antibiotic therapy should be given concurrently if indicated.

—Oxybutynin Cl should be stopped periodically to determine if patient still needs it.

WHAT THE PATIENT NEEDS TO KNOW:

—Take this drug as prescribed. Do not double up doses.

—These drugs may cause dry mouth, blurred vision, or drowsiness. Be careful while driving or performing hazardous tasks requiring alertness.

—Increase fluid intake to at least 2 quarts of water per day while taking this medication.

—You will need to have regular health checkups while taking this drug.

—If original symptoms do not resolve or you develop any new or troublesome symptoms, be certain to report them to your health care practitioner.

—Keep this medication out of the reach of children and all others for whom it is not prescribed.

EVALUATION:

ADVERSE REACTIONS: Flavoxate HCl: *Cardiovascular:* palpitations, tachycardia. *CNS:* confusion (especially in the elderly), dizziness, drowsiness, headache, hyperpyrexia. *Gastrointestinal:* dry mouth, nausea, vomiting. *Genitourinary:* dysuria. *Hematopoietic:* eosinophilia, leukopenia (rare). *Ophthalmologic:* blurred vision, changes in eye accommodation, increased ocular tension. *Other:* dermatoses, urticaria.

Oxybutynin Cl: *Cardiovascular:* palpitations, tachycardia. *CNS:* dizziness, drowsiness, insomnia, weakness. *Gastrointestinal:* bloating, constipation, dry mouth, nausea, vomiting. *Genitourinary:* impotence, urinary hesitancy, urinary retention. *Ophthalmologic:* blurred vision, cycloplegia, dilation of pupils, increased ocular tension. *Other:* decreased sweating, lactation suppression, urticaria, and other dermatoses.

OVERDOSAGE: Flavoxate HCl: Check with manufacturer (Smith Kline and French). Oxybutynin Cl: *Signs and symptoms:* Restlessness, excitement, psychotic behavior, flushing, fall in blood pressure, circulatory failure, paralysis, respiratory failure, and coma may all be seen. *Treatment:* Referral for gastric lavage. Physostigmine 0.5 to 2.0 mg IV (up to 5 mg) may be given. Ice or alcohol baths may be given to reduce fever. Sodium thiopental 2% slowly IV or 100 to 200 ml of 2% chloral hydrate by rectal infusion may be used to reduce excitement. Artificial respiration must be maintained if respiratory paralysis develops.

PARAMETERS TO MONITOR: Monitor for therapeutic effects (disappearance of symptoms or improved cystometric studies) and for aggravation of existing cardiac, renal, hepatic, prostatic, thyroid, or hiatal hernia problems. If adverse effects develop, alter or discontinue therapy.

EPHEDRINE SULFATE AND ATROPINE SULFATE

PRODUCTS (TRADE NAME):
Enuretrol (Available in 7.5 mg ephedrine sulfate and 0.15 mg atropine sulfate chewable tablets.)

DRUG SPECIFICS:
Ephedrine sulfate promotes continence through stimulation of the internal vesical bladder sphincter. Atropine sulfate increases bladder capacity through reduction of bladder pressure and decrease of bladder contractions. This product is used primarily for the control of nocturnal enuresis. It should not be given to patients with acute glaucoma, prostatic hypertrophy, hypersensitivity to parasympathetic depressants of sympathomimetic agents. Patients may complain of typical parasympathetic effects. Continue medication for a minimum of 4 to 6 weeks. If no response, gradually increase dosage to the limit of tolerance, when patient begins to complain of blurred vision, flushing, dryness of mouth, etc. If enuresis comes under control, gradually decrease dosage over a 2 week period.

ADMINISTRATION AND DOSAGE SPECIFICS:
Adults: Give 3 tablets morning and evening.
Children 11 to 15 years old: Give 2 tablets morning and evening.
Children 5 to 10 years old: Give 1 tablet morning and evening.

FLAVOXATE HCL

PRODUCTS (TRADE NAME):
Urispas (Available in 100 mg tablets.)

DRUG SPECIFICS:
At therapeutic levels this drug does not significantly alter blood serum or urinary values. Do not give to children under age 12.

ADMINISTRATION AND DOSAGE SPECIFICS:
Adults and children over 12 years: 1 to 2 tablets 3 to 4 times daily.

OXYBUTYNIN CHLORIDE

PRODUCTS (TRADE NAME):
   Ditropan (Available in 5 mg tablets; 5 mg/5 ml syrup.)
DRUG SPECIFICS:
   At therapeutic levels this drug does not significantly alter blood, serum or urinary values. Do not give to children under age 5.
ADMINISTRATION AND DOSAGE SPECIFICS:
   Adults: One tablet 2 to 3 times daily (maximum dose is one tablet four times daily.) One tsp (5 mg/5 ml syrup) may be given 2 to 3 times daily (with maximum 1 tsp four times daily.)
   Children over age 5 years: One tablet 2 times daily (maximum is one tablet 3 times daily), or one tsp (5 mg/ml syrup) 2 times daily (with maximum one tsp 3 times daily.)

Mary Ann Bolter

CHOLINERGIC STIMULANTS

ACTION OF THE DRUG: Cholinergic stimulants increase the tone of the detrusor muscle of the urinary bladder to produce contractions strong enough to initiate micturition.

ASSESSMENT:

   INDICATIONS: Cholinergic stimulants are used to prevent and treat post-operative urinary retention after mechanical obstruction has been excluded. They are also used for treating functional postpartum urinary retention and for neurogenic atony of the urinary bladder with retention.
   SUBJECTIVE: Patient may complain of "fullness or pressure" in suprapubic area, inability to void or feeling that even after voiding the bladder is not empty.
   OBJECTIVE: Examination may reveal distention of urinary bladder and decreased urinary output.

PLAN:

   CONTRAINDICATIONS: Bethanechol chloride should not be used in the presence of hypersensitivity to the drug, pregnancy, hyperthyroidism, peptic ulcer, latent or active bronchial asthma, marked bradycardia or hypotension, vasomotor instability, cornonary artery disease, epilepsy and parkinsonism. Do not use when the strength or integrity of the gastrointestinal or bladder wall is questionable or in the presence of mechanical obstruction.

Neostigmine methylsulfate should not be used in known hypersensitivity to the drug, peritonitis or mechanical obstruction of the gastrointestinal or urinary tract. Do not give to children.

WARNINGS: Bethanechol chloride sterile solution is for subcutaneous use only and should not be given intramuscularly or intravenously. Neostigmine methylsulfate should be used cautiously in patients with bronchial asthma, bradycardia, epilepsy, recent coronary occlusion, vagotonia, hypertension, cardiac arrhythmias or peptic ulcer.

PRECAUTIONS: The risk-benefit ratio must be considered in pregnant and nursing mothers. Patients receiving ganglionic blocking agents and bethanechol chloride may experience a critical fall in blood pressure. With bacteriuria, reflux infections may also develop. It is important to differentiate between myasthenic crisis and cholinergic crisis caused by overdosage of neostigmine methylsulfate, since they require different treatments.

IMPLEMENTATION:

DRUG INTERACTIONS: These products used with other cholinergics may increase the cholinergic effect and the potential for toxicity. Concurrent use with ganglionic blocking agents may produce a critical fall in blood pressure. Procainamide and quinidine antagonize the cholinergic effects.

ADMINISTRATION AND DOSAGE: Dosage must be individualized depending on the type and severity of the condition being treated. Give minimum effective dose.

IMPLEMENTATION CONSIDERATIONS:
—Obtain a complete health history, including the presence of hypersensitivity, underlying systemic disease, concurrent use of other medications and the possibility of pregnancy.
—If patient is confined to bed, make certain that bedpan is easily available.

WHAT THE PATIENT NEEDS TO KNOW:
—Take this medication exactly as ordered. If you miss a dose, take it as soon as you remember unless it is close to your next scheduled dose. Do not double doses.
—Bethanechol chloride tablets should be given on an empty stomach (1 hour before eating or 2 hours after eating) to decrease the possibility of nausea and vomiting.
—If you develop any unusual symptoms, report them to your health care provider.

EVALUATION:

ADVERSE REACTIONS: Bethanechol chloride: *Cardiovascular:* bradycardia, hypotension, tachycardia. *CNS:* headache, malaise, *EENT:* lacrimation, miosis. *Gastrointestinal:* abdominal cramps, belching, borborygmis, diarrhea, nausea, salivation, vomiting. *Genitourinary:* urinary urgency. *Other:* bronchoconstriction, flushing, sweating.

Neostigmine methylsulfate: *Cardiovascular:* bradycardia, hypotension. *CNS:* confusion, dizziness, muscle weakness, respiratory depression, sweating. *EENT:* miosis. *Gastrointestinal:* abdominal cramping, diarrhea, increased salivation, nausea, vomiting. *Other:* bronchospasm, muscle cramps.

OVERDOSAGE: *Signs and symptoms:* Problems result from parasympathetic stimulation: sensation of heat about the face, flushing, headache, malaise, colicky pain, diarrhea, nausea, belching, borborygmi, asthmatic attacks and fall in blood pressure. Problems may progress to respiratory paralysis and cardiac arrest. *Treatment:* Discontinue cholinergic drug. Specific antidote is atropine sulfate. Give 1 to 4 mg IV; repeat every 5 to 30 minutes as needed. Respiratory paralysis is not alleviated by atropine sulfate.

PARAMETERS TO MONITOR: Observe for signs of therapeutic effect, especially increased urinary output. Monitor intake and output. If patient has not voided within 1 hour after parenteral administration of drug, patient should be catheterized. Monitor vital signs and watch for signs and symptoms of adverse reactions to drug therapy.

BETHANECHOL CHLORIDE

PRODUCTS (TRADE NAME):

Bethanechol Chloride (Available in 5 mg, 10 mg, 25 mg and 50 mg tablets.) **Duvoid** (Available in 10 mg, 25 mg and 50 mg tablets.) **Myotonachol** (Available in 10 mg and 25 mg tablets.) **Urecholine** (Available in 5 mg, 10 mg, 25 mg and 50 mg tablets and injections.) **Vesicholine** (Available in 25 mg tablets.)

DRUG SPECIFICS:

Following administration of the tablet, the effects begin in 30-90 minutes and last for up to 6 hours. After subcutaneous injection, the effects occur within 5-15 minutes and last about 2 hours. Poor and variable absorption via the oral route requires larger oral doses. Oral and subcutaneous doses are not interchangeable.

ADMINISTRATION AND DOSAGE SPECIFICS:

Adults: 10 to 50 mg po, two to four times daily, or 5 mg SQ three to four times daily.

Children: 200 mcg (0.2 mg)/kg po three times daily, or 150 to 200 mcg (0.15 to 0.2 mg)/kg SQ three times daily.

NEOSTIGMINE METHYLSULFATE

PRODUCTS (TRADE NAME):
   Neostigmin Methylsulfate, Prostigmin (Available in 1:1000 and 1:4000 solutions for injection.)
DRUG SPECIFICS:
   The oral form of this drug is not used as a cholinergic stimulant for urinary tract problems. Parenteral dosage is not used for children with urinary tract problems. Atropine sulfate should be kept readily available when giving this drug parenterally.
ADMINISTRATION AND DOSAGE SPECIFICS:
   Prevention of postoperative urinary retention: 250 mcg (0.25 mg) IM or SQ immediately following surgery and repeated every 4 to 6 hours for 2-3 days.
   Treatment of urinary retention: 500 mcg (0.5 mg) IM or SQ repeated every 3 hours for at least 5 doses after the patient has voided or the bladder has been emptied.

Mary Ann Bolter

MISCELLANEOUS URINARY TRACT PRODUCTS

BASIC ALUMINUM CARBONATE GEL

ACTION OF THE DRUG: Basic aluminum carbonate gel binds dietary and gastrointestinal phosphates to lower serum phosphate. The elimination of phosphate is decreased in the urine and increased in the feces.

ASSESSMENT:

   INDICATIONS: This product is used in combination with a low-phosphate diet for the prophylaxis of urinary phosphate calculi. It is also used as an antacid.
   SUBJECTIVE: Patients may present with a history of phosphatic urinary calculi.
   OBJECTIVE: Phosphatic urinary calculi are found.

PLAN:

   WARNINGS: No more than 24 tablets, capsules or teaspoonfuls of basic aluminum carbonate gel should be taken in 24 hours. No more than 12 teaspoonfuls of the extra-strength solution should be taken in 24 hours.
   PRECAUTIONS: A lowered serum phosphate and a slightly elevated alkaline

phosphatase level may develop with continued overdosage and restriction of dietary phosphate and calcium. Use with care in the elderly. This product may cause constipation.

IMPLEMENTATION:

DRUG INTERACTIONS: Do not give concomitantly with any form of oral tetracycline therapy since absorption of tetracycline may be decreased.

PRODUCTS (TRADE NAME):

Basaljel (Available in dried basic aluminum carbonate gel equivalent to 608 mg dried aluminum hydroxide gel or in 500 mg aluminum hydroxide capsules or swallow tablets, suspension equivalent to 400 mg aluminum hydroxide/5 ml and extra-strength suspension equivalent to 1000 mg aluminum hydroxide/5 ml).

ADMINISTRATION AND DOSAGE: When given as prophylaxis or treatment of phosphatic renal calculi, a modified acid-ash diet is usually recommended. The dosage is higher than that given for antacid therapy. Usual adult dose is 15 to 30 ml of suspension in water or juice 1 hour after meals and at bedtime (for extra-strength suspension, give one third to one half of this dose), or two to six tablets or capsules 1 hour after meals and at bedtime.

IMPLEMENTATION CONSIDERATIONS:

—Obtain a complete health history, including presence of hypersensitivity, underlying systemic disease and concurrent use of other medications.

—Obtain baseline urinalysis, renal function tests, serum phosphate and alkaline phosphatase values, as well as serum calcium value.

—Patients with urinary calculi should increase fluid intake.

—Be alert for signs of urinary tract infections. These may be caused from trauma by calculi.

—A modified acid-ash diet may be needed in conjunction with drug therapy.

—If patient is on restricted sodium intake, monitor carefully.

—A mild, transient hypercalciuria may be present the first few weeks of therapy.

WHAT THE PATIENT NEEDS TO KNOW:

—Take this drug as prescribed. Do not double doses.

—You will need to be seen on a regular basis while on this therapy.

—Diet may be changed to lower the urinary pH. Milk and milk products, carbonated beverages, fruits and juices (except cranberries, prunes, plums) may be restricted. Fluid intake should be increased.

—All urine should be strained. Intake and output should be recorded.

—Liquid form of the drug should be shaken thoroughly before pouring.

—Inform your health care provider of any symptoms that develop while on this therapy.

EVALUATION:

ADVERSE REACTIONS: *Gastrointestinal:* anorexia, constipation, intestinal obstruction. *Other:* hypophosphatemia.

OVERDOSAGE: *Signs and symptoms:* Weakness, malaise, anorexia, bone pain, tremors, demineralization of bone (due to phosphate depletion) may develop. *Treatment:* Stop therapy and employ symptomatic measures as needed.

PARAMETERS TO MONITOR: Serum calcium, phosphate, alkaline phosphatase and other electrolyte levels should be obtained prior to initiation of therapy and periodically during prolonged therapy. A urinalysis should be ordered to check pH and to monitor for signs of stone formation and infection.

Mary Ann Bolter

SODIUM CELLULOSE PHOSPHATE

ACTION OF THE DRUG: Sodium cellulose phosphate binds calcium in an ion exchange of sodium for calcium. The calcium and cellulose phosphate complex is then excreted in the feces.

ASSESSMENT:

INDICATIONS: This relatively new product is used in the treatment of nephrolithiasis due to calcium oxalate or calcium phosphate. It is especially useful in patients with repeated problems with absorptive hypercalciuria type I. Long-term use reduces the incidence of stone formation in these patients.

SUBJECTIVE: History of repeated abdominal pain, stone passage or removal.

OBJECTIVE: Confirmation of calcium oxalate or calcium phosphate stones, through x-ray and assay. Normal serum calcium and phosphorus are present. Increased intestinal calcium absorption, hypercalciuria, normal urinary calcium during fasting, normal parathyroid function, no evidence of bone disease, and lack of renal leak or excessive skeletal mobilization of calcium also confirm the diagnosis.

PLAN:

CONTRAINDICATIONS: Medication should not be given with primary or secondary hyperparathyroidism, including renal hypercalciuria, enteric hyperoxaluria, normal or low intestinal absorption and renal excretion of calcium, hypomagnesiumic states, and evidence of bone disease such as osteoporosis, osteomalacia, or osteitis. Hypocalcemic states associated with hypoparathyroidism or intestinal malabsorption as also contraindications for this product.

WARNINGS: Safety has not been established for use in pregnant or breast-feeding women. Caution should also be used in giving to people for whom added sodium may pose a risk to circulatory or cardiac function.

PRECAUTIONS: Hyperparathyroid bone disease may be produced by stimulating parathyroid function when intestinal absorption of calcium is inhibited. This problem should be reduced when dosage is just sufficient to restore normal calcium absorption. Hyperoxaluria and hypomagnesiuria, magnesium depletion, depletion of trace metals (iron, zinc and copper), may also develop over time.

IMPLEMENTATION:

PRODUCTS (TRADE NAME):
Calcibind (Available in 2.5 gm powder.)
ADMINISTRATION AND DOSAGE: Mix each dose in a soft drink, fruit juice, or glass of water, and drink within 30 minutes of eating. Patients should be on a moderate calcium restricted diet.

Recommended initial dose is 5 gm three times daily with meals for patients with urinary calcium greater than 300 mg/day. When calcium declines to less than 150 mg/day, reduce dosage to 5 gm with supper and 2.5 gm with breakfast and lunch. Patients with controlled urinary calcium or levels between 200 and 300 mg/day should begin on 10 gm/day divided between three meals.

Magnesium supplements should be taken concomitantly according to the following schedule: Those receiving 15 gm of sodium cellulose phosphate/day should take 1.5 gm of magnesium gluconate before breakfast and again at bedtime. those taking 10 gm of sodium cellulose phosphate/day should take 1 gm of magnesium gluconate twice a day. Magnesium product should be taken at least 1 hour before or after the sodium cellulose phosphate and not at the same time.

IMPLEMENTATION CONSIDERATIONS:
—Obtain a thorough health history, including the presence of underlying disease, previous renal problems, and dietary patterns.
—Collect 24 hour urine calcium specimens in order to determine dosage requirements for individual patient.
—Encourage patient to adhere to a moderate calcium and sodium intake during therapy. Foods high in oxalate should be avoided, and fluid should be encouraged so that patient voids at least 2 quarts a day.

WHAT THE PATIENT NEEDS TO KNOW:
—Take this medication exactly as ordered.
—Report any new or troubling symptoms to your health care practitioner.
—Special attention to your diet will help this medication be more effective. A moderate calcium diet is recommended. Avoid eating dairy products, spinach, rhubarb, chocolate and brewed tea. Do not take vitamin C tablets. Do not add additional salt to your cooked or uncooked foods. Drink 2-3 quarts of water per day.
—You will need to return for periodic urine and blood evaluations while taking this medication.

EVALUATION:

ADVERSE REACTIONS: Some patients complain of diarrhea, loose bowel movements, dyspepsia, and the unpleasant taste of the drug.

PARAMETERS TO MONITOR: Complete physical and radiological studies should be obtained prior to beginning medication. Twenty-four-hour urinary calcium should be collected in order to determine dosage regimen. Once therapy has begun, parathyroid hormone (PTH) and calcium levels should be obtained at least once between the first two weeks to three months of treatment so therapy may be altered or discontinued if PTH levels increase. If urinary calcium does not fall to less than 30 mg/5 gm of sodium cellulose phosphate, the treatment should be considered ineffective and then terminated. Also end therapy if urinary oxalate exceeds 55 mg/day while dietary oxalate is moderately restricted.

Marilyn W. Edmunds

BIBLIOGRAPHY

Abruzzo, J. et al. Double-blind Study Comparing Piroxicam and Aspirin in the Treatment of Osteoarthritis, **American Journal of Medicine,** Feb. 16, 1982, 45–49.

Alpha Project Staff (ed), **Handbook of Non-Prescription Drugs.** (4th, 5th, 6th ed). Washington: American Pharmaceutical Association, 1977, 1978, 1979.

Albanese, Joseph A. **Nurses Drug Reference.** (1st and 2nd ed.), New York: McGraw Hill. 1979, 1981.

Albanese, Joseph A., and Bond, Thomas, **Drug Interactions: Basic Principles and Clinical Problems.** New York: McGraw Hill, 1978.

American Association of Pediatrics. **Report of Committee on Infectious Diseases.** (19th ed.), Evanston: A.A.P., 1982.

American Hospital Formulary Service. **Drug Information 84.** Washington, D.C.: American Society of Hospital Pharmacists, 1984.

American Medical Association. **AMA Drug Evaluations.** (4th ed.), Chicago: The Association, 1980.

American Thoracic Society: Guidelines for Short-Course Tuberculosis Chemotherapy, **American Review of Respiratory Disease.** 1980, 121, 613.

Anderson, J.L. Managing Cardiac Arrhythmias: An Empiric Approach, **Modern Medicine.** Nov. 1981, p. 78–94.

Arndt, Kenneth. **Manual of Dermatologic Therapeutics,** Boston: Little, Brown and Company, 1975.

Arndt, Kenneth, **Manual of Dermatologics with Essentials of Diagnosis,** (2nd ed.), Boston: Little, Brown and Company, 1978.

Asperheim, Mary and Eisenhower, Laurel. **The Pharmacologic Basis of Patient Care.** (4th ed.), Philadelphia: W.B. Saunders, 1981.

Avery, G.S. (ed.), **Drug Treatment: Principles and Practice of Clinical Pharmacology and Therapeutics.** New York: Adis Press, 1980.

Barker, Brian M., and Bender, David A. **Vitamins in Medicine.** Vol. 1 (4th ed.), London: William Heinemann Medical Books, Ltd., 1980.

Benenson, A.S. (ed.), **Control of Communicable Diseases in Man.** (13th ed.), Washington, D.C.: American Public Health Assoc., 1980.

Benitz, William E. **The Pediatric Drug Handbook.** Chicago: Year Book Medical Publishers, 1981.

Bergersen, B.S., **Pharmacology in Nursing.** St. Louis: C.V. Mosby, 1979.

Billups, Norman F. **American Drug Index.** (25th ed.), Pa: Lippincott, 1981.

Boedeker, Edgar and Dauber, James, **Manual of Medical Therapeutics.** Boston: Little, Brown and Co., 1976.

Bowman, W.C., and Rand, M.J., **Textbook of Pharmacology.** (2nd ed.), St. Louis: Blackwell Scientific Publications, 1980.

Braunwald, E. (ed.), **Heart Disease, A Textbook of Cardiovascular Medicine,** Vol. 1. Philadelphia: W.B. Saunders, 1980.

Bressler, Rubin and Bugdonoff, Morton. **The Physicians' Drug Manual.** New York: Doubleday and Co., Inc., 1981.

Brooks, S.M., (ed.), **Nurses' Drug Reference.** Boston: Little, Brown and Company, 1978.

Cheng, T., Thrombocytopenia Associated with Minidose Heparin Therapy, **Postgraduate Medicine,** December, 1981. 70, 73–78.

Clark, J.B., Queener, Sherry F., Karb, Virginia Burke. **Pharmacological Basis of Nursing Practice.** Philadelphia: J.B. Lippincott Co., 1976.

Clinical Anxiety/Tension in Primary Medicine: Proceedings of a Colloquim, Amsterdam: Excerpta Medica, 1979.

Cody, C.L., Baraff, L.J., Cherry, J.D., Marcy, S.M., & Manclark, C.R., Nature and Rates Associated with DTP and DT Immunization in Infants and Children. **Pediatrics.** November, 1981, 68 5, 650–659.

Compendium of Drug Therapy, New York: Biomedical Information Corporation, 1982.

Craig, C., and Buchanan, W. Antirheumatic Drugs: Clinical Pharmacology and Therapeutic Use **Drugs.** 1980, **20** 453–484.

Conn, H.F. (ed.), **Current Therapy 1981,** Philadelphia: W.B. Saunders, 1981, 1982.

Cutler, P. **Problem Solving in Clinical Medicine.** Baltimore: Williams and Wilkins Co, 1979.

DeGowan, Elmer L. and DeGowan, Richard L. **Bedside Diagnostic Examination.** (4th ed.), New York: MacMillan, 1981.

DeLoughery, M. Chronic Insomnia, **Nurse Practitioner,** Feb. 1981, 7 2

Derrick, F. Lower UTI's in Women, **Hospital Medicine.** 1981, 17 1, 35–38.

Diagnosis, Pennsylvania: Nursing 81 Books, 1981.

Diagnostic Standards and Classification of Tuberculosis and Other Mycobacterial Diseases,
New York: American Lung Assn., 1974.

Dickason, Elizabeth J., Schult, Martha Olsen., and Morris, Elaine Muller, Maternal and Infant Drugs
and Nursing Intervention. New York: McGraw-Hill Book, 1978.

DiPalma, Joseph R., (ed.). Practical Pharmacology for Prescribers. New Jersey: Medical Economics
Company, 1979.

Domonkos, A.N., Arnold, H.L., & Odom, R.B. Andrew's Diseases of the Skin. Philadelphia: W.B.
Saunders, 1982.

Dorland's Illustrated Medical Dictionary. Philadelphia: W.B. Saunders, 1974.

Drug Data: Proloprim/Trimpex. American Journal of Nursing. 1980, 80, 12, 2237–2239.

Drug Intelligence and Clinical Pharmacy, Vol. 15, Feb. 1981.

Drugs, Pennsylvania: Nursing 82 Books, 1982.

Drugs for Parasitic Infections, The Medical Letter, Jan. 22, 1982, 24.

Dukes, M.N.G., (ed.), Meyler's Side Effects of Drugs (9th ed.), Amsterdam: Excerpta Medica, 1980.

Dukes, M.N.G. Side Effects of Drugs Annual 4, 5, 6, Amsterdam: Excerpta Medica, 1980, 1981, 1982.

Dutt, W.W. and Stead, A.K. Chemotherapy of Tuberculosis for the 1980's, Primary Care 1980, 7 3,
513–527.

Dutt, W.W. and Stead, A.K. Managing and Preventing Drug-Resistant Tuberculosis, The Journal of
Respiratory Diseases. Nov–Dec, 1980, 12–18.

Dutt, W.W. and Stead, A.K. Modern Treatment of Tuberculosis. Drug Therapy. 1981, 11, 5, 85–99.

Fedson & Trenholme (eds). Infectious Disease, Primary Care: Clinics in Office Practice. 6 1, Philadelphia: Saunders, 1979.

Feigin, Ralph and Cherry, James D. (ed.), Textbook of Pediatric Infectious Diseases. 2 vols. Philadelphia: W.B. Saunders, 1981.

Feit, F. The Range of Supraventricular Tachycardias, Emergency Medicine. Feb. 28, 1982, 14, 4, 149–
175.

Flynn, K.T., Iron Deficiency Anemia Among the Elderly, Nurse Practitioner, November–December
1978, 20–24.

Frieson, W.T., Hekster, Y.A., Vree, T.B. Trimethoprim: Clinical Use and Pharmacokinetics, Drug Intelligence and Clinical Pharmacy. May 1981, 15 5, 325–329.

Fuller, E. Treating Ventricular Premature Beats, Patient Care, Feb 28, 1982, 55–71.

Gerald, Michael C. and O'Bannon, Freda V. Nursing Pharmacology and Therapeutics. New Jersey:
Prentice-Hall, Inc. 1981.

Gilman, A.G., Goodman, L.S., & Gilman, A. Goodman & Gilman's The Pharmacological Basis of
Therapeutics (6th ed.). New York: The MacMillan Co, 1980.

Gordon, Emmanuel. Immunoprophylaxis of Viral Hepatitis. Annals Emergency Medicine. November,
1981, 10, 216–221.

Gosselin, R., Hodge, A., Smith, R., Gleason, M. Clinical Toxicology of Commercial Products. (4th
ed.), Baltimore: Williams and Wilkins Co, 1976.

Govoni, Laura E., and Hayes, Janice E. Drugs and Nursing Implications. New York: Appleton-
Century-Crofts, 1978, 1982.

Groll, A.H., May, A.M., and Mulley, A.G. (ed.), Primary Care Medicine: Office Evaluation and
Management of the Adult Patient. Philadelphia: J.B. Lippincott, 1981.

Guthrie, D.W., Nursing Management of Diabetes Mellitus, St. Louis: C.V. Mosby, 1977.

Hahn, Anne Burgess, Barkin, R.L., & Oestreich, S.J.K. Pharmacology in Nursing, (15th ed.), St. Louis:
C.V. Mosby, 1982.

Halsey, J. et al. Benoxaprofen: Side Effect Profile in 300 patients., British Medical Journal. 1982, 284
5, 1365–1368.

Hanston, P.D. Drug Interactions. Philadelphia: Lea and Febiger, Co, 1979.

Harris, E., Sedative-Hypnotic Drugs, American Journal of Nursing. July, 1981, 1329–1334.

Harvey, A.M., Johns, R.J., McKusick, V.A., Owens, A.H., and Ross, R.S. The Principles and Practices
of Internal Medicine. New York: Appleton-Century-Crofts, 1975, 1980.

Hatcher, Robert A. & Stewart, Gary K. Contraceptive Technology 1980–1981. Irvington, 1980.

Heilmann, Klaus & Richardson, Kenneth T. Glaucoma: Conceptions of a Disease. Philadelphia: W.B.
Saunders, 1978.

Hollingsworth, James. Management of Rheumatoid Arthritis and Its Complications. Chicago: Year-
book Medical Publishers, Inc. 1978.

Hoole, A.J., Greenberg, R.A., & Pickard, C.G. Patient Care Guidelines for Family Nurse Practitioners. Boston: Little, Brown and Company, 1976.

Howry, Linda B. et al. Pediatric Medications. Philadelphia: J.B. Lippincott and Co., 1981.

Hudak, Carolyn M. et al. Clinical Protocols: A Guide for Nurses and Physicians. Philadelphia: J.B.
Lippincott Co., 1976.

Hunsberger, D., and Tackett M. **Family Centered Care of Children and Adolescents.** Philadelphia: W.B. Saunders, 1981.

Irons, Patricia Duggan, **Psychotropic Drugs and Nursing Interventions.** New York: McGraw Hill, 1978.

Isselbacher, K.J., Adams, R.D., Braunwald, E., Petersdorf, R.G. & Wilson, J.D. (eds.) **Harrison's Principles of Internal Medicine** (9th ed). New York: McGraw-Hill, 1980.

Johns, Marjorie, **Drug Therapy and Nursing Care,** New York: The MacMillan Company, 1979.

Kastrup, E. (ed.), **Facts and Comparisons.** St. Louis: Facts and Comparisons, Inc. 1980, 1981, 1982, 1983, 1984.

Kilo, Charles, The Use of Oral Hypoglycemic Agents, **Hospital Practice.** March, 1979, 45 3, 103–110.

Kirschenbaum, Harold and Rosenberg, Jack, What to Watch for with Coumadin, **R.N.** 1982, **45,** 10, 54–56.

Krupp, M.A. and Chatton, M.J. (eds.), **Current Medical Diagnosis and Treatment,** Los Altos, Ca.: Lange Medical Publications, 1981.

Lamy, Peter. **Prescribing for the Elderly.** Littleton, MA: PSG Publishing Co, Inc., 1980.

Leitch, C.J., and Tucker, R.V. (eds.), **Primary Care,** Philadelphia: F.A. Davis, 1978.

Lewis, Arthur J., (ed.), **Modern Drug Encyclopedia.** N.Y.: Yorke Medical Books, 1979.

Lewis, Arthur J., (ed.), **Modern Drug Encyclopedia and Therapeutic Index.** N.Y.: Yorke Medical Books, 1981.

Loebl, Suzanne, Spratto, George, and Heckheimer, Estelle, **The Nurses Drug Handbook** (2nd ed.). New York: Wiley Medical Company, 1982.

Long, James W. **Essential Guide to Prescription Drugs.** (2nd ed.), New York: Harper and Row, 1980.

Lubkin, Ilene. Evaluating Iron Deficiency Anemia, **The Nurse Practitioner.** October, 1982, **7,** 9.

J. and Sorensen, K.C., **Medical-Surgical Nursing.** Philadelphia: W.B. Saunders, 1980.

Lyle, W.H. Penicillamine, **Clinics in Rheumatic Disease.** 1979, 5 2 569–595.

Malseed, Roger T. **Pharmacology: Drug Therapy and Nursing Considerations.** Philadelphia: J.B. Lippincott, 1982.

Mandel, W.J. **Cardiac Arrhythmias: Their Mechanisms, Diagnosis, and Management.** Philadelphia: J.B. Lippincott, 1980.

Martin, **Drug Interactions Index 1978/1979,** Philadelphia: J.B., Lippincott Co, 1978.

Massoud, Neil. Update on the Treatment of Bacterial Urinary Tract Infections, **Drug Intelligence and Clinical Pharmacy,** Oct. 1981, **15,** 10, 738–748.

McEvoy, Gerald K. **The American Hospital Formulary Service.** Bethesda, Md: The American Society of Hospital Pharmacists, 1982.

Medication Teaching Manual: A Guide for Patient Counselling. (2nd ed.), Bethesda, Maryland: American Society of Hospital Pharmacists, 1980.

Melmon, K.L., & Morrelli, H.F. (ed.), **Clinical Pharmacology: Basic Principles in Therapeutics** (2nd ed.), New York: MacMillan, 1978.

Meyers, et. al. **Review of Medical Pharmacology.** (5th ed). Los Altos, Ca.: Lange Medical Publishers, 1976.

Michelson, E.L. Arrhythmias: The Benefits of Holter Monitoring, **Primary Cardiology,** March 1982.

Miller, D. Aspirin; A New Look, **U.S. Pharmacist,** Jan. 1982, pp. 43–53.

Miller, B.F. and Keane, C.B. **Encyclopedia and Dictionary of Medicine and Nursing.** Philadelphia: W.B. Saunders, 1972.

Modell, W. **Drugs of Choice.** Toronto: C.V. Mosby, Co. 1980.

Miller, Russell R., et al. (ed.), **Handbook of Drug Therapy.** N.Y.: Elsenier, 1979.

New Drugs: Trimethoprim Available Alone for Urinary Tract Infections, **Drug Therapy,** 1980, **10** 6, 22.

Newell, Frank W., **Opthalmology, Principles and Concepts.** (4th ed.), St. Louis: C.V. Mosby, 1978.

Nurse's Drug Alert, **American Journal of Nursing.** May, 1982, 837.

Nurses Guide to Drugs—Nursing '80's. Horsham: Intermed Communications, Inc., 1980.

Nademanee, K. and Singh, B.N. Advances in Antiarrhythmic Therapy, **Journal of the American Medical Association.** Jan 8, 1982, **247** 2, 217–222.

Neale, S. Verapamil for Tachycardia . . . and Much More? **Modern Medicine.** Nov. 1981.

Nursing 81 Drug Handbook Springhouse, Pennsylvania: Intermed Communication, Inc., 1981.

Nursing 82 Drug Handbook Springhouse, Pennsylvania: Intermed Communication, Inc., 1982.

Panwalker, A.P. Modern Management of UTI, **Drug Therapy.** 1981, **11** 4, 73–82.

Patterson, H.R., Gustafson, E.A., and Sheridan, E., **Falconer's Current Drug Handbook 1980–1982, 1983–1984.** Philadelphia: W.B. Saunders, 1980, 1982.

Peters, R.W., Paroxysmal Supraventricular Tachycardia, **Hospital Medicine.** April 1982.

Physicians Desk Reference. New Jersey: Medical Economics Company, 1980, 1981, 1982, 1983, 1984 editions.

Physicians Desk Reference for Nonprescription Drugs, 1980, 1981 edition.
Physicians Desk Reference for Ophthalmology, 1978/79, 1980/81 editions.
Pipes, Peggy L. **Nutrition in Infancy and Childhood.** (2nd ed.), St. Louis: C.V. Mosby, 1981.
Poe, William D., and Holloway, Donald A., **Drugs and the Aged.** New York: McGraw Hill, 1980.
Pyuria, **Hospital Medicine,** December 1979.
Rescind The Risks in Administering Anticoagulants, **Nursing '81,** October, 1981.
Rodman, Morton, J. and Smith, Dorothy, W. **Pharmacology and Drug Therapy in Nursing.** (2nd ed.), Philadelphia: J.B. Lippincott, 1979.
Romankiewicz, John A., Capelli, Ann, and Gotz, Vincent, **Handbook of Essential Drug Therapy for Critical Care Nurses.** Ill: Hamilton Press, 1980.
Rothermich, Norma. Chrysotherapy in Rheumatoid Arthritis, **Clinics in Rheumatic Disease.** August, 1979, **5** 2, 631–639.
Rubin, R.H. et. al. Trimethoprim-Sulfamethoxazole, **The New England Journal of Medicine.** 1980, **303,** 8, 426–431.
Russell, Helen, **Pediatric Drugs and Nursing Intervention.** New York: McGraw Hill, 1980.
Ryan, S., and Clayton, B., **Handbook of Practical Pharmacology.** St. Louis: C.V. Mosby, 1980.
Saherwhite, Terry K. Use of the Pneumococcal Vaccine, **American Family Physician.** November, 1981, **24,** 209–212.
Scheie, Howard & Alert, Daniel M., **Textbook of Opthalmology.** (9th ed.), Philadelphia: W.B. Saunders, 1977.
Schmidt, R.M. and Margolin, S. **Harper's Handbook of Therapeutic Pharmacology.** New York: Harper and Row, 1981.
Sheridan, E., Pattersen, H., Gustafson, E. **Falconer's The Drug, the Nurse, the Patient.** (5th, 6th, 7th ed.), Philadelphia: W.B. Saunders, 1978, 1980, 1982.
Shirley, Harry D. **Pediatric Dosage Handbook.** Washington, D.C.: American Pharmaceutical Company, 1980.
Shirkey, Harry D. ed. **Pediatric Therapy.** (6th ed.), St. Louis: C.V. Mosby, 1980.
Smith, D. **Medication Guide for Patient Counseling.** (2nd ed.), Philadelphia: Lea & Febiger, 1981.
Stead, William W., & Dutt, Asim K., Modern Treatment of Tuberculosis, **Drug Therapy,** May, 1981, 5, 85–99.
Stiehm, Richard and Fulginiti, Vincent (ed.), **Immunologic Disorders in Infants and Children** (2nd ed.), Philadelphia: W.B. Saunders, 1980.
Stiehm, Richard E. Standard and Special Human Immune Serum Globulins as Therapeutic Agents, **Pediatrics.** February, 1979, 63 301–319.
Swartz, Harry, **Prescriber's Handbook of Therapeutic Drugs.** Oradell, N.J.: Medical Economics, Co., 1981.
Tedford, Alberta A., and Van Hoozer, Helen L., **Pharmacology: A Self-Instructional Approach.** New York: McGraw Hill, 1980.
The Martindale Extra Pharmacopedia (27th ed.), The Council of the Pharmacologic Society of Great Britain, 1976–1977.
Thompson, L.W., & Edwards, L.M. Genitourinary Disorders, in Leitch, C.J., & Tinker, R.V., (eds). **Primary Care.** Philadelphia: F.A. Davis, Co., 1978.
Treating Respiratory Diseases in the Elderly, **Drug Therapy.** July, 1981.
Turner, R. Review of the Management of Rheumatoid Arthritis with Piroxicam. Advances in Arthritis Therapy: An International Review of Piroxicam, **Post Graduate Medicine.** April 1982, 42–48.
U.S.P. D.I.—United States Pharmacopeia Dispensing Information, Vol. I. Drug information for the Health Care Provider Vol II: Advice for the Patient. United States Pharmacopeial Convention, Inc. Rockville, Maryland, 1981, 1982, 1983 Editions.
Wang, Richard I.H., **Practical Drug Therapy.** Philadelphia: J.B. Lippincott Co., 1979.
Washington University School of Medicine, **Manual of Medical Therapeutics.** (23rd ed.), Boston: Little, Brown and Co, 1980.
Weiner, Howard L. & Levitt, Lawrence P., **Neurology for the House Officer.** (2nd ed.), Baltimore: Williams and Wilkins, 1978.
Wiener, Matthew R., Pepper, Ginette A., Kuhn-Weisman, Gail, and Romano, Joseph A. **Clinical Pharmacology and Therapeutics in Nursing.** New York: McGraw-Hill, 1979.
Worthington-Roberts, Bonnie S. **Contemporary Developments in Nutrition.** St. Louis: C.V. Mosby, 1981.
Wyngaarden, James B., & Smith, Lloyd H. Jr. (ed.), **Textbook of Medicine, Cecil** (16th ed.) Philadelphia: W.B. Saunders, 1982.
Yaffe, Sumner J., **Pediatric Pharmacology.** New York: Grune and Stratton, 1980.

APPENDIX

The Apothecary System

Volume

1 minim					
60 minims	1 fluidram				
480 minims	8 fluidrams	1 fluidounce			
7,680 minims	128 fluidrams	16 fluidounces	1 pint		
15,360 minims	256 fluidrams	32 fluidounces	2 pints	1 quart	
61,440 minims	1,024 fluidrams	128 fluidounces	8 pints	4 quarts	1 gallon

Weight

1 grain				
20 grains	1 scruple			
60 grains	3 scruples	1 dram		
480 grains	24 scruples	8 drams	1 ounce	
5,760 grains	288 scruples	96 drams	12 ounces	1 pound

The Metric System

The metric system is an international decimal system of weights and measures that originated in France. The United States Pharmacopeia (USP) adopted the metric system of weights and measures in 1890. Over the past decade the United States has been in the process of switching from the current system to the metric system. The gram, liter and meter represent the basic unit of weight, volume and length, respectively. The metric system is based on 10 and multiples of 10. All measurements are expressed in decimals. Subdivision of units of the metric system are expressed with Latin prefixes. Multiples of the metric unit are expressed with Greek prefixes.

Metric System Prefixes:

mega	1,000,000
myria	10,000
kilo	1,000
hecto	100
deka	10
unit (m, L, or g)	1
deci	0.1
centi	0.01
milli	0.001
micro	0.000001

Metric Units of Volume:

liter	L	1000 milliliters
milliliter	mL	0.001 liter
microliter	mcL	0.001 milliliter

Metric Units of Weight:

kilogram	kg	1,000 grams
hectogram	hg	100 grams
dekagram	dag	10 grams
gram	gm	
decigram	dg	0.1 gram
centigram	cg	0.01 gram
milligram	mg	0.001 gram
microgram	µg	0.001 milligram

Metric Units of Length and Area:

meter	m	
centimeter	cm	0.01 m
millimeter	mm	0.001 m
square meter	sqm	

Conversion Tables

1. To convert grams to milligrams (or liters to milliliters) move the decimal point three places to the right (e.g., 0.1 gm = 100 mg).
2. To convert milligrams to grams (or milliliters to liters) move the decimal point three places to the left (e.g., 1 mg = 0.001 gm).

Useful Equivalents

1 inch = 2.5 cm = 25.4 mm
1 grain (gr) = 65 mg
1 ounce (avoir) = 28.35 g
1 ounce (apoth) = 31.1 g
1 pound (avoir) = 7,000 gr (16 oz) = 453.59 g
1 pound (apoth) = 5,760 gr (12 gr) = 373.24 g
1 fluidounce = 30 ml
1 quart = 0.946 L; 946 ml
1 meter = 39.37 in; 3.3 ft; 1.1 yd
1 centimeter = 0.4 in
1 millimeter = 0.04 in
1 kilogram = 2.2 lb
1 gram = 15.4 gr
1 milligram = 1/65 gr
1 liter = 1.06 qt
1 milliliter = 16 minims

Household Equivalents

Measure	Apothecary	Metric
1 eyedropper drop	1 minim	0.06 ml
1 teaspoonful	1 fl dram	5 ml
1 dessert spoonful	2 fl dram	10 ml
1 tablespoonful	½ fl oz	15 ml
1 jigger	1½ fl oz	45 ml
1 cup (glass)	8 fl oz	240 ml
1 pint	2 cups	480 ml
1 quart	2 pints	960 ml

Pediatric Dosage Calculations

Pediatric doses may be calculated on the basis of the patient's age (least reliable but very common). Some of the more common rules for figuring dosage by age include:

Young's Rule: $\dfrac{\text{age in years}}{\text{age} + 12} \times \text{adult dose} = \text{approx dose}$

Fried's Rule: $\dfrac{\text{age in months}}{150} \times \text{adult dose} = \text{approx dose for patients under 1 year}$

Bastedo's Rule: $\dfrac{\text{age} + 3}{30} \times \text{adult dose} = \text{approx dose}$

Dilling's Rule: $\dfrac{\text{age}}{20} \times \text{adult dose} = \text{approx dose}$

Cowling's Rule: $\dfrac{\text{age at next birthday}}{24} \times \text{adult dose} = \text{approx dose}$

A second method for calculating pediatric doses uses the patient's weight (common and reliable). Some of the more common methods used for calculating dosage by weight include:

Dosage given in kg: Dose = dose per kg × weight of child in kilogram

Clark's Rule: $\dfrac{\text{wt of child in pounds}}{150} \times \text{adult dose} = \text{approx dose}$

A third method for calculating pediatric doses uses patient body surface area rules. This is the most reliable way.

Square meter dose: dose per square meter × surface area of child in square meters (from nomogram)

Clark's Rule: $\dfrac{\text{body surface area in square meters}}{1.73} \times \text{adult dose}$

Writing A Prescription

There are normally four parts to a prescription, which should be written legibly and politely:
1. The superscription includes the symbol Rx from the Latin recipe meaning "take."
2. The inscription specifies the ingredients and their quantities.
3. The subscription tells the pharmacist how to compound the medicine.
4. The signature, usually preceded by an S, represents the Latin signa meaning "mark." This includes what instructions are to be put on the outside of the package that direct the patient how and when to take the medicine and in what quantities. For example:

Superscription:	Rx:	
Inscription:		Hydrochlorthiazide 25 mg tablets
Subscription:		Dispense 50 tablets
Signature:	Sig:	Take 1 tablet each morning and evening with a full glass of orange juice. Please label.

Some other abbreviations used commonly in writing prescriptions are:

a.c.	before meals	omn. noct.	every night
aq.	water	p.c.	after meals
b.i.d.	twice a day	p.r.n.	as needed
caps	capsules	q.s.	a sufficient quantity
hora	an hour	q.i.d.	four times a day
h.s	at bedtime	q.	every
M.	mix	Rx	take a recipe
m.m. dict.	as directed	Sig.	directions
non. rep	do not repeat	statim	immediately
omn. hor.	every hour	t.i.d.	three times a day
omn. man.	every morning		

INDEX

This index lists all generic names, brand names and group names included in the book. Group names or major drug category headings appear in **bold type,** while generic names are printed in *italics.* Separate index entries are included when multiple forms of a product appear on different pages or when products are listed in more than one therapeutic group.

A

Accutane, 718
A'Cenol, 384
Aceta, 384
Acetaminophen, 382
Acetaminophen w/Codeine, 414
Acetazolamide
  Anticonvulsant, 444
  Diuretic, 327
  Ophthalmic, 697
Acetic Acid Otic, 1006
Acetohexamide, 815
Acetohydroxamic Acid, 1086
Acetospan, 796
Acetylsalicylic Acid, 438
Achromycin Ophthalmic, 72, 956
Achromycin IM, 72
Achromycin IV, 72
Achromycin V, 72
Achrostatin V, 73, 84
Acidifiers, Gastric
Acidifiers, Urinary, 1078
Acne Aid, 1012
Acne Aid Detergent Soap, 1011
Acnederm, 1016
Acne Products, 1010
Acne Products,
  Combinations, 1015
Acnomel, 1016
Acnophill, 1016
Acrisorcin, 1042
Actamine, 384
ACTH, 822
ACTH-Gel, 822
Acthar, 822
Actidil, 878
Actifed, 920
Active Immunizations, 157
Actrapid, 808
Acyclovir
  Parenteral, 133
  Topical, 1051
Adapin
  Antianxiety, 535
  Antidepressant, 555
Adenine Arabinoside, 962
Adolph's Salt Substitute, 764

Adrenalin Chloride
  Inhalant, 901
  Nasal Decongestant, 916
Adrenocortical Steroids
  Injection, 770
  Oral, 770
  Topical, 1016
Adrenergic Drugs
  Sympathomimetics, 897
Adsorbocarpine, 988
Advil, 431
Aerolate, 910
Aerolone, 903
Aerosporin, 65, 958, 1008
Afko-Lube, 666
Afrin, 917
Aftate, 1042
Agoral Plain, 672
A-hydroCort, 791
Akarpine, 988
AK-Cide, 998
AK-Con, 1000
AK-Dilate, 998
Akineton, 495
AK-Neo-Cort, 800
AK-Pentolate, 972
Akrinol, 1042
AK-Sulf, 958
AK-Taine, 949
Ak-Zol
  Anticonvulsants, 444
  Diuretic, 327
  Ophthalmic, 967
Alazide, 360
Albalon Liquifilm, 1000
Albalon-A Liquifilm, 1000
Albamycin, 50
Albuterol, 900
Alcaine, 949
Aldactazide, 360
Aldactone, 345
Aldomet, 292
Alermine, 877
Alersule, 926
Aliphatic Phenothiazine, 583
Alka-2, 629
Alkalinizers
  Systemic, 765
  Urinary, 1080

Alka-Seltzer, 439
Alkyalamine Antihistamines,
  876
Aller-Chlor, 877
Allerest, 921
Allerest Eye Drops, 1000
Allergesic, 921
Allerid-O.D.-8, 877
Allerid-O.D.-12, 877
Allerprop, 927
Allerstat, 921
Allopurinol, 366
Almocarpine, 988
Almora, 753
Alophen Pills, 677
Alpha Keri Oil, 1067
Alphalin Gelseals, 718
Alphamul, 676
Alpha-Redisol, 734
Alpha-Ruvite, 734
Alprazolam, 524
AlternaGEL, 628
Alu-Cap, 628
Aludrox, 633
Aluminum Acetate Solution,
  1069
Aluminum Carbonate Gel, 628,
  1113
Aluminum Hydroxide, 628
Aluminum Hydroxide Gel, 628
Aluminum Hydroxide Gel and
  Magnesium Hydroxide, 633
Aluminum Phosphate, 629
Alupent, 903
Alurate, 592
Alu-Tab, 628
AluWet Wet Dressing Crystals,
  1069
Amantadine HCl
  Antiparkinson Agent, 494
  Antiviral, 126
Ambesol, 1034
Ambodryl Kapseals, 879
Amcil, 54
Amcort, 797
Amebicides, 2
Amen, 859
Americaine,
  Anesthetic, 1034

1127